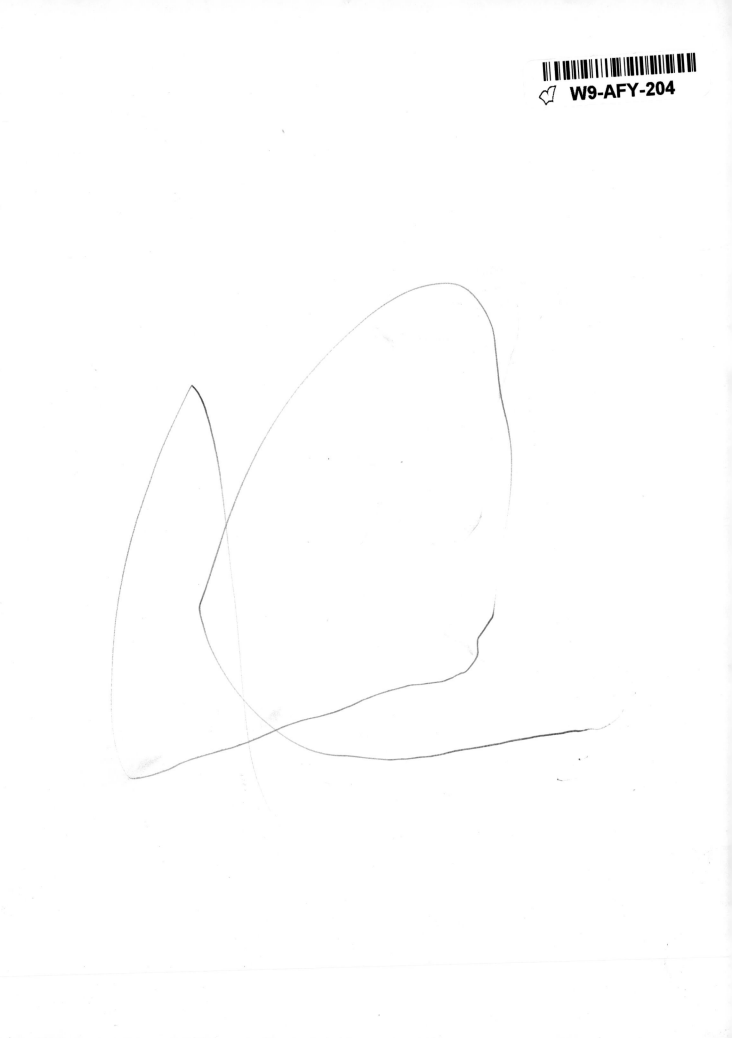

Clinical Practice
of the
Dental Hygienist

Clinical Practice
of the
Dental Hygienist

ESTHER M. WILKINS, B.S., R.D.H., D.M.D.

Department of Periodontology,
Tufts University, School of Dental Medicine,
Boston, Massachusetts

SIXTH EDITION

Lea & Febiger   Philadelphia • London

Lea & Febiger
200 Chester Field Parkway
Malvern, Pennsylvania   19355-9725
U.S.A.
(215) 251-2230
1-800-444-1785

Library of Congress Cataloging-in-Publication Data

Wilkins, Esther M.
    Clinical practice of the dental hygienist / Esther M. Wilkins.—
6th ed.
        p.   cm.
    Includes bibliographies and index.
    ISBN 0-8121-1181-8
    1. Dental hygiene. I. Title.
    [DNLM: 1. Dental Hygienists. 2. Preventive Dentistry. WU 90
W684c]
RK60.5.W5   1989
617.6′01—dc19
DNLM/DLC
for Library of Congress   89-2288
                                                              CIP

First Edition, 1959
    Reprinted 1962
Second Edition, 1964
    Reprinted 1966, 1968
Third Edition, 1971
    Reprinted 1972, 1973, 1975
Fourth Edition, 1976
    Reprinted 1977, 1979, 1980, 1981
Fifth Edition, 1982
    Reprinted 1983, 1984, 1986, 1988
Sixth Edition, 1989

Translations:
    Fourth Edition—
        Japanese Edition by Ishiyaku Publishers, Inc., Tokyo, Japan, 1986

Print No. 6   5   4   3   2

Preface

Significant advances have been made in research in the basic and clinical sciences that directly influence the recognition, prevention, and treatment of oral diseases. As the new research findings have been applied to preventive measures for the individual and the community, the oral health of the general public has improved. Consumer awareness of preventive measures has increased and is a welcome trend in oral health promotion. The dental hygienist has had, and will continue to have, an increasingly prominent place in the progress toward higher levels of oral health for the public.

Important aspects of contemporary health-care delivery are first, the role of self-care to be assumed by the patient, and second, the responsibility of the professional person to provide individualized instruction and treatment. To accomplish this, the dental hygienist must assess each patient's needs, plan and carry out the treatment program, and evaluate the effects of the treatment.

In *Clinical Practice of the Dental Hygienist*, the six parts and their respective chapters have been arranged in a general way to help dental hygienists proceed sequentially through logical steps in patient care. For each patient, observations are made and recorded and data assembled to evaluate the patient's oral condition. From the information gathered, the extent of oral disease is determined and the patient's treatment needs are outlined. Selective therapy can then be planned for the dental and periodontal problems that are amenable to resolution by dental hygiene care.

Implementation of the treatment plan involves the interaction of the dental team members, the patient, and where indicated because of age or general health status, the patient's family. Dental hygiene care may have short-term, intermediate, and long-term goals that may spread over a series of appointments and extend into a maintenance phase of care. The outcome of treatment is evaluated. Additional therapy may be indicated, and the maintenance program is introduced. At this stage, the objective is to prevent both the recurrence of disease and the initiation of new forms of oral disease.

The sixth edition of *Clinical Practice of the Dental Hygienist* has as its main objective to make available comprehensive information in a concise manner. Major reference sources are included that are fundamental to clinical dental hygiene practice. In addition, as in previous editions, specific chapters are devoted to material about patients with oral, systemic, physical, or other problems that require specialized knowledge and sometimes more skillful adaptations of the basic techniques. Although it is true that all dental hygiene care should be individualized, this text provides standard, commonly accepted procedures from general practice. Each dental hygienist will use professional clinical judgment in the selection and application of procedure for an individual patient.

In the preparation of this revised edition, new knowledge and concerns have led to modifications of many chapters as well as to the addition of new material. Two completely new chapters have been added: one to describe debonding, and the other to assist the practitioner in the care of the patient with alcoholism.

New and improved sections within existing chapters include information on transmissible diseases and infection control, contributing factors to periodontal diseases, probed attachment level, tooth fractures, microbiology of bacterial plaque, and new indices, particularly the Community Periodontal Index of Treatment Needs (CPITN) of the World Health Organization. In the area of prevention, new topics include the care of space maintainers and dental implants, eating disorders (anorexia nervosa and bulimia nervosa) and fluoride toxicity and safety.

The new edition offers several improvements over previous editions. New terminology has been introduced and all references and suggested readings have been updated. Many new illustrations and tables have been added to clarify content and enhance readability. A pronunciation guide for words listed in the Glossary has been added at the request of students. Every effort has been made to make the text as accurate and up-to-date as possible. This was accomplished through extensive reviews of the literature and through critiques provided by students, faculty members, and practicing professionals. Readers are encouraged to send in comments and recommendations for future editions.

Many chapters are currently used by dental and dental assisting students. Although intended primarily for members of the dental team, associates from other health professions also have found the book an excellent resource. The parts pertaining to prevention of oral disease have been widely used, as have the chapters in Part VI, in which discussions of the oral problems of physically and medically compromised patients provide information that can be integrated with nursing and medical care.

Beginning students use the book as a text and then, after graduation, as a reference source during practice. Many dental hygienists who have returned to practice after a leave of absence have found the book a practical aid to re-entry.

Personal integrity and competence in patient care are the foremost factors in assuring quality control within the dental hygiene profession. A principal goal of this book is to help each dental hygienist provide instructional and clinical services that will assure quality control for high standards of professional practice.

Boston, Massachusetts   Esther M. Wilkins

Acknowledgments

Many teachers, students, and dental hygiene practitioners have given ideas, information, and support during the preparation of this sixth edition of *Clinical Practice of the Dental Hygienist*. Using their insight, expertise, and experience, they have provided invaluable recommendations for changes and improvements and have helped to assure that current practices and professional standards are evident throughout the book.

Various chapters and sections have been read, criticized, and corrected by persons with specialized knowledge. The author is particularly grateful to those who reviewed whole chapters and clarified essential issues. Within that group are the following, whose multiple contributions apply to many different chapters or parts of chapters:

Suzanne Box, Cape Cod Community College, West Barnstable, Massachusetts;

Patricia Cohen, Canton, Massachusetts;

Tena McQueen, Columbus College, Columbus, Georgia;

Wana Milam, San Antonio, Texas;

Barbara Wilson, University of Rhode Island, Kingston, Rhode Island.

Others, whose time and efforts were devoted to specific chapters are, in the general order as the chapters appear in the book:

Infection Control: **Kathy Eklund,** Forsyth School for Dental Hygienists, Boston, Massachusetts, and **Barbara Brown,** University of Rhode Island

Personal, Medical, and Dental History: **Nancy Snyder Whitten,** University of Texas at San Antonio

Vital Signs: **Susan Ohman,** United States Veterans Administration, Department of Research and Development, Boston, Massachusetts

Section on Oral Cytology: **Dr. Arthur Miller,** Temple University Department of Pathology

Dental Radiographs: **Dorathea Foote,** Springfield Technical Community College, Springfield, Massachusetts

Bacterial Plaque and Other Soft Deposits: **Linda Hanlon,** Forsyth School for Dental Hygienists

Indices and Scoring Methods: **Sharon Gravois,** San Jose, California

Care of Dental Appliances: **Cynthia Biron,** New Hampshire Technical Institute

Section on Dental Implants: **Dr. Thomas Balshi,** Fort Washington, Pennsylvania; **Dr. Robert Chapman,** Tufts University School of Dental Medicine; and **Dr. Paul Schnitman,** Harvard University School of Dental Medicine

Section on Airpolisher: **Caren M. Barnes,** University of Alabama School of Dentistry

Debonding: **Marylou Everett-Gutmann,** Caruth School of Dental Hygiene, Dallas, Texas

Gerodontic Patient: **Yvonne Knazan,** University of Manitoba, Winnipeg, Manitoba

Care of Patients with Disabilities: **Janet Carroll-Memoli,** University of Bridgeport; **Barbara Brennan,** Grasso Center, Stratford, Connecticut; and **Charlotte Lawrence,** Ann Arbor, Michigan

Section on Autism: **Patricia Cowham,** Walsh School, Stratford, Connecticut

Section on Hearing Impairment: **Dr. Lottie L. Riekehof,** Gallaudet College, Washington, D.C.

Patient with Cardiovascular Disease: **Jeanne O'Leary Smith,** Middlesex Community College, Massachusetts

Section on Cardiac Pacemaker: **Patricia Griffiths,** Columbus, Ohio

Patient with Alcoholism: **Janet Carroll-Memoli,** University of Bridgeport

Emergency Care: **Susan Ohman,** United States Veterans Administration, Department of Research and Development, Boston, Massachusetts

The many new illustrations reflect the talent and expertise of artists **Amy Willcox** and **Paula Krick.** A special thanks goes to them for their patience and personal interest in improving the quality and consistency of the art.

Appreciation goes to the people at **Lea & Febiger,** particularly Tanya Lazar, Thomas Colaiezzi, and Raymond Kersey for their patience and cooperation in the preparation of this as well as other editions. Since the last edition, Lea & Febiger has celebrated its 200th year of publishing. The company is America's oldest publisher and is internationally famous for books in the health sciences. The publication of *Mouth Hygiene* by Alfred C. Fones in 1916 gave dental hygiene its first textbook. Since then, Lea & Febiger has retained leadership in publishing dental hygiene books. The significant impact of these books on dental hygiene education and, hence, on the dental hygiene profession is acknowledged with gratitude.

EMW

vii

Contents

I

Orientation to Clinical Dental Hygiene Practice

1 *The Professional Dental Hygienist*

The registered dental hygienist is a licensed, professional, oral health educator and clinician, who, as a co-therapist with the dentist, uses preventive, educational, and therapeutic methods for the control of oral diseases to aid individuals and groups in attaining and maintaining optimum oral health. The services of the dental hygienist are utilized in general and specialty dental practices, in the armed services, and in programs for research, professional education, public health, school health, industrial health, hospital, and institutional care.

I. Types of Services

The services the dental hygienist performs can be divided into three basic categories, namely, preventive, educational, and therapeutic. The three are inseparable and overlapping as patient care is planned and accomplished.

A. Preventive

Preventive services are the methods employed by the clinician and/or patient to promote and maintain oral health.[1]

Preventive services fall into two groups, primary and secondary. *Primary prevention* refers to measures carried out so that disease does not occur and is truly prevented. *Secondary prevention* involves the treatment of early disease to prevent further progress of potentially irreversible conditions which, if not arrested, may lead eventually to extensive rehabilitative treatment or loss of teeth.

An example of a primary preventive measure is the application of a topical agent for dental caries prevention. Removal of subgingival calculus and smoothing the root surface in a relatively shallow pocket is an example of a secondary prevention procedure in that the treatment of a small pocket contributes to the prevention of a deep pocket with marked bone loss.

B. Educational

Educational services are the strategies developed for an individual or for groups to elicit behaviors directed toward health.[1]

Educational aspects of dental hygiene service permeate the entire patient care system. The preparation for specific treatment, the success of treatment, and the long-term success of both preventive and therapeutic services depend on the patient's understanding of each procedure and daily care of the oral cavity.

C. Therapeutic

Therapeutic services are clinical treatments designed to arrest or control disease and maintain oral tissues in health.[1]

Dental hygiene treatment services are an integral part of the total treatment procedures. All scaling and root planing, along with the steps in postoperative care, are parts of the therapeutic phases in the treatment of periodontal diseases. Restorative procedures are involved in the treatment of dental caries.

II. Dental Hygiene Care

The term *dental hygiene care* is used to denote all integrated preventive and treatment services administered to a patient by a dental hygienist. This term is parallel to the commonly used term *dental care,* which refers to the services performed by the dentist.

Clinical services, both dental and dental hygiene, have limited long-range probability of success if the patient does not understand the need for cooperation in daily procedures of personal care and diet, and for regular appointments for professional care. Educational and clinical services are, therefore, mutually dependent and inseparable in the total dental hygiene care of the patient.

Dr. Alfred C. Fones, the "father of dental hygiene," emphasized the important role of education. In the first textbook for dental hygienists, he wrote:

> It is primarily to this important work of public education that the dental hygienist is called. She must regard herself as the channel through which dentistry's knowledge of mouth hygiene is to be disseminated. The greatest service she can perform is the persistent education of the public in mouth hygiene and the allied branches of general hygiene.[2]

Dental hygiene has been studied and the scope of practice has developed from Dr. Fones' original concept. Scientific information about the prevention of oral diseases has been advancing steadily. The public has become increasingly aware of the need for dental hygiene care and the importance of oral health instruction. The clinical practice of the dental hygienist integrates specific care with instructional services required by the individual patient.

A. Purposes in Planning Care

Planning dental hygiene care for a patient means preparing a schedule to guide the preventive, educational, and therapeutic activities prescribed by the dentist and delegated to the dental hygienist. Initially, the dental hygienist plays a major role in the collection of data to be used by the dentist in formulating the diagnosis on which the total treatment plan is based.

The dental hygienist must have a clear understanding of the patient's needs, the nature of the oral illness, and the principles relating to the treatment of the illness. The dental hygienist should be aware of the patient's emotional needs and psychological reactions to the oral conditions. It is important to create an atmosphere in which the patient can respond to instruction, carry out the necessary procedures to supplement professional treatment, and cooperate during dental and dental hygiene appointments for the specific services.

B. Role in Patient Care

The role of the dental hygienist is to implement and coordinate the treatment and preventive program prescribed for each patient. Specific clinical services are required, and the dental hygienist teaches, motivates, and guides the patient in the performance of measures for disease control. The success of each phase of treatment, whether periodontic, orthodontic, restorative, or prosthodontic, depends on the patient's cooperative daily performance of the recommended measures. Dental hygiene care as provided by the dental hygienist becomes an integral part of the total care of the patient.

In general, the sections of this book are arranged in an order to correspond with a sequence in which dental hygiene services may logically be performed.

Because much of the text is concerned with details of how to perform services for the patient, it is important to keep services and techniques in their proper perspective. Much more is involved in dental hygiene care than the performance of technical procedures.

C. The Challenge of Planning Patient Care

Advancement in dental science has made it imperative for the professional dental hygienist to be able to adapt dental hygiene care to changing concepts with understanding and flexibility. Dental hygiene care needs to be modified intelligently according to the patient, the oral condition and disease, and the personal problems.

Each patient is an individual with specific problems of oral care that need consideration. Good dental hygiene care is patient-centered.

The professional dental hygienist must be a self-directed person who can apply scientific knowledge to problem solving. The questions are the following: What is the status of this patient's oral health? Why and how did it happen? What can I do to supplement that which the dentist does for the patient? What can the patient learn to do as a result of my teaching and guidance? What will be the outcome?

In the effort to deliver more effective and comprehensive health service, a set pattern of dental hygiene care, one that was memorized or learned by rote, cannot always be used. Knowledge must be applied to meet the individual needs of each patient.

III. Special Practice Areas

A wide range of settings is available for the practice of a dental hygienist. Likewise, a wide range of patient problems brings out the need for specialized knowledge and skills.

There are eight areas of dentistry in which a dentist may conduct an ethical limited practice. They are the following: dental public health, endodontics, oral pathology, oral and maxillofacial surgery, orthodontics, pediatric dentistry (dentistry for children), periodontics, and prosthodontics.[3] Education and training for certification in the dental specialties require a minimum of 2 years of graduate or postgraduate study and the successful completion of written and practical examinations. Masters and doctoral degrees require 3 or more years beyond basic dental education.

Although dental hygienists have not been required to complete examinations for practice within a specialty, educational curricula exist for certain areas. For example, advanced degree programs to prepare for dental hygiene education or public health have been available for many years.

In other special areas, short-term courses have been developed, such as for instruction in the care of patients with disabilities. In-service training may be available in long-term care institutions, hospitals, and skilled nursing facilities. Some dental hygienists have learned how to practice in a specialty through private study, special conferences, and personal experience.

Dental hygienists are needed to practice with dentists in specialty areas, particularly orthodontics, pediatric dentistry, and periodontics. Others are involved in special clinics with a variety of health specialists, where patients with dental deformities, such as cleft lip and/or palate, or patients with oral cancer are under care. In other facilities, dental hygienists serve with a combined medical and dental team in the treatment of patients with severe systemic diseases, patients with physical, mental, or emotional handicapping conditions, or combinations of any of the problems mentioned.

FACTORS INFLUENCING CLINICAL PRACTICE

I. Legal

The law must be studied and respected by each dental hygienist practicing within the state, province, or country. Although the various practice acts have certain basic similarities, differences in scope and definition exist. Terminology varies, but each practice act regulates the patient services that may be delegated. Changes may be made from time to time.

II. Ethical

Professional people in the health services are set apart from others by virtue of the dignity and responsibility of their work. Service is the primary objective of the dental hygienist and is the reason for the existence of the profession. Others look to the professional person for leadership and expect more than ordinary demonstration of good human relations. Being professional requires interpersonal, professional, interprofessional, and community relationships of a high standard.

Dental Hygienists' Associations have defined principles of ethics for the professional dental hygienist. Figure 1-1 shows the Code of Ethics of the American Dental Hygienists' Association. Understanding of and loyalty to these principles is essential to successful practice.

PRINCIPLES OF ETHICS OF THE AMERICAN DENTAL HYGIENISTS' ASSOCIATION

Each member of the American Dental Hygienists' Association has the ethical obligation to subscribe to the following principles:

To provide oral health care utilizing highest professional knowledge, judgment, and ability.

To serve all patients without discrimination.

To hold professional patient relationships in confidence.

To utilize every opportunity to increase public understanding of oral health practices.

To generate public confidence in members of the dental health profession.

To cooperate with all health professions in meeting the health needs of the public.

To recognize and uphold the laws and regulations governing this profession.

To participate responsibly in this professional Association and uphold its purposes.

To maintain professional competence through continuing education.

To exchange professional knowledge with other health professions.

To represent dental hygiene with high standards of personal conduct.

Figure 1-1. Professional Code of Ethics

III. Personal

Each dental hygienist may represent the entire profession to the patient being served. The dental hygienist's expressed or demonstrated attitudes toward dentistry, dental hygiene, and other health professions, as well as toward health services and preventive measures, are apt to be reflected in the subsequent attitude of the patient toward other dental hygienists and dental hygiene care in general.

Members of health professions must exemplify the traits they hold as objectives for others if response and cooperation are to be expected. Many personal factors of general physical health, oral health, cleanliness, appearance, and mental health are to be considered. A few of these are mentioned below.

1. *General Physical Health.* Optimum physical health depends primarily on a well-planned diet, a sufficient amount of sleep, and an adequate amount of exercise.

   Because of the occupational hazards of dental personnel, routine examinations at least annually should include tests for hearing, sight, urinary mercury, and certain communicable diseases.[5,6] Immunizations are described on page 33.

2. *Oral Health.* The maintenance of a clean, healthy mouth demonstrates by example that the dental hygienist follows the teachings of the dental and dental hygiene professions relative to prevention and control of disease.

3. *Mental Health.* The mental health of the dental hygienist is reflected in interpersonal relationships and the ability to inspire confidence through a display of professional and emotional maturity. Adequate physical health, recreation, and participation in professional and community activities contribute to optimum mental health.

OBJECTIVES FOR PRACTICE

The hygienist's self-assessment is essential in attaining goals of perfection in service to the patient and assistance to the dentist in the total dental and dental hygiene care program. Personal objectives should be outlined and reviewed frequently in a plan for continued self-improvement.

The goal with respect to patients was included in the definition of the dental hygienist at the beginning of this chapter: *to aid individuals and groups in attaining and maintaining optimum oral health.* Other objectives are related to this primary one.

The professional dental hygienist will

A. Strive toward the highest degree of professional ethics and conduct.

B. Plan and carry out effectively the dental hygiene services essential to the total care program for an individual patient.

C. Apply knowledge and understanding of the basic

and clinical sciences in the recognition of oral conditions and prevention of oral diseases.

D. Apply scientific knowledge and skill to all clinical techniques and instructional procedures.

E. Recognize each patient as an individual and adapt techniques and procedures accordingly.

F. Identify and care for the needs of patients who have unusual general health problems that affect dental hygiene procedures.

G. Demonstrate interpersonal relationships that permit attending the patient with assurance and presenting dental health information effectively.

H. Provide a complete and personalized instructional service to help each patient to become motivated toward changes in oral health behavioral practices.

I. Practice safe and efficient procedures pertaining to the care and sterilization of instruments and to general clinical routines.

J. Apply a continuing process of self-development and self-evaluation in clinical practice throughout professional life.

  1. Be objective and critical of procedures used in order to perform the best possible service.

  2. Appreciate the need for acquiring new knowledge and skills by regular enrollment in continuing education courses.

FACTORS TO TEACH THE PATIENT

A. The role of the dental hygienist as a co-therapist in the dental profession.

B. The scope of service of the dental hygienist as defined by various practice acts.

C. The interrelationship of instructional and clinical services in dental hygiene care.

D. The individual's potential state of oral health and how it can be developed and maintained.

References

1. American Association of Dental Schools, Section on Dental Hygiene Education, Curriculum Guidelines Committee: Curriculum Guidelines for Clinical Dental Hygiene, *J. Dent. Educ., 49,* 832, December, 1985.
2. Fones, A.C., ed.: *Mouth Hygiene,* 4th ed. Philadelphia, Lea & Febiger, 1934, p. 248.
3. American Dental Association: *ADA Principles of Ethics and Code of Professional Conduct,* Chicago, American Dental Association, 1984.
4. American Dental Hygienists' Association, House of Delegates: *Professional Code of Ethics for the Dental Hygienist,* Revised November, 1974.
5. Gravois, S.L. and Stringer, R.B.: Survey of Occupational Health Hazards in Dental Hygiene, *Dent. Hyg., 54,* 518, November, 1980.
6. Goldman, H.S.: Hazards in the Dental Workplace. Prevention for the Dentist, *Clin. Prevent. Dent., 2,* 18, September-October, 1980.

Suggested Readings

Bird, L.P.: Dental Ethics: Where Science and Sensitivity Touch, *Spec. Care Dentist., 5,* 198, September-October, 1985.

Brownstone, E.: The Role of Dental Hygiene in Health Promotion, *Can. Dent. Hyg./Probe, 21,* 164, December, 1987.

Cohen, L., Labelle, A., Singer, J., Blandford, D., and Groeneman, S.: Prevalence of Nontraditional Dental Hygiene Practice, *J. Public Health Dent., 44,* 106, Summer, 1984.

Everett, M.S.: Orthodontic Specialization for Dental Hygienists, *Dent. Hyg., 59,* 400, September, 1985.

Forgay, M.G.E., Chairman, Working Group: The Practice of Dental Hygiene in Canada, *Can. Dent. Hyg., 20,* insert (i–xii) March, 1986.

Frazier, J.: Where Does Dental Hygiene Go From Here? *Dent. Hyg., 58,* 564, December, 1984.

Gallagher, D.: The Role of the Dental Hygienist in Achieving Health for All, *Can. Dent. Hyg./Probe, 21,* 119, September, 1987.

Ganssle, C.L. and Everett, M.S.: Dental Hygiene Utilization in Orthodontics, *Dent. Hyg., 57,* 17, November, 1983.

Giangrego, E., ed.: Dental Hygiene in a New Light, *J. Am. Dent. Assoc., 106,* 792, June, 1983.

Granger, B.: Legal Aspects of Dental Hygiene Practice, *Dent. Hyg., 54,* 337, July, 1980.

Jones, J.D. and Snyder, N.C.: Role of the Dental Hygienist in the Prosthodontic Practice, *J. Prosthet. Dent., 52,* 885, December, 1984.

Macdonald, G.: A Selected Review of Lawsuits Brought Against Dentists. Their Relevance to Dental Hygiene Practice, *Dent. Hyg., 60,* 358, August, 1986.

Newell, K.J., Young, L.J., and Yamoor, C.M.: Moral Reasoning in Dental Hygiene Students, *J. Dent. Educ., 49,* 79, February, 1985.

Pattison, A.M.: Can Dental Hygienists Affect the Periodontal Health of the Nation? An Assessment of The Future of Dental Hygiene, *J. Public Health Dent., 45,* 69, Spring, 1985.

Walsh, M.M.: Can Dental Hygienists Affect the Periodontal Health of the Nation? Trends and Potentials for Dental Hygiene, *J. Public Health Dent., 45,* 60, Spring, 1985.

Professionalism and Ethics

Fleming, W.C.: The Attributes of a Profession and Its Members. *J. Am. Dent. Assoc., 69,* 390, September, 1964.

Hine, M.K.: The Professional Concept—Its History and Meaning to Health Service, *J. Am. Coll. Dent., 37,* 19, January, 1970.

Jackson, E.: An Investigation of the Determinants of Professional Image, *Ann. Dent., 40,* 7, Summer, 1981.

MacQuarrie, E.E.: Factors in the Development of Professional Attitude. *J. Am. Dent. Hyg. Assoc., 45,* 86, March-April, 1971.

Motley, W.E.: *Ethics, Jurisprudence and History for the Dental Hygienist,* 3rd ed. Philadelphia, Lea & Febiger, 1983, 217 pp.

II

Preparation for Dental Hygiene Appointments

II

2 Infection Control: Transmissible Diseases

The transmission of disease is an insidious process. Infection and communicable diseases can lead to illness, disability, and loss of work time. In addition, other patients, family members, and community contacts become exposed and may become ill and lose productive time or suffer permanent aftereffects.

In dental and dental hygiene practice, the objective is to protect patients and dental personnel from acquiring infection in the environment of the office or clinic. Health services facilities, including dental facilities, must be places for the cure and prevention, not the dissemination of disease due to inadequate precautionary measures and habits of the professional personnel.

A group responsibility of a dental team is first to organize and maintain a system for the sterilization, disinfection, and care of instruments and equipment. The second step is to conduct all appointments in a manner that will prevent direct or indirect cross-infections between dental personnel and patients, and from one patient to another.

Pathogenic (disease producing), potentially pathogenic, or nonpathogenic microorganisms may be present in the oral cavity of each patient. Pathogenic organisms may be transient. Patients may be carriers of certain diseases. Inadvertent transmission to subsequent susceptible patients or to dental personnel may occur as a result of careless handwashing and unhygienic personal habits or by inadequate sterilization or handling of sterile instruments.

I. Microorganisms of the Oral Cavity

At birth the oral cavity is sterile, but within a few hours to one day a simple oral flora develops.[1] The microorganisms of the saliva in a mature mouth include over 40 species.[2] Most of the salivary bacteria come from the dorsum of the tongue, while some are from other mucous membranes. Much larger counts of total microorganisms are found in bacterial plaque and in periodontal pockets.

The intact mucous membrane of the oral cavity protects against infection to a degree. However, when the gingival tissues are manipulated during instrumentation, microorganisms can be introduced into the underlying tissues by way of the gingival sulcus or periodontal pocket.

II. Mechanisms for Transfer of Infectious Material

Recognition of the many possibilities for the transfer of infection in a dental office or clinic provides a basis for planning the system of sterilization, disinfection, and handling of instruments and equipment. The patient becomes the center of the many potential sources of infection as shown in figure 2–1. Several terms that apply to the transfer of infectious material are defined here.

A. Cross-contamination

Cross-contamination refers to the spread of microorganisms from one source to another: person to person, or person to an inanimate object and then to another person.

B. Direct Contact Transmission

When infection is spread from one person to another without an intermediate object, it is called direct contact.

C. Indirect Contact Transmission

Infection spread from one person to another person by way of an environmental surface, droplets, or other vehicle, is known as indirect contact.

D. Droplet Infection

Infection may be acquired by inhalation of droplets or aerosols that contain microorganisms or viruses from another person.

E. Vehicle

The term vehicle is used when referring to a substance or object that carries infectious material from one person to another, directly or indirectly. Saliva on the hands of a clinician or in the splatter from a patient's mouth is an example of the most common vehicle for cross-contamination in a dental setting.

AIRBORNE INFECTION

I. Microorganisms of the Air

A. Transmission

Transmission of microorganisms occurs by four general routes:
1. Droplets from patient to clinician or clinician to patient.
2. Hands and instruments that have made contact with the patient's oral cavity.

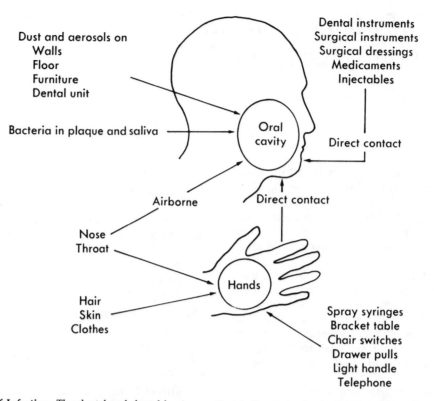

Dust and aerosols on
Walls
Floor
Furniture
Dental unit

Dental instruments
Surgical instruments
Surgical dressings
Medicaments
Injectables

Bacteria in plaque and saliva →

Oral cavity

Direct contact

Airborne

Direct contact

Nose
Throat

Hands

Hair
Skin
Clothes

Spray syringes
Bracket table
Chair switches
Drawer pulls
Light handle
Telephone

Figure 2–1. Sources of Infection. The dental and dental hygiene patient is the center for environmental, autogenous, and interpersonal transmission of infectious agents. (From Crawford, J.J., in Block, S.S.: *Disinfection, Sterilization, and Preservation,* 3rd ed. Philadelphia, Lea & Febiger, 1983.)

3. From the hands indirectly to other objects such as equipment or records. The organisms may then be picked up and brought to an oral cavity or skin break.

4. Organisms in air of the treatment area. The air provides another means for indirect transmission to a susceptible person, a subsequent patient, or a member of the dental team.

B. Dust-borne Organisms

Clostridium tetani (tetanus bacillus), *Staphylococcus aureus,* and enteric bacteria are among the organisms that may travel in the dust brought in from outside and that moves in and about dental treatment areas. When doors are opened and closed and people pass in and out, dust is set into motion that can settle on instruments, other objects, or people.

Infectious microorganisms also reach dust from the oral cavities of patients by way of large airborne particles, which are described as splatter further on. Dust-borne organisms can be sources of contamination for dental instruments and the hands of dental personnel.

Surface disinfection of all equipment contacted during a dental appointment contributes to control of dust-borne pathogens. Procedures

for surface disinfection are described on pages 53–54.

II. Aerosol Production[3]

Airborne particles are usually classified by size as either *aerosols* or *splatter.* They are constantly being produced.

A. Aerosols

An aerosol is an artificially generated collection of particles suspended in air and capable of causing an airborne infection. A particle of a true aerosol is less than 50 microns in diameter and nearly all are less than 5 microns. Aerosols are biologic contaminants that occur in solid or liquid form, are invisible, and remain suspended in air for long periods.

Aerosol particles that are 5 microns or smaller may be breathed deep into the lungs. Larger particles get trapped higher in the respiratory tree. The tiny particles may contain respiratory disease-producing organisms or traces of mercury or amalgam that collect in the lung because they are not biodegradable.

B. Splatter

Heavier, larger particles may remain airborne a relatively short time because of their own size and weight. They drop or splatter on objects, people, and the floor. The splatter is composed of particles greater than 50 microns in diameter.

In contrast to aerosols, splatter may be visible, particularly after it has landed on skin, hair, clothing, or environmental surfaces where gross contamination can result.

C. Origin

Aerosols and splatter are created during breathing, speaking, coughing, or sneezing. They are produced during all intraoral procedures, including examination and manual scaling. When produced by air-spray, air-water-spray, handpiece activity, or ultrasonic scaling, the number of aerosols increases to tremendous proportions.[3,4,5,6]

D. Contents

1. *Microorganisms.* An aerosol may contain a single organism or a clump of microorganisms adhered to a dust or debris particle. The organisms may be contained within a liquid droplet.

2. *Particles from Cavity Preparation.* Tooth fragments, microorganisms from saliva, plaque, and/or oropharynx/nasopharynx, oil from a handpiece, and water from the cooling equipment, may be in aerosols, following cavity preparation.

3. *Ultrasonic Scaling.* Great numbers of microorganisms have been found in the aerosols from ultrasonic scalers including *Staphylococcus aureus, albus,* and *pyogenes, Streptococcus viridans,* lactobacilli, Actinomyces, pneumococci, and diphtheroids.[5,6] Viruses also may be spread by ultrasonic instruments.

E. Concentration

Bacteria-laden aerosols and splatter are in greater concentration close to the scene of instrumentation; the quantity decreases with distance. The aerosols travel with air currents and, therefore, move from room to room.

III. Prevention of Transmission[3]

The control of airborne infection depends on elimination or limitation of the organisms at their source, interruption of transmission, and protection of the potentially susceptible recipient.

Carefully monitored procedures are necessary for all patients with or without a known serious communicable disease. A list of procedures appears on pages 56–57.

A. Limitation of Organisms

Organisms can be limited by postponement of elective treatment for a patient known to have specific communicable organisms in the oral cavity. Patients may be asked to change their appointments when they are suffering from respiratory or other communicable disease.

B. Preoperative Oral Hygiene Measures

Toothbrushing and using an antiseptic mouthrinse will reduce the numbers of bacteria contained in aerosols. Preparation of the patient is described on page 56.

C. Interruption of Transmission

1. Use rubber dam, high-volume evacuation, and manual instrumentation as much as possible.

2. Install air-control methods to supply adequate ventilation, filtration, and relative humidity.

3. Employ vacuum cleaning to remove dirt and microorganisms rather than dust-arousing housekeeping methods. The cleaner must have a filter to prevent the escape of organisms after they are suctioned.[7]

D. Clean Water

Run water through all tubings to handpieces, ultrasonic, and air/water spray for at least 2 minutes at the start of the day and at least 30 seconds after each appointment during the day. Contamination of splatter and aerosols will be reduced by this method.[8]

E. Protection of the Clinician

The use of masks and protective eyeglasses can prevent direct contact of splatter and aerosols with the faces of the dental team.

AUTOGENOUS INFECTION[9,10]

An autogenous infection is one that originates within a person when the normal defense mechanisms are modified. The microflora of the oral cavity may become pathogenic when, for example, the organisms are forced into the tissues during instrumentation.

I. Normal Defenses

The body responds to or resists bacterial and viral invasion in different ways, such as those listed below.

A. Nutritional Status

In health, disease is resisted; whereas in a deprived state, the body can be susceptible to infection.

B. Antibody Response

After certain types of infections, antibodies are produced that provide resistance against a second attack of the same organism.

C. Physical Barrier

The intact skin and mucous membranes serve as barriers to prevent microorganisms from invading susceptible tissues.

D. Defense Cell Reaction

Phagocytes and white blood cells, particularly polymorphonuclear leukocytes, respond to inflammation and collect at the site of infection to defend the body against disease.

II. Sources of Autogenous Infection

A. Bacteremia

Bacteremia is a condition in which bacteria or other microorganisms are in the bloodstream. In the oral cavity, bacteria can enter the blood by way of a break in the mucosa, or through a gingival or periodontal pocket. When scaling or other instrumentation is performed, the microbial flora is disturbed and may be forced into the underlying tissues.

B. Injection Site

An abscess can occur at the site of injection when microorganisms are picked up by the needle as it is carried to the injection site. Organisms from bacterial plaque or those residing on the mucosal surface can be carried into the underlying tissues as the needle is inserted.

III. Factors That Alter Normal Defenses

The patient's complete medical and dental history must be reviewed in order to identify specific problems and take necessary precautions. Examples of situations that alter the normal defenses are included under the topics below.

A. Abnormal Physical Conditions

A heart valve may be defective as a result of a congenital or acquired condition. Such a valve may be susceptible to infective endocarditis resulting from a bacteremia created during dental or dental hygiene instrumentation. Prevention of infective endocarditis is described on pages 686–687.

B. Systemic Diseases

Examples of systemic conditions in which susceptibility to infection is increased are diabetes mellitus, alcoholism, leukemia, glomerulonephritis, acquired immunodeficiency syndrome, and all causes of immunosuppression.

C. Drug Therapy

Certain drugs used in the treatment of systemic disease alter the body's defenses. Examples are steroids and chemotherapeutic agents that are immunosuppressive. Special precautions such as prophylactic antibiotics are needed to prevent infection.

D. Prostheses and Transplants

A patient with, for example, a joint replacement, cardiac prosthesis, ventriculoatrial shunt for hydrocephalus, or an organ transplant may require antibiotic premedication.

IV. Prevention of Autogenous Infection

A. Give Antibiotic Premedication

For the patient who is at risk for infection that may result from bacteremia, antibiotic premedication may be indicated. A list of patients who are medically compromised and potentially endangered during treatment appears on pages 85 and 91. For the American Heart Association recommendations for antibiotic premedication see page 91.

B. Lower the Surface Microbial Count

Suggested procedures for lowering the numbers of microorganisms at the treatment site just prior to treatment are described on page 56. They include bacterial plaque removal procedures, particularly toothbrushing and flossing, rinsing with an antibacterial rinse, and the application of a topical antiseptic. By lowering the numbers of surface microorganisms, the potential for autogenous infection is decreased.

C. Prepare an Injection Site[9,11]

After drying the tissue surface with a sterile sponge, a topical antiseptic is swabbed over the surface (page 56). Retraction should be maintained to prevent contact of other tissues or saliva.

Disposable needles are required for disease control. Particular care must be taken to avoid contacting the needle with anything prior to injection. Contact with a tooth or tissue can contaminate the needle with microorganisms, which can then be injected as the needle is inserted.

PATHOGENS TRANSMISSIBLE BY THE ORAL CAVITY

Selected pathogens that may be transmitted by way of the oral cavity with their disease manifestations, mode of transfer, incubation and communicability periods are listed in table 2–1. Several of the so-called "children's diseases" are included.

Tuberculosis, viral hepatitis, acquired immunodeficiency syndrome, and herpetic diseases will be described in detail in this chapter because of the special problems they create in personal and patient care. The general preventive measures described for these diseases should be applied during all appointments.

I. Oral Findings

The etiologic agents of many communicable diseases enter the body by way of the oral cavity. Many infectious diseases have specific oral manifestations from which the disease can be identified. Pathogens are often present within the oral cavity without producing oral signs or symptoms, a fact of particular importance to the total consideration of prevention of disease transmission.

When studying the diseases that may be acquired by members of the dental team from patients, consideration must be given to the tremendous loss of time and energy, and the potential long-range effect on, or permanent loss to, general health, that can result from illness.

II. Terminology

A few of the terms used in the study of disease transmission are defined here. Other words are defined as they are used in the text.

Incubation period: the time interval between the initial contact with an infectious agent and the appearance of the first sign or symptom of the disease.

Communicable period: the time during which an infectious agent may be transferred directly or indirectly from an infected person to another person. The communicable period may include or overlap the incubation period.

Carrier: a person who harbors a specific infectious agent in the absence of discernible clinical disease and serves as a potential source of infection. A carrier may be temporary or transient, or may be chronic.

Serum marker: a specific finding (such as an antibody or antigen) by blood laboratory analysis that identifies an existing disease state or stage.

Serologic diagnosis: the diagnosis of a disease by the serum markers of that specific condition.

Seroconversion: after exposure to the etiologic agent of a disease, the blood changes from negative ("seronegative") to positive ("seropositive") serum marker for that disease.

EIA or ELISA: an enzyme-linked immunosorbent assay laboratory test to detect antibody in the blood serum.

WB (Western Blot): a laboratory test for antibody that is more specific than the EIA, and is used to validate seropositive reactions to EIA.

Replication: the process by which viruses reproduce and multiply.

TUBERCULOSIS

Mycobacterium tuberculosis, the etiologic agent in tuberculosis, is a resistant organism that requires special consideration when sterilization and disinfection methods are selected and administered. Tuberculosis is a serious disease that can involve many months and years of lost time during the active stages of illness and the convalescence following. Clinical procedures must be planned to prevent exposure and infection from this debilitating disease.

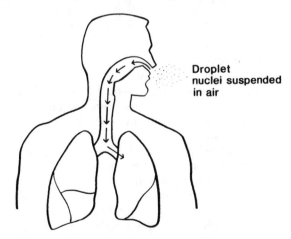

Droplet nuclei suspended in air

Figure 2–2. Droplet Nuclei. Many potentially pathogenic microorganisms are disseminated by aerosols and splatter. The primary mode of transmission of tubercle bacilli is by droplet nuclei breathed directly into the lung. (From McInnes, M.E.: *Essentials of Communicable Disease,* 2nd ed. St. Louis, The C.V. Mosby Co., 1975.)

Tuberculosis is a common communicable disease throughout the world. In the United States, it is no longer a leading cause of death as it was before preventive public health and medical measures were developed. Among reportable bacterial infections, however, it is still high.

I. Transmission

Tuberculosis is contracted by the inhalation of fresh droplets containing tubercle bacilli. The organisms are disseminated from sputum and saliva by coughing, breathing heavily, or sneezing (figure 2–2). During the use of ultrasonic and other handpieces, and water and air spray, aerosols are created that can carry the bacilli. Aerosol production was described on pages 10–11.

When the organisms are in tiny aerosols, they can pass readily into the lungs and the respiratory bronchioles. There, they can invade the tissue and establish an infection.

Transmission of tuberculosis is dependent on the following: (1) the degree to which the diseased person produces infectious droplets, (2) the amount and duration of exposure, and (3) the susceptibility of the recipient. Some patients are more contagious than others. Maximum communicability is usually just before the disease is diagnosed when the person may have a severe cough and other respiratory symptoms.

The tubercle bacillus may enter the body by ingestion or direct inoculation as well as by inhalation. Infection of the lungs is most common, but the tubercle bacillus also infects lymph nodes, meninges, kidneys, bone, skin, and the oral cavity.

A person may have or may have had an infection, and therefore have a positive tuberculin test. Many adults have positive tuberculin tests without ever having had disease symptoms.

II. Disease Process

A. Predisposing Factors

Any debilitating or immunosuppressive condition can predispose to invasion by the tubercle bacillus. Systemic conditions that may be related to lowered resistance to infection include diabetes, congenital heart disease, chronic lung disease, and alcoholism.

Tuberculosis is one of the opportunistic infections associated with the acquired immunodeficiency syndrome (page 23).[12]

B. Incubation Period

As shown in table 2–1, the incubation period may be as long as 6 months. After such an extended period, it is difficult or impossible to trace the origin of the disease.

C. Early Symptoms

In the early stages before marked symptoms appear, the patient may have a low-grade fever, loss of appetite, weight loss, and may tire easily. There may be a slight cough, and eventually spu-

Table 2–1. Infectious Diseases of Oral Transmission

Infectious Agent	Disease or Condition	Route or Mode of Transmission	Incubation Period	Communicable Period
Hepatitis A virus (HAV)	"Infectious" hepatitis Type A hepatitis	Fecal-oral Food, water, shellfish	2 to 6 weeks (average 28 to 30 days)	2 to 3 weeks before onset (jaundice) through 8 days after
Hepatitis B virus (HBV)	"Serum" hepatitis Type B hepatitis	Blood Saliva and all body fluids Sexual contact Perinatal	2 to 6 months (average 60 to 90 days)	Before, during, and after clinical signs Carrier state: indefinite
Delta agent Delta hepatitis virus (HDV)	Delta hepatitis	Coinfection with HBV Blood Sexual contacts Perinatal	2 to 10 weeks	All phases
Non-A, non-B hepatitis virus (HNANBV)	Non-A, non-B hepatitis (B-like)	Similar to HBV	2 to 6 months	Like HBV
	Epidemic Non-A, non-B (A-like)	Fecal-oral Contaminated water	15 to 64 days	Not known. May be like HAV
Human immunodeficiency virus (HIV)	Acquired immunodeficiency syndrome (AIDS)	Blood and blood products (infected IV needles) Sexual contact Transplacental and perinatal	3 months to 10 years 2 years for transfusion case	From asymptomatic through onset of opportunistic infections
Herpes simplex virus Type 1 (HSV-1) Type 2 (HSV-2)	Acute herpetic gingivostomatitis Herpes labialis Ocular herpetic infections Herpetic whitlow	Saliva Direct contact (lip, hand) Indirect contact (on objects, limited survival) Sexual contact	2 to 12 days	Labialis: one day before onset until lesions are crusted Acute stomatitis: 7 weeks after recovery Asymptomatic infection: with viral shedding Reactivation period: with viral shedding
Varicella-zoster virus (VZV)	Chickenpox Shingles	Direct contact Indirect contact Airborne droplet	2 to 3 weeks	5 days prior to onset of rash until crusting of vesicles
Epstein-Barr virus (EBV)	Infectious mononucleosis	Direct contact Saliva	4 to 6 weeks	Prolonged Pharyngeal excretion 1 year after infection

tum, indicating the possible presence of tubercle bacilli in the throat and saliva.

D. Later Symptoms

Definite temperature elevation, particularly in the afternoons, night sweats, weakness, and a persistent cough become apparent. Diagnosis is by chest radiograph and tuberculin testing.

E. Reinfection Tuberculosis

A focus of an infection may remain inactive and later produce a recurrence. Treatment of a primary infection may have been incomplete. Reactivity may be related to a debilitating condition or immunosuppression.

III. Clinical Management

A. Patient History

1. *Questions About Symptoms.* In early disease, there may not be a suspicion of tuberculosis to suggest a need for precautions to prevent personal exposure. Careful history-taking and review of previous histories for comparison may show the need to refer the patient to a physician.

2. *High-Incidence Groups.* Information may be available for specific residence groups. For example, in comparison to the prevalence of tuberculosis in the United States of approximately 9.3 cases per 100,000 population, the prevalence rate among Asian and Pacific Islander refugees was 49.6 per 100,000.[13] Preventive therapy has been administered to thousands of the refugees who have been exposed, as has treatment therapy for those with known active disease.

Table 2–1. Infectious Diseases of Oral Transmission (Continued)

Infectious Agent	Disease or Condition	Route or Mode of Transmission	Incubation Period	Communicable Period
Cytomegalovirus (CMV)	Neonatal cytomegalovirus infection Cytomegaloviral disease	Perinatal Direct contact (most body secretions) Blood transfusion	Inexact 3 to 8 weeks after transfusion	Months to years
Influenza viruses	Influenza	Nasal discharge Respiratory droplets	24 to 72 hours	3 days from clinical onset
Measles virus (Morbillivirus)	Rubeola (measles)	Direct contact Saliva Airborne droplet	8 to 13 days to fever, 14 days to rash	Few days before fever to 4 days after rash appears
Rubella virus (Togavirus)	Rubella (German measles)	Nasopharyngeal secretions Direct contact Airborne droplets	16 to 23 days	From 1 week to at least 4 days after rash appears Highly communicable
	Congenital rubella syndrome	Maternal infection first trimester		Infants shed virus for months after birth
Mumps virus (Paramyxovirus)	Infectious parotitis	Direct contact (saliva) Airborne droplet	2 to 3 weeks (average 18 days)	From 1 to 7 days before symptoms until 9 days after swelling
Poliovirus types 1, 2, 3	Poliomyelitis	Direct contact (saliva) Droplet Fecal-oral	7 to 14 days	Probably most infectious 7 to 10 days before and after onset of symptoms
Mycobacterium tuberculosis	Tuberculosis	Droplet nuclei Sputum Saliva	Up to 6 months	Long, repeated exposure usually needed
Treponema pallidum	Syphilis	Direct contact Transplacental	10 days to 10 weeks	Variable and indefinite May be 2 to 4 years
Neisseria gonorrhoeae	Gonorrhea	Direct contact Indirect (short survival of organisms)	2 to 9 days	During incubation Continued for months and years if untreated
Group A streptococci (Beta-hemolytic) Streptococcus pyogenes	Streptococcal sore throat Scarlet fever Impetigo Erysipelas	Respiratory droplets Direct contact	1 to 3 days	10 to 21 days, untreated Many nasal oropharyngeal carriers
Staphylococcus aureus Staphylococcus epidermidis	Abscesses Boils (furuncle) Impetigo Bacterial pneumonia	Saliva Exudates Nasal discharge	4 to 10 days Variable and indefinite	While lesions drain and carrier state persists

B. Extraoral and Intraoral Examination

Tuberculosis is primarily a lesion of the lungs, but any organ or tissue may be involved.

1. *Lymphadenopathy.* Regional lymph nodes may be enlarged.
2. *Oral Lesions.*[14] Oral lesions are relatively rare, but when they occur they are usually ulcers. They may be located on the soft or hard palate and, occasionally, on the tongue.

C. Patient Under Treatment

Chemotherapy can control the patient's contagious condition. Isoniazid is used for long periods, sometimes in combination with rifampin. After a few weeks from the beginning of therapy, bacilli in the sputum, the cough, and the infectivity are decreased.

VIRAL HEPATITIS

Hepatitis means inflammation of the liver. Viruses cause a variety of types of hepatitis. Some of the viruses have been specifically identified, and hepatitis A, hepatitis B, hepatitis D (delta), and hepatitis non-A, non-B are described in this section.

The incidence of hepatitis B has increased significantly over the past 20 years. It has been a serious occupational hazard for health-care workers. Among professional personnel, both medical and dental, the incidence has reached startling proportions, to the point where the use of strict sterilization of equipment and materials, aseptic techniques, and self-protection measures are mandatory. With the advent of the hepatitis B vaccine, immunization for health workers and other frequently exposed individuals is available.[15]

Table 2–2 lists the hepatitis terminology with abbreviations and significance.

HEPATITIS A[16]

Hepatitis A occurs much more frequently in children and young adults than in older adults. It is more severe in adults.

I. Transmission

A. Fecal–Oral Route

The most common transmission is through close contact in unsanitary conditions. Unwashed hands of an infected person can contaminate anything touched.

B. Waterborne and Food-borne

Epidemics may occur when sanitation is inadequate. Contaminated water may carry hepatitis A virus directly to those using the water, or it may contaminate shellfish grown in the water.

Infected food handlers can contaminate uncooked food or food handled after cooking.

C. Blood

In the earliest days of active disease, the blood contains transient hepatitis A viruses; however, transmission by blood transfusion is rare.

II. Disease Process

A. Incubation and Communicability

The incubation period is from 2 to 6 weeks, with an average of 30 days. During the 2- to 3-

Table 2–2. Viral Hepatitis: Common Abbreviations

Abbreviation	Term	Significance
HEPATITIS A		
HAV	Hepatitis A virus	Etiologic agent of type A hepatitis
anti-HAV	Antibody to hepatitis A virus	Immunity to infection
IgM anti-HAV	IgM antibody to hepatitis A	
HEPATITIS B		
HBV	Hepatitis B virus (Dane particle)	Etiologic agent of type B hepatitis
		HBV has 3 antigens (**s,c,e**)
HBsAg	Hepatitis B surface antigen (Australia antigen)	Indicates current HBV infection
		Serum marker in acute disease and carrier state
anti-HBs	Antibody to HBV surface antigen	Indicates
		(1) active immunity to HBV infection
		(2) passive immunity from HBIG
		(3) immune response from HBV vaccine
HBcAg	Hepatitis B core antigen	Marker for persistent infection
anti-HBc	Antibody to HBV core antigen	Indicates natural HBV exposure from past infection
HBeAg	Hepatitis B "e" antigen	Indicates high infectivity; persists into carrier state
anti-HBe	Antibody to HBV "e" antigen	Suggests low degree of infectivity
HEPATITIS D		
HDV	Delta virus	Etiologic agent of delta hepatitis; causes infection only in presence of HBV
delta-Ag (HD-Ag)	Delta antigen	Marker in early acute infection
anti-delta-Ag	Antibody to delta antigen	Indicates past or present infection with the delta virus
HEPATITIS NON-A, NON-B		
HNANBV	Unidentified agents of non-A, non-B	Etiologic agents of at least two types of hepatitis
Epidemic NANB	Epidemic non-A, non-B	Fecal-oral or waterborne hepatitis infection
IMMUNE GLOBULINS		
IG	Immune globulin	Contains antibodies to HAV; low titer antibodies to HBV
HBIG	Hepatitis B immune globulin	Contains high titer antibodies to HBV

week period before the onset of jaundice, the infection is communicable. Shortly after jaundice appears, the communicability begins to diminish. There is no carrier state.

B. Signs and Symptoms

The stages are defined by the incidence of jaundice, as preicteric (before jaundice appears) and icteric (while jaundice is present). Hepatitis A without jaundice (anicteric) is two to three times more prevalent than icteric. A diagnosis of hepatitis is not always made, because without jaundice, symptoms may resemble influenza or other diseases.

1. *Preicteric Phase.* Typically, there is an abrupt onset of an influenza-like illness, with fever, headache, fatigue, nausea, vomiting, and abdominal pain. The liver may be enlarged and tender to palpation.
2. *Icteric Phase.* Jaundice may appear in adults, but rarely in children. Other symptoms become prolonged, and the patient may be ill for a few days to a month. Occasionally, chronic hepatitis follows, but 85 to 90 percent of patients recover completely.

III. Immunity

Anti-HAV is usually detectable in the serum within 2 weeks of onset. Immunity to reinfection follows with recovery.

In addition to those who are known to have had the disease, many more people acquire immunity from undetected disease.

IV. Prevention

A. Sanitation and Personal Hygiene

Because the principal means of transmission is by way of the feces, prevention on that level is indicated.

1. Public health control of food handlers and of water contamination.
2. Personal hygiene control through scrupulous handwashing by a patient and all contacts, as well as by all health-care workers involved in patient care.

B. Application in Dental Setting

Instrument sterilization, use of disposable materials, and all related precautions for persons and objects contacted by the patient. Such procedures must be the same for all patients, because the presence of hepatitis A viruses is not usually known. Clinic procedures are described in Chapter 4.

V. Passive Immunization[17]

A. IG

Standard immune globulin (IG) is used for the prevention or modification of hepatitis A in a person known to be susceptible, who is accidentally exposed. Because the incubation period may be as short as 2 weeks, IG must be given within the first few days following exposure.

B. Indications

1. *Individual Exposure.* Exposure sufficient for the person to need IG requires close personal, physical contact, such as by the members of the patient's household and other intimate contacts.
2. *Institution for Custodial Care* (Examples: prisons, facilities for developmentally disabled). Hepatitis A may be endemic in certain institutions. IG may be used during outbreaks, for new admissions, and for all employees who have direct contact.
3. *Day-Care Centers.* When there is evidence of HAV transmission in a day-care center, particularly where children are in diapers, IG should be administered to staff, children, and family members with whom the children reside. Thorough handwashing after diaper changing is emphasized.
4. *Traveler to Endemic Area.* If a stay is to be longer than 3 months, and especially outside ordinary tourist routes, in a tropical area, or an area known to have endemic hepatitis A, IG may be indicated. A second dose may be recommended for a stay longer than 5 months. A subclinical infection may be acquired that would confer immunity.

HEPATITIS B[16,18]

Hepatitis B differs in many respects from hepatitis A, particularly in mode of transmission, the length of the incubation period, the onset, and the existence of a chronic carrier state. Hepatitis B occurs at any age. Figure 2–3 shows a diagram of the hepatitis B virus.

I. Transmission

The major sources of hepatitis B virus are patients with acute hepatitis B infection and symptomless chronic carriers.

A. Routes of Transmission

1. *Blood.* Parenteral inoculation is the usual mode of transfer. Blood transfusion from infected donors, use of contaminated instruments by medical and dental professionals, use of contaminated needles by drug abusers, and accidental self-inoculation by health-care workers are examples.

Testing of each unit of blood for HBsAg has been required for several years. Post-transfusion cases have been nearly eliminated.
2. *Other Body Fluids.* HBsAg has been found in nearly all body fluids including saliva, gingival sulcus fluid, semen, menstrual blood, tears, urine, sweat, and nasopharyngeal secretions. The transfer of disease may occur by oral

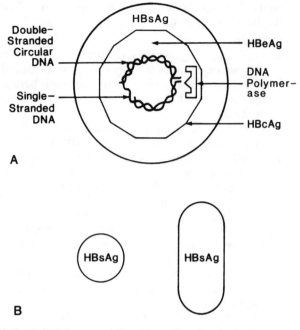

Figure 2–3. Diagram of the Hepatitis B Virus. A. The virus is composed of an outer component of HBsAg and an inner component of HBcAg. Inside the core particle is a single molecule of circular, partially double-stranded DNA, an endogenous DNA polymerase, and HBeAg. **B.** Spherical and tubular particles of HBsAg circulate in infected blood in great numbers. (Redrawn from Hoofnagle, J.H. and Schafer, D.F.: Serologic Markers of Hepatitis B Virus Infection, *Semin. Liver Dis.*, 6:1, Number 1, 1986.)

and sexual routes or other close physical contact. Salivary transmission by way of hands and aerosols is of particular importance to dental personnel.

3. *Perinatal Transmission.* An infected mother can transmit hepatitis B to her baby, especially when she has acute hepatitis during the third trimester of pregnancy. The baby can become a persistent carrier. The use of hepatitis B immune globulin (HBIG) and HB vaccine is recommended for postexposure prophylaxis.[19]

B. Individuals at Risk for Hepatitis B[17,20]

Risk populations are those that have an increased prevalence of infection, increased chances or likelihood of infection, and increased prevalence of disease carriers. High risk in HBV infection can be related to a variety of factors including occupation, place of residence, life style, confinement to an institution, other diseases and their treatments, and parenteral drug abuse. A person may belong to more than one of the risk groups listed here.

Health-care workers are included in the list; however, when they adhere to the use of protective barriers (gloves, masks, eyecoverings) and follow essential precautions for blood and other body fluid infection control, as well as having immunity following vaccination or acquired antibody to hepatitis B, they are really at a low risk.

1. Immigrants/refugees from areas of high endemic HBV.
2. Users of parenteral drugs (swapping contaminated needles).
3. Homosexually active males not using safe sex practices.*
4. Heterosexually active persons with multiple partners, including prostitutes, not using safe sex practices.*
5. Persons who have repeatedly contracted sexually transmitted diseases.
6. Clients and staff in institutions for the mentally retarded, current or former residents, particularly individuals with Down's syndrome.
7. Patients and staff in hemodialysis units.
8. Recipients of blood products used for treating clotting disorders, particularly before all blood was screened prior to 1985.
9. Patients with active or chronic liver diseases.
10. Health-care workers with frequent blood contact are at a higher risk than other health-care workers who have no or infrequent blood contact. Included are emergency room staff, hospital surgical staff, dental hygienists, dentists, blood bank and plasma fractionation workers.
11. Household contacts of HBV carriers.
12. Male prisoners.
13. Military populations stationed in countries with high endemic HBV.
14. Returned travelers from areas of endemic HBV who stayed longer than 3 months or who were treated medically by transfusion while there.
15. Morticians and embalmers.

II. Disease Process

A. Incubation and Communicability

The incubation period is longer than that for hepatitis A and ranges from 2 to 6 months, with an average of 60 to 90 days. The period of communicability varies, but HBsAg may be detected in the blood as early as 30 days after exposure to the disease.

The presence of serum HBsAg indicates communicability. HBsAg may no longer be detected in the blood from a few days to 3 months after the icteric or jaundice stage of illness.

B. Transient Subclinical Infection

The majority of patients do not have an icteric stage, but have subclinical disease. Many remain undiagnosed for hepatitis, but develop antibodies and permanent immunity.

The infection is transient because the individual has a rapid, strong immune response to the hepatitis virus, and the HBV is cleared before it can become established.

---

*"Safe sex practices" is meant to include barrier protection and no exchange of body fluids (saliva, semen, vaginal secretions), in accord with recommended guidelines.

C. Acute Type B Hepatitis[21]

Hepatitis B cannot be distinguished from other viral hepatitis infections on the basis of the clinical signs and symptoms. The onset or preicteric stage with fever, malaise, and influenza-like symptoms is typical of all types of acute viral hepatitis. The onset may be slower and more insidious for hepatitis B, and may include skin rash, itching, and joint pains.

The period of illness extends from 4 to 6 weeks for hepatitis A and usually longer for hepatitis B.

Convalescence begins with the disappearance of jaundice. During this period, serum antibody (anti-HBs) rises except in those who will become permanent carriers.

D. Carrier State

A chronic carrier of HBV is defined as an individual with the HBsAg marker in the blood serum for more than 6 months. From 5 to 10 percent of infected persons develop a chronic carrier state.

A carrier state may also result following a subclinical undiagnosed exposure and, therefore, be unknown to the individual. Many carriers eventually develop cirrhosis or cancer of the liver.

It is to be hoped that the HBsAg status of a patient can be determined so that dental and dental hygiene procedures can be carried out safely. However, as summarized on page 32, information from the most carefully prepared medical histories reveals only a proportion of the risk patients. For those patients who do not know their status, but who may be included in one of the high-risk groups, a diagnostic serologic test for HBsAg can be requested.

E. Immunity

The presence of anti-HBs in the serum shows that the person had a previous exposure to hepatitis B and is, therefore, immune to reinfection. The anti-HBs may be present, although unknown, because immunity may have been acquired following a subclinical, anicteric, or otherwise unrecognized case of hepatitis B. Pretesting for anti-HBs prior to vaccination for hepatitis may be indicated.

F. Disease Reporting

Physicians are responsible for having all cases of hepatitis they see classified and reported to the state or local health department. A report must also be made on any patient found to be HBsAg positive from testing requested by a dentist.

III. Clinical Management

A. Patient History

Selected questions should be asked to bring out the information needed when it is suspected that a patient may be in a risk group or may have had hepatitis B without knowing. Suggestions for questions are provided on page 32.

B. Sterilization and Barrier Techniques

Complete procedures for an appointment are shown on pages 53–58. Personal barrier techniques for gloves, glasses, masks, and clothing are indicated for all patients because it is not possible to determine the carrier state of all patients. It has been suggested that in a practice where 20 patients are treated daily, at least 1 hepatitis B carrier may come to that office in each 10 days.[20] All patients must be considered potential carriers.

PREVENTION OF HEPATITIS B

Hepatitis B viruses cause serious illness, including acute and chronic hepatitis, cirrhosis, and liver cancer, sometimes leading to disability and death. Hepatitis is the most critical occupational hazard for dental personnel because of their close association with the potentially infected body fluids of patients. Every health care individual should be immunized so that the possibilities of disease acquisition and transmission can be minimized.

I. Active Immunization: The Vaccines[17,19]

Two hepatitis B vaccines are available for pre- and postexposure prophylaxis. Both are administered intramuscularly in the deltoid arm muscle in 3 doses, the first at the outset, then at 1 and 6 months.

A. Plasma-derived HB Vaccine*

The original vaccine was prepared using purified and formalin-treated HBsAg from the plasma of chronic HBsAg carriers. In its preparation, the treatment steps inactivate all classes of viruses so that it becomes impossible to transmit any other disease.

B. Recombinant DNA HB Vaccine†

Recombinant DNA technology has been used to synthesize HBsAg in a culture of *Saccharomyces cerevisiae*, a yeast. The HBsAg is purified and sterilized.

C. Effectiveness

1. Both vaccines act in a comparable manner to stimulate antibody, and both convey the same degree of immunity.
2. In healthy 20- to 39-year-old adults, immunity is conferred in over 95 percent; in children, protective antibodies are shown in 99 percent.
3. Postvaccination testing for anti-HBs is recommended for a hemodialysis patient or other risk person having frequent exposure, including dental personnel.
4. Lower responses have been noted in older people, hemodialysis patients, and in people receiving the injection in the buttock rather than the deltoid muscle.[22]

---

*Heptavax, Merck Sharp & Dohme
†Recombivax HB, Merck Sharp & Dohme

5. The vaccines have no effect on a person who is already a carrier,[23] and no effect on a person who already has antibodies.
6. Immunization is not contraindicated during pregnancy, and it would be recommended for a woman in a risk group. An HBV infection during pregnancy can be severe, and the newborn can become a permanent carrier.[19]

D. Booster[19]
1. The higher initial peak of response usually means longer persistence of antibody.
2. A 7-year booster is suggested; however, the antibody level can be tested to determine individual needs.
3. For certain risk patients, particularly hemodialysis patients, semiannual antibody testing has been recommended.[19]

II. Postexposure Prophylaxis[17,19]

A. Indications for Prophylaxis
1. Newborn of HBsAg-positive mother.
2. Significant hepatitis B exposure to HBsAg-positive blood.
   a. Contaminated needlestick.
   b. Puncture wound from a contaminated sharp dental instrument.
   c. Contamination of mucous membrane or any open wound by saliva, blood, or aerosol spray.
3. Sexual exposure to an HBsAg-positive or suspected positive person.

B. Hepatitis B Immune Globulin (HBIG)
High-titer anti-HBs immune globulin (HBIG) has been available, following research over recent years. Its primary use is for postexposure prophylaxis.

IG, described for passive immunization for hepatitis A (page 17), contains low-titer anti-HBs of varying amounts. It is effective against HBV for preexposure prophylaxis to a lesser degree than HBIG, but should be used when HBIG is not available. IG is recommended when protection for exposure to non-A, non-B hepatitis (NANB) is needed.

C. Procedure for Newborn of HBsAg-Positive Mother
1. *Immediate Treatment:* HBIG and HBV vaccine intramuscularly within 7 days of birth and at 1 and 6 months.
2. *Effect:* the combined treatment prevents up to 94% of infants from developing a carrier state.[24]

D. Procedure for Needlestick or Wound from a Contaminated Instrument[17,19]
1. *Vaccinated Professional*
   a. Test for antibody unless adequate level has been shown within the past 12 months.
      b. Low antibody: HBIG and HBV-vaccine booster are indicated immediately (within 7 days).
2. *Not Vaccinated*
   a. Initiate HB vaccine series and obtain HBIG immediately (within 7 days).
   b. Test the source for HBsAg.

HEPATITIS D[17,25]

The delta hepatitis virus, also called the delta agent, cannot cause infection except in the presence of HBV infection. The diagram in figure 2–4 shows the delta antigen surrounded by HBsAg.

I. Transmission
Most frequently, the delta infection is superimposed on HBsAg carriers. It occurs primarily in persons who have multiple exposures to HBV, particularly patients with hemophilia and intravenous drug abusers.

Transmission is similar to that of HBV, that is, by way of direct inoculation of contaminated blood, illicit use of parenteral drugs, close personal contacts, and perinatal transfer.

II. Disease Process
Delta hepatitis is more severe and the mortality rate is greater than with hepatitis B. Infection can occur in the following ways:

A. Coinfection
Acute delta hepatitis occurring with acute HBV infection may lead to resolution of both types. Clearance of HBV may lead to clearance of delta virus.

B. Superinfection
Acute delta hepatitis is superimposed on an existing carrier HBV state. The HBV carrier state remains unchanged, and a delta carrier state may develop in addition.

C. Superimposition
Chronic delta hepatitis superimposes on the chronic HBsAg carrier.

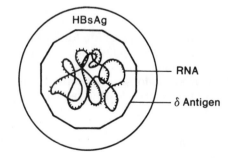

Figure 2–4. Diagram of the Hepatitis Delta Virus. The delta agent antigen is surrounded by the hepatitis B surface antigen. (Redrawn from Hoofnagle, J.H.: Type D Hepatitis and the Hepatitis Delta Virus, in Thomas, H.C. and Jones, E.A.: *Recent Advances in Hepatology.* Edinburgh, Churchill Livingstone, 1986.)

III. Prevention

All measures used to prevent hepatitis B will prevent delta hepatitis because HDV is dependent on the presence of HBV. Immunization with hepatitis B vaccine also protects the recipient from delta hepatitis infection.

HEPATITIS NON-A, NON-B[17]

When acute hepatitis cannot be attributed to A, B, D, or other known and identifiable viruses, the non-A, non-B category has been used. At least two and maybe more viruses with different modes of transmission have been classified as NANB. This group has also been referred to as Hepatitis C.

I. Classic Non-A, Non-B (B-Like)

Originally associated with therapeutic blood transfusions, this condition was termed "post-transfusion hepatitis." Cases of hepatitis following transfusions that could not be identified with hepatitis A or B were called non-A, non-B. This type is also found after parenteral drug abuse. It is uncommon in homosexuals.

The onset and symptoms of NANB are similar to those for all viral hepatitis. A carrier state develops more frequently than after hepatitis B.

II. Epidemic Non-A, Non-B (A-Like)

Another name for this type of hepatitis is enterically transmitted non-A, non-B (ET-NANB).[26,27] Large outbreaks have been reported associated with fecally contaminated water sources after heavy rains where sewage disposal was inadequate. Adults have been more affected than children, and the mortality rate in pregnant women has been high.

ACQUIRED IMMUNODEFICIENCY SYNDROME (AIDS)

The *acquired immunodeficiency syndrome* (AIDS) is a severe condition caused by infection with the *human immunodeficiency virus* (HIV). Infected patients may present with a variety of manifestations ranging from no symptoms to severe immunodeficiency and life-threatening secondary infectious diseases and cancers. Figure 2–5 illustrates the three general stages: asymptomatic infection, AIDS-related complex (ARC), and AIDS. During all stages, the serum test for HIV antibody is positive.

The HIV damages both the immune and the neurologic systems. Immunodeficiency results from the depletion of T4 helper/inducer lymphocytes. HIV is selective to the T4 lymphocyte and certain brain cells.

I. Terminology

AIDS: Acquired immunodeficiency syndrome.
ARC: AIDS-related complex.
HIV: Human immunodeficiency virus (previously called HTLV-III or LAV).
HIV Antibody: Indication of infection shown by blood test. It is the serum marker for HIV infection.
T4 Helper/Inducer (CD4): Thymus-derived lymphocyte (T cell) responsible for cell-mediated immunity.

II. Transmission

The AIDS virus has been found in most body fluids. Transmission has been demonstrated primar-

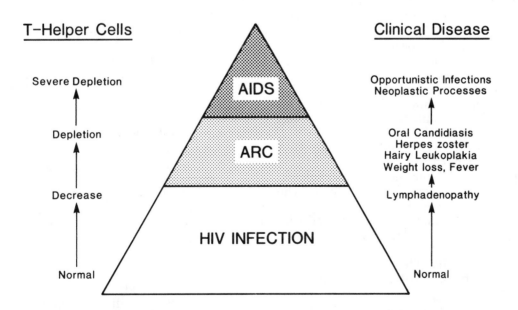

Figure 2–5. Stages of Infection with the Human Immunodeficiency Virus. (Adapted from *Etiology and Epidemiology of HTLV-III Related Disease*, Abbott Laboratories, North Chicago, Illinois, 1986.)

ids. Transmission has been demonstrated primarily by way of blood, semen, vaginal secretions, and breast milk.

A. Routes of Transmission

Sexual, blood, and perinatal contacts are the principal routes. For infection to occur, it is necessary for the HIV to enter the recipient's lymphocytes or brain cells by way of the bloodstream. The virus reaches the bloodstream by the following:

1. *Intimate Sexual Contact* (both homosexual and heterosexual). The virus from an infected person's blood, semen, or vaginal secretion enters the blood through tiny breaks in the rectum, vagina, or penis.
2. *Exposure to Infected Blood or Blood Products.*
   a. Inoculation during intravenous use of drugs: sharing of needles, syringes, or other invasive implements by drug users.
   b. Transfusion and use of blood products by patients with blood disorders; serologic testing of all donor blood has nearly eliminated the threat of infection from transfusion.
3. *Maternal Fetal or Perinatal Contact.*[28,29] Viruses can be transmitted across the placenta. Exposure to infection can occur in utero, during delivery, and after birth through breast milk or other close contact.

B. High Risk Individuals

1. Sexually active homosexual and bisexual men having multiple sex partners without using safe sex practices.*
2. Users or former users of intravenous drugs, particularly when contaminated needles are shared.
3. Recipients of blood transfusions or blood products prior to mandatory testing for HIV antibodies in 1985. This includes people with hemophilia or other coagulation disorders.
4. Male and female prostitutes who do not use safe sex practices.*
5. Health care workers who do not adhere to strict barrier procedures and do not follow essential blood and other body fluid precautions for infection control.
6. Females artificially inseminated with HIV-infected semen.
7. Recipients of HIV-infected organ transplants.
8. Steady sexual partners of all of the above who do not use safe sex practices.*
9. Steady sexual partners of those infected with AIDS or at high risk for AIDS who do not use safe sex practices.*
10. Infants born to HIV-infected mothers.
11. Infants fed breast milk from HIV-infected mothers.

---

*"Safe sex practices" is meant to include barrier protection and no exchange of body fluids (saliva, semen, vaginal secretions) in accord with recommended guidelines.

C. Serologic Tests for Antibodies[30]

Persons exposed to the HIV usually develop detectable antibody levels within 3 to 12 weeks. Antibody presence indicates infection, but there may be no clinical symptoms.

Blood banks are required to test all blood received for hepatitis B, syphilis, and the HIV antibody. Several tests have been used to detect the HIV antibody.[31] Frequently used tests have been the EIA (ELISA) and the WB (Western Blot) defined on page 13. When the test result is positive, the blood is rejected and the person is notified and counseled.

III. Disease Process[32,33]

A. Incubation Period

The incubation period ranges from 3 months to 10 years or more. An infection may be early and acute, or no symptoms may appear for several years. Infection with the HIV does not always lead to AIDS, but the infection remains and may be transmitted to others.

B. Disease Development

1. HIV enters by way of the blood and becomes bound by cellular receptors (CD4) on the surfaces of specific cells.
2. Target cells with CD4 include T-helper cells, macrophages, monocytes, natural killer cells, and certain neurons and glial cells of the brain.
3. The virus enters the cell; replication occurs after activation of the host cell.
4. Infectious viral particles are released; numbers of target cells are inactivated and decreased; the immune system is weakened.
5. HIV antibodies circulate in the bloodstream.

IV. Progression of Disease: Signs and Symptoms[33,34]

HIV infection can progress from initial exposure through primary (acute) infection, an asymptomatic stage, persistent generalized lymphadenopathy (PGL), to ARC, and finally, to AIDS. The course of the infection is shown in figure 2–6. Symptoms vary with individuals, and overlap of the stages is common.

A. Initial Stage: Primary HIV Infection

An acute infection may be experienced within 2 to 6 weeks following the initial exposure. Symptoms are usually not recognized as specific for HIV infection and may include the following:

1. Fever, rash, abdominal cramps, diarrhea.
2. Blood changes resembling infectious mononucleosis.

B. Asymptomatic Stage

Some patients go through a period of no apparent symptoms.

C. Persistent Generalized Lymphadenopathy (PGL)

PGL may last 3 months or longer, with or without fever.

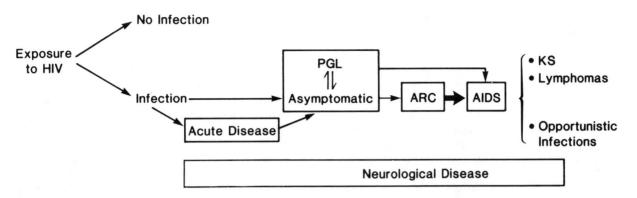

Figure 2–6. Course of Infection with Human Immunodeficiency Virus (HIV). ARC = AIDS-related complex; AIDS = Acquired immunodeficiency syndrome; PGL = Persistent generalized lymphadenopathy; KS = Kaposi's sarcoma. (From Seligmann, M., et al.: Immunology of Human Immunodeficiency Virus Infection and the Acquired Immunodeficiency Syndrome. *Ann. Intern. Med., 107,* 234, August, 1987.)

D. AIDS-Related Complex (ARC)

Both asymptomatic patients and those with PGL may progress to ARC with symptoms such as the following:

1. Long-lasting fever; night sweats.
2. Weight loss; chronic diarrhea; fatigue.
3. Oral conditions that may be among the first clinical signs of AIDS.

E. Head and Neck Findings in ARC and AIDS[35-38]

Nearly all HIV-infected patients will have head and/or neck manifestations. Certain oral findings have been identified as characteristic of HIV infection. The extra- and intraoral examination takes on special meaning in the recognition of disease symptoms; they may be the first recognizable symptoms.

1. *Lymphadenopathy*
2. *Infections*
   a. Fungal: Oral candidiasis appears in various forms, including the pseudomembranous type and angular cheilitis.
   b. Viral: Herpes simplex lesions, oral viral leukoplakia (hairy leukoplakia), oral lesions of chicken pox, verruca vulgaris, condyloma acuminatum, and cytomegalovirus ulcer may be seen.
   c. Bacterial: Necrotizing ulcerative gingivitis, accelerated gingivitis, and rapidly progressive periodontitis have occurred in otherwise well-kept mouths.
3. *Neoplasms*
   a. Kaposi's sarcoma: Reddish blue or purple lesions appear on the face and neck, and in the oral cavity on gingiva, palate, base of tongue, pharynx, and tonsils.
   b. Oral non-Hodgkin's lymphomas and squamous cell carcinomas may develop in HIV-infected patients.

F. Acquired Immunodeficiency Syndrome (AIDS)

AIDS is the end stage of HIV infection. Because of the wide variety of symptoms that may be present, the clinical and laboratory findings have been officially combined to provide a universal case definition. For the complete listing, the *Revision of the CDC Surveillance Case Definition for Acquired Immunodeficiency Syndrome*[39] should be consulted.

The generalized manifestations of the disease can be divided into opportunistic infections, neoplasms, encephalopathy, and the HIV wasting syndrome. Examples are listed.

1. *Opportunistic Infections.* Pneumocystis carinii pneumonia; candidiasis of the esophagus, trachea, bronchi, and/or lungs; herpesvirus infections; tuberculosis.
2. *Neoplasms.* Kaposi's sarcoma, primary lymphoma of the brain.
3. *HIV Encephalopathy.* Other names for this complication are HIV dementia and AIDS dementia. Disabling cognitive and/or motor dysfunction develops with symptoms of apathy, inability to concentrate, poor memory, and depression.
4. *HIV Wasting Syndrome ("slim" disease).* Long-term fever, marked weight loss, diarrhea, with chronic weakness are apparent, along with laboratory evidence of HIV infection.

V. AIDS in Children[40-42]

A percentage of patients with AIDS are children. Mortality is high, often as a result of overwhelming bacterial infections.

A. Primary Sources of Infection

1. Transfusion of infected blood or use of infected blood products.
2. Mother is infected or at a high risk for AIDS. A mother may have no symptoms and may never have been tested for antibody. A mother may be an intravenous drug abuser or have

heterosexual contacts with HIV-infected men not using safe sex practices.

B. Signs and Symptoms

1. *Children Infected In Utero.* Abnormal physical features that may result from exposure during early fetal development include microcephaly, slight obliquity of the eyes, flattened nasal bridge, and increased space between the eyes.

2. *Perinatal Problems.* A baby may be small, premature, fail to thrive, and have recurrent infections, particularly respiratory diseases. There may be lymphadenopathy, oral candidiasis, recurrent aphthous ulceration.

C. Test for Antibody

1. *Infant.* Whether the antibody test immediately after birth reveals infection depends on when the exposure to HIV occurred. Antibodies may not have developed if exposure to the virus was during the last trimester, during delivery, or during breast feeding.

2. *Mother.* Women of childbearing age who are at risk for HIV infection should be counseled and tested for antibody.[43] Pregnancy might be avoided, or if the woman is already pregnant, proper medical care could be advised.

VI. Clinical Management

A. Patient History

As described on page 32, patients may knowingly or unknowingly provide incorrect information about their health histories. A patient with AIDS may have been refused treatment elsewhere, and will not state the present condition for fear of another refusal.

Certain routine questions will reveal present or past symptoms of persistent infections, long-lasting fever, weight loss, and other characteristics of ARC or AIDS listed under IV above. Questions about other communicable diseases may provide symptoms of HIV infection.

When it is suspected that a patient may belong to one or more high-risk groups, direct, nonjudgmental questions may be asked relative to life style, sex orientation, intravenous drug use, and history of transfusions. A patient should be given to understand that such questions are routine office procedure, asked for the protection of all concerned.

B. Extraoral and Intraoral Examination

A thorough examination of the nodes, skin of the face and neck, oral mucous membranes, and throat of each patient should be routine at an initial appointment and at each maintenance recall. Because lymphadenopathy and certain oral conditions appear before other symptoms of ARC and AIDS, all findings must be carefully evaluated.

A follow-up procedure may be the preparation of a smear for confirmation of candidiasis infection.

C. Sterilization and Disinfection

Procedures for hepatitis B virus destruction are more than adequate for the HIV. Routine precautions must be observed for all patients (page 56) and special precautions applied as indicated (page 58).

Blood and semen are the primary vehicles for transmission. HIV has also been isolated from saliva, tears, and urine, but these have not yet been shown to be direct modes of transmission. Saliva may also contain blood.

D. Patient Factors

1. *Susceptibility.* As with all patients with immunosuppression, the AIDS patient has a high susceptibility to infection. Techniques and procedures for dental and dental hygiene therapy must eliminate possibilities for increasing the danger of infection in the patient.

2. *Stress.* A patient with advanced disease may have experienced loss of work and career, many hospitalizations, lack of support from family and friends because of fear of disease or social stigma, as well as loss of physical appearance and strength.[44] The professional person's attitude and conduct should reflect support, acceptance, and empathy.

E. Prevention

Until a vaccine is available, prevention depends on education to help people understand the modes of transmission of AIDS and how to identify and change risk behaviors. Dental personnel must keep well informed with accurate, current information in order to provide help and direction to patients.

HERPESVIRUS DISEASES

The herpesvirus infections represent a wide variety of disease entities that are highly infectious. Each virus is antigenically distinct. Herpesviruses produce diseases with latent, recurrent, and sometimes, malignant tendencies. For examples, herpes simplex type 2 has been implicated in cervical cancer and herpes simplex type 1 in oral cancer.

Immunosuppressed patients have more frequent and severe herpes infections. Herpesviruses are among the opportunistic organisms in acquired immunodeficiency syndrome (AIDS) (page 23).

I. Viruses: Abbreviations

Of the many herpesviruses, the four that cause diseases in humans are as follows:

VZV: Varicella-zoster virus
EBV: Epstein-Barr virus
CMV: Cytomegalovirus
HSV: Herpes simplex virus 1 (HSV-1) and 2 (HSV-2) *(Herpesvirus hominis)*

II. Viral Latency

A. Ganglia

The herpesviruses have the ability to travel along sensory nerve pathways to specific ganglia. The specific ganglia are usually the following:

1. Herpes simplex 1 (HSV-1) travels to the trigeminal nerve ganglion (figure 2–7).
2. Herpes simplex 2 (HSV-2) goes to the thoracic, lumbar, and sacral dorsal root ganglia.
3. Varicella-zoster (VZV) goes to the sensory ganglia of the vagal, spinal, or cranial nerves.

B. Primary Infection: Sequence of Events[45]

1. Exposure of person to the virus at the mucosal surface or abraded skin.
2. Replication begins in the cells of the dermis and epidermis.
3. Infection of sensory or autonomic nerve endings.
4. Virus travels along the nerve to the ganglion.
5. After primary disease resolves, the virus becomes latent in the ganglion.
6. Reactivation at a later date is precipitated by a stimulus such as sunlight, immunosuppression, infection, or stress (physical or emotional).
7. Virus transports along the nerve to the body surface where replication takes place and a lesion forms, usually in the same spot as the previous activation.

VARICELLA-ZOSTER VIRUS (VZV)[46]

Chickenpox (varicella) and shingles (herpes zoster) are caused by the same virus, the varicella-zoster.

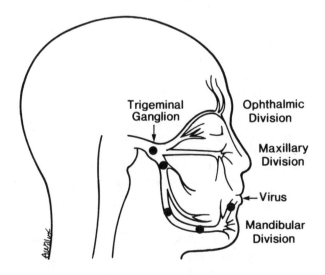

Figure 2–7. Latent Infection of Herpes Simplex Virus-I. Path of the virus traced from point of viral penetration on lip to establishment of latent infection in the trigeminal ganglion.

I. Chickenpox

A. Transmission

Chickenpox is a highly contagious disease transmitted by direct contact, droplet (possibly airborne), or by indirect contact with articles soiled by discharges from the vesicles and the respiratory tract.

B. Disease Process

Primarily a disease of children, it is occasionally found in adults not previously exposed. It is characterized by a maculopapular rash that becomes vesicular in a few days and then scabs. The lesions appear anywhere on the body, more abundantly on the covered than on the exposed parts. When oral lesions occur, they may spread into the upper respiratory tract.

If the itchy, crusted lesions of the skin are scratched, a secondary bacterial infection can result. Other complications are rare, but neurologic and ocular disorders are possible.

II. Shingles

A. Recurrent Infection

Chickenpox leaves a lasting immunity, but the VZV remains latent in the dorsal root ganglia. Reactivation at a older age may result from immunosuppression from drug therapy or from AIDS, and in people with advanced neoplastic disease.

B. Disease Process

Shingles consists of localized unilateral eruptions associated with the nerve endings of the area innervated by the infected sensory nerves. When the second division of the trigeminal nerve is involved, intraoral lesions may occur. Pain, burning, and itching are characteristic. Eye infections and complications of the lungs, central nervous system, liver, and pancreas have been secondary developments.

EPSTEIN-BARR VIRUS (EBV)

Infectious mononucleosis is caused by infection with the EBV. It has also been shown that the EBV replicates within the epithelial cells in hairy leukoplakia, the lesion associated with subsequent development of the acquired immunodeficiency syndrome (page 23).[47]

Infectious mononucleosis is generally a disease of adolescents and young adults. It is characterized by fever, lymphadenopathy, sore throat, and identified by specific atypical lymphocytes called mononucleosis cells.

The disease is transmitted orally by direct contact and by droplet. Viruses are excreted through the saliva even when the patient has no symptoms of disease, so there may be a long period of communicability or a lasting carrier state. EBV can remain latent and become reactivated, particularly when the immune system is compromised by disease or drug therapy.

CYTOMEGALOVIRUS (CMV)[48,49]

Cytomegalovirus infections appear in various forms. The most affected age groups are from 1 to 2 years and from 16 to 50 years. The infections are sometimes latent or subclinical in adults. CMV has been found in the tumor cells of Kaposi's sarcoma (page 23).

I. Transmission

A. Congenital and Neonatal

The virus from the mother's primary or recurrent infection may infect the infant in utero, in the birth canal, or through breast milk.

B. Direct Infections

The virus is excreted in urine, saliva, cervical secretions, and semen. Infection can result from the following:
1. Blood transfusion.
2. Graft transplant from a donor with latent infection.
3. Sexual transmission through semen, vaginal fluid, or saliva.
4. Respiratory droplet, especially among children. Children attending day care centers have a high prevalence of CMV infection.[50]

II. Disease Process

A. Infants

Cytomegalic inclusion disease in a fetus is the most severe form of the infection. Survivors may be premature, anemic, and have mental retardation, microcephaly, motor disabilities, deafness, and chronic liver disease.

B. Adult Infection

A mononucleosis-like syndrome may develop.

C. Immunosuppression and Debilitation

CMV, an opportunistic agent, is a common cause of both primary and reactivated infections in immunodeficient or immunosuppressed patients. Infection with CMV is a serious complication of the acquired immunodeficiency syndrome.

HERPES SIMPLEX VIRUS INFECTIONS[45,48,51]

Primary infection usually occurs in children but may occur at any age.[52] Antibodies (anti-HSV) are produced but do not guarantee immunity to recurrent herpes or to other herpesvirus infections.

Sulcular epithelium has been shown to serve as a reservoir for the viruses.[53] Anti-HSV is present in the gingival sulcus fluid.[54] The possibility exists that trauma to the oral area during a dental or dental hygiene appointment may bring about herpetic recurrence.[55,56]

Acyclovir, an antiviral drug, has been used in capsule, ointment, and intravenous forms in the treatment of HSV-1 and HSV-2. The best response has appeared to be when the drug was started during the prodromal stage.[57,58]

I. Primary Herpetic Gingivostomatitis

The primary infection may be asymptomatic. When clinical disease is evident, gingivostomatitis and pharyngitis are the most frequent manifestations, with fever, malaise, inability to eat, and lymphadenopathy for 2 to 7 days. Painful oral vesicular lesions may occur on the gingiva, mucosa, tongue, and lips. Both first-episode HSV-1 and HSV-2 can cause pharyngitis.

A patient may be a subclinical carrier, and reactivation from the trigeminal ganglia (figure 2–7) may by followed by asymptomatic excretion of the viruses in the saliva. On the other hand, reactivation may lead to herpetic ulcerations of the lip, the typical "cold sore."

II. Herpes Labialis (cold sore, fever blister)

Both HSV-1 and HSV-2 cause genital and oral-facial infections that cannot be distinguished clinically. Reactivations of oral-facial HSV-1 infections are more frequent than of oral-facial HSV-2 infections. Reactivations of genital HSV-2 are more frequent than of genital HSV-1 infections.[59]

Recurrent (HSV) lesions occur at or near the primary lesion at indefinite intervals. They are usually triggered by stress, sunlight, illness, or trauma. Not infrequently, they relate to the patient's dental appointment, when emotional stress and oral trauma may be involved.

A. Prodrome

Before the local lesion appears, there may be burning or slight stinging sensations with slight swelling as a forewarning or prodrome. Most frequently, the recurrent lesion is at the vermillion border of the lower lip; although less commonly, the lesions may occur intraorally on the gingiva or the hard palate.

B. Clinical Characteristics

A group of vesicles forms that will rupture and coalesce. Crusting follows, and healing may take up to 10 days. The lesions are infectious, with viral shedding. Care must be taken by the patient because autoinfection (to the eye, nose, or genitals, for example) is possible, as well as infection of others.

III. Herpetic Whitlow[60,61]

Herpetic whitlow is the herpes simplex infection of the fingers that results from the virus entering through minor skin abrasions. The most frequent location is around a fingernail, where cracks in the skin often occur. Figure 2–8 shows locations where whitlow has been observed.[62]

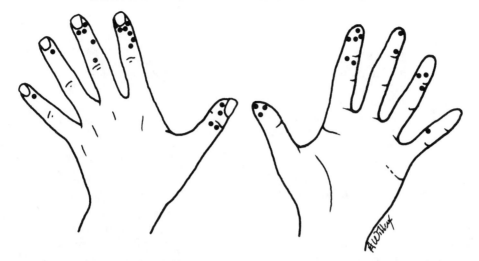

Figure 2–8. Locations of Herpetic Whitlow. Left hand of non-glove-wearing clinician shows frequent sites of herpetic whitlow. Fingers of the nonworking hand used to retract can be particularly vulnerable. (After Stern, H., Elek, S.D., Millar, D.M., and Anderson, H.F.: Herpetic Whitlow, A Form of Cross Infection in Hospitals, *Lancet, 2,* 871, November 21, 1959.)

A. Transmission

A whitlow may be a primary or recurrent infection of HBV-1 or HBV-2. Transmission results from direct contact with a vesicular lesion on a patient's lip or with saliva that contains the viruses. Members of the dental team who do not wear protective gloves will have whitlow on the index fingers and thumbs that are in close contact with the patient's saliva where instrumentation and retraction are performed.

Autoinfection from a lip or intraoral herpetic lesion is possible while nailbiting.

B. Disease Process

The whitlow usually starts suddenly as an area of irritation that becomes tender and painful. Groups of vesicles coalesce and the whole healing process may last up to 2 weeks. The lesions are infectious and transmissible even before the whitlow appears and is diagnosed.[63] Recurrences are not unusual.[61]

IV. Ocular Herpes[45,51]

Herpes simplex lesions in the eye can be a primary or recurrent infection of HSV-1 or HSV-2.

A. Transmission

1. Splashing saliva or fluid from a vesicular lesion directly into an unprotected eye.
2. Extension of infection from a facial lesion.
3. Infection of an infant's eye in utero or during birth.

B. Disease Process

Symptoms include fever, pain, blurring of vision, swelling, excess tears, and secondary bacterial infection. Herpes keratoconjunctivitis can cause deep inflammation and, when left untreated, is a leading cause of loss of sight.

CLINICAL MANAGEMENT[64,65]

I. Patient History

All patient histories must show experiences with herpesviruses. Terminology may be a problem, so terms such as "fever blisters" or "cold sores" need to be used to assure patient understanding.

II. Postpone Appointment with Patient with Active Lesion

A. Problems of Transmission: To be explained to patient

1. Contagiousness, with possible transmission to other patients.
2. Autoinoculation possible from instrumentation that can splash viruses to the patient's eye or extend lesion to nose.

B. Irritation to Lesions

Irritation to the lesions can prolong the course and increase the severity of the infection.

C. Prodromal State May Be the Most Contagious

The patient should be requested to call ahead to change an appointment when it is known that a lesion is developing.

III. Barrier and Other Techniques

All high-level techniques must be consistently applied for all patients because not all patients infected with a contagious disease will have clinically recognizable lesions. For certain lesions, the prodromal stage is the most infectious. Disposable and sterilizable materials should be used exclusively, not only when active lesions are present.

IV. Clinician with Herpetic Lesion

A. Herpetic Whitlow

Direct patient care should be avoided for the duration.[63] After the initial pain and soreness have lessened, careful and frequent handwashing and regloving can usually assure no transmission. Such procedures must be continued indefinitely, however, because lesions may recur. Double gloving may also be advised.

B. Herpes Labialis

Careful isolation, with a fresh mask worn for each patient and the mask changed should it become moist, is basic procedure.

FACTORS TO TEACH THE PATIENT

I. Reasons for postponing an appointment when a herpes lesion ("fever blister" or "cold sore") is present on the lip or in the oral cavity.
   A. Importance of not touching or scratching the lesion because of self-infection to fingers or eyes, for example.
   B. How the viruses can survive on objects and transfer infection to other people.

II. How to help by keeping the medical history up-to-date by informing of additional exposures and immunizations to communicable diseases for self and family members.

III. Preparation for a dental or dental hygiene appointment by thorough mouth cleaning with toothbrush and dental floss to lower the bacterial count for lessening aerosols in the treatment room.

References

1. Hardie, J.: Microbial Flora of the Oral Cavity, in Schuster, G.S., ed.: *Oral Microbiology and Infectious Disease,* 2nd Student edition. Baltimore, Williams & Wilkins, 1983, p. 162.
2. Ibid., p. 168.
3. Miller, R.L. and Micik, R.E.: Air Pollution and Its Control in the Dental Office, *Dent. Clin. North Am., 22,* 453, July, 1978.
4. Miller, R.L.: Generation of Airborne Infection—by High Speed Dental Equipment, *J. Am. Soc. Prev. Dent., 6,* 14, May/June, 1976.
5. Larato, D.C., Ruskin, P.F., and Martin, A.: Effect of an Ultrasonic Scaler on Bacterial Counts in Air, *J. Periodontol., 38,* 550, November-December, 1967.
6. Holbrook, W.P., Muir, K.F., MacPhee, I.T., and Ross, P.W.: Bacteriological Investigation of the Aerosol from Ultrasonic Scalers, *Br. Dent. J., 144,* 245, April 18, 1978.
7. Pokowitz, W. and Hoffman, H.: Dental Aerobiology, *N.Y. State Dent. J., 37,* 337, June-July, 1971.
8. Gross, A., Devine, M.J., and Cutright, D.E.: Microbial Contamination of Dental Units and Ultrasonic Scalers, *J. Periodontol., 47,* 670, November, 1976.
9. Crawford, J.J.: *Clinical Asepsis in Dentistry,* 4th ed. Mesquite, Texas, R.A. Kolstad, Publisher, 1987, pp. 11–13.
10. Whitacre, R.J., Robins, S.K., Williams, B.L., and Crawford, J.J.: *Dental Asepsis.* Seattle, Stoma Press, 1979, pp. 46–51.
11. Crawford, J.J.: Sterilization, Disinfection and Asepsis in Dentistry, in Block, S.S., ed.: *Disinfection, Sterilization, and Preservation,* 3rd ed. Philadelphia, Lea & Febiger, 1983, pp. 517–518.
12. Sunderam, G., McDonald, R.J., Maniatis, T., Oleske, J., Kapila, R., and Reichman, L.B.: Tuberculosis as a Manifestation of the Acquired Immunodeficiency Syndrome (AIDS), *JAMA, 256,* 362, July 18, 1986.
13. United States Department of Health and Human Services, Centers for Disease Control: Tuberculosis Among Asians/Pacific Islanders—United States, 1985, *MMWR, 36,* 331, June 5, 1987.
14. Schuster, G.S., ed.: *Oral Microbiology and Infectious Disease,* 2nd Student edition. Baltimore, Williams & Wilkins, 1983, pp. 300–302.
15. Szmuness, W., Stevens, C.E., Harley, E.J., Zang, E.A., Oleszko, W.R., William, D.C., Sadovsky, R., Morrison, J.M., and Kellner, A.: Hepatitis B Vaccine. Demonstration of Efficacy in a Controlled Clinical Trial in a High-Risk Population in the United States, *N. Engl. J. Med., 303,* 833, October 9, 1980.
16. Elvin-Lewis, M.: Viral Hepatitis: Hepatitis A, Hepatitis B and Hepatitis C (Non-A, Non-B), in Schuster, G.S., ed.: *Oral Microbiology and Infectious Disease,* 2nd Student edition. Baltimore, Williams & Wilkins, 1983, pp. 413–421.
17. United States Department of Health and Human Services, Immunization Practices Advisory Committee (ACIP): Recommendations for Protection Against Viral Hepatitis, *MMWR, 34,* 313, June 7, 1985.
18. Robbins, S.L., Cotran, R.S., and Kumar, V.: *Pathologic Basis of Disease,* 3rd ed. Philadelphia, W.B. Saunders Co., 1984, pp. 900–909.
19. United States Department of Health and Human Services, Centers for Disease Control: Protection Against Viral Hepatitis, *MMWR, 39,* 17, February 9, 1990.
20. Crawford, J.J.: *Clinical Asepsis in Dentistry,* 4th ed. Mesquite, Texas, R.A. Kolstad, Publisher, 1987, pp. 16–20.
21. Hoofnagle, J.H.: Acute Viral Hepatitis: Clinical Features, Laboratory Findings, and Treatment, in Berk, J.E., et al., eds.: *Bockus Gastroenterology,* 4th ed. Philadelphia, W.B. Saunders Co., 1985, p. 2856.
22. United States Department of Health and Human Services, Centers for Disease Control: Suboptimal Response to Hepatitis B Vaccine Given by Injection Into the Buttock, *MMWR, 34,* 105, March 1, 1985.
23. Dienstag, J.L., Stevens, C.E., Bhan, A.K., and Szmuness, W.: Hepatitis B Vaccine Administered to Chronic Carriers of Hepatitis B Surface Antigen, *Ann. Intern. Med., 96,* 575, May, 1982.
24. Stevens, C.E., Taylor, P.E., and Tong, M.J.: Yeast-recombinant Hepatitis B Vaccine: Efficacy With Hepatitis B Immune Globulin in Prevention of Perinatal Hepatitis B Virus Transmission, *JAMA, 257,* 2612, May 15, 1987.
25. Cottone, J.A.: Delta Hepatitis: Another Concern for Dentistry, *J. Am. Dent. Assoc., 112,* 47, January, 1986.
26. United States Department of Health and Human Services, Centers for Disease Control: Enterically Transmitted Non-A, Non-B Hepatitis—East Africa, *MMWR, 36,* 241, May 1, 1987.
27. United States Department of Health and Human Services, Centers for Disease Control: Enterically Transmitted Non-A, Non-B Hepatitis—Mexico, *MMWR, 36,* 597, September 18, 1987.
28. United States Department of Health and Human Services, Centers for Disease Control: Recommendtions for Assisting in the Prevention of Perinatal Transmission of Human T-Lymphotropic Virus Type III/Lymphadenopathy-Associated Virus and Acquired Immunodeficiency Syndrome, *MMWR, 34,* 721, December 6, 1985.
29. Pyun, K.H., Ochs, H.D., and Wedgewood, R.J.: Perinatal Infection with Human Immunodeficiency Virus. Specific Antibody Responses by the Neonate, *N. Engl. J. Med., 317,* 611, September 3, 1987.
30. United States Department of Health and Human Services, Centers for Disease Control: Recommendations for Prevention of HIV Transmission in Health-Care Settings, *MMWR, 36,* 2s, Supplement, August 21, 1987.
31. McDougal, J.S., Jaffe, H.W., Cabridilla, C.D., Sarngadharan, M.G., Nicholson, J.K.A., Kalyanaraman, V.S., Schable, C.A., Kilbourne, B., Evatt, B.L., Gallo, R.C., and Curran, J.W.: Screening Tests for Blood Donors Presumed to Have Trans-

mitted the Acquired Immunodeficiency Syndrome, *Blood, 65,* 772, March, 1985.

32. Reichart, P.A., Gelderblom, H.R., Becker, J., and Kuntz, A.: AIDS and the Oral Cavity. The HIV-infection: Virology, Etiology, Origin, Immunology, Precautions and Clinical Observations in 110 Patients, *Int. J. Oral Maxillofac. Surg., 16,* 129, April, 1987.

33. Seligmann, M., Pinching, A.J., Rosen, F.S., Fahey, J.L., Khaitov, R.M., Klatzmann, D., Koenig, S., Luo, N., Ngu, J., Riethmüller, G., and Spira, T.J.: Immunology of Human Immunodeficiency Virus Infection and the Acquired Immunodeficiency Syndrome, *Ann. Intern. Med., 107,* 234, August, 1987.

34. Bennett, J.A.: AIDS. What We Know About AIDS, *Am. J. Nurs., 86,* 1015, September, 1986.

35. Silverman, S., Migliorati, C.A., Lozada-Nur, F., Greenspan, D., and Conant, M.A.: Oral Findings in People With or at High Risk for AIDS: A Study of 375 Homosexual Males, *J. Am. Dent. Assoc., 112,* 187, February, 1986.

36. Silverman, S.: AIDS Update: Oral Findings, Diagnosis, and Precautions, *J. Am. Dent. Assoc., 115,* 559, October, 1987.

37. Schiødt, M. and Pindborg, J.J.: AIDS and the Oral Cavity. Epidemiology and Clinical Oral Manifestations of Human Immune Deficiency Virus Infection: A Review, *Int. J. Oral Maxillofac. Surg., 16,* 1, February, 1987.

38. Phelan, J.A., Saltzman, B.R., Friedland, G.H., and Klein, R.S.: Oral Findings in Patients With Acquired Immunodeficiency Syndrome, *Oral Surg. Oral Med. Oral Pathol., 64,* 50, July, 1987.

39. United States Centers for Disease Control, Council of State and Territorial Epidemiologists; AIDS Program, Center for Infectious Diseases: Revision of the CDC Surveillance Case Definition for Acquired Immunodeficiency Syndrome, *MMWR, 36,* 3s, Supplement, August 14, 1987.

40. Rubinstein, A. and Bernstein, L.: The Epidemiology of Pediatric Acquired Immunodeficiency Syndrome, *Clin. Immunol. Immunopathol., 40,* 115, July, 1986.

41. Klug, R.M.: AIDS Beyond the Hospital. Children with AIDS, *Am. J. Nurs., 86,* 1126, October, 1986.

42. Leggott, P.J., Robertson, P.B., Greenspan, D., Wara, D.W., and Greenspan, J.S.: Oral Manifestations of Primary and Acquired Immunodeficiency Diseases in Children, *Pediatr. Dent., 9,* 98, June, 1987.

43. United States Department of Health and Human Services, Centers for Disease Control: Public Health Service Guidelines for Counseling and Antibody Testing to Prevent HIV Infection and AIDS, *MMWR, 36,* 509, August 14, 1987.

44. Kopytko, T.K.: Who Are the AIDS Patients and Who Will Treat Them? *Dent. Hyg., 60,* 370, August, 1986.

45. Corey, L. and Spear, P.G.: Infections With Herpes Simplex Viruses, *N. Engl. J. Med., 314,* 686, March 13, 1986 (first part); *314,* 749, March 20, 1986 (second part).

46. Benenson, A.S., ed.: *Control of Communicable Disease in Man,* 14th ed. Washington, D.C., American Public Health Association, 1985, p. 69.

47. Greenspan, J.S., Greenspan, D., Lennette, E.T., Abrams, D.I., Conant, M.A., Petersen, V., and Freese, U.K.: Replication of Epstein-Barr Virus Within the Epithelial Cells of Oral "Hairy" Leukoplakia, An AIDS-associated Lesion, *N. Engl. J. Med., 313,* 1564, December 19, 1985.

48. Von Lichtenberg, F.: Viral, Chlamydial, Rickettsial, and Bacterial Diseases, in Robbins, S.L., Cotran, R.S., and Kumar, V.: *Pathologic Basis of Disease,* 3rd ed. Philadelphia, W.B. Saunders Co., 1984, pp. 284–288.

49. Benenson: op. cit., pp. 96–99.

50. Adler, S.P.: Molecular Epidemiology of Cytomegalovirus: Evidence for Viral Transmission to Parents from Children Infected at a Day Care Center, *Pediatr. Infect. Dis., 5,* 315, May-June, 1986.

51. Elvin-Lewis, M.: Herpesviruses: Herpes Simplex 1 and 2, *Herpesvirus simiae,* Varicella-Zoster Virus, Epstein-Barr Virus, and Cytomegalovirus, in Schuster, G.S., ed.: *Oral Microbiology and Infectious Disease,* 2nd Student edition. Baltimore, Williams & Wilkins, 1983, pp. 393–405.

52. Rees, T.D. and Matheson, B.R.: Primary Herpetic Gingivostomatitis in a 56-Year-Old Male, *Gerodontics, 2,* 28, February, 1986.

53. Zakay-Rones, Z., Ehrlich, J., Hochman, N., and Levy, R.: The Sulcular Epithelium as a Reservoir for Herpes Simplex Virus in Man, *J. Periodontol., 44,* 779, December, 1973.

54. Zakay-Rones, Z., Hochman, N., and Rones, Y.: Immunological Response to Herpes Simplex Virus in Human Gingival Fluid, *J. Periodontol., 53,* 42, January, 1982.

55. Rones, Y., Hochman, N., Ehrlich, J., and Zakay-Rones, Z.: Sensitivity of Oral Tissues to Herpes Simplex Virus—*in vitro, J. Periodontol., 54,* 91, February, 1983.

56. Ehrlich, J., Cohen, G.H., and Hochman, N.: Specific Herpes Simplex Virus Antigen in Human Gingiva, *J. Periodontol., 54,* 357, June, 1983.

57. Raborn, G.W., McGaw, W.T., Grace, M., Tyrrell, L.D., and Samuels, S.M.: Oral Acyclovir and Herpes Labialis: A Randomized, Double-blind, Placebo-controlled Study, *J. Am. Dent. Assoc., 115,* 38, July, 1987.

58. Schwandt, N.W., Mjos, D.P., and Lubow, R.M.: Acyclovir and the Treatment of Herpetic Whitlow, *Oral Surg. Oral Med. Oral Pathol., 64,* 255, August, 1987.

59. Lafferty, W.E., Coombs, R.W., Benedetti, J., Critchlow, C., and Corey, L.: Recurrences After Oral and Genital Herpes Simplex Virus Infection. Influence of Site of Infection and Viral Type, *N. Engl. J. Med., 316,* 1444, June 4, 1987.

60. Jones, J.G.: Herpetic Whitlow: An Infectious Occupational Hazard, *Aust. Dent. J., 31,* 214, June, 1986.

61. Merchant, V.A., Molinari, J.A., and Sabes, W.R.: Herpetic Whitlow: Report of a Case with Multiple Recurrences, *Oral Surg. Oral Med. Oral Pathol., 55,* 568, June, 1983.

62. Stern, H., Elek, S.D., Millar, D.M., and Anderson, H.F.: Herpetic Whitlow. A Form of Cross-infection in Hospitals, *Lancet, 2,* 871, November 21, 1959.

63. Manzella, J.P., McConville, J.H., Valenti, W., Menegus, M.A., Swirkosz, E.M., and Arens, M.: An Outbreak of Herpes Simplex Virus Type 1 Gingivostomatitis in a Dental Hygiene Practice, *JAMA, 252,* 2019, October 19, 1984.

64. Tolle, S.L.: Herpes, *RDH, 5,* 17, April, 1985.

65. McMechen, D.L. and Wright, J.M.: A Protocol for the Management of Patients With Herpetic Infections, *Dent. Hyg., 59,* 546, December, 1985.

Suggested Readings

Greenlee, J.S.: Microbiology and Prevention of Disease Transmission, in Darby, M.L. and Bushee, E.J., eds.: *Mosby's Comprehensive Review of Dental Hygiene.* St. Louis, The C.V. Mosby Co., 1986, pp. 280–296.

Leimone, C.A. and Marozzi, M.: The Transmission and Prevention of Hepatitis and Herpes in the Dental Office [An ADAA Continuing Education Course], *Dent. Assist., 53,* 21, November/December, 1984.

Rubinstein, L. and Singer, J.: Oral Herpes and Hepatitis B. The Dental Hygienist's Role in the Prevention of Disease Transmission, *Dent. Hyg., 60,* 500, November, 1986.

Silverman, S.: Infectious and Sexually Transmitted Diseases: Implications for Dental Public Health, *J. Pub. Health Dent., 46,* 7, Winter, 1986.

Aerosols

Ernst, R.C.: Biohazards in Dentistry. Part 1. Splatter and Aerosols, *Dent. Assist., 48,* 28, January/February, 1979.

Lu, D.P. and Zambito, R.F.: Aerosols and Cross Infection in Dental Practice—A Historic View, *Gen. Dent., 29,* 136, March-April, 1981.

Miller, R.L., Micik, R.E., Abel, C., and Ryge, G.: Studies on Dental Aerobiology: II. Microbial Splatter Discharged from the Oral Cavity of Dental Patients, *J. Dent. Res., 50,* 621, May-June, 1971.

Muir, K.F., Ross, P.W., MacPhee, I.T., Holbrook, W.P., and Kowolik, M.J.: Reduction of Microbial Contamination from Ultrasonic Scalers, *Br. Dent. J., 145,* 76, August 1, 1978.

Rosen, S., Scheid, R.C., Kim, C.K., Bright, J.S., Whitley, M.S., and Beck, F.M.: Potential Pathogens in Dental Aerosols. *Clin. Prevent. Dent., 5,* 17, November-December, 1983.

Hepatitis

Ahtone, J. and Goodman, R.A.: Hepatitis B and Dental Personnel: Transmission to Patients and Prevention Issues, *J. Am. Dent. Assoc., 106,* 219, February, 1983.

Alexander, R.E.: Hepatitis Risk: A Clinical Perspective, *J. Am. Dent. Assoc., 102,* 182, February, 1981.

Baker, C.H. and Hawkins, V.L.: Law in the Dental Workplace: Legal Implications of Hepatitis B for the Dental Profession, *J. Am. Dent. Assoc., 110,* 637, April, 1986.

Brown, B.S.: Non-A, Non-B Hepatitis: Implications for Health Care Professionals, *Horizons, 2,* 10, April, 1981.

Brown, B.S.: Viral Hepatitis B Perspectives: Past and Present, *Dent. Hyg., 55,* 22, October, 1981.

Brown, B.S.: Viral Hepatitis Update: Transmission and Outcome, *Dent. Hyg., 58,* 277, June, 1984.

Brown, B.S.: Hepatitis B: Eliminate the Risk, *Dent. Hyg., 60,* 172, April, 1986.

Cooley, R.L. and Lubow, R.M.: Hepatitis B Vaccine: Implications for Dental Personnel, *J. Am. Dent. Assoc., 105,* 47, July, 1982.

Cottone, J.A. and Goebel, W.M.: Hepatitis B: The Clinical Detection of the Chronic Carrier Dental Patient and the Effects of Immunization Via Vaccine, *Oral Surg. Oral Med. Oral Pathol., 56,* 449, October, 1983.

Falace, D.A. and Matheny, J.L.: Predictive Value of Epidemiologic Questioning in Hepatitis Screening, *J. Oral Med., 37,* 113, October-December, 1982.

Follett, E.A.C. and MacFarlane, T.W.: Infectivity in Hepatitis B Surface Antigen (Australia Antigen) Positive Patients, *Br. Dent. J., 150,* 92, February 17, 1981.

Goebel, W.M.: Hepatitis B Active and Passive Immunity, *J. Am. Dent. Assoc., 110,* 622, April, 1985.

Pollack, J.J., Andors, L., Gulumoglu, A., and Ells, P.F.: Direct Measurement of Hepatitis B Viral Antibody and Antigen Markers in Gingival Crevicular Fluid, *Oral Surg. Oral Med. Oral Pathol., 57,* 499, May, 1984.

Scully, C.: Hepatitis B: An Update in Relation to Dentistry, *Br. Dent. J., 159,* 321, November 23, 1985.

United States Department of Health and Human Services, Centers for Disease Control: Hepatitis B Associated With Jet Gun Injection, *MMWR, 35,* 373, June 13, 1986.

AIDS

American Dental Association, Council on Dental Therapeutics: *Facts About AIDS for the Dental Team.* Chicago, American Dental Association, 1986.

Andriolo, M., Wolf, J.W., and Rosenberg, J.S.: AIDS and AIDS-Related Complex: Oral Manifestations and Treatment, *J. Am. Dent. Assoc., 113,* 586, October, 1986.

Anneroth, G., Anneroth, I., and Lynch, D.P.: Acquired Immune Deficiency Syndrome (AIDS) in the United States in 1986: Etiology, Epidemiology, Clinical Manifestations, and Dental Implications, *J. Oral Maxillofac. Surg., 44,* 956, December, 1986.

Babajews, A., Poswillo, D.E., and Griffin, G.E.: Acquired Immune Deficiency Syndrome Presenting As Recalcitrant *Candida, Br. Dent. J., 159,* 106, August 24, 1985.

Barr, C.E., Torosian, J.P., and Quinones-Whitmore, G.D.: Oral Manifestations of AIDS: The Dentist's Responsibility in Diagnosis and Treatment, *Quintessence Int., 17,* 711, November, 1986.

Brown, B.S.: The Transmission and Manifestations of Acquired Immunodeficiency Syndrome (AIDS), *Dent. Hyg., 60,* 10, January, 1986.

Chandrasekar, P.H. and Molinari, J.A.: Oral Candidiasis: Forerunner of Acquired Immunodeficiency Syndrome (AIDS)? *Oral Surg. Oral Med. Oral Pathol., 60,* 532, November, 1985.

Cooley, R.L. and Lubow, R.M.: AIDS: An Occupational Hazard? *J. Am. Dent. Assoc., 107,* 28, July, 1983.

Fair, J.L., Crawford, J.J., and Forbes, E.A.: AIDS: A New Concern in Dentistry, *Dent. Hyg., 58,* 502, November, 1984.

Friedland, G.H. and Klein, R.S.: Transmission of the Human Immunodeficiency Virus, *N. Engl. J. Med., 317,* 1125, October 29, 1987.

Gerbert, B.: AIDS and Infection Control in Dental Practice: Dentists' Attitudes, Knowledge, and Behavior, *J. Am. Dent. Assoc., 114,* 311, March, 1987.

Goodwin, A.M.: Oral Manifestations of AIDS. An Overview, *Dent. Hyg., 61,* 304, July, 1987.

Greenspan, D.: Oral Viral Leukoplakia ("Hairy" Leukoplakia): A New Oral Lesion in Association with AIDS, *Compend. Contin. Educ. Dent., 6,* 204, March, 1985.

Greenspan, D., Greenspan, J.S., Pindborg, J.J., and Schiødt, M.: *AIDS and the Dental Team.* Chicago, Year Book Medical Publishers, 1986, 96 pp.

Hilgartner, M.W.: AIDS and Hemophilia, *N. Engl. J. Med., 317,* 1153, October 29, 1987.

Ho, D.D., Pomerantz, R.J., and Kaplan, J.C.: Pathogenesis of Infection with Human Immunodeficiency Virus, *N. Engl. J. Med., 317,* 278, July 30, 1987.

Kanas, R.J., Jensen, J.L., Abrams, A.M., and Wuerker, R.B.: Oral Mucosal Cytomegalovirus as a Manifestation of the Acquired Immune Deficiency Syndrome, *Oral Surg. Oral Med. Oral Pathol., 64,* 183, August, 1987.

Lozada, F., Silverman, S., Migliorati, C.A., Conant, M.A., and Volberding, P.A.: Oral Manifestations of Tumor and Opportunistic Infections in the Acquired Immunodeficiency Syndrome (AIDS): Findings in 53 Homosexual Men with Kaposi's Sarcoma, *Oral Surg. Oral Med. Oral Pathol., 56,* 491, November, 1983.

Marder, M.Z., Barr, C.E., and Mandel, I.D.: Cytomegalovirus Presence and Salivary Composition in Acquired Immunodeficiency Syndrome, *Oral Surg. Oral Med. Oral Pathol., 60,* 372, October, 1985.

Mitsuya, H. and Broder, S.: Strategies for Antiviral Therapy in AIDS, *Nature, 325,* 773, February 26, 1987.

Neupert, A.H.: AIDS and the Dental Team, *Dent. Hyg., 61,* 314, July, 1987.

Parker, M.E.: Acquired Immune Deficiency Syndrome. Implications for Dental Hygiene Practice, *Dent. Hyg., 59,* 312, July, 1985.

Petit, J.-C., Ripamonti, U., and Hille, J.: Progressive Changes of Kaposi's Sarcoma of the Gingiva and Palate. Case Report in an AIDS Patient, *J. Periodontol., 57,* 159, March, 1986.

Scully, C., Cawson, R.A., and Porter, S.R.: Acquired Immune Deficiency Syndrome: Review, *Br. Dent. J., 161,* 53, July 19, 1986.

Starr, C.: Dental Implications for Patients with Acquired Immune Deficiency Syndrome, *Gen. Dent., 35,* 22, January-February, 1987.

Tolle, S.L.: AIDS—Implications for Dental Hygienists, *RDH, 5,* 21, March, 1985.

United States Department of Health and Human Services, Centers for Disease Control: Immunization of Children Infected with Human T-Lymphotropic Virus Type III/Lymphadenopathy-Associated Virus, *MMWR, 35,* 595, September 26, 1986.

United States Department of Health and Human Services, Centers for Disease Control: Classification System for Human Immunodeficiency in Children Under 13 Years of Age, *MMWR, 36,* 225, April 24, 1987.

Winkler, J.R. and Murray, P.A.: Periodontal Disease. A Potential Intraoral Expression of AIDS May Be Rapidly Progressive Periodontitis, *Calif. Dent. Assoc. J., 15,* 20, January, 1987.

Wofford, D.T. and Miller, R.I.: Acquired Immune Deficiency Syndrome (AIDS): Disease Characteristics and Oral Manifestations, *J. Am. Dent. Assoc., 111,* 258, August, 1985.

Wormser, G.P., Joline, C., and Duncanson, F.: Needle-stick Injuries During the Care of Patients with AIDS, *N. Engl. J. Med., 310,* 1461, May 31, 1984.

Herpes

Cawson, R.A.: Update on Antiviral Chemotherapy: The Advent of Acyclovir, *Br. Dent. J., 161,* 245, October 11, 1986.

George, D.I. and Heinz, R.O.: Dental Considerations of Herpesvirus Infections, *Compend. Contin. Educ. Dent., 5,* 569, July/August, 1984.

Longenecker, S.A. and Beck, F.M.: Herpetic Whitlow: An Occupational Hazard, *Dent. Hyg., 55,* 16, October, 1981.

McMechen, D.L. and Wright, J.M.: A Protocol for the Management of Patients with Herpetic Infections, *Dent. Hyg., 59,* 546, December, 1985.

Mintz, G.A. and Rose, S.L.: Diagnosis of Oral Herpes Simplex Virus Infections: Practical Aspects of Viral Culture, *Oral Surg. Oral Med. Oral Pathol., 58,* 486, October, 1984.

Pallasch, T.J., Joseph, C.E., and Gill, C.J.: Acyclovir and Herpes-virus Infections, A Review of the Literature, *Oral Surg. Oral Med. Oral Pathol., 57,* 41, January, 1984.

Rowe, N.H., Shipman, C., and Drach, J.C.: Herpes Simplex Virus Disease: Implications for Dental Personnel, *J. Am. Dent. Assoc., 108,* 381, March, 1984.

Rowe, N.H., Heine, C.S., and Kowalski, C.J.: Herpetic Whitlow: An Occupational Disease of Practicing Dentists, *J. Am. Dent. Assoc., 105,* 471, September, 1982.

Saginur, R. and Hardie, J.: Herpes Simplex in the Dental Office, *Can. Dent. Assoc. J., 52,* 700, August, 1986.

Zysset, M.K., Carlson, R.D., Montgomery, M.T., and Redding, S.W.: Undiagnosed Oral Herpes in Immunosuppressed Patients, *J. Oral Med., 41,* 70, April-June, 1986.

3 Infection Control: Barriers for Patient and Clinician

MEDICAL HISTORY

The content and various types of patient histories are described extensively in Chapter 6. Items from the histories that call for immediate application are described beginning on page 83. One of the items for immediate attention relates to the patient's status relative to infectious disease.

Before an oral examination or any clinical procedure is performed, screening for possible contagious disease is needed. Prevention of cross-contamination begins at the very start of the appointment, even prior to seating the patient.

I. Key Questions to Include in a History

Questions concerning a basic history of past disease and current disease that is under treatment are typically included in a medical history. For a patient who gives no history of certain communicable diseases, or is uncertain, additional leading questions are needed to determine possible exposure.

In the case of hepatitis B, for example, questions can be included that may reveal those individuals who have a high risk potential as listed on page 18. When infection is suspected, the antigen test for HBsAg and other serologic tests can be requested.

Examples of questions that may be used to supplement a basic history questionnaire are suggested here:

1. What vaccinations have you had? Have you had hepatitis vaccine? When was your last booster for tetanus?
2. Do you know what type of hepatitis you had? How old were you when you had hepatitis? What caused the hepatitis? Did other people have hepatitis at the same time?
3. Have you had or do you have liver disease, hepatitis, chronic diarrhea, or jaundice?
4. Have you had close contact at home or socially with anyone with hepatitis, especially during the past 6 months?
5. Have you received blood products, a transfusion, kidney dialysis, or hemodialysis?
6. Have you ever had a test for hepatitis or AIDS? Have you ever had your blood refused for donation to a blood bank?
7. Have you ever had to stay in a hospital or other institution for a long period of time?
8. Are you a health-care professional exposed to hepatitis patients?
9. Have you traveled or lived in any other countries for 3 months or longer? Were you ill while there, and did you require hospitalization and/or blood transfusions?
10. Have you recently had any unexpected weight loss and tiredness?
11. Have you recently had night sweats or a slight fever?

II. Limitations of a Medical History

For the safety of the patient and the dental health team, correct and current information about communicable diseases is vital. Problems arise because a patient does not always have or give complete information about past disease and present status of communicability. Frequently, the word of the patient is all that is available, and consultation with the patient's physician is needed for confirmation and supplementation.

Studies have been conducted to determine the reliability of the medical history as a means of identifying patients likely to transmit hepatitis.[1,2,3] In the research, by comparing serologic test findings with data from medical histories provided by patients, it was found that comprehensive questioning for a dental and medical history is insufficient to identify all patients who carry HBsAg. Many patients did not know that they had had hepatitis at all, and others who knew they had had hepatitis had no knowledge of whether they had type A, type B, type D, or non A, non B (NANB).[1,2,3] As described on page 19, individuals can become carriers of hepatitis B surface antigen (HBsAg) following a subclinical case that was not diagnosed as hepatitis.

Dental personnel are placed in a hazardous position. When a patient's history does not provide the necessary information, serologic testing is advisable, at least for individuals in one of the risk groups (page 18).

III. Use of the Medical History

A. Screen All Patients

All patients should be checked for potential communicable disease before any clinical instrumentation for examination or treatment is performed. Avoid exposure to an unknown infectious disease by wearing mask, glasses, and gloves. Other basic precautions are listed on pages 56–58.

B. New Patient
1. Obtain a complete medical history; supplement it with information from the patient's physician as indicated.
2. Request serologic or other laboratory tests; plan future appointment after information is returned.

C. Current Patient on Recall or Continuing Care
1. Update the patient history regularly.
2. Avoid exposure to current infectious disease by rescheduling after the communicability period. Common cold, influenza, and other respiratory diseases may be more serious than initially realized.
3. Request periodic laboratory tests as changes in the disease history occur.

D. Emergency Patient
1. Complete the medical history.
2. Follow precautions with strict barrier protection procedures when the patient status is not known and when immediate pain-relieving treatment is required.

PERSONAL PROTECTION OF THE DENTAL TEAM

The continuing health and productivity of dental health personnel depend to a large degree on the control of cross-contamination. Loss of work time, personal suffering, long-term systemic effects, and even exclusion from continued practice are possible results from communicable diseases. The only safe procedure is to practice defensively at all times, with specific precautions for personal protection.

In this section, topics include immunizations and periodic tests, clothing, barriers to infectious microorganisms such as face mask, eyeglasses, personal hygiene, handwashing, gloves, and habits.

IMMUNIZATIONS AND PERIODIC TESTS

Dental personnel in a hospital setting are subject to the rules and regulations for all hospital employees. Policies usually require certain immunizations for new employees if written proof of vaccinations is not available and tests for antibodies prove to be negative.

In private dental practices, individual initiative is required to maintain standards of safety for all dental team members. All staff members should be well aware of the signs and symptoms of diseases that are occupational hazards. All must be encouraged to seek early diagnosis and treatment of a seemingly minor condition that could be the initial symptom of a more serious communicable disease.

At the time of employment, it is reasonable for a dentist-employer to request of employees a record of current immunizations and their most recent updating, as well as specific tests, such as for tuberculosis

(Mantoux test) and hepatitis B (serum HBsAg and anti-HBs). Immunization for rubella is particularly important for female employees of child-bearing age.

Following are listed the infectious diseases for which immunization is usually provided during infancy and childhood. Booster or reimmunization requirements are specific for each disease and apply throughout life.

I. Immunizations
A. Basic Schedule
The immunization schedule for infants and children may include protection against poliomyelitis, diphtheria, tetanus, pertussis (whooping cough), measles, mumps, and rubella (German measles).[4]

B. Booster and Reimmunization
Each agent requires booster or reimmunization on a specific plan, which may range from 1 to 10 years, or reimmunization only upon intimate contact or exposure. The needs differ in different climates, countries, and locations. Persons moving or traveling need to become aware of specific precautions.

For tetanus boosters, intervals of 10 years are indicated.[5] If an injury occurs, however, a booster should be given on the day of the injury.

The booster for hepatitis B has been advised at an interval of 5 years. A serum anti-HBs evaluation may be used to check the titer, because the 5-year plan is only an average recommendation (page 20).

C. Other Immunizations
Annual influenza immunization can provide needed protection for health personnel. Pneumococcal vaccine is recommended for susceptible groups at certain intervals. Hepatitis vaccine is essential for health professionals.

II. Management Program
A. Recommended Tests
1. Annual tuberculin test (Mantoux); chest radiograph as indicated.
2. Periodic throat culture for possible hemolytic streptococcus carrier.
3. Serologic test for herpes simplex virus I (HSV-1) antibodies to determine susceptibility to primary HSV.[6]

B. Obtaining Tests
Obtain tests promptly when exposed to certain infectious diseases and seek prophylactic immunization as indicated and available.

C. Written Records
Keep written records of immunizations, boosters, and reimmunizations; plan for regular follow-up. When the status of current immunizations is known, time is saved by not needing a susceptibility test prior to initiating passive immunizations when accidental exposure occurs.

CLINICAL ATTIRE

The wearing apparel of clinicians and their assistants is vulnerable to contamination from splash, splatter, aerosols, and patient contact. The gown or uniform should be designed and cared for in a manner that will minimize cross-contamination.

I. Strict Aseptic Procedures

In a *strict aseptic* technique, with the highest level of asepsis (page 43), one-use gowns and other attire may come from sterile packages. Also in strict aseptic technique, the use of coverings for hair, beards, and shoes becomes part of customary routines.

Procedures for use when treating a patient with active symptoms of a known contagious disease, such as one who has active tuberculosis or one who is a hepatitis B carrier, are outlined on page 58.

II. Sterile-Clean Procedure

When a *sterile-clean* technique is followed in routine practice, personal hygiene and cleanliness do not differ from that in the strict aseptic technique.

A. Gown, Uniform, or Scrubsuit

Gowns, uniforms, or scrubsuits are expected to be clean and maintained as free as possible from contamination. Wearing clinic coats over street clothes cannot be recommended because of the exposure of the street clothes to infectious material.

1. *Solid, Closed Front.* The garment should be closed at the neck. The fabric should be able to be washed commercially and withstand washing with bleach.
2. *No Pockets.* Pockets are too readily available for placing contaminated objects such as writing implements or keys. Gloved hands, prepared for patient treatment, must be kept from touching objects or being placed in pockets.
3. *Long Sleeves.* Hand, wrist, and forearm washing and scrubbing are necessary in preparation for gloving. Long sleeves with fitted cuffs permit protective gloves to extend over the cuffs.

B. Hair and Head Covering

Hair must be worn off the shoulders and back. When longer, it should be held within a head cover. Because the hair is exposed to much contamination, an appropriate head cover is advised when using handpieces, ultrasonic, or airbrasive instruments.

C. Protection of Uniform

A plastic, washable or a disposable apron may be used when clinical services are performed that usually involve blood, splatter, or aerosols.

D. Outside Wear

Clinic uniforms and shoes should not be worn outside the clinic practice setting.[7] When clinic clothing is worn outside, it carries contamination from, and brings contamination into, the treatment area.

Another problem is that contamination is taken into the home when uniforms are worn to and from the work area. When laundered at home, the items from a dental office or clinic should be kept separate and treated with household bleach for disinfection.

USE OF FACE MASK

In the attempt to prevent airborne infections, it has been common practice to wear a mask when either the patient or the operator is known to have an acute respiratory infection. Such a practice has its own value, but does not take into account the fact that many diseases are transmissible during the incubation period when no clinical signs are apparent.

Dispersion of particles of debris, polishing agents, calculus, and water, all of which are contaminated by the patient's oral flora, occurs regularly during all instrumentation. The greatest aerosols are created following the use of a handpiece, prophylaxis angle, or ultrasonic scaler. Evidence of the spread of particles appears on the splashed face, glasses, and uniform, and on the coverall placed over the patient for protection from the spray. Aerosol production was described on pages 10–11.

I. Mask Efficiency

A. Essential Characteristics

Undesirable characteristics that minimize the comfort with which a mask will be worn are the ability to create irritation to the nose, heat leading to perspiration, and pressure or a tight feeling about the ears and face, which may leave marks on the face. Unfortunately, discomfort is a common reason for neglect in wearing a mask that can make an important contribution to the total disease control plan.

The shape, material, and degree of absorption will influence the efficiency of a mask. A scientifically effective mask will

1. Prevent inward and outward passage of microorganisms.
2. Filter particles produced during dental and dental hygiene procedures.
3. Have minimal marginal leakage.

B. Materials

Various materials have been used for masks, including gauze and other cloth, plastic foam, fiberglass, synthetic fiber mat, and paper. In one research study, foam, paper, and cloth were found to be the least adequate filters of aerosols, whereas glass fiber and synthetic fiber mat were shown to be the most effective.[8,9]

II. Use of a Mask

Wearing a mask and protective glasses is required for all appointments (figure 3–1).

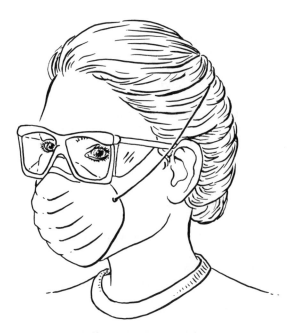

Figure 3–1. Face Mask with Protective Glasses. Minimal barrier protection for all professionals includes face mask, eyeglasses, and gloves.

A. Tie on the mask before a scrub or handwash.
B. Use a fresh mask for each patient. When a mask becomes wet it should be changed, because a wet mask is no longer an effective barrier.
C. Keep the mask on after completing a procedure, while still in the presence of aerosols. Particles under 5 micrometers remain suspended longer (up to 24 hours) than larger particles and can be inhaled directly into terminal lung alveoli. Removal of a mask in the treatment room immediately following the use of aerosol-producing procedures permits direct exposure to airborne organisms.

USE OF PROTECTIVE EYEGLASSES

Eye protection during dental and dental hygiene appointments for the dental team members and patients is necessary to prevent physical injuries and infections of the eyes. A list of measures for eye accident prevention is included on page 735 in conjunction with emergency treatment.

Severe and disabling eye accidents and infections have been reported.[10,11,12] Eye involvement may lead to pain, discomfort, loss of work time, and, in certain instances, permanent injury. Accidents can occur at any time, and as with most accidents, they occur when least prepared for or expected.

Eye infections can follow the accidental dropping of an instrument on the face or the splashing of various materials from a patient's oral cavity into the eye. Contamination can be introduced from saliva, plaque, carious material, and pieces of old restorative materials during cavity preparation, bacteria-laden

calculus during scaling, and any other microorganisms contained in aerosols or splatter as described on page 10. An aerosol created by an ultrasonic scaler can be heavily contaminated with oral microorganisms.

Careful, deliberate techniques and instrument management, with evacuation and other procedures for the control of oral fluids, contribute to the prevention of accidents and infections of the eyes. All measures described for prevention of airborne disease transmission by aerosols and splatter apply to eye protection (page 11). The most effective defense is the use of protective eyeglasses by all concerned, dental team and patients.

I. Indications for Use of Eyeglasses
A. Dental Team Members

Glasses should be worn at all times (figure 3–1). For dental personnel who do not require corrective lens for vision, protective glasses with clear lens should become a routine part of clinical dress.

If glasses are intended to be worn only when a handpiece, ultrasonic instrument, or other aerosol-producing instrument is used, they can easily be forgotten or misplaced. Even without power-driven instruments, pieces of calculus and splatter from air and water spray can reach the eyes.

B. Patients

Protective eye coverage is recommended for each patient at each appointment. The patient's medical history should reflect types of eye surgery, implants, or other special concerns. Contact lens should be removed.

Patients with their own prescription lens may prefer to wear them, but for the safety of the patient's glasses, the use of the protective glasses provided in the office or clinic is advisable.

II. Protective Glasses
A. General Features of Acceptable Glasses
1. Wide coverage, preferably with side shields, to protect around the eye.
2. Shatterproof; made of strong, sturdy plastic.
3. Light weight.
4. Flexible and with rounded smooth edges to prevent discomfort if pressed against the nose or ears.
5. Easily disinfected
   a. Surface areas should be smooth to prevent accumulation of infectious material.
   b. Frames and lens should not be damaged or distorted by the disinfectant used.
6. Lens color. A clear or lightly tinted lens rather than very dark for a patient will permit the dental team members to watch the patient's reactions and maintain contact and response.
7. Protection against glare. Certain patients may request tinted lens or prefer to wear their own

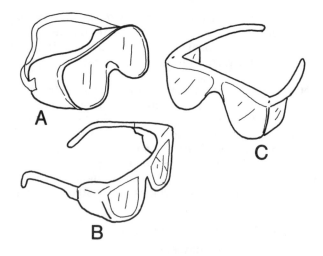

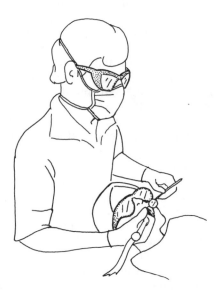

Figure 3–2. Protective Eye Wear. Protective cover for both patient and clinician may be **A.** goggles-style, or **B.** and **C.** glasses with side shields.

sunglasses when their eyes are especially sensitive to the dental light.

B. Types of Glasses

Many styles, including regular glasses shapes and those described below, have been used.

1. *Goggles* (figure 3–2A). Shielding on all sides of the glasses may give the best protection, provided they fit closely around the edges. Goggle-style coverage is especially necessary for protection during laboratory work.

2. *Glasses with Side Shields* (figure 3–2B and C). A side shield can provide added protection. For the member of the dental team, it may be possible to wear this type over regular prescription glasses.

3. *Glasses with Curved Frames.* When the sides of the glasses are curved back, they may pro-

vide a protection somewhat similar to those with the side shield.

4. *Postmydriatic Spectacles Used by Ophthalmologist.* Disposable glasses are available that are made of flexible plastic. They may be especially useful for patients with a known communicable disease or carrier state.

5. *Child-Sized.* Child-sized sunglasses and children's play spectacles have been used.

C. Availability

Several pairs of goggles or glasses are maintained to facilitate cleaning and disinfection after each use.

III. Suggestions for Clinical Application

A. Patient Instruction

A patient who has not been asked to wear protective glasses before needs a simple explanation of the reasons for the glasses.

B. Contact Lens

1. Dental team members who wear contact lens should always wear protective glasses over them.

2. Patients with contact lens should be asked to remove them and then use the protective glasses that are provided.

C. Care of Protective Glasses

1. Run glasses under water stream to remove abrasive particles. Rubbing an abrasive agent over the plastic lens will create scratches.

2. Immerse in 2% alkaline glutaraldehyde for disinfection (pages 51–52).[13]

3. Rinse thoroughly after immersion because glutaraldehyde is irritating to eyes and skin.

4. Check periodically for scratches on the lens, and replace appropriately.

HAND CARE

Hands, through direct contact with a patient's saliva, become contaminated and therefore are sources for cross-infection. Cross-infection can be at least partially controlled by making a conscious effort to keep the gloved hands from touching objects other than the instruments and disinfected parts of equipment prepared for the immediate patient.

I. Bacteriology of the Skin[14]

A. Resident Bacteria

Large numbers of relatively stable bacteria inhabit the surface epithelium or deeper areas in the ducts of skin glands or depths of hair follicles; they are ultimately shed with the exfoliated surface cells, or with excretions of the skin glands. They may be altered by newly introduced pathogens, or reduced by washing. They tend to be less susceptible to destruction by disinfection procedures.

B. Transient Bacteria

These reflect continuous contamination by routine contacts: some bacteria are pathogens and may act temporarily as residents, may be washed away, or in the event that a skin break exists, may cause an autogenous infection. Most transients can be removed with soap and water by washing 5 to 10 minutes.

II. Handwashing Principles

A. Rationale

Effective and frequent handwashing can reduce the overall bacterial flora of the skin and prevent the organisms acquired from a patient from becoming skin residents. It is impossible to sterilize the skin, but every attempt must be made to reduce the bacterial flora to a minimum.

B. Purposes

The objective of all scrub procedures is to reduce the bacterial flora of the hands to an absolute minimum. An effective scrub procedure can be expected to accomplish the following:

1. Remove surface dirt and transient bacteria.
2. Dissolve the normal greasy film on the skin.
3. Rinse and remove all loosened debris and microorganisms.
4. With a long-acting antiseptic, provide disinfection.

C. Hand Care

1. Maintain clean, smoothly trimmed, short fingernails with well-cared-for cuticles to prevent breaks where microorganisms can enter.
2. Remove hand and wrist jewelry at the beginning of the day. Microorganisms can become lodged in crevices of rings, watchbands, and watches, where scrubbing is impossible.
3. After hand washing, don gloves. Never expose open skin lesions or abrasions to a patient's oral tissues and fluids. The use of gloves is described on pages 39–40.
4. Keep gloved hands away from face, hair, clothing (pockets), dental chair, operating stool (manipulate by foot action), telephone, patient records, and other objects that cannot be sterilized or disinfected.

III. Facilities

A. Sink

1. Use a sink with a foot pedal for water-flow control to avoid contamination from faucet handles.
2. Adaptation for regular sink: turn on water at the beginning and leave on through the entire procedure. Turn faucets off with the towel after drying hands.
3. Use a sink of sufficient size so that contact with the inside of the wash basin can be avoided easily. A sink cannot be sterilized and is highly contaminated.
4. Prevent contamination of uniform by not leaning against the sink.
5. Use a separate area and sink reserved for instrument washing. Contaminated instruments should be removed from the treatment room prior to preparation for the next patient.

B. Soap

1. Use a liquid surgical scrub containing an antimicrobial agent. Povidone-iodine (iodophore) has a broad spectrum of action. Chlorhexidine preparations are used extensively to provide rapid disinfection and a cumulative, persistent (residual) action.
2. Apply from a foot- or knee-activated dispenser to avoid contamination to and from a hand-operated dispenser or cake soap.[15]
3. Do not substitute the use of foam hand preparations, alcohol wipes, or other substitutes for handwashing, because many pathogenic microorganisms cannot be destroyed by disinfecting preparations. Rinsing is a very important part of the hand-washing procedure.

C. Scrub Brushes

1. Clean brushes with a detergent, and sterilize after each use.
2. Avoid over-vigorous use of a brush, to minimize skin abrasion. Skin irritation and abrasion can leave openings for additional cross-contamination.
3. Disposable sponges are available commercially and may be preferred when a scrub brush is traumatic to the skin.
4. Identify brushes by label or color-code for handwashing to prevent mixing with instrument scrub brushes; however, both types will be sterilized. Handwashing and instrument cleaning should be accomplished at separate sinks.

D. Towels

1. Obtain towel from a dispenser that requires no contact except with the towel itself, which hangs down from the container (figure 3–3).
2. When a cloth towel is used, it must be used for only one patient.

IV. Methods of Handwashing

The three methods that will be described here are called the *short scrub, short standard handwash,* and the *surgical scrub.* Handwashing techniques are usually defined by numbers of latherings and rinsings, whereas scrub techniques are completed in time periods or by specific numbers of scrub brush strokes.[16]

The two commonly used systems for scrub techniques are the "stroke-count" method and the "time" method. In the *stroke-count* method, a specific number of brush strokes is applied to each surface, and each finger and part of the hand is considered to have four surfaces. In the *time* method each surface is scrubbed for a certain number of seconds.

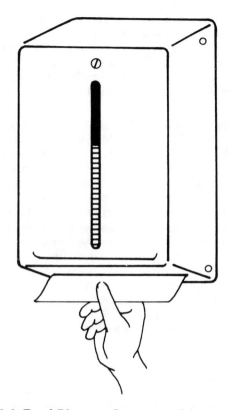

Figure 3–3. Towel Dispenser. Correct type of dispenser that requires no contact except with the towel itself, hanging down from the container.

When learning to perform a scrub, it is helpful to combine the stroke-count and the time methods, to assure complete coverage and to develop a sequence of performance that can be completed in a minimum of time.

A. Short Scrub

The short scrub is recommended for the beginning of the day just prior to the first patient appointment, and just prior to the first appointment of the second half of the day. It is also used following an appointment for a patient with a known communicable disease, and following any major interruption that may have caused unusual contamination.

When the time method is used, a short scrub may vary from a minimum of 3 minutes to 5 minutes. Approximately one half of the time is used for scrubbing each hand. For a 3-minute scrub, the time may be divided as follows:[16]

> Nails and fingertips
>   1/2 minute (15 seconds each hand)
> Fingers and hands
>   1 1/2 minutes (45 seconds each hand)
> Wrists and forearms
>   1 minute (30 seconds each hand)

The procedure outlined below may be expected to take 3 minutes when 5 stroke-counts are applied to each surface.

1. Don eyeglasses and mask and fix hair securely back. Remove watch and all jewelry.
2. Wash hands and arms briefly, using surgical scrub soap. Leave water running at a moderate speed that will not allow splashing from base and sides of sink.
3. Clean under finger nails with orangewood stick from sterile package. Orangewood stick and scrub brush may be packaged together for sterilization.
4. Rinse from fingertips to hands, wrists to elbows. Keep hands higher than elbows through the entire procedure.
5. Lather hands and arms again. Leave the soap lather on the hands and arms during the scrub to increase exposure time to the antimicrobial ingredient of the scrub soap.
6. Remove scrub brush from the previously opened sterile package; apply several measures of soap. Note the time, and start scrubbing in an orderly sequence without returning to areas already scrubbed.
7. First hand
   a. Brush back and forth across nails and finger tips five times.
   b. Begin with the thumb, use small circular strokes (five strokes each area) on each side of thumb and each finger, then palm, and back of hand. Extend fingers to gain access to each crevice and line.
   c. Scrub wrist on all sides and move to forearm.
   d. When completed, rinse well, from fingertips on up the arm; let water run off at the elbow.
8. Rinse the brush and transfer to other hand; repeat entire procedure.
9. Rinse brush and drop it into the sink.
10. Rinse the hand and arm generously and thoroughly to wash away all transient microorganisms.
11. Dry hands
    a. Take care not to recontaminate hands while drying them.
    b. Use a separate paper towel for each hand.
    c. Cloth towel: use one end of a large towel for one hand and the other end for the other hand, taking care not to drag the towel over unwashed parts or clothing. Two small towels may be used, one for each hand.
12. Don gloves (page 40).

B. Short Standard Handwash

Handwashing is used after the first glove removal and before and after each succeeding glove application. It is the general procedure for all times except those indicated under the short scrub technique.

Handwashing is considered the most important single procedure for the prevention of cross-contamination and is a basic requirement before and after hospital patient care.

1. Don eyeglasses and mask and fix hair securely back. Remove watch and all jewelry.
2. Use comfortably warm water and surgical scrub soap.
3. Lather hands, wrists, and forearms quickly, rubbing all surfaces vigorously. Interlace fingers and rub back and forth with pressure.
4. Rinse thoroughly, running the water from fingertips down the hands. Keep water running.
5. Repeat 2 more times. One lathering for 3 minutes is less effective than 3 short latherings and rinsing 3 times in 30 seconds. The lathering serves to loosen the debris and microorganisms and the rinsings wash them away.
6. Use paper towels for drying, taking care not to recontaminate.

C. Surgical Hand Scrub

Each hospital or oral surgery clinic will have rules and regulations for scrub procedures. These should be posted over the scrub sinks.

A surgical scrub performed as the initial scrub of a day should be 10 minutes and subsequent scrubs may be 3 to 5 minutes. Following a contagious or isolated patient, the scrub should be at least 5 minutes.[16]

The outline for a long scrub presented below is similar to the short scrub described previously. The major differences are in the number of strokes when the stroke-count method is used and the longer time spent.

1. Don eyeglasses, mask, and hair and beard coverings. Make sure hair is completely covered. Remove watch and jewelry.
2. Open sterile brush package to have ready.
3. Wash hands and arms over the elbows, using surgical soap to remove gross surface dirt before using the scrub brush. Lather vigorously with strong rubbing motions, 10 on each side of hands, wrists, arms. Interlace the fingers and thumbs to clean the proximal surfaces.
4. Rinse thoroughly from fingertips across hands and wrists. Hold hands higher than elbows throughout the procedure. Leave water running.
5. Use orangewood stick or file from the sterile package to clean nails. Rinse.
6. Lather the hands and arms and leave the lather on during the scrub to increase the exposure time to the antimicrobial ingredient.
7. Apply surgical soap, and begin the brush procedure. Note the time, and scrub in an orderly sequence without returning to areas previously scrubbed.
8. First hand and arm
   a. Brush back and forth across nails and fingertips, passing the brush under the nails (30 seconds).
   b. Fingers and hand. Use small circular strokes on all sides of the thumb and each finger, overlapping strokes for complete coverage (2½ minutes).
   c. Continue to wrist. Apply more soap to maintain a good lather (2 minutes for wrist and forearm).
   d. When arm is completed over the elbow, leave lather on.
9. Repeat on other arm. Some systems require the use of a second sterile brush for the second hand. When this is so, discard the first brush into the proper container and obtain second brush.
10. At one half of scrub time, rinse hands and arms thoroughly, first one and then the other, starting at the fingertips and letting water pass down over the arm.
11. Lather and repeat to, but not over, the elbows.
12. At end of time (or counts), rinse thoroughly, each arm separately, from fingertips. When a sterile towel is available for drying, apply towel from fingertips to elbow without reapplying to hand area.
13. Hold hands up and clasped together. Proceed to dressing area for gowning and gloving.

V. Gloves

The wearing of gloves is part of the total plan for control of cross-contamination and protection of the clinician. Unseen blood from a patient can be impacted and retained under the fingernails for 5 or more days after exposure during an appointment.[17] Hepatitis virus is known to be resistant to drying and might be retained under a fingernail with blood and saliva. Even scrubbing cannot remove all microorganisms from under nails.[18]

Tiny cuts and abrasions cannot be seen or felt.[17] Protective gloves are needed at all times.

A. Types of Gloves

1. *General Use Gloves*
   a. Material. Latex and vinyl non-sterile gloves are available. Latex gloves may be of single or double thickness.
   b. Surface. Gloves are available powdered or unpowdered. Powdered gloves have either cornstarch or an antimicrobial agent.
   c. Sizes. Ambidexterous gloves are made in small, medium, large, or extra large in boxes of 100.
   d. Use. The general use gloves are commonly referred to as "examination" gloves, but they are suitable for procedures that do not require a strict sterile regimen. Wearing two pairs or "double gloving" is useful in high-risk situations.
2. *Sterile Individually Paired Gloves.* Packaged and sealed in sterile pairs by hand size, they are prepared for procedures requiring a sterile technique. They have commonly been referred

to as "surgeon's gloves" but they also have special use where high-risk patients are being treated.

3. *Utility Gloves.* Non-lined heavy utility gloves are indicated for all instrument handling during clean-up and preparation for sterilization, as well as unit preparation and surface disinfection (see figure 4–1, page 44).

B. Procedures for Use of Gloves

1. *Hand Scrub Before Donning Gloves.* Because gloves are susceptible to tears and pinholes from instrument sticks, infection can be introduced inadvertently. In addition, bacteria may multiply profusely under gloves, where a warm damp medium is provided. Long fingernails under gloves are a potential cause of breaks in the gloves.[16]

2. *Torn, Cut, or Punctured Glove.* Remove immediately, wash hands thoroughly, and don new gloves.

3. *Hand Wash Before Glove Removal.* Before removing gloves, lather and rinse thoroughly to
   a. Reduce possible contamination to hands during removal and disposal.
   b. Reduce contamination in the waste, particularly following a patient known to have a communicable disease.

TECHNICAL HINTS

I. Determine, preferably by group discussion of the entire clinic or office personnel, the policy and procedures for infection control, and record in an Office Procedures Manual.
   A. Outline the emergency procedures to follow when accidentally exposed to a communicable disease.
   B. List sources with addresses and telephone numbers of all barrier materials.
   C. Orient new personnel to the procedures in the manual.
   D. Update information regularly from research readings and information from continuing education programs.
II. Small abrasions or cracks of the fingers should be covered with a clear liquid bandage for safety under gloves.

FACTORS TO TEACH THE PATIENT

I. Importance of the patient's complete history in the protection of both the patient and the professional person.
II. Necessity for use of barriers (face mask, eyeglasses, and gloves) by the clinician for the benefit of the patient.
III. Eye protection for the patient.

References

1. Tullman, M.J. and Boozer, C.H.: Past Infection with Hepatitis B Virus in Patients at a Dental School, *J. Am. Dent. Assoc.,* *97,* 477, September, 1978.
2. Goebel, W.M.: Reliability of the Medical History in Identifying Patients Likely to Place Dentists at an Increased Hepatitis Risk, *J. Am. Dent. Assoc.,* *98,* 907, June, 1979.
3. Tullman, M.J., Boozer, C.H., Villarejos, V.M., and Feary, T.W.: The Threat of Hepatitis B from Dental School Patients, A One-year Study, *Oral Surg. Oral Med. Oral Pathol.,* *49,* 214, March, 1980.
4. United States Department of Health and Human Services, Immunization Practices Advisory Committee (ACIP): New Recommended Schedule for Active Immunization of Normal Infants and Children, *MMWR,* *35,* 577, September 19, 1986.
5. Benenson, A.S., ed.: *Control of Communicable Disease in Man,* 14th ed. Washington, D.C., American Public Health Association, 1985, pp. 384–388.
6. Brooks, S.L., Rowe, N.H., Drach, J.C., Shipman, C., and Young, S.K.: Prevalence of Herpes Simplex Virus Disease in a Professional Population, *J. Am. Dent. Assoc.,* *102,* 31, January, 1981.
7. Federation Dentaire Internationale, Commission on Dental Practice: Technical Report: Recommendations for Hygiene in Dental Practice, *Int. Dent. J.,* *29,* 72, March, 1979.
8. Micik, R.E., Miller, R.L., and Leong, A.C.: Studies on Dental Aerobiology: III. Efficacy of Surgical Masks in Protecting Dental Personnel from Airborne Bacterial Particles, *J. Dent. Res.,* *50,* 626, May-June, 1971.
9. Miller, R.L. and Micik, R.E.: Air Pollution and Its Control in the Dental Office, *Dent. Clin. North Am.,* *22,* 453, July, 1978.
10. Colvin, J.: Eye Injuries and the Dentist, *Aust. Dent. J.,* *23,* 453, December, 1978.
11. Cooley, R.L., Cottingham, A.J., Abrams, H., and Barkmeier, W.W.: Ocular Injuries Sustained in the Dental Office: Methods of Detection, Treatment, and Prevention, *J. Am. Dent. Assoc.,* *97,* 985, December, 1978.
12. Hartley, J.L.: Eye and Facial Injuries Resulting from Dental Procedures, *Dent. Clin. North Am.,* *22,* 505, July, 1978.
13. Gleason, M.J. and Molinari, J.A.: Stability of Safety Glasses During Sterilization and Disinfection, *J. Am. Dent. Assoc.,* *115,* 60, July, 1987.
14. Altemeier, W.A.: Surgical Antiseptics, in Block, S.S., ed.: *Disinfection, Sterilization, and Preservation,* 3rd ed. Philadelphia, Lea & Febiger, 1983, pp. 493–495.
15. Crawford, J.J.: Sterilization, Disinfection and Asepsis in Dentistry, in Block, S.S.: *Disinfection, Sterilization, and Preservation,* 3rd ed. Philadelphia, Lea & Febiger, 1983, pp. 515–516.
16. Hooley, J.R. and Phillips, R.E.: The Operating Room, in Hooley, J.R. and Daun, L.G.: *Hospital Dental Practice.* St. Louis, The C.V. Mosby Co., 1980, pp. 192–214.
17. Allen, A.L. and Organ, R.J.: Occult Blood Accumulation Under the Fingernails: A Mechanism for the Spread of Bloodborne Infection, *J. Am. Dent. Assoc.,* *105,* 455, September, 1982.
18. Parker, M.E. and Williams, H.: Cross-infection and Cross-contamination. The Relationship Between Subungual Bacteria and Fingernail Length, *Dent. Hyg.,* *61,* 68, February, 1987.

Suggested Readings

American Association of Public Health Dentistry, Ad Hoc Committee on Infectious Diseases: The Control of Transmissible Diseases in Dental Practice: A Position Paper of the American Association of Public Health Dentistry, *J. Public Health Dent.,* *46,* 13, Winter, 1986.
American Dental Association: The Health of the Dental Professional, *J. Am. Dent. Assoc.,* *114,* 514, April, 1987.
Boyer, E.M., Elton, J., and Preston, K.: Precautionary Procedures. Use in Dental Hygiene Practice, *Dent. Hyg.,* *60,* 516, November, 1986.
LeClair, J.M., Freeman, J., Sullivan, B.F., Crowley, C.M., and Gold-

mann, D.A.: Prevention of Nosocomial Respiratory Syncytial Virus Infections through Compliance with Glove and Gown Isolation Precautions, *N. Engl. J. Med., 317,* 329, August 6, 1987.

Macdonald, G.: Hazards in the Dental Workplace, *Dent. Hyg., 61,* 212, May, 1987.

Underhill, T.E., Terezhalmy, G.T., and Cottone, J.A.: Prevention of Cross-infections in the Dental Environment, *Compend. Contin. Educ. Dent., 7,* 260, April, 1986.

Immunizations

Elvin-Lewis, M., Storch, G.A., and Parker, M.: Control of a Rubella Outbreak in a Dental School Population, *J. Am. Dent. Assoc., 108,* 783, May, 1984.

Heggie, A.D.: Immunization Against Communicable Diseases, *U.S. Navy Med., 77,* 26, March–April, 1986; *77,* 20, May–June, 1986.

LaForce, F.M.: Immunizations, Immunoprophylaxis, and Chemoprophylaxis to Prevent Selected Infections, *JAMA, 257,* 2464, May 8, 1987.

Parker, M.E. and Wooten, R.K.: Assessment of Immunologic Status Among Dental Hygiene Students. Implications for Practice, *Dent. Hyg., 60,* 210, May, 1986.

United States Department of Health and Human Services, Centers for Disease Control: Immunization Practices in Colleges—United States, *MMWR, 36,* 209, April 17, 1987.

Windom, R.E.: Adult Immunization Should Be Routine, Too (Editorial), *Pub. Health Rep., 102,* 245, May–June, 1987.

Personal Barriers

Brantley, C.F., Heymann, H.O., Shugars, D.A., and Vann, W.F.: The Effect of Gloves on Psychomotor Skills Acquisition Among Dental Students, *J. Dent. Educ., 50,* 611, October, 1986.

Casey, D.M. and Casey, E.P.: Patient Eye Protection in the Dental Office, *N.Y. State Dent. J., 45,* 460, November, 1979.

Craig, D.C. and Quayle, A.A.: The Efficacy of Face-masks, *Br. Dent. J., 158,* 87, February 9, 1985.

Chernosky-Adshead, M. and Derouen, A.S.: Guarding Against Eye Injuries, *RDH, 4,* 30, January/February, 1984.

Field, E.A. and Martin, M.V.: Handwashing: Soap or Disinfectant? *Br. Dent. J., 160,* 278, April 19, 1986.

Folk, J.C. and Lobes, L.A.: Intraocular Complications (Letter to Editor), *J. Am. Dent. Assoc., 102,* 161, February, 1981.

Furuhashi, M. and Miyamae, T.: Effect of Pre-operative Hand Scrubbing and Influence of Pinholes Appearing in Surgical Rubber Gloves During Operation, *Bull. Tokyo Med. Dent. Univ., 26,* 73, June, 1979.

Gobetti, J.P., Cerminaro, M., and Shipman, C.: Hand Asepsis: The Efficacy of Different Soaps in the Removal of Bacteria from Sterile, Gloved Hands, *J. Am. Dent. Assoc., 113,* 291, August, 1986.

Gregg, B. and Davies, J.: Malpractice. A Case for Safety Glasses, *Can. Dent. Assoc. J., 52,* 583, July, 1986.

Mitchell, R., Cumming, C.G., MacLennan, W.D., Ross, P.W., Peutherer, J.F., and Baxter, P.M.K.: The Use of Operating Gloves in Dental Practice, *Br. Dent. J., 154,* 372, June 11, 1983.

Olsen, R.A. and Olsen, D.B.: Hospital Protocol for Inpatients and Outpatients, *Spec. Care Dentist, 7,* 257, November–December, 1987.

Peters, E., Gardner, D.G., Altini, M., and Crooks, J.: Granular Cell Reaction to Surgical Glove Powder, *J. Oral Pathol., 15,* 454, September, 1986.

Pippin, D.J., Verderame, R.A., and Weber, K.K.: Efficacy of Face Masks in Preventing Inhalation of Airborne Contaminants, *J. Oral Maxillofac. Surg., 45,* 319, April, 1987.

Rustage, K.J., Rothwell, P.S., and Brook, I.M.: Evaluation of a Dedicated Dental Procedure Glove for Clinical Dentistry, *Br. Dent. J., 163,* 193, September 19, 1987.

Skaug, N.: Micropunctures of Rubber Gloves Used in Oral Surgery, *Int. J. Oral Surg., 5,* 220, October, 1976.

Uldricks, J.M., Caccamo, P., Beck, F.M., and Schmakel, D.: Effects of Surgical Gloves on Preclinical Scaling Skills, *J. Dent. Educ., 49,* 316, May, 1985.

Wilson, M.P., Gound, S., Tishk, M., and Feil, P.: Gloved Versus Ungloved Dental Hygiene Clinicians, *Dent. Hyg., 60,* 310, July, 1986.

4 Infection Control: Clinical Procedures

The success of a planned system for control of disease transmission depends on the cooperative effort of each member of the dental health team. The objective should be to provide the highest level of sterile procedures possible and practical that will ensure a safe environment for both patient and professionals.

When a patient is known to have a condition that involves communicable pathogenic microorganisms, special precautions must be taken before instruments and other nondisposable items are used for another patient. The presence of disease-producing organisms is not always known; therefore, application of protective, preventive procedures is needed prior to, during, and following *all* patient appointments.

Basic factors involved in the conduct of safe practice include the material in Chapter 3 and the following, to be described in this chapter:
1. Treatment room features.
2. Sterilization and disinfection
   a. Preparation
   b. Methods and equipment
3. Preparation for appointment.
4. Unit water lines.
5. Environmental surfaces.
6. Care of sterile instruments.
7. Patient preparation.
8. Summary of procedures for the prevention of disease transmission.

TREATMENT ROOM FEATURES[1,2,3]

The current design of many treatment rooms may not be conducive to ideal planning for infection control. Changes can be made in routines so that updated, preferred systems can be adapted. When renovations or a new dental office or clinic are anticipated, plans must reflect the most advanced knowledge available relative to safety and disease control.

A partial list of notable features is included here. The objective is to have materials, shapes, and surface textures that facilitate the use of infection control measures.
1. UNIT
   —Designed for easy cleaning and disinfection, with smooth, uncluttered surfaces.
   —Removable hoses that can be cleaned and disinfected.
   —Hoses that are not mechanically retractable, but are straight, not coiled, with round smooth outer surfaces.
   —Syringes with removable autoclavable tips.
   —Handpieces with anti-retraction valves.
   —Handpieces that can be autoclaved.
2. DENTAL CHAIR
   —Controls all foot-operated. If hand-operated, must have overlay to cover buttons (switches) that can be removed for disinfection.
   —Surface and finish of easily cleaned plastic that will withstand chemical disinfection without discoloring; cloth upholstery to be avoided.
3. LIGHT
   —Foot-activated switches.
   —Removable handle for sterilization.
4. OPERATING STOOL
   —Smooth, plastic material that will be easily disinfected with minimum of seams and creases.
   —Foot-operated controls. If hand-operated, must have a barrier cover for the control.
5. FLOOR
   —Carpeting should be avoided.
   —Floor covering should be smooth, easily cleaned, nonabsorbent.
6. SINK
   —Wide and deep enough for effective hand-washing to the elbows.
   —Water and soap with electronic, knee, or foot-operated controls.
   —Separate room or area for contaminated instrument care.
7. SUPPLIES
   —All possible disposable.
8. WASTE
   —Receptacle with opening large enough to prevent contact with sides when material is dropped in.
   —Heavy-duty plastic bag liner to be sealed tightly for disposal.
   —Small receptacle bag near operating area to receive contaminated sponges and other waste. Small bag to be tied tightly for disposal in large waste receiver.

TERMINOLOGY FOR ASEPTIC TECHNIQUE

Clarification of terms is important to understanding the objectives to be attained in the use of various methods applied for the control of disease transmission. In addition to the procedures described here, other terms are defined in the glossary.

I. Sterilization

The process by which all forms of life, including bacterial spores and viruses, are destroyed by physical or chemical agents.

II. Disinfection

Any process, chemical or physical, by means of which pathogenic agents or disease-producing microorganisms can be destroyed. *Disinfectants* are applied to inanimate objects in contrast to *antiseptics*, which are applied to living tissues. Disinfectants are categorized by their biocidal activity as high level, intermediate level, or low level.

A. High Level

High-level disinfectants inactivate spores and all forms of bacteria, fungi, and viruses. High-level disinfection is the same as sterilization.

B. Intermediate Level

Intermediate-level disinfectants inactivate all forms of bacteria, fungi, and viruses, but do not destroy spores.

C. Low Level

Low-level disinfectants inactivate vegetative bacteria and certain lipid-type viruses, but do not destroy spores, tubercle bacilli, or non-lipid viruses.

III. Sanitization

The process by which the number of organisms on inanimate objects is reduced to a safe level. It does not imply freedom from microorganisms, and generally refers to a cleaning process.

IV. Surface Disinfection

The process by which microorganisms that contaminate environmental surfaces of implements and equipment are removed by vigorous scrubbing with a germicidal disinfectant.

V. Contamination

The presence of microorganisms on a body surface or on inanimate articles or substances.

VI. Aseptic Technique

The use of aseptic technique refers to procedures carried out in the absence of pathogenic microorganisms, techniques that avoid contamination of patients, and the careful use of sterilized instruments and materials to avoid contamination.

A. Sepsis

A condition in which disease-producing (pathogenic) microorganisms are present.

B. Asepsis

A condition in which living pathogenic microorganisms are absent.

C. Chain of Asepsis

A chain of asepsis means a procedure that avoids transfer of infection. "Chain" implies that each step, related to the previous one, continues to be carried out without the presence of pathogenic microorganisms.

D. Strict Aseptic Technique

Procedures used during strict aseptic technique are similar to those used in a hospital operating room, conducted with the highest level of asepsis for the treatment area, and the personal cleanliness of the clinicians and their auxiliaries, all of whom should be properly vaccinated. Clinician's hair and feet are covered. A surgical hand scrub is used before donning gloves and gowns from sterilized packages.

E. Sterile-Clean Technique

For dental and dental hygiene appointments, a sterile-clean technique is practiced routinely. Sterilization of instruments and other nondisposable items is the same as for a strict aseptic technique. Clinicians and their assistants must exercise consistent barrier techniques with maximum usage of protective eyewear, face mask, and gloves, as described in Chapter 3.

PREPARATION FOR INSTRUMENT STERILIZATION

A consistent system for the removal of used instruments and equipment from the treatment area at the completion of a patient appointment should be worked out to assure safety measures against self-contamination. Cycling to keep used instruments in one area and sterile trays or packages in another can be planned. A good rule is to learn the most effective method of preventing cross-contamination, and then always to follow that method without exception.

I. Handling

A. Preventive Aspects

Wear glasses and mask while cleaning instruments. Heavy-duty household gloves should be worn (figure 4–1). A transfer or handling forceps may be kept especially for use during the handling of nonsterile instruments.

During processing for cleaning and sterilization, careless handling of instruments with delicate working ends, such as scalers and explorers, can lead to fracture of the tips. Rubbing or rough contact of blades or tips with other instruments contributes to their dullness. Pressure or bending will distort various instruments.

To prevent rusting or discoloration, instruments should be cleaned as soon as possible after use. Even stainless steel can acquire a tarnish that

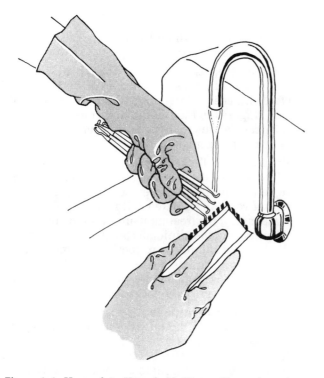

Figure 4–1. Heavy-duty Household Gloves. Heavy duty gloves should be worn to prevent hand injuries while instruments are being cleaned and prepared for sterilization as well as while preparing the treatment area prior to seating the patient. (From Torres, H.O. and Ehrlich, A.: *Modern Dental Assisting*, 3rd ed. Philadelphia, W.B. Saunders Co., 1985)

is difficult to remove. If there is an unavoidable delay, or when instruments are accumulated to be cared for after a series of appointments, they should be rinsed with cold water to remove blood and debris and then immersed in a disinfectant.

B. Sharp Instruments

During careful handling, prevention of injury to the hands is particularly important. An uncapped needle must not be left on the instrument tray where accidental injury can occur. After they have been used, disposable needles and blades should be placed directly into puncture-resistant containers made for that purpose.[4]

When a needle is reserved for administering multiple injections during an appointment, great care must be exercised to prevent needlestick. The needle may be recapped by laying the cap on the tray and sliding the needle into it or by holding the cap with a forceps or needlestick shield (figure 4–4, page 57).

II. Manual Cleaning

A. Pre-clean

Soak in disinfectant, then scrub to remove blood and debris. Avoid splashing, because splatter can contain blood, saliva, or other contaminated material.

B. Dismantle Instruments

Dismantle instruments with detachable parts, such as the porte polisher or a mouth mirror with handle, and open instruments with joints, such as scissors.

C. Clean by Scrub Technique

1. Apply a solvent to remove greases or oils left by dental materials.
2. Scrub with a stiff brush with detergent and running water to remove all particles of dried blood or debris. Hold the item low in the sink.
3. Use a detergent, not ordinary soap.
   a. Soap can form insoluble alkalies in hard water that can enmesh and protect the bacteria from the sterilizing effect later.
   b. Cake soap can harbor microorganisms and become a potential source of transfer.
   c. Avoid use of abrasives because they may roughen the instrument surface and affect the stainless properties of the metal.
4. Apply individual measures for problem areas, such as grooves and joints where debris can collect and harden; for example, the mouth mirror with grooves at the attachment of the shank as well as around the mirror rim.

D. Rinse

Rinse in hot water to remove all detergent.

E. Dry

1. Purposes
   a. To prevent instrument discoloration if there is an interval before sterilization.
   b. Water will dilute the pre-autoclaving emulsion or disinfection solution.
2. Air dry. Prevents need for extra handling.
3. Dry carefully with paper towels when time does not permit air drying.

F. Care of Scrub Brushes

1. Wash contaminated brushes in detergent, rinse thoroughly, and sterilize.
2. Label brushes to prevent inadvertent mixing with hand-scrubbing brushes.

III. Ultrasonic Cleaning

Ultrasonic cleaning prior to sterilization is safer than manual cleaning. Risk of injury to hands and of infection is not as great.

Manual cleaning of instruments is a difficult and time-consuming procedure with numerous disadvantages. When ultrasonic equipment is adjusted for optimum performance and those using it are properly informed and adhere to the manufacturer's instructions, the quality of cleaning is much better than by the hand-scrub technique. *Ultrasonic processing is not a substitute for sterilization: it is only a cleaning process.*

A. Advantages

Benefits from the use of ultrasonic cleaning include the following:

1. Increased efficiency in obtaining a high degree of cleanliness.
2. Reduced potential danger to clinician from direct contact with hepatitis viruses and other pathogens.
3. Improved effectiveness for disinfection.
4. Elimination of possible dissemination of microorganisms through release of aerosols and droplets, which can occur during the scrubbing process.
5. Penetration into areas of the instruments where the bristles of a brush are too coarse to contact.
6. Removal of tarnish.

B. Principles of Action

Ultrasonic vibrations initiate cavitation in the cleansing solution. Cavitation means that minute bubbles are generated that expand until they are unstable, then collapse by bursting inward. This creates minute vacuum areas that are responsible for the cleaning process by dislodging, dispersing, or dissolving the material that has adhered to the surface of the instrument.

Cleaning is accomplished by both the physical agitation and chemical dissolution. Soluble material goes into solution and heavier material sinks to the bottom of the cleaning tank.

C. Procedure

1. Select the proper agent from the various concentrates available from the manufacturers. Selection is based on the specific use; for example, one solution is prepared for general instrument cleaning and another for removal of denture stains.
2. Wear heavy-duty rubber gloves to protect against infection and chemicals.
3. Place instruments in the carrier tray or basket and submerge in the solution.
   a. Guard against overloading and crowding, which can prevent the solution from reaching all surfaces.
   b. Open jointed instruments; dismantle detachable parts.
   c. Space instruments to avoid contacts between easily damaged surfaces, which may lead to bending or dulling.
   d. Do not mix various metals in the same bath; for example, separate stainless steel, aluminum, copper, and brass.
4. Time from 1 to 10 minutes, depending on the unit, the solution, and the material being treated. Consult manufacturer's chart.
5. Remove, drain, then rinse thoroughly with warm water.
6. Dry in air thoroughly.

D. Care of Unit

Change solution for each use to maintain its efficiency.

1. The solution does not contain a disinfectant and becomes heavily contaminated.
2. The unit should be kept covered to prevent contamination from air and splatter.
3. Empty container after each use, and disinfect.

IV. Packaging

A. Methods

There are several ways of arranging instruments and equipment for sterilization after manual and/or ultrasonic cleaning. Preset trays or packages can be preplanned to contain all the items usually needed for a particular appointment.

Each tray or package should be marked for identification of contents: for example, *Adult Scaling and Root Planing, Examination,* or *Preventive Maintenance with Topical Fluoride.*

Chemical indicator tape is used to seal all packages. The chemical, usually in the form of a series of stripes, changes color during the sterilization process. The change of color means that the temperature reached a designated height required for penetration and that the contact time was adequate (figure 4–2). Distinct black stripes should appear. A lighter color change may be a warning signal that the autoclave function should be checked.

Indicator tape does not serve to test for true sterilization. A biologic indicator in the form of microbial spores must be used to test each sterilizer routinely.[5,6]

The striped indicator tape is left on the sealed package and thereby serves to identify those packages ready for use.

Following are suggested methods for instrument arrangement for sterilization:

1. They may be placed on an open tray, which fits into a see-through autoclave bag to be sealed with indicator tape before sterilizing.
2. They may be arranged in perforated trays with fitted covers. The covered tray is wrapped with special autoclave paper and sealed with indicator tape.
3. They may be packaged in various types of bags available commercially. The packaging material must permit steam or gas penetration. Acceptable and unacceptable wrappers will be listed as each of the sterilizing methods is described. A package is sealed to preserve the sterile state and not opened until ready to be used.

B. Suggestions for Packaging

1. Insert a sharp tip into a small piece of a cotton roll.
   a. to protect the sharp tip from damage by other instruments.
   b. to prevent it from puncturing a bag or wrapper during sterilization. A punctured package can no longer be considered sterile.

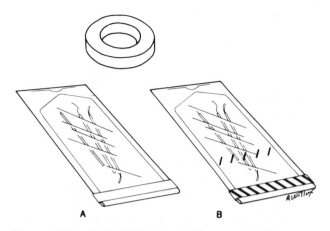

Figure 4–2. Process Indicator Tape. A. Before autoclaving, **B.** After autoclaving. The change of color in the stripes indicates that the package has been subjected to the proper temperature for sterilization. A biologic indicator is also needed periodically to determine that the autoclave is functioning properly and that sterilization is actually taking place.

2. Place a strip of sterilizer indicator tape inside each package on the instruments to show that the package contents have been raised to the proper temperature for sterilization and that the wrapper did not hinder penetration.
3. Label and date each package. To prevent puncturing the bag while writing, the label should be placed before loading the bag.
4. Seal each package securely by folding the material twice and sealing with indicator tape.
5. Gauze sponges, cotton rolls, and other accessories can be packaged in small lots for individual appointments.
6. Extra instruments to replace a dulled or dropped instrument, or to supplement when a particular problem requires a special instrument, are sterilized separately in labeled wrappers and kept sealed in a convenient place within reach of the operating position.

STERILIZATION[7,8,9]

I. Approved Methods

Each of the methods listed here will be described in detail in the sections following.
A. Moist heat: steam under pressure.
B. Dry heat.
C. Chemical vapor.
D. Ethylene oxide gas.
E. Chemical sterilant (immersion).

II. Selection of Method

All materials and items cannot be treated by the same system of sterilization. Supplement with disposable one-use products when sterilization is not possible.

The method for sterilization that is selected must provide complete destruction of all microorganisms, viruses, and spores, and yet must not damage the instruments and other materials treated. In addition, the procedures must not be complex, with many chances for errors in the processing.

Careful, specific use of sterilizing equipment in accord with the manufacturer's specifications is necessary. Incomplete sterilization is most frequently due to inadequate preparation of the materials to be sterilized, misuse of the equipment, or inadequate maintenance.

MOIST HEAT: STEAM UNDER PRESSURE

Destruction of microorganisms by heat takes place as a result of inactivation of essential cellular proteins or enzymes. Moist heat causes coagulation of protein.

I. Use

Moist heat may be used for all materials except oils, waxes, and powders that are impervious to steam, or materials that cannot be subjected to high temperatures.

II. Principles of Action

A. Sterilization is achieved by action of heat and moisture; pressure serves only to attain high temperature.
B. Sterilization depends on the penetrating ability of steam.
   1. Air must be excluded, otherwise steam penetration and heat transfer are prevented.
   2. Space between objects is essential to assure access for the steam.
   3. Materials must be thoroughly cleaned, because adherent material can provide a barrier to the steam.
   4. Air discharge occurs in a downward direction; load must be arranged for free passage of steam toward bottom of autoclave.

III. Preparation of Materials

Linens are laundered; instruments are scrubbed or cleaned in ultrasonic cleaner and dried.

A. Protection of Metal Instruments from Corrosion
   Use a corrosion inhibitor such as 2% sodium nitrite.[10] Immerse, drain, and wrap or place in tray. This procedure is needed primarily for carbon steel instruments.

B. Wrapping
   Bundles may be made with paper, muslin, see-through plastic and paper bags, or metal trays. Steam will not penetrate closed metal containers, canvas, or aluminum foil.

   Seal with autoclave tape; do not use pins for fastening paper because the pinholes leave openings for contamination. Label with date and list of contents.

C. Autoclave Tape

Bundle is sealed with tape that develops colored stripes at 121° C (250° F). The tape serves as a chemical monitor to identify packages that have been put through the sterilizer[5] (figure 4–2).

D. Autoclave Bags

They should not be overloaded.

E. Packing Autoclave

Pack loosely to permit steam to reach all instruments in all packages; place jars or tall vessels on their sides to permit air to leave as steam enters.

IV. Operation

Follow manufacturer's specifications for use of autoclave.

The two ranges generally used when instruments are treated are described here.

A. Standard Procedure

121° C (250° F) at 15 pounds pressure for 15 minutes after the meters show that proper pressure and temperature have been reached. Use 30 minutes for heavy loads to assure penetration.

B. "Flash" Treatment

132° C to 135° C (270° F) at 30 pounds pressure for 3 minutes (unwrapped) or 7 minutes (wrapped) has been used for light loads; however, there is a greater chance for error in that an object might not heat through. Certain materials and metals cannot withstand the higher temperature. This is not a recommended procedure.

V. Cooling

A. Dry Materials

Release steam pressure, turn operating valve, and open the door; required time for drying, about 15 minutes.

B. Liquids

Reduce chamber pressure slowly at an even rate over 10 to 12 minutes to prevent boiling or escape of fluids into the chamber; preferable to turn off the autoclave and let the pressure fall before opening the door. Check heat sensitivity of each solution and avoid prolonged exposure, as indicated.

VI. Care of Autoclave

A. Daily

Maintain proper level of distilled water; wash trays and interior surfaces of chamber with water and a mild detergent; clean removable plug, screen, or strainer.

B. Weekly

Flush chamber discharge system with an appropriate cleaning solution such as hot trisodium phosphate or a commercial cleaner.

VII. Biologic Indicator or Spore Test[5,6]

The chemical indicator color change or monitor is related to temperature, not time (figure 4–2). For a real test of sterilization, a daily or weekly spore test is recommended for clinics and hospitals; whereas a weekly or monthly test may be sufficient for a smaller practice, depending on the amount of use. A spore test should also be made on a new machine, following repairs, and when there is a change of the personnel who operate the equipment.

Ampules contain living resistant spores plus a color indicator. An ampule is placed in the center of a package between instruments and that package placed in the middle of a load of packages to be autoclaved. After sterilization has been completed by the usual time-temperature, the ampule and one that was not autoclaved are incubated according to the manufacturer's instructions. Nonautoclaved spores will change the color indicator, whereas the autoclaved spores will not germinate. Certain companies provide spore strips that are returned to the company for culturing. The delay in incubation during mailing could alter bacterial growth.

VIII. Evaluation of Steam Under Pressure

A. Advantages

1. All microorganisms, spores, and viruses destroyed quickly and efficiently.
2. Wide variety of materials may be treated; most economical method of sterilization.

B. Disadvantages

1. May corrode carbon steel instruments if precautions are not taken.
2. Unsuitable for oils or powders that are impervious to heat.

DRY HEAT

The action of dry heat is oxidation.

I. Use

A. Primarily for materials that cannot safely be sterilized with steam under pressure.
B. Oils and powders when they are thermostabile at the required temperatures.
C. For small metal instruments enclosed in special containers or that might be corroded or rusted by moisture, such as endodontic instruments.

II. Principles of Action

A. Sterilization is achieved by heat that is conducted from the exterior surface to the interior of the object; the time required to penetrate varies among materials.
B. Sterilization can result when the whole material is treated for a sufficient length of time at the specified temperature: therefore, timing for sterilization must start when the entire contents of the sterilizer have reached the peak temperature needed for that load.
C. Oil, grease, or organic debris on instruments in-

sulates and protects microorganisms from the sterilizing effect.

III. Preparation of Materials

A. Instruments

Instruments, glassware, or other materials must be thoroughly cleaned and dried to prevent corrosion.

B. Packaging

Small packages permit greater access to the heat. Materials that may be used for packaging are paper bags, muslin towels, aluminum trays, pans, or aluminum foil.

C. Packing the Sterilizer

Allow space for access to heat around each item; never load to the limit.

IV. Operation[8]

A. Temperature

160° C (320° F) held for 2 hours; 170° C (340° F) for 1 hour. Timing must start after the desired temperature has been reached.

B. Penetration Time

Heat penetration varies with different materials, and the nature and properties of various materials must be considered.

C. Care

Care must be taken not to overheat because certain materials can be affected: temperatures over 160° C (320° F) may destroy the sharp edges of cutting instruments; over 170° C, paper and cotton materials will begin to scorch.

D. Spore Tests

Procedures for testing sterilization are similar to those for a steam autoclave, but spores of different microorganisms are used.[5]

V. Evaluation of Dry Heat

A. Advantages

1. Useful for materials that cannot be subjected to steam under pressure.
2. When maintained at correct temperature, it is well suited for sharp instruments.
3. No corrosion as found with steam under pressure.

B. Disadvantages

1. Long exposure required; penetration slow and uneven.
2. High temperatures critical to certain materials.

CHEMICAL VAPOR STERILIZER[11]

A combination of alcohols, formaldehyde, ketone, water, and acetone heated under pressure produces a gas that is effective as a sterilizing agent.

I. Use

Chemical vapor sterilization cannot be used for materials or objects that can be altered by the chemicals that make the vapor or that cannot withstand the high temperature. Examples are low-melting plastics, liquids, or heat-sensitive handpieces.

II. Principles of Action

Microbial and viral destruction results from the permeation of the heated formaldehyde and alcohol. Heavy, tightly wrapped or sealed packages would not permit the penetration of the vapors.

III. Preparation of Materials

A. Protection from Corrosion

Rusting is not to be expected if instruments are dried before they are placed in the sterilizer.

B. Wrapping

1. Penetration into and around the instruments is necessary. Sealed tubes or jars or multiple thick cloth wrappings would hinder the circulation of the vapor.
2. Acceptable for packaging are paper and perforated metal trays, covered with autoclave paper and sealed with autoclave tape. Plastic bags compatible with the gases as advised by the manufacturer may also be used.
3. Instruments may be placed on a sterilizer tray without wrapping when the sterilized materials will be used directly and, therefore, do not need the protection of a wrapper.

IV. Operation

A. Temperature

127° to 132° C (260° to 270° F) with 20 to 40 pounds pressure in accord with the manufacturer's directions.

B. Time

Minimum of 20 minutes after the correct temperature has been attained. Time should be extended for a large load or a heavy wrap.

V. Cooling at the Completion of the Cycle

Instruments are dry. Larger instruments may need a short period for cooling.

VI. Care of Sterilizer

Depending on the amount of use, refilling will be needed by at least every 30 cycles. In accord with manufacturer's instructions, the condensate tray is removed, the exhausted solution emptied, and the tray cleaned.

VII. Spore Test for Sterilization

A spore test strip is placed inside a typical package on a regular basis; weekly, in a busy clinical situation. Procedures are similar to those described previously for a steam autoclave. Each type of sterilizer requires selected types of organisms in the spore test strip.

VIII. Evaluation of Chemical Vapor Sterilizer

A. Advantages
1. Corrosion- and rust-free operation for carbon steel instruments.
2. Ability to sterilize in a relatively short total cycle.
3. Ease of operation and care for the equipment.

B. Disadvantages
1. Adequate ventilation is needed; cannot use in a small room.
2. Slight odor, which is rarely objectionable.

ETHYLENE OXIDE[12]

Gaseous sterilization using ethylene oxide is not commonly found in a private dental office or clinic, but rather in hospitals and larger clinics. As compact units are developed, ethylene oxide will be more widely used in dentistry.

I. Use

Nearly all materials, whether metal, plastic, rubber, or cloth, can be sterilized in ethylene oxide with little or no damage to the material.

II. Principles of Action

Ethylene oxide vapor is effective against all types and forms of microorganisms provided sufficient time is allowed.

III. Preparation of Materials

A. Instruments
Instruments must be completely cleaned and dried.

B. Wrapping
1. Penetration around and on all surfaces is necessary for sterilizing action. Sealed metal containers are not acceptable for packaging.
2. Acceptable for packaging are paper, and perforated trays with covers, covered with autoclave paper and sealed with autoclave tape.

IV. Operation

Specific operation is related to the type of equipment. Operation in a well-ventilated room is necessary. Overnight processing is usually the most practical.

A. Time and Temperature
The time may vary from 2 to 12 hours, depending on both the temperature and the concentration of ethylene oxide used.

B. Aeration After Completion of the Cycle
Plastic and rubber products need to be aerated at least 24 hours. Metal instruments can be used immediately.

V. Spore Test

Effectiveness of sterilization must be tested regularly. A system similar to that described for steam autoclave is used, but does not contain the same types of spores.

VI. Evaluation of Ethylene Oxide

A. Advantages
1. Many types of materials can be sterilized with minimum or no damage to the material itself. There is no damage to the finest instruments.
2. Low temperature for operation.

B. Disadvantages
1. High cost of the equipment.
2. Problems of dispersement of gaseous exhaust. Need for planned and tested ventilation.
3. Increased time of operation.
4. Gas absorption requires airing of plastic, rubber, and cloth goods for several hours.

CHEMICAL STERILANTS (IMMERSION)

Immersion in a chemical sterilant is used only for items that cannot be sterilized by heat. When ethylene oxide sterilizers are available, many of the items may be treated by that method.

Chemicals used for immersion sterilization have been approved by the Environmental Protection Agency (EPA) and the American Dental Association (ADA) and meet the criteria listed on page 50. Manufacturer's instructions must be followed explicitly. A chemical may require only 10 to 30 minutes for disinfection, whereas the same chemical at the same or different concentrations may require from 6¾ to 10 hours for sterilization. Temperature may also be a factor.

Instruments cannot be packaged, so maintenance of strict asepsis is not possible after chemical sterilization. Also, because of toxic effects to skin and mucosa, the chemical must be rinsed away with sterile water and dried before use on a patient.

Information about the categories, action, uses, and other factors regarding chemical sterilants will be described in the next section.

CHEMICAL DISINFECTANTS

Disinfection does not accomplish complete destruction of all forms of microorganisms; therefore, it is not a substitute for sterilization. The object is to reduce the level of microbial contamination to a safe level. The term decontamination may also be applied.

The properties of an ideal disinfectant are shown in Table 4–1.

I. Uses

A. Environmental Surfaces Disinfection
Following each appointment, the treatment area is cleaned and disinfected (pages 53–55).

Table 4–1. Properties of an Ideal Disinfectant*

1. **Broad spectrum:**
   Should always have the widest possible antimicrobial spectrum.

2. **Fast acting:**
   Should always have a rapidly lethal action on all vegetative forms and spores of bacteria and fungi, protozoa, and viruses.

3. **Not affected by physical factors:**
   Active in the presence of organic matter—such as blood, sputum, and feces.

   Should be compatible with soaps, detergents, and other chemicals encountered in use.

4. **Nontoxic**

5. **Surface compatibility:**
   Should not corrode instruments and other metallic surfaces.

   Should not cause the disintegration of cloth, rubber, plastics, or other materials.

6. **Residual effect on treated surfaces**

7. **Easy to use**

8. **Odorless:**
   An inoffensive odor would facilitate its routine use.

9. **Economical:**
   Cost should not be prohibitively high.

*Molinari, J.A., Gleason, M.J., Cottone, J.A., and Barrett, E.D., Comparison of Dental Surface Disinfectants, *Gen. Dent.*, 35, 171, May–June, 1987.

B. Holding Solution

After use, instruments are placed in a disinfecting solution until cleaning and preparation for sterilization can be accomplished. An appropriate container such as a flat basin can be kept near the treatment area so that instruments may be placed directly into the disinfectant after the final use. This has particular application during extended procedures when debris can dry on instruments.[13]

C. Dental Laboratory Impressions and Prostheses

Impressions can be carriers of infectious material to a dental laboratory, and completed prostheses must be disinfected before delivery to a patient.[14,15,16] Additional references may be found with the Suggested Readings at the end of Chapter 10.

II. Principles of Action

A. Disinfection is achieved by coagulation, precipitation, or oxidation of protein of microbial cells or denaturation of the enzymes of the cells.

B. Disinfection depends on the contact of the solution at the known effective concentration for the optimum period of time.

C. Items must be thoroughly cleaned and dried, be-cause action of the agent is altered by foreign matter and dilution.

D. A solution has a specific shelf life, use life, and re-use life. Some may be altered by changes in pH, or the active ingredient may decrease in potency. Check manufacturer's directions.

III. Criteria for Selection of a Chemical Agent

The objective is to select a product that is effective in the control of microorganisms and practical to use. Properties of an ideal disinfectant are shown in table 4–1.

The manufacturer's informational literature and container labels must provide facts about the product that assure its effectiveness. After the product has been selected, it is the responsibility of the dental personnel to use it as directed to obtain the best possible infection control. When the label has insufficient information, the manufacturer should be contacted and instructions obtained.

The criteria should include at least the following:
A. EPA approval.
B. ADA approval.
C. Chemicals must be tuberculocidal, bacteriocidal, virucidal, and fungicidal.
D. Label must state
   1. Effectiveness and stability expressed by
      a. Shelf life: the expiration date indicating the termination of effectiveness of the unopened container.
      b. Use life: the time the product is active after mixing but before it is used.
      c. Re-use life: the time a product is effective as it is being used. When not specified, the re-use life should be considered 1 day.
   2. Directions for activation (mixing proportions).
   3. Type of container for storage and place (conditions such as heat and light).
   4. Directions for use
      a. Pre-cleaning and drying of items to be submerged.
      b. Time/temperature ratio.
   5. Instructions for disposal of used solution.
   6. Warnings; cautions
      a. Toxic effects (i.e., eyes, skin).
      b. Specific directions for emergency care in the event of an accident (e.g., splash in eye).

IV. Preparation of Materials

A. Scrub thoroughly or use ultrasonic cleaner (pages 44–45) to eliminate organic matter (blood, debris, oil, grease), which interferes with the action of the chemical. Use wire brush for grooved metal instruments such as files or burs.

B. Rinse thoroughly to eliminate soap or detergent that is incompatible with the chemical.

C. Dry thoroughly. Dilution of the chemical solution will lessen or eliminate its effect. Place on paper towels to blot dry.

V. Operation

A. Place instruments in solution and immerse completely; solution must contact all parts. Care must be taken to prevent overloading.
B. Temperature: usually room temperature.
C. Time: follow manufacturer's instructions. Time varies from 30 minutes to 10 hours.
D. Do not add other instruments without starting timing over again.
E. When time is complete, drain the instruments, remove with sterile transfer forceps, and dry with a sterile towel. When a solution is known to be irritating to tissue or distasteful, instruments should be rinsed with sterile water to remove the chemical before using in a patient's mouth.

VI. Care of Equipment

A. Keep the container covered to prevent contamination of the solution from dust- or airborne microorganisms.
B. Clean the container and change the solution daily in accord with manufacturer's directions to maintain its cleanliness, proper dilution, and potency in accord with the use life of the chemical.

RECOMMENDED CHEMICAL DISINFECTANTS

The agents that have been shown adequate for use in dentistry are glutaraldehydes, iodophores, chlorine compounds, and synthetic phenolics. These will be described below. Table 4–2 shows the dilution and required time of immersion for disinfection and sterilization.

Alcohols and quaternary ammonium compounds are not approved for instrument or environmental surface disinfection. The alcohols, ethanol and isopropanol, have been widely accepted and used for the preparation of the skin prior to injections or blood-taking procedures. The use of alcohol for this purpose is as a cleansing action; the length of time involved is not enough for antibacterial effect.[17]

I. Glutaraldehydes[14,18]

As shown in table 4–2, the three types of glutaraldehydes are the alkaline, acid, and neutral preparations.

A. Action

They are high-level disinfectants and act to kill microorganisms by damaging their proteins and nucleic acids.

Table 4–2. Chemical Sterilizing/Disinfecting Agents*

Chemical Classification	Disinfectant	Sterilant
Glutaraldehydes		
Glutaraldehyde 2% neutral	full strength 10 minutes	full strength 10 hours
Glutaraldehyde 2% alkaline	full strength 10–90 minutes† 20–25° C†	full strength 10 hours 20/25° C†
Glutaraldehyde 2% alkaline with phenolic buffer	1:16 dilution 10 minutes 20° C	full strength 6¾ hours 20° C
Glutaraldehyde 2% acidic	1:4 dilution† 30 minutes 20° C	full strength 10 hours 25° C
Chlorines		
Chlorine dioxide	4:1:1 dilution 2 minutes 20° C	4:1:1 dilution 6 hours 20° C
Sodium hypochlorite 5.25% household bleach	1:10 dilution 10 minutes 20° C	‡
Iodophors		
Iodophor (1% available iodine)	1:213 dilution 10 minutes 20° C	‡
Combination Phenolics		
o-phenylphenyl 9% with o-benzyl-p-chlorophenol 1%	1:32 dilution 10 minutes 20° C	‡

*Data from American Dental Association, Council on Dental Therapeutics
†Commercial products vary. Follow manufacturer's instructions.
‡Not effective as a sterilant
 Temperature: 20° C = 68° F (room temperature)
            25° C = 77° F

B. Preparation

The solutions become activated when the components of the two containers are mixed. The manufacturers' labels must show shelf use and re-use life, because the various preparations differ.

C. Limitations

1. Caustic to skin: use forceps and gloves.
2. Irritating to eyes: need protective glasses.
3. Corrosive to some metal instruments.
4. Items must be rinsed in sterile water after removal from immersion bath.
5. Not used as a surface disinfectant because of toxic effects of fumes; surfaces wiped with glutaraldehyde should have residual film wiped off with sterile water.

II. Chlorine Compounds

A. Action

Chlorine compounds have been used in a variety of ways for disinfection. Their use in water purification is well known. Solutions of sodium hypochlorite are used in cleaning dentures (page 346). Microorganisms are destroyed primarily by oxidation of microbial enzymes and cell wall components.

B. Chlorine Dioxide[18]

The use life of chlorine dioxide is only one day, so new preparations must be made. The preparation is economical and generally nontoxic, but corrosive to non-stainless steel instruments.

C. Sodium Hypochlorite

Daily fresh solutions are needed because sodium hypochlorite tends to be unstable. Use distilled water for mixing to improve the stability. The solutions can harm the eyes, skin, and clothing, and corrode certain instruments; and the strong odor may be offensive. In spite of certain disadvantages, it is widely used, recommended by the Centers for Disease Control,[19] and economical.

III. Iodophors

A. Action

Iodine is released slowly from the iodophor compound, and creates a disinfecting action as a broad-spectrum antimicrobial.

Povidone-iodine preparations are widely used in the forms of surgical scrubs, liquid soaps, mouthrinse, and surface antiseptics prior to hyperdermic injection.

B. Environmental Surface Disinfectant

Concentrated solutions of iodophor contain less free iodine; therefore, the correct dilution for hard-surface disinfection is 1 part iodophor concentrate to 213 parts soft or distilled water. Hard water inactivates iodophors. The solution changes from amber to clear as it loses its activity.

IV. Combination Phenolics (synthetic)

A. Action

High concentration phenols act as protoplasmic poisons that destroy the cell wall and precipitate the protein. The lower concentrations used as surface disinfectants inactivate enzyme systems.

B. Use

Although a 10-minute disinfecting time is designated, the regulation for approval of the products containing the phenolics requests an immersion time of 20 minutes when the presence of tuberculosis is a risk.[20]

BOILING WATER DISINFECTION[21]

I. Use

Boiling water may be used to disinfect metal instruments, glassware, or other materials that can be subjected to water.

II. Principles of Action

A. Disinfection is accomplished by heat.
B. Objects must be completely submerged for a sufficient length of time.
C. Bactericidal effect is increased by the addition of an alkali such as 2% sodium carbonate.
D. Distilled water should be used to supply the boiler.

III. Preparation of Materials

A. Scrub thoroughly, or use ultrasonic cleaner (pages 44–45).
B. Disassemble or open jointed instruments.
C. Arrange items carefully in metal basket of boiler to protect delicate and sharp edges and provide access of the boiling water; instruments must be completely submerged.

IV. Operation

A. Minimum of 30 minutes at boiling (100° C or 212° F at sea level).
B. When instruments are added to those already boiling, the time cycle must start again.
C. An increase of heat does not increase the temperature of boiling water. Action is more vigorous and evaporation is increased.
D. Instruments should be removed with sterile transfer forceps while hot and dried promptly to prevent rusting.

V. Care of Unit

To decrease corrosive action on instruments and the formation of scaly deposit on the sides of the unit, use distilled water and add an antirust agent such as trisodium phosphate, sodium carbonate, or borax. Daily cleaning is necessary for units in constant use. Add a small amount of acetic acid (vinegar) and boil for 10 minutes to loosen the scale, then apply scrub brush and water, and rinse before filling.

VI. Evaluation

A. Advantages

A relatively short time is required for disinfection, and the preparation of materials is simple.

B. Disadvantages

1. Resistance of certain organisms.
2. Reduction in sharpness of instruments.
3. Corrosion of certain metals.

UNIT WATER LINES

High counts of microorganisms have been found in the waterline tubings after overnight standing. Tests have been made on tubings to handpieces, water syringes, and ultrasonic scalers. When the lines were flushed for 2 minutes, the microbial counts were reduced.[22]

Contaminated water should not be used for surgical purposes or during the irrigation of pocket areas, because infective microorganisms can be introduced. If contaminated water were directed forcefully into a pocket, microorganisms could enter the tissue and bacteremia result.

I. Procedures for Clinical Use

A. Flush all water lines at least 5 to 6 minutes at the beginning of each day.
B. Operate handpieces and waterspray over a sink or cuspidor for 30 seconds before and 30 seconds after each patient appointment.

II. Water Retraction System

To correct saliva and debris suck-back in the water line of a handpiece, the water retraction valve should be removed and a check valve or antiretractor valve installed.[23] Originally, handpieces were made with a retraction valve to prevent dripping when the instrument was turned off. Material sucked into the line, possibly filled with microorganisms including hepatitis viruses, tubercle bacilli, and other pathogens, will then be discharged when the handpiece is used for the succeeding patient.

PREPARATION FOR APPOINTMENT

The cleanliness and neatness of the treatment room reflect the character and conscientiousness of the dental personnel. The patient, with limited knowledge of dental science, may judge the ability of the dental personnel by the appearance of the office or clinic.

The patient's attitude is important, but more important is the relationship of cleanliness to the presence of microorganisms and the need for performing techniques in a situation that minimizes cross-contamination.

The orderliness and immaculate cleanliness of the treatment rooms result from continuing care. An excellent test for the effects of care and any minor oversights is for the dentist or dental auxiliary to sit in the dental chair occasionally and look around at what the patient sees from that vantage point.

I. Objectives

Effective care of instruments and equipment contributes to the following:
A. Control of disease transmission by way of environmental surfaces.
B. An increase in the working efficiency of the office personnel.
C. An atmosphere of cleanliness and orderliness that will contribute to the patient's well-being.
D. An increase in the patient's confidence in the ability of the dental personnel.
E. The maintenance of the working efficiency of office equipment and instruments
   1. To prolong their span of usefulness.
   2. To contribute to patient safety (see Cardiac Pacemaker, pages 692–694).
F. A decrease in the occurrence of unpleasant odors in the office.

II. Environmental Surfaces

The preparation of environmental surfaces for an appointment is, in reality, the disinfection after the previous appointment. Indeed, at the end of the final appointment of a day, the steps for disinfection should be carried out so that splatter and microorganisms are not left to dry on the contaminated surfaces overnight.

During appointments, the dental furniture, equipment, and the room fixtures may become contaminated by the contact of the hands of members of the dental team carrying saliva, blood, bacterial plaque, and other potentially infectious material from the patient's oral cavity (figure 2–1, page 10). In addition, aerosols and splatter created during the treatment procedures are spread throughout the area.

Pathogenic as well as other organisms can survive on environmental surfaces. Transfer of microorganisms is, therefore, possible from one patient to a subsequent patient by contact with a chair arm, headrest, or other surface. A patient may use a telephone that was previously contaminated by the hands of the dental personnel. Hepatitis B viruses can remain active for transmission for days to weeks, depending on the environmental conditions.

III. Planning for Decontamination

To decontaminate the treatment room when time between appointments is limited requires an efficient procedural system and an effective disinfecting agent. When a dentist uses several treatment rooms, preparation time can be a designated part of the rotating system. Dental hygienists frequently are confined to one room, so that a continuing orderly arrangement for decontamination is necessary.

Planning for a system of disinfection can be accomplished by first making a list of all the surfaces contacted during a usual appointment. Each contact can then be placed in one of the categories listed below. The list can be studied for possible changes to increase efficiency, save time, and decrease cross-contamination.

A. Unnecessary Hand Contacts

Only contacts essential to the service to be performed should be made. Planning ahead to have materials ready so that cabinet knobs or drawer handles do not have to be contacted is an example.

B. Sterilizable Items

Removable tips for air and water that can be cleaned and sterilized are examples. Handpieces and prophylaxis angles that can be sterilized are important additions to the list. Several handpieces are needed for rotation. Much time is saved, and the instrument used is safer.

C. Disposable Items

Disposable items should be used wherever possible.

D. Items That May Be Covered

Coverings, particularly plastic-backed patient napkins, and clear plastic wrap or bags can prevent contamination from reaching surfaces. Covers for light handles, counter tops, x-ray cone, and water faucet are examples. Care must be taken when removing the covers not to contaminate the object beneath.

E. Items That Require Chemical Disinfection

Objects and surfaces that cannot be included in one of the above categories must be treated with a chemical disinfectant. If the material is not compatible with the chemical action of the disinfectant, a substitute item, which is either disposable or coverable, will be needed.

IV. Disinfection of Environmental Surfaces

A. Agent

1. *Preparation.* The approved effective agents were described on pages 51–52 and in table 4–2.
2. *Action.* The effectiveness of the disinfection procedure is the result of two actions, which are the physical rubbing and removal of contaminated material and the chemical inactivation of the living microorganisms.
3. *Care of Solution.* Do not store gauze sponges in the solution.

B. Procedure[24]

1. Wash gloved hands before starting the disinfecting process. Wear heavy-duty household gloves (figure 4–1).
2. Use several large gauze sponges or paper towels. Small sponges are time wasting. A disinfectant-soaked sponge in each hand can decrease the time of doing certain objects, and contaminated objects such as tubings can be held with one sponge while scrubbing with the other sponge.

Spraying a disinfectant must be followed by vigorous scrubbing. When applied only by spray without scrubbing, the agent does not penetrate or remove the film of microorganisms. Scrub the disinfectant over the entire surface with attention to irregularities where contaminated material can aggregate.

3. Spray again and spread. Leave the surface wet.

C. Surfaces to Disinfect[24,25]

The list of surfaces will vary from one clinic or office to another because of different equipment and availability of sterilizable and disposable items. The list must include all surfaces that are contacted if they are not sterilized, covered, or disposable. A typical list of surfaces would include the following:

1. All hose ends (e.g., saliva ejector, evacuator, handpiece, ultrasonic).
2. Non-sterilizable air/water syringe (removable tip is sterilized or disposable).
3. Forked holder for hanging suction device, handpiece, or air/water syringe.
4. Bracket tray, Mayo stand, or other instrument tray holder (will be covered).
5. Control knobs and switches (including dental chair, light, ultrasonic unit).
6. Cuspidor. A cuspidor will require special handling.
   a. Use paper towels to first wash with soap and water.
   b. Rinse off the soap.
   c. Disinfect first the outside, then the inside.
   d. Discard sponges and towels used.
   e. Wash hands before going on to other items.
7. Headrest (after disinfection, place the headrest disposable cover).
8. Dental chair arms. When of a color that may become stained by an iodine preparation, alcohol may be used, followed by placing a plastic or paper cover.
9. Sink
   a. Manually operated faucets. Scrub with disinfectant and then cover handles.
   b. Manually operated soap dispenser. Scrub with disinfectant and then cover release knob with plastic.
   c. Rim of sink. The outer rim where clothes may contact should be scrubbed with disinfectant.
10. Radiographic equipment. All contact areas should be scrubbed, including control knobs, machine head and cone, and film dispenser.

Plastic covers may be placed over the head and cone. Nondisposable film holder must be sterilized.

11. **Inhalant anesthetic masks and tubing.** These must be sterilized by autoclave, ethylene oxide, or at least thoroughly washed, rinsed, and dried before immersing in a chemical sterilant.

12. **Miscellaneous items.** Other materials and equipment that will be contacted should be included on the list of items to be treated during disinfection of environmental surfaces. The stethoscope endpiece is an example.

CARE OF STERILE INSTRUMENTS

After the effort has been made to sterilize and disinfect, procedures are then conducted to prevent contamination and to control the transfer of pathogenic microorganisms. Although a strict procedure for sterile technique such as is practiced in a hospital operating room would be difficult or even impossible in a dental office, it is possible to preserve the chain of sterility through effective handling and storage procedures.

I. Tray Preparation

The instrument tray is reserved for sterile instruments. Other equipment that has been disinfected needs its own special area. Educational devices and materials that are neither sterile nor disinfected are kept apart.

The tray is disinfected (if not a sterilizable tray) and covered over the rims. Currently available plastic-back towels, which are also used for a patient's clip-on napkin, are useful for the tray cover. The plastic back aids to keep liquid contaminants from leaking through and contaminating the tray underneath. A paper tray liner is placed on the open towel to receive the sterilized instruments.

II. Handling Instruments and Materials

A. Opening a Sterile Package

1. Do not open a sterile package until ready to use.
2. Touch only the outer surfaces of the wrapper.
3. Cloth wrapper can be laid back to become the sterile instrument tray cover, with contents exposed on the top.
4. Paper container is opened by tearing off an end and sliding the sterile instruments onto the prepared tray cover.

B. Transfer Forceps

When a transfer forceps is to be used, it must be sterilized for each patient. A transfer forceps container must also be sterilized after each use.

C. Transfer of Sterile Items from a Closed Container

1. Hold cover of container in nondominant hand in a downward direction while using a sterile forceps to remove the item from the inside (figure 4–3). Return cover promptly.
2. When it is necessary to place the cover down, turn it up with the sterile inside surface away from the tabletop to prevent contamination to the inner surface.

III. Storage

Instruments stored without sealed wrappers are only momentarily sterile because of airborne contamination. Unwrapped items must be stored in a closed cabinet wrapped in clean towels.

Labeled, sterilized, and sealed packages are stored unopened in clean, dry cabinets or drawers. Paper-wrapped packages must be handled carefully to prevent tearing. All stored packages should be dated and used in rotation.

Packages wrapped and sealed in paper do not usually need re-sterilizing for 14 days. Plastic or nylon with tape or heat seal may be expected to remain sterile longer. However, the expected shelf life before resterilizing depends on the area surrounding the stored packages. A closed, protected area without exposure, such as a cabinet or drawer that can be disinfected routinely, is preferred.

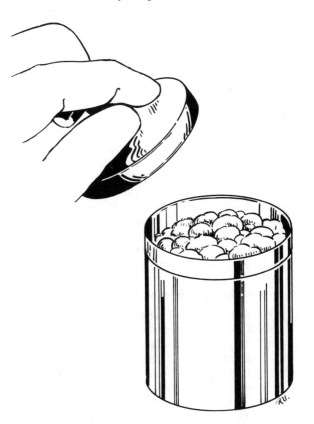

Figure 4–3. Handling Sterilized Supplies. When the cover is removed from a container of sterile supplies, the cover is held with the inner surface downward as shown. When the cover must be placed on the table, the cover is turned over and the outer surface only is in contact with the table top to prevent contamination to the inner surface. Items are removed from the container with a sterile forceps.

PATIENT PREPARATION

The use of preoperative rinsing and toothbrushing has been shown to lower the numbers of oral bacteria and, therefore, to lower the numbers of infected aerosols created during instrumentation.

Oral procedures that require penetration of tissues, such as giving anesthesia by injection or scaling and root planing subgingival pocket surfaces, can introduce bacteria into the tissues and hence into the blood stream. Enough organisms injected into the tissue could multiply and create an abscess. Because of natural resistance, the body can handle and destroy invading microorganisms, provided the numbers can be kept to a minimum. Autogenous infection was described on page 11.

Practical procedures for the preparation of a patient include preoperative oral hygiene measures and the application of a surface disinfectant. These contribute to the prevention of disease transmission.

I. Preoperative Oral Hygiene Measures

A. Toothbrushing

Toothbrushing disturbs and removes microorganisms. When a patient is being trained in bacterial plaque control measures and needs supervision at each appointment, a double purpose can be accomplished. Demonstration of plaque removal from the teeth, tongue, and gingiva contributes to surface degerming prior to treatment procedures.

B. Rinsing

The numbers of bacteria on the gingival or mucosal surfaces can be reduced by the use of an antiseptic mouthrinse. In studies using povidone-iodine mouthrinse, the bacterial counts on mucosal surfaces were reduced before and during scaling and gingivectomy.[26,27] Aerosol contamination was also reduced.[28,29] Reduction of surface and total bacteria in the oral cavity during oral procedures can contribute to surgical cleanliness and more favorable healing after treatment.

II. Application of a Surface Disinfectant

A. Prior to Injection of Anesthetic[30]

As a needle is introduced into the mucosa for penetration to deeper tissues, microorganisms on the surface can be carried into the tissue (page 12). During positioning of the instrument for injection, the needle might accidentally contact a tooth surface and pick up some plaque, which could be carried to and into the injection site.

To decrease the risk of introducing septic material into the soft tissue, an antiseptic should be applied prior to the injection.
1. Dry the surface (sponge).
2. Apply antiseptic (swab).
3. Apply topical anesthetic (swab).

B. Prior to Scaling and Other Dental Hygiene Instrumentation

1. *Instrumentation* in the sulcus or pocket and around the gingival margin can create breaks in the tissue where bacteria can enter. Subgingival instrumentation in a pocket with broken down sulcular epithelium can contribute to the entrance of bacteria into the underlying tissues. Local infection or bacteremia can be created.
2. *Procedure.* Dry the surface and swab the area prior to instrumentation. Use the antiseptic solution to irrigate the sulci and pockets carefully to prevent forcing the solution into the tissues. Research has shown povidone-iodine to be an effective prophylactic germicide for this purpose.[26]

UNIVERSAL PROCEDURES FOR THE PREVENTION OF DISEASE TRANSMISSION

Basic procedures for clinical management are listed here. For many items, a detailed description has been provided in Chapter 3 or Chapter 4.

I. Patient Factors

A. Prepare a comprehensive patient history. Refer patients suspected of carrying infectious disease for laboratory tests available for symptomless carriers.
B. Request diagnostic tests for patients who may be carriers of hepatitis B, syphilis, or tuberculosis.
C. Avoid elective procedures for a patient suffering from a communicable disease, such as a respiratory infection, or who has an open lesion on or about the lips or oral tissues. When emergency care must be provided, precautions and strict adherence to environment, personal barriers, and sterilization factors are needed.
D. Have the patient rinse with germicidal mouthrinse to reduce the numbers of oral microorganisms.
E. Provide protective eyeglasses.

II. Clinic Preparation

A. Run water through all water lines including the air/water syringe, handpieces, and ultrasonic unit for 5 to 6 minutes at the start of the day and at least 30 seconds before and after each use during the day.
B. Cover or disinfect all environmental surfaces that may be touched during the appointment. Make an orderly sequence for surface disinfection.
C. Sterilize instruments and all other equipment that can be sterilized by one of the methods for complete sterilization. Use specific sterilization procedures for all patients, not only those suspected or known to have an existing communicable disease or to be in a carrier state.

III. Factors for the Dental Team

A. Have medical examinations; keep immunizations up to date; have appropriate testing on a periodic basis.

B. Always use mask, protective eyeglasses, gloves, and a clean, closed-front uniform.

C. Wash hands using a short scrub at the start of the day and handwashes with three latherings and thorough rinsings before and after donning gloves.

D. Develop habits that minimize contacts with switches and other parts of the dental unit, dental chair, light, and operating stool, and avoid all possible environmental contacts unrelated to the procedure at hand.

IV. Treatment Factors

A. Hypodermic Needles

1. Use disposable injection needles and other disposables when treatment involves penetration of tissue.

2. Use a needlestick shield to prevent accidental penetration or self-inoculation (figure 4–4).

3. Place used needles into a puncture-resistant container.

4. Dispose of all partially emptied carpules of anesthetics.

B. Aerosol Control

Use manual instruments to minimize use of instruments and procedures that create aerosols (handpiece, prophylaxis angle, ultrasonic scaler, air/water spray). Control the spread of microorganisms over the room, people, equipment, and other objects. Use rubber dam for applicable procedures.

C. Removable Oral Appliances

Routinely, gloves should be worn to receive a septic appliance from a patient. Place appliance in a disposable cup and cover with a disinfectant. Use a fresh solution of .05% iodophor in water, or a 1:5 dilution of 5% sodium hypochlorite. Clean by ultrasonics.

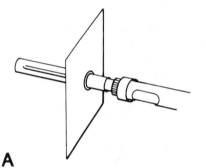

A

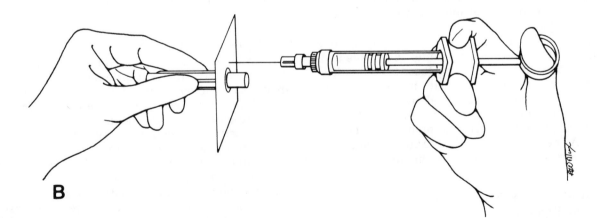

B

Figure 4–4. Needlestick Shield. To prevent needlestick injury, needles should be promptly discarded into a puncture-resistant container. When multiple injections will be required, a needlestick shield inserted on the needle cap **(A)** can be used to guard the fingers during recapping **(B)**.

When a lathe is used for cleaning the denture, wear goggles and a mask and use a sterile rag-wheel and fresh pumice. Pumice is used only once and caught on a disposable paper liner in the dustbin and discarded.

V. Post-Treatment

A. Fold tray cover over instruments to transport them to the sterilization area. Use heavy household gloves to handle used instruments.

B. Follow routines on pages 43–46 to disinfect, clean in ultrasonic cleaner, and prepare for sterilization.

C. Contaminated waste is secured in plastic disposal bags. See *Technical Hints* at the end of the chapter for Guidelines.

D. Disinfect safety glasses for patient and dental team members.

SUPPLEMENTAL PRECAUTIONS AND PROCEDURES FOR INFECTIOUS PATIENTS[31,32,33]

Universal infection control procedures are necessary for all patients. When a patient is in the active stages of a communicable disease, is ill and debilitated, a strict aseptic technique is indicated (page 43). The patient, particularly one with a suppressed immune system, may be very susceptible to infection.

Many of the required procedures for maximum prevention that are listed below are similar to the procedures of the daily routine but are applied with increased intensity.

All dental personnel should be immunized against HBV, rubella, and all communicable diseases for which vaccines are available (page 33). Members of the dental team who have immunity to the communicable disease of the particular patient, should be trained to take over the appointments for the special carrier patients. Without the threat of personal exposure, attention can be concentrated on control of transmission to other members of the team and to subsequent patients.

Whether or not any team member has immunity, rehearsals of the proper procedures are needed. A list of the items to receive covers, those to be avoided, and others to maintain in sterile packages can be placed in a procedures manual along with other office or clinic policies. Drawings, flow charts, and other descriptive material can be prepared as specific guides. As new research findings and new materials become available, the procedures manual can be revised.

I. Clinical Features Essential to Maximum Precautions

A. Enclosed, confined treatment area.

B. Removal from the room of all equipment and materials that will not be used at this time.

C. Adequate sterilization equipment and approved disinfectant solution.

D. Unit with smooth plastic hoses.

E. Handpiece water lines with antiretraction valves installed (page 53).

F. Handpieces and air/water syringe that can be steam autoclaved or sterilized in gas (ethylene oxide).

G. All possible disposable items available.

II. Preparation of Treatment Area

A. Schedule the patient for the last appointment of the day to allow time for room decontamination and preparation for the next appointment in that room.

B. Materials and all necessities should be readied and in the treatment room to prevent the need for any traffic. Only those attending the patient should be allowed in the room.

C. Disinfect and drape all environmental surfaces
  1. Cover the entire dental chair. A drape of disposable plastic such as is used by painters for drop cloths is suggested.
  2. Bracket, light handles, and other smaller items may be covered with clear plastic wrap or bags.
  3. Hand controls can be covered with clear plastic taped on; they can be operated through the plastic. Hand controls of unit, light, dental chair, x-ray machine, viewbox, all are included.
  4. Cover x-ray machine, head, position-indicating device and time control switch. Operate control through the cover.

D. Use disposable materials wherever possible.

E. Sterilized instruments, handpieces, air/water syringe, and all tips are readied. Extra packages of sterile scalers and curets are available to open when instruments are dulled, to prevent need for sharpening equipment.

F. Place available radiographs on viewbox and cover radiographs and viewbox with transparent plastic.

III. Preparation of the Dental Team

Even the dental hygienist who routinely does not have the help of a dental assistant should not attempt treatment for a maximum precautions patient alone. Appointment management can be greatly improved when two people work together, and strict asepsis can be maintained with increased efficiency.

A. Wear a gown with cuffs that gloves can overlap or that is disposable. Operating-room-style hair cover can also be obtained.

B. Wear protective glasses with side shields (see figure 3–2 B or C). For those who require prescription eyeglasses, protective glasses should be placed over them.

C. Wear two pairs of surgical gloves, donned after a scrub procedure. Care must be taken during instrumentation to avoid procedures that can injure the hands or cut the gloves.

D. Wear double tie-on masks. Facial hair must be covered.

IV. Patient Preparation

A. Cover the patient's hair with a disposable cap.
B. Use a long disposable drape to cover the patient's clothes.
C. Provide protective disposable eyeglasses.
D. Have the patient rinse for 30 to 60 seconds with a germicidal mouthrinse.

V. Treatment Factors

A. Avoid use of aerosol-producing handpieces, especially the ultrasonic and airbrasive.
B. In all procedures, touch only areas draped or otherwise covered.
C. Use a disposable radiographic film holder (pages 131, 132, and figure 9–7).
D. Use disposable trays for making impressions. Disinfect the impression by immersion in an accepted product.[34] Rinse before taking to the laboratory. Stone models can be sterilized with ethylene oxide.

VI. Post-treatment

A. Place instruments directly in the sterilizer without cleaning them. After sterilization, they will be ready to clean, package, and sterilize again.
B. Place all disposable contaminated covers, sponges, gloves, and other materials into a bag for direct incineration, or sterilize them.
C. Disinfect all surfaces not draped but touched. Disinfect twice and keep the surfaces wet for 30 minutes.
D. Disinfect all eyeglasses in an accepted 2% glutaraldehyde solution.[35]
E. Wash face, hands, and exposed arms by lathering and rinsing three times, using a disinfectant-containing soap.

TECHNICAL HINTS

I. Cleaning the Face

Check and clean the exposed parts of the face not covered by mask or eyeglasses, where splatter collects, as an aid to disease control as well as for general sanitation. The face should be cleaned several times each day, and washed before eating. When washing the face, an effort should be made not to spread splatter material into the eyes or the mouth.

II. Smoking and Eating

Smoking or eating should not be permitted in treatment areas.

III. Toys

Select toys and other reception area items that can be cleaned and disinfected.

IV. Handpiece Maintenance

Keep records of handpiece purchase, maintenance, and other information pertinent to longevity and effectiveness. Maintain a sufficient number of handpieces to permit rotation and routine sterilization.

V. Sterilization Monitoring

Keep a written record of dates when processing tests and biologic monitor tests were performed for each sterilizer. Indicate advance dates for the next testing clearly on a calendar or other reference point. Tests made weekly should be performed on the same day to simplify remembering.

VI. Office Policy Manual

Include in the clinic or office policy manual outlines of procedures to follow for special precautions, such as for a patient who is a hepatitis carrier. Addresses for sources of various materials can be kept in a special reference section of the manual. Emergency procedures to follow when accidentally exposed should also be defined clearly (Passive Immunization, page 20).

VII. Disposal of Waste

A. Regulations

Investigate the regulations of each town or city sanitation division for rules concerning disposal of contaminated waste. The safety of the workers has been protected in many areas by the refusal to pick up bags of waste from hospitals and dental clinics unless the contents of the bags have been pre-sterilized.

B. Guidelines[36]

Disposable materials such as gloves, masks, wipes, paper drapes, or surfacecovers that are contaminated with blood or body fluids should be carefully handled and discarded in sturdy, impervious plastic bags in order to minimize human contact. Blood, suctioned fluids, or other liquid waste may be carefully poured into a drain that is connected to a sanitary sewer system in compliance with applicable local regulations. Sharp items, such as needles and scalpel blades, should be placed intact into puncture-resistant containers before disposal in plastic bags.

Human tissue may be handled in the same manner as sharp items. Such contaminated solid wastes can then be disposed of according to the requirements established by local or state environmental regulatory agencies and published recommendations. Infectious medical waste, including tissues and culture media, should be handled in a manner consistent with local regulations before disposal.

Liquid chemicals should be carefully poured into a drain connected to a sewer while flushing with copious amounts of water unless labeling or local regulations prohibit such a practice. Disposal methods for solid chemicals vary with the type of chemical and local regulations governing waste management practices (from American Dental Association, Council on Dental Therapeutics).

VIII. Sources for Test Materials

Biologic Monitors and Chemical Indicators

AMSCO Medical Products Division *(Spordi)*
American Sterilizer Company
2820 West 23rd Street
Erie, Pennsylvania 16512

Dental Products Division/3M *(Attest)*
3M Center Bldg. 225-5 South
St. Paul, Minnesota 55144

MDT Corporation *(Spor-test)*
15025 South Main Street
Gardena, California 90248

Sybron Corporation *(Unispore)*
Medical Products Division
P.O. Box 23077
Rochester, New York 14692

FACTORS TO TEACH THE PATIENT

I. Facts about the normal oral flora and the factors that influence an increased number of bacteria on the tongue, mucosa, and in the plaque.

II. Methods for personal daily control of the oral bacteria through plaque control and tongue brushing.

III. Reasons for preoperative brushing, flossing, and rinsing.

IV. Method for thorough rinsing (page 329).

References

1. United States Veterans Administration: *Symposium in Infection Control in Dental Practice.* Washington, D.C., Office of Dentistry, Veterans Administration Central Office, January, 1987, pp. 26–28.
2. Runnells, R.R.: *Infection Control in the Wet Finger Environment,* 1st ed. Salt Lake City, Publishers Press, 1984, pp. 119–125.
3. Crawford, J.J.: *Clinical Asepsis in Dentistry,* 4th ed. Mesquite, Texas, R.A. Kolstad, Publisher, 1987, pp. 32–34.
4. United States Department of Health and Human Services, Centers for Disease Control: Recommendations for Prevention of HIV Transmission in Health-care Settings, *MMWR, 36,* 6S, Supplement 2S, August 21, 1987.
5. Runnells, R.R. and Schmoegner, J.C.: The Need to Monitor Use and Function of Sterilizers, *Dent. Surv., 56,* 20, October, 1980.
6. Watkins, B.J.: Sterilizer Monitoring: An Essential Component of Sterilization Procedures, *Compend. Contin. Educ. Dent., 8,* 476, June, 1987.
7. American Dental Association, Council on Dental Materials, Instruments, and Equipment: *Dentist's Desk Reference,* 2nd ed. Chicago, American Dental Association, 1983, pp. 390–401.
8. Molinari, J.A.: Sterilization and Disinfection, in Schuster, G.S., ed.: *Oral Microbiology and Infectious Disease,* 2nd Student edition. Baltimore, Williams & Wilkins, 1983, pp. 67–84.
9. Crawford: op. cit., pp. 40–46.
10. Bertolotti, R.L. and Hurst, V.: Inhibition of Corrosion During Autoclave Sterilization of Carbon Steel Dental Instruments, *J. Am. Dent. Assoc., 97,* 628, October, 1978.
11. Harvey Chemiclave, MDT Corporation, Box 3957, 15025 South Main Street, Gardena, California, 90248.
12. Caputo, R.A. and Odlaug, T.E.: Sterilization with Ethylene Oxide and Other Gases, in Block, S.S.: *Disinfection, Sterilization, and Preservation,* 3rd ed. Philadelphia, Lea & Febiger, 1983, pp. 47–62.
13. Runnells: op. cit., p. 106.
14. American Dental Association, Council on Dental Therapeutics and Council on Prosthetic Services and Dental Laboratory Relations: Guidelines for Infection Control in The Dental Office and the Commercial Dental Laboratory, *J. Am. Dent. Assoc., 110,* 969, June, 1985.
15. Kahn, R.C., Lancaster, M.V., and Kate, W.: The Microbiologic Cross-contamination of Dental Prostheses, *J. Prosthet. Dent., 47,* 556, May, 1982.
16. Minagi, S., Yano, N., Yoshida, K., and Tsuru, H.: Prevention of Acquired Immunodeficiency Syndrome and Hepatitis B. II: Disinfection Method for Hydrophilic Impression Materials, *J. Prosthet. Dent., 58,* 462, October, 1987.
17. Requa, B.S. and Holroyd, S.V.: *Applied Pharmacology for the Dental Hygienist.* St. Louis, The C.V. Mosby Co., 1982, p. 120.
18. United States Air Force Dental Investigation Service: *USAF Dental Service Infection Control Program,* Dental Items of Significance #22, May 1986, USAF School of Aerospace Medicine/NGD, Brooks AFB Texas, pp. 22–26.
19. United States Department of Health and Human Services, Centers for Disease Control: Recommended Infection-control Practices for Dentistry, *MMWR, 35,* 237, April 18, 1986.
20. American Dental Association, Council on Dental Therapeutics: Acceptance of OMNI-II Disinfectant for Instruments and Equipment, *J. Am. Dent. Assoc., 110,* 394, March, 1985.
21. Nolte, W.A., ed.: *Oral Microbiology,* 4th ed. St. Louis, The C.V. Mosby Co., 1982, pp. 58–60.
22. Gross, A., Devine, M.J., and Cutright, D.E.: Microbial Contamination of Dental Units and Ultrasonic Scalers, *J. Periodontol., 47,* 670, November, 1976.
23. Bagga, B.S.R., Murphy, R.A., Anderson, A.W., and Punwani, I.: Contamination of Dental Unit Cooling Water with Oral Microorganisms and Its Prevention, *J. Am. Dent. Assoc., 109,* 712, November, 1984.
24. Crawford: op. cit., pp. 27–34.
25. Runnells: op. cit., pp. 61–68.
26. Randall, E. and Brenman, H.S.: Local Degerming with Povidone-iodine. I. Prior to Dental Prophylaxis, *J. Periodontol., 45,* 866, December, 1974.
27. Brenman, H.S. and Randall, E.: Local Degerming with Povidone-iodine. II. Prior to Gingivectomy, *J. Periodontol., 45,* 870, December, 1974.
28. Litsky, B.Y., Mascis, J.D., and Litsky, W.: Use of Antimicrobial Mouthwash to Minimize the Bacterial Aerosol Contamination Generated by the High-speed Drill, *Oral Surg. Oral Med. Oral Pathol., 29,* 25, January, 1970.
29. Wyler, D., Miller, R.L., and Micik, R.E.: Efficacy of Self-administered Preoperative Oral Hygiene Procedures in Reducing the Concentration of Bacteria in Aerosols Generated During Dental Procedures, *J. Dent. Res., 50,* 509, March-April, 1971.
30. Malamed, S.F.: *Handbook of Local Anesthesia,* 2nd ed. St. Louis, The C.V. Mosby Co., 1986, p. 118.
31. Crawford: op. cit., pp. 54–55.
32. United States Air Force Dental Investigation Service: op. cit., pp. 11–12.
33. Runnells: op. cit., pp. 39–41.
34. American Dental Association, Council on Dental Materials, Instruments, and Equipment, Council on Dental Practice, and Council on Dental Therapeutics: Infection Control Recommendations for the Dental Office and the Dental Laboratory, *J. Am. Dent. Assoc., 116,* 241, February, 1988.
35. Gleason, M.J. and Molinari, J.A.: Stability of Safety Glasses During Sterilization and Disinfection, *J. Am. Dent. Assoc., 115,* 60, July, 1987.
36. American Dental Association, Council on Dental Therapeutics: Guidelines for Disposal of Waste Material, American Den-

tal Association, 1987 House of Delegates, Las Vegas, Nevada, October 10–13, 1987.

Suggested Readings

Colchamiro, E.K.: The Control of Infections in the Dental Operatory, *Compend. Contin. Educ. Dent., 7,* 394, June, 1986.

Connor, J.P. and Edelson, J.G.: Needle Tract Infection, *Oral Surg. Oral Med. Oral Pathol., 65,* 401, April, 1988.

Cooley, R.L., Stilley, J., and Lubow, R.M.: Formaldehyde Emitted by Chemical Vapor Sterilizers, *Oral Surg. Oral Med. Oral Pathol., 57,* 28, January, 1984.

Crawford, J.J.: Sterilization, Disinfection, and Asepsis in Dentistry, in Block, S.S.: *Disinfection, Sterilization, and Preservation,* 3rd ed. Philadelphia, Lea & Febiger, 1983, pp. 505–523.

Crawford, J.J.: State-of-the-Art: Practical Infection Control in Dentistry, *J. Am. Dent. Assoc., 110,* 629, April, 1985.

Doundoulakis, J.H.: Surface Analysis of Titanium After Sterilization: Role in Implant-tissue Interface and Bioadhesion, *J. Prosthet. Dent., 58,* 471, October, 1987.

Fitzgibbon, E.J., Bartzokas, C.A., Martin, M.V., Gibson, M.F., and Graham, R.: The Source, Frequency and Extent of Bacterial Contamination of Dental Unit Water Systems, *Br. Dent. J., 157,* 98, August 11, 1984.

Gorman, S.P. and Scott, E.M.: A Comparative Evaluation of Dental Aspirator Cleansing and Disinfectant Solutions, *Br. Dent. J., 158,* 13, January 5, 1985.

Greenlee, J.S.: Review of Currently Recommended Aseptic Procedures. I. Dental Operatory Contamination, *Dent. Hyg., 57,* 22, November, 1983; II. Dental Instrument Preparation, *Dent. Hyg., 57,* 12, December, 1983; III. Radiographic Equipment and Dental Professional Preparation, *Dent. Hyg., 58,* 74, February, 1984.

Hedtke, M.: An Introduction to Microbiology and Sterilization in the Dental Office, *Dent. Assist., 52,* 25, September/October, 1983.

Jakush, J., ed.: Infection Control in the Dental Office: A Realistic Approach, *J. Am. Dent. Assoc., 112,* 458, April, 1986.

Littner, M.M., Kaffe, I., and Tamse, A.: Occupational Hazards in the Dental Office and Their Control. I. Measures for Controlling Infections, *Quintessence Int., 14,* 67, January, 1983.

Maloney, J.M. and Kohut, R.D.: Infection Control. Barrier Protection and the Treatment Environment, *Dent. Hyg., 61,* 310, July, 1987.

Martin, M.V.: The Significance of the Bacterial Contamination of Dental Unit Water Systems, *Br. Dent. J., 163,* 152, September 5, 1987.

Mills, S.E., Lauderdale, P.W., and Mayhew, R.B.: Reduction of Microbial Contamination in Dental Units with Povidone-iodine 10%, *J. Am. Dent. Assoc., 113,* 280, August, 1986.

Nixon, A.D., Law, R., Officer, J.A., Cleland, J.F., and Goldwater, P.N.: Simple Device to Prevent Accidental Needle-prick Injuries, *Lancet, 1,* 888, April 19, 1986.

Palenik, C.J. and Miller, C.H.: The Dental Assistant as an Infection Control Officer, *Dent. Assist., 55,* 11, November/December, 1986.

Scarlett, M.I. and Furman, L.J.: Infection Control. Risk Assessment and Management for the Dental Health Professional, *Dent. Hyg., 61,* 300, July, 1987.

Shovelton, D.S.: The Prevention of Cross-infection in Dentistry, *Dental Health (London), 22,* 8, Number 2, 1983.

Stern, K.: Asepsis and Sterilization—Update for Practitioners, *RDH, 6,* 20, March-April, 1986.

United States Department of Health and Human Services, Centers for Disease Control: Recommended Infection-control Practices for Dentistry, *MMWR, 35,* 237, April 18, 1986.

United States Department of Health and Human Services, Centers for Disease Control: Recommendations for Prevention of HIV Transmission in Health-care Settings, *MMWR, 36,* 3S, Supplement 2S, August 21, 1987.

Survival of Microorganisms

Allen, A.L. and Organ, R.J.: Occult Blood Accumulation Under the Fingernails: A Mechanism for the Spread of Blood-borne Infection, *J. Am. Dent. Assoc., 105,* 455, September, 1982.

Barnett, M.L., Baker, R.L., and Olson, J.W.: Material Adherent to Probes During a Periodontal Examination, *J. Periodontol., 53,* 446, July, 1982.

Bean, B., Moore, B.M., Sterner, B., Peterson, L.R., Gerding, D.N., and Balfour, H.H.: Survival of Influenza Viruses on Environmental Surfaces, *J. Infect. Dis., 146,* 47, July, 1982.

Caughman, W.F., O'Connor, R.P., Volkmann, K.R., Schuster, G.S., and Caughman, G.B.: Visible-light-curing Devices: A Potential Source of Disease Transmission, *Oper. Dent., 12,* 10, Winter, 1987.

D'Hondt, D.G., Pape, H., and Loesche, W.J.: Reduction of Contamination on the Dental Explorer, *J. Am. Dent. Assoc., 104,* 329, March, 1982.

Mintz, G.A., Klocko, K., Cutarelli, P., and Kumar, M.L.: Survival of Herpes Simplex Virus on Dental Handpieces, *J. Oral Med., 40,* 158, July-September, 1985.

Powell, G.L., Fenn, J.P., and Runnells, R.: Hydrocolloid Conditioning Units: A Potential Source of Bacterial Cross Contamination, *J. Prosthet. Dent., 58,* 280, September, 1987.

Thomas, L.E., Sydiskis, R.J., DeVore, D.T., and Krywolap, G.N.: Survival of Herpes Simplex Virus and Other Selected Microorganisms on Patient Charts: Potential Source of Infection, *J. Am. Dent. Assoc., 111,* 461, September, 1985.

Chemical Agents

Balanyk, T.E.: Chemical Sterilizing/Disinfecting Solutions, *Oral Health, 77,* 41, May, 1987.

Doherty, M.E. and Sampson, T.C.: The Glutaraldehyde Advantage, *RDH, 5,* 18, April, 1985.

Kolstad, R. and Petit, H.: A Safe, Effective Germicide-deodorizer for Removable Appliances, *J. Clin. Orthod., 17,* 56, January, 1983.

Molinari, J.A., Gleason, M.J., Cottone, J.A., and Barrett, E.D.: Comparison of Dental Surface Disinfectants, *Gen. Dent., 35,* 171, May-June, 1987.

Myklebust, S.: Comparative Antibacterial Effectiveness of Seven Hand Antiseptics, *Scand. J. Dent. Res., 93,* 546, December, 1983.

Petit, H., Kolstad, R., and Chu, S.: Disinfection of Removable Appliances, *J. Clin. Orthod., 19,* 293, April, 1985.

Rudd, R.W., Senia, E.S., McCleskey, F.K., and Adams, E.D.: Sterilization of Complete Dentures With Sodium Hypochlorite, *J. Prosthet. Dent., 51,* 318, March, 1984.

Spire, B., Montagnier, L., Barré-Sinoussi, F., and Chermann, J.C.: Inactivation of Lymphadenopathy Associated Virus by Chemical Disinfectants, *Lancet, 2,* 899, October 20, 1984.

United States National Institute for Occupational Safety and Health, Centers for Disease Control: Symptoms of Irritation Associated with Exposure to Glutaraldehyde—Colorado, *MMWR, 36,* 190, April 3, 1987.

Warfield, D.K. and Bryington, S.Q.: Ultrasonic Potentiation of the Sporicidal Activity of Glutaraldehyde, *Oral Surg. Oral Med. Oral Pathol., 53,* 342, April, 1982.

Instruments and Handpieces

Cooley, R.L., Stilley, J., and Lubow, R.M.: Mercury Vapor Produced During Sterilization of Amalgam-contaminated Instruments, *J. Prosthet. Dent., 53,* 304, March, 1985.

Cooley, R.L., Barkmeier, W.W., and Wayman, B.E.: Sterilization and Disinfection of Dental Burs, *Gen. Dent., 30,* 508, November-December, 1982.

Eakle, W.S., Kao, R.T., Gordon, M., and Pelzner, R.B.: Microbiological Assessment of Ultraviolet Sterilization of Dental Handpieces, *Clin. Prevent. Dent., 8,* 10, March-April, 1986.

Edwardsson, S., Svensäter, G., and Birkhed, D.: Steam Sterilization of Air Turbine Dental Handpieces, *Acta Odontol. Scand., 41,* 322, Number 6, 1983.

Johnson, G.K., Perry, F.U., and Pelleu, G.B.: Effect of Four Anticorrosive Dips on the Cutting Efficiency of Dental Carbide Burs, *J. Am. Dent. Assoc., 114,* 648, May, 1987.

Martin, M.V. and Bartzokas, C.A.: The Boiling of Instruments in General Dental Practice: A Misnomer for Sterilisation, *Br. Dent. J., 159,* 18, July 6, 1985.

Neal, R.G., Craig, R.G., and Powers, J.M.: Effect of Sterilization and Irrigants on the Cutting Ability of Stainless Steel Files, *J. Endodont., 9,* 93, March, 1983.

Samit, A. and Dodson, R.: Instrument-marking Tapes: An Unnecessary Hazard, *J. Oral Maxillofac. Surg., 41,* 687, October, 1983.

Scheid, R.C., Kim, C.K., Bright, J.S., Whitely, M.S., and Rosen, S.: Reduction of Microbes in Handpieces by Flushing Before Use, *J. Am. Dent. Assoc., 105,* 658, October, 1982.

Von Krammer, R.: The Dentist's Health: High-speed Rotary Equipment as a Risk Factor, *Quintessence Int., 16,* 367, May, 1985.

Walsh, M.M.: The Effect of Various Sterilizing Wraps on the Corrosion of Instruments During Autoclaving, *Dent. Hyg., 53,* 504, November, 1979.

Wirthlin, M.R., Shklair, I.L., Northerner, R.A., Shelton, S.W., and Bailey, G.L.: The Performance of Autoclaved High-speed Dental Handpieces, *J. Am. Dent. Assoc., 103,* 584, October, 1981.

Young, S.K., Graves, D.C., Rohrer, M.D., and Bulard, R.A.: Microwave Sterilization of Nitrous Oxide Nasal Hoods Contaminated with Virus, *Oral Surg. Oral Med. Oral Pathol., 60,* 581, December, 1985.

Orthodontics

Campbell, P.M. and Phenix, N.: Sterilization in the Orthodontic Office, *J. Clin. Orthod., 20,* 684, October, 1986.

Kirchhoff, S.T., Sekijima, R.K., Masunaga, M.I., and Alizadeh, C.M.: Sterilization in Orthodontics, *J. Clin. Orthod., 21,* 327, May, 1987.

Matlack, R.E.: Instrument Sterilization in Orthodontic Offices, *Angle Orthod., 49,* 205, July, 1979.

Mulick, J.F.: Upgrading Sterilization in the Orthodontic Practice, *Am. J. Orthod., 89,* 346, April, 1986.

Payne, G.S.: Sterilization and Disinfection in the Orthodontic Office: A Practical Approach, *Am. J. Orthod., 90,* 250, September, 1986.

Singer, J.: Occupational Health Hazards in the Orthodontic Office, *Am. J. Orthod., 86,* 518, December, 1984.

Starnbach, H. and Biddle, P.: A Pragmatic Approach to Asepsis in the Orthodontic Office, *Angle Orthod., 50,* 63, January, 1980.

Dental Laboratory Hygiene

Engelmeier, R.L.: Autoclavable Custom-made Metal Impression Trays to Improve Infection Control, *J. Prosthet. Dent., 58,* 121, July, 1987.

Henderson, C.W., Schwartz, R.S., Herbold, E.T., and Mayhew, R.B.: Evaluation of the Barrier System, An Infection Control System for the Dental Laboratory, *J. Prosthet. Dent., 58,* 517, October, 1987.

Herrera, S.P. and Merchant, V.A.: Dimensional Stability of Dental Impressions After Immersion Disinfection, *J. Am. Dent. Assoc., 113,* 419, September, 1986.

Holt, R.A., Stratton, R.J., and Donoghue, T.: Prevention of Cross-contamination During Immediate Denture Delivery, *Quintessence Int., 16,* 787, November, 1985.

Kwok, W.M. and Ralph, W.J.: The Use of Chemical Disinfectants in Dental Prosthetics, *Aust. Dent. J., 29,* 180, June, 1984.

Merchant, V.A., Herrera, S.P., and Dwan, J.J.: Marginal Fit of Cast Gold MO Inlays from Disinfected Elastomeric Impressions, *J. Prosthet. Dent., 58,* 276, September, 1987.

Radue, J.T., Unger, J.W., and Molinari, J.A.: Avoiding Cross-contamination in Immediate Denture Treatment, *J. Prosthet. Dent., 49,* 576, April, 1983.

Thomasz, F.G.V., Chong, M.P., and Tyas, M.J.: Virucidal Chemical Glutaraldehyde on Alginate Impression Materials, *Aust. Dent. J., 31,* 295, August, 1986.

Williams, H.N., Falkler, W.A., Hasler, J.F., and Libonati, J.P.: The Recovery and Significance of Nonoral Opportunistic Pathogenic Bacteria in Dental Laboratory Pumice, *J. Prosthet. Dent., 54,* 725, November, 1985.

5 *Patient Reception and Positioning in the Dental Chair*

The patient's well-being is the all-important consideration throughout the appointment. At the same time, the clinician must function effectively and efficiently by applying work simplification principles to reduce stress and fatigue.

The physical arrangement and interpersonal relationships provide the setting for specific services to be performed. The patient's presence in the office or clinic is an expression of confidence in the dentist and the dental hygienist. This confidence is inspired by the reputation for professional knowledge and skill, the appearance of the office, and the action of the workers in it.

I. Preparation for the Patient

A. Treatment Area

The procedures for the prevention of disease transmission were described in Chapters 3 and 4. The requirements for precautions for all patients whether or not the presence of a communicable disease is known are listed on page 56.

1. *Environmental Surfaces.* All contact areas must be thoroughly disinfected or covered to control cross-contamination. Appointment preparation was described on pages 53–55.
2. *Instruments.* Packaged instruments remain sealed until the start of the appointment.
3. *Equipment.* Prepare and make ready other materials that will be used, such as for the determination of blood pressure and patient instruction. Anticipate specific needs for assessment procedures for a new patient.

B. Records

By leaving the record open for possible reference, the need for handling the record after hand scrubbing and gloving for instrumentation may be avoided. Radiographs can be placed on the viewbox and the light left on.

1. Review the patient's medical and dental history for pertinent appointment information and need for updating.
2. Read previous appointment case records to focus the current treatment needs.
3. Anticipate examination procedures and new record making for a new patient.

C. Position Chair

1. Upright, in low position.
2. Chair arm adjusted for access.
3. Pre-adjustment of traditional chair when size

of patient is known, will contribute to ease while making final adjustments.

D. Clear Path

Clear pathway to chair of obstacles: rheostat, operating stool.

II. Patient Reception

A. Introductions

1. The dental assistant or the dentist may introduce the new patient to the dental hygienist, but more frequently, a self-introduction is in order. The patient is greeted by name and the hygienist's name is clearly stated, for example, "Good morning, Mrs. Smith; I am Miss Jones, the dental hygienist." Wearing a name-tag for the patient's convenient observation is helpful.
2. Procedure for introducing the patient to others:
   a. A lady's name always precedes a gentleman's.
   b. An older person's name precedes the younger person's (when of the same sex and when the difference in age is obvious).
   c. In general, the patient's name precedes that of a member of the dental personnel.
3. An older patient is not called by the first name except at the patient's request.

B. Procedures

1. Invite patient to be seated.
   a. For the average patient, stand ready to adjust the chair.
   b. Assist the elderly, the infirm, or very small children; guide into the chair by supporting the patient's arm.
2. Assist with wheelchair. Bring wheelchair adjacent to the dental chair and provide assistance when indicated. Wheelchair transfers and assistance for a patient with a walker or crutches are described on pages 615–617.
3. Place handbag within the patient's view.
4. Apply drape and napkin. An elderly patient may need a blanket. Stabilization aids for patients with handicaps are described on pages 617–618.
5. Receive removable prosthetic appliances and place in water in a protective container.
6. Provide protective eyeglasses. For information about the types and care of protective eye-

glasses, see pages 35–36. When a patient removes personal corrective eyeglasses to substitute those provided by the office or clinic, make sure the personal glasses are placed in their case in a safe place.

POSITION OF THE CLINICIAN

The adjustment for the position of the patient is contingent upon the position of the clinician. Attention to the patient's comfort must always be foremost, but when the working arrangement is considered, it is realistic to remember that the patient's position will be assumed for a relatively short time compared with that of the clinician, who may conduct a major portion of a full day's professional activity in close proximity to the chairside. The patient, therefore, is positioned so that a thorough, biologically oriented service may be performed conveniently and efficiently within a reasonable length of time.

I. Objectives

Objectives concern the health of the clinician, the service to be performed, and the effect on the patient. The *preferred* working position is one that will attempt to accomplish the following:

A. Contribute to rather than detract from the health of the clinician.
B. Provide physical comfort and mental tranquility.
C. Apply principles of body mechanics that will reduce fatigue and maintain stamina for prolonged periods of peak efficiency.
D. Contribute to ease and efficiency of performance, which will produce complete, thorough results for effective treatment; this, in turn, will have long-range benefits for the patient.
E. Transmit to the patient a sense of well-being, security, and confidence, as well as a need for cooperation with dental personnel.
F. Develop better patient-clinician relationships because of greater comfort, lessened physical stress, and reduced appointment time.
G. Be flexible in relation to individual needs of patients with special health problems, where limitations of physiologic or pathologic conditions require variations in chair positions.
H. Be flexible in relation to studying and utilizing, where applicable, new concepts of patient care and new developments in dental equipment that will contribute to all objectives of service.

II. The Seated Clinician

In keeping with current concepts, it is expected that an operating stool will be used. Benefits can result that relate to general health, productivity, and the manner in which work is accomplished.

A. Characteristics of an Acceptable Operating Stool[1]

1. *Base.* Broad and heavy for stability, with no fewer than four casters. A stool with five casters has greater stability.

2. *Mobility.* Completely mobile; not connected to other dental equipment; built with free-rolling casters; without tipping hazards.
3. *Seat.* Relatively large to provide complete body support; padded firmly, yet not too hard; without a welt on the leaning edge that could dig into the upper part of the thigh.
4. *Height.* Adjustable to provide exactly the correct level for the individual so that feet can be flat on the floor and thighs parallel with the floor.
5. *Assistant's Stool.* Needs additional support at the base, with at least five casters recommended for maximum stability; should be freely adjustable for height. A footrest is needed at the base of the chair, because the assistant is positioned 4 to 6 inches higher than the clinician, and generally, the feet could not reach the floor.

B. Use of the Operating Stool

Once the operating stool is adjusted for the individual, it does not need changing, unless other personnel also use it. Once adjusted, the height remains constant, and other dental equipment is arranged to accommodate for optimum usage. Positioning that incorporates principles of good body mechanics benefits both the clinician and the patient. Basic positioning includes the following features related to posture and the field of operation.

1. Feet are flat on the floor; thighs parallel with the floor (figure 5–1A).
2. Back is straight; head is relatively erect; shoulders are relaxed and parallel with floor.
3. Body weight is completely supported by the chair; balancing on the edge of the stool should be avoided (figure 5–1B).
4. Eyes are directed downward in a manner that

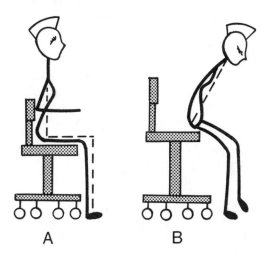

Figure 5–1. Use of Operating Stool. A. Correct position, with feet flat on the floor, thighs parallel with floor, and body weight supported by the stool. **B.** Incorrect position, with seat high, body balanced on the edge of the stool, and back bent forward.

prevents neck strain and eye strain; it is not necessary to bend the head.

5. Operating distance from the patient's mouth to the eyes of the clinician should be 14 to 16 inches.

6. With elbows close to the sides, the field of operation (patient's mouth) is adjusted to elbow height.

III. The Standing Clinician

As in the seated position, the standing posture also requires application of principles of good body mechanics.

A. Distribution of Balance

1. Both feet are flat on the floor with toes forward.
2. Back is straight; head relatively erect; shoulders relaxed and parallel with floor.
3. Weight is centered over the balls of the feet and distributed evenly to both feet; knees are slightly flexed.

B. Relation to Field of Operation

1. With elbows close to the sides, the field of operation (patient's mouth) is adjusted to elbow height.
2. Eyes are directed downward in a manner that prevents neck strain and eye strain; it is not necessary to bend the head.
3. Operating distance from the patient's mouth to the eyes of the clinician should be 14 to 16 inches.

POSITION OF THE PATIENT

Once the height of operation is established by the height of the clinician's elbow, dental chair positioning relates directly to the type of dental chair. The sequence of procedures for effective, efficient adjustment of the traditional or conventional dental chair and of the contoured chair is outlined here.

I. General Positions

Four commonly used body positions are shown in figure 5–2. Body positions are of extreme importance during emergency care; they are identified in Table 60–1, with outlines for emergency procedures.

A. Upright

This is the initial position from which chair adjustments are made.

B. Semi-upright

A patient with certain types of cardiovascular or respiratory diseases may need to be in a semi-upright position for dental and dental hygiene procedures.

C. Supine

The patient is flat, with the head and feet on the same level.

D. Trendelenburg

The patient is in supine and tipped back and down 35 to 45 degrees so that the heart is higher than the head.

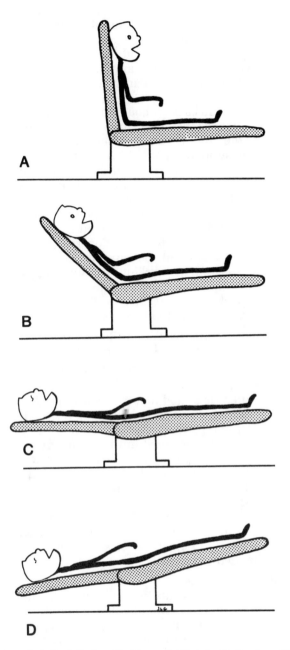

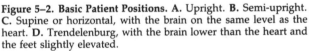

Figure 5–2. Basic Patient Positions. A. Upright. **B.** Semi-upright. **C.** Supine or horizontal, with the brain on the same level as the heart. **D.** Trendelenburg, with the brain lower than the heart and the feet slightly elevated.

II. Contoured Dental Chair

A contoured chair provides complete body support for the patient, which increases patient relaxation. The clinician can be in a comfortable working position with good access, light, and visibility, which in turn, contribute to an efficient performance.

In a supine position, a patient is ideally situated for support of the circulation. Rarely could a patient faint while lying in a supine position.

A. Characteristics of a Contoured Chair for Efficient Utilization

1. Provides complete body support.
2. Seat and leg support move as a unit; back and headrest move as a unit; both are power controlled.
3. Has a thin back without protruding adjustment devices so that the chair may be lowered close to the clinician's elbow height.
4. Has supports that hold the patient's arms as the chair is lowered into the supine position; otherwise the hands hang down or the patient must hold them up forcibly.
5. Chair base should be as shallow as possible to permit the chair to be lowered as close to the floor as needed for correct operating position.
6. Chair base should be power driven with pedal access from the working position on the dental operating stool. The controls for the back and seat should be readily available to both the assistant and clinician.

B. Prepositioning for Patient Reception

1. Chair at low level; back upright.
2. Chair arm raised on side of approach.

C. Adjustment Steps

1. Patient is seated first with back upright.
2. Chair seat and foot portion are raised first to help the patient settle back.
3. Backrest is lowered until the patient reaches the supine position for maxillary instrumentation. For mandibular teeth, adjust chair back to a 20-degree angle with the floor (figure 5–3).
4. Patient is requested to slide up until the head is at the upper edge of the backrest and on the side next to the clinician. Note patient's head position in figure 5–4, shown for a right-handed clinician.

D. Final Adjustment

1. Lower or raise the total chair until the field of operation (patient's mouth) is at the clinician's elbow when the shoulder is relaxed.
2. Clinician's positions can be designated by the hours of a clock around the patient's head. Noon, or 12:00, is at the top, over the patient's forehead as shown in figure 5–4.

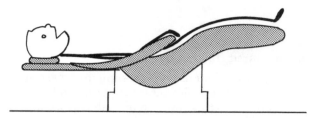

Figure 5–3. Contoured Chair. For instrumentation in the maxillary arch, the patient is in supine position, with the back of the chair nearly parallel with the floor and the feet slightly higher than the head. For mandibular teeth, adjust the chair back to a 20-degree angle with the floor.

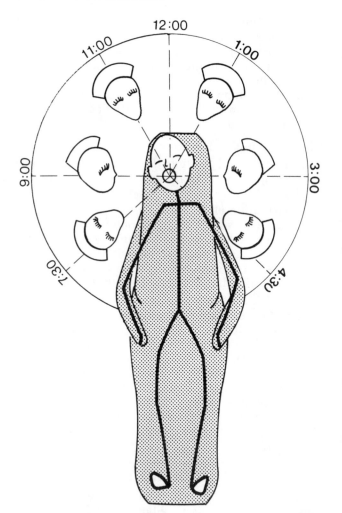

Figure 5–4. Operating Positions. The patient's head is placed at the upper edge of the backrest or headrest on the side next to the clinician as shown here for the right side. The right-handed clinician is positioned between 7:30 and 12:00; whereas the left-handed clinician is positioned between 12:00 and 4:30 for side-front, side, or side-back.

a. Right-handed clinician: positioned for instrumentation between 7:30 and 12:00.
b. Left-handed clinician: positioned between 12:00 and 4:30.

E. Conclusion of Appointment

1. Raise backrest slowly.
2. Tilt chair forward.
3. Request that patient sit in an upright position briefly, to avoid effects of postural hypotension.

III. Traditional Dental Chair

The back of the chair is adjusted first, then the headrest; the chair is inclined, to adjust the seat; and finally, the whole chair is lowered or raised to bring the field of operation to the correct level and angulation. For most patients, the footrest remains in a constant position, but it should be adjusted to meet individual needs.

A. Prepositioning for Patient Reception
1. Seat parallel with floor.
2. Back slightly inclined back and away from the upright position.
3. Headrest tilted back to prevent its bumping the patient during seating.

B. Backrest
1. Raise or lower until the curvature of the chair back corresponds with the curvature in the middle of the patient's back.
2. When correctly positioned, the top border of many traditional chairs will be at a level approximating the lower third of the patient's scapulae. Other chairs have taller backs that may reach nearer the upper third of the scapulae.

C. Headrest
1. Request the patient to hold the head erect with chin slightly up.
2. Bring the headrest to a position almost touching the back of the head under the occipital protuberances before securing it.

D. Chair Seat
1. Incline the whole chair back as a unit. For the correct position, usually the chair will be tilted as far as it will go.
2. The "V" formed between the seat and the back prevents the patient from sliding forward (figure 5–5A).

E. Final Adjustment
1. *The Seated Clinician*
   a. Lower the chair to its lowest level and incline the chair back as far as it will go.
   b. To lower the field of operation further, it may be necessary to lower the back of the chair.
2. *The Standing Clinician.* With the chair inclined as far back as possible, raise or lower the whole chair until the patient's mouth is at elbow height of the clinician.
3. *Basic Position of the Patient.* When correctly positioned, the spinal cord of the patient should be straight from the brain to the hips. An imaginary straight line can be drawn from the top of the ear to the hips to test this.

F. Effects of Chair Maladjustment
1. *Backrest Too Low or Too High.* Curvature of the spine will cause muscle tension and restlessness, and the patient will attempt to slide into a more comfortable posture out of appropriate operating position.
2. *Headrest Too High or Too Far Forward.* Chin moves toward chest, making it difficult to maintain accessibility and visibility; clinician must lean forward and bend neck sidewards (figure 5–5B).
3. *Headrest Too Low or Too Far Back.* Patient's neck muscles can be stretched and become fatigued; swallowing may be difficult; patient will slide down (figure 5–5C).
4. *Chair Seat Parallel with Floor.* Patient will slide forward and down (figure 5–5B).

IV. Chair Position for Small Child

A. Traditional Chair
1. Use a portable seat or a large, firm cushion to raise seat level.
2. Cover the seat with a cloth to protect the finish from the child's shoes, or the child's shoes can be removed.
3. Lower back and headrest to lowest levels with back at right angles to chair seat.
4. Incline chair back.
5. Final adjustment: child's head will rest as near the headrest as possible; legs may be crossed to give support.

B. Contoured Chair
Adjustment the same as for an adult. Child will slide up so that the head is near the top of the backrest and on the side toward the clinician (figure 5–4).

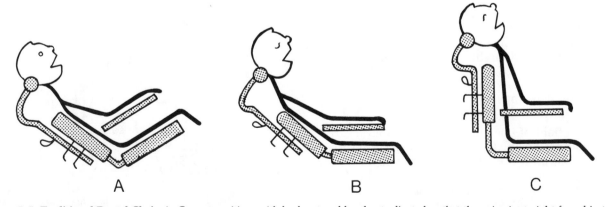

A   B   C

Figure 5–5. Traditional Dental Chair. A. Correct position, with backrest and headrest adjusted so that the spine is straight from hip to top of head and the whole chair is tilted back. **B.** Incorrect position, with headrest too far forward and chair seat flat, which encourages the patient to slide forward. **C.** Incorrect position, with headrest too far back.

FUNCTIONAL FACTORS

I. Lighting

During treatment, visibility of specific areas of the oral cavity is prerequisite to thoroughness without undue trauma to the tissues. With inadequate light, inefficiency increases and leads to prolonged treatment time, which reduces patient cooperation.

The position of the dental light or lights and the intensity of the beam affect the illumination. A study of the treatment room can be made that includes measurement of the total light at the patient's face in working position. Selection of an operating light that meets certain standards can assure intensity sufficient for good visibility and yet safe for the eyes.

A. Dental Light: Suggested Features

1. The light should be readily adjustable both vertically and horizontally and the beam capable of being focused.
2. The size must be small enough so that it may be brought close to the treatment area without being in the way, blocking the room light, or being a hazard for movement of people in its vicinity.
3. Intensity of room light should be sufficient to prevent a marked contrast between it and the illuminating beam of the dental light. An all-luminous ceiling contributes to evenly distributed room lighting.

B. Dental Light: Location

1. *Attachment.* The most versatile arrangement is a ceiling-mounted light on a track, which permits the light to move over a range from behind a supine patient's head to a position in front of the patient's chin.
2. *Dual Lighting.* With a supine patient position in a contoured chair, advantages to the use of two operating lights have been demonstrated. One light directed from the front of the patient may be attached to the dental chair or unit; the other light mounted on a ceiling track as described above.

C. Dental Light: Adjustment

Direct the light first on the napkin under the patient's chin, then rotate the light up to the mouth to avoid flashing light in the patient's eyes.

II. Working Positions

A. Objectives

1. The field of operation should be seen clearly without having to assume body positions that are harmful if held over long periods.
2. When an assistant participates, the field of operation must be accessible and visible to both clinician and dental assistant.
3. Instruments and equipment must be within reach without stretching.

B. Clinician without Assistant

1. Arrange necessary items for immediate access without leaving operating stool.
2. Cervical tray may be used and positioned conveniently around the patient.
3. Height of tray for instruments should be at or slightly below the elbow, so that no effort need be expended when instruments are changed.

C. Clinician with Assistant

1. Position of assistant: seated with eye level 4 to 6 inches above the clinician's eye level and facing toward the head of dental chair (figure 5–6).
2. Assistant applies principles of good body mechanics: body weight supported by operating stool; feet are rested on the base of the operating stool.
3. Instruments and other essential materials are kept within arm's length and the portable cabinet with sterilized prepared tray is in front of the dental assistant.[2]
4. Four-handed dentistry procedures are practiced with instrument transfers and evacuation during clinical procedures.[3]

TECHNICAL HINTS

I. The face of the clinician should not be in close proximity to that of the patient. If it is difficult to keep working distance at 14 to 16 inches, an eye examination may be indicated.

II. Keep body contact at a minimum. A good clinician does not lean on the patient, rest the forearms on the patient's shoulders, or rest the hands on the patient's face or forehead. Unnecessary contact can be very unpleasant to certain patients, and, more importantly, it contributes to disease transmission.

III. Conditions that contraindicate use of the supine position include congestive heart disease, cerebrovascular insufficiency, and any condition associated with breathing difficulty such as emphysema, severe asthma, or sinusitis.

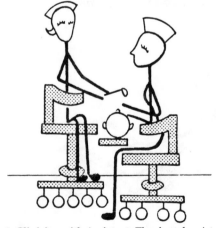

Figure 5–6. Clinician with Assistant. The dental assistant is seated with eye level 4 to 6 inches higher than the clinician's. The sterile tray is placed on a portable cabinet in front of the assistant within easy reach for passing instruments.

FACTORS TO TEACH THE PATIENT

I. Orientation of patients, particularly previous patients, is important when changes in equipment and operating procedures are introduced.

II. Give specific instruction on the parts of a dental chair or other equipment that will be of concern to the patient to prevent embarrassment or adverse reactions.

References

1. Sinnett, G.M. and Wuehrmann, A.H.: The Dental Operatory of the Future, in Peterson, S., ed.: *The Dentist and His Assistant,* 3rd ed. St. Louis, The C.V. Mosby Co., 1972, pp. 392–401.

2. Sinnett, G.M., McDevitt, E.J., Robinson, G.E., and Wuehrmann, A.H.: Four-handed Dentistry: a New Mobile Dental Cabinet Design, *J. Am. Dent. Assoc., 78,* 305, February, 1969.

3. Torres, H.O.: Concepts and Practice of Four-handed, Six-handed, and Team Dentistry, in Darby, M.L. and Bushee, E.J., eds.: *Mosby's Comprehensive Review of Dental Hygiene.* St. Louis, The C.V. Mosby Co., 1986, pp. 619–636.

Suggested Readings

American Dental Association, Council on Dental Materials, Instruments, and Equipment: *Dentist's Desk Reference: Materials, Instruments and Equipment,* 2nd ed. Chicago, American Dental Association, 1983, pp. 378–389.

Armstrong, M.: Occupational Health Hazards for Dental Hygienists, *Can. Dent. Hyg. (Probe), 20,* 99, September, 1986.

Colangelo, G., Hobart, D.J., and Belenky, M.M.: Human Performance in Dentistry: Preferred Operator Posture and Position (Abstract), *J. Dent. Educ., 51,* 61, January, 1987.

Cunningham, M.A., Sharp, J.D., and Field, H.M.: Teaching Dental Students a Proper Way of Introducing Patients to Instructors, *J. Dent. Educ., 48,* 518, September, 1984.

Cutler, M. and Cutler, J.: Office Space and Facilities, in Clark, J.W., ed.: *Clinical Dentistry,* Volume 5, Chapter 24. Philadelphia, J.B. Lippincott Co., 1987.

Gildersleeve, J.R., Hardage, J.L., and Young, J.M.: Dental Fiberoptic Handpieces: Recommendations for Proper Use, *J. Am. Dent. Assoc., 114,* 200, February, 1987.

Gravois, S.L. and Stringer, R.B.: Survey of Occupational Health Hazards in Dental Hygiene, *Dent. Hyg., 54,* 518, November, 1980.

Hardage, J.L., Gildersleeve, J.R., and Rugh, J.D.: Clinical Work Posture for the Dentist: An Electromyographic Study, *J. Am. Dent. Assoc., 107,* 937, December, 1983.

Nield, J.S. and Houseman, G.A.: *Fundamentals of Dental Hygiene Instrumentation,* 2nd ed. Philadelphia, Lea & Febiger, 1988, Chapter 2.

Pruitt, C.O.: Exercises for Prevention and Alleviation of Back Pain, *Gen. Dent., 36,* 199, May-June, 1988.

Rankin, J.A. and Harris, M.B.: Patients' Preferences for Dentists' Behaviors, *J. Am. Dent. Assoc., 110,* 323, March, 1985.

Rasmus, B.J. and Wulf, B.R.: Work Simplification for the Dental Hygienist, *Educ. Dir. Dent. Aux., 5,* 11, August, 1980.

Scanlan, D.: A Dental Chair Modification for Children, *Can. Dent. Assoc. J., 45,* 165, April, 1979.

Smith, A.A., Heuer, G.A., and Kaminski, R.A.: Dental Equipment Selection, in Clark, J.W., ed.: *Clinical Dentistry,* Volume 5, Chapter 25. Philadelphia, J.B. Lippincott Co., 1987.

Wilson, M.P.: Oh My Aching Back: The Unnecessary Occupational Hazard, *RDH, 6,* 44, November/December, 1986.

Young, J.M., Satrom, K.D., and Berrong, J.M.: Intraoral Dental Lights: Test and Evaluation, *J. Prosthet. Dent., 57,* 99, January, 1987.

Four-handed Procedures

Castano, F.A. and Alden, B.A., eds: *Handbook of Expanded Dental Auxiliary Practice,* 2nd ed. Philadelphia, J.B. Lippincott Co., 1980, pp. 27–42.

Paul, J.E.: *A Manual of Four-handed Dentistry,* Chicago, Quintessence Publishing Co., 1980, 154 pp.

Robinson, G.E.: Utilization of Dental Auxiliaries, in Clark, J.W., ed.: *Clinical Dentistry,* Volume 5, Chapter 31. Philadelphia, J.B. Lippincott Co., 1987.

Robinson, G.E., McDevitt, E.J., Sinnett, G.M., and Wuehrmann, A.H.: *Four-handed Dentistry Manual,* 2nd ed. Birmingham, University of Alabama, School of Dentistry, 1971.

Torres, H.O. and Ehrlich, A.: *Modern Dental Assisting,* 3rd ed. Philadelphia, W.B. Saunders Co., 1985, pp. 346–386.

III

Patient Evaluation

DIAGNOSTIC WORK-UP

Before treatment begins, information must be obtained about the patient's general and oral health, from which a diagnosis and treatment plan can be formulated. The gathering, organizing, and assembling of all data from observations, patient questioning, and clinical and radiographic examination may be called a *diagnostic work-up.* Basically, it is a collection of all pertinent facts and materials for the dentist to use during diagnosis and treatment planning and for use during all treatment as a guide.

The chapters in this section, *Patient Evaluation,* include descriptions for the preparation of materials that make up a diagnostic work-up. While specific parts of the work-up are prepared, comments on or reactions to any findings must be withheld until after the diagnosis and treatment plan are finalized by the dentist. Even a simple, well-intentioned remark can be misleading to the patient and create misunderstandings that can be difficult to clarify later.

I. Parts of a Diagnostic Work-up

A. Basic Procedures

The essential information for assessment of a patient prior to formulation of the diagnosis and treatment plan by a dentist is derived from the following:
1. Patient histories (personal, medical, and dental).
2. Determination of vital signs.
3. Extraoral and intraoral examination.
4. Radiographic survey.
5. Study casts.
6. Examination of the gingival and periodontal tissues, including clinical signs of disease involvement, pocket measurement and charting, and mobility evaluation.
7. Examination of the teeth to determine and record deposits, restorations, carious lesions, structural defects, pulp vitality, and occlusion factors.

B. Diagnostic Work-up for Preventive Treatment Plan

A preventive program is planned to meet individual needs. Therefore, information to be obtained depends on the particular oral problems and could include:
1. Dental or periodontal indices.
2. Dietary analysis.
3. Caries activity test.

C. Additional Procedures

In addition to the basic procedures, other parts of a diagnostic work-up will be selected depending on the individual needs of a patient, as well as the specialty area and special emphasis of the dentist. Selection of procedures to be used may be influenced by the age group to which the patient belongs.

Certain procedures may be of an emergency examination category. For example, if during the intraoral examination of the oral mucosa a suspicious lesion was found for which a biopsy was indicated, such a diagnostic procedure would take precedence over any other.

In accord with the policy or special request of the dentist, a diagnostic work-up may include some or all of the following:
1. Photographs.
2. Biopsy or cytologic smear.
3. Tests for suspected systemic conditions such as bleeding tendencies, sickle cell anemia, or diabetes.
4. Special consultations with or referrals to a physician.

II. Purposes

The diagnostic work-up can benefit the patient, aid the dentist, and provide an overall perspective from which a patient-oriented dental hygiene care program can be formulated. Basic objectives of a diagnostic work-up are to
A. Organize information and materials for the den-

tist to use while making the diagnosis and outlining the treatment plan for the patient.

B. Aid the dental hygienist in
1. Planning dental hygiene preventive care and instruction for the patient.
2. Guiding techniques during dental hygiene appointments.
3. Correlating dental hygiene care with dental care.

C. Provide a permanent, documented, continuing record of the patient's oral and general health for
1. Evaluating the response to treatment, which may be compared with future observations at maintenance appointments.
2. Protecting the dental practice in case of misunderstandings or evidence in legal matters should questions arise.

D. Increase the scope of contribution of the dental hygienist to comprehensive patient care by the dental health team.

EXAMINATION PROCEDURES

A specific objective of patient examination as a part of the total diagnostic work-up is the recognition of deviations from normal, that may be signs and symptoms of disease. The importance of careful, thorough examination cannot be overstressed. Concentration and attention to detail are necessary in order that each slight deviation from normal may be entered on the record for review by the dentist. Signs and symptoms of disease are the deviations from normal that must be recorded.

I. Signs and Symptoms

A. Sign

A *sign* is any abnormality that may be indicative of a deviation from normal or of disease that is discovered by a professional person while examining a patient. A sign is an objective symptom.

Examples of signs are changes in color, shape, or consistency of a tissue not observable by the patient. Other signs are findings revealed by the use of a probe, explorer, radiograph, or vitality tester of the dental pulp.

B. Symptom

A *symptom* is also any departure from the normal that may be indicative of disease. Symptoms may be subjective or objective.
1. *Subjective symptom*: when observed by the patient. Examples are pain, tenderness, or itching.
2. *Objective symptom*: when observed by the professional person during an examination. As described above, objective symptoms are frequently called *signs*.

C. Pathognomonic Signs and Symptoms

Some signs and symptoms are general and may occur during various disease states. An increase in body temperature, for example, accompanies many infections.

Other signs and symptoms are *pathognomonic*, which means that the sign or symptom is unique to a particular disease and can be used to distinguish that disease or condition from other diseases or conditions.

II. Types of Examination

A. Complete

A complete examination means that a thorough, comprehensive diagnostic work-up is prepared.

B. Screening

Screening implies a brief examination, using only parts of the complete diagnostic work-up. Screening is used for initial evaluation and classification. In a community health program, when a survey of a population is made to single out people with a particular condition, it is called screening.

C. Limited

A limited examination is usually made for an emergency. It may be used in the management of acute conditions.

D. Follow-up

A follow-up examination is a type of limited examination. It is used to observe the effects of treatment after a period of time during which the tissue or lesion can recover and heal. Indications of the need for additional or alternate treatment are apparent at a follow-up examination.

E. Maintenance

An examination is made after a specified period of time following the completion of treatment and the restoration to health. A maintenance examination is a complete examination with a comprehensive diagnostic work-up.

III. Examination Methods

A patient is examined by various visual, tactile, manual, and instrumental methods. General types are defined briefly here, and other specific methods are found throughout the book as they apply to a certain area under consideration.

A. Visual Examination
1. *Direct Observation.* Visual examination is made in a systematic order to note surface appearance (color, contour, size, etc.) and to observe movement and other evidence of function.
2. *Radiographic Examination.* The use of radiographs can reveal deviations from the normal not noticeable by direct observation.
3. *Transillumination.* A strong light directed through a soft tissue or a tooth to enhance examination is especially useful for detecting

irregularities of the teeth and locating calculus.

B. Palpation

Palpation is examination using the sense of touch through tissue manipulation or pressure on an area with the fingers or hand. The method used depends on the area to be investigated. Types of palpation are described on page 104.

C. Instrumentation

Examination instruments such as the explorer and probe are used for specific examination of the teeth and periodontal tissues. They are described in detail on pages 192–194 and 202–204.

D. Percussion

Percussion is the act of tapping or striking a surface or tooth with the fingers or an instrument. Information about the status of health of the part is determined either by the response of the patient or by the sound. Example: A metal mirror handle is used to tap each tooth successively. When a tooth is known to be painful to movement, percussion should be avoided.

E. Electrical Test

An electrical pulp vitality tester is used to detect the presence or absence of vital pulp tissue. The technique for use is described on pages 222–223.

F. Auscultation

Auscultation is the use of sound. An example is the sound of clicking or snapping of the temporomandibular joint when the jaw is moved.

TOOTH NUMBERING SYSTEMS

The three tooth designation systems in general use are the *Universal* or *Continuous Numbers 1 through 32* as adopted by the American Dental Association;[1] the *F.D.I. Two-digit,* adopted by the Federation Dentaire Internationale;[2] and the *Palmer* or *Quadrant Numbers 1 through 8.*[3] Because different systems are used in dental offices and clinics, it is necessary to be familiar with all of them.

I. Continuous Numbers 1 Through 32

This tooth numbering method is referred to as the *universal* or *ADA* system.

A. Permanent Teeth

Start with the right maxillary third molar (Number 1) and follow around the arch to the left maxillary third molar (16); descend to the left mandibular third molar (17), and follow around to the right mandibular third molar (32). Figure III–1 shows the crowns of the teeth with the corresponding numbers.

B. Primary or Deciduous Teeth

Use continuous upper case letters A through T in the same order as described for the permanent teeth: right maxillary second molar (A) around to left maxillary second molar (J); descend to left mandibular second molar (K), and around to the right mandibular second molar (T).

II. F.D.I. Two-Digit

The *FDI* system is also called the *International.*

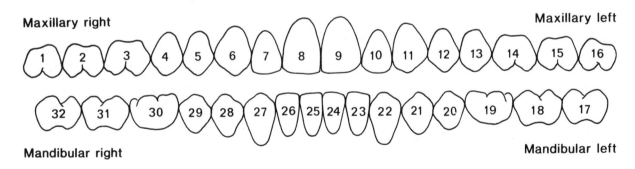

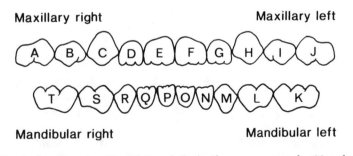

Figure III–1. Universal Tooth Numbering (American Dental Association). *Above,* permanent dentition designated by numbers 1 through 32, starting at the maxillary right with 1 and following around to maxillary left third molar (number 16) to the left mandibular third molar (number 17) and around to the right mandibular third molar (number 32). *Below,* primary teeth are designated by letters in the same sequence.

A. Permanent Teeth

Each tooth is numbered by the quadrant (1 to 4) and by the tooth within the quadrant (1 to 8).

1. *Quadrant Numbers*
   1 = Maxillary right
   2 = Maxillary left
   3 = Mandibular left
   4 = Mandibular right
2. *Tooth Numbers Within Each Quadrant.* Start with number 1 at the midline (central incisor) to number 8, third molar. Figure III–2 shows each tooth number in the four quadrants.
3. *Designation.* The digits are pronounced separately. For example, "two-five" (25) is the maxillary left second premolar, and "four-two" (42) is the mandibular right lateral incisor.

B. Primary or Deciduous Teeth

Each tooth is numbered by quadrant (5 to 8) to continue with the permanent quadrant numbers. The teeth are numbered within each quadrant (1 to 5).

1. *Quadrant Numbers*
   5 = Maxillary right
   6 = Maxillary left
   7 = Mandibular left
   8 = Mandibular right
2. *Tooth Numbers Within Each Quadrant.* Number 1 is the central incisor, and number 5 is the second primary molar.
3. *Designation.* The digits are pronounced separately. For example, "eight-three" (83) is the mandibular right primary canine, and "six-five" (65) is the maxillary left second primary molar.

III. Quadrant Numbers 1 Through 8

Names to identify this method are the *Palmer system* or *Set-square.*

A. Permanent Teeth

With Number 1 for each central incisor, the teeth in each quadrant are numbered to 8, the third molar (figure III–3). To identify individual teeth, horizontal and vertical lines are used, drawn to indicate the quadrant. For example, the left maxillary first pre-molar is ⌊4, the right mandibular first and second molars are 76⌉. An entire quadrant may be represented by the use of the letter Q, for example the maxillary right quadrant is Q⌋.

B. Primary or Deciduous Teeth

Upper case letters A through E are used instead of the numbers. Examples are the mandibular left canine ⌈C, and the maxillary right first primary molar D⌋.

References

1. American Dental Association: System of Tooth Numbering and Radiograph Mounting, Approved by the American Dental Association House of Delegates, Miami Beach, Florida, October, 1968.
2. Fédération Dentaire Internationale: Two-digit System of Designating Teeth, *Int. Dent. J., 21,* 104, March, 1971.
3. American Dental Association: Proceedings of Dental Societies, *Dent. Cosmos., 12,* 522, October, 1870.
4. Palmer, C.: Palmer's Dental Notation, *Dental Cosmos., 33,* 194, 1891.

Suggested Readings

Allen, D.L, McFall, W.T., and Jenzano, J.W.: *Periodontics for the Dental Hygienist,* 4th ed. Philadelphia, Lea & Febiger, 1987, pp. 93–136.

PERMANENT TEETH

Maxillary right								Maxillary left							
18	17	16	15	14	13	12	11	21	22	23	24	25	26	27	28
48	47	46	45	44	43	42	41	31	32	33	34	35	36	37	38
Mandibular right														Mandibular left	

PRIMARY TEETH

Maxillary right					Maxillary left				
55	54	53	52	51	61	62	63	64	65
85	84	83	82	81	71	72	73	74	75
Mandibular right					Mandibular left				

Figure III–2. International Tooth Numbering (Fédération Dentaire Internationale). Each quadrant is numbered 1 through 4, with number 1 on maxillary right, number 2 on maxillary left, number 3 on mandibular left, number 4 on mandibular right. Each tooth in a quadrant is numbered 1 through 8 from the central incisor. Quadrants of the primary dentition are numbered from 5 through 8. It is a two-digit system.

PERMANENT TEETH

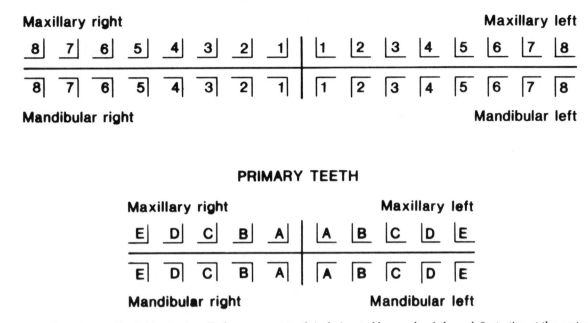

Maxillary right   **Maxillary left**

8 | 7 | 6 | 5 | 4 | 3 | 2 | 1 | 1 | 2 | 3 | 4 | 5 | 6 | 7 | 8

8 | 7 | 6 | 5 | 4 | 3 | 2 | 1 | 1 | 2 | 3 | 4 | 5 | 6 | 7 | 8

Mandibular right   **Mandibular left**

PRIMARY TEETH

Maxillary right   **Maxillary left**

E | D | C | B | A | A | B | C | D | E

E | D | C | B | A | A | B | C | D | E

Mandibular right   **Mandibular left**

Figure III–3. Palmer System Tooth Numbering. Each permanent tooth is designated by number 1 through 8, starting at the central incisor of each quadrant. Quadrants are designated by horizontal and vertical lines. Primary teeth are identified by the letters A through E, starting at the central incisor.

American Dental Association, Council on Dental Care Programs: Code on Dental Procedures and Nomenclature, *J. Am. Dent. Assoc., 114,* 373, March, 1987.

Carranza, F.A.: *Glickman's Clinical Periodontology,* 6th ed. Philadelphia, W.B. Saunders Co., 1984, pp. 493–530.

Goldman, H.M. and Cohen, D.W.: *Periodontal Therapy,* 6th ed. St. Louis, The C.V. Mosby Co., 1980, pp. 303–377.

Kerr, D.A., Ash, M.M., and Millard, H.D.: *Oral Diagnosis,* 6th ed. St. Louis, The C.V. Mosby Co., 1983, pp. 3–13, 77–81.

Krysinski, Z.: The Three-digit System of Designating Supernumerary Teeth, *Quintessence Int., 17,* 127, February, 1986.

Sandham, J.A.: The FDI Two-digit System of Designating Teeth, *Int. Dent. J., 33,* 390, December, 1983.

Dental Photography

Bengel, W.: Standardization in Dental Photography, *Int. Dent. J., 35,* 210, September, 1985.

Brackett, W.W.: Dental Photography: Getting Started, *Compend. Contin. Educ. Dent., 7,* 297, April, 1986.

Dankoski, E. and Painter, L.: An Author's Guide to Controlling the Photograph. Good, Consistent Results Require Consistent Conditions, *J. Prosthet. Dent., 56,* 133, August, 1986.

Freehe, C.L.: Photography in Dentistry: Equipment and Technique, *Dent. Clin. North Am., 27,* 3, January, 1983.

Gordon, P.D.: Principles of Close-up Photography, *Br. Dent. J., 162,* 229, March 21, 1987.

Gordon, P. and Wander, P.: Techniques for Dental Photography, *Br. Dent. J., 162,* 307, April 25, 1987.

Wander, P.A.: The Applications of Photography in General Practice, *Br. Dent. J., 162,* 195, March 7, 1987.

Woodall, I.R., Dafoe, B.R., Young, N.S., Weed-Fonner, L., and Yankell, S.L.: *Comprehensive Dental Hygiene Care,* 2nd ed. St. Louis, The C.V. Mosby Co., 1985, pp. 271–291.

6 Personal, Medical, and Dental History

For safe, scientific dental and dental hygiene care, a meaningful, complete patient history is necessary. The history directs and guides steps to be taken in preparation for, during, and following appointments.

At least a part of the history is needed before oral examination procedures with periodontal probe and explorer are carried out. The use of instruments that would manipulate the soft tissue around the teeth may be contraindicated in certain instances until after a medical consultation to determine whether protective, precautionary measures are needed.

When a question exists about the medical history as described by the patient or when an unusual or abnormal condition is observed, consultation with the patient's physician or referral for examination of the patient who does not have a physician is mandatory. Even emergency treatment such as for the relief of pain should be postponed tentatively or kept to a minimum until the patient's status is determined.

The significance of the history cannot be overestimated. Oral conditions reflect the general health of the patient. Dental procedures may complicate or be complicated by existing pathologic or physiologic conditions elsewhere in the body. General health factors influence response to treatment, such as tissue healing, and thereby affect the outcomes that may be expected from oral care.

The state of the patient's health is constantly changing. Therefore, the history represents the period in the patient's life in which the history was made. With successive appointments, the history must be reviewed and considered along with other new findings.

I. Purposes of the History

Carefully prepared personal, medical and dental histories are used in comprehensive patient care to

A. Provide information pertinent to the etiology and diagnosis of oral conditions and the total treatment plan.

B. Reveal conditions that necessitate precautions, modifications, or adaptations during appointments to assure that dental and dental hygiene procedures will not harm the patient and that emergency situations will be prevented.

C. Aid in the identification of possible unrecognized conditions for which the patient should be referred for further diagnosis and treatment.

D. Permit appraisal of the general health and nutri-

tional status, which in turn, contributes to the prognosis of success in patient care and instruction.

E. Give insight into emotional and psychologic factors, attitudes, and prejudices, which may affect present appointments as well as continuing care.

F. Document records for reference and comparison over a series of appointments, for periodic follow-up.

G. Furnish evidence in legal matters should questions arise.[1]

II. History Preparation

The general methods in current use for obtaining a health history are the *interview*, the *questionnaire*, or a combination of the two. There are several systems for obtaining the history.

A. Alternative Appointment Procedures

1. *Complete history* made at the initial visit: may be a combination of interview and questionnaire.

2. *Brief history* of vital items obtained at the initial visit; complete history obtained at a succeeding appointment.

   a. Purposes of brief history: to prepare for emergency care and to learn of any condition that may contraindicate instrumentation in and around the gingival sulcus during dental and periodontal examinations.

   b. Brief history may be in the form of a questionnaire; an interview for follow-up provides opportunity for individual evaluation.

3. *Self-history* prepared at home: the history form may be mailed to the patient in advance or given at the first appointment to complete and bring in at the second appointment. Such a form might include some checking, as in a questionnaire, and some space to allow free expression by the patient.

B. Record Forms

1. *Types.* Many varying forms are in current use. Forms are available commercially or from the American Dental Association,[2] but many dentists and dental hygienists prefer to prepare their own and have a form printed to their specifications.

2. *Characteristics of an Adequate Form.* The number of items or questions included is not necessarily indicative of the value of the form. The extensive and involved form may be as practical or impractical as the brief checklist that permits no detailed description. Success in use depends on function and a clear common understanding of the meaning of the recorded information to all who will refer to it.

Some characteristics of an adequate form are that it should

a. Provide for convenient notation of important details in a logical sequence.

b. Permit quick identification of special needs of a patient when the history is reviewed prior to each appointment.

c. Allow ample space to record the patient's own words whenever possible in the interview method, or for self-expression by the patient on a questionnaire.

d. Have space for notes concerning attitudes and knowledge as stated or displayed by the patient during the history-taking or other later appointments.

e. Be of a size consistent with the complete patient record forms for filing and ready availability.

C. Introduction to the Patient

The patient needs to realize why the information requested in the histories is essential before treatment can be undertaken. Dental personnel must convey the idea that oral health and general health are interrelated, without creating undue alarm concerning potential ill effects or harmful sequelae from required treatment.

For building rapport, children may participate in their history preparation, but most of the information will need to be supplied by a parent. The signature of the responsible adult on the record is advisable.

D. Limitations of a History[3,4]

Many patients cannot or will not provide complete or, in certain cases, correct information when answering medical or dental history questions. There may be problems related to the method of obtaining the histories, how the questions are worded, or an inadvertent lack of neutrality in the attitude of the person preparing the history. Some patients may have difficulty in comprehending a self-administered test, or there may be a language barrier.

Where the questionnaire is completed may influence answers. A crowded reception area where other patients can see the form and the checks made does not provide sufficient privacy.

Another reason for inaccuracy or incompleteness is that patients may not understand a relationship between certain diseases or conditions and having dental treatment. Information may seem irrelevant, so it is withheld. Occasionally, a patient will not want to tell about a condition that may be embarrassing to discuss. The patient may fear refusal of treatment, particularly if there had been previous experiences in other dental practices.

Studies conducted to determine the reliability of a medical history in identifying patients who are positive for hepatitis B antigen were described on page 32.

III. The Questionnaire

Positive findings on a completed questionnaire need supplementation in a personal interview. A questionnaire by itself cannot be expected to satisfy the overall purposes of the history, but can be adapted best to phases of the personal history, some aspects of the dental history, and factual information in the medical history.

A. Types of Questions

The Health Questionnaire available from the American Dental Association (figure 6–1) provides useful examples of questions essential to patient evaluation.[2]

1. *System-oriented.* Direct questions or topics to check whether the patient has had a disease of, for example, the digestive system, respiratory system, or urinary system may be used. The questions may contain references to body parts, for example the stomach, lungs, kidneys. Questions can then be directed to the specific disease state and the dates and duration.

2. *Disease-oriented.* A typical set of questions for the patient to check may start with "Do you have, or have you had, any of the following diseases or problems?" A listing under that question contains items such as diabetes, asthma or rheumatic fever arranged alphabetically or grouped by systems or body organs.

Follow-up questions can determine dates of illness, severity, and outcome. Suggested questions for determining information related to communicable diseases were listed on page 32.

3. *Symptom-oriented.* In the absence of previous or current disease states, questions may lead to a suspicion of a condition, which, in turn, can provide an opportunity to recommend and encourage the patient to schedule an examination by a physician. Samples of the symptom-oriented question appear in figure 6–1; for example, "Are you thirsty much of the time?" Does your mouth frequently become dry?" or "Do you have to urinate (pass water) more than six times a day?" the positive answers for which could lead to tests for diabetes detection.

B. Advantages of a Questionnaire

1. Broad in scope: useful during the interview to identify positive areas that need additional clarification.
2. Time saving.
3. Consistent: all selected questions are included, and none omitted because of time or other factors.
4. Patient has time to think over the answers: not under pressure, nor under the eyes of the interviewer.
5. Patient may write information that might not be expressed directly in an interview.
6. Legal aspect of a written record with patient's signature.

C. Disadvantages of a Questionnaire (if used alone without a follow-up interview)

1. Impersonal: no opportunity to develop rapport.
2. Inflexible: no provision for additional questioning in areas of specific importance to an individual patient.

IV. The Interview

In long-range planning for the patient's health, much more is involved than asking questions and receiving answers. The rapport established at the time of the interview contributes to the continued cooperation of the patient.

A. Participants

The interviewer is alone with the patient or parent of the child patient. The history should never be taken in a reception area when other patients are present.

B. Setting

1. A consultation room or office is preferred; the patient should be away from the atmosphere of the treatment room where thoughts may be on the techniques to be performed.
2. Treatment room may be the only available place where privacy is afforded.
   a. Seat patient comfortably in upright position.
   b. Turn off running water and dental light, and close the door.
   c. Sit on operating stool to be at eye level with the patient.

C. Pointers for the Interview

Interviewing involves communication between individuals. Communication implies the transmission or interchange of facts, attitudes, opinions, or thoughts, through words, gestures, or other means. Through tactful but direct questioning, communication can be successful and the patient will give such information as is known. Frequently, the patient is unaware of a health problem.

The attitude of the dental personnel should be one of friendly understanding, reassurance, and acceptance. Genuine interest and willingness to listen when a patient wishes to describe symptoms or complaints not only aids in establishing the rapport needed, but frequently provides insight into the patient's real attitudes and prejudices. By asking simple questions at first, and more personal questions later after rapport has developed, the patient will be more relaxed and frank in answering.

Self-confidence and gentle efficiency on the part of the interviewer help to give the patient a feeling of confidence. Skill is required, because tact, ingenuity, and judgment are taxed to the fullest in the attempt to obtain both accurate and complete information from the patient.

D. Interview Form

The interviewer may use a structured form with places to check and fill in or record on blank sheets from questions created from a guide list of essential topics. Either may involve reference to the positive or negative answers on a previously completed questionnaire. Familiarity with the items on the history will permit the interviewer to be direct and informal without reading from a fixed list of topics, a method that may lack the personal touch necessary to gain the patient's confidence. When appropriate, the patient's own words are recorded.

E. Advantages of the Interview

1. Personal contact contributes to development of rapport for future appointments.
2. Flexibility for individual needs: details obtained can be adapted for supplementary questioning.

F. Disadvantages of Interview

1. Time-consuming when not prefaced with questionnaire.
2. Unless a list is consulted, items of importance may be omitted.
3. Patient may be embarrassed to talk about personal conditions and may hold back significant information.

V. Items Included in the History

Information obtained by means of the history is directly related to how the goals of dental and dental hygiene care can and will be accomplished. In tables 6–1, 6–2, and 6–3, items are listed with possible medications and other treatments the patient may have or has had, along with suggested influences on appointment procedures. Objectives for the items to include in the various parts of the history are listed on pages 82 and 83.

In specialized practices, objectives may require increased emphasis on certain aspects. The age group most frequently served would influence the material needed. Parental history and pre- and postnatal information may take on particular significance for the

Medical History

Date _____

Name _____   Address _____
      Last   First   Middle   Number, Street

City _____ State _____ Zip Code _____ Home _____ Business _____
                                             Phone   Phone

Date of Birth _____ Sex _____ Height _____ Weight _____ Occupation _____

Social Security No. _____ Single _____ Married _____ Name of Spouse _____

Closest Relative _____   Phone _____

If you are completing this form for another person, what is your relationship to that person? _____

Referred by _____

In the following questions, circle yes or no, whichever applies. Your answers are for our records only and will be considered confidential.

1. Are you in good health? . . . . Yes   No
2. Has there been any change in your general health within the past year? . . . . Yes   No
3. My last physical examination was on _____
4. Are you now under the care of a physician? . . . . Yes   No
   If so, what is the condition being treated? _____
5. The name and address of my physician is _____
   _____
   _____
6. Have you had any serious illness or operation? . . . . Yes   No
   If so, what was the illness or operation? _____
7. Have you been hospitalized or had a serious illness within the past five (5) years? . . . . . . Yes   No
   If so, what was the problem? _____
8. Do you have or have you had any of the following diseases or problems?
   a. Damaged heart valves or artificial heart valves, including heart murmur . . . . Yes   No
   b. Congenital heart lesions . . . . Yes   No
   c. Cardiovascular disease (heart trouble, heart attack, coronary insufficiency, coronary occlusion, high blood pressure,
      arteriosclerosis, stroke) . . . . Yes   No
      1. Do you have pain in chest upon exertion? . . . . Yes   No
      2. Are you ever short of breath after mild exercise? . . . . Yes   No
      3. Do your ankles swell? . . . . Yes   No
      4. Do you get short of breath when you lie down, or do you require extra pillows when you sleep? . . . . Yes   No
      5. Do you have a cardiac pacemaker? . . . . Yes   No
   d. Allergy . . . . Yes   No
   e. Sinus trouble . . . . Yes   No
   f. Asthma or hay fever . . . . Yes   No
   g. Hives or a skin rash . . . . Yes   No
   h. Fainting spells or seizures . . . . Yes   No
   i. Diabetes . . . . Yes   No
      1. Do you have to urinate (pass water) more than six times a day? . . . . Yes   No
      2. Are you thirsty much of the time? . . . . Yes   No
      3. Does your mouth frequently become dry? . . . . Yes   No
   j. Hepatitis, jaundice or liver disease . . . . Yes   No
   k. Arthritis . . . . Yes   No
   l. Inflammatory rheumatism (painful swollen joints) . . . . Yes   No
   m. Stomach ulcers . . . . Yes   No
   n. Kidney trouble . . . . Yes   No
   o. Tuberculosis . . . . Yes   No
   p. Do you have a persistent cough or cough up blood? . . . . Yes   No
   q. Low blood pressure . . . . Yes   No
   r. Venereal disease . . . . Yes   No
   s. Epilepsy . . . . Yes   No
   t. Psychiatric problems . . . . Yes   No
   u. Cancer . . . . Yes   No
   v. AIDS or other immunosuppressive disorders . . . . Yes   No
   w. Other _____

B500   (over)

Figure 6–1. Health Questionnaire. From Council on Dental Therapeutics, American Dental Association. Reprinted by permission.

9. Have you had abnormal bleeding associated with previous extractions, surgery, or trauma? . . . . Yes No
    a. Do you bruise easily? . . . . Yes No
    b. Have you ever required a blood transfusion? . . . . Yes No
    If so, explain the circumstances _____

10. Do you have any blood disorder such as anemia? . . . . Yes No

11. Have you had surgery, x-ray or drug treatment for a tumor, growth, or other condition of your head or neck? . . . . . Yes No

12. Are you taking any drug or medicine?. . . . . Yes No
    If so, what? _____

13. Are you taking any of the following:
    a. Antibiotics or sulfa drugs . . . . Yes No
    b. Anticoagulants (blood thinners) . . . . Yes No
    c. Medicine for high blood pressure . . . . Yes No
    d. Cortisone (steroids). . . . . Yes No
    e. Tranquilizers . . . . Yes No
    f. Antihistamines . . . . Yes No
    g. Aspirin . . . . Yes No
    h. Insulin, tolbutamide (Orinase) or similar drug. . . . . . Yes No
    i. Digitalis or drugs for heart trouble . . . . Yes No
    j. Nitroglycerin . . . . Yes No
    k. Oral contraceptive or other hormonal therapy . . . . . . Yes No
    l. Other _____

14. Are you allergic or have you reacted adversely to:
    a. Local anesthetics . . . . Yes No
    b. Penicillin or other antibiotics. . . . . Yes No
    c. Sulfa drugs . . . . Yes No
    d. Barbiturates, sedatives, or sleeping pills . . . . Yes No
    e. Aspirin . . . . Yes No
    f. Iodine. . . . . Yes No
    g. Codeine or other narcotics . . . . Yes No
    h. Other _____

15. Have you had any serious trouble associated with any previous dental treatment? . . . . Yes No
    If so, explain _____

16. Do you have any disease, condition, or problem not listed above that you think I should know about? . . . . Yes No
    If so, explain _____

17. Are you employed in any situation which exposes you regularly to x-rays or other ionizing radiation? . . . . Yes No

18. Are you wearing contact lenses? . . . . Yes No

19. Have you had anything to eat or drink in the last 4 hours?. . . . . Yes No

20. Are you wearing removable dental appliances? . . . . Yes No

Women

21. Are you pregnant? . . . . Yes No

22. Do you have any problems associated with your menstrual period? . . . . Yes No

23. Are you nursing? . . . . Yes No

Chief Dental Complaint

I certify that I have read and understand the above. I acknowledge that my questions, if any, about the inquiries set forth above have been answered to my satisfaction. I will not hold my dentist, or any other member of his/her staff, responsible for any errors or omissions that I may have made in the completion of this form.

_____
Signature of Patient

_____
Signature of Dentist

American Dental Association

Figure 6–1. (Continued)

treatment of a small child; in a pedodontist's practice, a special form could be devised to include all essential items.

Insight and awareness shown while preparing the patient history depend on background knowledge of the manifestations of systemic diseases and the medications for various conditions.

A. Personal History (table 6–1)

The basic objectives in gathering personal information about the patient are
1. Data essential for appointment planning and business aspects.
2. Approval of care of a minor and other legal aspects.

3. Patient's physician: for consultation relative to interrelations between general and oral health.

B. Dental History (table 6–2)

The dental history should contribute to knowledge of
1. The immediate problem, chief complaint, cause of present pain, or discomfort of any kind in the oral cavity.
2. The previous dental care as described by the patient, including extent of restorative and prosthetic replacement, as well as any adverse effects.
3. The attitude of the patient toward oral health

Table 6–1. Items for the Personal History

Items to Record in Patient History	Considerations	Influences on Appointment Procedures
1. Name Addresses: Residence and Business Telephone Numbers Sex Marital Status For Child: Name of Parent or Guardian For Parent: Ages and Sex of Children	Accurate recording necessary for business aspects of dental practice	Aids in establishing rapport Instruction applicable to entire family Advice concerning fluorides for children
2. Birthdate	Whether of age or a minor Oral conditions related to age changes; diseases, healing, and other possible characteristics	Approval of parent or guardian necessary for care of minor or person with a mental handicap; signature must be obtained Approach to patient instruction
3. Birthplace and Residence in Early Years	Presence of fluoride in drinking water Food and eating patterns Conditions endemic to certain areas	Effects of fluoride on teeth Instruction in dietary needs adapted to cultural practices
4. Occupation: Present and Former Spouse's Occupation For Children: Parent's Occupation	May be a factor in etiology of certain diseases, dental stains, occlusal wear May affect diet, oral habits, general health	Instruction applied to specific needs Dexterity in use of self-care devices related to dexterity gained from occupation Influence on oral care of entire family For child: which parent will supervise and assist child in oral care
5. Physician	Name, address, and telephone number For consultation	Consultation indicated: (1) for condition that may require premedication (2) when disease symptoms are suspected but patient does not state (3) in an emergency
6. Referred by and Address	To whom to send referral acknowledgment and appreciation	Contribution to rapport with patient Patient referred by another patient may have concept of the office procedures

and care of the mouth as may be indicated by previous periodic dental and dental hygiene treatments.

4. The personal daily care exercised by the patient as evidence of knowledge of the purposes of continuing care and of the value placed on the teeth and their supporting structures.

C. **Medical History** (table 6–3)

Objectives of the medical history are to determine whether the patient has or has had any conditions in the following categories:

1. Diseases that may contraindicate certain kinds of dental and dental hygiene treatment.
   Examples. Leukemia, because of lowered resistance to infection; uncontrolled hypertension, with blood pressure reading 180/105 or greater; congestive heart failure, which requires treatment before stressful procedures, particularly surgery, can be performed.

2. Diseases that require special precautions or premedication prior to treatment.
   Examples. Antibiotic coverage for patient with a history of rheumatic fever or congenital heart defect, to prevent infective endocarditis; possible need for increased sedation in patients subject to convulsions to prevent a seizure if treatment is to be stressful.

3. Diseases under treatment by a physician require medicating drugs that may influence or contraindicate procedures of the dental or dental hygiene appointments.
   Examples. Tranquilizers in daily use could contraindicate premedication with sedatives; anticoagulant therapy requires consultation with physician; antihypertensive drugs may alter the choice of general or local anesthetic used.

4. Allergic or untoward reactions to drugs.
   Examples. All drugs that may possibly be used or recommended to the patient for postoperative care should be checked with the patient as to previous use and reaction.

5. Diseases and drugs with manifestations in the mouth.
   Examples. Hematologic disorders; phenytoin-induced gingival overgrowth.

6. Communicable diseases that endanger the dental personnel.
   Examples. Active tuberculosis; viral hepatitis; herpes; syphilis.

7. Physiologic state of the patient.
   Examples. Pregnancy; puberty; menopause.

VI. Review of History

Updating the history at each maintenance appointment is essential. Changes in health status revealed by interim medical examinations or evidenced by reported illness or hospitalizations must be recorded and considered during continuing treatment.

Following a review of the previously recorded history, questions can be directed to the patient to compare the present condition with the previous one and to determine at least the following:

A. Interim illnesses: changes in health.

B. Visits to physician: reasons and results.

C. Laboratory tests performed and the results: blood, urine, or other analyses.

D. Current medications.

E. Changes in the oral soft tissues and the teeth, observed by the patient.

IMMEDIATE APPLICATIONS OF PATIENT HISTORIES

Together with information from all other parts of the diagnostic work-up, the patient histories are essential for the preparation of the treatment plan. Treatment planning for an individual patient is described on pages 292–293.

Immediate evaluation of the histories is necessary before proceeding to succeeding steps in the preparation of materials for the complete diagnostic work-up. Any one of the objectives for the medical history could alter the procedures to be accomplished.

The list that follows is not intended to be exhaustive, but rather suggestive. From these items, it is expected that the dental personnel will be alerted to precautions that may be needed.

I. Medical Consultation

Dentist and physician need to consult relative to the patient's current therapy and medications or to the patient's past health status that can influence present dental treatment needs.[5]

A. **Telephone or Personal Contact**

Immediate consultation may be needed so that urgent treatment may proceed. Follow-up in writing is essential because without legal record of the advice or decision, a misunderstanding by the patient could result.

B. **Written Request**

A letter of formal request is the preferred procedure. A prepared form can be developed with spaces to fill in the specific questions and space in the lower half for the physician or the assistant completing confidential information from the patient's medical record to provide the necessary directions.

C. **Referrals**

1. Patient should be referred for medical examination when signs of a possible disease condition are apparent.

2. Patient should be referred for laboratory tests when recent test results are not available or follow-up tests are needed.

II. Communicable Disease

A history of communicable disease, either past or current, usually requires additional questioning of

Table 6–2. Items for the Dental History

Items to Record in the History	Considerations	Influences on Appointment Procedures
1. Reason for Present Appointment	Chief complaint in patient's own words Pain or discomfort Onset, symptoms, duration of an acute condition	Need for immediate treatment Attitude toward dentistry and preventive care
2. Previous Dental Appointments	Date last treatment Services performed Regularity	Patient knowledge concerning regular dental care Cooperation anticipated
3. Anesthetics Used	Local, general Adverse or allergic reactions	Choice of anesthetic
4. Radiation History	Date most recent survey Availability from previous dentist Amount of exposure considered with exposure for medical purposes	Amount of exposure: limitations Patient's appreciation for need and use of radiographs
5. Family Dental History	Parental tooth loss or maintenance	Attitude toward saving teeth and preventive dentistry
6. Previous Treatment	Type of treatment; frequency maintenance appointments Whether referred to specialist	Attitude toward specialized care Previous familiarity with role of dental hygienist
A. Periodontal	History of acute infection (necrotizing ulcerative gingivitis, page 481) Surgery; postoperative healing	Attitude toward self-care and disease control
B. Orthodontic	Age during treatment; completion Previous problem Habit correction	For current treatment, consultation with orthodontist needed to determine instructions
C. Endodontic	Dates, etiology	Periodic recheck
D. Prosthodontic	Types of prostheses	Care of prostheses and abutment teeth
E. Other	Extent of restorations	Understanding of prevention
7. Injuries to Face or Teeth	Causes and extent Fractured teeth or jaws	Limitation of opening Special care during healing (pages 597–599)

the patient. The limitations and problems related to information provided by the patient were discussed on page 32.

III. Radiation

When a patient is receiving radiation therapy or has had recent radiation for other purposes, a complete oral radiographic survey may be contraindicated. Conference with the physician or oncologist involved may be necessary to determine the quantity of radiation received.

IV. Prophylactic Premedication

Patients susceptible to infective endocarditis must have antibiotic premedication prior to any tissue manipulation that could create a bacteremia. Other patients who may need prophylactic premedication are those with marked reduced capacity to resist infection.

Tissue manipulation, particularly the use of a probe and an explorer subgingivally, must be withheld until the risk has been determined, the condition has been discussed with the patient's physician, and the prescription obtained. Bacteremia created by instrumentation is described on page 456 and infective endocarditis on pages 685–687.

The American Heart Association and the American Dental Association recommend that risk patients must have antibiotic premedication for all dental procedures likely to induce gingival bleeding.[6,7] The dental hygienist has a legal, moral, and ethical responsibility to prevent infective endocarditis and

Table 6–2. *Continued*

Items to Record in the History	Considerations	Influences on Appointment Procedures
8. Temporomandibular Joint	History of injury, discomfort, disease, dislocation Previous treatment	Effect on opening; accessibility during instrumentation
9. Habits	Clenching, bruxism, doodling Mouth breathing Biting objects: fingernails, pipe stem, thread, other Cheek or lip biting Patient awareness of habits	Tension of patient Instruction relative to effects of habits
10. Tobacco Use	Form of tobacco, amount used Frequency Knowledge of effects on oral tissues	Instruction concerning oral effects Need for frequent observation to detect tissue changes if patient continues at same rate Dental stains; dentifrice selection
11. Fluorides	Systemic, topical, dates Residences during tooth development years Amount of fluoride in drinking water	Current preventive procedures and need for reevaluation

12. Plaque Control Procedures	Toothbrushing: current procedures
	  Type of brush (manual or powered)
	  Texture of bristles
	  Frequency of use
	  Age of brush; frequency of having a new brush
	Dentifrice
	  Name
	  How selected; reason
	Additional cleansing devices and frequency of use
	  Dental floss
	  Water irrigation
	  Perio-aid, rubber tip, or other
	Mouthrinse or other agents: frequency, purpose
	Source of instruction in care of oral cavity
		Present practices and previous instruction
		New instruction needed; reception by patient
		Relation of techniques to prevention of dental caries and periodontal infections
		Supervision of child by parent: current practices
		Problems of habit change

other infections that can result from dental hygiene therapy.[8]

It is not possible to define specific recommendations for all patients who will need antibiotic premedication. Practitioners must use clinical judgment and the advice of the patient's physician to determine the need for preventive antibiotics. The lists below are not intended to be all-encompassing, but represent summaries of the common conditions for which consideration must be given.

A. Indications for Prophylactic Premedication: Cardiac-Related Conditions

1. Congenital heart disease; most congenital cardiac malformations.
2. Rheumatic heart disease.
3. Rheumatic fever and other febrile diseases that predispose to valvular damage. When a patient has a heart murmur, it may be necessary to determine from the patient's physician whether the murmur is considered functional or organic. As advised by the physician, a functional murmur may not require premedication, whereas an organic murmur that is based on a defect in the structure of the heart does require antibiotic coverage.[9]
4. Prosthetic cardiac valves. Patients with vascular autografts generally do not need antibiotic premedication,[10] whereas those with prosthetic valves are very susceptible to infective endocarditis.[11]
5. Previous history of infective endocarditis.
6. Indwelling transvenous cardiac pacemaker.

(continued on page 91)

Table 6–3. Items for the Medical History

Item to Record in History	Considerations	Possible Medications and Treatment Modalities	Influences on Appointment Procedures
1. General Health and Appearance	Disabilities Overall impression of well-being Patient's appraisal of own health		Response, cooperation and attitude to expect during appointments
2. Medical Examination	Date most recent examination Reason for the examination Tests performed; results Anticipated surgery	New prescriptions received Previous prescriptions continued	Verification with physician for added information Need for superior state of oral health in advance of surgery (1) when long recovery is expected and patient may miss maintenance appointments (2) prior to transplant, heart surgery, or prosthesis
3. Major Illnesses, Hospitalizations, Operations	Causes of illness Type and duration of treatment Anesthetics used Convalescence Course of healing: normal, not normal	Medications, treatments	Influence of illnesses on health and care of the oral cavity Anesthetic choice Expected outcome from gingival treatment
4. Age Factors	Problems of health in different age groups Geriatric: multiple disease entities. Patient may need to bring the containers for identification of their medications		Effects on dental and dental hygiene procedures and personal care
5. Height and Weight	Weight changes over past years or months Obesity Undernourishment Child growth pattern	"Diet pills" Substance abuse	Marked weight change may be a symptom of undiagnosed disease; suggest referral for medical examination Influence on dietary instructions for oral health
6. Medications Prescribed by Physician	Reasons: relation to dental care Frequency Patient's regularity of taking Sugar content of liquid medicines, threatening to dental caries (also true of over-the-counter [OTC] items)	List all drugs by name Ask patient for drugs, medicine, injections, tonics, vitamins, pills, capsules, to get a complete answer	Consultation with physician concerning adjustments in dosage for dental or dental hygiene appointments Indications for premedication Side effects of drugs
7. Self-Medication	Type, frequency OTC preparations Substance abuse	Pain relievers Sleeping tablets Cough syrup Antacids Cathartics Vitamins	Information not revealed by patient could complicate treatment Lack of interest in oral health, only pain relief
8. Familial Medical History	Predisposition to certain diseases (example: diabetes) History of diseases that occur in the family	Cultural beliefs about medications	May help patient seek medical examination when symptom suggests possible disease

Table 6–3. *Continued*

Item to Record in History	Considerations	Possible Medications and Treatment Modalities	Influences on Appointment Procedures
9. Daily Diet	Recommendations of patient's physician, past and present Vitamin supplements Appetite Regularity of meals Food likes and dislikes	Vitamin supplements	Instructions to be given relative to oral health Prognosis for healing after treatment Need for dietary review and analysis

10. Alcohol Consumption	Frequency
	Amount
	Substance abuse
		Recovering alcoholic:
		  May be taking disulfiram, vitamins
		  Must avoid all alcohol-containing preparations, including commercial mouthrinses.
			Excessive use: effect on anesthesia; increased healing time
			Poor nutritional state is common; lack of oral care
			May result in poor patient cooperation

11. Allergies	Determine substances to which the patient is allergic:
	  Anesthetics
	  Penicillin
	  Medicaments
	  Foods
	  Iodine
		Antihistamines
		Inhalers
		Decongestants
		Steroids
			Preparation for emergency
			Xerostomia
			Avoid use of substances to which the patient is allergic
			Consider allergies when planning dietary recommendations

12. Arthritis	Joint pain Immobility Temporomandibular joint involvement	Aspirin Nonsteroidal anti-inflammatory drugs Corticosteroids Total joint replacements	Antibiotic premedication Dental chair adjustment
13. Blood Disorder	Type and duration of disease Leukemia: remission thrombocytopenia	Vitamins Minerals: Iron (iron-deficiency anemia) Folic acid supplement (sickle cell anemia) Antineoplastic drugs	Consultation with physician Need for high level of oral health Antibiotic premedication Immunosuppression Increased bleeding Oral lesions
14. Bleeding	Bleeding associated with previous dental appointments History of disorder with coagulation problem History of transfusions or other blood products Check use of aspirin (relation to bleeding tendency) Laboratory tests for bleeding time, coagulation may be needed	Anticoagulant Hemophilia factor replacement	Antibiotic premedication Emergency prevention through pre-appointment precautions Avoid tissue trauma May need to apply dressing after scaling to provide pressure Special measures for hemophilia (pages 710–712)
15. Cancer	Head and neck radiation effects on oral cavity, salivary glands Dental and dental hygiene therapy updated before start of surgery, radiation therapy, or immunosuppression Blood count prior to dental and dental hygiene therapy.	Radiation therapy Fluoride therapy: daily topical application Antineoplastic drugs alkylating agents, antimetabolites, antibiotics, plant alkaloids, steroids	Antibiotic premedication Bleeding; infection; poor healing response Avoid trauma to tissues Effect on oral radiographic survey: prevention of overexposure Dental caries: preventive measures Xerostomia: substitute saliva

(continued next page)

Table 6–3. *Continued*

Item to Record in History	Considerations	Possible Medications and Treatment Modalities	Influences on Appointment Procedures
16. Cardiovascular diseases	Consultation with physician Refer for examination when patient seems unsure of problem	Cardiac glycosides Antiarrhythmics Antianginals Antihypertensives Anticoagulants	Minimize stress Premedication for stress Ascertain that medications have been taken
Congenital Heart Disease Rheumatic Heart Disease	Susceptibility to infective endocarditis Type of problem; date of rheumatic fever	Antibiotic (prevent recurrence of rheumatic fever)	Antibiotic premedication required
Hypertension	Symptom of other disease state Monitoring blood pressure for each appointment Anesthesia: limit epinephrine or omit as recommended by physician	Diuretics Antiadrenergic agents Vasodilators Angiotensin-converting enzyme inhibitors	Postural hypotension (raise dental chair slowly) Xerostomia: saliva substitute and fluoride rinse may be needed
Angina Pectoris	Prepare for symptoms: have ready amyl nitrite vaporole or nitroglycerin tablets	Amyl nitrite, nitroglycerin, or other antianginal drugs	Allay fears and prevent stress
Heart Diseases	History of disease Symptoms of fatigue, shortness of breath, or cough Consult with physician	Glycosides (digitalis) Anticoagulants Antiarrhythmic drugs Pacemaker	Short, more frequent appointments Change dental chair slowly Patient with breathing problem (sleeps with 2 or more pillows) may need semi-upright position Bleeding tendency associated with anticoagulant Avoid ultrasonic (pacemaker) Antibiotic premedication usually indicated
Surgically Corrected Cardiovascular Lesions	Type, date of operation Consultation with physician Before surgical procedure, when possible: the patient needs complete oral evaluation and corrective dental work done, and needs motivation to high level of oral personal care daily	No tobacco use Anticoagulants	Antibiotic premedication vital for synthetic valves or other replacements, indefinitely Autogenous graft (by-pass) needs antibiotic first 6 months Gingival bleeding can be expected
Cerebrovascular Accident (Stroke)	Date of onset; residual disabilities Speech, vision, mental function	No tobacco; low-salt diet Anticoagulants Antihypertensives Vasodilator Steroid Anticonvulsant	Gingival bleeding likely when anticoagulants are used Adapt procedures for physical disability
17. Communicable Diseases	History of diseases; immunizations Present disease; communicability Residences or extended trips in countries with high endemic incidence of certain diseases Risk group factor	Immunizations	Laboratory test requests when unknown disease or carrier state suspected Routine sterilization, barrier techniques for all

Table 6–3. *Continued*

Item to Record in History	Considerations	Possible Medications and Treatment Modalities	Influences on Appointment Procedures
17. continued Hepatitis B	Jaundice history Clarification of type of hepatitis Laboratory clearance	Vaccine for HBV	Postpone appointment if physician's certificate needed
Tuberculosis	Active or passive Cough Duration of disease	Isoniazid (INH)	Active: requires hospital sterile procedures Length of treatment: infectivity diminished after few months of treatment
Sexually-transmitted Diseases (STDs)	May not obtain history of STDs Oral and pharyngeal lesions may be present	Antibiotics	Infectiousness diminishes with antibiotic therapy for gonorrhea and syphilis Refer to physician and postpone treatment when lesions or other signs suggest infection Caution for risk from previously treated diseases
Herpes	Lesions can be transmitted readily	Nondefinitive; symptomatic and palliative treatment Acyclovir	Postpone routine care when oral lesions are present
AIDS	Risk group identification Oral manifestations	Wide variety of opportunistic infections and complications require variety of drugs	Complete sterilization and barrier procedures as for all communicable diseases
18. Diabetes Mellitus	Uncontrolled: requires antibiotic premedication Undiagnosed: excess thirst, appetite, and urination Family incidence: help in finding susceptible, undiagnosed Severe advanced diabetes: complications (vision, kidney, cardiovascular, nervous system)	IDDM (Insulin-dependent): Insulin NIDDM (Non-insulin dependent): Diet control Hypoglycemics	Prepare for emergency: insulin Appointment time related to insulin therapy and mealtime Avoid tissue trauma Need frequent maintenance appointments Periodontal disease accelerated Referral for tests for suspected undiagnosed
19. Ears	Deafness or degree of hearing impairment Infections, operations, ringing, dizziness, balance	Treatment for infection Hearing aid	Adaptations for communication and plaque control instruction
20. Endocrine	Age-group relation to certain conditions Growth, development Menstruation, menopause	Thyroid hormone supplement Antithyroid Estrogen/progestin Oral contraceptives Corticosteroids	Emphasis on high level of plaque control Any patient taking steroids may need antibiotic premedication for appointments Monitor blood pressure
21. Epilepsy	Type, frequency of seizures precipitating factors Preparation for emergency seizure	Anticonvulsant Sedative	Minimize stress Medications make patient drowsy, less alert Valproic acid requires bleeding time pre-operatively

(continued next page)

Table 6–3. *Continued*

Item to Record in History	Considerations	Possible Medications and Treatment Modalities	Influences on Appointment Procedures
22. Eyes	Disturbance of vision Purpose for corrective eyeglasses or contact lens Manifestations of systemic disease	Eyedrops (e.g., glaucoma)	Remove contact lens Protective eyewear during appointment Adaptations for communication with limited sight
23. Gastrointestinal	Nature and treatment of the disease Diet restrictions prescribed by physician	Antacids Antidiarrheal Laxatives Antispasmodics	Patient instruction in accord with prescribed diet and medication Xerostomia
24. Kidney	Renal disease; kidney stones Hemodialysis: hypertension anemia hepatitis carrier Transplant: hypertension hepatitis	Salt restriction Many drugs are nephrotoxic Immunosuppressive drugs	Antibiotic premedication Monitor blood pressure Bleeding tendency Poor healing Susceptibility to infection Limited stress toleration
25. Liver	History of jaundice, hepatitis Impaired drug metabolism Cirrhosis: history of alcoholism	Nutritional emphasis Abstinence from alcohol	Laboratory test for hepatitis Bleeding problems
26. Mental, Psychiatric	Emotional problems hinder oral care	Antipsychotic drugs Antianxiety drugs Tranquilizers Antidepressants Antiparkinsonism drugs	Limited stress tolerance Xerostomia (side effect)
27. Physical Activity	Overall health consciousness	Good health habits Regular exercise Basic 4 diet	Contribute to cooperative attitude in maintaining oral health
28. Physical Disabilities	Extent, cause, duration Type of treatment related to individual condition (Chapter 54) Consultation with physician or medical specialist	Pain reliever Muscle relaxant Anticonvulsant	Adjustment of physical arrangements Wheelchair accessibility and transfer Adaptations of techniques and instruction Antibiotic premedication for certain conditions: Examples: prosthetic joint replacement, shunt
29. Pregnancy	Month, parturition date Possible oral manifestations History of previous pregnancies Iron deficiency anemia	Iron	Adjust physical position for comfort Frequent appointments for maintaining high level of oral hygiene
30. Respiration	Breathing problems Persistent cough Cough up blood Chest pain Precipitation of asthmatic attack	Codeine cough syrup Antihistamine Bronchial dilators Expectorants Decongestants Steroids	Dental chair position Ultrasonic and airbrasive contraindicated Anesthesia choice No aerosol agents

7. Mitral valve prolapse with insufficiency.
8. Surgically constructed systemic-pulmonary shunts.

B. Other Indications for Prophylactic Premedication

1. Reduced capacity to resist infection.
   a. Corticosteroid or other immunosuppressive therapy.
   b. Anticancer chemotherapy.
   c. Blood diseases, especially acute leukemia, agranulocytosis, and sickle cell anemia.
2. Uncontrolled, unstable diabetes mellitus. Controlled diabetes can be treated as normal (page 721).
3. Grossly contaminated traumatic facial injuries and compound fractures.
4. Renal transplant and hemodialysis; glomerulonephritis or other active renal disorder.[12,13]
5. Prosthetic joint replacement.[14,15,16]

V. Prophylactic Antibiotic Regimens[6,7]

The American Heart Association's recommended regimens are divided into *Standard* and *Special* as summarized in table 6–4.

The *Standard* regimen is generally used, except for patients at high or very high risk for endocarditis (for examples, those with prosthetic heart valves or surgically constructed systemic-pulmonary shunts) when it is advised that parenteral antibiotic be administered. Other *Special* regimen patients include those allergic to penicillin.

Patients with problems of delayed healing may require additional doses of antibiotic. It has been shown that bacteremia rarely persists more than about 15 minutes after the instrumentation is terminated. It has also been shown that the incidence of bacteremia is less when the periodontal tissues are maintained in optimum health.

TECHNICAL HINTS

I. Date all records.
II. Keep permanent records in ink.
III. Provide a specific line on a health history form for the signature of the patient.[1] The completed history for a minor should be signed by a parent or guardian.
IV. All information obtained for a patient history must be maintained in strictest confidence.
V. For patients with special health problems that require premedication or other adaptation of procedure, some type of coded tab can be used to alert all dental personnel to check the medical history prior to each appointment.
VI. Analyze the usefulness of items on the patient history form periodically and plan for revision as scientific research reveals new information that must be applied.
VII. A medical history update wall plaque is avail-

Table 6–4. Summary of Recommended Antibiotic Regimens for Dental Procedures

STANDARD REGIMEN	
For dental procedures that cause gingival bleeding	Penicillin V 2 g orally 1 hour before, then 1 g 6 hours after initial dose. For patients unable to take oral medications, 2 million units of aqueous penicillin G intravenously or intramuscularly 30–60 minutes before a procedure and 1 million units 6 hours after initial dose may be substituted.

SPECIAL REGIMENS	
Parenteral regimen for use when maximal protection desired (for example, for patients with prosthetic valves)	Ampicillin 1–2 g intramuscularly or intravenously, plus gentamicin 1.5 mg/kg intramuscularly or intravenously, one-half hour before procedure, followed by 1 g oral penicillin V 6 hours after initial dose. Alternatively, the parenteral regimen may be repeated once 8 hours after initial dose
Oral regimen for penicillin-allergic patients	Erythromycin 1 g orally 1 hour before, then 500 mg 6 hours after initial dose
Parenteral regimen for penicillin-allergic patients	Vancomycin 1 g intravenously slowly over 1 hour, starting 1 hour before. No repeat dose is necessary

NOTE: Pediatric doses: Ampicillin 50 mg/kg per dose; erythromycin 20 mg/kg for first dose, then 10 mg/kg; gentamicin 2.0 mg/kg per dose; penicillin V full adult dose if greater than 60 lb (27 kg), one-half adult dose if less than 60 lb (27 kg); aqueous penicillin G 50,000 units/kg (25,000 units/kg for follow-up); vancomycin 20 mg/kg per dose. The intervals between doses are the same as for adults. Total doses should not exceed adult doses. (Reproduced with permission. From *Prevention of Bacterial Endocarditis*. American Heart Association)

able for posting in an appropriate place in a dental office or clinic. It reads: *Please Advise Us of Any Change in Your Medical History Since Your Last Visit.* It is available from the American Dental Association, Order Department, 211 East Chicago Avenue, Chicago, Illinois 60611

FACTORS TO TEACH THE PATIENT

I. The need for obtaining the personal, medical, and dental history prior to performance of dental and dental hygiene procedures and the need for keeping the histories up to date.

II. The relationship between oral health and general physical health.

III. The interrelationship of medical and dental care.

IV. Advantages of cooperation in furnishing information that will help dental personnel to interpret observations accurately and to assure the dentist that the correct diagnosis and treatment plan have been made.

V. All patients who require antibiotic premedication need special attention paid to (1) the importance of preventive dentistry, (2) the imperative need for regular dental care, and (3) the necessity for taking the prescribed prescription one hour before the appointment will start.

References

1. Sheppard, G.A.: Medical-legal Considerations, in Malamed, S.F.: *Handbook of Medical Emergencies in the Dental Office,* 2nd ed. St. Louis, The C.V. Mosby Co., 1982, pp. 55–65.
2. American Dental Association, Form B-500, Medical History, Order Department, 211 East Chicago Avenue, Chicago, Illinois 60611.
3. Brady, W.F. and Martinoff, J.T.: Validity of Health History Data Collected from Dental Patients and Patient Perception of Health Status, *J. Am. Dent. Assoc., 101,* 642, October, 1980.
4. Goebel, W.M.: Reliability of the Medical History in Identifying Patients Likely to Place Dentists at an Increased Hepatitis Risk, *J. Am. Dent. Assoc., 98,* 907, June, 1979.
5. Chiodo, G.T. and Rosenstein, D.I.: Consultation Between Dentists and Physicians, *Gen. Dent., 32,* 19, January-February, 1984.
6. Shulman, S.T., Amren, D.P., Bisno, A.L., Dajani, A.S., Durack, D.T., Gerber, M.A., Kaplan, E.L., Millard, H.D., Sanders, W.E., Schwartz, R.H., and Watanakunakorn, C.: Prevention of Bacterial Endocarditis. A Statement for Health Professionals by the Committee on Rheumatic Fever and Infective Endocarditis of the Council on Cardiovascular Disease in the Young, *Circulation, 70,* 1123A, December, 1984.
7. American Dental Association, Council on Dental Therapeutics: Prevention of Bacterial Endocarditis: A Committee Report of the American Heart Association, *J. Am. Dent. Assoc., 110,* 98, January, 1985.
8. Shannon, S.A.: Infective Endocarditis. What Every Dental Hygienist Should Know, *Dent. Hyg., 59,* 552, December, 1985.
9. Little, J.W. and Falace, D.A.: *Dental Management of the Medically Compromised Patient,* 2nd ed. St. Louis, The C.V. Mosby Co., 1984, p. 63.
10. Lindemann, R.A. and Henson, J.L.: The Dental Management of Patients with Vascular Grafts Placed in the Treatment of Arterial Occlusive Disease, *J. Am. Dent. Assoc., 104,* 625, May, 1982.
11. Baumgartner, J.C. and Plack, W.F.: Dental Treatment and Management of a Patient with a Prosthetic Heart Valve, *J. Am. Dent. Assoc., 104,* 181, February, 1982.
12. Naylor, G.D., Hall, E.H., and Terezhalmy, G.T.: The Patient with Chronic Renal Failure Who Is Undergoing Dialysis or Renal Transplantation: Another Consideration for Antimicrobial Prophylaxis, *Oral Surg. Oral Med. Oral Pathol., 65,* 116, January, 1988.
13. Heard, E., Staples, A.F., and Czerwinski, A.W.: The Dental Patient with Renal Disease: Precautions and Guidelines, *J. Am. Dent. Assoc., 96,* 792, May, 1978.
14. Mulligan, R.: Late Infections in Patients with Prostheses for Total Replacement of Joints: Implications for the Dental Practitioner, *J. Am. Dent. Assoc., 101,* 44, July, 1980.
15. Jacobsen, P.L. and Murray, W.: Prophylactic Coverage of Dental Patients with Artificial Joints: A Retrospective Analysis of Thirty-three Infections in Hip Prostheses, *Oral Surg. Oral Med. Oral Pathol., 50,* 130, August, 1980.
16. Howell, R.M. and Green, J.G.: Prophylactic Antibiotic Coverage in Dentistry: A Survey of Need for Prosthetic Joints, *Gen. Dent., 33,* 320, July-August, 1985.

Suggested Readings

Brady, W.F. and Martinoff, J.T.: Diagnosed Past and Present Systemic Disease in Dental Patients, *Gen. Dent., 30,* 494, November-December, 1982.

Derouen, A.S. and Adshead, M.C.: Passing the Medical History Legal Test, *RDH, 5,* 36, January, 1985.

Fay, J.T. and O'Neal, R.B.: Dental Responsibility for the Medically Compromised Patient, *J. Oral Med., 39,* 12, January-March; *39,* 115, April-June; *39,* 148, July-September; *39,* 218, October-December, 1984.

Friedlander, A.H.: The Dental Management of Depressed Patients, *Spec. Care Dentist., 7,* 65, March-April, 1987.

Griffiths, R.H.: Report of the President's Conference on the Examination, Diagnosis, and Management of Temporomandibular Disorders, *J. Am. Dent. Assoc., 106,* 75, January, 1983.

Halstead, C.L., Blozis, G.G., Drinnan, A.J., and Gier, R.E.: *Physical Evaluation of the Dental Patient,* St. Louis, The C.V. Mosby Co., 1982, pp. 27–44.

Haugejorden, O. and Nielsen, W.A.: Experimental Study of Two Methods of Data Collection by Questionnaire, *Community Dent. Oral Epidemiol., 15,* 205, August, 1987.

Kerr, D.A., Ash, M.M., and Millard, H.D.: *Oral Diagnosis,* 6th ed., St. Louis, The C.V. Mosby Co., 1983, pp. 34–67.

Langlais, R.P., Bricker, S.L., Cottone, J.A., and Baker, B.R.: *Oral Diagnosis, Oral Medicine and Treatment Planning.* Philadelphia, W.B. Saunders Co., 1984, pp. 11–31.

Little, J.W. and Falace, D.A.: *Dental Management of the Medically Compromised Patient,* 2nd ed. St. Louis, The C.V. Mosby Co., 1984, pp. 28–64.

McCarthy, F.M.: A New Patient-administered Medical History Developed for Dentistry, *J. Am. Dent. Assoc., 111,* 595, October, 1985.

Nery, E.B., Meister, F., Ellinger, R.F., Eslami, A., and McNamara, T.J.: Prevalence of Medical Problems in Periodontal Patients Obtained from Three Different Populations, *J. Periodontol., 58,* 564, August, 1987.

Palchick, Y.S.: Obtaining a Practical Case History and Examination, *Dent. Clin. North Am., 27,* 505, July, 1983.

Parnell, A.G.: The Medically Compromised Patient, *Int. Dent. J., 36,* 77, June, 1986.

Petersen, J.K.: Complications in Patients on Therapeutic Drugs, *Int. Dent. J., 36,* 83, June, 1986.

Romriell, G.E. and Streeper, S.N.: The Medical History, *Dent. Clin. North Am., 26,* 3, January, 1982.

Scully, C. and Boyle, P.: Reliability of a Self-administered Questionnaire for Screening for Medical Problems in Dentistry, *Community Dent. Oral Epidemiol., 11,* 105, April, 1983.

Snyder, N.C.: *Dental Hygiene Clinical Applications in Pharmacology.* Philadelphia, Lea & Febiger, 1987, pp. 129– 239.

Sonis, S.T., Fazio, R., Setkowicz, A., Gottlieb, D., and Vorhaus, C.: Comparison of the Nature and Frequency of Medical Problems Among Patients in General, Specialty and Hospital Dental Practices, *J. Oral Med., 38,* 58, April-June, 1983.

Steffen, R., Rickenbach, M., Wilhelm, U., Helminger, A., and Schär, M.: Health Problems After Travel to Developing Countries, *J. Infect. Dis., 156,* 84, July, 1987.

Stout, F. and Doering, P.: The Problematic Drug History, *Dent. Clin. North Am., 27,* 387, April, 1983.

Terezhalmy, G.T.: Proceedings of the American Academy of Oral Medicine. The Medical History, *J. Oral Med., 37,* 141, October-December, 1982.

Antibiotic Premedication

Brooks, S.L.: Survey of Compliance with American Heart Association Guidelines for Prevention of Bacterial Endocarditis, *J. Am. Dent. Assoc., 101,* 41, July, 1980.

Carroll, G.C. and Sebor, R.J.: Dental Flossing and Its Relationship to Transient Bacteremia, *J. Periodontol., 51,* 691, December, 1980.

Cawson, R.A.: Infective Endocarditis as a Complication of Dental Treatment, *Br. Dent. J., 151,* 409, December 15, 1981.

Crespi, P.V. and Friedman, R.B.: Dental Examination Guidelines for Children Requiring Infective Endocarditis Prophylaxis, *J. Am. Dent. Assoc., 111,* 931, December, 1985.

Durack, D.T., Kaplan, E.L., and Bisno, A.L.: Apparent Failures of Endocarditis Prophylaxis. Analysis of 52 Cases Submitted to a National Registry, *JAMA, 250,* 2318, November 4, 1983.

Ehrmann, E.H.: Infective Endocarditis and the Dentist, *Aust. Dent. J., 31,* 351, October, 1986.

Gaidry, D., Kudlick, E.M., Hutton, J.G., and Russell, D.M.: A Survey to Evaluate the Management of Orthodontic Patients with a History of Rheumatic Fever or Congenital Heart Disease, *Am. J. Orthod., 87,* 338, April, 1985.

Holbrook, W.P., Willey, R.F., and Shaw, T.R.D.: Prophylaxis of Infective Endocarditis Problems in Practice, *Br. Dent. J., 154,* 36, January 22, 1983.

Jacobson, J.J., Millard, H.D., Plezia, R., and Blankenship, J.R.: Dental Treatment and Late Prosthetic Joint Infections, *Oral Surg. Oral Med. Oral Pathol., 61,* 413, April, 1986.

Jacobson, J.J. and Mathews, L.S.: Bacteria Isolated from Late Prosthetic Joint Infections: Dental Treatment and Chemoprophylaxis, *Oral Surg. Oral Med. Oral Pathol., 63,* 122, January, 1987.

Jaspers, M.T. and Little, J.W.: Prophylactic Antibiotic Coverage in Patients with Total Arthroplasty: Current Practice, *J. Am. Dent. Assoc., 111,* 943, December, 1985.

Kaiser, A.B.: Antimicrobial Prophylaxis in Surgery, *N. Engl. J. Med., 315,* 1129, October 30, 1986.

Kilmartin, C. and Munroe, C.: The Dental Management of the Cardiac Patient Requiring Antibiotic Prophylaxis, *Can. Dent. Assoc. J., 52,* 77, January, 1986.

Kilmartin, C. and Munroe, C.: Prophylactic Antibiotic Coverage and the Cardiac Patient. How to Identify the "At Risk" Patient, *Can. Dent. Assoc. J., 52,* 71, January, 1986.

Little, J.W.: Prevention of Bacterial Endocarditis in Dental Patients, *Gen. Dent., 35,* 382, September-October, 1987.

Littner, M.M., Kaffe, I., Tamse, A., and Buchner, A.: New Concept in Chemoprophylaxis of Bacterial Endocarditis Resulting from Dental Treatment, *Oral Surg. Oral Med. Oral Pathol., 61,* 338, April, 1986.

Sadowsky, D. and Kunzel, C.: Clinician Compliance and the Prevention of Bacterial Endocarditis, *J. Am. Dent. Assoc., 109,* 425, September, 1984.

Slots, J., Rosling, B.G., and Genco, R.J.: Suppression of Penicillin-resistant Oral Actinobacillus Actinomycetemcomitans with Tetracycline. Considerations in Endocarditis Prophylaxis, *J. Periodontol., 54,* 193, April, 1983.

Sullivan, B.V. and Blong, M.A.: The Cardiac Patient. Chemoprophylaxis Considerations, *Dent. Hyg., 60,* 462, October, 1986.

Zysset, M.K., Montgomery, M.T., Redding, S.W., and Dell'Italia, L.J.: Systemic Lupus Erythematosus: A Consideration for Antimicrobial Prophylaxis, *Oral Surg. Oral Med. Oral Pathol., 64,* 30, July, 1987.

Interview

Chambers, D.W. and Abrams, R.G.: *Dental Communication.* Norwalk, Connecticut, Appleton-Century-Crofts, 1986, pp. 147–159.

Croft, J.J.: Interviewing in Physical Therapy, *Physical Therapy, 60,* 1033, August, 1980.

Enelow, A.J. and Swisher, S.N.: *Interviewing and Patient Care,* 3rd ed. New York, Oxford University Press, 1986.

Holli, B.B. and Calabrese, R.J.: *Communication and Education Skills: The Dietitian's Guide.* Philadelphia, Lea & Febiger, 1986.

Langlais, R.P., Bricker, S.L., Cottone, J.A., and Baker, B.R.: *Oral Diagnosis, Oral Medicine and Treatment Planning.* Philadelphia, W.B. Saunders Co., 1984, pp. 23–31.

7 Vital Signs

The vital signs are the body temperature, pulse and respiratory rates, and blood pressure. Table 7–1 summarizes the normal values for adults.

Recording vital signs contributes to the proper systemic evaluation of a patient in conjunction with the complete medical history. Treatment planning and appointment sequencing are directly influenced by the findings. Proficiency in determination of the vital signs is essential for monitoring during emergency treatment (see Chapter 60).

Abnormal vital signs must be regarded with suspicion, because they may indicate undetected systemic problems. For example, a patient's life may be saved because of medical treatment initiated as a result of a high blood pressure determination during a dental hygiene appointment.

When vital signs are not within normal range, they are called to the dentist's attention. The patient should be informed and the findings discussed with a physician. When the patient does not have a personal physician, a recommendation for referral for additional diagnostic procedures is indicated.

BODY TEMPERATURE

While preparing the patient history and making the extraoral and intraoral examinations, the need for taking the temperature may become apparent, or the dentist may have requested the procedure in conjunction with current oral disease. When the temperature is to be taken along with the other vital signs, the pulse and respiratory rates are determined concurrently, while the thermometer is in the patient's mouth.

A temperature above the normal range can indicate the presence of infection. Patients can have an elevated body temperature due to oral causes such as an apical or periodontal abscess or acute pericoronitis. Determination of the temperature of a patient with an oral infection may be necessary for diagnosis and treatment planning.

For the protection of the health of the personnel in the dental office or clinic, to prevent loss of working time because of illness, as well as for the protection of subsequent patients who may be indirectly exposed, it is important to detect the presence of a systemic, contagious condition. Screening for elevated temperature among patients may have particular significance during certain seasons or epidemics. When a definite increase in temperature is found,

Table 7–1. Adult Vital Signs

Vital Sign	Values of Significance in Dental and Dental Hygiene Appointments	
Body Temperature (oral)	Normal 37.0° C (98.6° F) Normal range 35.5° to 37.5° C (96.0° to 99.5° F)	
Pulse Rate	Normal range 60 to 100 per minute	
Respiration	Normal range 14 to 20 per minute	
Blood Pressure	**Diastolic Blood Pressure** (mm. Hg)	**Category**
	<85	Normal blood pressure
	85 to 89	High normal blood pressure
	90 to 104*	Mild hypertension
	105 to 114†	Moderate hypertension
	>115‡	Severe hypertension
	Systolic Blood Pressure (mm. Hg) With diastolic blood pressure<90	
	<140	Normal blood pressure
	140 to 159*	Borderline isolated systolic hypertension
	>160†	Isolated systolic hypertension

*Confirm promptly (not to exceed 2 months)
†Refer promptly to source of care (not to exceed 2 weeks)
‡Refer immediately to a source of care
Data from The 1988 Report of the Joint National Committee on Detection, Evaluation, and Treatment of High Blood Pressure. U.S. Department of Health and Human Services National Institutes of Health.

the patient can be dismissed by the dentist to prevent further contamination of the office or clinic. The patient can be advised to seek medical care.

I. Maintenance of Body Temperature

A. Normal
1. *Adult.* The normal average temperature is 37.0° C (98.6° F) as illustrated in figure 7–1. The normal range is from 35.5° to 37.5° C (96.0° to 99.5° F).
2. *Children.*[1] There is no appreciable difference between boys and girls. Average temperatures are as follows:
   a. First year: 37.3° C (99.1° F).
   b. Fourth year: 37.5° C (99.4° F).
   c. Fifth year: 37° C (98.6° F).
   d. Twelfth year: 36.7° C (98.0° F).

B. Temperature Variations
1. *Fever (pyrexia).* Values over 37.5° C (99.5° F).
2. *Hyperthermia.* Values over 41.0° C (105.8° F)
3. *Hypothermia.* Values below 35.5° C (96.0° F).

C. Factors that Alter Body Temperature
1. *Time of Day.* Highest in late afternoon and early evening; lowest during sleep and early morning.
2. *Temporary Increase.* Exercise, hot drinks, smoking, or application of external heat.
3. *Pathologic States.* Infection, dehydration, hyperthyroidism, myocardial infarction, tissue injury from trauma.
4. *Decrease*: Starvation, hemorrhage, or physiologic shock.

II. Methods of Determining Temperature

A. Oral
Most commonly used.
1. *Indications for Use.* An oral thermometer is used for the patient who
   a. Can follow instructions.
   b. Can keep the mouth closed to hold the thermometer.
   c. Will not bite or otherwise break the thermometer (which could happen with small children or confused patients of any age).

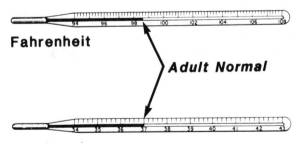

Fahrenheit

Adult Normal

Centigrade

Figure 7–1. Thermometers. Centigrade and Fahrenheit thermometers compared. Adult normal temperature is shown at 37.0° Centigrade and 98.6° Fahrenheit.

d. Has no mouth injuries or problems breathing through the nose.
2. *Contraindications.* The oral thermometer cannot be used for a patient who is unconscious, confused, irrational or restless; infants or small children; or a patient with a very dry mouth.

B. Rectal
Generally applicable when the oral thermometer is contraindicated.

C. External
Axillary and groin positions are the least accurate; but occasionally, the oral or rectal methods are impossible to use.

D. Types of Thermometers
1. *Mercury-column Clinical Thermometer.* Consists of a bulb containing mercury, which, when heated by the body temperature, expands and rises in the hollow center of the glass stem. The bulb of the oral thermometer is usually tapered, whereas the rectal thermometer has a blunt, round mercury bulb.
2. *Electronic.* Some hospitals use electronic thermometers, which require less time for taking the temperature, are more easily cared for because of their disposable tips, and which decrease the possibility of cross-contamination.

E. Comparison of Readings
Rectal readings are about 1 degree above oral readings, and oral readings are about 1 degree above axillary or groin readings.

III. Procedure

A. Equipment
Clinical thermometer, tissues, clock or watch with second hand, sheath.

B. Prepare Patient
1. Tell patient what is to be done.
2. Wait 15 minutes for the patient who has just had a hot or cold beverage or has smoked within 10 minutes, because the surface temperature of the oral mucosa can alter the accuracy of the thermometer reading.

C. Prepare the Thermometer
1. Hold the thermometer only by the stem, never by the bulb.
2. Wipe with a tissue.
3. Check the reading: it must be below 35.6° C (96° F).
4. Shake down the mercury level if not already below 35.6° C (96° F). The thermometer maintains the highest temperature previously registered, and remains there until the force of shaking lowers the mercury level.
   a. Move away from furniture or other hard objects to prevent accidental forceful contact of the thermometer.
   b. Grasp stem firmly and shake with a firm, even, downward motion one or two times.

c. Recheck the reading and reshake if indicated.
5. Place the thermometer into a thermometer sheath (a disposable cover available from a medical supply) to prevent contact with the patient's oral microflora. Figure 7–2 illustrates the procedure for preparation of a sheath.

D. Take the Temperature
1. Insert the bulb under the patient's tongue, with the stem outside the mouth.
2. Instruct patient to hold the thermometer gently with the lips, to avoid biting, and to breathe through the nose.
3. Observe watch or other timer, and remove thermometer after 3 clocked minutes.

E. Read and Record
1. Stand with back to light source and hold the thermometer by the stem at eye level to read.
2. Roll the thermometer slowly between the fingers to find the solid column of mercury.
3. Read at the point where the mercury ends. Each long line represents a degree of temperature, and short lines between are at two-tenths (0.2) of a degree.
4. Retake the temperature when the reading is unusually high or low.

a. Reshake the mercury column down.
b. Watch the patient to make certain that the thermometer is in position during the 3 minutes.
5. Record date, time of day, and temperature on the patient's record.
6. Inform the dentist of a temperature over 37.5° C (99.5° F).

F. Care of the Thermometer
1. *Disposable Thermometer Sheath.* Remove and dispose in waste.
2. *Conventional*
   a. Wash with soap and slightly warm water; rinse with clear cool water; dry. Hot water can raise the temperature and force the mercury to break the thermometer.
   b. Soak in disinfectant solution, completely covered.
   c. Rinse with water and dry before placing in container or using again. Container should be sterilizable.

IV. Care of Patient with Temperature Elevation[2,3]

A. Temperature Over 41.0° C (105.8° F)
1. Treat as medical emergency.
2. Transport to a hospital for medical care.

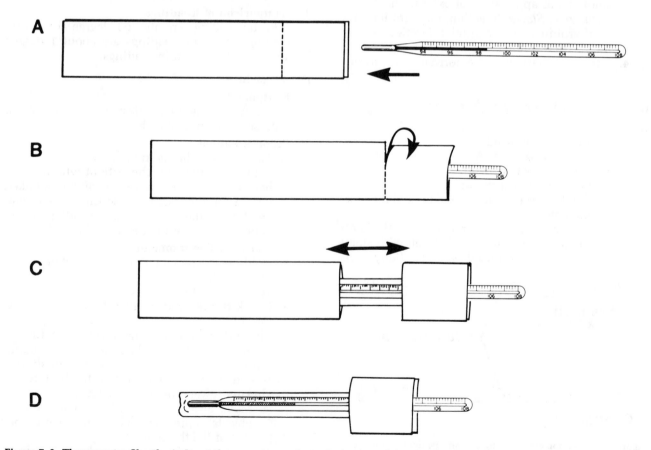

Figure 7–2. Thermometer Sheath. A. Insert thermometer gently to the bottom of the sheath. **B.** Tear at dotted line by twisting. **C.** Pull apart, holding by the small section of cover. **D.** Sheathed thermometer is ready for insertion under patient's tongue.

B. Temperature 37.6° to 41.0°C (99.6° to 105.8°F)
1. Check possible temporary or factitious cause, such as hot beverage or smoking, and observe patient while repeating the determination.
2. Review the dental and medical history.
3. Call to the attention of the dentist.
4. Provide no elective care when there are signs of respiratory infection or other possible communicable disease.

PULSE

The pulse is the intermittent throbbing sensation felt when the fingers are pressed against an artery. It is the result of the alternate expansion and contraction of an artery as a wave of blood is forced through the heartbeat. The pulse rate or heart rate is the count of the heartbeats. Irregularities of strength, rhythm, and quality of the pulse should be noted while counting the pulse rate.

I. Maintenance of Normal Pulse

A. Normal Pulse Rates
1. *Adults.* There is no absolute normal. The adult range is 60 to 100 beats per minute, slightly higher for women than for men.
2. *Children.*[1] The pulse or heart rate falls steadily during childhood.
   a. In utero—150 beats per minute (bpm).
   b. At birth—130 bpm.
   c. Second year—105 bpm.
   d. Fourth year—90 bpm.
   e. Tenth year—70 bpm.

B. Factors That Influence Pulse Rate
An unusually fast heartbeat (over 150 beats per minute in an adult) is called *tachycardia*; an unusually slow beat (below 50) is *bradycardia.*
1. *Increased Pulse.* Caused by exercise, stimulants, eating, strong emotions, extremes of heat and cold, and some forms of heart disease.
2. *Decreased Pulse.* Caused by sleep, depressants, fasting, quieting emotions, and low vitality from prolonged illness.
3. *Emergency Situations.* Listed in table 60–1, pages 747–754.

II. Procedure for Determining Pulse Rate

A. Sequence
The pulse rate is conveniently obtained at the same time that the thermometer is in the patient's mouth to determine body temperature. Respirations are counted immediately following the pulse rate.

B. Sites
The pulse may be felt at several points over the body. The one most commonly used is on the radial artery at the wrist and is called the *radial pulse* (figure 7–3). Other sites convenient for use in a dental office or clinic are the *temporal* artery

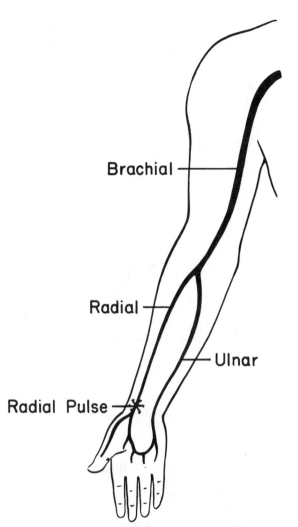

Figure 7–3. Arteries of the Arm. Note location of radial pulse. The brachial pulse may be felt just before the brachial artery branches into the radial and ulnar arteries.

on the side of the head in front of the ear, or the *facial* artery at the border of the mandible.

The carotid pulse is used during cardiopulmonary resuscitation (pages 741–742 and figure 60–6).

C. Prepare the Patient
1. Tell the patient what is to be done.
2. Have the patient in a comfortable position with arm and hand supported, palm down.
3. Locate the radial pulse on the thumb side of the wrist with the tips of the first three fingers (figure 7–4). Do not use the thumb because it contains a pulse that may be confused with the patient's pulse.

D. Count and Record
1. When the pulse is felt, exert light pressure and count for 1 clocked minute. Use the second hand of a watch or clock. Check with a repeat count.
2. While taking the pulse, observe the following:

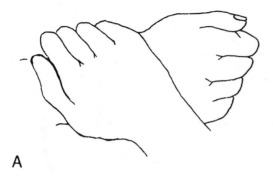

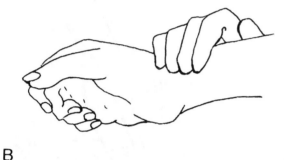

A

B

Figure 7–4. Determination of Pulse Rate. A. Correct position of hands. **B.** The tips of the first three fingers are placed over the radial pulse located on the thumb side of the ventral surface of the wrist.

    a. Rhythm: regular, regularly irregular, irregularly irregular.

    b. Volume and strength: full, strong, poor, weak, thready.

3. Record on patient's record: date, pulse rate, other characteristics.

4. Call unusual findings to the dentist's attention. A pulse rate over 90 should be considered abnormal for an adult and over 120 abnormal for a child.

RESPIRATION

The function of respiration is to supply oxygen to the tissues and to eliminate carbon dioxide. Variations in normal respirations may be shown by characteristics such as the rate, rhythm, depth, and quality and may be symptomatic of disease or emergency states.

I. Maintenance of Normal Respirations

A respiration is one breath taken in and let out.

A. Normal Respiratory Rate

1. *Adults.* The adult range is from 14 to 20 per minute, slightly higher for women.

2. *Children.*[1] The respiratory rate decreases steadily during childhood. Averages are
    a. First year—30 per minute
    b. Second year—25 per minute

    c. Eighth year—20 per minute
    d. Fifteenth year—18 per minute

B. Factors That Influence Respirations

Many of the same factors that influence pulse rate also influence the number of respirations. A rate of 12 per minute or fewer is considered subnormal for an adult; over 28 is accelerated; and rates over 60 are extremely rapid and dangerous.

1. *Increased Respiration.* Caused by work and exercise, excitement, nervousness, strong emotions, pain, hemorrhage, shock.

2. *Decreased Respiration.* Caused by sleep, certain drugs, pulmonary insufficiency.

3. *Emergency Situations.* Listed in table 60–1, pages 747–754.

II. Procedures for Observing Respirations

A. Determine Rate

1. Make the count of respirations immediately after counting the pulse.

2. Maintain the fingers over the radial pulse.

3. Respirations must be counted so that the patient is not aware, as the rate may be voluntarily altered.

4. Count the number of times the chest rises in 1 clocked minute. It is not necessary to count both inspirations and expirations.

B. Factors to Observe

1. *Depth.* Describe as shallow, normal, or deep.

2. *Rhythm.* Describe as regular (evenly spaced) or irregular (with pauses of irregular lengths between).

3. *Quality.* Describe as strong, easy, weak, or labored (noisy). Poor quality may have an effect on body color; for example, a bluish tinge of the face or nailbeds may mean an insufficiency of oxygen.

4. *Sounds.* Describe deviant sounds made during inspiration, expiration, or both.

5. *Position of Patient.* When the patient assumes an unusual position to secure comfort during breathing or prefers to remain seated upright, mark records accordingly.

C. Record

Record all findings on the patient's record.

D. Notify

Call to the attention of the dentist any unusual findings.

BLOOD PRESSURE

Information about the patient's blood pressure is essential during dental and dental hygiene appointments because special adaptations may be needed. Screening for blood pressure in dental offices has been shown to be an effective health service for all ages.

Cardiovascular diseases are described in Chapter 56, and the causes, predisposing factors, and treatment of hypertension on pages 687–688. That information can be a helpful introduction and is recommended for reading in conjunction with this section on the techniques for obtaining blood pressure.

I. Components of Blood Pressure

Blood pressure is the force exerted by the blood on the blood vessel walls. When the left ventricle of the heart contracts, blood is forced out into the aorta and travels through the large arteries to the smaller arteries, arterioles, and capillaries. The pulsations extend from the heart through the arteries and disappear in the arterioles. During the course of the cardiac cycle, the blood pressure is changing constantly.

A. Systolic Pressure

Systolic pressure is the peak or the highest pressure. It is caused by ventricular contraction. The normal systolic pressure is less than 140 mm. Hg.

B. Diastolic Pressure

Diastolic pressure is the lowest pressure. It is the effect of ventricular relaxation. The normal diastolic pressure is less than 85 mm. Hg.

C. Pulse Pressure

The pulse pressure is the difference between the systolic and the diastolic pressures. The normal or safe difference is less than 55 mm. Hg.

II. Blood Pressure Classification

Table 7–1 (page 94) includes the classification for blood pressure in adults. Normal average blood pressure in mm. Hg at different ages is as follows:[4]

Age	Mean Systolic	Mean Diastolic
1 month	80	46
3 years	100	67
6 years	100	56
9 years	107	57
12 years	115	59
18 and over	140 or less	85 or less

III. Factors That Influence Blood Pressure

A. Maintenance of Blood Pressure

Blood pressure depends on
1. Force of the heart beat (energy of the heart).
2. Peripheral resistance; condition of the arteries; changes in elasticity of vessels, which may occur with age.
3. Volume of blood in the circulatory system.

B. Factors That Increase Blood Pressure

1. Exercise, eating, stimulants, and emotional disturbance.
2. Menopause: In general, women have recorded blood pressure 4 to 5 mm. Hg less than men until menopause, when there is usually an abrupt rise to slightly more than the male average.

C. Factors That Decrease Blood Pressure:

1. Fasting, rest, depressants, and quiet emotions.
2. Emergencies: fainting, blood loss, shock.

IV. Equipment for Determining Blood Pressure

The mercury manometer is usually considered the most reliable recorder of blood pressure. Electronic devices are available, but additional research is needed before their reliability can be fully assured. Another type is the aneroid, which has a round gauge. It requires frequent calibration.

A. Sphygmomanometer (blood pressure machine)

Consists of an *inflatable cuff* and *two tubes,* one connected to the *pressure hand control bulb,* and the other to the *pressure gauge.*

1. *Cuff*
   a. Material. The cuff is made of a nonelastic material and is fastened by a velcro overlap. The inflatable bladder is located within the material of the cuff.
   b. Size. The diameter of the arm, not the age of the patient, determines the size of the cuff selected. There are four cuff sizes available: child size, regular adult, large adult, and thigh. The thigh size is needed for grossly obese persons.
   c. Dimension. The cuff width that is used should be 20 percent greater than the diameter of the arm to which it is applied (figure 7–5). It should cover approximately two thirds of the upper arm.

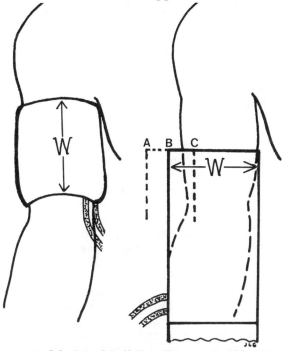

Figure 7–5. Selection of Cuff Size. The correct width (W) is 20 percent greater than the diameter of the arm where applied. **A.** Too wide, **B.** correct width, **C.** too narrow.

When a cuff is too narrow, the blood pressure reading will be too high; when the cuff is too wide, the reading will be too low.[5]

2. *Mercury Manometer*
   a. Gauges are marked with long lines at each 10 mm. Hg, with shorter lines at 2-mm. intervals between each long line.
   b. The level of the column of mercury of the manometer should be at eye level for accurate reading and must not be tilted.

B. Stethoscope (a listening aid that magnifies sound)

Consists of an *endpiece* that is connected by tubes to carry the sound to the *earpieces.*
1. *Types of Endpieces.* Bell-shaped or flat (diaphragm): the bell shape is used for medical examinations, particularly for chest examination.
2. *Care of Earpieces.* Clean by rubbing with gauze sponge moistened in disinfectant.

V. Procedure for Determining Blood Pressure

A. Prepare Patient
1. Tell patient briefly what is to be done. Detailed explanations should be avoided because they may excite the patient and change the blood pressure.
2. Seat patient comfortably, with the arm slightly flexed, with palm up and the whole forearm supported on a level surface at the level of the heart.
3. Use either arm unless otherwise indicated, for example, by a handicap. Repeat blood pressure determinations should be made on the same arm, because there may be as much as 10 mm. Hg difference between arms.
4. Take pressure on bare arm, not over clothing. A tight sleeve should be loosened.

B. Apply Cuff
1. Apply the completely deflated cuff to the patient's arm, supported at the level of the heart. It has been shown that when the arm rests on the arm of a dental chair, higher than the heart, the diastolic pressure shows a small but significant increase.[6]
2. Place the portion of the cuff that contains the inflatable bladder directly over the brachial artery. The cuff may have an arrow to show the point that should be placed over the artery. The lower edge of the cuff is placed 1 inch above the antecubital fossa (figure 7–6). Fasten the cuff evenly and snugly.
3. Adjust the position of the gauge for convenient reading but so that the patient cannot see the mercury.
4. Palpate 1 inch below the antecubital fossa to locate the brachial artery pulse (figure 7–3). The stethoscope endpiece will be placed over the spot where the brachial pulse is felt.

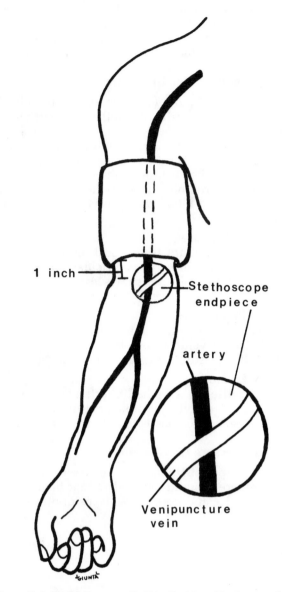

Figure 7–6. Blood Pressure Cuff in Position. The lower edge of the cuff is placed approximately 1 inch above the antecubital fossa. The stethoscope endpiece is placed over the palpated brachial artery pulse point approximately 1 inch below the antecubital fossa and slightly toward the inner side of the arm.

5. Position the stethoscope earpieces in the ears, with the tips directed forward.

C. Locate the Radial Pulse (figures 7–3 and 7–4)
Hold the fingers on the pulse.

D. Inflate the Cuff
1. Close the needle valve (air lock) attached to the hand control bulb firmly but so it may be released readily.
2. Pump to inflate the cuff until the radial pulse stops. Note the mercury level at which the pulse disappears.

3. Look at the dial, and pump to 20 or 30 mm. Hg beyond where the radial pulse was no longer felt. This is the maximum inflation level (MIL). It means that the brachial artery is collapsed by the pressure of the cuff and no blood is flowing through.

Unless the MIL is determined, the level to which the cuff is inflated will be arbitrary. Excess pressure can be very uncomfortable for the patient.

E. Position the Stethoscope Endpiece

Place the endpiece over the palpated brachial artery, 1 inch below the antecubital fossa, and slightly toward the inner side of the arm (figure 7–6). Hold lightly in place.

F. Deflate the Cuff Gradually

1. Release the air lock slowly (2 to 3 mm. per second) so that the dial drops very gradually and steadily.
2. Listen for the first sound: *systole* ("tap tap"). Note the number on the dial that is the *systolic pressure*. This is the beginning of the flow of blood past the cuff.
3. Continue to release the pressure slowly. The sound will continue, first becoming louder, then diminishing and becoming muffled, until finally disappearing. Note the number on the dial where the last distinct tap was heard. That number is the *diastolic pressure.*
4. Release further (about 10 mm.) until there is a cessation of all sounds. That is the second diastolic point. In some clinics and hospitals, the last sound is taken as the diastolic pressure.
5. Let the rest of the air out rapidly.

G. Repeat for Confirmation

Wait 30 seconds before inflating the cuff again. More than one reading is needed within a few minutes to determine an average and assure a correct reading.

H. Record

1. Write date and arm used.
2. Record blood pressure as a fraction, for example 120/80. When both diastolic points are recorded, it can be written 120/80/72.

I. Notify

Call to the prompt attention of the dentist any unusual variation from normal or from previous readings noted in the patient's permanent record.

VI. Blood Pressure Follow-Up Criteria[7]

Table 7–1 (page 94) provides a summary of recommendations at each level of blood pressure findings. Dental personnel have an obligation to advise and *refer for further evaluation.* Diagnosis of hypertension would never be made or treatment started on the basis of an isolated reading.

When the blood pressure is within normal range (140/85), it should be rechecked within 2 years. Rechecking within 1 year rather than 2 is recommended for persons at increased risk for hypertension. The risks include family history, weight gain, obesity, black race, use of oral contraceptives, and excessive alcohol consumption.

TECHNICAL HINTS

I. When a patient's sleeve is drawn back for blood pressure determination, observe the sleeve and the arm for small blood stains or evidence of an injection, which may reveal a mainliner drug addict. The patient may request, even insist, that a particular arm be used. When suspicion of drug abuse has been previously aroused because of physical observation or items in a medical history, determine the blood pressure on both arms to permit observation. Tell the patient that the pressure should always be measured on both sides.

II. Sources of Materials

National High Blood Pressure Education Program
High Blood Pressure Information Center
120/80 National Institutes of Health
Bethesda, Maryland 20205

American Heart Association
7320 Greenville Avenue
Dallas, Texas 75231

FACTORS TO TEACH THE PATIENT

I. How vital signs can influence dental and dental hygiene appointments.

II. The importance of having a blood pressure determination at regular intervals.

III. For patient diagnosed as hypertensive: encourage regular continuing use of prescription drugs for control of high blood pressure.

References

1. Silver, H.K.: Growth and Development, in Kempe, C.H., Silver, H.K., and O'Brien, D., eds: *Current Pediatric Diagnosis and Treatment,* 8th ed. Los Altos, California, Lange Medical Publications, 1984, pp. 20–24.
2. Soltero, D.J. and Whitacre, R.J.: *Vital Signs.* Seattle, Instructional Services, 1978, 48 pp.
3. McCarthy, F.M.: Vital Signs—the Six-Minute Warnings, *J. Am. Dent. Assoc., 100,* 682, May, 1980.
4. Lum, G.M., Todd, J.K., and O'Brien, D.: Kidney and Urinary Tract, in Kempe, C.H., Silver, H.K., and O'Brien, D., eds: *Current Pediatric Diagnosis and Treatment,* 8th ed. Los Altos, California, Lange Medical Publications, 1984, p. 595.
5. Geddes, L.A. and Whistler, S.J.: The Error in Indirect Blood Pressure Measurement with the Incorrect Size of Cuff, *Am. Heart J., 96,* 4, July, 1978.
6. Beck, F.M., Weaver, J.M., Blozis, G.G., and Unverferth, D.V.: Effect of Arm Position and Arm Support on Indirect Blood Pressure Measurements Made in a Dental Chair, *J. Am. Dent. Assoc., 106,* 645, May, 1983.
7. United States Department of Health and Human Services, National High Blood Pressure Coordinating Committee: *The 1988 Report of the Joint National Committee on Detection, Evaluation, and Treatment of High Blood Pressure.* NIH Pub-

lication Number 84–1088, 1988, National Heart, Lung, and Blood Institute, National High Blood Pressure Education Program, 120/80 National Institutes of Health, Bethesda, Maryland 20205.

Suggested Readings

American Academy of Oral Medicine, Special Committee For Clinical Investigation: Vital Signs, *J. Oral Med., 39,* 122, April-June, 1984.

Barsley, R.E. and Phillips, J.H.: Evaluating Venous Pulse and Pressure to Screen for Cardiovascular Disorders, *Compend. Contin. Educ. Dent., 5,* 311, April, 1984.

Beck, F.M. and Weaver, J.M.: Blood Pressure and Heart Rate Responses to Anticipated High-stress Dental Treatment, *J. Dent. Res., 60,* 26, January, 1981.

DiAngelis, N. and Leupker, R.V.: The Effect of the Dental Setting on Blood Pressure Measurement, *Am. J. Public Health, 73,* 1210, October, 1983.

Halstead, C.L., Blozis, G.G., Drinnan, A.J., and Gier, R.E.: *Physical Evaluation of the Dental Patient.* St. Louis, The C.V. Mosby Co., 1982, pp. 74–81.

Ramaprasad, R., Carson, P.H., Congdon, E.B., Barta, P.J., and Ziskin, L.Z.: Dentists and Blood Pressure Measurement: A Survey of Attitudes and Practice, *J. Am. Dent. Assoc., 108,* 767, May, 1984.

Segal, H., Katcher, A.H., and Kieval, R.: Talking and Blood Pressure During Dental Treatment, *Gen. Dent., 33,* 336, July-August, 1985.

Singer, J., Meiller, T.F., and Rubenstein, L.: Blood Pressure Fluctuations During Dental Hygiene Treatment, *Dent. Hyg., 57,* 24, August, 1983.

United States Department of Health and Human Services, National Heart, Lung, and Blood Institute's Task Force on Blood Pressure Control in Children: Report of the Second Task Force on Blood Pressure Control in Children—1987, National Heart, Lung and Blood Institute, 7550 Wisconsin Avenue, Bethesda, Maryland, 20892.

8 Extraoral and Intraoral Examination

A careful overall observation of each patient and a thorough examination of the oral cavity and adjacent structures is essential to total evaluation prior to treatment. A variety of lesions may be observed for which the patient may or may not report subjective symptoms. Recognition, treatment, and follow-up of specific lesions may be of definite significance to the present and future general and oral health of the patient.

Despite the occurrence of many seemingly minor lesions, the danger of oral malignancies remains a definite possibility. In the United States, approximately four percent of all male cancers and two percent of female cancers occur in the area of the oral cavity.[1] Every effort must be made to detect potentially cancerous lesions early.

Each area of the mucous membrane must be examined, and minor deviations from normal must be given prompt attention. A life may depend on an oral examination. Routine examination for each new patient and at each maintenance appointment provides a realistic approach to the control of oral disease.

The oral tissues are sensitive indicators of the general health of the individual. Changes in these structures may be the first indication of subclinical disease processes in other parts of the body.

Although not legally permitted to diagnose, the dental hygienist has the responsibility to observe, record, and call to the attention of the dentist deviations from the normal appearance of the oral cavity. Prerequisite to accomplishing this are knowledge and understanding of the normal morphology, anatomy, and physiology of the oral cavity and the surrounding area, which can be applied in the intelligent recognition of oral conditions.

OBJECTIVES

A thorough examination is essential to the total care of the patient as suggested by the following objectives:

I. To observe the patient overall as well as all areas in and about the oral cavity and to record and call to the attention of the dentist those areas that appear to deviate from normal and that may be evidence of disease.

II. To screen each patient at least annually to detect lesions that may be pathologic, particularly cancer.

III. To recognize a need for postponement of the current appointment because of evidence of communicable disease or in deference to the need for urgent medical consultation and/or treatment.

IV. To prevent the development of advanced, irreversible, or untreatable oral disease by early recognition of initial lesions.

V. To identify suspected conditions that require additional testing and referral for medical evaluation.

VI. To recognize the need for other diagnostic aids that the dentist may use or may direct the dental hygienist to use.

VII. To identify extraoral and intraoral deviations from normal that are related to and for which dental hygiene care and instruction may need special adaptations.

VIII. To provide a means of comparison of individual oral examinations over a series of maintenance appointments, and thus to determine the effects of dental and dental hygiene care and the success of patient instruction.

IX. To provide information for continuing records of the patient's diagnosis and treatment plan for legal purposes.

COMPONENTS OF EXAMINATION

The current concept of patient care is that the total patient is being treated, not only the oral cavity, and particularly not only the teeth and their immediately surrounding tissues. The examination must be, therefore, an all-inclusive one to include any detectable physical, mental, or psychologic influences of the whole patient on the oral health.

Certain parts of the examination may be carried out by the dentist. Other parts will be delegated to the dental hygienist. Thorough examination must become a routine part of each patient appointment if treatment for the control and prevention of oral diseases is to be effective.

Emphasis must be placed on patient and clinician protection from the spread of communicable disease. Therefore, examinations are made using basic gloves, mask, and protective eyeglasses.

I. Preparation for Examination

A. Patient Preparation

1. Review the patient's health histories and other parts of the records.

2. Examine radiographs on viewbox.

3. Explain the procedures to be performed.

B. Instruments and Equipment

Mouth mirror	Gloves
Probe and explorer	Mask
Cotton pliers	Protective eyeglasses
Sponges	Hand mirror for patient
Tongue depressor	

II. Methods of Examination

The various examination methods were described on pages 72–73. The extraoral and intraoral examination is accomplished primarily by direct observation and palpation, but other methods are also used.

A. Direct Observation

Patient position, optimum lighting, and effective retraction for accessibility contribute to the accuracy and completeness of the examination. Visual examination is made in conjunction with other methods.

B. Palpation

Gloved hands are used to move or press tissue to detect changes in consistency and size. Types of palpation include the following:

1. *Digital.* Use of a single finger. Example: index finger applied to inner border of the mandible beneath the canine-premolar area to determine the presence of a torus mandibularis.

2. *Bidigital.* Use of finger and thumb of the same hand. Example: palpation of the lips (figure 8–1).

3. *Bimanual.* Use of finger or fingers and thumb from each hand applied simultaneously in coordination. Example: index finger of one hand palpates on the floor of the mouth inside, while a finger or fingers from the other hand press on the same area from under the chin externally (figure 8–2).

4. *Bilateral.* The two hands are used at the same time to examine corresponding structures on opposite sides of the body. Comparisons may

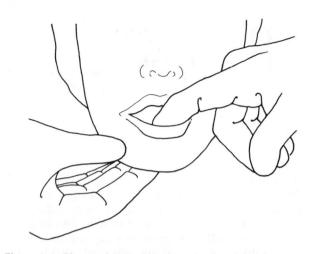

Figure 8–2. Bimanual Palpation. Examination of the floor of the mouth by simultaneous palpation with fingers of each hand in apposition.

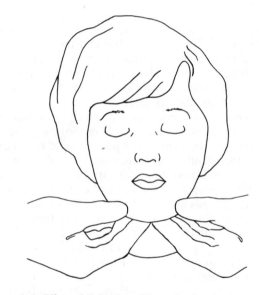

Figure 8–3. Bilateral Palpation. Bilateral palpation is used to examine corresponding structures on opposite sides of the body.

be made. Example: fingers placed beneath the chin to palpate the submandibular lymph nodes (figure 8–3).

SEQUENCE OF EXAMINATION

A recommended order for examination is outlined in table 8–1, in which factors to consider during appointments are related to the actual observations made and recorded. The sequence presented in table 8–1 is adapted from the *Oral Cancer Examination Procedure* available from the American Cancer Society.[2]

I. Systematic Sequence for Examination

The advantages of following a routine order for examination include the following:

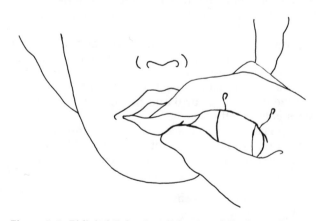

Figure 8–1. Bidigital Palpation. Palpation of the lip to illustrate the use of a finger and thumb of the same hand.

A. Minimal possibility of overlooking an area and missing details of importance.

B. Increased efficiency and conservation of time.

C. Maintenance of a professional atmosphere, which will inspire the patient's confidence.

II. Steps for Thorough Examination (table 8–1)

A. Extraoral

1. Observe patient during reception and seating to note physical characteristics and abnormalities, and make an overall appraisal.
2. Observe head, face, eyes, and neck, and evaluate the skin of the face and neck.
3. Palpate the salivary glands and lymph nodes. Figure 8–4 shows the location of the major lymph nodes of the face, oral regions, and neck.
4. Examine mandibular movement and palpate the temporomandibular joint.

B. Intraoral

1. Make a preliminary examination of the lips and intraoral mucosa, using a mouth mirror or a tongue depressor. Never retract directly with ungloved fingers in the event of an open lesion that may be communicable.
2. View and palpate lips, labial and buccal mucosa, and mucobuccal folds.
3. Examine and palpate the tongue, including the dorsal and ventral surfaces, lateral borders, and base. Retract to observe posterior third: first to one side then the other (figure 8–5).
4. Observe mucosa of the floor of the mouth. Palpate the floor of the mouth (figure 8–2).
5. Examine hard and soft palates, tonsillar areas, and pharynx. Use mirror to observe oropharynx, nasopharynx, and larynx.
6. Note amount and consistency of the saliva and evidences of dry mouth.

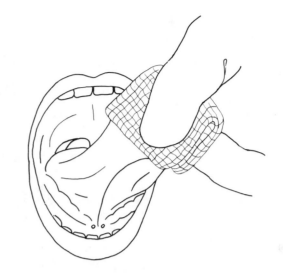

Figure 8–5. Examination of the Tongue. To observe the posterior third of the tongue and the attachment to the floor of the mouth, hold the tongue with a gauze sponge, retract the cheek and move the tongue out, first to one side and then the other, as each section of the mucosa is carefully examined.

DESCRIPTION OF OBSERVATIONS

I. Record Form

A. Contain adequate space for complete descriptions of lesions observed; not merely a check sheet.

B. Contain spaces for successive examinations at follow-up and maintenance appointments.

II. Information to Record

A complete description of each finding includes the location, extent, size, color, surface texture or configurations, consistency, morphology, and history.

A. Location and Extent

When a lesion is first seen, its location is noted in relation to adjacent structures. A printed diagram of parts of the oral cavity drawn into the record form can be a valuable aid for marking the location (figure 8–6). Descriptive words to define the location and extent include the following:

1. *Localized.* Lesion limited to a small focal area.
2. *Generalized.* Involves most of an area or segment.
3. *Single Lesion.* One lesion of a particular type with a distinct margin.
4. *Multiple Lesions.* More than one lesion of a particular type. Lesions may be
   a. Separate: discrete, not running together; may be arranged in clusters.
   b. Coalescing: close to each other with margins that merge.

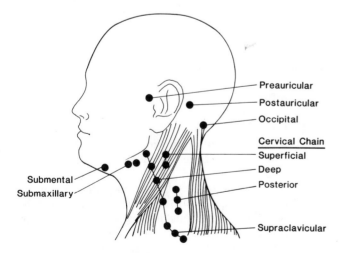

Preauricular
Postauricular
Occipital
Cervical Chain
Superficial
Deep
Posterior
Supraclavicular
Submental
Submaxillary

Figure 8–4. Lymph Nodes. The location of the major lymph nodes into which the vessels of the facial and oral regions drain.

Table 8–1.　Extraoral and Intraoral Examination

Order of Examination	To Observe	Influences on Appointments
1. Overall Appraisal of Patient	Posture, gait General health status; size Hair; scalp Breathing; state of fatigue Voice, cough, hoarseness	Response, cooperation, attitude toward treatment Length of appointment
2. Face	Expression: evidence of fear or apprehension Shape; twitching; paralysis Jaw movements during speech Injuries; signs of abuse	Need for alleviation of fears Evidence of upper respiratory or other infections Enlarged masseter muscle (related to bruxism)
3. Skin	Color, texture, blemishes Traumatic lesions Eruptions, swellings Growths	Relation to possible systemic conditions Need for supplementary history Biopsy or other treatment Influences on instruction in diet
4. Eyes	Size of pupil (figure 8–10) Color of sclera Eyeglasses (corrective) Protruding eyeballs	Dilated pupils or pinpoint may result from drugs, emergency state (Table 60–1, pages 747–754) Eyeglasses essential during instruction Hyperthyroidism
5. Nodes (palpate) (figure 8–4) a. Pre- and postauricular b. Occipital c. Submental; submaxillary d. Cervical chain e. Supraclavicular	Adenopathy; lymphadenopathy Induration	Need for referral Medical consultation Coordinate with intraoral examination
6. Temporomandibular Joint	Limitations or deviations of movement Tenderness; sensitivity Crepitation	Disorder of joint; limitation of opening Discomfort during appointment and during personal plaque control
7. Lips a. Observe closed, then open b. Palpate (figure 8–1)	Color, texture, size Cracks, angular cheilosis Blisters, ulcers Traumatic lesions Irritation from lip-biting Limitation of opening; muscle elasticity; muscle tone Evidences of mouthbreathing Induration	Need for further examination: referral Immediate need for postponement of appointment when a lesion may be communicable or could interfere with procedures Care during retraction Accessibility during intraoral procedures Patient instruction: dietary; special plaque control for mouthbreather
8. Breath Odor	Severity Relation to oral hygiene, gingival health	Possible relation to systemic condition Alcohol use history; special needs

(continued on next page)

B. History

Questions directed to the patient provide necessary information in the management of an oral lesion. Because alarming the patient must be avoided, judgment is needed for selecting the appropriate time to obtain the history of a lesion.

1. Whether the lesion is known or not known to the patient.
2. Duration; changes in size and appearance.
3. Symptoms.

C. Physical Characteristics

1. *Size.* Record length and width in millimeters. The height of an elevated lesion may be significant. Use a probe to measure as shown in figure 8–7.
2. *Color.* Red, pink, white, and red and white are the most commonly seen. Other more rare lesions may be blue, purple, gray, yellow, black, or brown.[3]
3. *Surface Texture.* A lesion may have a smooth or an irregular surface. The texture may be papillary, verrucous or wart-like, fissured, corrugated, or crusted. Other descriptive terms are defined later in IV, page 109.
4. *Consistency.* Lesions may be soft, spongy, resilient, hard, or indurated.

Table 8–1. *Continued*

Order of Examination	To Observe	Influences on Appointments
9. Labial and Buccal Mucosa Left and right examined systematically a. Vestibule b. Mucobuccal folds c. Frena d. Opening of Stenson's duct e. Palpate cheeks	Color, size, texture, contour, Abrasions, traumatic lesions, cheekbite Effects of tobacco use Ulcers, growths Moistness of surfaces Relation of frena to free gingiva Induration	Need for referral, biopsy, cytology Frena and other anatomic parts that need special adaptation for radiography or impression tray Avoid sensitive areas during retraction
10. Tongue a. Dorsal surface b. Lateral borders c. Base of tongue (Retract, see figure 8–5)	Shape: normal, asymmetric Color, size, texture, consistency Fissures; papillae Coating Lesions: elevated, depressed flat Induration	Need for referral, biopsy, cytology Need for instruction in tongue cleaning
11. Floor of Mouth a. Ventral surface of tongue b. Palpate (figure 8–2) c. Duct openings d. Mucosa, frena e. Tongue action	Varicosities Lesions: elevated, flat, depressed, traumatic Induration Limitation or freedom of movement of tongue Frena; tonguetie	Large muscular tongue influences retraction, gag reflex, accessibility for instrumentation Film placement problems
12. Saliva	Quantity; quality (thick, ropy) Evidences of dry mouth: lip wetting Tongue coating	Reduced in certain diseases, by certain drugs Special dental caries control program Influence on instrumentation Need for saliva substitute
13. Hard Palate	Height, contour, color Appearance of rugae Tori, growths, ulcers	Need for referral, biopsy, cytology Signs of tongue thrust, deviate swallow Influence on radiographic film placement
14. Soft Palate, Uvula	Color, size, shape Petechiae Ulcers, growths	Referral, biopsy, cytology Large uvula influences gag reflex
15. Tonsillar Region, Throat	Tonsils: size and shape Color size, surface characteristics Lesions, trauma	Referral, biopsy, cytology Enlarged tonsils encourage gag reflex Throat infection, a sign for appointment postponement (refer to history)

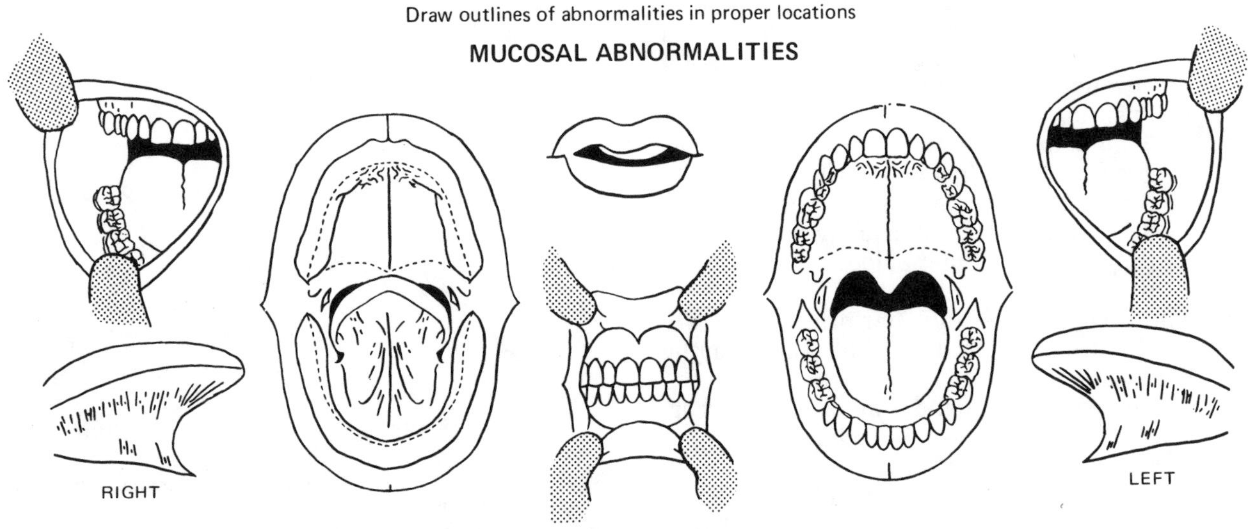

Draw outlines of abnormalities in proper locations

MUCOSAL ABNORMALITIES

RIGHT   LEFT

Figure 8–6. Record Form for Clinical Findings. As part of a clinical examination record form, deviations from normal can be drawn to show the location and relative size. (Courtesy, University of Southern California School of Dentistry.)

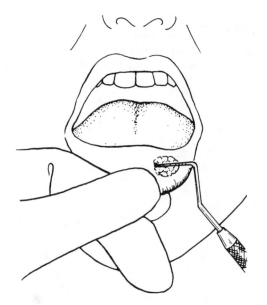

Figure 8–7. Use of Probe to Measure a Lesion. In addition to the exact location, the width and length of a lesion should be recorded. Using the probe provides a convenient method.

III. Morphologic Categories[4,5]

Most lesions can be classified readily as *elevated*, *depressed*, or *flat*, as they relate to the normal level of the skin or mucosa. Tables 8–2, 8–3, and 8–4 break down the terms used for describing lesions in each category. Terms used in the tables are defined here.

A. Elevated Lesions (table 8–2)

An elevated lesion is one that is above the plane of the skin or mucosa. Elevated lesions are considered *blisterform* or *nonblisterform*.

1. *Blisterform.* Blisterform lesions contain fluid and are usually soft and translucent. They may be vesicles, pustules, or bullae.
    a. Vesicle. A vesicle is a small (less than 5 mm. wide), circumscribed lesion with a thin surface covering. It may contain serum or mucin and appear white.
    b. Pustule. A pustule may be more or less than 5 mm. in diameter. It contains pus. Pus gives the pustule a yellowish color.
    c. Bulla. A bulla is large (more than 5 mm.). It is filled with fluid, usually mucin or serum, but may contain blood. The color depends on the fluid content.
2. *Nonblisterform.* Nonblisterform lesions are solid and do not contain fluid. They may be papules, nodules, tumors, or plaques.

Papules, nodules, and tumors are also characterized by the base or attachment. The *pedunculated* lesion is attached by a narrow stalk or pedicle, and the *sessile* lesion has a base as wide as the lesion itself (figure 8–8).

a. Papule. A papule is a small (pinhead to 5 mm. in diameter), solid lesion that may be pointed, rounded, or flat-topped.
b. Nodule. A nodule is larger than a papule (greater than 5 mm. but less than 2 cm.).
c. Tumor. A tumor is greater than 2 cm. in width. In this context, "tumor" means a general swelling or enlargement, and does not refer to neoplasm, either benign or malignant.
d. Plaque. A plaque is a slightly raised lesion with a broad, flat top. It is usually larger than 5 mm. in diameter, with a "pasted on" appearance.

B. Depressed Lesions (table 8–3)

A depressed lesion is one that is below the level of the skin or mucosa. The outline may be regular or irregular, and there may be a flat or a raised border around the depression. The depth is usually described as superficial or deep. A deep lesion is greater than 3 mm. deep.

1. *Ulcer.* Most depressed lesions are ulcers and represent a loss of continuity of the epithelium. The center is often gray to yellow, surrounded by a red border. An ulcer may result from the rupture of an elevated lesion (vesicle, pustule, or bulla).
2. *Erosion.* An erosion is a shallow, depressed lesion that does not extend through the epithelium into underlying tissue.

C. Flat Lesions (table 8–4)

A flat lesion is on the same level as the normal skin or oral mucosa. Flat lesions may occur as single or multiple lesions and have a regular or irregular form.

A *macule* is a circumscribed area not elevated above the surrounding skin or mucosa. It may be identified by its color, which contrasts with the surrounding normal tissues.

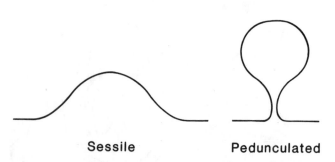

Sessile   Pedunculated

Figure 8–8. Attachment of Nonblisterform Lesions. The *sessile* lesion has a base as wide as the lesion itself; the *pedunculated* lesion is attached by a narrow stalk or pedicle.

Table 8–2. Descriptive Terminology for Elevated Lesions

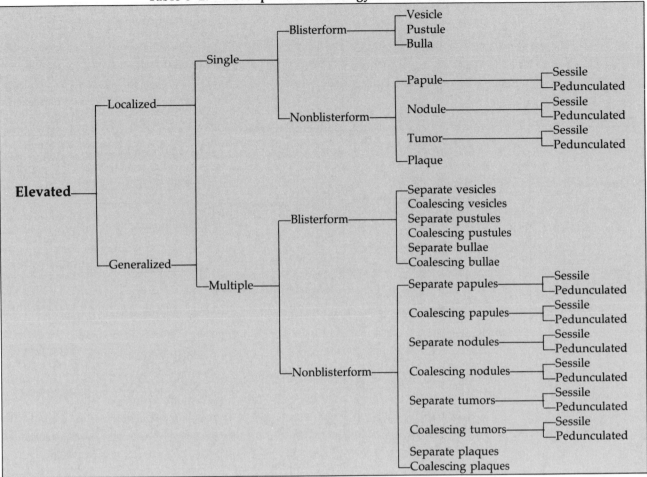

Adapted from McCann, A.L. and Wesley, R.K.: A Method for Describing Soft Tissue Lesions of the Oral Cavity, *Dent. Hyg.,* *61,* 219, May, 1987, with permission of the authors.

IV. Other Descriptive Terms

A. **Crust:** an outer layer, covering, or scab that may have formed from coagulation or drying of blood, serum, or pus, or a combination. A crust may form after a vesicle breaks; for example, the skin lesion of chicken pox is first a macule, then a papule, then a vesicle, and then a crust.

B. **Erythema:** red area of variable size and shape.

C. **Exophytic:** growing outward.

D. **Indurated:** hardened.

E. **Papillary:** resembling a small nipple-shaped projection or elevation.

F. **Petechiae:** minute hemorrhagic spots of pinhead to pinpoint size.

G. **Pseudomembrane:** a loose membranous layer of exudate, containing organisms, precipitated fibrin, necrotic cells, and inflammatory cells, produced during an inflammatory reaction on the surface of a tissue.

H. **Polyp:** any mass of tissue that projects outward or upward from the normal surface level.

I. **Punctate:** marked with points or dots differentiated from the surrounding surface by color, elevation, or texture.

J. **Torus:** bony elevation or prominence usually found on the midline of the hard palate (torus palatinus) and the lingual surface of the mandible (torus mandibularis) in the premolar area.

K. **Verrucous** (verrucose): rough, wart-like.

ORAL CANCER

The objective is to detect cancer of the mouth at the earliest possible stage. Discovered early, it is likely to have a high survival rate; whereas, when a cancer extends into adjacent structures and to the lymph nodes of the neck, the prognosis is less favorable.

Because the early lesions are generally symptomless, they may go unnoticed and unreported by the patient. Observation by the dentist or dental hygienist, therefore, is the principal method for the control of oral cancer. The first step in accomplishing this is to examine the entire face, neck, and oral mucous

Table 8–3.   Descriptive Terminology for Depressed Lesions

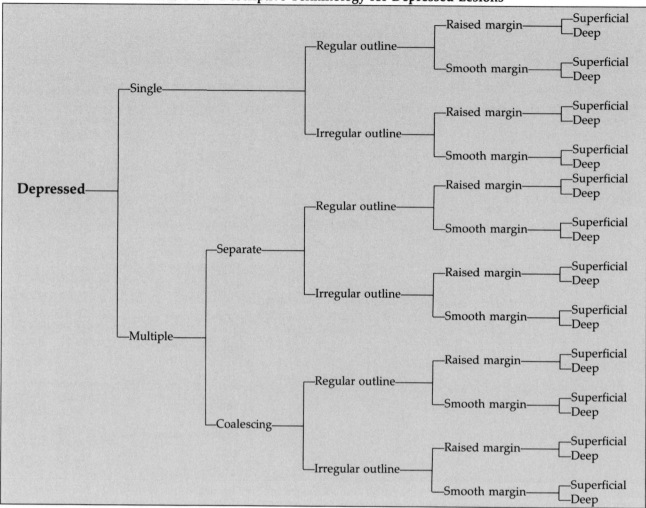

Adapted from McCann, A.L. and Wesley, R.K.: A Method for Describing Soft Tissue Lesions of the Oral Cavity, *Dent. Hyg.,* *61,* 219, May, 1987, with permission of the authors.

Table 8–4.   Descriptive Terminology for Flat Lesions

Adapted from McCann, A.L. and Wesley, R.K.: A Method for Describing Soft Tissue Lesions of the Oral Cavity, *Dent. Hyg.,* *61,* 219, May, 1987, with permission of the authors.

membrane for each patient at the initial examination and at each maintenance appointment.

The dental hygienist needs to know how to conduct the oral examination, where oral cancer occurs most frequently, what an early cancerous lesion may look like, and what to do when such a lesion is found.

I. Location

Tumors may arise at any site in the oral cavity. The most common sites are the floor of the mouth, lateral parts of the tongue, the lower lip, and the soft palate complex.

Although patients may be instructed in self-examination to watch for changes in oral tissues, it is difficult for a person to see his or her own tissues, particularly the entire floor of the mouth and base of the tongue, by the usual mirror and lighting systems available in a private home. Self-examination should be routinely supplemented with professional examination.

II. Appearance of Early Cancer

Early oral cancer takes many forms and may resemble a variety of common oral lesions. All types should be looked at with suspicion. Five basic forms are listed here.

A. White Areas

These may vary from filmy, barely visible changes in the mucosa to heavy, thick, heaped up areas of dry white keratinized tissue. Fissures, ulcers, or areas of induration in a white area are most indicative of malignancy.

A leukoplakia is a white patch or plaque that cannot be characterized as any other disease and is not associated with any physical or chemical causative agent except the use of tobacco.

B. Red Areas

Lesions of red, velvety consistency, sometimes with small ulcers, should be identified.

The term erythroplakia is used to designate lesions of the oral mucosa that appear as bright red patches or plaques that cannot be characterized as any specific disease.

C. Ulcers

These may be with flat or raised margins that may appear similar to traumatic ulcers. Palpation may reveal induration.

D. Masses

Papillary masses, sometimes with ulcerated areas, occur as elevations above the surrounding tissues. Other masses may occur below the normal mucosa and may be found only by palpation.

E. Pigmentation

This appears as brown or black pigmented areas located on mucosa where pigmentation does not normally occur.

III. Procedure for Follow-up of a Suspicious Lesion

As designated by the dentist, a lesion may be biopsied immediately, a cytologic smear may be obtained, or the patient may be referred for additional diagnosis and biopsy.

A. Biopsy

1. *Definition.* Biopsy is the removal and examination, usually by microscope, of a section of tissue or other material from the living body for the purposes of diagnosis. A biopsy is either *excisional,* when the entire lesion is removed, or *incisional,* when a representative section from the lesion is taken.
2. *Indications for Biopsy*[6,7]
   a. Any unusual oral lesion that cannot be identified with clinical certainty must be biopsied.
   b. Any lesion that has not shown evidence of healing in 2 weeks should be considered malignant until proven otherwise.
   c. A persistent, thick, white, hyperkeratotic lesion and any mass (elevated or not) that does not break through the surface epithelium should be biopsied.
   d. Any tissue surgically removed should be biopsied.

B. Cytologic Smear

1. *Definition.* The cytologic smear technique is a diagnostic aid in which surface cells of a suspicious lesion are removed for microscopic evaluation.
2. *Indications for Smear Technique*[6]
   a. In general, a lesion for which a biopsy is not planned may be examined by smear. An exception is a keratotic lesion that is not suitable for exfoliative cytology.
   b. A lesion that looks like potential cancer should be examined by smear if the patient refuses to have a biopsy specimen taken. A positive report from a smear should convince the patient of the need for treatment or biopsy.
   c. The smear technique is used for follow-up examination of patients with oral cancer treated by radiation. The treated tissue may heal inadequately and cause persistent ulceration.
   d. Cytology is useful for identifying *Candida albicans* organisms in patients with suspected candidiasis (moniliasis).
   e. In mass screening programs for cancer detection, smears may be taken. However, all lesions of high suspicion should be referred for biopsy.
   f. Research studies to show changes in surface cells, for example the effects of topical agents, may use a smear technique.

3. *Limitations of Smear Technique*
   a. When a clear-cut lesion, recognized as pathologic, is present, treatment must not be delayed by waiting for cytologic smear analysis.
   b. The smear detects only surface lesions.
   c. It is difficult or impossible to scrape deep enough to obtain representative cells from a heavily keratinized lesion.
   d. Except for candidiasis, treatment cannot be determined by smear technique results only. After a positive smear, a biopsy is needed for definitive diagnosis.
   e. Because research has shown that the smear technique is not diagnostically reliable (there can be "false negatives," which turn out to be positive biopsies), a negative report should not be considered conclusive.

EXFOLIATIVE CYTOLOGY

Stratified squamous cells are constantly growing toward the epithelial surface of the mucous membrane where they are exfoliated. Exfoliated cells and cells beneath them are scraped off, and when prepared on a slide, changes in the cells can be detected by staining and studying them microscopically. The malignant cells stain differently than normal cells and take on unusual, abnormal forms.

I. Procedure

A. Materials

Gauze sponges
Glass microscopic slides with frosted end
Plain lead pencil
Paper clips
Blade to scrape lesion (flexible metal spatula)
Fixative (70% alcohol)
Protective mailing container
History form or data sheet

B. Steps

1. *Prepare Materials.* Write the patient's name on the frosted ends of two glass slides (two for each lesion) in pencil, and place a paper clip on the end of one slide to prevent contact between the slides when packaged for mailing to the laboratory.
2. *Prepare the Lesion.* Irrigate the surface to remove debris. Wipe the surface gently with a wet gauze sponge as needed to remove debris or blood. Do not dry.
3. *Scrape the Lesion.* Use a flexible metal spatula. Scrape the entire surface of the lesion firmly several times (all strokes in the same direction) (figure 8–9A). When a wooden tongue depressor is used, it must be wet before taking the sample so the material will not be absorbed into the wood.
4. *Smear the Glass Slide.* Spread the collected material on the glass slide. Start at the center

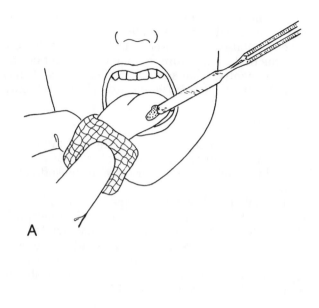

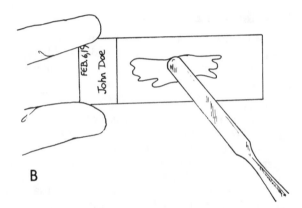

Figure 8–9. Oral Cytology Technique. A. Tongue is held out with gauze sponge while a metal spatula is used to scrape a lesion. **B.** Collected material is spread evenly on a glass slide. See text for details.

of the clear end of the slide and smear evenly across the surface. Cover an area approximately 20 mm. wide. Handle all glass slides by their edges to prevent finger prints or other contamination (figure 8–9B).

5. *Fix the Cells.* Immediately, to prevent drying of the cells, place the slide on a flat surface and flood with generous drops of 70% alcohol or use prepared commercial fixative spray.
6. *Obtain Second Smear.* Duplicate previous smear technique. Apply fixing agent immediately.
7. *Complete the Fixation.* Leave slides for 30 minutes. After 20 minutes, tip the slide to let remaining alcohol run off. Air dry where dust or other foreign material cannot contaminate the smear.
8. *Prepare History or Data Sheet.* Basic information includes the following:
   Dentist: name and address.

Patient: name and address.

Lesion: description (size, color, location, shape, consistency, and duration).

Other related clinical findings or pertinent history.

9. *Prepare for Mailing.* Wrap slides to prevent breakage. Pack with the history or data sheet. Mailing containers, provided by most laboratories, provide specific instructions.

II. Laboratory Report

The pathologist makes the microscopic examination and classifies the specimen in one of the following categories:

Unsatisfactory	Slide is inadequate for diagnosis. The specimen may have been too thick or thin, or the cells may have dried before fixation. Another smear should be made promptly.
Class I	Normal.
Class II	Atypical, but not suggestive of malignant cells.
Class III	Uncertain (possible for cancer).
Class IV	Probable for cancer.
Class V	Positive for cancer.

III. Follow-up

A. Report of Class IV or V
Refer for biopsy.

B. Report of Class III
Re-evaluate clinical findings; biopsy usually indicated.

C. Report of Class I or II
1. The patient must not be dismissed until the lesion has healed.
2. When lesion persists, the dentist will either re-evaluate the clinical findings and request a repeat cytologic smear or perform a biopsy.

D. Negative Report
Either biopsy or smear requires careful follow-up when a negative report is obtained for an oral lesion that appears suspicious by clinical examination. It is possible to have a false negative report; that is, a malignancy may be present, but the sample examined in the smear or biopsy may not have included cancerous cells.

SPECIAL APPLICATIONS FOR THE EXTRAORAL AND INTRAORAL EXAMINATION

In Part VI of this book, many types of patients with special needs for adapted techniques are described. Some of them have general physical and oral characteristics that can be identified during an extraoral and intraoral examination. Facial and oral tissue examinations for pathology apply to all patients.

With certain patients, the recognition of particular characteristics has another dimension, which may have social and legal implications. One example is the group of intraoral and extraoral signs that may reveal a child who is a victim of abuse or neglect. The physical or emotional abuse, neglect, or exploitation of the elderly has also become a problem of growing significance.[8]

Another patient who may not be identified by questions from a medical and dental history is a substance abuser. A variety of treatment problems are related to the care of a patient who misuses drugs. Identification of the patient's addiction can be essential to successful treatment. Characteristics for recognition of certain special patients are described here.

CHILD ABUSE AND NEGLECT

Recognition of a child who has been abused or neglected should be important to the entire dental team. There is a need to be aware of the problem of child abuse, to be able to identify and report suspected cases, and document the injuries observed for future reference and comparison.

During the extraoral and intraoral examination, various findings may lead to a suspicion of child abuse. Head, facial, or oral trauma occurs in 50 to 65 percent of child abuse cases.[9] Some of the patients may be seen in dental offices or clinics, whereas others are taken to a hospital emergency clinic because other serious bodily injuries have been inflicted.

Children ranging from infants through teenagers are involved. Several thousands a year die as a result of the severe physical damage inflicted, while others suffer permanent brain damage or physical deformities.

I. Definitions[10,11]

Maltreatment of children may be categorized as abuse and neglect.

A. Abuse
Abuse refers to nonaccidental physical, sexual, or emotional acts against a child by a parent or caretaker that are beyond the acceptable norms of child care. Characteristically, the injury is more severe than might be expected from the explanation provided by the parent or caretaker.

B. Neglect
Child neglect can be defined as the failure of a parent or other person legally responsible for the child to provide for basic needs at an adequate level of care. Basic needs include food, clothing, health care, safety, and education.

C. Dental Neglect
Dental neglect is defined as the failure of the parent or guardian to seek treatment for visually apparent, untreated dental caries, oral infections and/or oral pain, or failure of the parent or guard-

ian to follow through with treatment once informed that the above condition(s) exists.[12]

II. Recognition[13,14,15]

Recognition of signs of suspected neglect or abuse is the first step toward protection of the child. As the child enters the reception area and then goes into the treatment room, identifiable characteristics may be displayed that are suggestive of abuse.

A. General Signs

1. Behavioral. An abused child may be very fearful and cry excessively, show no fear at all, or appear unhappy and withdrawn. The child may act differently when the parent is present than when alone, which may provide clues to the type of relationship that exists. Frequently, evidence exists of developmental delays, including those of language or motor skills.
2. Overall appearance.
   a. Failure to thrive; malnutrition.
   b. Uncleanliness and other signs of lack of care.
   c. Clothing with long sleeves and long pants even in warm weather, which may suggest that bruises and lacerations are being covered.
3. Abrasions and lacerations of varying degrees of healing; inconsistent with explanations given by the parent.
4. Burns, bite marks, trauma to the eyes, external ears, or the neck.

B. Oral Signs

1. Bruised and swollen lips; scars on lips may show previous trauma.
2. Abrasions at the corners of the mouth, such as from a gag tied around the head.
3. Lacerations of lingual and labial frena, possibly from forced feeding, or related to external traumatic blows.
4. Teeth
   a. Avulsed, fractured, darkened.
   b. Radiograph: signs of fractures in different degrees of healing.
5. Jaw fracture.
6. Tongue injuries: evidence of scarring and recent healing.
7. Signs of dental neglect.
   a. Untreated disease, including rampant caries, pain, inflammation, bleeding gingiva.
   b. Lack or irregularity of professional care. Appointments may have been primarily for tooth removal.

C. Parental Attitude

Parents who abuse their children are frequently immature and not prepared to accept the responsibilities of parenting. On the other hand, they may have been abused by their own parents. Drug abuse and alcoholism are sometimes involved.

Child abuse is very complex. A few of the possible parental attitudes and behavior patterns are mentioned here.

1. Disinterest or denial in relationship to the child; may be critical, scolding, or belittling in front of others, including dental personnel.
2. Lack of interest in proposed dental and dental hygiene treatment plan, with a tendency to want only pain relief for the child. Such an attitude may not be shown toward other children in the family.
3. Unavailable for consultation. Does not usually accompany the child for dental appointments, but sends the child with another sibling.
4. Provides inconsistent information about the sources and causes of damaged teeth, bruises, or other signs of trauma.

III. Reporting

Professional people have a particular responsibility to report suspected child abuse to the proper authorities. Each state in the United States has laws defining and governing child abuse and neglect. In certain states, the failure to report can lead to legal involvement. The failure to recognize and act in behalf of the child may be dangerous, even fatal, for the child involved.

SUBSTANCE ABUSE

It is usually not possible to determine from a patient's medical and dental histories whether the patient uses alcohol and/or unprescribed drugs regularly, perhaps to the level of dependency. The general categories of the drugs of abuse are listed with examples in table 8–5, along with their "street" names. When a history is being prepared, more information may be obtained about drug use if the common street names of products are used. Problems related to the use of alcohol and alcoholism are considered in Chapter 59.

Patients who use drugs recreationally may "premedicate" themselves when a stressful situation such as a dental appointment is anticipated. Because the day-to-day use of drugs varies, questioning at each appointment may be necessary to prevent complications.

When no information is provided by the patient, awareness by dental personnel of the characteristics that suggest the possible use of drugs is important. A few of the common features that may aid in general identification are included in this section. Certain precautions must be taken during patient care.

I. Definitions[16,17]

A. Drug

A drug is a chemical substance used for diagnosis, prevention, or treatment of disease. Drugs are classified by biochemical action, physiologic effect, or the organ system involved.

Table 8–5. Categories of Substances of Abuse with Street Names

Drug Category	Examples	Street Names
Opioids Analgesics	Heroin Morphine	H, Horse, junk, smack, Harry, chip, skag, hard or heavy goods M, white stuff, Miss Emma, hocus, monkey
Central Nervous System Depressants Sedative-Hypnotics Anti-anxiety	Barbiturates Alcohol Diazepam (Valium)	Goofballs, barbs, peanuts, downers, candy, yellows, yellow jackets, reds, red birds, red devils, blue devils, blue heavens, double trouble
Central Nervous System Stimulants	Amphetamines Cocaine Freebase cocaine	Bennies, peaches, splash, speed, crystal, uppers C, coke, Charlie, Cadillac, gold dust, stardust, joy powder, snow Crack
Hallucinogens	LSD (d-lysergic acid diethylamide) Mescaline	Acid, cubes, cupcake, blue dragon, sunshine Big chief, buttons, mesc
Phencyclidines	Phencyclidine Ketamine	Hog, angel dust, peace pill, PCP PCE
Cannabinoids	Marijuana Hashish	Grass, pot, hemp, Mary Jane, weed Cigarettes: joint, reefer, roach Hash, soles
Inhalants	Acetone (paint thinner, model cement) Benzene (adhesives, gasoline) Ethyl acetate (paint thinner) Nitrous oxide (anesthetic, propellant)	

B. Substance Abuse

Substance or drug abuse is the regular use of a drug other than for its accepted medical purpose or in doses greater than considered appropriate.

C. Chemical Dependence

Dependence refers to the interaction between a drug and the individual in which there is a compulsion to take the drug to obtain its effects and/or to avoid the discomforts of withdrawal.

D. Physical Dependence

Physical dependence results when the drug becomes necessary for continued body functioning. An altered physiologic state has developed from repeatedly increasing drug concentrations.

E. Psychologic Dependence

Psychologic dependence refers to the state of mind in which the individual believes the drug is required for maintaining well-being.

F. Tolerance

The state of tolerance means that there is a need for increased amounts of the drug to achieve the same effect.

G. Withdrawal (Abstinence) Syndrome

A group of signs and symptoms, both physiologic and psychologic, occurs on abrupt discontinuation of drug use.

II. Recognition[18,19]

There are many addictive drugs, each with characteristic effects on the user. Specific identification is usually difficult or impossible without information from the patient. Physical and behavioral factors that are common signs of drug abuse are listed below.

A. General Signs

1. Personal appearance
   a. Careless in appearance with apparent lack of interest in dress and personal hygiene; particularly a person who previously was neatly dressed.
   b. Wears long sleeves to cover needle marks.
   c. May have small blood stains on clothes or skin left from previous injections.
   d. Dramatic weight loss.
2. Eyes
   a. Wears sunglasses to conceal dilated or constricted pupils, eye redness, or to avoid bright light because of eye sensitivity.
   b. Pupils dilated (amphetamine, LSD, cocaine, marijuana) (figure 8–10).
   c. Pupils constricted (heroin, morphine, methadone).
   d. Red, inflamed, bloodshot (marijuana).
3. Needle marks on arms. These may be noted

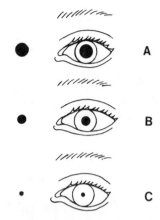

Figure 8–10. Examination of the Pupils. A. Dilated, occurs in shock, heart failure, and other emergencies, and in the use of hallucinogens and amphetamines; **B.** Normal; **C.** Pinpoint, occurs in drug use of morphine and related drugs, heroin, barbiturates. (Adapted from *American National Red Cross, Standard First Aid and Personal Safety.*)

when sleeve is raised to determine the blood pressure.

    4. Unusual behavior[20]
      a. Sneezing; itching.
      b. Tendency to gaze into space; moodiness.
      c. Drowsiness; yawning; may sleep long hours.
      d. Appearance of intoxication without odor of alcohol; slurred speech.
      e. Changes in habits, attitudes, and efficiency or irregular attendance at appointments by a previously conscientious, regular patient.
    5. Possession of pills, capsules.
    6. Hallucinations or convulsions; indicate need for immediate medical emergency care.

B. Oral Characteristics[21,22,23,24]
    1. Poor oral hygiene; lack of personal care or interest in care; diet high in cariogenic substances.
    2. Higher incidence of periodontal infections than peers. Gingival lesions may result from direct application of cocaine.[25,26]
    3. High dental caries incidence with open rampant carious lesions and tooth loss; few if any restorations. The abuse of analgesic drugs, which reduce pain, helps the addict to become indifferent to pain.
    4. Drug-induced xerostomia may relate to high incidence of dental caries.

III. Appointment Factors

A. Drug Effects
    Possible drug interactions should be checked. For example, epinephrine-containing products should not be used when treating habitual marijuana users.[27] Methadone masks the effects of narcotics, so other drugs must be used for pain relief.[28]

Local anesthesia is less frequently successful in addicts than in non-addicts.[29]

B. Postponement of Appointment
    When a patient is under the influence of a drug, only limited procedures should be performed. Not advised are procedures requiring anesthesia or those that involve soft tissue healing.

C. Prophylactic Antibiotic Premedication[20]
    For addicts who inject their drugs, antibiotic premedication has been advised. People who abuse intravenous substances frequently share needles and syringes. Therefore, a greater risk from bacteremia exists. See page 91 for the regimen.

    Many intravenous drug abusers use prophylactic antibiotics regularly to prevent infections.[30] Specific history questions can be directed to obtain this information.

D. Increased Disease Incidence
    There is a high incidence of hepatitis B carriers among addicts who inject their drugs (page 18). Intravenous drug abusers represent one of the highest risk groups for Acquired Immunodeficiency Syndrome (AIDS).[31]

E. Attempt of Addicts to Obtain Prescriptions
    Addicts frequently use dentists to obtain prescriptions of various pain-relieving drugs. By having a toothache, refusing to have the tooth removed but needing pain relief, a prescription can be obtained. Prescription pads should be kept out of sight, as addicts have been known to steal a pad and forge the dentist's signature.

    Drugs kept in the dental office or clinic should be locked in a place inaccessible and unknown to patients to prevent theft. Drugs kept for emergency purposes are described on page 737.

TECHNICAL HINTS

  I. Wear protective gloves when making an intraoral examination to avoid contact with contagious lesions.
  II. Learn the state and community regulations for reporting suspected child abuse and the specific agency that should receive the report. Keep telephone numbers readily available.

FACTORS TO TEACH THE PATIENT

  I. Reasons for a careful extraoral and intraoral examination at each recall.
  II. A method for self-examination. Examination should include the face, neck, lips, gingiva, cheeks, tongue, palate, and throat. Any changes should be reported to the dentist and the dental hygienist.
  III. The Warning Signs of Oral Cancer

A. A swelling, lump, or growth anywhere; with or without pain.
B. White scaly patches, or red velvety areas.
C. Any sore that does not heal promptly (within two weeks).
D. Numbness or tingling.
E. Excessive dryness or wetness.
F. Prolonged hoarseness, sore throats, persistent coughing, or the feeling of a "lump in your throat."
G. Difficulty with swallowing.
H. Difficulty in opening your mouth.

IV. General dietary and nutritional influences on the health of the oral tissues.

V. How the oral cavity tends to reflect the general health.

References

1. Cancer Statistics, 1988, *CA, 38,* 5, January/February, 1988.
2. Engelman, M.A. and Schackner, S.J.: *Oral Cancer Examination Procedure.* Published by Oral Cancer Prevention and Detection Center, St. Francis Hospital, Poughkeepsie, N.Y. Distributed by American Cancer Society, New York.
3. Halstead, C.L., Blozis, G.G., Drinnan, A.J., and Gier, R.E.: *Physical Evaluation of the Dental Patient.* St. Louis, The C.V. Mosby Co., 1982, p. 53.
4. McCann, A.L. and Wesley, R.K.: A Method for Describing Soft Tissue Lesions of the Oral Cavity, *Dent. Hyg., 61,* 219, May, 1987.
5. Halstead, Blozis, Drinnan, and Gier: op. cit., pp. 46–53.
6. Alling, C.C.: History and Examination of the Patient, in Wood, N.K. and Goaz, P.W.: *Differential Diagnosis of Oral Lesions,* 3rd ed. St. Louis, The C.V. Mosby Co., 1985, pp. 26–27.
7. Kerr, D.A., Ash, M.M., and Millard, H.D.: *Oral Diagnosis,* 6th ed. St. Louis, The C.V. Mosby Co., 1983, pp. 296–301.
8. Felder, R., Helm, A., and Koenig, V.: Elder Abuse, *Gerodontics, 2,* 127, August, 1986.
9. Becker, D.B., Needleman, H.L., and Kotelchuck, M.: Child Abuse and Dentistry: Orofacial Trauma and Its Recognition by Dentists, *J. Am. Dent. Assoc., 97,* 24, July, 1978.
10. American Medical Association, Council on Scientific Affairs: AMA Diagnostic and Treatment Guidelines Concerning Child Abuse and Neglect, *JAMA, 254,* 796, August 9, 1985.
11. Schmitt, B.D.: Types of Child Abuse and Neglect: An Overview for Dentists, *Pediatr. Dent., 8,* 67, May, 1986.
12. American Academy of Pediatric Dentistry, Board of Directors: Definition of Dental Neglect, Adopted November 13, 1983.
13. Giangrego, E., ed.: Child Abuse: Recognition and Reporting, *Spec. Care Dentist., 6,* 62, March-April, 1986.
14. Kittle, P.E., Richardson, D.S., and Parker, J.W.: Examining for Child Abuse and Child Neglect, *Pediatr. Dent., 8,* 80, May, 1986.
15. Schmitt, B.D.: Physical Abuse: Specifics of Clinical Diagnosis, *Pediatr. Dent., 8,* 83, May, 1986.
16. Requa, B.S. and Holroyd, S.V.: *Applied Pharmacology for the Dental Hygienist.* St. Louis, The C.V. Mosby Co., 1982, pp. 284–285.
17. Aston, R.: Drug Abuse, in Neidle, E.A., Kroeger, D.C., and Yagiela, J.A.: *Pharmacology and Therapeutics for Dentistry,* 2nd ed. St. Louis, The C.V. Mosby Co., 1985, p. 674.
18. Rosenbaum, C.H.: Did You Treat a Drug Addict Today? *Int. Dent. J., 31,* 307, December, 1981.
19. Aston, R.: Drug Abuse. Its Relationship to Dental Practice, *Dent. Clin. North Am., 28,* 595, July, 1984.
20. Rosenbaum, C.H.: Dental Precautions in Treating Drug Addicts: A Hidden Problem Among Teens and Preteens, *Pediatr. Dent., 2,* 94, June, 1980.
21. Shapiro, S., Pollack, B.R., and Gallant, D.: The Oral Health of Narcotic Addicts, *J. Public Health Dent., 30,* 244, Fall Issue, 1970.
22. Shapiro, S., Pollack, B.R., and Gallant, D.: Periodontal Disease in Narcotic Addicts, *J. Dent. Res., 49,* 1556, November-December, 1970.
23. Scheutz, F.: Dental Health in a Group of Drug Addicts Attending an Addiction-Clinic, *Community Dent. Oral Epidemiol., 12,* 23, February, 1984.
24. Rosenstein, D.I.: Effect of Long-term Addiction to Heroin on Oral Tissues, *J. Public Health Dent., 35,* 118, Spring, 1975.
25. Dello Russo, N.M. and Temple, H.V.: Cocaine Effects on Gingiva (Letters to the Editor), *J. Am. Dent. Assoc., 104,* 13, January, 1982.
26. Gargiulo, A.V., Toto, P.D., and Gargiulo, A.W.: Cocaine Induced-Gingival Necrosis, *Periodont. Case Rep., 7,* 44, Number 2, 1985.
27. Horowitz, L.G. and Nersasian, R.R.: A Review of Marijuana in Relation to Stress-response Mechanisms in the Dental Patient, *J. Am. Dent. Assoc., 96,* 983, June, 1978.
28. Rosenstein, D.I. and Stewart, A.V.: Dental Care for Patients Receiving Methadone, *J. Am. Dent. Assoc., 89,* 356, August, 1974.
29. Scheutz, F.: Drug Addicts and Local Analgesia–Effectivity and General Side Effects, *Scand. J. Dent. Res., 90,* 299, August, 1982.
30. Schaffer, S.R. and Schaffer, S.K.: Use of Prophylactic Antibiotics by Drug Users, *JAMA, 252,* 1410, September 21, 1984.
31. Friedland, G.H., Harris, C., Butkus-Small, C., Shine, D., Moll, B., Darrow, W., and Klein, R.S.: Intravenous Drug Abusers and the Acquired Immunodeficiency Syndrome (AIDS). Demographic, Drug Use, and Needle-sharing Patterns, *Arch. Intern. Med., 145,* 1413, August, 1985.

Suggested Readings

Antoon, J.W. and Miller, R.L.: Aphthous Ulcers—A Review of the Literature on Etiology, Pathogenesis, Diagnosis, and Treatment, *J. Am. Dent. Assoc., 101,* 803, November, 1980.

Bouquot, J.E.: Common Oral Lesions Found During a Mass Screening Examination, *J. Am. Dent. Assoc., 112,* 50, January, 1986.

Bouquot, J.E. and Gundlach, K.K.H.: Odd Lips: The Prevalence of Common Lip Lesions in 23,616 White Americans Over 35 Years of Age, *Quintessence Int., 18,* 277, April, 1987.

Davis, C.C., Hlava, G.L., and Sprague, W.G.: Preliminary Evaluation of Extraoral and Intraoral Lesions, *Dent. Hyg., 56,* 44, January, 1982.

Davis, C.C., Sprague, W.G., and Hlava, G.L.: Preliminary Evaluation of Oral Lesions: What Is This Exophytic Mass on the Gingiva? *Dent. Hyg., 58,* 217, May, 1984.

Dorey, J.L. and Hubbard, F.: Examining the Soft Tissues in Routine Dental Hygiene Practice, *Can. Dent. Hyg., 18,* 37, Summer, 1984.

Eversole, L.R., Silverman, S., Tolley, P., and Polly, M.: The Dental Hygienist as a Comprehensive Head and Neck Cancer Screener, *Educ. Dir. Dent. Aux., 5,* 25, December, 1980.

Giunta, J.L.: *Oral Pathology,* 2nd ed. Baltimore, Williams & Wilkins, 1984, pp. 70–110, 132–136.

Goltry, R.R. and Ayer, W.A.: Head, Neck, and Oral Abnormalities in Dentists Participating in the Health Assessment Program, *J. Am. Dent. Assoc., 112,* 338, March, 1986.

Grushka, M.: Clinical Features of Burning Mouth Syndrome, *Oral Surg. Oral Med. Oral Pathol., 63,* 30, January, 1987.

Halstead, C.L., Blozis, G.G., Drinnan, A.J., and Gier, R.E.: *Physical Evaluation of the Dental Patient.* St. Louis, The C.V. Mosby Co., 1982, pp. 45–73.

Hlava, G., Sprague, W.G., and Davis, C.: Preliminary Evaluation of Extraoral and Intraoral Lesions, *Dent. Hyg., 56,* 44, February, 1982.

Mashberg, A.: Final Evaluation of Tolonium Chloride Rinse for Screening of High-risk Patients with Asymptomatic Squamous Carcinoma, *J. Am. Dent. Assoc., 106,* 319, March, 1983.

Shugar, M.A., Nosal, P., and Gavron, J.P.: Technique for Routine Screening for Carcinoma of the Base of Tongue, *J. Am. Dent. Assoc., 104,* 646, May, 1982.

Skinner, R.L., Davenport, W.D., and Weir, J.C.: A Survey of Biopsied Oral Lesions in Pediatric Dental Patients, *Pediatr. Dent., 8,* 163, June, 1986.

Tolle, S.L. and Allen, D.S.: Oral Cancer Self-examination. The Dental Hygienist's Role, *Dent. Hyg., 59,* 356, August, 1985.

Weidman, B. and Warman, E.: Lymph Nodes of the Head and Neck, *J. Oral Med., 35,* 39, April-June, 1980.

Weir, J.C., Davenport, W.D., and Skinner, R.L.: A Diagnostic and Epidemiologic Survey of 15,783 Oral Lesions, *J. Am. Dent. Assoc., 115,* 439, September, 1987.

White, B.A., Lockhart, P.B., Connolly, S.F., and Sonis, S.T.: The Use of Infrared Thermography in the Evaluation of Oral Lesions, *J. Am. Dent. Assoc., 113,* 783, November, 1986.

Wright, J.M.: Oral Manifestations of Drug Reactions, *Dent. Clin. North Am., 28,* 529, July, 1984.

Wong, P.N.C.: Secondary Syphilis with Extensive Oral Manifestations, *Aust. Dent. J., 30,* 22, February, 1985.

Child Abuse

Bowen, P.L.: Child Neglect Identification: The Hygienist and Child Advocacy, *Dent. Hyg., 54,* 71, February, 1980.

Cahan, W.G.: Opinion. Abusing Children by Smoking, *CA, 37,* 31, January, 1987.

Casamassimo, P.S.: Child Sexual Abuse and the Pediatric Dentist, *Pediatr. Dent., 8,* 102, May, 1986.

Dubowitz, H. and Newberger, E.: Sequelae of Reporting Child Abuse, *Pediatr. Dent., 8,* 88, May, 1986.

Fontana, V.J.: A Physician's View of Responsibility in Reporting Child Abuse, *Spec. Care Dentist., 6,* 55, March-April, 1986.

Kempe, C.H., Silverman, F.N., Steele, B.F., Droegemueller, W., and Silver, H.K.: The Battered Child Syndrome, *JAMA, 181,* 17, July 7, 1962.

Kittle, P.E., Richardson, D.S., and Parker, J.W.: Two Child Abuse/Child Neglect Examinations for the Dentist, *J. Dent. Child., 48,* 175, May-June, 1981.

Marinelli, R.D.: Detecting and Reporting Child Abuse is Your Obligation, *RDH, 3,* 13, September/October, 1983.

McNeese, M.C. and Hebeler, J.R.: The Abused Child. A Clinical Approach to Identification and Management, *CIBA Clinical Symposia, 29,* Number 5, 1977, 36 pp.

Mundie, G.E.: The Importance of a Team Approach When Identifying and Treating Child Maltreatment: A Personal View. *Spec. Care Dentist., 6,* 58, March-April, 1986.

Needleman, H.L.: Orofacial Trauma in Child Abuse: Types, Prevalence, Management, and the Dental Profession's Involvement, *Pediatr. Dent., 8,* 71, May, 1986.

Polk, K.K., Carlin, S.A., and Lee, M.M.: Are Dental Hygiene Educators Teaching Hygienists to Detect Child Abuse, *Educ. Dir. Dent. Aux., 9,* 30, September, 1984.

Primosch, R.E. and Young, S.K.: Pseudobattering of Vietnamese Children (cao gio), *J. Am. Dent. Assoc., 101,* 47, July, 1980.

Regis, J.D.: Early Detection of Child Maltreatment, *Dent. Hyg., 59,* 62, February, 1985.

Schuman, N.J. and Hamilton, R.L.: Discovery of Child Abuse with Associated Dental Fracture in a Hospital-affiliated Clinic: Report of a Case With A Four-year Follow-up, *Spec. Care Dentist., 2,* 250, November-December, 1982.

Sims, A.P.T.: Non-accidental Injury in the Child Presenting as a Suspected Fracture of the Zygomatic Arch, *Br. Dent. J., 158,* 292, April 20, 1985.

Symons, A.L., Rowe, P.V., and Romaniuk, K.: Dental Aspects of Child Abuse: Review and Case Reports, *Aust. Dent. J., 32,* 42, February, 1987.

Drug Abuse

American National Red Cross: *Advanced First Aid and Emergency Care,* 2nd ed. New York, Doubleday, 1982, Chapter 8.

Arthur, M.S. and Roth-Schechter, B.F.: Drug Abuse, in Holroyd, S.V. and Wynn, R.L.: *Clinical Pharmacology in Dental Practice,* 3rd ed. St. Louis, The C.V. Mosby Company, 1983, pp. 411–422.

Brunswick, A.F. and Messeri, P.: Drugs, Lifestyle and Health: A Longitudinal Study of Urban Black Youth, *Am. J. Public Health, 76,* 52, January, 1986.

Chiodo, G.T. and Rosenstein, D.I.: Cocaine Use and Dental Treatment, *Gen. Dent., 34,* 218, May-June, 1986.

Friedlander, A.H. and Mills, M.J.: The Dental Management of the Drug-dependent Patient, *Oral Surg. Oral Med. Oral Pathol., 60,* 489, November, 1985.

Gillespie, J., Kronish, A.D., and Dubin, R.: Anesthetic Management for Dentistry in Patients on Methadone Maintenance, *Anesth. Prog., 27,* 85, May-June, 1980.

Isaacs, S.O., Martin, P., and Washington, J.A.: Phencyclidine (PCP) Abuse. A Close-up Look at a Growing Problem, *Oral Surg. Oral Med. Oral Pathol., 61,* 126, February, 1986.

Isaacs, S.O., Martin, P., and Willoughby, J.H.: "Crack" (an Extra Potent Form of Cocaine) Abuse: A Problem of the Eighties, *Oral Surg. Oral Med. Oral Pathol., 63,* 12, January, 1987.

Mittleman, R.E. and Wetli, C.V.: Death Caused by Recreational Cocaine Use. An Update, *JAMA, 252,* 1889, October 12, 1984.

Scheutz, F.: Dental Habits, Knowledge, and Attitudes of Young Drug Addicts, *Scand. J. Soc. Med., 13,* 35, Number 1, 1985.

Scheutz, F.: Five-year Evaluation of a Dental Care Delivery System for Drug Addicts in Denmark, *Community Dent. Oral Epidemiol., 12,* 29, February, 1984.

Scheutz, F.: Drug Addicts and Local Analgesia—Effectivity and General Side Effects, *Scand. J. Dent. Res., 90,* 299, August, 1982.

Schwartz, R.H. and Hawks, R.L.: Laboratory Detection of Marijuana Use, *JAMA, 254,* 788, August 9, 1985.

Shiloah, J., Lee, W.B., and Binkley, L.H.: Self-inflicted Oral Injury to Secure Narcotic Drugs, *J. Am. Dent. Assoc., 108,* 977, June, 1984.

Wilford, B.B., ed.: *Drug Abuse: A Guide for the Primary Care Physician.* Chicago, American Medical Association, 1981, pp. 21–84.

Young, B.F.: Drug Abuse. What Dental Professionals Should Know, *Dent. Hyg., 60,* 546, December, 1986.

9 *Dental Radiographs*

Radiographs are an essential adjunct to other means of oral diagnosis for treatment planning in the complete care program for a patient. The dentist is responsible for determining the need for radiographs and the number and type to be prepared. Excessive exposure of a patient to low levels of ionizing radiation from dental radiation cannot be justified. Designation of the number and types of dental exposures must be made selectively.

Preparation of radiographs may be one of the first procedures to be accomplished for a patient, following a partial or complete history and a preliminary extraoral and intraoral examination. The radiographs are then available for use during the subsequent complete oral examination and charting. Later, during dental hygiene treatment appointments, the radiographs serve to guide instrumentation and to aid in patient instruction.

The objective in radiography is to use techniques that require the least amount of radiation exposure possible to produce radiographs of the greatest interpretive value. The first consideration is to limit the number of exposures to those that have been determined necessary for the specific requirements of the patient. Quality assurance then can be accomplished by application of known safety measures for the patient and clinician, through analysis of techniques to prevent a need for excess numbers of retakes, through monitoring equipment and processing practices, and through continuing study to keep informed of research developments.[1]

This chapter is designed to serve as a summary of terminology, fundamentals of x-ray production, techniques of exposure and processing, safety factors, analysis of the completed radiograph, and suggestions for patient instruction. A comprehensive bibliography is provided to allow additional study.

TERMS USED IN RADIOGRAPHY*

I. Radiology

Radiology is that branch of medicine dealing with the diagnostic and therapeutic applications of ionizing radiation.

*All definitions in this chapter are taken from or adapted from and in accord with the *Glossary of Dental Radiology,* 2nd ed. prepared by the Committee on Nomenclature, American Academy of Dental Radiology, 1978.

II. Radiation

Radiation is the emission and transmission of energy through space or a material medium in the form of waves; for example, electromagnetic waves. **Ionizing radiation** is any electromagnetic or particulate radiation capable of producing positively and negatively charged ions, directly or indirectly, in its passage through matter.

III. Radiography

The art or science of making radiographs is known as radiography.

IV. Radiograph

A radiograph is an image or picture produced on a radiation-sensitive film emulsion by exposure to ionizing radiation directly through an area or region or substance of interest, followed by chemical processing of the film (noun). To make a radiograph (verb).

V. Types of Radiation

A. Primary

Radiation coming directly from the target of the anode of an x-ray tube is called primary radiation. Except for the useful beam, most of this radiation is absorbed in the tube housing.

B. Useful Beam

The useful beam is that part of the primary radiation that is permitted to emerge from the tube housing as limited by the aperture, lead-lined position-indicating device (PID), or other collimating method.

C. Leakage

Radiation is called leakage radiation when it escapes through the protective shielding and housing of the x-ray tube.

D. Secondary

Radiation emitted by any matter being irradiated with x-rays is known as secondary.

E. Scattered

Scattered radiation during the passage through a substance has been deviated in direction and may have been modified with an increase in wavelength. It is one form of secondary radiation.

F. Stray

Stray radiation is used in a broad sense to include all radiation emitted in directions other than that of the useful beam; for example, leakage radiation, secondary radiation, or scattered radiation.

VI. Irradiation

Irradiation refers to the exposure of material to x-ray or other radiation. One speaks of radiation therapy, but of irradiation of the patient.

ORIGIN AND CHARACTERISTICS OF X-RAY

X-rays were first discovered by Wilhelm C. Roentgen in 1895, who called them x rays after the mathematical symbol "x" for an unknown. "Roentgen rays" is a term often applied to mechanically generated x-rays.

Professor Roentgen used a Crookes tube; it was not until 1913 that William D. Coolidge designed a tube in which electricity was used instead of gas. Modern x-ray tubes have the same principles of construction as the Coolidge tube. The historical development of the science of radiology and radiography provides a realistic monument to the early researchers and their efforts.[2]

I. Definition and Properties of X-Ray

A. X-Ray

Electromagnetic, ionizing radiation of very short wavelength, resulting from the bombardment of a material (usually tungsten) by highly accelerated electrons in a high vacuum.

B. Properties
1. Short wavelength
   a. Hard x-rays: shorter wavelengths, high penetrating power.
   b. Soft x-rays: relatively longer wavelengths, relatively less penetrating; more likely to be absorbed into the tissue through which the x-rays pass.
2. Speed of travel same as visible light.
3. Power to penetrate opaque substances.
4. Invisible.
5. Ability to affect the emulsion of a photographic film.
6. Ability to produce fluorescence on contact with certain crystals.
7. Ability to stimulate or destroy living cells.

II. How X-Rays are Produced[3,4,5,6]

With reference to the definition of x-ray above, essential to x-ray production are (1) a source of electrons, (2) a high voltage to accelerate the electrons, and (3) a target to stop the electrons. The parts of the tube and the circuits within the machine are designed to provide these.

A. The X-Ray Tube (figure 9–1)
1. *Protective Tube Housing.* X-ray tube enclosure that reduces the primary radiation to permissible exposure levels; highly vacuated glass tube surrounded by a specially refined oil with high insulating powers.
2. *Cathode* (−)
   a. Tungsten filament, which is heated to give off a cloud of electrons.
   b. Molybdenum cup around the filament to focus the electrons toward the anode.
3. *Anode* (+)
   a. Copper arm containing a tungsten button, the target, positioned opposite the cathode.
   b. Focal spot: that part of the target on the anode bombarded by the focused electron stream when the tube is energized.
4. *Aperture.* Where the useful beam emerges from the tube; covered with a permanent seal of glass or aluminum.

B. Circuits
1. Low voltage filament circuit.
2. High voltage cathode-anode circuit.

C. Transformers
1. *Autotransformer.* A voltage compensator that corrects minor variations in line voltage.
2. *Step-down Transformer.* Decreases the line voltage to approximately 3 volts to heat the filament and form the electron cloud.
3. *Step-up Transformer.* Increases the current (110 volts) to 65,000 to 90,000 volts to give electrons the required high speed to produce x-ray particles.

D. Machine Control Devices
Machines vary, but in general, in operating an x-ray machine there are four factors to control: the line switch (to electrical outlet), the kilovoltage, the milliamperage, and the time. Certain machines operate at a standard kilovoltage (for example, 65 kVp) and milliamperage (10 mA), whereas others permit a range of selection.
1. *Voltage Control* (may be 1 or 2 meters, depending on the machine).
   a. Circuit voltmeter; registers line voltage before voltage is stepped up by the transformer (with alternating current, this is 110 volts); or may register the kilovoltage that will result after step-up.
   b. KVp (kilovoltage peak) selector: to change the line voltage to a selected kilovoltage (65 to 90 kVp).
2. *Milliamperage Control.* Milliammeter: to select the actual current through the tube circuit used during the time of exposure (10 to 20 mA).
3. *Time Control*
   a. X-ray timer: a time switch mechanism used to complete the electrical circuit so that x-rays will be produced for a predetermined time.
   b. Mechanical timer: spring-activated device; range from ¼ to 10 or 15 seconds; does not

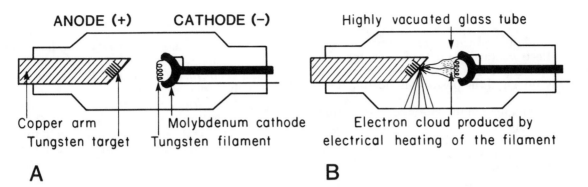

ANODE (+) **CATHODE (−)**

Copper arm
Tungsten target

Molybdenum cathode
Tungsten filament

A

Highly vacuated glass tube

Electron cloud produced by
electrical heating of the filament

B

Figure 9–1. X-Ray Tube. **A.** Inactive. **B.** In function. Highly accelerated electrons are propelled from the cathode to the anode. X-rays are produced as the electrons strike the tungsten target.

reset itself; will not accommodate new high-speed film and techniques.

  c. Electronic timer: vacuum tube device; will reset itself automatically to the last-used exposure time. The timer is calibrated in seconds, with 60 *impulses* in each second (in a 60-cycle AC current).

E. Steps in the Production of X-Rays[4,6]

1. Tungsten filament is heated and a cloud of electrons is produced.
2. Difference in electrical potential is developed between the anode and the cathode.
3. Electrons are attracted to the anode from the cathode at high speed during the intervals of the alternating current, when the anode is charged positive and the cathode, negative. (During the alternating half of the cycle, the electrons are attracted back into the filament in a self-rectifying tube.)
4. Curvature of the molybdenum cup controls the direction of the electrons and causes them to be projected on the focal spot.
5. Reaction of the electrons as they strike the tungsten target: loss of energy.
   a. Approximately 1 percent of the energy of electrons is converted to electromagnetic energy of an x-ray (larger percent at higher kilovoltages).
   b. Approximately 99 percent of the energy is converted to heat, which is dissipated through the copper anode and oil of the protective tube housing.
6. X-rays leave the tube through the aperture to form the useful beam.

FACTORS THAT INFLUENCE THE FINISHED RADIOGRAPH

As the beam leaves the x-ray tube it is collimated, filtered, and allowed to travel a designated source-film (or focal spot-film) distance before reaching the film of a selected speed. The quality or diagnostic usefulness of the finished radiograph as well as the total exposure of the patient and operator are influenced by the *collimation, filtration, source-film distance, film speed, kilovoltage, and milliampere seconds.*

Film processing (pages 141–144) also influences directly the quality of the radiograph and indirectly the total exposure, because re-exposure would be necessary should the film be rendered inadequate during processing.

I. Characteristics of an Acceptable Radiograph

A. All Parts of the Image

Shown as close to their natural size and shape as possible with a minimum of distortion and superimposition.

B. Area to be Examined

Shown completely with sufficient surrounding tissue included to provide for comparative interpretation.

C. Highest Film Quality

1. *Density.* The degree of darkening of exposed and processed x-ray film.
2. *Contrast.* The visual differences in density between adjacent areas on the radiograph.
3. *Definition.* The property of the projected images relating to their sharpness, distinctness, or clarity of outline.

II. Collimation[7,8]

Collimation is the technique or mechanism for controlling the size and shape of the beam of radiation emitted through the aperture of the tube. A *collimator* is a diaphragm or system of diaphragms made of an absorbing material designed to define the dimensions and direction of a beam of radiation.[9]

A. Purposes

1. Eliminate peripheral or more divergent radiation.
2. Minimize exposure to patient's face.
3. Minimize secondary radiation, which can fog the film and expose the bodies of patient and clinician.

B. Methods

1. *Diaphragm.* A diaphragm usually is made of lead and pierced with a central aperture of the smallest practical diameter for making radiographic exposure; it is located between the x-ray tube and the position-indicating device (PID).

   a. Recommended thickness of lead: ⅛ inch.

   b. Recommended size of aperture: to permit a diameter of the beam of radiation equal to 2¾ inches at the end of the PID next to the patient's face.

   c. Use of rectangular collimation: As shown in figure 9–2, a patient receives much less unnecessary radiation with the use of a rectangular PID, because the size of the beam is greatly reduced. When a rectangular diaphragm is used, it should be approximately 1½ × 2 inches at the skin. A rectangular diaphragm must be rotated to accommodate for films positioned horizontally or vertically.

Rectangular collimation has been shown to reduce the exposure and absorbed dose in the bone marrow of the head and neck areas by as much as 60 percent.[9]

2. *Lead-lined Cylindrical PID* (position-indicating device).*

3. *Cylindrical Scatterguard.* A steel cylinder inserted by the manufacturer into the center of the PID where the PID attaches to the aperture of the tube head to prevent scatter rays from reaching parts of the film not being exposed by the primary x-ray beam.[10]

C. Relation to Techniques

The dimensions of the largest periapical film are 1¼ by 1⅝ inches. Precise angulation techniques are required to eliminate "cone-cut" of

---

*The PID was formerly called the "cone" or "plastic cone." Research has shown that the PID must be a lead-lined, open-ended cylinder to prevent secondary radiation.

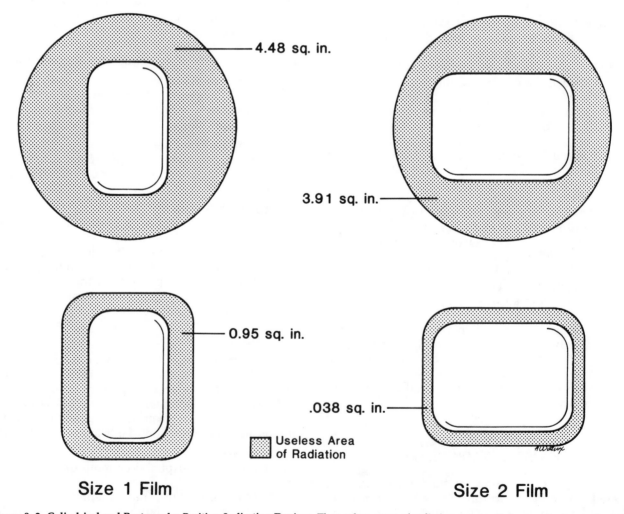

4.48 sq. in.

3.91 sq. in.

0.95 sq. in.

.038 sq. in.

▨ Useless Area of Radiation

Size 1 Film   **Size 2 Film**

Figure 9–2. Cylindrical and Rectangular Position-Indicating Devices. The useless areas of radiation are greatly lessened when rectangular collimation is used. The patient can be spared exposure to excess radiation. (Redrawn from Shannon, S.A.: Rectangular versus Cylindrical Collimation. *Dent. Hyg., 61,* 173, April, 1987; copyright 1987 by the American Dental Hygienists' Association.)

film,* particularly when rectangular collimation is used.

III. Filtration[7,8]

Filtration is the insertion of layers of aluminum for selective removal of x-rays of longer wavelengths from the primary beam.

A. Purpose

To minimize exposure of the patient's skin to unnecessary radiation that will not reach and expose the film.

B. Methods

1. *Inherent Filtration.* Includes the glass envelope encasing the x-ray tube, the glass window in the tube housing, and the insulating oil surrounding the tube.
2. *Added Filtration.* Thin, commercially pure aluminum disks inserted between the lead diaphragm and the x-ray tube.
3. *Total Filtration.* The sum of inherent and added filtration.
   a. Recommended total: equivalent of 0.5 mm. (below 50 kVp); 1.5 mm. (50 to 70 kVp); and 2.5 mm. (over 70 kVp) of aluminum.
   b. Check the inherent filtration of the individual x-ray machine; then add a sufficient amount of commercially pure aluminum to bring the total to the recommended level.

C. Disadvantage of Added Filtration

Some secondary radiation is produced, which scatters in all directions.

IV. Kilovoltage

A. Amount of Kilovoltage

Determines the quality of the x-radiation.

1. Kilovoltage creates a difference in potential between the anode and the cathode for the production of x-rays.
2. The higher the kilovoltage, the greater the acceleration of the electrons, the greater the force with which they bombard the target; therefore, the shorter the wavelength.
3. The shorter the wavelength, the greater the penetrating power at the skin surface.

B. Use of High Kilovoltage (90 kVp)[7]

1. Density of the finished radiograph increases with increased kilovoltage (other factors remaining constant).
2. To maintain the proper film density, the milliampere seconds must be decreased as the kVp is increased.
3. Variation in contrast
   a. Low kilovoltage: high contrast, with sharp black-white differences in densities be-

tween adjacent areas, but small range of distinction between subject thicknesses recorded.
   b. High kilovoltage: low contrast, with wide range of subject thicknesses recorded; greater range of densities from black to white (more gray tones), which, when examined under proper viewing conditions, provide more interpretive details.
4. Advantages
   a. Permits shorter exposure time.
   b. Reduces exposure to tissues lying in front of the film packet.
5. Disadvantages
   a. Increased radiation to tissues outside the edges of the film.
   b. More internal scattered radiation at 90 kVp than at 65 kVp once the primary beam has hit the film; but more scatter at the face with 65 kVp.

V. Milliampere Seconds

A. Milliamperage

The measure of the electron current passing through the x-ray tube; it regulates the heat of the filament, which determines the number of electrons available to bombard the target.

B. Quantity of Radiation

Quantity of radiation is expressed in milliampere seconds (mAs).
1. MAs are the milliamperes multiplied by the exposure time in seconds.
2. Example: at 10 milliamperes for one-half second, the exposure of the film would be 5 mAs.

C. Radiographic Density

Radiographic density increases with increased milliamperage and/or time of exposure (other factors remaining constant).

VI. Distance

Several distances are involved in x-ray film exposure. The source-surface, the source-film, and the object-film distances must be considered for film placement. In addition, there is the distance the clinician stands from the patient's head during film exposure, which is outlined on page 126 in connection with safety factors.

A. Object-Film Distance

In a technique where x-ray films are placed against the teeth being radiographed, the object-film distance is negligible. Close adaptation of the film to the tooth is essential to obtain a sharp image when an 8-inch source-film distance is utilized.

With the paralleling or right-angle technique and use of a longer source-film distance (16 to 20 inches), object-film distance is increased for most radiographs. A collimated beam and increased

---

*"Cone-cut" refers to an error of technique that results when the PID is not angled for the beam of radiation to cover completely the film being exposed. The term "cone-cut" is still commonly used and is used in this chapter.

source-film distance compensate to preserve definition and film quality.

B. Source-Film Distance

The PID on the x-ray machine is designed to indicate the direction of the central axis of the x-ray beam and to serve as a guide in establishing a desired source-surface and source-film distance. Techniques using 8- and 16-inch source-film distances are common.

The source-film distance is the sum total of the distance from the source to the PID within the tube housing, the length of the position-indicating device (PID), and the distance from the end of the PID (at the face) to the film. Directions in technique call for lightly touching the skin with the end of the PID to standardize the source-film distance.

Principles related to source-film distance are as follows:

1. The intensity of the x-ray beam varies inversely as the square of the source-film distance. Example: if a film of the same speed were used at a 16-inch source-film distance as at 8 inches, with all other factors such as kVp and mAs remaining constant, the film at 16 inches would require 4 times the exposure (time) to maintain the same density in the finished radiograph.
2. The exposure decreases as the distance increases: when the distance is made twice as great, the radiation-exposure to the patient is reduced to one-fourth.
3. To maintain film density when distance is increased, an increase in mAs, kVp, or film speed is required.

C. Advantages in the Use of an Extended Source-Film Distance

1. Definition or distinctness and clarity of detail improve (because the image is produced by the more central rays).
2. Enlargement or magnification of image decreases (because at shorter distances the outer, more divergent rays tend to enlarge or magnify the image).
3. Skin exposure of the patient is reduced.
4. Less tissue is within the primary beam of radiation, because less spreading of the x-ray beam occurs.

VII. Films[11]

With optimum filtration, collimation, and fast film, the skin dose to the face can be reduced significantly. Within recent years, the manufacture of very slow-speed films has been discontinued, the speed of many films has been doubled, and the use of higher speed films has gained increasing acceptance by the dental profession.

A. Film Composition

A film is a thin, transparent sheet of cellulose acetate or similar material coated on one or both sides with an emulsion sensitive to radiation and light.

1. *Emulsion.* Gelatin containing a suspension of countless tiny crystals of silver halide salts.
2. *Film Packet.* Small, light-proof, moisture-resistant, sealed paper envelope containing an x-ray film (or two), and a thin sheet of lead foil.
   a. Two-film packet: useful for processing one film differently than the other to make diagnostic comparisons; for sending to specialist to whom patient may be referred; for legal evidence.
   b. Purpose of lead foil backing: to prevent exposure of the film by scattered radiation that could enter from back of packet, and to protect the patient's tissues lying in the path of the x-ray.

B. Film Speed

Film speed or film emulsion speed refers to the sensitivity of the film to radiation exposure. The speed is the amount of exposure required to produce a certain image density.

1. *Factors Determining*
   a. Grain size: the smaller the grain size, the slower the film speed.
   b. Use of double or single emulsion: slower have single, on one side only. Nearly all present-day films have two emulsions.
2. *Classification.* Films have been classified by the American National Standard Institute (ANSI) in cooperation with the American Dental Association (ADA). The ANSI/ADA Specification Number 22 designates six groups, A through F. Speed groups A, B, and C, the slowest, are associated with excess radiation exposure and are not used. Only film speeds D or faster are used for dental purposes. E film requires up to one-half the exposure time used for D film.

EXPOSURE TO RADIATION

Several factors influence the biologic effects of radiation, including the quality of the radiation, the chemical composition of the absorbing medium, the tissues irradiated, the dose (total and rate per unit of time), the blood supply to the tissues, and the size of the area exposed. Generally, radiation of a specific area is less harmful than whole-body radiation. Biologic effects of radiation are either somatic (of the general body cells) or genetic (heritable changes, chiefly mutations, produced by the absorption of ionizing radiation by reproductive cells).

I. Ionization

The phenomenon of separation of electrons from molecules that changes their chemical activity is called ionization. The organic and inorganic compounds that make up the human body may be altered by exposure to ionizing radiation. The biologic effects following irradiation are secondary effects in that they result from physical, chemical, and biologic action set in motion by the absorption of energy from radiation.

II. Permissible Exposure

A. Exposure

A measure of the x-radiation to which a person or object, or a part of either, is exposed at a certain place; this measure is based on its ability to produce ionization.

1. *Threshold Exposure.* The minimum exposure that will produce a detectable degree of any given effect.
2. *Entrance or Surface Exposure.* Exposure measured at the surface of an irradiated body, part, or object. It includes primary radiation and backscatter from the irradiated underlying tissue. The term skin exposure is used with reference to the exposure measured at the center of an irradiated skin surface area.
3. *Erythema Exposure.* The radiation necessary to produce a temporary redness of the skin. The exposure required varies with the quality of the radiation to which the skin is exposed.

B. Exposure Units[12,13]

The International Commission on Radiation Units and Measurements recommended the adoption of new units of absorbed dose expressed in *joules*/kilogram (1 rad = 0.01 j/kg). The new units are shown in table 9–1.

The new unit of measurement is the *gray* (Gy). An absorbed dose of 1 gray is equal to 1 j/kg; therefore, an absorbed dose of 1 Gy is equal to 100 rads.

The new unit of biologic equivalence is the *sievert* (Sv). 1 Sv = 100 rem.

C. Dose

The radiation dose is the amount of energy absorbed per unit mass of tissue at a site of interest. The gonadal dose is the dose of radiation absorbed by the gonads.

D. Permissible Dose

The amount of radiation that may be received by an individual within a specified period with-out expectation of any significantly harmful result is called the *permissible dose.*

Assumptions on which permissible doses are calculated include the following:

1. That no irradiation is beneficial.
2. There is a dose below which no somatic change will be produced.
3. Children are more susceptible than older people.
4. There is a dose below which, even though it is delivered before the end of the reproductive period, the probability of genetic effects will be slight.

E. Radiation Hazard

A condition under which persons might receive radiation in excess of the maximum permissible dose. Exposure would be a risk in an area where x-ray equipment is being used or where radioactive materials are stored.

F. National Council on Radiation Protection and Measurements[14]

1. Limits for dentists and dental personnel (table 9–2).
2. Limits for patients: Exposure to x-ray radiation shall be kept to the minimum level consistent with clinical requirements. This limitation is determined by the professional judgment of the dentist.
3. ALARA concept: Radiation exposures must be kept **As Low As Reasonably Achievable.** This concept is accepted and enforced by all regulatory agencies.

III. Sensitivity of Cells[15,16]

A. Factors Affecting

1. *Maturity of Cell.* Immature cells are most sensitive.
2. *Reproductive Capacity.* Rapidly reproducing cells are more sensitive; most sensitive when undergoing mitosis.
3. *Metabolism.* Cells are more sensitive in periods of increased metabolism.

B. Radiosensitive Tissues

Blood-forming tissues, reproductive cells, lymphatic tissues, young bone tissue, and skin are the most radiosensitive.

Table 9–1. Radiation Units

Definition	Traditional Unit	S.I. Unit*	Equivalent
Unit of Radiation Exposure	Roentgen (R)	Coulomb per kilogram (C/kg)	1 R = 2.58 × 10⁻⁴ C/kg
Unit of Absorbed Dose	Rad	Gray (Gy)	100 rad = 1 Gy
Unit of Dose Equivalent	Rem	Sievert (Sv)	100 rem = 1 Sv
Unit of Radioactivity	Curie (Ci)	Becquerel (Bq)	1 Ci = 3.7 × 10¹⁰ Bq

*S.I. (System International) is from the French *Système International d'Unités*

Table 9–2. Maximum Permissible Dose Equivalent Values (MPD)* to Whole Body, Gonads, Blood-Forming Organs, Lens of Eye[14]

Average Weekly Exposure†	Maximum 13-week Exposure	Maximum Yearly Exposure	Maximum Accumulated Exposure‡
0.1 R	3 R	5 R	5(N-18)R§

*Exposure of persons for dental or medical purposes is not counted against their maximum permissible exposure limits.
†Used only for the purpose of designating radiation barriers.
‡When the previous occupational history of an individual is not definitely known, it shall be assumed that the full dose permitted by the formula 5(N-18) has already been received.
§N = Age in years and is greater than 18. The unit for exposure is the roentgen (R).

C. Radioresistant Tissues

Most glandular tissues, muscle tissue, nerve tissue, and mature bone tissue are radioresistant.

D. Tissue Reaction

1. *Latent Period.* Lapse between the time of exposure and the time when effects are observed. (May be as long as 25 years or relatively short, as in the case of the production of a skin erythema.)
2. *Cumulative Effect*
   a. Amount of reaction depends on dose: reaction is less when radiation is received in fractional doses than in one large dose.
   b. Partial or total repair will occur as long as destruction is not complete.
   c. Some irreparable damage may be cumulative as, little by little, more radiation is added (examples: hair loss, skin lesions, falling blood count).

RULES FOR RADIATION PROTECTION

Dental X-ray Protection prepared by the National Council on Radiation Protection and Measurements[14] provides specific information about radiation barriers, film speed group rating, film badge service sources, x-ray equipment data, and operating procedure regulations.

In the application of procedures for protecting the clinician and the patient from excessive radiation, particular attention should be paid to unnecessary radiation that may result from the need for an unusual number of retakes because of inadequate technical procedures. Perfecting techniques contributes to the accomplishment of minimum exposure for maximum safety.

I. Protection of Clinician

A. Protection from Primary Radiation

1. Stand behind a protective barrier.
2. Avoid the useful beam of radiation.
3. Never hand-hold the film during exposure.
4. Fluorescent mirrors shall not be used in dental examination.

B. Protection from Leakage Radiation

1. Do not hand-hold the tube housing or the position-indicating device of the machine during exposures.
2. Test machine for leakage radiation. Surpak is a film device for surveying dental x-ray machines, which can be obtained at no cost from a State Health Department. The survey determines the size of the beam, the output of the machine, the total filtration, the beam symmetry, and the presence of leakage radiation occurring in a forward direction.

C. Protection from Secondary Radiation

The major sources of secondary radiation are the filter and the irradiated soft tissues of the patient. Formerly when a pointed plastic cone was used for the PID, the cone was a major source of scatter radiation. Other sources may be the leakage from the tube housing, or furniture and walls where the primary beam may contact. Methods of protection are related to these sources.

1. *Minimization of Total X-Radiation*
   a. Use high-speed films. When attempting to use high-speed films with older x-ray machines, the original mechanical timers may prove inadequate. Replacement timers are available.
   b. Replace older x-ray machines with modern shockproof equipment.
2. *Collimation of Useful Beam.* Use diaphragms or PIDs to collimate the useful beam to an area no larger than 2.75 inches in diameter at the patient's skin. Rectangular collimation has been shown to be more effective than round (figure 9–2, page 122).
3. *Type of Position-Indicating Device.* Use an open-ended, shielded (lead-lined) cylinder.
4. *Position of Clinician While Making Exposures.* The clinician shall stand behind the patient's head behind the major sources of secondary radiation, to prevent direct exposure.
   a. Exposure of the region of the central incisors: stand at a 45-degree angle to the path of the central ray. This position is approximately behind either the left or the right ear of the patient (figure 9–3).
   b. Exposure of other regions: stand behind the patient's head and at an angle of 45 degrees to the path of the central ray of the x-ray beam.
5. *Distance*
   a. Safety increases with distance. A long cord on the timer permits greater freedom of movement.
   b. The clinician shall stand as far as practical from the patient, at least 6 feet, outside the

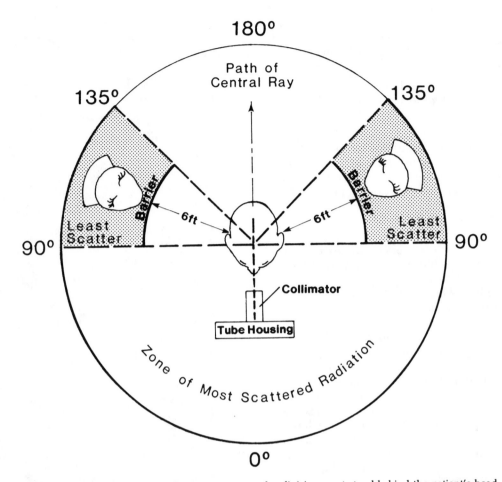

Figure 9–3. Safe Position for Clinician. While making an exposure, the clinician must stand behind the patient's head, at an angle of 45 degrees to the central ray, and at least 6 feet away.

path of the useful beam, and behind a suitable barrier.

c. When space limitations within the dental office prevent occupying the safer positions listed above, the clinician should step out of the room and stand behind a thick wall.

D. Monitoring

Monitoring refers to the periodic or continuous determination of the amount of ionizing radiation or radioactivity present at a given location, usually for considerations of health protection.

The amount of x-ray radiation that reaches the dental personnel can be measured economically with a film badge. Badges can be obtained from one of several laboratories. The film badge is worn on the clothing for 1, 2, or 4 weeks and is then returned by mail to the laboratory where it was purchased. At the laboratory, the film in the badge is carefully processed and its exposure evaluated. The amount of radiation recorded by the film badge is a measure of the exposure of

the wearer, who is notified by mail of the amount of exposure.

II. Protection of Patient

A. Films
Use high-speed films.

B. Collimation
Use diaphragms and open-ended, shielded (lead-lined), rectangular cylinder to collimate the useful beam.

C. Filtration
Use filtration of the useful beam to recommended levels (page 123).

D. Processing
Process films according to the manufacturer's directions. When a choice of two periods of development is offered, the exposure of the patient can be reduced if the longer development time is employed.

E. Film Size
Use the largest intraoral film that can be skillfully placed in the mouth. Maximum coverage is

provided in this manner with one exposure, whereas two exposures may be required if smaller films are used to examine the same area of the mouth. This factor is especially important when examining the mouths of children.

F. Total Exposure

Do not expose the patient unnecessarily. There must be a good and valid reason for each exposure.

G. Patient Body-shields

The use of leaded body-shields for each patient is required by law in many states and countries. The purpose of the shield is to absorb scattered rays. Shields contain the equivalent of 0.25 or 0.3 mm. lead thickness.

1. *Leaded Apron*
    a. Types
        i. General body coverage with extensions over the shoulders and down over the gonadal area.
        ii. Body coverage, with cervical thyroid collar attached.
        iii. Body coverage, with added coverage for the patient's upper back for wear during panoramic radiography.
    b. Care. Leaded aprons and collars should not be folded. If folded and creased, cracks eventually can develop and decrease the effective protection as well as decrease the length of usefulness of the apron. A hanging device or hooks on the wall near the dental chair can provide a convenient arrangement for keeping the apron flat (figure 9–4). Disinfecting the apron is facilitated.
2. *Thyroid Cervical Collar.* Thyroid cancer can result from long-term exposure of the gland to x-rays.[17] The gland should be covered during dental radiographs throughout life. Figure 9–5 shows the position of a thyroid collar over the neckline of a body apron. The gland is positioned over the trachea approximately halfway between the chin and the clavicles.

H. High Voltage

The use of high voltages has been overemphasized. High voltages permit shorter exposure times and reduce the exposure of tissues lying in front of the film packet, but the exposure of the gonads and the tissues lying behind the film packet can increase with increased voltage.

RADIOGRAPHY APPOINTMENT

I. Preliminary Preparation

A. Attention to Infection Control

1. *Surface Disinfection* of patient's surroundings includes wiping the parts of the x-ray machine that are to be handled, in addition to the customary preparation of equipment (pages

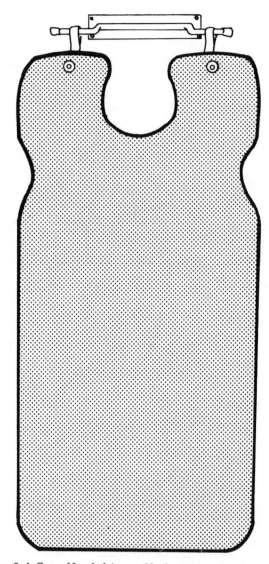

Figure 9–4. Care of Leaded Apron. Hooks or a hanging device near the x-ray machine where the apron can be kept will prevent cracks and prolong the usefulness of the apron.

53–55). Cross contamination by contact of the hands of the clinician with the radiographic equipment has been demonstrated.[18]

2. *Analysis of Procedures* to provide as aseptic a technique as possible. Use of instruments that can be sterilized or items that are disposable and eliminating contacts contributes to a safer routine. Certain film holders minimize finger contact with a patient's oral cavity.

3. *High-risk Patient.* Apply intensive care as described on pages 58–59. Film can be pre-wrapped and sealed in plastic autoclave bagging material before insertion into the oral cavity, and transfer of the film for processing can be accomplished without contamination of the darkroom facility.[19]

4. *Clinician Preparation.* Gloves, glasses, and

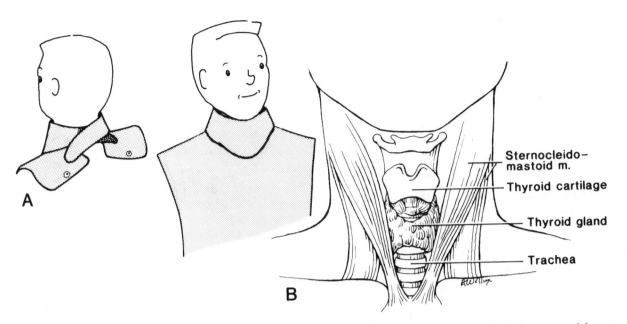

Figure 9–5. Thyroid Cervical Collar. A. Thyroid collar in position, covering the neck and overlapping the leaded apron used for general body coverage. Velcro tabs facilitate overlap fastening at back of neck. Collars are available in child and adult sizes. **B.** The thyroid gland is located over the trachea approximately half way between the chin and the clavicles. Drawing shows anatomic relationship to the sternocleidomastoid muscle.

mask should be worn as for all clinic procedures.

B. Patient Preparation
1. Provide oral antiseptic rinse to minimize microbial count.
2. Remove eyeglasses and removable dental prostheses.
3. For panoramic radiography, earrings are removed.

C. Review Medical and Dental History
1. Obtain information about previous radiation.
2. Apply appropriate precautions.

D. Oral Examination
1. *Purpose.* To determine necessary adaptations during film placement.
2. *Factors of Particular Interest*
   a. Position of teeth and edentulous areas.
   b. Apparent size of teeth as compared with average size of teeth.
   c. Accessibility: height and shape of palate, flexibility of muscles of orifice, floor of the mouth, possible gag reflex, size of tongue.
   d. Unusual features: tori, sensitive areas of the mucous membranes.

II. Patient Cooperation: Prevention of Gagging[20]

Gagging may be the result of psychologic or physiologic factors. It presents some problem in the placement of all films for molar radiographs and may be initiated in the patient who ordinarily does not gag if techniques are not carried out efficiently. Many of the factors related to the prevention of gagging may be applied for the comfort and cooperation of all patients.

A. Causes of Gagging
1. *Hypersensitive Oral Tissues,* particularly of posterior region of oral cavity.
2. *Anxiety and Apprehension*
   a. Fear of unknown, of the film touching a sensitive area.
   b. Previous unpleasant experiences with radiographic techniques.
   c. Failure to comprehend the clinician's instructions.
   d. Lack of confidence in the clinician.
3. *Techniques.* Film moved over the oral tissues or retained in the mouth longer than necessary.

B. Preventive Procedures
1. Inspire confidence in ability to perform the service.
2. Alleviate anxiety; explain procedures carefully.
3. Place film firmly and positively without sliding the film over the tissue.
4. Use a film holder on which the patient can bite to distract from the procedure.
5. Instruct patient to breathe through the nose with quick, short breaths during film placement and to hold the breath during exposure.
6. Use a premedicating agent prescribed by the dentist.
7. Use a topical anesthetic.
   a. Cold water or ice cube held in the mouth for a short time before film placement dulls the sensory nerve endings.

b. Salt: one-half teaspoonful placed on the tongue has an anesthetic effect. It may be swallowed or rinsed after radiographs are made.

c. Prepared topical anesthetics, in the form of an ointment (applied with cotton swab), troche, or rinse can give up to 20 minutes of surface anesthesia (pages 469–470).

TECHNIQUES FOR FILM PLACEMENT AND ANGULATION OF RAY

The characteristics of the acceptable finished radiograph have been listed (page 121), and certain technical factors, including collimation, filtration, kilovoltage, milliampere seconds, distance, and films have been described. For consideration next in the procedure for preparation of radiographs is the placement of the film and the angulation of the useful beam.

Basic intraoral techniques for periapical, bitewing, and occlusal radiographs are included in this chapter. The principles and uses of panoramic radiographs are also described.

Two fundamental periapical techniques are used in practice: the *paralleling* or right-angle and the *angle bisection*. The paralleling technique is sometimes referred to as the "long" or "extension cone" and the angle bisection as the "short cone" technique.

Clinicians vary in their application of the principles of the two techniques. Basically, the primary ray should pass through the region to be examined and the film should be placed in relation to the ray so that all parts of the image are shown as close to their natural size and shape as possible with a minimum of distortion in the finished radiograph.

As with other techniques, the development of a systematic procedure is essential. A comfortable, smooth operation saves time and energy for both patient and clinician, increases the confidence of the patient, and allows for consistency in technique, which produces consistent results. A basic objective during radiographic technique is to minimize the length of time the film packet remains in the patient's mouth.

I. Film Selection for Intraoral Surveys

A. Periapical
1. *Purpose.* To obtain a view of the entire tooth and its periodontal supporting structures.
2. *Films*
   a. Child size: Number 0 (1.0) ($\frac{7}{8}$ × $1\frac{3}{8}$ inches) for primary teeth and small mouths.
   b. Anterior: Number 1 (1.1) ($\frac{15}{16}$ × $1\frac{9}{16}$ inches) for anterior regions where width of arch makes positioning of standard film difficult or impossible.
   c. Standard: Number 2 (1.2) ($1\frac{1}{4}$ × $1\frac{5}{8}$ inches) may be used for all positions.
3. *Number of Films Used in a Complete Survey.*

For the adult mouth, it varies from 14 to 30, depending on the clinician's preferences, objectives for showing specific areas, anatomy of the patient's mouth, and the size of the films used. For children see page 140.

B. Bitewing (Interproximal)
1. *Purpose.* To show the crowns of the teeth, the alveolar crest, and the interproximal area.
2. *Films with Tab Attached*
   a. Anterior teeth ($\frac{15}{16}$ × $1\frac{9}{16}$ inches): three films are usually used.
   b. Adult posterior teeth, standard film size: four films, one for molar region and one for premolar, each side.
   c. Child posterior teeth, with first permanent molar erupted, standard size film; one on each side.
   d. Adult posterior teeth using longer, narrower film: Number 3 ($1\frac{1}{16}$ × $2\frac{1}{8}$ inches) designed to include molars and premolars; one on each side.
3. *Commercial Tabs.* To be attached to standard or child-sized films: two types, one a loop to slide over the film packet and the other with an adhesive to attach directly to the film packet.

C. Occlusal
1. *Purpose.* To show large areas of the maxilla, mandible, or floor of the mouth.
2. *Film.* Number 4 ($2\frac{1}{4}$ × 3 inches) for use in self packet or in intraoral cassette.
3. *Standard Film.* ($1\frac{1}{4}$ × $1\frac{5}{8}$ inches) for child or individual areas of adult.

II. Definitions and Principles Related to Techniques

A. Planes
1. *Sagittal or Median.* The plane that divides the body in the midline into right and left sides.
2. *Occlusal.* The mean occlusal plane represents the mean curvature from the incisal edges of the central incisors to the tips of the occluding surfaces of the third molars. The occlusal plane of the premolars and first molar may be considered as the mean occlusal plane.

   When it is specified in techniques that the occlusal plane of the teeth being radiographed shall be parallel to the floor, at least three head positions are involved for the maxillary: for anterior teeth, the head must be tipped forward; for premolars, held at the mean occlusal plane; and for molars, tipped back.

B. Angulation
1. *Horizontal.* The angle at which the central ray of the useful beam is directed within a horizontal plane. Inadequate horizontal angulation results in overlapping or superimposition of parts of adjacent teeth in the radiograph.
2. *Vertical.* The plane at which the central ray of

the useful beam is directed within a vertical plane. Less vertical angulation than necessary results in *elongation;* and more angulation than necessary creates *foreshortening* of the image.

C. Long Axis of a Tooth

The long axis can be represented by an imaginary line passing longitudinally through the center of the tooth.

Because of marked variations in tooth position and root curvature, estimation of the long axis of a tooth is difficult. Clinically, it can be considered that the long axis of a posterior tooth is at right angles to the occlusal surface plane. For single-rooted teeth, the long axis would ordinarily pass from the center of the incisal edge to the tip of the apex, but it is not possible to observe this during clinical examination. It must be remembered that the line from the incisal edge to the cervical third on the labial surface should not be confused with the long axis.

PERIAPICAL SURVEY: PARALLELING TECHNIQUE

The paralleling or right-angle technique is based on the principles that *the film is placed as nearly parallel to the long axis of the tooth as the anatomy of the oral cavity will permit and the central ray is directed at right angles to the film.* In figure 9–6 A, the parallel relationship of the film with the long axis of the tooth and the right-angle direction of the central ray are shown.

The distance between the crown of the tooth and the film is increased to attain parallelism. In the majority of positions for individual films, the edge of the film against the soft tissues is approximately in the same position on the palate or the floor of the

mouth as when the film is placed against and close to the tooth, for example, in the angle-bisection technique. In other words, the distance between the root apex and the film is not materially different in the paralleling technique from that in the angle-bisection technique. Figure 9–6 A and B shows the comparative projection of the parts of the tooth on the film to produce the image in the radiograph.

I. Patient Position

As long as the film is parallel to the long axis of the tooth and the central ray is directed at right angles to the film, the head may be in any position convenient to the clinician and comfortable for the patient. Slight modification of positioning may be needed for making radiographs in a supine position.[21,22]

New x-ray units have been developed in which an extra-long arm permits equal ease of angulation whether the patient is in an upright or a supine position. With the use of the supine patient position, less radiation to body areas below the neck has been demonstrated.[23]

The use of a film holder (fig. 9–7) facilitates obtaining the correct angulation of the ray, because the PID for the central ray can be lined up with the part of the film holder that extends from between the teeth and that is designed to be at right angles to the film.

For the inexperienced clinician, horizontal angulation may be visualized more readily when the occlusal plane of the teeth being radiographed is parallel with the floor and the sagittal plane is perpendicular to the floor.

II. Film Placement

A. Film Position and Angulation of the Central Ray

Instructions for film placement and angulation are included in this section. In addition to the references associated with specific parts of this

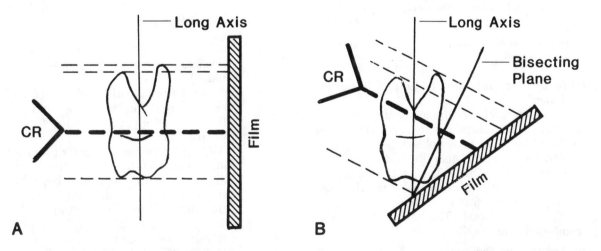

Figure 9–6. Comparison of Paralleling and Angle Bisection Techniques. A. Paralleling technique. The film is parallel with the long axis of the tooth and the central ray (CR) is directed perpendicularly both to the film and the long axis of the tooth. **B.** Angle bisection. The central ray (CR) is directed perpendicularly to an imaginary line that bisects the angle formed by the film and the long axis of the tooth.

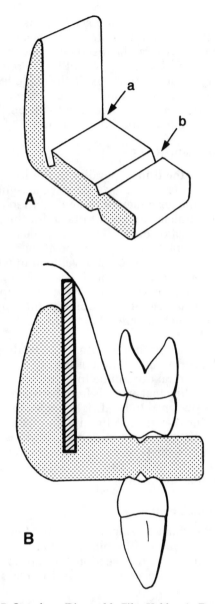

Figure 9–7. Styrofoam Disposable Film Holder. A. Empty holder to show *a*, slot for insertion of the film, and *b*, break-off point to shorten the bite surface for use in the mandibular posterior positions. **B.** Film placement for maxillary molar radiograph for patient with a high palatal vault.

section, further study may be helpful to perfect techniques.[24,25]

1. *Basic Principles* for film placement and angulation of the central ray are shown in figures 9–8 and 9–9. The image objective in the completed radiograph is also illustrated.
2. *Horizontal Angulation.* The ray is directed approximately at the center of the film and through the interproximal area.
3. *Vertical Angulation.* The ray is directed at right angles to the film.

B. Film Positioning Devices

1. *Purposes.* The use of a beam-guiding, field-size-limiting film-holding instrument pro-

vides important advantages, including dose reduction, film quality, and consistently adequate diagnostic radiographs without frequent retakes. Sanitation is improved, and lack of need for patient involvement in holding films is helpful.

2. *Characteristics.* An effective film positioning device has characteristics such as the following:
   a. Adaptable to all necessary positions for obtaining diagnostic radiographs of the entire dental arches.
   b. Weight and other properties that do not hinder placement or holding, without requiring the patient to hand-hold the device.
   c. Comfortable for the patient during the necessary time interval.
   d. Simplicity of placement; minimal complexity for learning.
   e. Aid in alignment of x-ray beam for correct exposure of film.
   f. Disposable or conveniently sterilized. To this end, more than one device should be maintained to permit sterilization between patients.

3. *Types*[26,27]
   a. *Hemostat* is inserted through a rubber bite block and film is positioned and held in claws of the hemostat. The film is positioned in the mouth and held by the patient biting on the bite block.
   b. *Bite blocks:* plastic or wooden (short and long for different areas of the mouth).
   c. *Styrofoam disposable film holder* (Stabe).[28] Simple, comfortable, lightweight device; assists in beam alignment by the end that protrudes after the teeth are closed down to hold the device in place (figure 9–7).
   d. *Precision x-ray device:* has a facial shield attached to the bar, which holds the film in position parallel to the shield. A rectangular hole in the shield permits the passage of only those x-rays that will reach the film. (Distributed by the Precision X-ray Company.)
   e. *Snap-A-Ray:* plastic film holder with two ends for positioning anterior and posterior films. It is held between the teeth. (Rinn Corporation.)
   f. *X-C-P (X-tension C-one P-aralleling):* has an adjustable circular ring that permits film alignment with the primary beam by bringing the open end of the cone in contact with the ring.[24] (Rinn Corporation.)
   g. *V.I.P. (Versatile Intraoral Positioner):* film-holding, beam-directing, with a target attachment for alignment of the open-end tube. It is called versatile because it has holders to accommodate three film sizes

PARALLELING TECHNIQUE
Maxillary

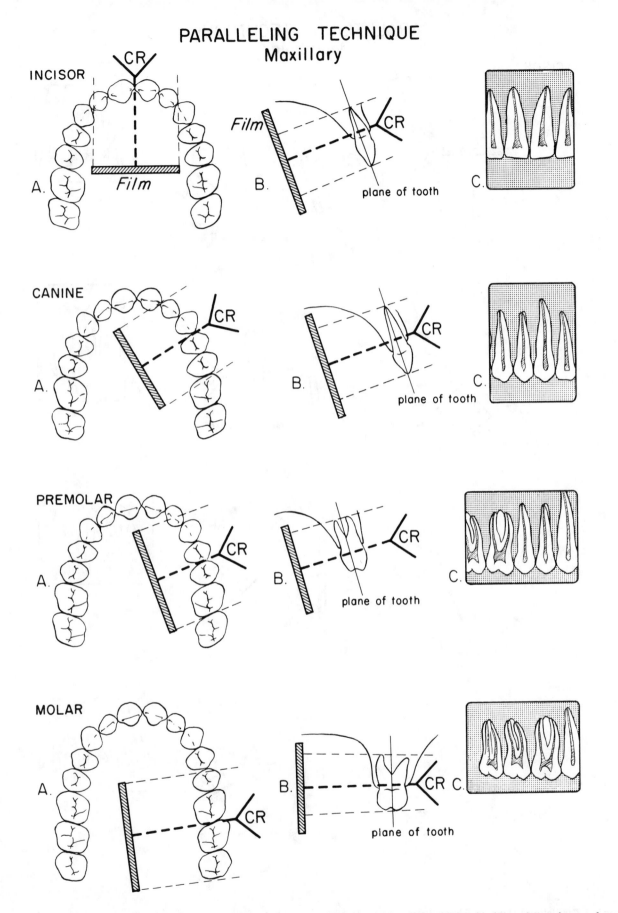

INCISOR

CR

Film

Film

CR

plane of tooth

A.   B.   C.

CANINE

CR

CR

plane of tooth

A.   B.   C.

PREMOLAR

CR

CR

plane of tooth

A.   B.   C.

MOLAR

CR

CR

plane of tooth

A.   B.   C.

Figure 9–8. Paralleling Technique. Film positioning for the four major maxillary positions. Two additional radiographs are frequently made centered at the right and left lateral incisors. **A.** Horizontal angulation, with film placed parallel to the long axes of the teeth; central ray (CR) directed parallel with a line through the interproximal space. **B.** Vertical angulation, with central ray (CR) directed at right angles to the film. **C.** Image objective for the completed radiograph.

PARALLELING TECHNIQUE
Mandibular

INCISOR

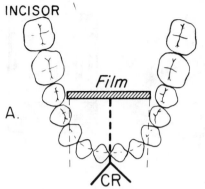 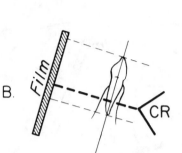 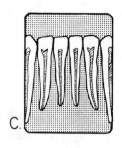

A. B. C.

Film

CR

plane of tooth

CANINE

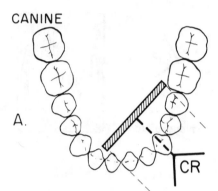 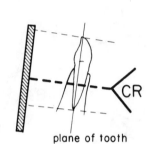 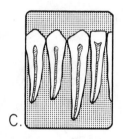

A. B. C.

CR

plane of tooth

PREMOLAR

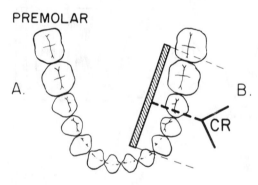 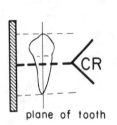 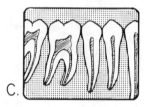

A. B. C.

CR

plane of tooth

MOLAR

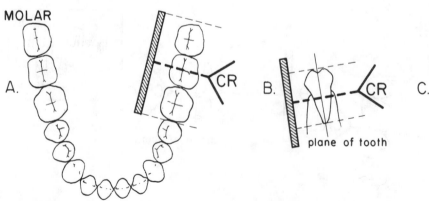 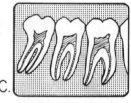

A. B. C.

CR

plane of tooth

Figure 9–9. Paralleling Technique. Film positioning for the four major mandibular positions. Additional radiographs may be made centered at the lateral incisors. **A.** Horizontal angulation, with film placed parallel to the long axes of the teeth; central ray (CR) directed through the interproximal space. **B.** Vertical angulation, with central ray (CR) directed at right angles to the film. **C.** Image objective for the completed radiograph.

and it can be used for periapical and bite-wing surveys. (UP-RAD Corporation.)

4. *Supplements*
   a. Removable denture may be needed in place in opposite jaw to stabilize a film holder.
   b. A cotton roll between the film holder or bite block and the biting surface can aid in paralleling when teeth are short and/or the palatal vault is low.

III. Paralleling Technique: Advantages

A. Accuracy
The paralleling technique gives truer size and shape of dental structures with less distortion than when angle bisection is used.
1. Facial and lingual aspects can be shown in proper relation to each other.
2. Zygomatic bone can be shown in its normal position above the root apices of the molars and premolars.

B. Bitewing Radiographs May Not Be Required
In a complete survey, the right-angle view of proximal surfaces in paralleling technique radiographs is the same as in the bitewing. Time and effort as well as radiation to patient may be saved.

C. Simpler to Perform
Bisection of the angle between the long axis and the film in the bisection technique can be difficult to visualize.

D. Horizontal Ray Direction
No rays are directed toward the thyroid; whereas with angle bisection, several radiographs require a relatively steep vertical angulation.

E. Less Scattered Radiation[29]
Less scattered radiation reaches the walls of the treatment room when the extension paralleling technique is used. The beam is more closely collimated.

BITEWING SURVEY

The bitewing or interproximal survey is used as an adjunct to the periapical survey. It has been used at the time of the maintenance appointment to detect proximal surface caries.

As with all other radiographic surveys, a bitewing survey should be made only when a need is demonstrated for specific diagnostic purposes.

When the angle-bisection technique is used for the periapical radiographs, the bitewing survey is essential, because an accurate view of all proximal surfaces cannot otherwise be obtained. The angulation for the bitewing radiographs is based on the same principle as that for periapical surveys made with the paralleling or right-angle technique.

I. Preparation for Film Placement

A. Patient Position
1. *Traditional.* Sagittal plane perpendicular to the floor and occlusal plane parallel with the floor.
2. *Patient in Supine Position.* The planes are reversed in their relation to the floor.

B. Vertical Angulation
Set at +10 degrees.

C. Patient Instruction
Request patient to practice closing on posterior teeth prior to positioning film for posterior bitewings, and edge-to-edge (figure 15–3 page 228) for anterior.

II. Film Placement and Central Ray Angulation

Figure 9–10 shows in diagram form the position of the molar bitewing film in relation to the teeth, the horizontal and vertical angulation, and the image objective for both the premolar and molar completed radiographs when standard film is used.

A. Position of Film
1. *Molar* (standard film). Mesial border of film at mesial of maxillary second premolar or more distal as needed to include the distal surface of the third molar when it is erupted and in position.
2. *Premolar* (standard film). Mesial border of film at center or mesial of maxillary canine.
3. *Anterior.* Center of film at mesial surface of maxillary canine for the two lateral bitewings: center of film at midline for central bitewing.

B. Position of Directing Cone
With the vertical angulation at +10 degrees, the horizontal angulation is adjusted to direct the central ray to the center of the film. The ray must pass through the interproximal space or parallel to a line through the interproximal space.

C. Maintain Film Flat During Exposure
Although slight curving of the film may be needed for certain patients, depending on the oral anatomy and tissue sensitivity, the basic rule is to keep the film as flat as possible to prevent distortion.

PERIAPICAL SURVEY: ANGLE-BISECTION TECHNIQUE

The angle-bisection technique is based on the geometric principle that *the central ray is directed perpendicularly to an imaginary line that is the bisector of the angle formed by the long axis of the tooth and the plane of the film.* Figure 9–6 B illustrates in diagram form the relationship of the long axis of the tooth, the film, and the bisector of the angle formed by these two.

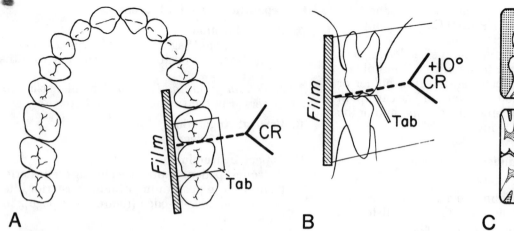
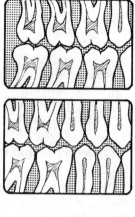

A   B   C

Figure 9–10. Bitewing Radiograph. A. Film position showing horizontal angulation for molar bitewing, with central ray (CR) directed through the interproximal space to the center of the film. **B.** Vertical angulation set at +10 degrees. **C.** Image objective for molar (above) and premolar (below) regions.

I. Patient Position

A. Traditional
1. *Sagittal Plane.* Perpendicular to the floor.
2. *Occlusal Plane.* Parallel with the floor.

B. Patient in Supine Position
The planes are reversed in their relation to the floor.

II. Film Placement and Position

Instructions for film placement and angulation are included in this section. Additional references will be helpful in studying and perfecting techniques.[24,25]

A. Basic Considerations
1. *Center of Film.* At center of teeth being radiographed. The exception to this rule is the maxillary canine film, which is placed slightly distal to accommodate film positioning.
2. *Border of Film.* Located ⅛ to ¼ inches beyond the occlusal or incisal surface.
3. *Film Must Be Kept as Flat as Possible.* A cotton roll may be used with the anterior and maxillary molar films to aid in accomplishing this.

B. Film Position in Relation to Angulation of the Central Ray
Figures 9–11 and 9–12 show the position of the individual films, the horizontal and vertical angulations, and the image objective in the completed radiograph.

III. Direction of the Central Ray

A. Direct the Ray Through the Apical Third of the Teeth Being Radiographed
1. *Maxillary.* To determine location of the apices of the teeth, draw an imaginary line from the ala of the nose to the tragus of the ear, and the apices will be approximately at that level.
2. *Mandibular.* Apices are located approximately ½ inch above the lower border of the mandible.

B. Horizontal Angulation
The ray should pass through the interproximal or parallel to a line through the interproximal space, at approximately the center of the area being radiographed.

C. Vertical Angulation
Bisect the angle formed by the film and the long axes of the teeth, and direct the ray perpendicular to this line.

D. Average Angles for Vertical Angulation
1. *Uses*
   a. For the anatomically ideal mouth: it would be expected that the average angle and the angle determined by the bisection principle would be the same.
   b. As a point from which to begin when bisecting the angle: usually the angle of the bisection would be within 5 to 10 degrees of the average angle.
   c. As a time saver in angle-bisection technique: prior to placing the film in the patient's mouth, the PID is positioned at the average angle to facilitate angulation and prevent undue discomfort on the part of the patient.
2. *The Average Angles*

Maxillary		Mandibular	
Central	+ 40–45	*Central*	− 15–20
Canine	+ 45–50	*Canine*	− 20–25
Premolar	+ 30–35	*Premolar*	− 10–15
Molar	+ 20–25	*Molar*	− 5– 0

OCCLUSAL SURVEY

The use of occlusal films is particularly important for observing areas that cannot be completely or conveniently shown on other films, in cases where positioning periapical films is difficult or impossible, to supplement the angulation provided by other films

BISECTING ANGLE TECHNIQUE
Maxillary

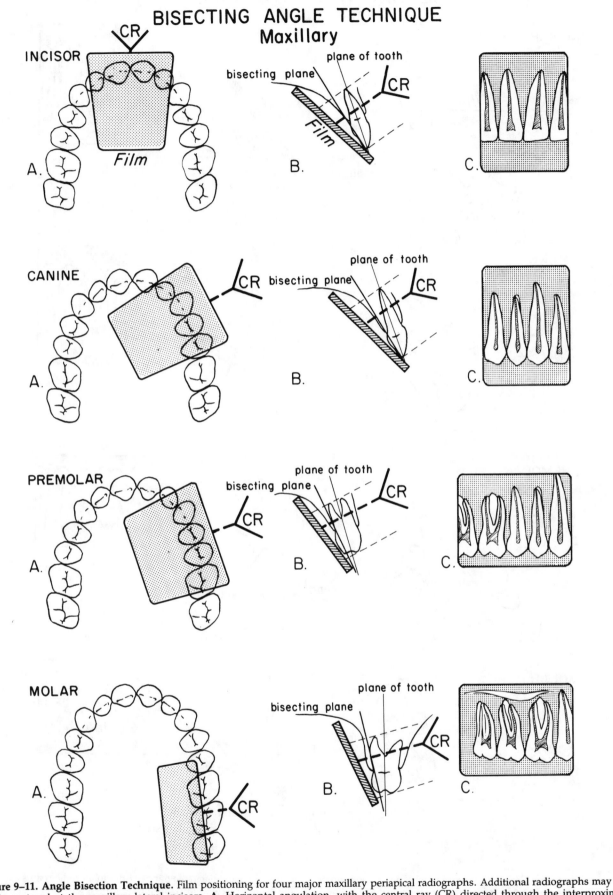

Figure 9–11. Angle Bisection Technique. Film positioning for four major maxillary periapical radiographs. Additional radiographs may be made centered at the maxillary lateral incisors. **A.** Horizontal angulation, with the central ray (CR) directed through the interproximal space. **B.** Vertical angulation, with central ray (CR) directed perpendicularly to the bisector of the angle formed by the film and the long axes of the teeth. **C.** Image objective for the completed radiograph.

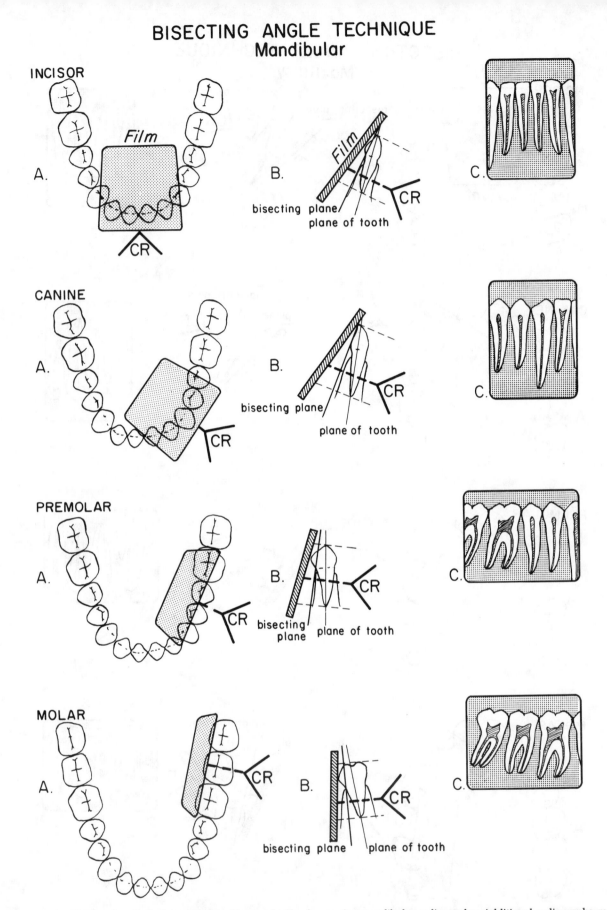

BISECTING ANGLE TECHNIQUE
Mandibular

INCISOR

A.

Film

CR

B.

Film

bisecting plane
plane of tooth

CR

C.

CANINE

A.

B.

bisecting plane

plane of tooth

CR

C.

PREMOLAR

A.

B.

bisecting plane

plane of tooth

CR

C.

MOLAR

A.

CR

B.

bisecting plane

plane of tooth

CR

C.

Figure 9–12. Angle Bisection Technique. Film positioning for the four major mandibular radiographs. Additional radiographs may be centered at the right and left incisors. **A.** Horizontal angulation, with the central ray (CR) directed through the interproximal space. **B.** Vertical angulation, with central ray (CR) directed perpendicularly to the bisector of the angle formed by the film and the long axes of the teeth. **C.** Image objective for the completed radiograph.

for such conditions as fractures, impacted teeth, or salivary duct calculi, and as a specific part of a complete survey for edentulous or very young patients.

The central midline films for maxillary and mandibular are described in this section. A variety of positions for the occlusal films is possible, depending on the area to be examined. Additional references will be helpful as a guide.[30,31]

I. Maxillary Midline

A. Position of Patient's Head

The line from the tragus of the ear to the ala of the nose is parallel with floor.

B. Position of Film

The emulsion side is toward the palate; posterior border of film is brought back close to third molar region; film is held between the teeth with edge-to-edge closure.

C. Angulation

The PID is directed toward the bridge of the nose at a 65-degree angle.

D. Exposure

Consult chart of film manufacturer's specifications for exposure related to source-film distance, kilovoltage, and milliamperage. When a cassette is used, exposure time is reduced, an advantage in prevention of movement of the film.

II. Mandibular Midline

A. Position of Patient's Head

The head is tilted directly back.

B. Position of Film

The emulsion side is toward the floor of the mouth, the posterior border of the film is in contact with the soft tissues of the retromolar area, and the film is held between the teeth in an edge-to-edge bite.

C. Angulation

For the incisal region, the PID is pointed at the tip of the chin at an angle of approximately 55 degrees. For the floor of the mouth, the PID is directed from under the chin, perpendicular to the film.

D. Exposure

Consult chart of film manufacturer's specifications.

PANORAMIC RADIOGRAPHS

Panoramic radiography refers to techniques that produce films showing large areas of the maxillary and mandibular arches with adjacent structures on one or more extraoral films. This type of radiograph is a supplement to a periapical survey but not a substitute because of less sharpness and detail in the panoramic radiograph. The derived benefit must be weighed against the additional exposure to a wide area of tissues outside the oral tissues.

I. Types of Panoramic Techniques[32,33]

A. Tomography or Curved-Surface Laminography

Lamina means layer, and in this technique, a single layer of the teeth and surrounding structures appears in the radiograph. Other structures do not appear superimposed as they do in traditional extraoral techniques. The head is stabilized with a chin support or one of several types of head holders characteristic of each machine. Two methods are used in laminography.

1. Film and x-ray source rotate around the patient's head. Examples are the Panorex (S.S. White), Panelipse II (General Electric), and the Orthopantograph (Siemens).
2. Patient is rotated between the x-ray source and the film. An example is the Rotagraph (Watson, England).

B. Still-Picture Technique

An intraoral fine-focus x-ray tube is placed within the patient's mouth.

1. Film in cassette is molded to the face, using separate films for the mandible and the maxilla. An example is the Status-X (Siemens).
2. Head and film positioners are used to make a series of lateral jaw radiographs. An example is the Orthoramix (Dental Corporation of America) which attaches to a conventional x-ray machine. With the Orthoramix, four overlapping exposures are made to cover the entire maxillary and mandibular arches.

II. Uses

Because definition and detail are inferior to periapical radiographs and because distortion occurs, panoramic radiographs provide an overall view, not a detailed one. They do not show proximal carious lesions except for large cavities, which can be seen by direct examination. They are also inadequate for examination of periodontal supporting structures.

Routine use of panoramic radiographs for patients seeking general oral care cannot be recommended.[34,35] Possible uses are listed here.

A. Oral Pathology

The area surveyed in oral examination increases with the use of a panoramic radiograph, but the number of pathologic lesions found has been shown to be small.[34] Rarely is it possible to base a diagnosis on a panoramic radiograph alone.[36]

B. Edentulous Patient

A panoramic survey prior to making complete dentures can usually provide sufficient information for most patients.[37]

C. Orthodontics

The overall view of growth and development at the beginning of orthodontic observation, diagnosis, and treatment, and during the treatment, to assess periodic progress, can be helpful to the orthodontist.

D. Patients for Whom Conventional Radiographs Cannot Be Used

For patients with handicaps or systemic conditions that hinder cooperation, such as patients with trismus, temporomandibular joint disability, Parkinson's disease, facial paralysis, intermaxillary fixation, or with facial trauma, when examination may not be possible by intraoral techniques.

III. Limitations

A. Inferiority of Definition and Detail

Causes of poor definition are
1. Use of intensifying screens.
2. Increased object-film distance.
3. Movement of x-ray tube and film.

B. Distortion

1. Magnified images are produced because of increased film-object distance.
2. Overlapping. In periapical techniques, each film is angulated with the central ray so that when a tooth is out of line, adjustment is made to prevent overlapping. With panoramic technique, the head and teeth remain fixed, and the ray and film are positioned for the average only.

IV. Technique[32]

Learning to use panoramic equipment is not difficult. Each machine has its own characteristics that can be learned readily from the manufacturer's instructions.

A. Patient Preparation

The use of a leaded apron with a collar or a separate thyroid shield is important.[36,38,39,40] A special shield for panoramic radiography is available with coverage over the shoulders and part way down the back.[40]

B. Film

Film sizes are usually either 5 × 12 or 6 × 12 inches. Speed film should be used to minimize radiation. The new master-control panoramic radiography can be performed at 4 mA for increased patient safety, compared with 8 mA of previous machines.

C. Processing

Regular processing solutions are used for panoramic film. Special film holders may be obtained.

CHILD PATIENT SURVEY

For all ages, the frequency of making radiographic surveys as well as the selection of type, size, and number of films to be used is based on individual patient evaluation. The objective is to minimize exposure of children to radiation. Low levels of x-radiation are associated with the induction of cancer, and children are more sensitive than adults.[36]

The need for radiographs in a healthy child is limited when the oral cavity appears free from disease as shown by direct clinical examination.[41] A specific rule of frequency for making complete surveys is not in keeping with current knowledge of radiation hygiene and safety.

With consideration of risk and benefit, five categories have been suggested for which radiographs may be indicated. These are the detection of congenital dental anomalies in the mixed dentition of children undergoing complete dental care or needing orthodontic treatment; detection of proximal surface dental caries when close contacts do not permit direct examination; third molar evaluation; infection; and trauma to the teeth or jaws.[36]

In addition, periodontal radiographic evaluation may be needed after probing reveals the presence of bone loss and periodontal pockets. Prepubertal periodontitis, although relatively rare, may be generalized or localized and may be evident as early as 4 years of age. Severe bone destruction is characteristic.[42]

The aim for a young child is to make as thorough a clinical evaluation of the teeth and the surrounding structures as possible. The real need for radiographs can then be determined.

I. Primary Dentition

When radiographs are indicated, various combinations of periapical, bitewing, occlusal, panoramic, and extraoral films have been recommended by the specialists.[43,44,45] Film size is suggested that will be consistent with the size of the mouth, the cooperation of the patient, and the ability of the clinician. Examples of number and size of films for three effective surveys are listed here.

A. Occlusal views of anterior maxillary and mandibular (standard film) and posterior bitewings (child or adult anterior film); total of four films.
B. Occlusal views of anterior maxillary and mandibular and maxillary posterior (standard film), posterior bitewings (child or standard film), and extraoral lateral jaw films (5 × 7 inches).
C. Periapical views for each posterior quadrant and one each for anterior (child size film); total of six films.

II. Mixed Dentition (6 to 9 Years)

When a complete survey is determined necessary, 12 to 14 exposures using standard film are suggested. These include two posterior bitewings, four molar (to include first permanent and primary molars), four canine, and two or four incisor periapical views.

III. Technique with Children[46]

A. Use of Leaded Apron and Thyroid Collar

Children are more susceptible than adults to low-level radiation.

B. Orientation to Lessen Apprehension

1. For a young child's first visit to the dental office, making the radiographic survey may be

a necessary first procedure. When the child is not able to cooperate, the survey may be delayed until the second or even the third visit except in an emergency.

2. Explain procedures carefully; rehearse to show what is to be done; repeat instructions with each film placement.

C. Sequence

Make the easiest, most comfortable exposures first (extraoral, panoramic, occlusal).

D. Periapical Films

Use film holder.

EDENTULOUS SURVEY

I. Types of Surveys

Periapical, occlusal, and panoramic surveys have been used alone and together for edentulous patients. The periapical series, usually of 14 films, has been shown to be the most complete and accurate for diagnosis. Radiographic examination of an edentulous mouth is frequently used to detect residual pathologic conditions, foreign bodies, and retained teeth or root tips prior to denture construction.

In research to compare three techniques—panoramic; two occlusal films, one maxillary and one mandibular; and a 14-film periapical survey—total residual and potential disease was found in 37 percent of the periapical surveys, 17 percent of the occlusal radiographs, and 31 percent of the panoramic.[47] A detailed review of the retained root tips in the same study proved that the occlusal films were of little value, whereas the periapical survey revealed 115 tips to only 71 in the panoramic.[48] The research makes it clear that panoramic and occlusal films by themselves cannot be relied on to provide complete information.

II. Techniques for Periapical Survey

A. Film Placement

1. *Paralleling Technique.* A film holder adjusted to provide a wider biting area is needed.
   a. Rubber bite block on a hemostat: turn bite block around so that the broader dimension is in the vertical plane.
   b. Film holder can be padded with cotton rolls.
2. *Angle Bisection Technique.* Use cotton rolls to aid in positioning the films, and increase the angulation to accommodate flattened film.

B. Exposure Time

The time is reduced by approximately 25 percent.[49]

PARACLINICAL PROCEDURES

Supplemental to the chairside clinical procedures are the processing of the films and the mounting of radiographs for diagnostic and clinical use. Standard procedures are outlined in the following sections.

I. Definition

Film processing is the chemical transformation of the latent image, produced in a film emulsion by exposure to radiation, into a stable image visible by transmitted light. The usual procedure is basically a selective reduction of affected silver halide salts to metallic silver grains (development), followed by the selective removal of unaffected silver halide (fixation), washing to remove the processing chemicals, and drying.

II. Infection Control

Personnel of each office or clinic need to work out a specific protocol appropriate to the facility and the type of processing used. Suggested ideas for consideration are proposed here.

A. Films become covered with saliva and should be confined to a disposable cup after exposure.

B. Gloved hands fresh from the patient's film positioning should not contact walls, doors, or light switches when transporting the cup of contaminated exposed films to the darkroom.

C. In the darkroom, films can be opened carefully and "spilled" out of their wrapping onto a clean paper bench cover. Gloves can then be changed before placing the films on the processing rack or in the automated processor slot.

D. Wrappers are placed directly in a specific waste receiver that will be tied up for disposal without further contact.

E. Generous use of disinfectant on environmental surfaces is important.

CONVENTIONAL PROCESSING

Standardization of processing procedure goes hand in hand with standardized exposure techniques if consistently acceptable radiographs are to be prepared. Processing should be treated as an exacting chemical operation in which each step has specific objectives for the finished product. Fast and extra-fast film are even more sensitive to variations in temperature, light, and processing chemicals than are the medium and slow film formerly in general use; hence, the need for fastidious attention to detail.

I. Essentials of an Adequate Darkroom

Cleanliness and orderliness are mandatory. Because the films are handled in near darkness, materials must be available at the fingertips and each piece of equipment must be kept in its own place.

The work area must be free from chemicals, water, dust, and other substances that can contaminate the film either by splashing or direct contact should a film touch the bench. The processing room should not be used as a storage room or for other dental procedures in which dust or fumes might be produced.

Convenience and ease in carrying out precision techniques can be provided through good planning for the location and arrangement of equipment.

A. **Lighting**
 1. *Darkroom Completely Void of White Light*
  a. Find and eliminate all possible light leaks.
  b. Do not use fluorescent overhead light because of afterglow.
 2. *Safelight*
   By following a manufacturer's instructions on a film package, the correct and safe lighting can be used. Different films require different light filters. A 7.5-watt bulb is used in a light fixture 4 feet above the working surface, and a filter selected for the light in accord with the type of film.
  a. Filter Type GBX-2 (red filter) designed for both intraoral and extraoral film.
  b. Filter Type ML-2 (orange filter) is for intraoral films only.
 3. *Safe Lighting Test[50]*
  a. Unwrap a film in totally dark darkroom.
  b. Place film on work tabletop and place a coin on the film.
  c. Turn on safelight and leave for maximum amount of time (such as 5 minutes) typical of that required when preparing a survey to be processed.
  d. Turn off safelight, remove coin, process film.
  e. Observe the radiograph: if any evidence exists of a light circle where the coin was placed, the darkroom safelight is excessive.
 4. *Lock on Door of Darkroom.* A signal light should be on the outside to show that the room is in use.

B. **Basic Equipment and Facilities**
 1. *Tanks* for developer and fixer with water bath between
  a. Removable tanks made of stainless steel with joints welded and polished to prevent reactions with the processing chemicals.
  b. Close-fitting, light-proof cover for tank.
  c. Stirring paddles identified specifically for developer and fixer.
  d. Water bath with connecting water flow and temperature control indicator.
  e. Floating tank thermometer (kept in developer tank).
 2. *Workbench.* Covered with linoleum or Formica for easy cleaning.
 3. *Drying Facilities.* Rod to hold hangers over drip pan; electric fan to facilitate drying.
 4. *Utility Sink.*
 5. *Interval Timing Clock.*
 6. *Storage Area* beneath workbench for materials to change solutions.

 7. *Waste Receiver.* Conveniently located for ready disposal of film wrappers to prevent losing films in midst of paper wrappers.

C. **Care of Solution**
 1. *Factors Affecting Life of Solution*
  a. Original quality (care in preparation).
  b. Age.
  c. Care received (temperature, whether kept covered, contamination).
  d. Number of films processed.
 2. *Changing Solutions.* At least every 3 weeks.
 3. *Preparation of New Solution*
  a. Tanks must be thoroughly scrubbed with water and a soft brush and then thoroughly rinsed.
  b. Label tanks as well as stirrers and mixing jars to prevent possibility of interchange.
  c. Follow manufacturer's specifications and directions precisely.

D. **Protection of Solution**
 1. *Use Same Position for Tank Cover* so that same cover routinely is used for the same solution.
 2. *Purposes for Covering Tanks*
  a. Prevent evaporation: which can change the concentration of the solutions and lower the level so the top film on rack is not covered during processing.
  b. Prevent oxidation: reduces useful life of solution.
  c. Prevent contamination: dust, drippings.
 3. *Temperature.* Keep cool when not in use: heated solutions can oxidize rapidly.
 4. *Replenisher.* Between changing of solutions, freshness may be maintained by replenishment according to manufacturer's specifications.

II. **Processing**

A. **Preparation**
 1. Stir solutions and check temperature of solutions and water bath: all should be 20° C (68° F) (within 2°)
  a. Lower temperatures: chemical reactions too slow.
  b. Higher temperatures: cause fogging and may soften the emulsion.
 2. Check cleanliness of workbench and film racks; wash hands to prevent film contamination.
 3. Plan number of films to be processed so that facilities will not be overcrowded: films must hang individually, out of possible contact with other films, sides of tanks, or wall in drying area.
 4. Prepare labels for identification of radiographs.
 5. Extinguish white lights; turn on safelight; lock door.
 6. Load film hangers

a. Hold film by edges to avoid finger marks, scratches, or bending.

b. Clip firmly; test by pulling gently on film.

B. Developing

1. Set timer. (Refer to time-temperature chart provided by the film manufacturer.*)
2. Completely immerse rack with films in developer; turn on timer.
3. Agitate racks (without splashing) to eliminate air bubbles and assure contact of solution with all film surfaces.
4. When timer rings, remove racks to water or to a stop bath.

C. Rinsing

1. Immerse in freely running water for at least 30 seconds: agitate to provide contact of water with film.
2. Stop bath: a 10% acetic acid may be preferred in place of running water: immerse for 30 to 45 seconds.
3. Remove and drain for several seconds to prevent carrying an excess of water or acetic acid to the fixing bath.

D. Fixing

1. Immerse completely; set and start timer.
2. Agitate racks to remove air bubbles and assure contact of the solution with all parts of the film surfaces.
3. Clearing time: time needed for complete disappearance of white or milky opaqueness.
4. Total fixing time: minimum of twice clearing time
   a. Check manufacturer's specifications.
   b. Minimum of 10 minutes and maximum of 1 hour are safe; excess time will produce a light radiograph.
5. Wet readings can be made after fixing 2 to 3 minutes. Rinse in water before taking to the viewbox. Return to the fixer for completion of the fixing process.

E. Washing

1. Place in running water bath for minimum of 20 minutes.
2. Temperature: 20° C (68° F)
   a. Too warm: gelatin will swell, thus hindering diffusion.
   b. Drastic temperature changes cause reticulation (network of wrinkles or corrugations in the emulsion); retake necessary.

F. Drying

1. Drain off water and place in dryer.
2. Radiographs become brittle when left in a heated drying cabinet too long.

---

*The time-temperature method of processing is the only way to be assured of dependable results. Processing by the "visual inspection" method is not recommended because of the lack of standardization.

III. How the Image is Produced

A. The Chemistry of Processing

1. Film emulsion contains crystals of silver halides (bromide and iodide).
2. X-ray exposure changes the silver halides to silver and halide ions.
3. Developer reacts with the halide ions, leaving only the metallic silver in a specific arrangement corresponding with the radiolucency and radiopacity of the tissue being radiographed.
4. Fixer removes only those crystals of silver halide that were not affected by the action of the x-rays. Fixer has no affect on the black metallic silver produced by the developer.
5. End result: a negative, showing various degrees of lightness and darkness (microscopic grains of black metallic silver).

B. Developer Action

1. Purpose: to remove the halides from the metallic silver.
2. Constituents
   a. Developing agents (reducers): *elon* brings out detail and *hydroquinone* reacts slowly and brings out contrast.
   b. Preservative: sodium sulfite: to protect the developing agents from oxidizing rapidly in air.
   c. Restrainer: potassium bromide: inhibits the fogging tendency of the solution and slows the reaction of the reducers.
   d. Activator (alkali): sodium carbonate: initiates the action of the reducers with the halides.
3. Transfer to water bath at completion of developing time: if racks are shaken or allowed to drip over the developer, the solution falling back into the tank will be highly oxidized, which will shorten the life of the solution.

C. Rinsing Purposes

1. To stop the developing process.
2. To remove the developing solution from the emulsion to reduce carry-over of alkaline developer to the acid fixing bath.
3. To preserve the acidity of the fixer, and hence, make a more efficient, longer lasting fixing bath.

D. Fixer Action

1. *Purpose:* To remove the undeveloped halide salts.
2. *Constituents*
   a. Fixing agent: sodium thiosulfate ("hypo"): to dissolve the silver halides.
   b. Acidifer: acetic acid: to neutralize the alkali from the developer.
   c. Hardener: potassium alum: to shrink and harden the emulsion.
   d. Preservative: sodium sulfite: to counteract

surface oxidation and stabilize the solution.

E. Washing Purpose
To remove residual chemicals from the negative.

AUTOMATED PROCESSING

Film selection varies: certain film can be processed by manual or automated means only, whereas other film may be processed by either. Generally, film that may be processed by either method requires more exposure of the patient to radiation.[51]

I. Objectives and Advantages

Although cost and maintenance factors may be greater than with a traditional darkroom procedure, an automated and/or rapid processing machine has advantages, including those listed below.
A. Conservation of time by dental personnel.
B. Finished radiographs in 5 to 8 minutes, depending on the machine used. Some have dryers.
C. Consistency of results through automated control of temperature and time.
D. Radiographs available for immediate use during diagnosis, which is particularly important in emergencies, during endodontic therapy, and certain surgical procedures.

II. Principles of Operation

Manufacturer's instructions must be followed and routine care and cleaning attended to for maintenance of equipment.

Automated or accelerated processing (or both) is accomplished by one or a combination of the following:

A. Automated Film Transport

Rollers or tracks are used to carry the film through developing, washing, and fixing, then washing again, and finally, forced drying. Certain machines produce wet films and do not have hot-air drying chambers. The various machines available are built to carry different sizes of film. Some machines may process only standard intraoral films, whereas others may also accommodate extraoral sizes.

B. High Temperature

Increased temperature decreases processing time. Special solutions are needed for the rapid processors, because with conventional solutions the excess temperature causes deterioration and fogging of the film. Solution temperatures in the automated and rapid processors may be from 17° to 38° C (62° to 100° F), and with drying temperatures up to 65° C (150° F), the total processing and drying may take about 5 minutes.

C. Use of Special Films and Processing Solutions

1. *Concentrated Processing Solution.* Solutions with increased chemical reactivity decrease developing time. In one type of machine, a combined developer-fixer is used that eliminates the need for film to pass through two solutions. The diagnostic quality of the film is generally less with the special solutions.
2. *Films.* Films with special emulsions have been developed that process best at higher temperatures and with the special processing solutions.

D. Agitation

Mechanically controlled movement of the film and/or movement of the solution is built into some units to provide fresh solution continuously at the film surface. This decreases the processing time.

ANALYSIS OF COMPLETED RADIOGRAPHS

The completed radiographs are mounted and examined at a viewbox with an adequate light source. Interpretation of radiographs is difficult for the dentist and the determination of a pathologic condition requires keen evaluation, but to attempt to base interpretation on inadequate, insufficient radiographs is guesswork rather than true, timely diagnosis.

I. Use of Reference Radiographs[52]

The characteristics of acceptable finished radiographs (page 121) serve as the basis for analysis. Nothing less than the ideal should satisfy, and errors must be studied so that techniques can be improved for future surveys.

A. Available Ideal Radiographs

1. Tape a periapical or bitewing radiograph to a viewbox for continuing reference and comparison.
2. Note changes in density, contrast, or other feature so that techniques can be adjusted.
3. Use information to determine the need for changes in processing solutions and timing.

B. Complete Surveys

Examples of ideal surveys for periapical, bitewing, panoramic, edentulous, pediatric of various ages, or other special radiographs can be maintained for study and review. New staff members can benefit by learning what is expected.

II. Mounting

A. Legibly mark the mount with the name of patient, date, name of dentist; printing is preferred.
B. Handle radiographs only by the edges with clean, dry hands, or wear clean cotton gloves.
C. Keep films clean, free from dust, liquids, or other contaminants.
D. Place a clean, dry towel or paper in front of the illuminator where mounting is to be done; arrange radiographs on this or mount one by one directly as they are removed from the rack.
E. The embossed dot near the edge of the negative

is the guide to mounting: the depressed side of the dot is on the lingual side.

F. Identify individual negatives by the teeth and other anatomic landmarks.

G. Approved mounting system:[53] looking at the teeth from outside the mouth, the teeth are viewed and mounted in the same manner as the approved numbering system (figure III–I, page 73).

III. Anatomic Landmarks

A. Definition

An anatomic landmark is an anatomic structure, the image of which may serve as an aid in the localization and identification of the regions portrayed by a radiograph. The teeth are the primary landmarks.

B. Landmarks That May Be Seen in Individual Radiographs

1. *Maxillary Molar.* Maxillary sinus, zygomatic process, zygomatic (malar) bone, hamular process, coronoid process of the mandible, maxillary tuberosity.
2. *Maxillary Premolar.* Maxillary sinus.
3. *Maxillary Canine.* Maxillary sinus, junction of the maxillary sinus and nasal fossa (Y-shaped, radiopaque).
4. *Maxillary Incisors.* Incisive foramen, nasal septum and fossae, anterior nasal spine (V-shaped), median palatine suture, symphysis of the maxillae.
5. *Mandibular Molar.* Mandibular canal, internal oblique line, external oblique ridge, mylohyoid ridge.
6. *Mandibular Premolar.* Mental foramen.
7. *Mandibular Incisors.* Lingual foramen, mental ridge, genial tubercles, symphysis of the mandible. Nutrient canals are seen most frequently in this radiograph.

IV. Identification of Inadequacies in Radiographs

Inadequacies are related to film placement, angulation, exposure, processing, care and handling of the film, and, indeed, any step in the entire procedure. Errors appear as problems of inadequate density, contrast, incomplete or distorted images, fogging, artifacts, or stains. Table 9–3 outlines the more common inadequacies and their causes, the keys to correction.

V. Interpretation

Radiographs are used in conjunction with clinical examination for a complete program of treatment. Periodic radiographs permit continuing evaluation. As part of the permanent record, radiographs help to document the oral condition for comparative purposes as well as legal.

The quality of the radiographs determines their usability for diagnostic interpretation. Techniques for the preparation of radiographs must be perfected in order that radiographs have maximum interpretability with minimum radiation exposure of the patient.

A. Prerequisites for Interpretation[54]

1. *Mounting.* Mount radiographs in an opaque mount to prevent light between each radiograph from creating glare and producing a blinding effect.
2. *Viewbox.* Use an adequately lighted viewbox. Dimmed room light improves visibility for contrasting radiolucent and radiopaque areas.

   Holding the radiographs up to view by window, room, or unit light is inadequate and only gross interpretation can be accomplished. When a viewbox is larger than the mount used, cover the edges to block out peripheral light.
3. *Hand Magnifying Glass.* Examine radiographs on a viewbox through a magnifying glass. A viewbox is available with a built-on magnifying glass.

B. Systematic Examination

1. Observe one radiographic feature at a time. Examine all of the radiographs for that feature, rather than taking each radiograph separately to find everything. It is important to note comparisons for each change over the entire survey.
2. When examining a particular tooth, compare the appearance of that tooth in each radiograph in which it appears, including bitewings. At different angulations, different findings may become apparent.

C. Coordination with Clinical Examination

A description of radiographic examination of the teeth may be found on page 220 and of the periodontal tissues, on page 207. Correlation of radiographic findings with the clinical examination, using probe and explorer, is basic to an understanding of the true oral condition of the patient.

TECHNICAL HINTS

I. Holding Film

Never hold a film in a patient's mouth during exposure.

II. Question Radiation Exposure

Inquire whether the patient is receiving or has recently received radiation treatment. It may be necessary to minimize the number of exposures. The patient's physician should be consulted.

III. Film Placement

Dot on film packet is placed toward the occlusal surface or incisal edge to prevent the embossed dot

Table 9–3.   Analysis of Radiographs: Causes of Inadequacies

	Inadequacy	*Cause: Factors in Correction*
Image	Elongation	Insufficient vertical angulation
	Foreshortening	Excessive vertical angulation
	Superimposition (overlapping)	Incorrect horizontal angulation (central ray not directed through interproximal space)
	Partial image	Cone-cut (incorrect direction of central ray or incorrect film placement)
		Incompletely immersed in processing tank
		Film touched other film or side of tank during processing
	Blurred or double image	Patient, tube, or packet movement during exposure
		Film exposed twice
	Stretched appearance of trabeculae or apices	Bent film
	No image	Machine misfunction from time-switch to wall-plug
		Failure to turn on the machine
		Film placed in fixer before developer
Density	Too dark	Excessive exposure
		Excessive developing
		Developer too warm
		Unsafe safelight
		Accidental exposure to white light (may be completely black)
	Too light	Insufficient exposure
		Insufficient development or excessive fixation
		Solutions too cool
		Use of old, contaminated, or poorly mixed solutions
		Film placement: leaded side toward teeth
		Film used beyond expiration date
Fog	Chemical fog	Imbalance or deterioration of processing solutions
	Light fog	Unintentional exposure to light to which the emulsion is sensitive, either before or during processing
		(1) Unsafe safelight
		(2) Darkroom leak
		(3) Holding unprocessed films too close to the safelight
		(4) Exposed to safelight longer than $2\frac{1}{2}$ minutes
	Radiation fog	Improper storage of unused film
		Film exposed prior to processing
Reticulation	(puckered or pebbly surface)	Sudden temperature changes during processing, particularly from warm solutions to very cold water
Artifacts	Dark lines	Bent or creased film
		Static electricity
		(1) Film removed from wrapper with excessive force
		(2) Wrapper sticking to film, when opened with wet fingers, or if there was excessive moisture from patient's mouth
		Fingernail used to grasp film during opening
	Herringbone pattern (light film)	Packet placed in mouth backwards with foil next to teeth
Discoloration	Stains and spots	Unclean film hanger
		Splatterings of developer, fixer, dust
		Finger marks
		Insufficient rinsing after developing before fixing
		Splashing dry negatives with water or solutions
		Air bubbles adhering to surface during processing (insufficient agitation)
		Overlap of film on film in tanks or while drying
		Paper wrapper stuck to film (film not dried when removed from patient's mouth)
	At later date after storage of completed radiographs	Incomplete processing or rinsing
		Storage in too warm a place
		Storage near chemicals

on the film from superimposing over the image on the negative.

IV. Check State Radiation Protection Laws

Many states have regulations concerning x-ray unit registration, inspection, safety requirements, and limitations for use of x-rays.

V. Record in Patient's Permanent Record

A. Radiation Services Exposure Record

A continuing record for each patient is kept to show number of exposures and the area.

B. Patient Signature

When a patient refuses to have radiographs made, record this in the patient's permanent record. Obtain patient's signature to a statement indicating such refusal in the event a legal issue should arise related to an operation performed.

VI. Who Owns Dental Radiographs?

They are part of the dentist's record and remain as professional property, the same as do other parts of the case record.[55] The first rule is never to give radiographs to a patient. If they are to be loaned to another dentist, they should be sent or delivered directly, preferably with a letter indicating, if known, when they will next be needed and should be returned. When possible, a duplicate set can be made by using a two-film packet. It is also possible to duplicate the mounted set so that the originals can be kept with the patient's complete record.

VII. Film Storage

Film should always be stored in a clean, cool, dry place. Keep in lead-lined container. Watch expiration dates. Store oldest film in front for next use. Purchase as needed, not in excess quantity.

VIII. Study Informational Sheets

It is important to study the informational sheets provided in the film package. This applies particularly when a new brand of film is being used.

IX. Stain Removal from Clothes

A. Do not launder before spot removal.
B. Commercially prepared spot removers are available from dental supply companies.
C. Removal of spots in nylon materials
  1. Prepare solution containing
    Sodium hypochlorite   ½ oz. (15 ml)
      (5% solution)
      (household bleach)
    Acetic acid   ½ oz. (15 ml)
      (5% solution)
      (household vinegar)
    Water at about 38° C (100° F)   1 gal (3.8 L)
  2. Soak the stained portion in the solution for 5 to 10 minutes, then soak in *fresh* fixer.
  3. Rinse thoroughly in plain water. Dry.

X. X-ray Film Contamination by Stannous Fluoride

Stannous fluoride can cause artifacts on a finished radiograph. When radiographs are to be made and stannous fluoride solution is to be applied topically, it is recommended that the radiographs be made first.

FACTORS TO TEACH THE PATIENT

I. When the Patient Asks About the Safety of Radiation

Patients ask questions about safety factors, and occasionally, a patient may refuse to have any radiographs made. The patient must be reassured with confidence, be instructed as to why radiographs are necessary at this time, and be informed about how modern equipment and techniques are in accord with minimum radiation standards.

A. Adapt the answer to the patient. Certain patients have more fear; others have more knowledge about x-rays. If the clinician expresses confidence, this aids in allaying fears. Hesitation increases the patient's doubt.
B. Radiographs are essential to diagnosis and treatment. Without the information provided, the dentist can only guess at conditions not visible clinically.
C. The benefits resulting from the intelligent use of x-rays outweigh any possible negative effects.
D. Modern x-ray machines are equipped for safety. For the patient who understands, details about filtration, collimation, film speed, and short exposure times can be explained.

II. Educational Features in Dental Radiographs

(Avoid diagnosis. For teaching, it may be advisable to use radiographs of someone other than the patient.)
A. Position of unerupted permanent teeth in relation to primary teeth.
B. Detection of early carious lesions not visible by clinical examination.
C. Effects of loss of teeth and the importance of having replacements.
D. Periodontal changes and other pathologic conditions appropriate to an individual patient.

References

1. American Dental Association, Council on Dental Materials, Instruments, and Equipment: Recommendations in Radiographic Practices: An Update, 1988: *J. Am. Dent. Assoc., 118,* 115, January, 1989.
2. Glenner, R.A.: 80 Years of Dental Radiography, *J. Am. Dent. Assoc., 90,* 549, March, 1975.
3. Manson-Hing, L.R.: *Fundamentals of Dental Radiography,* 2nd ed. Philadelphia, Lea & Febiger, 1985, pp. 1–15.

4. Wuehrmann, A.H. and Manson-Hing, L.R.: *Dental Radiology,* 5th ed. St. Louis, The C.V. Mosby Co., 1981, pp. 4–21.

5. Edwards, C., Statkiewicz-Sherer, M.A., and Ritenour, E.R.: *Radiation Protection for Dental Radiographers.* Denver, Colorado, Multi-Media Publishing, 1984, pp. 13–26.

6. Barr, J.H. and Stephens, R.G.: *Dental Radiology: Pertinent Basic Concepts and Their Applications in Clinical Practice.* Philadelphia, W.B. Saunders Co., 1980, pp. 27–42.

7. Wuehrmann and Manson-Hing: op. cit., pp. 35–53, 76–85.

8. Edwards, Statkiewicz-Sherer, and Ritenour: op. cit, pp. 129–144.

9. White, S.C. and Rose, T.C.: Absorbed Bone Marrow Dose in Certain Dental Radiographic Techniques, *J. Am. Dent. Assoc., 98,* 553, April, 1979.

10. de Lyre, W.R.: *Essentials of Dental Radiography for Dental Assistants and Hygienists,* 2nd ed. Englewood Cliffs, New Jersey, Prentice-Hall, 1980, pp. 77–78, 391.

11. Manson-Hing: op. cit., pp. 16–19.

12. International Commission on Radiation Units and Measurements (ICRU): Radiation Quantities and Units, ICRU Report Number 33, Washington, D.C., 1980.

13. Edwards, Statkiewicz-Sherer, and Ritenour: op. cit., pp. 33–44.

14. National Council on Radiation Protection and Measurements: *Dental X-Ray Protection.* NCRP Report Number 35, March 9, 1970, 50 pp.

15. Manson-Hing: op. cit., pp. 99–105.

16. Edwards, Statkiewicz-Sherer, and Ritenour: op. cit., pp. 69–116.

17. Herrmann, H.J. and Myall, R.W.T.: Observations on the Significance of the Thyroid Gland to the Dentist, *Spec. Care Dentist., 3,* 13, January–February, 1983.

18. White, S.C. and Glaze, S.: Interpatient Microbiological Cross-Contamination after Dental Radiographic Examination, *J. Am. Dent. Assoc., 96,* 801, May, 1978.

19. Ash, J.L., LaTurno, S.A.L., and Corcoran, J.F.: The Use of a Sealed Plastic Bag for Radiographic Film to Avoid Cross-Contamination, *J. Endod., 10,* 512, October, 1984.

20. Langland, O.E.: Radiologic Examination, in Clark, J.W., ed.: *Clinical Dentistry,* Volume 1, Chapter 4. Philadelphia, J.B. Lippincott Co., 1984, pp. 14–15.

21. Park, J.K.: Radiographic Technique in the Contour Dental Chair, *J. Am. Dent. Hyg. Assoc., 46,* 351, September-October, 1972.

22. Venokur, P.C., Einbender, S., and Myers, B.S: Modified X-Ray Technique for Dentistry with Patients in the Supine Position, *Oral Surg. Oral Med. Oral Pathol., 38,* 148, July, 1974.

23. Baum, A.T. and Morgan, E.: Reduction of X-Ray Dose by Variable Rectangular Collimation and Reflex Optical Direction of Dental X-Ray Beams and by Supine Position of the Patient, *J. Am. Dent. Assoc., 85,* 1091, November, 1972.

24. Eastman Kodak Company: *X-Rays in Dentistry.* Rochester, Eastman Kodak Company, 1985, pp. 18–69.

25. Manson-Hing: op. cit., pp. 45–67.

26. Manson-Hing: op. cit., pp. 73–78.

27. Pitts, N.B.: Film-holding, Beam-aiming and Collimating Devices as an Aid to Standardization in Intra-oral Radiography: A Review, *J. Dent., 12,* 36, March, 1984.

28. Stabe Disposable Periapical X-Ray Filmholder, Greene Dental Products, Division of Rinn Corporation, 1212 Abbott Drive, Elgin, Illinois 60123-1819.

29. Reid, J.A. and MacDonald, J.C.F.: Use and Workload Factors in Dental Radiation-Protection Design, *Oral Surg. Oral Med. Oral Pathol., 57,* 219, February, 1984.

30. Manson-Hing: op. cit., pp. 129–133.

31. Eastman Kodak Company: op. cit., pp. 40–51.

32. Manson-Hing: op. cit., pp. 149–163.

33. Eastman Kodak Company: op. cit., pp. 92–97.

34. White, S.C. and Weissman, D.D.: Relative Discernment of Lesions by Intraoral and Panoramic Radiography, *J. Am. Dent. Assoc., 95,* 1117, December, 1977.

35. Stephens, R.G., Kogon, S.L., Reid, J.A., and Ruprecht, A.: A Comparison of Panorex and Intraoral Surveys for Routine Dental Radiography, *Can. Dent. Assoc. J., 43,* 281, June, 1977.

36. Valachovic, R.W. and Lurie, A.G.: Risk-Benefit Considerations in Pedodontic Radiology, *Pediatr. Dent., 2,* 128, June, 1980.

37. Perrelet, L.A., Bernhard, M., and Spirgi, M.: Panoramic Radiography in the Examination of Edentulous Patients, *J. Prosthet. Dent., 37,* 494, May, 1977.

38. Block, A.J., Goepp, R.A., and Mason, E.W.: Thyroid Radiation Dose during Panoramic and Cephalometric Dental X-Ray Examinations, *Angle Orthod., 47,* 17, January, 1977.

39. Myers, D.R., Shoaf, H.K., Wege, W.R., Carlton, W.H., and Gilbert, M.A.: Radiation Exposure during Panoramic Radiography in Children, *Oral Surg. Oral Med. Oral Pathol., 46,* 588, October, 1978.

40. Whitcher, B.L., Gratt, B.M., and Sickles, E.A.: A Leaded Apron for Use in Panoramic Dental Radiography, *Oral Surg. Oral Med. Oral Pathol., 49,* 467, May, 1980.

41. White, G.E. and Tsamtsouris, A.: The Use and Abuse of Radiographs of the Primary Dentition, *Quintessence Int., 8,* 59, August, 1977.

42. Page, R.C., Bowen, T., Altman, L., Vandesteen, E., Ochs, H., Mackenzie, P., Osterberg, S., Engel, L.D., and Williams, B.L.: Prepubertal Periodontitis. I. Definition of a Clinical Disease Entity, *J. Periodontol., 54,* 257, May, 1983.

43. Howard, H.E.: Rethinking Pedodontic Radiology, ASDC *J. Dent. Child., 48,* 192, May-June, 1981.

44. White, S.C.: Radiation Exposure in Pediatric Dentistry: Current Standards in Pedodontic Radiology with Suggestions for Alternatives, *Pediatr. Dent., 3,* 441, Special Issue 2, 1982.

45. Nowak, A.J. and Miller, J.W.: High-yield Pedodontic Radiology, *Gen. Dent., 33,* 45, January-February, 1985.

46. Manson-Hing: op. cit., pp. 171–174.

47. Scandrett, F.R., Tebo, H.G., Miller, J.T., and Quigley, M.B.: Radiographic Examination of the Edentulous Patient. Part I. Review of the Literature and Preliminary Report Comparing Three Methods, *Oral Surg. Oral Med. Oral Pathol., 35,* 266, February, 1973.

48. Scandrett, F.R., Tebo, H.G., Quigley, M.B., and Miller, J.T.: Radiographic Examination of the Edentulous Patient. Part II. Differences in Number and Location of Root Fragments, *Oral Surg. Oral Med. Oral Pathol., 35,* 872, June, 1973.

49. de Lyre: op. cit., pp. 278–286.

50. Manson-Hing: op. cit., pp. 24, 208–209.

51. American Dental Association, Council on Dental Materials, Instruments, and Equipment: Recommendations for Radiographic Darkrooms and Darkroom Practices, *J. Am. Dent. Assoc., 104,* 886, June, 1982.

52. American Academy of Dental Radiology, Quality Assurance Committee: Recommendations for Quality Assurance in Dental Radiography, *Oral Surg. Oral Med. Oral Pathol., 55,* 421, April, 1983.

53. American Dental Association: System of Tooth Numbering and Radiograph Mounting, Approved by the American Dental Association House of Delegates, October, 1968.

54. Welander, U., McDavid, W.D., Higgins, N.M., and Morris, C.R.: The Effect of Viewing Conditions on the Perceptibility of Radiographic Details, *Oral Surg. Oral Med. Oral Pathol., 56,* 651, December, 1983.

55. Terezhalmy, G.T. and Bottomley, W.K.: General Legal Aspects of Diagnostic Dental Radiography, *Oral Surg. Oral Med. Oral Pathol., 48,* 486, November, 1979.

Suggested Reading

American Association of Dental Schools, Section on Oral Radiology: Curricular Guidelines for Clinical Competency by Dental Auxiliaries in Dental Radiography, *J. Dent. Educ., 48,* 217, April, 1984.

Brooks, S.L.: A Study of Selection Criteria for Intraoral Dental Radiography, *Oral Surg. Oral Med. Oral Pathol., 62,* 234, August, 1986.

Douglass, C.W., Valachovic, R.W., Wijesinha, A., Chauncey, H.H., Kapur, K.K., and McNeil, B.J.: Clinical Efficacy of Dental Radiography in the Detection of Dental Caries and Periodontal

Diseases, *Oral Surg. Oral Med. Oral Pathol., 62*, 330, September, 1986.

Edwards, C.: Radiation Protection for Dental Professionals. An ADAA Continuing Education Course, *Dent. Assist., 54*, 13, November-December, 1985.

Farman, A.G., Grammer, S., Hunter, N., and Baker, C.: Survey of Radiographic Requirements and Techniques in United States Dental Assisting Programs, 1982, *Oral Surg. Oral Med. Oral Pathol., 56*, 430, October, 1983.

Farman, A.G., Hunter, N., and Grammer, S.: Radiology Requirements in United States Dental Hygiene Programs, *Oral Surg. Oral Med. Oral Pathol., 60*, 341, September, 1985.

Galal, A., Manson-Hing, L., and Jamison, H.: A Comparison of Combinations of Clinical and Radiographic Examinations in Evaluation of a Dental Clinic Population, *Oral Surg. Oral Med. Oral Pathol., 60*, 553, November, 1985.

Gofman, J.W.: Ionizing Radiation: Concepts for the Dental Assistant, *Dent. Assist., 51*, 17, July-August, 1982; Part II, *51*, 17, September-October, 1982; Part III, *51*, 21, November-December, 1982.

Gregg, B.G.E.: Radiation in Dentistry. Dental "X-Ray" Risks in Perspective, *Can. Dent. Hyg., 20*, 15, March, 1986.

Osman, F., Scully, C., Dowell, T., and Davies, R.: Reasons for Taking Radiographs in General Dental Practice, *Community Dent. Oral Epidemiol., 14*, 146, June, 1986.

Scaramucci, M.K.: Radiology Credentialing: An Overview, *Educ. Dir. Dent. Aux., 10*, 12, September, 1985.

Silverstein, S.J. and Stokes, A.N.S.: Dental X-Ray Exposure in a Group of New Zealand Children, *Community Dent. Oral Epidemiol., 11*, 283, October, 1983.

Shwartz, M., Pliskin, J.S., Gröndahl, H.-G., and Boffa, J.: The Frequency of Bitewing Radiographs, *Oral Surg. Oral Med. Oral Pathol., 61*, 300, March, 1986.

Smith, N.J.D.: The Ionising Radiations Regulations 1985, *Br. Dent. J., 160*, 135, February 22, 1986.

Stephens, R.G., Kogon, S.L., and Reid, J.A.: Prescription Radiography. A New Concept for Radiation Protection in Dental Practice, *Can. Dent. Assoc., J., 51*, 672, September, 1985.

Torres, H.O. and Ehrlich, A.: *Modern Dental Assisting*, 3rd ed. Philadelphia, W.B. Saunders Co., 1985, pp. 387–461.

Weems, R.A., Manson-Hing, L.R., Jamison, H.C., and Greer, D.F.: Diagnostic Yield and Selection Criteria in Complete Intraoral Radiography, *J. Am. Dent. Assoc., 110*, 333, March, 1985.

Exposure Control

Gelskey, D.E. and Baker, C.G.: The ALARA Concept. Population Exposures from X Rays in Dentistry—As Low as Reasonably Achievable? *Can. Dent. Assoc., J., 50*, 402, May, 1984.

Canadian Dental Association: Guidelines for the Control of Radiation in the Dental Office, *Can. Dent. Assoc. J., 50*, 14, January, 1984.

Colquitt, W.N. and Richards, A.G.: An Old/New Idea for Reducing Exposure to X-Rays, *Oral Surg. Oral Med. Oral Pathol., 54*, 597, November, 1982.

Kaffe, I., Littner, M.M., Schlezinger, T., and Segal, P.: Efficiency of the Cervical Lead Shield During Intraoral Radiography, *Oral Surg. Oral Med. Oral Pathol., 62*, 732, December, 1986.

Kircos, L.T., Lorton, L., and Angin, L.L.: Order of Magnitude Dose Reduction in Intraoral Radiography, *J. Am. Dent. Assoc., 114*, 344, March, 1987.

Richards, A.G. and Colquitt, W.N.: Reduction in Dental X-Ray Exposures During the Past 60 Years, *J. Am. Dent. Assoc., 103*, 713, November, 1981.

Sikorski, P.A. and Taylor, K.W.: The Effectiveness of the Thyroid Shield in Dental Radiology, *Oral Surg. Oral Med. Oral Pathol., 58*, 225, August, 1984.

Techniques

Choksi, S.K.: Modification Designed to Improve Instruction in Intraoral Dental Radiography, *Oral Surg. Oral Med. Oral Pathol., 59*, 653, June, 1985.

Crandell, C.E.: Diagnostic Quality Control: The Missing Link in Dental Radiology Quality Assurance, *Oral Surg. Oral Med. Oral Pathol., 62*, 212, August, 1986.

Diehl, R., Gratt, B.M., and Gould, R.G.: Radiographic Quality Control Measurements Comparing D-speed Film, E-speed Film, and Xeroradiography, *Oral Surg. Oral Med. Oral Pathol., 61*, 635, June, 1986.

Fletcher, J.C.: A Comparison of Ektaspeed and Ultraspeed Films Using Manual and Automatic Processing Solutions, *Oral Surg. Oral Med. Oral Pathol., 63*, 94, January, 1987.

Frommer, H.H. and Jain, R.K.: A Comparative Clinical Study of Group D and E Dental Film, *Oral Surg. Oral Med. Oral Pathol., 63*, 738, June, 1987.

Gould, R.G. and Gratt, B.M.: Technical Aspects of a Dedicated Quality-control System for Dental Radiology, *Oral Surg. Oral Med. Oral Pathol., 56*, 437, October, 1983.

Hardman, P.K., Rios-Reyes, I.C., Kassebaum, D.K., and Taylor, T.S.: Vertical Bone Height: A Comparison of Bitewing Techniques, *Gen. Dent., 34*, 124, March-April, 1986.

Hardman, P.K., Tilmon, M.F., and Taylor, T.S.: Radiographic Solution Contamination, *Oral Surg. Oral Med. Oral Pathol., 63*, 733, June, 1987.

Horton, P.S., Sippy, F.H., Kohout, F.J., Nelson, J.F., and Kienzle, G.C.: A Clinical Comparison of Speed Group D and E Dental X-Ray Films, *Oral Surg. Oral Med. Oral Pathol., 58*, 104, July, 1984.

Kaffe, I., Gordon, M., Laufer, B., and Littner, M.M.: Detection of Proximal Carious Lesions: Two-film Versus Four-film Bitewing Radiography, *Oral Surg. Oral Med. Oral Pathol., 57*, 567, May, 1984.

Kaffe, I. and Gratt, B.M.: E-speed Dental Films Processed with Rapid Chemistry: A Comparison with D-speed Film, *Oral Surg. Oral Med. Oral Pathol., 64*, 367, September, 1987.

Keur, J.J.: Radiographic Localization Techniques, *Aust. Dent. J., 31*, 86, April, 1986.

McDonald, S.P.: A Method to Reduce Interproximal Overlapping and Improve Reproducibility of Bitewing Radiographs for Use in Clinical Trials, *Community Dent. Oral Epidemiol., 11*, 289, October, 1983.

Nery, E.B., Olson, J.W., Henkin, J.M., and Kalbfleisch, J.H.: Film-Holder Device for Radiographic Assessment of Periodontal Tissues, *J. Periodont. Res., 20*, 97, January, 1985.

Nysether, S. and Hansen, B.F.: Errors on Dental Bitewing Radiographs, *Community Dent. Oral Epidemiol., 11*, 286, October, 1983.

Ponce, A.Z., McDavid, W.D., Underhill, T.E., and Morris, C.R.: Use of E-speed Film with Added Filtration, *Oral Surg. Oral Med. Oral Pathol., 61*, 297, March, 1986.

Sewerin, I.P.: Mechanically Induced Images on Dental X-Ray Film, *Oral Surg. Oral Med. Oral Pathol., 63*, 241, February, 1987.

Shannon, S.A.: Rectangular Versus Cylindrical Collimation. A Study of Cone Cuts on Radiographs, *Dent. Hyg., 61*, 172, April, 1987.

Short, T.: Back to the Basics in Bitewing Radiology, *RDH, 1*, 22, March, 1981.

Stephens, R.G., Kogon, S.L., Wainwright, R.J., and Reid, J.A.: Information Yield from Routine Bitewing Radiographs for Young Adults, *Can. Dent. Assoc. J., 47*, 247, April, 1981.

Updegrave, W.J.: Right Angle Dental Radiography Described, Simplified and Standardized (Part I), *Compend. Cont. Educ. Dent., 2*, 379, November-December, 1981.

Valachovic, R.W., Reiskin, A.B., and Kirchhof, S.T.: A Quality Assurance Program in Dental Radiology, *Pediatr. Dent., 3*, 26, March, 1981.

Infection Control

Bernhardt, H. and Matick, H.G.: Systemic Investigation of Hygiene in the Darkroom and at the Radiography Chair, *Quintessence Int., 14*, 455, April, 1983.

Jones, G.A.: Intraoral X-Ray Film Holders and Infection Control in U.S. Dental Schools, *J. Dent. Educ., 49*, 656, September, 1985.

United States Air Force, Dental Investigation Service: *USAF Dental Service Infection Control Program*, Dental Items of Significance No. 22, May 86, USAF School of Aerospace Medicine/NGD, Brooks AFB, Texas, pp. 15–16.

United States Veterans Administration: *Symposium in Infection Control in Dental Practice.* Washington, D.C. Office of Dentistry, V.A. Central Office, January, 1987, pp. 13–14.

Gagging Patient

Hoad-Reddick, G.: Gagging: A Chairside Approach to Control, *Br. Dent. J., 161,* 174, September 6, 1986.

Ramsey, D.S., Weinstein, P., Milgrom, P., and Getz, T.: Problematic Gagging: Principles of Treatment, *J. Am. Dent. Assoc., 114,* 178, February, 1987.

Sewerin, I.: Gagging in Dental Radiography, *Oral Surg. Oral Med. Oral Pathol., 58,* 725, December, 1984.

Wilks, C.G.W. and Marks, I.M.: Reducing Hypersensitive Gagging, *Br. Dent. J., 155,* 263, October 22, 1983.

Children

Balis, S.: Error and Accuracy Rates of Panoramic Radiography as a Screening Method for Mass Surveying of Children, *J. Public Health Dent., 41,* 220, Fall, 1981.

Kronmiller, J.E., Nirschl, R.F., and Zullo, T.G.: An Evaluation of Pit and Fissure Caries and Caries Experience as Selection Criteria in Bitewing Examinations for Children, *ASDC J. Dent. Child., 53,* 184, May-June, 1986.

Locht, S.: Four-intraoral Film Radiographic Examination on Children Imparting Less Radiation than Pantomography, *Scand. J. Dent. Res., 90,* 69, February, 1982.

Myers, D.R.: Dental Radiology for Children, *Dent. Clin. North Am., 28,* 37, January, 1984.

White, S.C.: Radiation in Dentistry for Children, *J. Pedod., 8,* 242, Spring, 1984.

White, S.C.: Radiation Safety for Children, *Int. Dent. J., 32,* 259, September, 1982.

White, S.C.: Radiation in Pediatric Dentistry: Current Standards in Pedodontic Radiology with Suggestions for Alternatives, *Pediatr. Dent., 3,* 441, Special Issue, 1982.

Panoramic Radiography

Bankvall, G. and Hakansson, H.A.R.: Radiation-absorbed Doses and Energy Imparted from Panoramic Tomography, Cephalometric Radiography, and Occlusal Film Radiography in Children, *Oral Surg. Oral Med. Oral Pathol., 53,* 532, May, 1982.

Barrett, A.P., Waters, B.E., and Griffiths, C.J.: A Critical Evaluation of Panoramic Radiography as a Screening Procedure in Dental Practice, *Oral Surg. Oral Med. Oral Pathol., 57,* 673, June, 1984.

Bean, L.R. and Akerman, W.Y.: Intraoral or Panoramic Radiography? *Dent. Clin. North Am., 28,* 47, January, 1984.

Ewen, K.: Must the Vertebrae be Protected during Panoramic Radiography? *Quintessence Int., 14,* 341, March, 1983.

Farman, A.G., Phelps, R., and Downs, J.B.: Artifact or Pathosis? Problem-solving for Panoramic Dental Radiology, *Quintessence Int., 14,* 55, January, 1983; Part II, *14,* 209, February, 1983.

Forsgren, L. and Julin, P.: Radiation Dose Reduction in Panoramic Radiography. Orthopantomograph Model OP 3 Modified for Rare Earth Intensifying Screens, *Swed. Dent. J., 6,* 225, Number 6, 1982.

Garcia, R.I., Valachovic, R.W., and Chauncey, H.H.: Longitudinal Study of the Diagnostic Yield of Panoramic Radiographs in Aging Edentulous Men, *Oral Surg. Oral Med. Oral Pathol., 63,* 494, April, 1987.

Gratt, B.M., White, S.C., Packard, F.L., and Petersson, A.R.: An Evaluation of Rare-Earth Imaging Systems in Panoramic Radiography, *Oral Surg. Oral Med. Oral Pathol., 58,* 475, October, 1984.

Hassen, S.M. and Manson-Hing, L.R.: A Study of the Zone of Sharpness of Three Panoramic X-Ray Machines and the Effect of Screen Speed on the Sharpness Zone, *Oral Surg. Oral Med. Oral Pathol., 54,* 242, August, 1982.

Hurlburt, C.E. and Coggins, L.J.: Rare Earth Screens for Panoramic Radiography, *Oral Surg. Oral Med. Oral Pathol., 57,* 451, April, 1984.

Jones, J.D., Seals, R.R., and Schelb, E.: Panoramic Radiographic Examination of Edentulous Patients, *J. Prosthet. Dent., 53,* 535, April, 1985.

Keur, J.J.: A Rare Earth Screen-Film System for Dental Panoramic Radiography, *Aust. Dent. J., 28,* 105, April, 1983.

Kogan, S.L. and Stephens, R.G.: Selective Radiography Instead of Screening Pantomography—A Risk/Benefit Evaluation, *Can. Dent. Assoc. J., 48,* 271, April, 1982.

Lloyd, P.M. and Gambert, S.R.: Periodic Oral Examinations and Panoramic Radiographs in Edentulous Elderly Men, *Oral Surg. Oral Med. Oral Pathol., 57,* 678, June, 1984.

Locht, S.: Dose Reduction in Pantomography of Children By Means of Reduction of Irradiated Area, *Community Dent. Oral Epidemiol., 11,* 180, June, 1983.

Matteson, S.R.: Theory of Pantomographic Imaging, Normal Radiographic Anatomy, and Developmental Abnormality Interpretation, *Dent. Radiog. Photog., 57,* 3, Numbers 1–4, 1985.

McDavid, W.D., Tronje, G., Welander, U., and Morris, C.R.: Effects of Errors in Film Speed and Beam Alignment on the Image Layer in Rotational Panoramic Radiography, *Oral Surg. Oral Med. Oral Pathol., 52,* 561, November, 1981.

Ponce, A.Z., McDavid, W.D., Lundeen, R.C., and Morris, C.R.: Adaptation of the Panorex II for Use with Rare Earth Screen-Film Combinations, *Oral Surg. Oral Med. Oral Pathol., 61,* 645, June, 1986.

Schiff, T., D'Ambrosio, J., Glass, B.J., Langlais, R.P., and McDavid, W.D.: Common Positioning and Technical Errors in Panoramic Radiography, *J. Am. Dent. Assoc., 113,* 422, September, 1986.

Stenström, B., Rehnmark-Larson, S., Julin, P., and Richter, S.: Radiation Shielding in Dental Radiography, *Swed. Dent. J., 7,* 85, Number 3, 1983.

Stephens, R.G. and Reid, J.A.: The Extraoral Lateral Oblique Radiograph: A Radiation-efficient Replacement for the Pantomograph, *Can. Dent. Assoc. J., 49,* 483, July, 1983.

Valachovic, R.W., Douglass, C.W., Reiskin, A.B., Chauncey, H.H., and McNeil, B.J.: The Use of Panoramic Radiography in the Evaluation of Asymptomatic Adult Dental Patients, *Oral Surg. Oral Med. Oral Pathol., 61,* 289, March, 1986.

White, S.C., Forsythe, A.B., and Joseph, L.P.: Patient-selection Criteria for Panoramic Radiography, *Oral Surg. Oral Med. Oral Pathol., 57,* 681, June, 1984.

Wright, S.M.: The Radiographic Examination of Edentulous Patients, *J. Prosthet. Dent., 50,* 164, August, 1983.

10 *Study Casts*

As accurate reproductions of the teeth, gingiva, and adjacent structures, study casts can be useful and frequently indispensable adjuncts in the care of a patient. The study casts, radiographs, and clinical examination with recordings and chartings, together with the medical and dental histories, are utilized in the diagnosis, total treatment planning, treatment, and subsequent maintenance by the dentist and the dental hygienist.

I. Purposes and Uses of Study Casts

A. To serve as a permanent record of the patient's present condition.
B. To give sharper delineation and corroboration of the observations made during the oral examination.
C. To observe normal conditions, the variations of and departures from the normal at the outset of treatment, and, by comparison with subsequent periodic casts, to compare and evaluate certain aspects of treatment.
D. During charting of the teeth, to note missing teeth, anomalies of size, shape, or number, partial eruption, tooth positions such as drifting, tilting, and open or closed spacing, and other factors.
E. During examination of the occlusion, to observe the static relations (Angle's classification, malrelations of groups of teeth, and malpositions of individual teeth; pages 226–231) and other features such as wear patterns and the effects of premature loss of teeth.
F. During periodontal charting, to record anatomic features such as the position, size, and shape of the gingiva and interdental papillae, and the position of freni.
G. To be an effective visual aid to use when the oral conditions are explained and the dental and dental hygiene treatment plan is presented; to enable the patient to visualize and understand the need for the specific care outlined.
H. To serve as a guide to clinical treatment procedures.
I. To supplement clinical observations in the selection of an oral disease and plaque control program for the patient's own treatment, and to serve as a visual aid in teaching aims and procedures of the recommended measures to the patient.

II. Terms Used*

A. **Cast** (also called a model)
   Positive likeness of some desired form.

B. **Study Cast or Diagnostic Cast**
   Positive likeness of part or parts of the oral cavity for the purpose of study and treatment planning.

C. **Impression**
   An imprint or negative likeness of the teeth and/or edentulous areas where the teeth have been removed, made in a plastic material that becomes relatively hard or set while in contact with the tissues. Impressions are named or classified by the type of material used to make the impression, such as reversible or irreversible hydrocolloid, plaster, or wax.

D. **Interocclusal Record**
   A record of the positional relation of the opposing teeth or jaws to each other made in a plastic material such as wax.

III. Steps in the Preparation of Study Casts

The steps noted here are detailed in the sections following.

A. **Clinical Procedures**
   1. Assemble materials and equipment.
   2. Prepare the patient.
   3. Select and prepare the impression trays.
   4. Make the mandibular impression.
   5. Make the maxillary impression.
   6. Make the interocclusal record for occluding the casts.

B. **Paraclinical Procedures**
   1. Assemble materials and equipment.
   2. Prepare the impressions for pouring.
   3. Pour the casts.
   4. Trim and finish the casts.
   5. Polish the casts.

CLINICAL PREPARATION

The need for and uses of study casts are explained to the patient when the steps in diagnosis and treatment planning are outlined. As with any procedure

*Definitions are taken or adapted from and in accord with the *Glossary of Prosthodontic Terms*, 5th ed., Journal of Prosthetic Dentistry, *58*, 717, December, 1987.

not familiar to the patient, an explanation is in order. The reactions of patients who have had an impression made previously may range from indifference to dread, and the conversation and approach can be directed accordingly.

When the radiographic survey has been made for the new patient prior to the study casts, it will have been determined whether precautions to prevent gagging require special application. With all patients, a calm approach, an exhibition of confidence, a direct and efficient procedure, and a gentle handling of the patient's oral tissues will increase rapport and contribute to a satisfactory result.

I. Assemble Materials and Equipment

A. Coverall (plastic drape), towel, and mouthrinse.
B. Impression trays
   1. Perforated type generally used: small, medium, and large sizes are available.
   2. Care of trays: for use in the patient's mouth; trays must be disposable or clean, shiny, and sterilized metal.
C. Mixing bowl: clean, dry, flexible rubber or plastic with smooth, unscratched surface.
D. Spatula: clean, dry, stiff, with a smooth, rounded end that will reach every part of the bowl without scraping or cutting its surface.
E. Saliva ejector.
F. Dental materials
   1. Wax for preparation of tray rim: soft utility wax.
   2. Alginate: irreversible hydrocolloid with manufacturer's measurer.
   3. Soft baseplate wax.
G. Water thermometer.

II. Clinician Preparation

Eyeglasses, mask, and gloves should be worn as for all clinic procedures.

III. Prepare the Patient

A. Antibiotic Premedication

Research has not demonstrated the production of bacteremia following an impression using irreversible hydrocolloid.[1] When a high-risk patient has moderate to severe periodontitis with mobile teeth, however, clinical judgment must be used when deciding on the need for antibiotic premedication.

Impressions can be planned for an appointment when the patient is protected and has received antibiotic coverage for other procedures. The medical and dental histories must be reviewed for all possible precautionary needs.

B. Explain the Procedure to be Performed

The material has a slight, pleasant flavor; it may feel cold when first placed.

C. Position the Patient

Position the patient upright for maximum visibility and accessibility and to minimize gagging. Stabilize the patient's head on the headrest.

D. Receive Removable Appliances

Provide a container with water in which the patient can place removable oral appliances.

E. Drape the Patient

Drape patient with a protective coverall and towel.

F. Examine the Oral Cavity

Note labially and buccally displaced teeth, height of palate, undercut areas, mandibular tori, and other factors that may influence the size or preparation of the impression tray and the procedures to be carried out during impression making.

G. Free the Mouth of Debris

1. Spray proximal areas; use dental floss.
2. When excess, tenacious debris is present, plaque control instruction should be started so that debris and plaque can be removed during brushing by the patient.

H. Request Patient to Use Mouthrinse

1. To aid in the removal of saliva and debris and lessen the numbers of surface microorganisms.
2. To lower the surface tension; aids in preventing bubbles in the impression.
3. To provide a pleasant taste and feeling for the patient.
4. To distract an anxious patient while the trays are being prepared.

I. Dry the Teeth

Use a cotton roll or compressed air stream to remove saliva from the teeth to prevent irregularities in the surface of the study cast.

J. Prevent Gagging

1. Approach with confidence to reassure the patient.
2. Work as quickly and efficiently as possible.
3. Use a topical anesthetic (pages 468–470)
   a. Cold water or an ice cube held in the mouth has some anesthetic effect.
   b. Salt: a small amount (¼ teaspoon) on the tongue to swallow just before the tray is to be inserted may relieve tissue reactions.
   c. Apply topical anesthetic to posterior palatal area, or patient may rinse with a commercial topical agent. A spray topical preparation is contraindicated because of proximity to throat where coughing may be initiated.
4. Technique considerations
   a. Avoid excessive impression material in the tray.
   b. Seat the maxillary tray from posterior to anterior as described in II., A., 3., a., b. (page 156).
   c. Instruct patient to breathe deeply through

the nose before the tray is inserted and to continue after insertion; bring head forward.

PREPARATION OF IMPRESSION TRAYS

I. Selection of Proper Size and Shape
A. Width
1. Objectives: to allow an adequate thickness of impression material on the facial and lingual surfaces of each tooth to provide strength and rigidity to the impression.
2. Tray flanges may be spread to accommodate for extra width in the molar regions, particularly lingual to the mandibular molars in the mylohyoid region.
3. When a tooth is in prominent labio-, bucco-, or linguoversion, a minimum thickness of ⅛ to ¼ inch is suggested, but even then the fragility of the impression material in that area is increased.
4. The tray that is too wide may appear in correct relation to the facial surfaces but may impinge on the lingual or palatal cusps of molars.

B. Length
1. Objective: to allow coverage of the retromolar area of the mandible and the tuberosity of the maxilla.
2. Anteriorly there should be at least ¼ inch clearance labial to the most protruded incisor without impingement on lingual or palatal gingiva.

II. Maxillary Tray Try-in
A. Position of Clinician: side back of patient.
B. Retraction
1. With index finger of nondominant hand retract the patient's lip and cheek.
2. At the same time, use the side of the tray to distend the other side of the patient's mouth to gain entry (figure 10–1).

C. Insertion
1. With a rotary motion, insert the tray.
2. Orient the tray beneath the arch and center it, using the tray handle and the midline (usually between the central incisors and in line with the middle of the nose) as guides for positioning.
3. Bring the front of the tray to a position ¼ inch labial to the most labially inclined incisor.
4. Seat the tray by bringing the posterior up before the anterior; retract the lip as the anterior is brought into place.

D. Evaluation
Evaluate the size of the tray: gently lower the front of the tray while holding the posterior border in place (figure 10–2) and examine the relationship of the posterior border to the most pos-

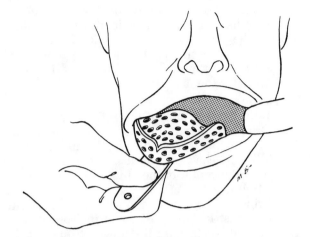

Figure 10–1. Maxillary Tray Insertion. The patient's lip and cheek are retracted with the fingers of the nondominant hand, while the side of the tray is used to distend the other lip and cheek to gain entry. The tray is inserted with a rotary motion. The procedure for the mandibular tray is similar.

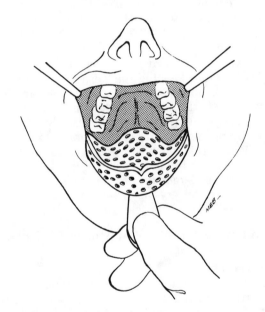

Figure 10–2. Selection of Impression Tray. To determine adequate coverage, the posterior border of the tray is held in position while the front of the tray is lowered to observe the relationship of the posterior border to the maxillary tuberosity areas to be covered by the impression. The mandibular tray position is examined by lifting the tray to observe coverage of the retromolar areas.

terior molars and the tuberosity areas to determine whether the coverage will be ample. By moving the tray up and down it is possible to observe the relation to the facial surfaces of all teeth, malaligned teeth, protuberances, and other features to assay the space allowed for the impression material.

III. Mandibular Tray Try-in
A. Position of Clinician: at side front of patient.
B. Retraction

1. With index and middle fingers of nondominant hand, retract the patient's lip and cheek.
2. At the same time, use the side of the tray to distend the side of the mouth to gain entry, similar to the procedure illustrated in figure 10–1 for the maxillary tray.

C. Insertion
1. With a rotary motion insert the tray.
2. Orient the tray over the dental arch and center it, using the tray handle and the midline (usually between the central incisors and in line with the center of the chin) as guides for positioning.
3. Bring the tray rim to about ¼ inch anterior to the most labially positioned incisor; instruct the patient to raise the tongue to permit the lingual flange of the tray to pass by the lateral borders of the tongue without interference.
4. As the tray is lowered, retract the cheeks in the posterior regions to make certain the buccal mucosa is not caught beneath the edge of the tray; hold the lip out to ascertain that there is clearance to the base of the vestibule.

D. Evaluation
1. Evaluate the size of the tray. Lift the tray handle while keeping the posterior in position, similar to the procedure illustrated in figure 10–2 for the maxilla, to determine whether the coverage will be ample posteriorly to include the retromolar areas and laterally to allow for ¼ inch thickness of impression material on the facial and lingual aspects of the teeth.
2. Reselect larger or smaller trays as indicated and repeat try-in. When in doubt, use the larger tray rather than the smaller.

IV. Application of Wax Rim Around Borders of Trays (Beading)

A. Purposes
1. To position the loaded trays without the metal rims causing discomfort to the soft tissues.
2. To seat the vestibular periphery firmly into position with reduced pressure on the displaced tissues.
3. To prevent penetration of the incisal or occlusal surfaces through the impression material and thus prevent a defective cast.
4. To provide a slight undercut at the rim as an aid in the retention of the alginate in the tray during placement and removal.
5. To create a posterior palatal seal to aid in preventing excess material from passing into the throat.

B. Procedure
1. Attach a strip of soft utility wax firmly around the entire periphery of each tray (figure 10–3).
2. Mandibular tray: add extra layers from canine to canine labially and notch the wax, to fit about the labial frenum.

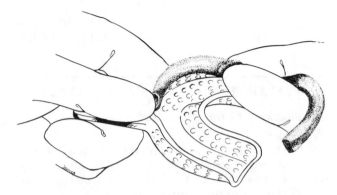

Figure 10–3. Beading the Tray. A strip of soft utility wax is applied around the periphery of each tray.

3. Maxillary tray
   a. Add extra layers as needed to extend the tray into the vestibule above the anterior teeth and notch the wax to fit about the labial frenum (figure 10–4).
   b. Apply extra thickness across the posterior palatal seal area.
   c. When a patient has a high palatal vault, apply extra wax to support the impression material in that area.
4. Try the rimmed trays in the mouth and examine by retraction of the lips and cheeks and by use of a mouth mirror for lingual areas; hold the tray in position.
5. Characteristics of the completed molding: when the tray is held firmly, the wax contacts all borders of the mucous membrane, displaces the soft tissue outward and upward, and the teeth do not touch the tray.

THE IMPRESSION MATERIAL

I. Factors Related to the Impression Material That Contribute to a Satisfactory Impression

Texts on dental materials should be reviewed for complete information about the irreversible hydrocolloids.[2,3,4] Properties related to the clinical procedures essential to making an accurate impression are listed here.

A. Powder
The alginate material deteriorates on standing, particularly at higher temperatures and humidity.
1. Keep metal container tightly closed; store in a cool place.
2. Use individually sealed packages to eliminate the problem of heat and moisture.
3. Individual package may be refrigerated in hot weather, provided the powder is used immediately on opening. If left exposed, water condenses on the powder. The bulk container cannot be refrigerated for that reason.

B. Water
Temperature controls gelation time.
1. At room temperature, 20° to 21° C (68° to 70°

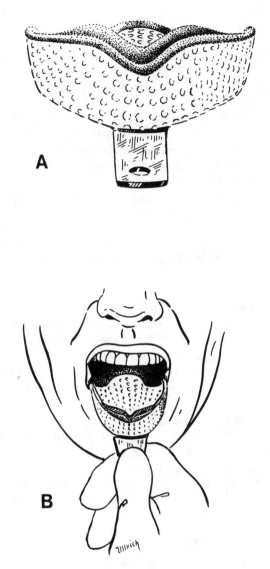

Figure 10–4. Check the Beading Wax. A. Tray with double layer of beading wax about the labial frenum. The extra wax extends the tray, protects the soft tissue from the metal rim, and provides a more complete impression of the area. **B.** Try-in after beading. The wax should contact all borders of the mucous membrane, displace the soft tissue outward, and prevent the teeth from contacting the tray.

F), an ideal gelation time between 3 to 4 minutes provides adequate working time.
2. Temperature of the water should be measured with a thermometer at the time of mixing.
3. Control in hot, humid weather: use cooler water and refrigerate the bowl and spatula.

C. Strength and Quality
The strength and quality of the finished impression depend on the following factors:
1. Powder-water ratio accurately weighed and measured.
2. Spatulation (1 minute) to allow chemical reactions to proceed uniformly.
3. Holding the impression material in position

for an optimum period (2 clocked minutes after the mix on the spatula has lost its stickiness). The elasticity of most alginates improves with time; therefore, a superior reproduction can be obtained by waiting. Distortion can result when the impression is left in the mouth too long.

D. Surface Accuracy
The cast must be poured immediately to prevent loss of water from the impression. Permanent distortion can result.

II. Mixing the Impression Material
Follow manufacturer's specifications precisely: total time lapse for mixing and insertion is approximately 2 minutes.
A. Place measured water 20° to 21° C (68° to 70° F, measured with a thermometer) in a clean, dry mixing bowl.
B. Sprinkle measured powder (from individually sealed package or premeasured from large container) into the water.
C. Quickly incorporate the powder and water, using a clean, dry, stiff spatula.
D. Mix for 1 minute (clocked) vigorously, incorporating powder into the water, until a smooth, creamy mix is obtained.

III. Tray Preparation
The mandibular impression is made first to introduce the patient to the procedure in an area where discomfort or gagging may be the least likely.

A. Working Time
The working time is 30 seconds.

B. Filling the Tray
1. Fill the tray from one end to the other, being careful not to trap air bubbles.
2. Adapt the material to the tray thoroughly; press slightly through the perforations in the tray.
3. Do not overload; fill to a level just below the edge of the wax rim.
4. Wet index finger with cold water and pass lightly over the surface of the impression material; smooth the surface and make a slight indent where the teeth will insert.

C. Excess Material
Quickly gather the excess material from the bowl and bring the material on the spatula near to patient.

THE MANDIBULAR IMPRESSION

I. Precoat Potential Areas of Air Entrapment
This prevents air bubbles in the finished impression.
A. Take a small amount of impression material from the spatula on the index finger.

B. Apply quickly with a positive pressure to
1. Undercut areas, such as distal surfaces of teeth adjacent to edentulous areas, cervical areas of erosion or abrasion, or gingival surfaces of fixed partial dentures.
2. Vestibular areas, particularly anterior areas about the freni.
3. Occlusal surfaces.

II. Insertion of Tray

A. Steps
1. Follow the procedure for try-in of mandibular tray described on pages 153–154, III. Briefly, from the front of the patient, retract patient's lip and cheek with fingers of nondominant hand; use side of tray to distend the other lip and cheek; rotate the tray into position, center it over the teeth, introduce the tray ¼ inch anterior to the labial surface of the most anterior incisor. Instruct patient to raise tongue while tray is lowered; retract cheeks and lip to clear the way for impression material to reach the base of the vestibule.
2. Seat the tray directly downward with a slight vibratory motion to aid in filling all crevices between the teeth.
3. Instruct the patient to extrude the tongue briefly to mold the lingual borders of the impression.
4. Apply equal bilateral pressure firmly, holding the middle fingers over the premolar regions and using the thumbs to support the mandible; or, if equal pressure can be maintained with one hand, place an index finger over the patient's premolar area on one side and the middle finger over the opposite side, with the thumb under the edge of the mandible for stabilization. Mold cheeks around buccal.
5. Saliva ejector: when the impression tray is held with one hand or when assistance is available, a saliva ejector may be slipped in over the tray and then removed before the tray is removed.

B. Setting Time
When the leftover material on the spatula has lost its surface stickiness (tackiness), the impression is held in position 2 more clocked minutes.

III. The Completed Impression

A. Removal of Impression
1. Hold tray with thumb and fingers.
2. Retract cheek and lip with fingers and release the edge of the impression by depressing the buccal mucosa.
3. Do not rock the impression back and forth to release it because these movements may cause permanent distortion of the final impression.
4. Remove the impression with a sudden jerk or snap.

B. Rinse
Rinse under cool running water to remove saliva. Rinse carefully to prevent splashing contaminated saliva or blood over surroundings.

C. Examine and Evaluate the Impression
Observe surface detail, proper extension over retromolar area, and the peripheral roll (rounded border of the impression) generally.

D. Repeat Procedure When Necessary
Correct mistakes, rather than be satisfied with a substandard impression.

E. Wrap Mandibular Impression in a Wet Towel
while making the maxillary impression.

THE MAXILLARY IMPRESSION

I. Preparation

A. Request Patient to Rinse
To clear particles left from the mandibular impression and to relax the oral muscles.

B. Examine the Maxillary Teeth
Teeth should be examined for particles of mandibular impression material: remove. Request patient to use mouthrinse.

C. Prepare the Alginate
Fill the tray as described previously for the mandibular impression.

D. Precoat Undercut Areas
Precoat undercut areas, vestibular areas, and occlusal surfaces (see procedure for mandibular impression).

II. Insertion of Tray

A. Steps
1. Follow the procedure for insertion of maxillary tray described on page 153. Briefly, from the side back position, retract the patient's lip with the fingers of the nondominant hand; use side of tray to distend the lip and cheek; insert the tray with a rotary motion; center it over the teeth, using the small gap in the red wax border to relate to the labial frenum.
2. Introduce the material to the teeth so that the wax rim is about ¼ inch labial to the most labially inclined incisor.
3. Seat the tray
   a. Seat the tray from posterior to anterior to direct the impression material forward and thus prevent irritation to the soft palate area.
   b. Retract the lip and bring the tray to place with a slight vibratory motion to allow the material to flow into crevices and proximal areas.
   c. The middle finger of each hand is placed over the premolar region to support and

guide the tray; the index fingers and thumbs hold the lip out.

d. Request the patient to form a tight "O" with the lips to mold the impression material.

e. Maintain equal pressure on each side of the tray throughout the setting of the alginate. If assistance is available or if the pressure to hold the tray can be maintained with one hand, a saliva ejector can be inserted.

B. Setting Time

When the material on the spatula has lost its surface stickiness, the impression is held in place for 2 more clocked minutes.

III. The Completed Impression

A. Remove Impression

Hold the tray handle with the thumb and fingers of the dominant hand and retract the opposite lip and cheek with the fingers of the other hand. Elevate the cheek over the edge of the impression to break the seal, and remove the impression with a sudden jerk.

B. Rinse

Rinse under cool running water to remove saliva. Rinse carefully to prevent dissemination of contaminated saliva and blood.

C. Examine

Examine surface detail and proper extension to include tuberosity areas and a complete reproduction of the height of the vestibule.

D. Repeat Procedure When Necessary

Repeat procedure rather than be satisfied with a substandard impression.

E. Wrap Impression in a Damp Towel

This is to prevent dehydration and distortion; however, impressions should be poured promptly.

F. Check Manufacturer's Specifications

Check for use of a fixative.

IV. Disinfection of Impressions

To prevent cross-contamination during laboratory procedures, impressions should be immersed in an approved disinfectant after rinsing. The dimensional stability of some impression materials may be affected by certain disinfectants, so research and manufacturer's information must be heeded.[5,6] Iodophore and glutaraldehyde solutions have been used.[7,8]

When impressions are to be sent to a laboratory, they should be isolated in a package. If the patient was known to be at high risk for a communicable disease, the laboratory must be notified so that appropriate precautions can be taken.[5]

A list of infection control references is provided in the suggested readings at the end of the chapter.

THE INTEROCCLUSAL RECORD (WAX BITE)

I. Purposes

A. To relate the maxillary and mandibular casts correctly. Many, if not most, maxillary and mandibular casts will orient to each other readily in only one position, but when there are problems such as openbite, crossbite, edentulous areas, end-to-end, or edge-to-edge relations that may interfere with direct occlusion of the casts, a wax bite is generally needed.

B. To place between the casts during trimming and storage to prevent breakage of teeth.

II. Procedure

A. Have patient practice opening and closing on the posterior teeth to assure that the correct position can be obtained easily.

B. Ask patient to rinse with cold water.

C. Shape a double layer of soft baseplate wax in the form of the arch, warm slightly over a gas burner or soften in warm water, and place over the maxillary occlusal surfaces.

D. Request patient to close; press the wax against the facial surfaces of the teeth to shape it accurately to the arch.

E. Remove carefully to prevent distortion; chill in cold water.

PARACLINICAL PROCEDURES

Supplemental to the chairside clinical procedures is the laboratory work involved in the production of the study casts from the impressions. These duties may be the responsibility of the dental laboratory technician or other dental auxiliary, as directed by the dentist.

The most frequent error in the use of the alginates for impressions is delay in pouring the cast. Undue dehydration or water loss from the alginate will cause permanent distortion, an uneven surface, and hence an inaccurate cast. Regard for the sensitive properties of the dental materials, precision and practice in laboratory procedures, and pride in the production of neat, smooth, well-proportioned study casts determine the finished product's appearance, usefulness, and accuracy.

I. Equipment and Materials

A. Mixing bowl: clean, dry, flexible rubber or plastic, with smooth, unscratched surface.

B. Spatula: clean, dry, stiff, with a smooth, rounded end that will reach every part of the bowl without scraping or cutting its surface.

C. Plaster knife: sharp.

D. Vibrator.

E. Mechanical mixer.

F. Model-base formers, glass or ceramic slab, wax paper or other nonabsorbent-surfaced material.

G. Dental materials
 1. Baseplate wax (and wax spatula).
 2. White dental stone.
H. Water at room temperature, with measuring container.
 I. Model trimmer.
 J. Compass or dividers.
K. Plastic ruler.
L. Waterproof sandpaper.
M. Soap solution.

II. Preparation of the Impressions

A. Rinse impressions under cool running water; shake out excess water gently and apply gentle blast of compressed air.
B. Mandibular: create an artificial floor of the mouth in the impression to facilitate pouring and trimming of the cast.
 1. Trim the lingual impression material all around so that the height is consistent from the occlusal and incisal surfaces to the base of the impression.
 2. Using alginate
  a. Mix a small portion of alginate.
  b. Hold the mandibular impression upright in the nondominant hand, with the middle and ring fingers extended from under the tray into the tongue area.
  c. Apply alginate over the fingers to form a flat bridge slightly above the lingual flanges of the impression.
  d. Smooth the surface with a finger moistened with cool water; hold until the alginate sets.
  e. When assisted at the chair, the floor for the mandibular impression can be made while the maxillary impression is being held for setting. There is usually sufficient alginate mixed with that for the maxillary impression to use for this purpose.
 3. Using baseplate wax
  a. Cut a piece of baseplate wax to the shape of the lingual periphery of the impression.
  b. Seal into place with a warm spatula, taking care that no heat is applied to the anatomic portions of the impression.
  c. Cool under running water.

III. Mixing the Stone

A. Factors Related to Dental Stone That Contribute to a Successful Cast

Texts on dental materials should be reviewed for complete information about gypsum products.[9,10,11] Some pertinent properties are listed here as reference points.
 1. *Dental Stone.* Sensitive to changes in the relative humidity of the atmosphere.
  a. Store in airtight container; close soon after use; do not let water enter the container.

  b. Keep the spoon or scoop used to remove the powder clean and dry.
 2. *Water.* Controls the strength, rigidity, and hardness of the cast.
  a. Temperature: generally, cooler water decreases the setting time and warmer water increases it.
  b. Quantity: follow manufacturer's proportions exactly. Increasing the water over the specifications prolongs the setting time and reduces the strength.
 3. *Spatulation.* Prolonged or very rapid mixing can hasten the chemical reaction and shorten the setting time.

B. The Mix

 1. Measure the water and powder by the manufacturer's specifications.
  a. White stone is generally preferred for study casts. Plaster produces a cast more susceptible to breakage.
  b. Ratio of 30 to 40 ml. water to 100 g. stone.
 2. Place measured water (room temperature) in a clean, dry, mixing bowl.
 3. Sift in the powder gradually to prevent air trapping and to allow each particle to become wet.
 4. Wait briefly until all powder is wet, then vibrate to release large bubbles.
 5. Spatulation: with clean, stiff spatula.
  a. Hand spatulate for not less than 30 and not more than 60 seconds.
  b. Contact the entire inner surface of the bowl so no powder is left unincorporated.
  c. Do not whip or beat because this encourages bubble formation.
  d. Vibrate during and after spatulation to remove bubbles.
  e. Mechanical mixer or vacuum mixer may be used when available.
 6. Result: smooth, homogeneous, creamy mix.

IV. Pouring the Cast

The finished cast will have two connected parts, the anatomic portion and the base or art portion (see figure 10–6, page 160).

A. Pouring the Anatomic Portion

 1. Shake water out of the impression.
 2. Hold the impression tray by the handle and press handle against the vibrator.
 3. With a small amount of stone mix on the end of the spatula, start at one posterior corner and allow the mix to flow through the impression. Use small amounts and vibrate continually.
  a. Tip the impression so the material will pass into the tooth indentations and flow slowly down the side, across the occlusal surface or the incisal edge and up the other side of the impression of each tooth.
  b. Air will be trapped if the process is hurried

or if too large a quantity of mix is poured in at one time without attentive control of the flow.

4. When all tooth indentations are covered, add larger amounts of mix to fill the impression slightly over the periphery. Vibrate.

B. One-Step Method for Forming the Base of the Cast

1. Fill rubber model-base former with the remainder of the mix, or form a mass of stone on a glass or ceramic slab or other nonabsorbable surface (wax paper on a smooth surface). Add excess stone at the heel areas.

2. Invert the poured impression onto the base
   a. Use a slight back-and-forth motion to secure the two parts together.
   b. Common error: inverting the impression before the stone is firm. The mix can flow out of the impression.

3. Adjust tray to proper position
   a. Occlusal plane (at premolars) should be parallel with the base of the model-base former or tabletop.
   b. Midline (anterior as judged by handle of impression tray) centered at the midline of the model-base former.
   c. Accommodate position so that a tooth in labio- or buccoversion will not protrude over the trimming line of the art portion (see figure 10–6).

4. Add stone on peripheral and heel areas to provide a smooth surface; remove excess so that wax periphery of the tray is visible. When excess stone above the edge of the tray rim is permitted to set, it is difficult to separate the tray, and the use of a knife to carve the excess from the tray may damage the cast.

5. Final set occurs within 1 hour. Separate 1 hour after pouring to prevent damage to the surface of the cast.

C. Other Methods for Forming the Base of the Cast

1. *Two-step or Double-pour.* Both maxillary and mandibular impressions are poured and left upright (Step IV., A., 1. through 4.). Stone is then prepared separately for the bases, and the model-base formers are filled or the mass is placed on the smooth nonabsorbent surface.

   The impression is inverted and held on the surface of the new stone while the sides and periphery are shaped and smoothed. An advantage to this method is that there is no danger of inverting the poured impression too soon. If the cast is turned before it starts to set, the unset stone can fall away from the occlusal and incisal portions and leave bubbles in strategic places.

2. *Boxing Technique.* The object is to form a wall around the impression before pouring to provide a shape for the base as well as to prevent the need for inverting the poured impression. A strip of utility (beading) wax is attached slightly below the periphery of the impression and completely around the impression. Boxing wax or baseplate is applied around the strip of utility wax and attached to it by means of a warm spatula at a height that allows for proper thickness of the final cast, about ½ inch. Care must be taken not to displace the impression dimensionally or to touch the anatomic portions with the warm spatula. Pouring is carried out as described previously.

   Work-model formers with side walls to provide the boxing effect are available. Such a mold has a slot through the rubber where the handle of the impression tray can be inserted.

V. Separation of the Impression and the Cast

A. Objective: to remove tray and impression material without breaking the teeth.

B. When model-base former is used, remove it first.

C. Cut away stone from the periphery to free the margin of the tray.

D. Remove the tray by itself.

E. Cut the impression material along the line of the occlusal surfaces and peel off the impression material (with care not to scratch the stone cast during cutting).

F. Direct removal: when the teeth are in reasonably normal alignment, the tray and the impression material may be removed with a straight pull after first releasing the anterior portion by a slight downward and forward movement. When this method is used, do not apply lateral pressures or rock the tray back and forth, because it is easy to break the teeth by using such forces.

G. Trimming is started promptly, or if delayed, the cast must be thoroughly soaked in water before trimming.

TRIMMING THE CASTS

The exact proportions of the study casts and the steps required to accomplish the trimming and finishing depend on several factors. These include the measurements of the patient's dental arches, the positions of the teeth, and the preferences of the dentist. Development of a routine, systematic procedure for trimming can lead to the production of consistent, attractive, and useful diagnostic casts.

The method described here is dependent on the use of a precision-type model trimmer. No specific directions are provided for the use of angulators that are available to fit on the table of the model trimmer to give average set angles for trimming the margins of the casts; when these are available, directions are usually supplied by the manufacturer.

When a mechanical model trimmer is not available, greater skill must be developed to produce well-proportioned and smooth casts. The use of the

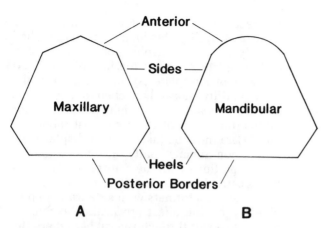

Figure 10–5. Base Shapes for Finished Study Casts. Maxillary and mandibular casts are trimmed at the labeled areas. See text for procedures.

model-base formers or a boxing method can be developed to a higher degree of precision. Trimming with a plaster knife must be started as soon as the impression is separated. Plaster files are available to aid in cutting the borders of the base.

Before the step-by-step description of the trimming procedure, an outline of the characteristics of the finished casts is provided as an overall guide.

I. Objectives: Characteristics of the Finished Casts

A. Overall Base Shape (figure 10–5).

B. Proportions

Approximately one-third art portion and two-thirds anatomic (figure 10–6 A).

C. Bases

The mean occlusal plane of the related casts is parallel with both bases, which are parallel with each other (figure 10–6 A).

D. Posterior Borders

1. At a right angle with the bases (figure 10–6 B).
2. Maxillary and mandibular posterior borders

are in the same plane; when standing on their posterior borders, the casts will rest together in natural intercuspation (figure 10–6 B).
3. Posterior borders are perpendicular to the median line from the incisors through the palate (maxillary, figure 10–7 A) and the middle of the tongue (mandibular, figure 10–7 B).

E. Sides

Symmetrical angulation with posterior border and heel cuts (figure 10–7); parallel with a line through the central grooves of the premolars of the same side.

F. Heels

Make ½ inch cuts parallel with the mesiodistal plane of the opposite canine (figure 10–7).

G. Anterior

Mandibular is shaped in an arc, maxillary in a point, with the cuts extending from the canine area (figure 10–7).

H. Borders

1. *Posterior.* Should include retromolar area and tuberosity (figure 10–7).
2. *Sides.* Should be ¼ to ⁵⁄₁₆ inch from bony protuberance over premolars and molars; anatomy of mucobuccal fold included in the cast.
3. *Anterior.* Should be ¼ to ⁵⁄₁₆ inch from the most protruded tooth or from the depth of the mucobuccal fold, whichever is most labial.

I. Surfaces of the Cast

Smooth and polished with air bubbles removed or filled.

II. Preliminary Steps to Trimming the Cast

A. Casts must be wet: soak at least 5 minutes.
B. Remove bubbles of stone on or about the teeth with a small sharp instrument; use care not to scar the cast.
C. Level down excess stone that is distal to the

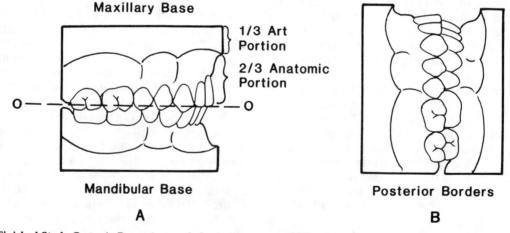

Figure 10–6. Finished Study Casts. A. Proportions and planes. The *art* portion is one third and the anatomic portion two thirds of the total height of the cast. Note parallelism of the maxillary and mandibular bases with the mean occlusal plane (0–0). **B.** Posterior borders are at right angles to the bases. When the maxillary and mandibular casts are placed on their posterior borders, the teeth will intercuspate exactly.

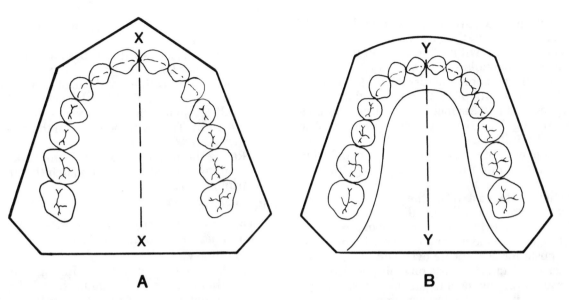

Figure 10–7. Occlusal Views of Finished Casts. A. Maxillary. **B.** Mandibular. The posterior border is perpendicular to the median line from the incisors through the palate (X–X) and the middle of the tongue (Y–Y). The tuberosity of the maxilla and the retromolar areas of the mandible are preserved.

retromolar area and tuberosity so casts may be occluded. Do not shorten the cast anteriorly-posteriorly at this time.

D. Trim casts conservatively on the sides to make a smooth surface for marking.

III. Trimming the Bases

A. Objectives
1. To make bases parallel with the mean occlusal plane and to each other.
2. To make correct proportions for the height of the casts: art portion one-third and anatomic portion two-thirds (figure 10–6 A).

B. Mandibular Cast Is Trimmed First
1. Measure the greatest height of the anatomic portion (usually this is from the tip of the canine to the depth of the vestibule) with a plastic ruler (figure 10–8).
2. Divide by two: this will be the height of the art portion.
3. Add the measured height of the anatomic por-

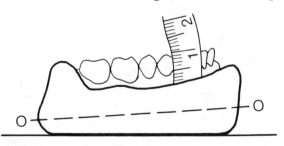

Figure 10–8. Trimming the Base. Measure the anatomic portion at its greatest height, which is usually from the tip of the canine to the depth of the vestibule. Note ruler in position. One half of the measurement is the height of the art portion. The trimming line (0–0) is parallel with the mean occlusal plane. See text for details.

tion to the height of the art portion for the total height of the cast. Set compass or dividers at this measurement.

4. Place the cast teeth down on a flat surface and mark a line around the art portion at the height calculated in step 3. This line should be parallel with the occlusal plane (line 0–0 in figure 10–8). Trim the cast at the line.

C. Maxillary Cast
1. Measure the greatest depth of the anatomic portion (usually at the canine) and divide by two to obtain the height of the art portion.
2. Relate the two casts (use the wax bite if necessary) and place the mandibular base on the flat surface.
3. Measure from the base of the mandibular cast to the highest point of the maxillary anatomic portion (usually in the vestibule over the canine), and add this figure to the height of the maxillary art portion calculated in step 1 above.
4. Set the compass at this measurement and mark a line around the maxillary cast at the total height. The line must be parallel with the base of the mandibular cast and with the occlusal plane. Trim.

IV. Posterior Borders

A. Select the longest cast to trim first by measuring from the incisors to points distal to the retromolar and tuberosity areas.

B. On the longest cast, place the tip of the compass at the gingival border behind the midline anteriorly (usually this is between the central incisors) and mark an arc ¼ inch distal to the tuberosity (if the maxillary cast) or retromolar area (if the mandibular cast) on each side.

C. Intersect the arc with a line through the central grooves of the molars (figure 10–9 A).

D. Connect the two points across the back of the cast (0–0 in figure 10–9 A). Check that this line is perpendicular to the median line from the incisors through the palate or the tongue (X–Y in figure 10–9 B).

E. With the base of the cast flat on the model trimmer table, trim on the line marked for the posterior border.

F. For the shorter cast, relate the two casts with the wax bite and place flat on the base of the first trimmed cast. Bring them carefully to the cutting surface of the model trimmer, and trim until the two posterior borders are even and parallel.

G. Check by placing the casts on their posterior borders and bringing them together. They should relate in their natural intercuspation (figure 10–6 B).

V. Sides and Heels

A. Select the widest cast to trim first: casts are usually widest at the molar region.

B. Mark with ruler two symmetrical lines ¼ inch buccal from the buccal bony prominence at the premolar regions and parallel with lines through the central grooves of the premolars (figure 10–10 A).

1. Check that the lines form equal angles with the posterior border.

2. Before trimming, make certain that the lines when cut would not remove any vestibular anatomy.

3. Trim the sides with the base flat on the model trimmer table.

C. Mark trimming lines for the heels: cuts are ½ inch wide and parallel with a line through the mesiodistal plane of the opposite canine (figure 10–10 B). Trim with base flat on the model trimmer table.

D. Relate the opposite cast with the wax bite and trim the sides and heels to match the previously trimmed cast.

VI. Anterior

The maxillary cast is trimmed to a point and the mandibular cast is rounded (figure 10–5).

A. Maxillary

1. A ruler can be used to draw guidelines for trimming on each side of the midline to the canine areas. Note the broken lines in figure 10–11 A. The lines should be ¼ inch labial to the depth of the mucobuccal fold (vestibule) or to the most labially inclined tooth.

2. Before trimming, check that both sides of the cast will be the same length from the intersection of the front cut to the heels.

B. Mandibular

1. Sketch the shape of an arc from canine to canine to conform generally with the curvature of the anterior teeth and approximately ¼ inch labial to the depth of the mucobuccal fold or the most labially inclined or positioned tooth (figure 10–11 B).

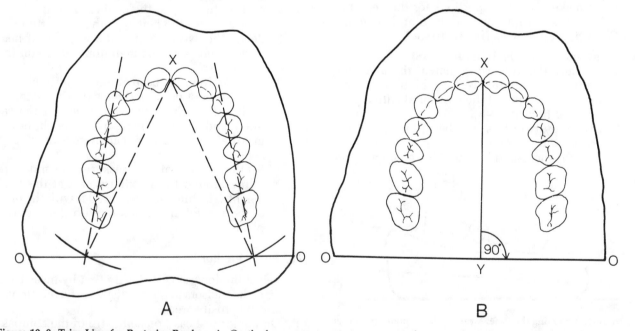

A   B

Figure 10–9. Trim Line for Posterior Borders. A. On the longest cast, use a compass to draw arcs from the anterior midline point (X) to ¼ inch distal to the tuberosity (maxilla) or retromolar area (mandible). Intersect the arc with a line through the central grooves of the molars and connect the two points across the cast (0–0). **B.** Check that the 0–0 line is perpendicular to the median line from the incisors through the palate or tongue (X–Y) before trimming.

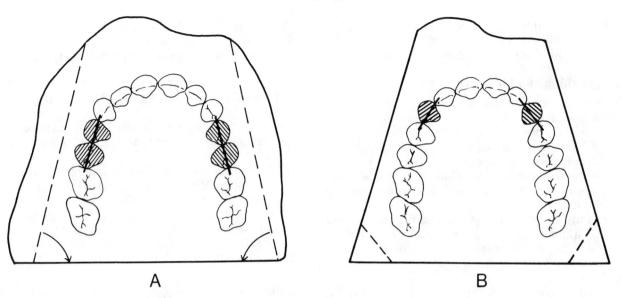

Figure 10–10. Trim Lines for Sides and Heels. A. On the widest cast, the trim lines for the sides are drawn parallel with lines through the central grooves of the premolars. The two symmetrical lines form equal angles with the posterior border of the cast. **B.** Mark trim lines for heels ¼ inch wide and parallel with lines through the mesiodistal plane of the opposite canine. The lines are symmetrical with each other and form equal angles with the posterior border.

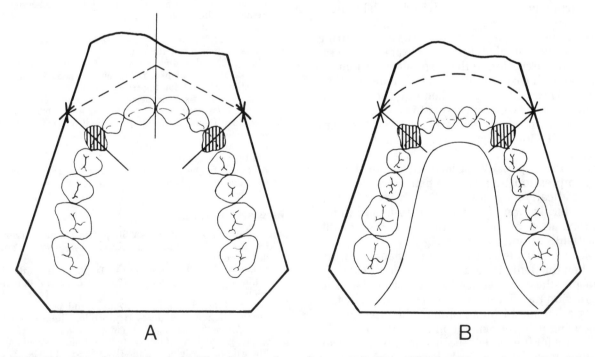

Figure 10–11. Trim Lines for Anterior. A. Maxillary lines are drawn from opposite the middle of each canine to meet in a point at the midline and approximately ¼ inch labial to the most labially positioned tooth. **B.** Mandibular line forms an arc drawn from the middle of each canine approximately ¼ inch labial to the most labially positioned tooth.

2. Before trimming, check that both sides of the cast will be the same length from the intersection of the front cut to the heels.

VII. Finishing and Polishing

A. Trim rough edges and margins of both casts and the lingual portion of the mandibular cast to even off irregularities and make the depth of the vestibule visible. Remaining bubbles are removed.

B. Use waterproof sandpaper and a plaster smoothing stone to remove marks left by the model trimmer on the art portion. Sandpaper is not used on the anatomic portion.

C. Fill any holes in the wet casts with stone applied with a spatula to the flat surfaces of the art portion or a camel's hair brush to the anatomic portion. Smooth off excess.

D. Finish and polish
1. Allow casts to dry thoroughly for 2 to 3 days.
2. Smooth the art portion with fine sandpaper.
3. Soak in heated soap solution for 30 to 60 minutes. Concentrated model gloss soap is available commercially.
4. Rub with chamois, cotton, or a soft cloth.
5. Talc or baby talcum powder with olive oil may be used, followed by rubbing with a chamois or soft cloth.

TECHNICAL HINTS

I. Safety Factors[12]
A. Wear protective eyeglasses while handling powdered dental materials or using a model trimmer. Goggles are advised for laboratory procedures (see figure 3–2, page 36).
B. Do not agitate powders unnecessarily during mixing. Inhaled dust particles can cause serious irritation to the respiratory system.

II. Label each cast with the patient's name and the date. These may be inscribed into the posterior border of the cast before soaping and polishing.

III. Boxes of an appropriate size are available commercially for storage of one or more pairs of casts.

IV. Note in the patient's permanent record the size of impression tray used. When casts are made periodically for follow-up, time is saved both in the sterilization of all sizes for try-in and in the preparation of the wax rim in advance of the patient's appointment.

V. Make duplicate cast for the permanent record when the dentist uses the original for the design of prosthesis or fabrication of a secondary impression tray. The duplicate cast is made by taking a laboratory impression of the original and pouring it in the same manner as the original.

VI. To care for the model trimmer, following its use, allow motor to run until clear water is flowing through and all particles of stone or plaster have been washed away.

VII. Replace scratched mixing bowls.

VIII. Sterilize aluminum impression trays. Clean completely to prepare for sterilization.

FACTORS TO TEACH THE PATIENT

I. Importance and purposes of study casts. Reasons for comparative casts following treatment or at a later date.

II. Use of the casts of other patients to show effects of treatment or what can happen if the prescribed treatment is not carried out.

III. Areas that present difficulty in the plaque control and oral physical therapy program: use of devices can be demonstrated on the patient's own study cast.

References

1. Stankewitz, C.G., Carpenter, W.M., and Kate, W.: Bacteremia Associated with Irreversible Hydrocolloid Dental Impressions, *J. Prosthet. Dent., 44,* 251, September, 1980.
2. American Dental Association, Council on Dental Materials, Instruments and Equipment: *Dentist's Desk Reference: Materials, Instruments, and Equipment,* 2nd ed. Chicago, American Dental Association, 1983, pp. 227–229.
3. Craig, R.G., ed: *Restorative Dental Materials,* 7th ed. St. Louis, The C.V. Mosby Co., 1985, pp. 255–261.
4. Phillips, R.W.: *Skinner's Science of Dental Materials,* 8th ed. Philadelphia, W.B. Saunders Co., 1982, pp. 126–136.
5. American Dental Association, Council on Dental Materials, Instruments, and Equipment, Council on Dental Practice, and Council on Dental Therapeutics: Infection Control Recommendations for the Dental Office and the Dental Laboratory, *J. Am. Dent. Assoc., 116,* 241, February, 1988.
6. United States Department of Health and Human Services: Recommended Infection-Control Practices for Dentistry, *MMWR, 35,* 237, April 18, 1986.
7. Crawford, J.: *Clinical Asepsis in Dentistry,* 4th ed. Mesquite, Texas, R.A. Kolstad, 1987, p. 37.
8. Minagi, S., Fukushima, K., Maeda, N., Satomi, K., Ohkawa, S., Akagawa, Y., Miyake, Y., Suginaka, H., and Tsuru, H.: Disinfection Method for Impression Materials: Freedom from Fear of Hepatitis B and Acquired Immunodeficiency Syndrome, *J. Prosthet. Dent., 56,* 451, October, 1986.
9. American Dental Association, Council on Dental Materials, Instruments, and Equipment: op. cit., pp. 250–252.
10. Craig: op. cit., pp. 303–317.
11. Phillips: op. cit., pp. 63–89.
12. American Dental Association, Council on Dental Materials, Instruments, and Equipment: op. cit., p. 49.

Suggested Readings

Carlin, S.A. and Oertling, K.: A Simplified Guide to Trimming Esthetically Appealing Diagnostic Casts, *J. Prosthet. Dent., 53,* 882, June, 1985.
Hansen, C.A.: A Method to Eliminate Trapping Air in the Palate While Making Impressions, *J. Prosthet. Dent., 55,* 405, March, 1986.
Johnson, G.H. and Craig, R.G.: Accuracy and Bond Strength of Combination Agar/Alginate Hydrocolloid Impression Materials, *J. Prosthet. Dent., 55,* 1, January, 1986.
LeCompte, E.J. and Whitford, G.M.: The Biologic Availability of Fluoride from Alginate Impressions and APF Gel Applications in Children, *J. Dent. Res., 60,* 776, April, 1981.
Strang, R.H.W. and Thompson, W.M.: *A Textbook of Orthodontia,* 4th ed. Philadelphia, Lea & Febiger, 1958, pp. 786–798.

Torres, H.O. and Ehrlich, A.: *Modern Dental Assisting,* 3rd ed. Philadelphia, W.B. Saunders Co., 1985, pp. 474–489.

Woodall, I.R., Dafoe, B.R., Young, N.S., Weed-Fonner, L., and Yankell, S.L.: *Comprehensive Dental Hygiene Care,* 2nd ed. St. Louis, The C.V. Mosby Co., 1985, pp. 238–270.

Woodward, J.D., Morris, J.C., and Khan, Z.: Accuracy of Stone Casts Produced by Perforated Trays and Nonperforated Trays, *J. Prosthet. Dent., 53,* 347, March, 1985.

Infection Control

Durr, D.P. and Novak, E.V.: Dimensional Stability of Alginate Impressions Immersed in Disinfecting Solutions, *J. Dent. Child., 54,* 45, January-February, 1987.

Firtell, D.N., Moore, D.J., and Pelleu, G.B.: Sterilization of Impression Materials for Use in the Surgical Operating Room, *J. Prosthet. Dent., 27,* 419, April, 1972.

Herrera, S.P. and Merchant, V.A.: Dimensional Stability of Dental Impressions after Immersion Disinfection, *J. Am. Dent. Assoc., 113,* 419, September, 1986.

Leung, R.L. and Schonfeld, S.E.: Gypsum Casts as a Potential Source of Microbial Cross-contamination, *J. Prosthet. Dent., 49,* 210, February, 1983.

Merchant, V.A., McNeight, M.K., Ciborowski, C.J., and Molinari, J.A.: Preliminary Investigation of a Method for Disinfection of Dental Impressions, *J. Prosthet. Dent., 52,* 877, December, 1984.

Moore, T.C., Smith, D.E., and Kenny, G.E.: Sanitization of Dentures by Several Denture Hygiene Methods, *J. Prosthet. Dent., 52,* 158, August, 1984.

Radue, J.T., Unger, J.W., and Molinari, J.A.: Avoiding Cross-contamination in Immediate Denture Treatment, *J. Prosthet. Dent., 49,* 576, April, 1983.

Rowe, A.H.R. and Forrest, J.O.: Dental Impressions. The Probability of Contamination and a Method of Disinfection, *Br. Dent. J., 145,* 184, September 19, 1978.

Rudd, R.W., Senia, E.S., McCleskey, F.K., and Adams, E.D.: Sterilization of Complete Dentures with Sodium Hypochlorite, *J. Prosthet. Dent., 51,* 318, March, 1984.

Storer, R. and McCabe, J.F.: An Investigation of Methods Available for Sterilizing Impressions, *Br. Dent. J., 151,* 217, October 6, 1981.

Wakefield, C.W.: Laboratory Contamination of Dental Prostheses, *J. Prosthet. Dent., 44,* 143, August, 1980.

Williams, H.N., Falkler, W.A., and Hasler, J.F.: *Acinetobacter* Contamination of Laboratory Dental Pumice, *J. Dent. Res., 62,* 1073, October, 1983.

Williams, H.N., Falkler, W.A., Smith, A.G., and Hasler, J.F.: The Isolation of Fungi from Laboratory Dental Pumice, *J. Prosthet. Dent., 56,* 737, December, 1986.

Safety Factors

Brune, D. and Beltesbrekke, H.: Dust in Dental Laboratories. Part III: Efficiency of Ventilation Systems and Face Masks, *J. Prosthet. Dent., 44,* 211, August, 1980.

Brune, D. and Beltesbrekke, H.: Levels of Airborne Particles Resulting from Handling Alginate Impression Material, *Scand. J. Dent. Res., 86,* 206, May, 1978.

Knibbs, P.J. and Piney, M.D.: An Assessment of the Relative Dustiness of Different Alginate Impression Materials Under Simulated Working Conditions, *Br. Dent. J., 158,* 171, March 9, 1985.

Mack, P.J.: Inhalation of Alginate Powder During Spatulation, *Br. Dent. J., 146,* 141, March 6, 1978.

Setcos, J.C., Vrijhoef, M.M.A., Blumershine, R., and Phillips, R.W.: Airborne Particles from Alginate Powders, *J. Am. Dent. Assoc., 106,* 355, March, 1983.

11 *The Gingiva*

The true test of successful treatment, the real evaluation of the effects of scaling and related instrumentation, is the *health* of the gingival tissues. The objective of all treatment is to bring the diseased gingiva to a state of health that can be maintained by the patient. To do this, the first thing is to learn to recognize normal healthy tissue; to observe certain characteristics of color, texture, and form; to test for bleeding; and to apply this knowledge to the treatment and supervision of the patient's gingiva until health is attained.

An outline of the clinical features of the periodontal tissues in health and disease is included in this chapter. It is expected that complete information about the gross and microscopic anatomy of the periodontium and periodontal pathology will have been studied or will be studied in preparation for clinical practice. Textbooks and other references are listed in *Suggested Readings* at the end of the chapter for review.

OBJECTIVES

The ultimate objective is that the dental hygienist's knowledge and skill in examination and evaluation of the periodontal tissues is applied in patient care so that each patient attains and maintains optimum oral health. The dental hygienist knows when the treatment provided by dental hygiene services is definitive in restoring health and when additional treatment is needed. The patient can be properly informed so that complete treatment can be provided.

Specific objectives for the dental hygienist are to be able to

I. Recognize normal periodontal tissues.
II. Know the features of the periodontal tissues that must be examined for a complete assessment.
III. Recognize the basic signs of periodontal infections and classify them by type and degree of severity.
IV. Identify the dental hygiene treatment and instruction needed.
V. Outline the patient's preventive periodontal program (page 297).

THE FIELD OF OPERATION

The techniques of dental hygiene are applied directly to the teeth, the gingiva, and the gingival sul-

cus. Detailed knowledge and understanding of the anatomy and normal clinical appearance of the field of operation are prerequisite to meaningful examination and treatment.

I. The Teeth
A. Clinical Crown

The part of the tooth above the attached periodontal tissues. It can be considered the part of the tooth where clinical techniques are applied (figure 11–1).

B. Clinical Root

The part of the tooth below the base of the gingival sulcus or periodontal pocket. It is the part of the root to which periodontal fibers are attached.

C. Anatomic Crown

The part of the tooth covered by enamel.

D. Anatomic Root

The part of the tooth covered by cementum.

II. Oral Mucosa

The lining of the oral cavity, the oral mucosa is a mucous membrane composed of connective tissue covered with stratified squamous epithelium. There are three divisions or categories of oral mucosa.

A. Masticatory Mucosa

1. Covers the *gingiva* and the *hard palate*, the areas used most during the mastication of food.

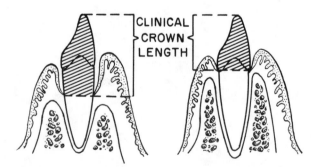

Figure 11–1. Clinical Crown. The clinical crown is the part of the tooth that is above the attached periodontal tissue. **Left,** When the periodontal pocket depth is increased, the clinical crown extends to a position at which the clinical crown length is greater than the clinical root length. The clinical root is that part of the tooth with attached periodontal tissues. **Right,** When the attachment is at the cementoenamel junction, the clinical crown and the anatomic crown are the same.

2. Except for the free margin of the gingiva, the masticatory mucosa is firmly attached to underlying tissues.
3. The epithelial covering is generally keratinized.

B. Lining Mucosa
1. Covers the *inner surfaces of the lips and cheeks, the floor of the mouth, the under side of the tongue, the soft palate, and the alveolar mucosa.*
2. These tissues are not firmly attached to underlying tissue.
3. The epithelial covering is not generally keratinized.

C. Specialized Mucosa
1. Covers the *dorsum* (upper surface) *of the tongue.*
2. Anterior part is composed of many papillae; some contain tastebuds.

III. The Periodontium

The periodontium is the functional unit of tissues that surrounds and supports the tooth. The four parts are the gingiva, periodontal ligament, cementum, and bone; the last three make up the attachment apparatus.

A. Gingiva
The part of the masticatory mucosa that surrounds the necks of the teeth and is attached to the teeth and the alveolar bone.

B. Periodontal Ligament
Connective tissue fibers that surround the root and connect the tooth and bone. The fibers that are inserted into the tooth on one side and the bone on the other side are called *Sharpey's fibers.*

C. Cementum
The calcified tissue that covers the root and attaches the fibers of the periodontal ligament to the tooth.

D. Alveolar Bone
The bone of the mandible and the maxilla that surrounds the roots of the teeth to support them. Periodontal ligament fibers are attached to the bone.

THE GINGIVA AND RELATED STRUCTURES

The gingiva is made up of the free gingiva, the attached gingiva, and the interdental gingiva or interdental papilla.

I. Free Gingiva (Marginal Gingiva)

The free gingiva is closely adapted around each tooth. It connects with the attached gingiva at the free gingival groove and attaches to the tooth at the coronal portion of the junctional epithelium (figure 11–2).

A. Free Gingival Groove
1. A shallow linear groove that demarcates the free from the attached gingiva. Generally, about one third of the teeth show a visible gingival groove when the gingiva is healthy.[1]

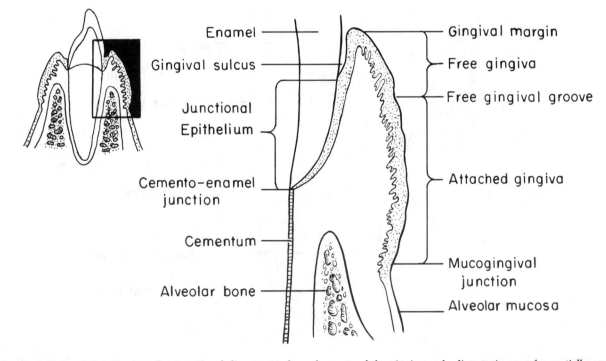

Figure 11–2. Parts of the Gingiva. Cross-sectional diagram to show the parts of the gingiva and adjacent tissues of a partially erupted tooth. Note that the junctional epithelium is on the enamel.

2. In the absence of disease and pocket formation, the gingival groove runs somewhat parallel with and about 0.5 to 1.5 mm. from the gingival margin,[2] and is approximately at the level of the bottom of the gingival sulcus.

B. Oral Epithelium (outer gingival epithelium, figure 11–3)
1. Covers the free gingiva from the gingival groove over the gingival margin.
2. Composed of keratinized stratified squamous epithelium.

C. Gingival Margin (gingival crest, margin of the gingiva, or free margin)
1. It is the edge of the gingiva nearest the incisal or occlusal surface.
2. Marks the opening of the gingival sulcus.

D. Gingival Sulcus (crevice)
1. It is the crevice or groove between the free gingiva and the tooth.
2. Boundaries (figure 11–3)
   a. Inner: tooth surface. May be the enamel, cementum, or part of each, depending on the position of the junctional epithelium.
   b. Outer: sulcular epithelium.
   c. Base: coronal margin of the attached tissues. The base of the sulcus or pocket is also called the "depth of the sulcus" or the "bottom of the pocket."
3. Sulcular epithelium: the continuation of the oral epithelium covering the free gingiva. Sulcular epithelium is not keratinized.
4. Depth of sulcus: healthy sulci are shallow and

may be only 0.5 mm. The average depth of the healthy sulcus is about 1.8 mm.[3]
5. Gingival sulcus fluid (sulcular fluid, crevicular fluid).
   a. A serum-like fluid seeps from the connective tissue through the epithelial lining of the sulcus or pocket.
   b. Occurrence: slight to none in a normal sulcus; increased with inflammation. It is part of the local defense mechanism and is able to transport antibodies and certain systemically administered drugs.

II. Junctional Epithelium (Attachment Epithelium)

A. Description

The junctional epithelium is a cuff-like band of stratified squamous epithelium that is continuous with the sulcular epithelium and completely encircles the tooth. It is triangular in cross section, widest at the junction with the sulcular epithelium, and narrowing down to the width of a few cells at the apical end.

The *epithelial attachment* is the inner part of the junctional epithelium adjacent to the tooth. It is attached to the tooth by hemidesmosomes and the basement lamina.

B. Size

The junctional epithelium may be up to 15 or 20 cells thick where it joins the sulcular epithelium and tapers down to 1 or 2 cells thick at the apical end. The length ranges from 0.25 to 1.35 mm.

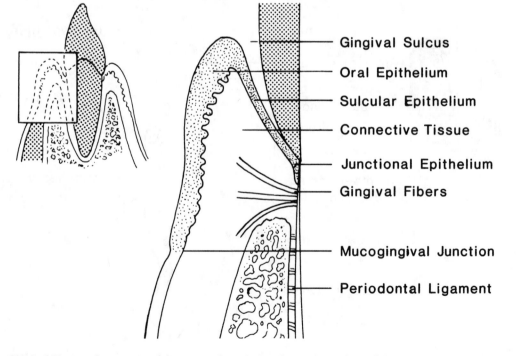

— Gingival Sulcus

— Oral Epithelium

— Sulcular Epithelium

— Connective Tissue

— Junctional Epithelium

— Gingival Fibers

— Mucogingival Junction

— Periodontal Ligament

Figure 11–3. The Gingival Tissues. Cross-sectional diagram to show the histologic relationships of the oral, sulcular, and junctional epithelia and the connective tissue.

C. Position

1. As the tooth erupts, the attachment is on the enamel; during eruption, the epithelium migrates toward the cementoenamel junction (figure 11–4).
2. At full eruption, the attachment is on the cementum where it becomes firmly attached.
3. With wear of the tooth on the incisal or occlusal surface and in disease, the attachment migrates along the root surface (figure 11–4 E).

D. Relation of Crest of Alveolar Bone to the Attached Gingival Tissue

The distance between the base of the attachment and the crest of the alveolar bone is approximately 1.0 to 1.5 mm. This distance is maintained in disease when the epithelium moves along the root surface and horizontal bone loss occurs.

E. Attachment of the Epithelium to the Tooth Surface

An adhesive, organic, mucopolysaccharide substance secreted by the epithelial cells provides a seal at the base of the sulcus and along the border of the junctional epithelium and the tooth surface.

III. Interdental Gingiva (Interdental Papilla)

A. Location

The interdental gingiva occupies the interproximal area between two adjacent teeth. The tip and lateral borders are continuous with the free gingiva, while other parts are attached gingiva.

B. Shape

1. Varies with spacing or overlapping of the teeth: the interdental gingiva may be flat or saddle-shaped when there are wide spaces between the teeth, or tapered and narrow when the teeth are crowded or overlapped.
2. Between anterior teeth: pointed, pyramidal.
3. Between posterior teeth
   a. Flatter than anterior papillae, which is

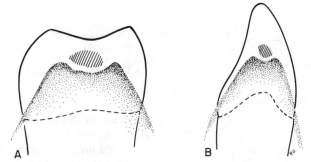

Figure 11–5. Col. A col is the depression between the lingual or palatal and the facial papillae under the contact area. The contact area is represented by the striped lines. **A.** Mesial of mandibular molar to show wide col area. **B.** Mesial of mandibular incisor to show a narrow col. The col deepens when gingival enlargement occurs.

caused by wider teeth, wider contact areas, and flattened interdental bone.
   b. Two papillae, one facial and one lingual, connected by a col, are found when teeth are in contact.

C. Col

1. A col is the depression between the lingual or palatal and facial papillae that conforms to the proximal contact area (figure 11–5).
2. The center of the col area is not usually keratinized, which makes it more susceptible to disease. Most periodontal infection begins in the col area.

IV. Attached Gingiva

A. Extent

1. The attached gingiva is continuous with the oral epithelium of the free gingiva and is covered with keratinized stratified squamous epithelium.
2. Maxillary palatal gingiva is continuous with the palatal mucosa.
3. Mandibular facial and lingual gingiva, and maxillary facial gingiva: the attached gingiva is demarcated from the alveolar mucosa by the mucogingival junction.

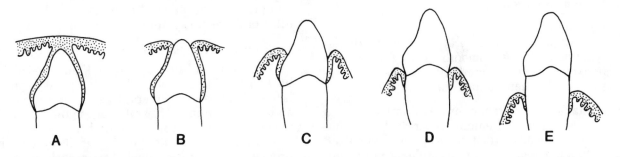

Figure 11–4. Tooth Eruption and the Gingiva. **A.** Before eruption, the oral epithelium covers the tooth. **B.** As the tooth emerges, the reduced epithelium joins the oral epithelium as the gingival sulcus is formed. **C.** Partial eruption with the junctional epithelium along the enamel. **D.** Eruption complete, with junctional epithelium at the cementoenamel junction. **E.** From disease or other cause, the attachment migrates along the root surface, exposing the cementum.

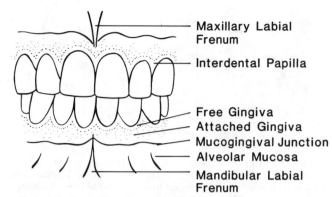

Maxillary Labial Frenum
Interdental Papilla
Free Gingiva
Attached Gingiva
Mucogingival Junction
Alveolar Mucosa
Mandibular Labial Frenum

Figure 11–6. Parts of the Gingiva. The mucogingival junction for each arch is shown in relation to the attached gingiva, alveolar mucosa, and labial anterior frena.

B. Attachment

Firmly bound to the underlying cementum and alveolar bone.

C. Shape

Follows the depressions between the eminences of the roots of the teeth.

D. Mucogingival Junction

1. *Appearance.* The mucogingival junction appears as a scalloped line that marks the connection between the attached gingiva and the alveolar mucosa.

   A contrast can be seen between the pink of the keratinized, stippled, attached gingiva and the darker alveolar mucosa.

2. *Location.* A mucogingival line is found on the facial surface of all quadrants and on the lingual surface of the mandibular arch. There is no alveolar mucosa on the palate. The palatal tissue is firmly attached to the bone of the roof of the mouth. There are three mucogingival lines: facial mandibular, lingual mandibular, and facial maxillary. In figure 11–6, the facial maxillary and mandibular mucogingival junctions are shown in relation to the attached gingiva and the alveolar mucosa.

V. Alveolar Mucosa

A. Description

Movable tissue loosely attached to the underlying bone. It has a smooth, shiny surface with nonkeratinized, thin epithelium. Underlying vessels may be seen through the epithelium.

B. Frena (singular: frenum or frenulum)

1. *Description.* A frenum is a narrow fold of mucous membrane that passes from a more fixed to a movable part; for example, from the gingiva to the lip, cheek, or undersurface of the tongue. A frenum serves to check undue movement.

2. *Locations*
   a. Maxillary and mandibular anterior frena: at midlines between central incisors. Figure 11–6 shows diagrammatically the location of the anterior frena.
   b. Lingual frenum: from undersurface of the tongue.
   c. Buccal frena: in the canine-premolar areas, both maxillary and mandibular.

3. Attachment of frena in relation to the attached gingiva
   a. May be closely associated with the mucogingival junction.
   b. When the attached gingiva is narrow or missing, the frena may pull on the free gingiva and displace it laterally. A "tension test" is used to locate frenal attachments and check the adequacy of the attached gingiva (page 199).

THE RECOGNITION OF GINGIVAL AND PERIODONTAL DISEASES

The recognition of normal gingiva, gingival infections, and deeper periodontal involvement depends on a disciplined, step-by-step examination. To recognize the signs of disease, a basic examination must include clinical observation for gingival tissue changes, bleeding, exudate, pockets, furcation involvement, mucogingival involvement, occlusion factors, tooth mobility, and a radiographic examination.

It is also necessary to know the extent of the disease. *Gingival diseases* are confined to the gingiva; whereas *periodontal diseases* include all parts of the periodontium, namely, the gingiva, periodontal ligament, bone, and cementum.

Patients may or may not have specific symptoms to report because periodontal diseases are insidious in development. Symptoms the patient notices or feels may include bleeding gingiva, sometimes only while brushing, sometimes with drooling at night, or sometimes spontaneously. Other possible symptoms are sensitivity to hot and cold, tenderness or discomfort while eating or some pain after eating, food retained between the teeth, unpleasant mouth odors, chronic bad taste, or a feeling that the teeth are loose. Most of these are symptoms of advanced disease.

I. Clinically Normal

The terms "clinically normal" or "clinically healthy" may be used to designate gingival tissue that is a shade of pale or coral pink varied by complexion and pigmentation; has a knife-edged gingival margin that adapts closely around the tooth; is stippled; firm; has minimal sulcus depth with no bleeding when probed. Although "normal" varies with anatomic, physiologic, and other factors, general characteristics form a baseline for a contrast in the recognition of disease.

II. Causes of Tissue Changes

Disease changes produce alterations in the color, size, position, shape, consistency, surface texture, bleeding readiness, and exudate production.

To understand the changes that take place in the gingival tissues during the transition from health to disease, it is necessary to have a clear picture of what bacterial plaque is, the role of plaque microorganisms in the development of disease, and the inflammatory response by the body.

When the products of the plaque microorganisms cause breakdown of the intercellular substances of the sulcular epithelium, injurious agents can pass into the connective tissue where an inflammatory response is initiated. An inflammatory response means that there is increased blood flow, increased permeability of capillaries, and increased collection of defense cells and tissue fluid. It is these changes that produce the tissue alterations such as color, size, shape, and consistency that are described in the next section.

III. Descriptive Terminology

The degree of severity and distribution of a change should be noted when examining the gingiva. When a deviation from normal affects a single area, it can be designated by the number of the adjacent tooth and the surface of the tissue involved, namely, facial, lingual, mesial, or distal. Teeth numbering systems are described on pages 73–75.

A. Severity

Severity is expressed as slight, moderate, or severe.

B. Distribution

Terms used for describing distribution are as follows:

1. *Localized.* Localized means that the gingiva is involved only about a single tooth or a specific group of teeth.
2. *Generalized.* Generalized means that the gingiva is involved about all or nearly all of the teeth throughout the mouth. A condition may also be generalized throughout a single arch, the maxillary or mandibular.
3. *Marginal.* A change that is confined to the free or marginal gingiva. This is specified as either localized or generalized.
4. *Papillary.* A change that involves a papilla but not the rest of the free gingiva around a tooth. A papillary change may be localized or generalized.
5. *Diffuse.* When the attached gingiva is involved as well as the free gingiva, it is referred to as a diffuse change. A diffuse condition is most frequently localized, rarely generalized.

IV. Early Recognition of Tissue Changes

Marked changes, such as moderate to severe generalized redness, enlargement, sponginess, deep pockets, and definite mobility, are relatively easy to detect even with limited experience, provided there is good light and accessibility for vision. In contrast, when changes are subtle, localized about one or a few teeth, and of a lesser degree of severity, more skillful application of knowledge is needed.

Early recognition of gingival and periodontal disease prevents neglect of conditions that can develop into severe disease. Treatment is less complicated, and the success of treatment and recovery to healthy tissue is predictable when early recognition makes early treatment possible.

THE GINGIVAL EXAMINATION

The examination of the gingiva includes evaluation of the color, size, shape, consistency, surface texture, position, mucogingival junctions, bleeding, and exudate. These are summarized in table 11–1, which is a clinical reference chart (pages 174–175).

I. Color

A. Signs of Health

1. *Pale Pink.* Darker in people with darker complexions.
2. *Factors Influencing Color*
   a. Vascular supply.
   b. Thickness of epithelium.
   c. Degree of keratinization.
   d. Physiologic pigmentation: melanin pigmentation occurs frequently in Negroes, Orientals, Indians, and Caucasians of Mediterranean countries.

B. Changes in Disease

1. *In Chronic Inflammation.* Dark red, bluish red, magenta, or deep blue.
2. *In Acute Inflammation.* Bright red.
3. *Extent.* Deep involvement can be expected when color changes extend into the attached gingiva or from the marginal gingiva to the mucogingival junction or over into alveolar mucosa.

II. Size

A. Signs of Health

1. *Free Gingiva.* Flat, not enlarged; fits snugly around the tooth.
2. *Attached Gingiva*
   a. Width of attached gingiva varies among patients and among teeth for an individual, from 1 to 9 mm.[4]
   b. Wider in maxilla than mandible: broadest zone related to incisors, narrowest at the canine and premolar regions.

B. Changes in Disease

1. *Free Gingiva and Papillae.* Become enlarged. This may be localized or limited to specific areas or generalized throughout the gingiva. The col deepens as the papillae increase in size.

2. *Attached Gingiva.* Decreases in amount as the pocket deepens. How to measure the amount of attached gingiva is described on page 200.

C. Enlargement from Drug Therapy

Certain drugs used for specific systemic therapy cause, as a side effect, gingival enlargement. Examples of the drugs are phenytoin, cyclosporin, and nifedipine.[5] They are described on page 186 along with other contributing factors to disease development.

III. Position

The *actual* position of the gingiva is the level of the attached periodontal tissue. It is not directly visible, but can be determined by probing.

The *apparent* position of the gingiva is the level of the gingival margin or crest of the free gingiva, which is seen by direct observation.

A. Signs of Health

In an adult, for the fully erupted tooth, the apparent position of the gingival margin is normally at the level of, or slightly below, the enamel contour or prominence of the cervical third of a tooth.

B. Changes in Disease

1. *Effect of Gingival Enlargement.* When the gingiva enlarges, the gingival margin may be high on the enamel, partly or nearly covering the anatomic crown.
2. *Effect of Gingival Recession*
   a. Definition. Recession is the exposure of root surface that results from the apical migration of the junctional epithelium (figure 11–7).

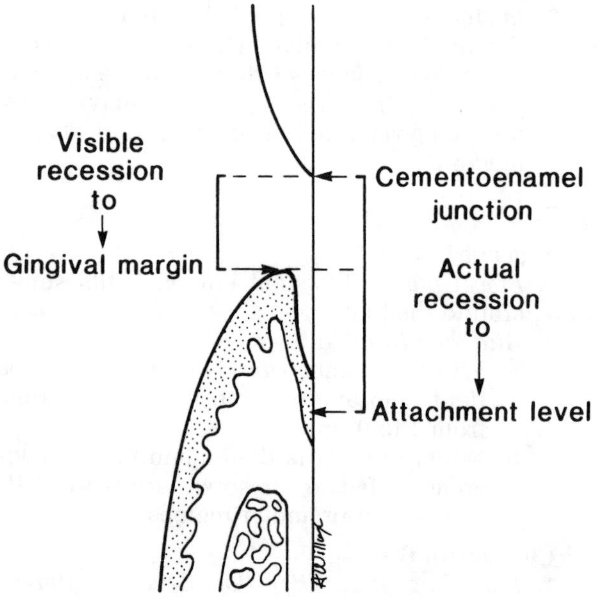

Figure 11–7. Gingival Recession. Left, Clinically visible recession of the gingival margin with root surface apparent to the eye. **Right,** The actual recession exposes the root surface as the periodontal attachment migrates along the root surface.

   b. Actual recession. The actual recession is shown by the position of the attachment level. The "receded area" is from the cementoenamel junction to the attachment.
   c. Apparent recession. The apparent recession is the exposed root surface that is visible on clinical examination. It is seen from the gingival margin to the cementoenamel junction.
   d. Localized recession (figure 11–8). A localized recession may be narrow or wide, deep or shallow. The root surface is denuded, and the apparent recession may extend to or through the mucogingival junction.
   e. Measurement. Both actual and apparent recession can be measured with a probe from the cementoenamel junction. Total recession is the actual and apparent added together.

IV. Shape (Form or Contour)

A. Signs of Health

1. *Free Gingiva*
   a. Follows a curved line around each tooth; may be straighter along wide molar surfaces.
   b. The margin is knife-edged or slightly rounded on facial and lingual gingiva; closely adapted to the tooth surface.
2. *Papillae*
   a. Teeth with contact area: facial and lingual gingiva are pointed or slightly rounded papillae with a col area under the contact (figure 11–5).
   b. Spaced teeth (with diastemas): interdental gingiva is flat or saddle-shaped (figure 12–4D, page 187).

B. Changes in Disease

1. *Free Gingiva.* Rounded or rolled.
2. *Papillae.* Blunted, flattened, bulbous, cratered (figure 11–9, page 176).
3. *Festoon ("McCall's festoon").* An enlargement of the marginal gingiva with the formation of a lifesaver-like gingival prominence. Frequently, the total gingiva is very narrow, with associated apparent recession as shown in figure 11–9D.
4. *Clefts*
   a. "Stillman's cleft" (figure 11–10, page 176). A localized recession may be V-shaped, apostrophe-shaped, or form a slit-like indentation. It may extend several millimeters toward the mucogingival junction or even to or through the junction.
   b. Floss cleft. A cleft created by incorrect floss positioning appears as a vertical linear or V-shaped fissure in the marginal gingiva.[6,7] It usually occurs at one side of an inter-

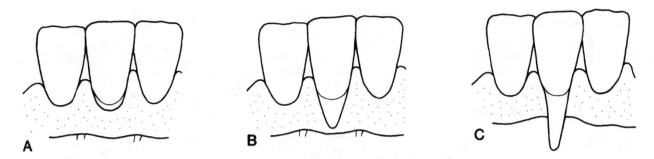

Figure 11–8. Localized Recession. A single tooth may show narrow or wide, deep or shallow recession. **A.** Wide, shallow. **B.** Wide, deep, with narrow attached gingiva. **C.** Narrow, deep, with missing attached gingiva.

dental papilla. The injury can develop when dental floss is curved repeatedly in an incomplete "C" around the line angle so the floss is pressed across the gingiva. Correct flossing positioning is shown in figure 23–1 on page 319.

V. Consistency

A. Signs of Health
1. Firm when palpated with the side of a blunt instrument (probe).
2. Attached gingiva is bound down firmly to the underlying bone.

B. Changes in Disease
1. *To Determine Consistency.* Gently press side of probe on free gingiva. Soft, spongy gingiva dents readily; firm, hard tissue resists.
2. *Soft Spongy Gingiva.* Related to acute stages of inflammation with increased infiltration of fluid and inflammatory elements. The tissue appears red, may be smooth and shiny with loss of stippling, has marginal enlargement, and bleeds readily on probing.
3. *Firm, Hard Gingiva.* Related to chronic inflammation with increased fibrosis. The tissue may appear pink and well stippled. Bleeding, when probed, usually occurs only in the deeper part of a pocket, not near the margin.
4. *Retraction of the Margin Away from the Tooth.* Normally, the free gingiva fits snugly about the tooth. When the margin tends to hang slightly away or is readily displaced with a light air blast, it means that the gingival fibers that support the margin have been destroyed.

VI. Surface Texture

A. Signs of Health
1. *Free Gingiva.* Smooth.
2. *Attached Gingiva.* Stippled (minutely "pebbled" or "orange peel" surface).
3. *Interdental Gingiva.* The free gingiva is smooth; the center portion of each papilla is stippled.

B. Changes in Disease
1. *Inflammatory Changes.* May be loss of stippling, with smooth, shiny surface.

2. *Hyperkeratosis.* May result in a leathery, hard, or nodular surface.
3. *Chronic Disease.* Tissue may be hard and fibrotic, with a normal pink color, and have normal or deep stippling.

VII. Bleeding

A. Signs of Health
1. No bleeding spontaneously or on probing.
2. Healthy tissue does not bleed.

B. Changes in Disease
1. Bleeding occurs spontaneously or when pockets are probed.
2. Sulcular epithelium becomes diseased *pocket epithelium.* The ulcerated pocket wall bleeds readily on gentle probing. Development of inflammation and pocket formation are described on pages 181–182.

VIII. Exudate

A. Signs of Health
There is no exudate except slight gingival sulcus fluid (page 168). Gingival sulcus fluid cannot be seen by direct observation.

B. Changes in Disease
1. *Suppuration.* Formation or secretion of pus.
2. *White Fluid.* May appear at the entrance to the pocket or may be squeezed out of the pocket by light finger pressure on the external wall of the pocket. Pus is a semifluid, creamy, yellow-white product of inflammation composed mainly of leukocytes and serum.
3. *Amount of Exudate.* Related to the severity of the acute inflammation, not to the depth of the pocket.

IX. The Gingiva of Young Children[8]

A. Signs of Health
1. *Primary Dentition*
   a. Color: pink or slightly red.
   b. Shape: thick, rounded, or rolled.
   c. Consistency: firm, but not tightly adapted to the teeth; it may be easily displaced with a light air jet.

Table 11–1.   Examination of the Gingiva. Clinical Reference Chart

	Appearance in Health	*Changes in Disease Clinical Appearance*	*Causes for Changes*

Color	Uniformly pale pink or coral pink
	
	Variations in pigmentation related to complexion, race
		Acute: bright red	Inflammation:
			  capillary dilation
			  increased blood flow

		Chronic: bluish pink, bluish red pink	Vessels engorged Blood flow sluggish Venous return impaired Anoxemia Increased fibrosis
		Attached gingiva: color change may extend to the mucogingival line	Deepening of pocket, mucogingival involvement

Size	Not enlarged
	
	Fits snugly around the tooth
		Enlarged	Edematous:
			  inflammatory fluid
			  cellular exudate
			  vascular engorgement
			  hemorrhage
			
			Fibrotic:
			  new collagen fibers

Shape	Marginal gingiva:
	  knife-edged, flat
	  follows a curved line about the tooth
	Papillae:
	(1) normal contact:
	    papilla is pointed and pyramidal; fills the interproximal area
	(2) space (diastema) between teeth: gingiva is flat or saddle-shaped
		Marginal gingiva:
		  rounded
		  rolled
		
		Papillae:
		  bulbous
		  flattened
		  blunted
		  cratered
			Inflammatory changes:
			  edema or fibrosis
			
			Bulbous with gingival enlargement (see edematous and fibrotic, above)
			
			Cratered in necrotizing ulcerative gingivitis

Consistency	Firm Attached gingiva firmly bound down	Soft, spongy: dents readily when pressed with probe Associated with red color, smooth shiny surface, loss of stippling, bleeding on probing	Edematous: fluid between cells in connective tissue
		Firm, hard: resists probe pressure Associated with pink color, stippling, bleeding only in depth of pocket	Fibrotic: collagen fibers

Table 11-1. Examination of the Gingiva. Clinical Reference Chart *Continued*

	Appearance in Health	*Changes in Disease* *Clinical Appearance*	*Causes for Changes*
Surface Texture	Free gingiva: smooth Attached gingiva: stippled	Acute condition: smooth, shiny gingiva Chronic: hard, firm, with stippling, sometimes heavier than normal	Inflammatory changes in the connective tissue; edema, cellular infiltration Fibrosis
Position of Gingival Margin	Fully erupted tooth: margin is 1–2 mm. above cemento-enamel junction, at or slightly below the enamel contour	Enlarged gingiva: margin is higher on the tooth, above normal, pocket deepened Recession: margin is more apical; root surface is exposed	Edematous or fibrotic Junctional epithelium has migrated along the root; gingival margin follows
Position of Junctional Epithelium	During eruption: along the enamel surface Fully erupted tooth: the junctional epithelium is at the cementoenamel junction	Position, determined by use of probe, is on the root surface	Apical migration of the epithelium along the root
Mucogingival Junctions	Make clear demarcation between the pink, stippled, attached gingiva and the darker alveolar mucosa with smooth shiny surface	No attached gingiva: (1) color changes may extend full height of the gingiva; mucogingival line obliterated (2) Probing reveals that the bottom of the pocket extends into the alveolar mucosa (3) Frenal pull may displace the gingival margin from the tooth	Deepening of the pocket Apical migration of the junctional epithelium Attached gingiva decreases with pocket deepening Inflammation extends into alveolar mucosa
Bleeding	No spontaneous bleeding or upon probing	Spontaneous bleeding Bleeding on probing: Bleeding near margin in acute condition; bleeding deep in pocket in chronic condition	Degeneration of the sulcular epithelium with the formation of pocket epithelium Blood vessels engorged Tissue edematous
Exudate	No exudate on pressure	White fluid, pus, visible on digital pressure Amount not related to pocket depth	Inflammation in the connective tissue Excessive accumulation of white blood cells with serum and tissue fluid makes up the exudate (pus)

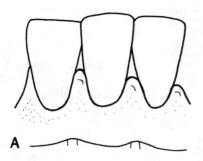

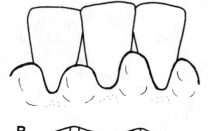

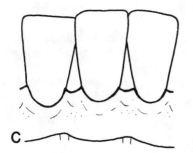

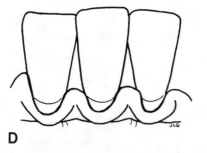

Figure 11–9. Gingival Shape or Contour. A. Blunted papillae. **B.** Bulbous papillae. **C.** Cratered papillae. **D.** Rolled, life-saver-shaped "McCall's festoons."

d. Surface texture: may or may not have stippling; high percentage of patients has shiny gingiva.

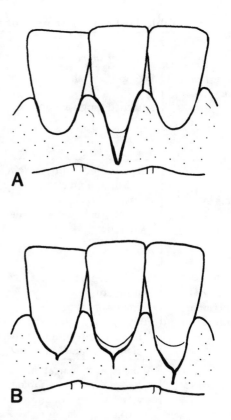

Figure 11–10. Gingival Clefts. A. V-shaped Stillman's cleft. **B.** Slit-like Stillman's clefts of varying degrees of severity in relation to the mucogingival junction.

    e. Width of attached gingiva in children ages 3 to 5: between 1 and 6 mm.[4]
    f. Interdental gingiva.
      i. Anterior: diastemas are frequently present and the papillae are flat or saddle-shaped; when teeth are in contact, the usual pyramid is present (page 169).
      ii. Posterior: col between facial and lingual papillae when teeth are in contact (figure 11–5).
2. *Mixed Dentition*
    a. Constant state of change related to exfoliation and eruption.
    b. Free gingiva may appear rolled or rounded, slightly reddened, shiny, and with a lack of firmness.
    c. Position: the gingiva covers a varying portion of the anatomic crown, depending on the stage of eruption (figure 11–4).

B. Changes in Disease

Examination of the periodontal tissues of a child is not different from that of an adult. A complete examination is necessary, including probing around each tooth.

Gingivitis affects over 80 percent of young

children[9] and increases in prevalence until a high of over 90 percent can be found in the 9- to 14-year-old group.

Although relatively rare, periodontitis can occur in primary dentition. Prepubertal periodontitis is described on page 180, in table 12–1.

Mucogingival problems occur in children.[10] The recognition of deficiencies of attached gingiva has particular significance for the child who will need orthodontic treatment.

X. The Gingiva after Periodontal Surgery

The characteristics of "normal healthy gingiva" take on different dimensions for the patient who has completed treatment for pockets, bone loss, and other signs of a periodontal disease. The junctional epithelium will be apical to the cementoenamel junction. After healing, the sulcus depth will be within normal range and no bleeding should occur when probed.

Depending on the exact treatment performed, examination will show changes from the initial evaluation. For example, where the initial examination showed a deficiency of attached gingiva with frenal pull, mucogingival surgery may have been designed and treatment satisfactorily completed to create new attached gingiva. With each maintenance appointment a thorough, careful examination is necessary to control factors that may permit recurrence of disease.

FACTORS TO TEACH THE PATIENT

I. Characteristics of normal healthy gingiva.
II. The significance of bleeding: healthy tissue does not bleed.
III. Relationship of findings during a gingival examination to the personal daily care procedures for disease control.
IV. The special attention needed for an area of gingival recession to prevent abrasion, inflammation, and further involvement.
V. How the method of brushing, stiffness of toothbrush filaments, abrasiveness of a dentifrice, and pressure applied during brushing, can be factors in gingival recession.
VI. Eight Warning Signs of Periodontal Disease*
  1. Gums that bleed when you brush your teeth.
  2. Gums that are red, swollen, or tender.
  3. Gums that have pulled away from the teeth.
  4. Pus between the teeth and gums when the gums are pressed.
  5. Permanent teeth that are loose or separating.
  6. Any change in the way your teeth fit together when you bite.
  7. Any changes in the fit of your partial dentures.
  8. Bad breath.

*From *Periodontal Disease. Don't Wait Till It Hurts.* American Dental Association, Catalog #W121. Order Department, 211 E. Chicago Avenue, Chicago, Illinois 60611.

References

1. Ainamo, J. and Löe, H.: Anatomical Characteristics of Gingiva. A Clinical and Microscopic Study of the Free and Attached Gingiva, *J. Periodontol., 37,* 5, January-February, 1966.
2. Orban, B.: Clinical and Histologic Study of the Surface Characteristics of the Gingiva, *Oral Surg. Oral Med. Oral Pathol., 1,* 827, September, 1948.
3. Bhaskar, S.N., ed.: *Orban's Oral Histology and Embryology,* 10th ed. St. Louis, The C.V. Mosby Co., 1986, p. 316.
4. Bowers, G.M.: A Study of the Width of Attached Gingiva, *J. Periodontol., 34,* 201, May, 1963.
5. Butler, R.T., Kalkwarf, K.L., and Kaldahl, W.B.: Drug-induced Gingival Hyperplasia: Phenytoin, Cyclosporin, and Nifedipine, *J. Am. Dent. Assoc., 114,* 56, January, 1987.
6. American Academy of Periodontology: *Glossary of Periodontic Terms, J. Periodontol.,* p. 5, 12, Supplement, November, 1986.
7. Hallman, W.W., Waldrop, T.C., Houston, G.D., and Hawkins, B.F.: Flossing Clefts. Clinical and Histologic Observations, *J. Periodontol., 57,* 501, August, 1986.
8. Carranza, F.A.: *Glickman's Clinical Periodontology,* 6th ed. Philadelphia, W.B. Saunders Co., 1984, pp. 291–308.
9. World Health Organization: *Epidemiology, Etiology, and Prevention of Periodontal Diseases.* WHO Technical Report Series Number 621, Geneva, World Health Organization, 1978, 60 pp.
10. Maynard, J.G. and Ochsenbein, C.: Mucogingival Problems, Prevalence and Therapy in Children, *J. Periodontol., 46,* 543, September, 1975.

Suggested Readings

Abrams, K., Caton, J., and Polson, A.: Histologic Comparisons of Interproximal Gingival Tissues Related to the Presence or Absence of Bleeding, *J. Periodontol., 55,* 629, November, 1984.

Ainamo, A., Ainamo, J., and Poikkeus, R.: Continuous Widening of the Band of Attached Gingiva From 23 to 65 Years of Age, *J. Periodont. Res., 16,* 595, November, 1981.

Allen, D.L., McFall, W.T., and Jenzano, J.W.: *Periodontics for the Dental Hygienist,* 4th ed. Philadelphia, Lea & Febiger, 1987, pp. 6–29.

Bergstrom, J.: The Topography of Papillary Gingiva in Health and Early Gingivitis, *J. Clin. Periodontol., 11,* 423, August, 1984.

Carranza, F.A.: *Glickman's Clinical Periodontology,* 6th ed. Philadelphia, W.B. Saunders Co., 1984, pp. 3–39.

Goldman, H.M. and Cohen, D.W.: *Periodontal Therapy,* 6th ed. St. Louis, The C.V. Mosby Co., 1980, pp. 1–49.

Grant, D.A., Stern, I.B., and Listgarten, M.A., eds.: *Periodontics,* 6th ed. St. Louis, The C.V. Mosby Co., 1988, pp. 3–75.

Kennedy, J.E., Bird, W.C., Palcanis, K.G., and Dorfman, H.S.: A Longitudinal Evaluation of Varying Widths of Attached Gingiva, *J. Clin. Periodontol., 12,* 667, September, 1985.

Kisch, J., Badersten, A., and Egelberg, J.: Longitudinal Observation of "Unattached," Mobile Gingival Areas, *J. Clin. Periodontol., 13,* 131, February, 1986.

Lang, N.P., Joss, A., Orsanic, T., Gusberti, F.A., and Siegrist, B.E.: Bleeding on Probing. A Predictor for the Progression of Periodontal Disease? *J. Clin. Periodontol., 13,* 590, July, 1986.

Melfi, R.C.: *Permar's Oral Embryology and Microscopic Anatomy,* 8th ed. Philadelphia, Lea & Febiger, 1988, pp. 217–231.

Mukherjee, S.: The Significance of Crevicular Fluid, *Compend. Contin. Educ. Dent., 6,* 611, September, 1985.

Smith, R.G.: A Longitudinal Study into the Depth of the Clinical Gingival Sulcus of Human Canine Teeth During and After Eruption, *J. Periodont. Res., 17,* 427, July, 1982.

Takei, H.H.: The Interdental Space, *Dent. Clin. North Am., 24,* 169, April, 1980.

Tintari, C.R.: Junctional Epithelium: A Literature Review, *Quintessence Int., 14,* 327, March, 1983.

Wennström, J.L.: Lack of Association Between Width of Attached Gingiva and Development of Soft Tissue Recession, *J. Clin. Periodontol., 14,* 181, March, 1987.

Gingiva of Children

Bimstein, E., Machtei, E., and Eidelman, E.: Dimensional Differences in the Attached and Keratinized Gingiva and Gingival Sulcus in the Early Permanent Dentition: A Longitudinal Study, *J. Pedod., 10,* 247, Spring, 1986.

Garcia-Godoy, F. and Locker, D.: Gingival Sulcus Depth in the Young Permanent Dentition, *J. Pedod., 8,* 178, Winter, 1984.

Keszthelyi, G. and Szabo, I.: Attachment Loss in Primary Molars, *J. Clin. Periodontol., 14,* 48, January, 1987.

Kleiner, R. and Garcia-Godoy, F.: Gingival Sulcus Depth in the Primary Dentition, *J. Pedod., 6,* 288, Summer, 1982.

Maynard, J.G. and Wilson, R.D.: Diagnosis and Management of Mucogingival Problems in Children, *Dent. Clin. North Am., 24,* 683, October, 1980.

Sanchez, M.C. and Tsamtsouris, A.: Mucogingival Defects in the Pedodontic Patient, *J. Pedod., 8,* 227, Spring, 1984.

Stoner, J.E. and Mazdyasna, S.: Gingival Recession in the Lower Incisor Region of 15-year-old Subjects, *J. Periodontol., 51,* 74, February, 1980.

Tenenbaum, H. and Tenenbaum, M.: A Clinical Study of the Width of the Attached Gingiva in the Deciduous, Transitional and Permanent Dentitions, *J. Clin. Periodontol., 13,* 270, April, 1986.

Tsamtsouris, A. and Saadia, A.M.: Gingivitis in Children, *J. Pedod., 5,* 173, Winter, 1981.

12 *Disease Development and Contributing Factors*

Early in the process of case assessment in preparation for treatment planning, the presence and severity of periodontal infection must be determined. Is the patient's disease limited to the gingival tissue without loss of periodontal attachment? Does the patient have bone loss, pocket formation, or other signs of periodontitis? Where is the attachment level? Is altered cementum exposed within the pockets?

When the disease is limited to the gingiva, the next question is: can the disease be reversed by having the patient follow daily disease-control self-treatment methods supplemented by professional scaling? On the other hand, if there is apical positioning of the periodontal attachment, accompanied by other indications of periodontitis, will conservative procedures of scaling, root planing, and gingival curettage provide sufficient professional treatment or will more complex periodontal therapy be required?

The dental hygienist needs to understand what can be accomplished by dental hygiene therapeutic procedures and when the patient will require more advanced therapy by a dentist or a periodontist in order to bring the oral tissues to a state of maximum health. It is not always possible to determine when additional therapy will be required until after the initial steps have been completed and a reevaluation has been made. When the initial treatment program is presented to the patient, it should be made clear that a reevaluation will be necessary.

CLASSIFICATION OF PERIODONTAL DISEASE

Gingivitis means inflammation of the gingival tissues. *Periodontitis* is the extension of the inflammation into the connective tissue and bone surrounding the teeth, which leads to progressive destruction of the periodontium.

Periodontal disease is not a single pathologic entity. It is a term used to describe a variety of inflammatory and degenerative diseases that affect the supporting structures of the teeth. A widely used system for classifying the types and severity of periodontal diseases is the one prepared by the American Academy of Periodontology as shown in Table 12–1.[1]

In this chapter, gingival and periodontal pockets and their formation will be described in preparation for clinical examination. Contributing factors in disease development to be observed for charting and recording will be outlined.

GINGIVAL AND PERIODONTAL POCKETS

A pocket is a diseased sulcus. It is the presence or absence of disease and the level of attachment on the tooth that distinguish a pocket from a sulcus, and not only the depth as measured with a probe. A pocket has an *inner wall, the tooth surface,* and an *outer wall, the sulcular* or *pocket epithelium* of the free gingiva. The two walls meet at the base of the pocket. The base of the pocket is the coronal margin of the attached periodontal tissues.

Histologically, the base of a healthy sulcus is the coronal border of the junctional epithelium, whereas the base of a pocket (diseased sulcus) may be at the coronal border of the connective tissue attachment. Research has shown that during probing of a healthy sulcus the end of the probe is near the level of the junctional epithelium. When periodontal disease is present, the position of the probe tip varies depending on the degree of inflammation and adjacent connective tissue destruction.[2]

I. Types of Pockets

Pockets are divided into *gingival* and *periodontal* types to clarify the degree of anatomic involvement. They are then further categorized by their position in relation to the alveolar bone; that is, whether their pocket base is suprabony or intrabony (figure 12–1).

A. Gingival Pocket

1. Definition: a pocket formed by gingival enlargement without apical migration of the junctional epithelium (figure 12–1B).
2. Other names: pseudopocket, false pocket, relative pocket.
3. The margin of the gingiva has moved toward the incisal or occlusal without the deeper periodontal structures becoming involved.
4. The tooth wall is enamel.
5. During eruption, the base of the pocket is at various levels along the enamel. The base of the pocket of a fully erupted tooth is near the cementoenamel junction (figure 11–4, page 169).
6. All gingival pockets are suprabony; that is, the base of the pocket is coronal to the crest of the alveolar bone.

B. Periodontal Pocket

1. Definition: a pocket formed as a result of disease or degeneration that caused the junctional

Table 12–1. Classification of Periodontal Diseases*

I. GINGIVAL DISEASE

A. *Gingivitis*—inflammation of the gingiva characterized clinically by changes in color, gingival form, position, surface appearance, and presence of bleeding and/or exudate. The most common cause of gingivitis is bacterial plaque.

1. Nonspecific gingivitis—the most common form of gingivitis. It is caused by dental plaque bacteria and their products.

2. Acute necrotizing ulcerative gingivitis (ANUG)—an infection which first affects the interdental papillary area and is characterized by necrosis and pseudomembrane formation.

B. *Manifestations of systemic diseases and hormonal disturbances*—associated with viral diseases including acute herpetic gingivostomatitis, blood dyscrasias including leukemia, autoimmune diseases such as pemphigus, and metabolic diseases such as diabetes. In some types of gingival disease modification of the sex hormones is considered to be either the initiating or complicating factor.

C. *Drug associated*—gingival inflammation and/or enlargement resulting from plaque-associated gingivitis complicated by systemic drug administration. Dilantin hyperplasia is a common example.

D. *Miscellaneous gingival changes associated with various etiologies*—includes all other pathologic and physiologic alterations in the gingival tissue. Changes include atrophy, cyst formation, hyperplasia, neoplasia, and degeneration and may be due to heredity, growth and development, infection, irritation, or trauma.

II. MUCOGINGIVAL CONDITIONS—changes in the position and relationship of the gingiva and gingival margin to the alveolar mucosa. It includes gingival recession and aberrant frena and/or muscle attachments.

III. PERIODONTITIS

A. *Adult Periodontitis*

1. Slight—progression of the gingival inflammation into the deeper periodontal structures and alveolar bone crest, with slight bone loss. The usual periodontal probing depth is 3 to 4 mm with slight loss of connective tissue attachment and slight loss of alveolar bone.

2. Moderate—a more advanced state of the above condition, with increased destruction of the periodontal structures and noticeable loss of bone support possibly accompanied by an increase in tooth mobility. There may be furcation involvement in multirooted teeth.

3. Advanced—further progression of periodontitis with major loss of alveolar bone support usually accompanied by increased tooth mobility. Furcation involvement in multirooted teeth is likely.

4. Rapidly progressive—includes several unclassified types of periodontitis characterized either by rapid bone and attachment loss, or slow but continuous bone and attachment loss, and resistance to normal therapy. It is usually associated with gingival inflammation and continued pocket formation.

B. *Juvenile periodontitis* (JP)—found in children and young adults. All forms usually progress at a rapid rate.

1. Prepubertal—an uncommon disease manifested by the formation of pockets and destruction of the alveolar bone around some, but not all, of the deciduous teeth. Onset may occur during, or immediately after, the eruption of the primary teeth. This disease may be present in either a generalized or localized form.

2. Generalized (GJP)—circumpubertal or postpubertal. An inflammatory process of the connective tissue and the bone surrounding the teeth, leading to progressive destruction of these tissues. Destruction may be cyclical with exacerbations and remissions. Increased pocket probing depth and loss of attachment are found.

3. Localized (LJP)—A specific periodontitis thought to be associated with one or more of the following: infection with *Actinobacillus actinomycetemcomitans*, heredity, or abnormalities in white blood cell function. Bone loss pattern has a predilection for the permanent central incisors and first molars.

C. *Periodontal abscess*—the result of the closure of the orifice of a deep periodontal pocket with the development of a localized acute infection, often accompanied by severe bone destruction.

IV. PATHOLOGY ASSOCIATED WITH OCCLUSION

Trauma from occlusion—tissue injury to the periodontal attachment apparatus caused by excessive occlusal forces. The most recognized etiologic factor is bruxism (clenching and grinding of the teeth). It may be associated with disorders of the temporomandibular joints.

V. OTHER CONDITIONS OF THE ATTACHMENT APPARATUS—includes all pathologic processes of the periodontium including infection, abrasion, trauma, and cystic, degenerative, or neoplastic changes.

*American Academy of Periodontology, *Current Procedural Terminology for Periodontics*, 5th ed. 1987.

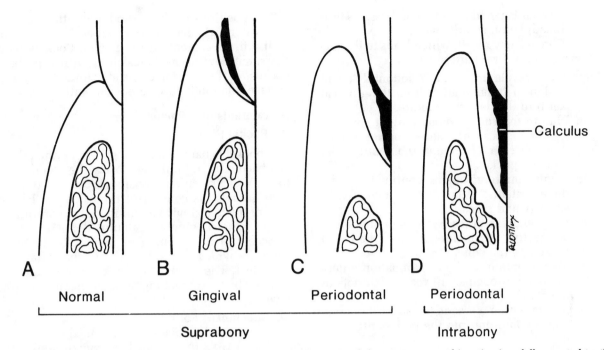

Figure 12-1. Types of Pockets. A. Normal relationship of the gingival tissue and the cementoenamel junction in a fully erupted tooth. **B.** Gingival pocket showing attachment at the cementoenamel junction and the pocket formed by enlarged gingival tissue. There is no bone loss. **C.** Periodontal pocket showing attachment on cementum with root surface exposed. Gingival tissue has enlarged. **D.** Periodontal intrabony pocket with the bottom of the pocket within the bone. See the text for further description of each type of pocket.

epithelium to migrate apically along the cementum.

2. Other names: true pocket, absolute pocket.
3. The periodontal deeper structures (attachment apparatus) are involved; that is, the cementum, periodontal ligament, and bone.
4. The tooth wall is cementum or partly cementum and partly enamel.
5. The base of the pocket is on cementum at the level of attached periodontal tissue.
6. Periodontal pockets may be suprabony or intrabony.
   a. Suprabony: pocket in which the base of the pocket is coronal to the crest of the alveolar bone (figure 12-1C).
   b. Intrabony: pocket in which the base of the pocket is below or apical to the crest of the alveolar bone (figure 12-1D). "Intra" means located within the bone. The term "infrabony" is used in some texts. "Infra" means under or beneath.

II. Pocket Formation

A. Steps in the Development of a Gingival Pocket
1. Microorganisms of plaque produce harmful substances: enzymes and toxins.
   a. Plaque collects at and below the gingival margin.
   b. Bacterial products (enzymes and toxins) cause breakdown of epithelial intercellular substances, which leads to ulceration of the sulcular epithelium.

c. Widening of intercellular spaces permits injurious agents to penetrate into the connective tissue beneath the epithelium.
2. Inflammatory reaction in the connective tissue
   a. Dilation and increased permeability of capillaries with increased blood flow results in redness of tissue and bleeding when probed.
   b. Increased numbers of inflammatory cells collect for defense: primarily lymphocytes, plasma cells, polymorphonuclear leukocytes, and macrophages. An exudate may be produced in an acute stage.
   c. Edema from the leakage of fluid into the tissues results in an increase in size and alteration in shape of the gingival tissue.
3. Gingival pocket formation
   a. Junctional epithelium does not move at the base of the pocket.
   b. Increased depth is due to the enlarged gingiva.
4. Reversible: when plaque is controlled and calculus that is harboring plaque is removed, the number of microorganisms is reduced and the irritant is removed. The inflammation then subsides and the enlargement can decrease.
5. Continued exposure to plaque organisms means continued inflammatory reaction and increased pocket depth.
6. Chronic gingivitis develops
   a. Destruction (inflammation) and healing

(new collagen fibers and blood vessels produced) go on simultaneously.

    b. Fibrosis may result, which leads to the formation of firm hard gingiva.

B. Steps in the Development of a Periodontal Pocket

  1. Extension of inflammation from the gingival pocket into the deeper structures.

    a. Plaque microorganisms collect in large numbers because plaque control procedures were ineffective in the depth of the gingival pocket.

    b. Plaque microorganisms continue to produce irritants: inflammation increases in severity and spreads.

    c. Inflammation spreads through the loose connective tissue along (beside) the blood vessels to the bone.[3]

    d. Most commonly, the inflammation enters the bone through small vessel channels in the alveolar crest.

    e. Inflammation spreads through the bone marrow and out into the periodontal ligament.

  2. Progressive destruction of connective tissue fibers under the base of the sulcus at the apical border of the junctional epithelium.

    a. Undermining destruction: epithelium migrates along the root surface.

    b. Coronal portion of the junctional epithelium becomes detached.

    c. Because the epithelial cells must be living to migrate, the junctional epithelium usually remains partially intact and does not have the severe ulcerations or other destructive changes that occur in the pocket epithelium.

  3. Exposed cementum where the fibers were attached becomes altered.[4] Changes occur chemically, physically, and in permeability. Bacterial and inflammatory products from the periodontal pocket become incorporated. The diseased cementum contains endotoxin.

  4. Pocket becomes progressively deepened as the migration of epithelium continues toward the apex of the tooth.

    a. Pocket retains plaque microorganisms and is not cleanable by the patient.

    b. Plaque retention leads to calculus formation.

TOOTH SURFACE POCKET WALL

I. Tooth Structure Involved

A sulcus or a pocket has a gingival side, which is the sulcular epithelium, and a tooth side. In gingival pockets, the tooth surface wall is enamel; whereas, in periodontal pockets the tooth surface wall is either cementum or a combination of cementum and enamel.

The positions of the periodontal attachment and gingival margin determine whether the tooth surface wall will be cementum or enamel. Pockets may be the same depth when measured with a probe, but because of the location of the attachment on the tooth surface, the tooth surface pocket wall varies.

II. Contents of a Pocket

A. Pocket Size

A pocket is narrow and the pocket epithelial lining is adjacent to and follows closely the contour of the tooth. When calculus deposits are present, the pocket wall follows the contour of the calculus. The firmness of the free gingiva is influential in confining and shaping the subgingival calculus deposit.

Access of the opening of the pocket to the oral cavity provides an opportunity for bacterial plaque to collect. The deeper the pocket, the less it can be cleaned by toothbrushing or other plaque control devices.

B. Substances Found

Subgingival plaque is described in Chapter 16. Table 16–2 (page 238) lists content and features of subgingival plaque and the periodontal pocket.

The following may be inside a pocket in contact with the tooth surface on one side and on the surface of the pocket epithelium on the other.

  1. Microorganisms and their products: enzymes, endotoxins, and other metabolic products.

  2. Calculus deposits and other rough areas covered with bacterial plaque.

  3. Gingival sulcus fluid.

  4. Desquamated epithelial cells.

  5. Leukocytes: numbers increase with increased inflammation in the tissues.

  6. Purulent exudate made up of living and broken down leukocytes, living and dead microorganisms, and serum.

III. Nature of the Tooth Surface

Knowledge of the characteristics and quality of the tooth surface pocket wall is of prime importance in instrumentation. During the examination of the tooth surface with probe and explorer, the various irregularities that can occur must be differentiated. How the irregularities came into existence is important for interpretation and understanding.

A. Pocket Development Factors

  1. The pocket deepens as a result of continuing action of the irritants and destructive agents from bacterial plaque.

  2. The periodontal ligament fibers become detached and the junctional epithelium migrates apically.

  3. The cementum becomes exposed to the open pocket and the oral fluids.

  4. Physical, structural, and chemical changes alter the cementum.

  5. Surface changes occur as a result of the ex-

change of minerals with oral fluids and exposure to plaque bacteria and their products. On different surfaces of the same teeth or different teeth in the same mouth, any of the following can occur[5]:

   a. Hypermineralization of the surface cementum increases with time.
   b. Demineralization.
   c. Calculus formation.
   d. Plaque and debris collection.

B. Tooth Surface Irregularities

Surface irregularities are detected supragingivally by drying the surface with air and observing under adequate direct or indirect light, followed by the use of an explorer as needed.

Subgingivally, examination is dependent, for the most part, on tactile and auditory sensitivity transmitted by a probe and an explorer. Causes of surface roughness include the following:

1. *Enamel Surface*
   a. Structural defects: cracks, grooves.
   b. Dental caries, demineralization.
   c. Calculus deposits and heavy stain deposits.
   d. Erosion, abrasion.
   e. Pits and irregularities from hypoplasia.

2. *Cementoenamel Junction.* Cementum overlaps enamel in 60 to 65 percent of teeth; cementum and enamel meet directly in 30 percent; or there may be a small zone of dentin between, in 5 to 10 percent.[6] The relationships of enamel and cementum at the cementoenamel junction are shown in figure 12–2.

   Despite the differences, the junction is usually smooth or with a slight groove, except when cementum is worn away by abrasion. Abrasion may undermine the enamel.

3. *Cemental Surface*
   a. Diseased altered cementum.
   b. Cemental resorption.
   c. Cemental caries.
   d. Abrasion.

   e. Calculus.
   f. Deficient or overhanging filling.
   g. Grooves from previous incomplete instrumentation.

4. *The Cementum.* The cementum varies in thickness.[7,8] It is thickest around the apical third of the tooth where it may be 200 to 600 μm (0.2 to 0.6 mm.). It is thinnest at the cervical third next to the cementoenamel junction where it may be only 20 to 50 μm (0.02 to 0.05 mm.).

An objective of root planing is to remove the thin layer of diseased altered cementum, because the toxic materials in the altered cementum may prevent the adjacent gingival soft tissue from returning to health. The instrumentation for root planing is described in Chapter 33.

COMPLICATIONS OF POCKET FORMATION

I. Furcation Involvement

Furcation involvement means that the pocket and bone loss have extended into the furcation area, or furca, the area between the roots of a multirooted tooth. Furcation involvement, however incipient it may appear to be in a radiograph or by probing, indicates progressive periodontal disease.

A. Types of Furcations

Furcation involvement is usually classified by the amount of a furcation that has been exposed by periodontal bone destruction.

The three general classes, as shown in figure 12–3, are as follows:

Class I. Early, beginning involvement. A probe can enter the furcation area and the anatomy of the roots on either side can be felt by moving the probe from side to side. Figure 33–2C illustrates this on page 457.

Class II. Moderate involvement. Bone has been destroyed to an extent that permits a probe to

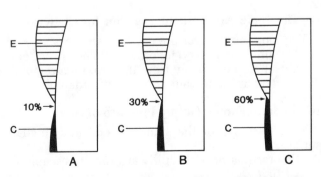

Figure 12–2. Cementoenamel Junction. The possible relationships of the enamel and the cementum at the cementoenamel junction. A. The cementum and the enamel do not meet and there is a small zone of dentin exposed in 10% of teeth. B. The cementum meets the enamel in approximately 30% of teeth. C. The cementum overlaps the enamel in about 60% of teeth.

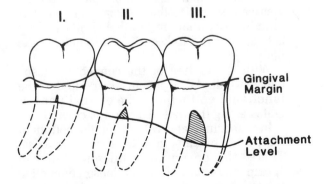

Figure 12–3. Classification of Furcations. I. Early, beginning involvement. II. Moderate involvement, in which the furcation can be probed but not through and through. III. Severe involvement, when the bone between the roots is destroyed and a probe can be passed through.

enter the furcation area but not to pass through between the roots.

Class III. Severe involvement. A probe can be passed between the roots through the entire furcation.

B. Clinical Observations
1. When the gingiva over the furcation has not receded, the following may be seen:
   a. The furcation is covered by the gingival tissue pocket wall.
   b. No differences in color, size, or other tissue changes may exist to differentiate the area from adjacent gingiva; but when color changes do exist, they provide clues to supplement probe examination.
2. When the gingiva over a molar buccal furcation is receded, the root division may be seen directly.

C. Detection
A suggested procedure for probing furcations is described on page 199. Radiographic examination of furcation areas may be studied on page 208.

II. Mucogingival Involvement

When a pocket extends to or beyond the mucogingival junction and into the alveolar mucosa, it is described as *mucogingival involvement.* There is no attached gingiva in the area, and a probe can be passed through the pocket and beyond the mucogingival junction into the alveolar mucosa (figure 13–9, page 200).

A. Significance of Attached Gingiva
1. *Functions of Attached Gingiva*
   a. Give support to the marginal gingiva.
   b. Withstand the frictional stresses of mastication and toothbrushing.
   c. Provide attachment or a solid base for the movable alveolar mucosa for the action of the cheeks, lips, and tongue.
2. *Barrier to Passage of Inflammation.* Without attachment, the inflammation from the pocket area can extend to the alveolar mucosa. The junctional epithelium (epithelial attachment) acts as a barrier to keep infection outside the body.

   With destruction of the connective tissue and periodontal ligament fibers under the junctional epithelium, the epithelium migrates along the root. A pocket is created.

   In mucogingival involvement, the bottom of the pocket extends into the alveolar mucosa. There, the unconfined inflammation can spread more rapidly in the loose connective tissue.

B. Clinical Observations
Color changes, tension test, and probe measurements are used during assessment. These are described on pages 199–200.

1. *Width of Attached Gingiva.* A narrow zone of gingiva from gingival margin to mucogingival junction, caused by recession or occurring naturally without recession, is more susceptible to developing mucogingival involvement because there is less attached gingiva at the start.
2. *Base of Pocket at Mucogingival Junction.* When the probe measures only 1 to 2 mm. and there is no bleeding on probing but the tip of the probe is at the mucogingival junction, the area should be charted and reevaluated at each successive maintenance review. Such an area needs specific instruction in plaque control procedures for preventive maintenance.

   When an area of minimal attached gingiva (1 to 2 mm.) will be placed under stress by restorative, prosthetic, or orthodontic treatment procedures, an assessment should be made of the need for periodontal treatment to increase the zone of attached gingiva.

SELF-CLEANSING MECHANISMS

The teeth, by their anatomy, alignment, and occlusion, and the gingiva, tongue, cheeks, and saliva function in a relationship called the self-cleansing mechanism of the oral cavity. A review of the self-cleansing mechanisms during and following mastication is included here to relate the natural processes to the deviating influences to be described in the next section.

The steps below are described for food particles, but the same processes apply to any substances that enter the mouth and influence oral cleanliness and the formation of deposits on the teeth.

I. Food Enters the Mouth

It is carried by the tongue, assisted by the lips and cheeks, to the occlusal surfaces for grinding.
A. Salivary flow increases as a result of sensory reflex stimulation.
B. Saliva begins lubrication of food and oral tissues.

II. The Teeth Are Brought Together for Chewing

The food moves over the occlusal surfaces.
A. Marginal ridges tend to force particles toward occlusal surfaces, away from the proximal region.
B. Contact areas prevent entrance interdentally.

III. Food Is Forced Out by Pressure of Bite

Food passes over the smooth facial and lingual surfaces.
A. Embrasures provide spillways for the escape of particles.
B. Cervical enamel ridges deflect particles away from the free gingiva onto the attached gingiva.
C. Gingival crest prevents retention of particles by being positioned at a point below the height of contour of the cervical enamel ridge, by its knife-

edge shape, and by its close adherence to the tooth surface.

D. Interdental papilla fills the interproximal area and prevents particles from entering.

IV. Food Particles Are Brought Back by the Tongue to the Occlusal Surfaces for Additional Chewing

The process is repeated until the food is ready for swallowing.

A. Salivary flow continues to be stimulated by repeated masticatory movements.

B. Saliva moistens food and oral mucosa and thus reduces the adhering capacity of the food.

V. Food Particles Remaining on the Teeth Are Removed

A. Tip of tongue explores and attempts to dislodge remaining particles.

B. Lips and cheeks in conjunction with tongue aid in natural rinsing process by forcing saliva over and between the teeth.

C. Saliva continues to flow in increased amounts during rinsing and swallowing of particles, then gradually returns to its normal flow.

VI. Factors Affecting Self-Cleansing

Self-cleansing is influenced by the physical characteristics of the teeth and gingiva as described in the next section. It is seriously influenced by xerostomia (page 187), because without lubrication, bacteria collect and multiply.

A. Congenital Malformations
1. Tongue: tonguetie; macroglossia.
2. Lips: short upper lip, unusually small orifice.

B. Muscle Tone and Action
1. Paralysis.
2. Neuromuscular diseases (pages 662–669).

CONTRIBUTING FACTORS IN DISEASE DEVELOPMENT

Bacterial plaque is the primary etiologic factor in the development of gingival and periodontal diseases. A variety of other factors predispose to the retention of bacterial deposits and hence to the development of disease in the soft tissues. Factors described in this section that relate to microbial plaque retention apply also to dental caries development. Dental caries is described on page 216.

Although debris can be cleared away by self-cleansing, bacterial plaque adheres firmly to the tooth surface and cannot be removed completely by self-cleansing.

Retentive areas relate to rough surfaces of teeth and restorations, tooth contour and position, and gingival size, shape, and position. Iatrogenic causes, that is, factors created by professionals during patient treatment or neglect of treatment, are significant. Factors

of mastication, saliva, the tongue, cheeks, lips, and oral habits contribute as well as external factors such as diet, smoking, and personal plaque control techniques.

The patient's study casts can be especially useful for observing the physical factors. Irregularities, contour, position, malocclusion, and contact areas of the teeth, as well as features of the gingiva, may be partially or wholly noted.

The patient's history may contribute and provide insight into why certain irregularities exist. Problem areas can be explained to the patient by demonstration on the study casts. Changes in the patient's habits and daily personal care routine may be made.

I. Definitions

Complicating factors to disease development may be etiologic, predisposing, or contributing. These are delineated as follows:

1. *Etiologic Factor.* A factor that is the actual cause of a disease or condition.
2. *Predisposing Factor.* A factor that renders a person susceptible to a disease or condition.
3. *Contributing Factor.* A factor that lends assistance to, supplements, or adds to a condition or disease.

Etiologic, predisposing, and contributing factors may be local or systemic, defined as follows:

1. *Local Factor.* A factor in the immediate environment of the oral cavity or specifically in the environment of the teeth or periodontium.
2. *Systemic Factor.* A factor that results from a general physical or mental disease or condition.

II. Dental Factors

A. Tooth Surface Irregularities
Pellicle and plaque microorganisms attach to defective or rough surfaces including the following:
1. Pits, grooves, cracks.
2. Calculus.
3. Exposed altered cementum with irregularities (page 183).
4. Dental caries and demineralization.
5. Iatrogenic
   a. Rough or grooved surfaces left after scaling.
   b. Inadequately polished dental restorations.

B. Tooth Contour
Altered shape may interfere with self-cleansing mechanisms and make personal care procedures difficult.
1. Congenital abnormalities
   a. Extra or missing cusps.
   b. Bell-shaped crown with prominent facial and lingual contours tends to provide deeper retentive area in cervical third.
2. Teeth with flattened proximal surfaces have

faulty contact with adjacent teeth, thus permitting debris to wedge between.

3. Occlusal and incisal surfaces altered by attrition interrupt normal excursion of food during chewing. Marginal ridges have worn down.

4. Areas of erosion and abrasion (figures 14–3 and 14–4, pages 213, 216).

5. Carious lesions.

6. Heavy calculus deposits: plaque retained on rough surface.

7. Restorations: overcontoured and undercontoured (figure 41–2, page 529).

C. Tooth Position

1. Malocclusion: irregular alignment of a single tooth or groups of teeth leave areas conducive to collection of microorganisms for plaque formation.
   a. Crowded or overlapped.
   b. Rotated.
   c. Deep anterior overbite
      i. Mandibular teeth force food particles against maxillary lingual surface (figure 15–9, page 228).
      ii. Lingual inclination of mandibular teeth allows maxillary teeth to force food particles against mandibular facial gingiva.

2. Tooth adjacent to edentulous area may be inclined or migrated; contact missing.

3. Opposing tooth missing: tooth may extrude beyond the line of occlusion.

4. Related to eruption
   a. Incomplete eruption: below line of occlusion.
   b. Partially erupted impacted third molar.

5. Lack of function or use of teeth eliminates or decreases effectiveness of natural cleansing.
   a. Lack of opposing teeth.
   b. Open bite.
   c. Marked maxillary anterior protrusion.
   d. Crossbite with limited lateral excursion.
   e. Unilateral chewing.

6. Food impaction
   a. Defined: food impaction is the forceful wedging of food into the periodontium by occlusal forces.
   b. Created by the combined effect of tooth contour, missing proximal contact, proximal carious lesions, irregular marginal ridge relationship, inclination related to loss of adjacent tooth, and a plunger cusp from the opposite arch (figure 12–4A).

7. Defective contact area
   a. Restoration: margin is faulty, and the contact area is missing, improperly located, or unnaturally wide.
   b. Inclined tooth: irregular marginal ridge relation (figure 12–4C).
   c. Missing, unrestored contact (figure 12–4B).

D. Dental Appliances

1. Orthodontic appliances provide retentive areas.

2. Fixed partial denture with deficient margin of an abutment tooth or an unusually shaped pontic (figures 25–1 and 25–2, page 355).

3. Removable partial denture: inadequately adapted clasps.

III. Gingiva

A. Position: deviations from normal provide retentive areas.

1. Receded: normal depressed area is left at cementoenamel junction.

2. Enlarged: extended to or over the height of contour.

3. Reduced height of interdental papilla leaves open interdental area.

4. Tissue flap over occlusal of erupting tooth.

5. Periodontal pocket
   a. Free gingiva cannot adhere to tooth.
   b. Shape of pocket conducive to bacterial plaque collection.
   c. Depth of pocket not available to toothbrush and cleaning aids.
   d. Calculus provides rough retentive surface.

B. Size and Contour

1. Deviation of shape of enlarged gingiva: rolled, bulbous, cratered.

2. Combined with presence of irregular restorations or dental appliance can result in marked plaque retention.

C. Effect of Mouth Breathing

Dehydration of oral tissues in anterior region leads to changes in size, shape, surface texture, and consistency.

D. Effect of Certain Drugs

Medications for specific systemic conditions can lead to gingival enlargement.[9] The enlarged tissue encourages bacterial plaque retention, thus increasing the potential for periodontal infections.

1. *Phenytoin-induced Gingival Enlargement.* Phenytoin is a drug used to control seizures (pages 642–644).

2. *Cyclosporin-induced Gingival Enlargement.* Cyclosporin is an immunosuppressant drug used for patients with organ transplants to prevent rejection.

3. *Nifedipine-induced Gingival Enlargement.* Nifedipine is used in the treatment of angina and ventricular arrhythmias.

IV. Other Factors

A variety of factors may predispose or contribute to the progression of periodontal infections. Some of the items listed here may have an indirect effect, whereas others have a direct effect on the oral tissues.

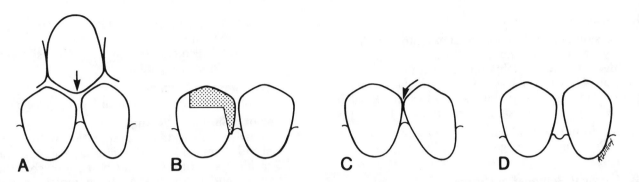

Figure 12–4. Effect of Tooth Position. A. Food impaction area shown by plunger cusp (with arrow), directing pressure between lower teeth with open contact area. **B.** Inadequate restoration without proximal contact and with overhang. **C.** Tipped tooth leaving irregular marginal ridge relation. **D.** Open contact with saddle-shaped gingival margin.

A. Personal Oral Care
1. Neglect can lead to generalized bacterial plaque accumulation and disease promotion.
2. Faulty plaque control techniques. Incorrect use of brush, abrasive dentifrice, and the effects of other harmful, detrimental procedures are described on page 313.

B. Diet and Eating Habits
1. Soft foods tend to adhere more than fibrous, firm foods.
2. Cariogenic food selection.
3. Masticatory deficiencies limit diet selection. Missing teeth, ill-fitting partial dentures, and various occlusal deficiencies alter diet selection and eating habits.

C. Tobacco
1. Smokers, especially cigarette users, have increased calculus and debris. An association between poor oral hygiene and tobacco use has been shown.[10]
2. Smokeless tobacco. Users of smokeless tobacco products have oral effects including predisposition to oral cancer. Periodontal lesions with severe recession and root exposure occur at the site where the quid is held.[11,12]

D. Individual Characteristics
1. *Awareness of Oral Cleanliness.* Cleansing habits, including both self-cleansing mechanisms and mechanical plaque removal, depend in part on an individual's perception and feeling of debris through taste and tongue activity.
2. *Psychogenic Factors*[13]
   a. Stress has been considered a predisposing factor in the development of necrotizing ulcerative gingivitis (page 482).
   b. Fear and anxiety decrease salivary flow with an effect on the lubrication of the oral mucosa and the self-cleansing effect on the teeth and gingiva.

E. Systemic Factors
1. Systemic factors do not have a direct etiologic effect in the initiation of periodontal infection.
2. Pocket formation or other symptoms of periodontal infection are not a result of any systemic disease.
3. Systemic conditions, especially when changes in immune factors occur, can influence the *severity* and *rate of development* of periodontal disease as well as the response to healing.
   a. An altered exaggerated response to bacterial plaque irritants can occur.
   b. Alteration of healing capacity and lowered resistance to infection can influence the outcome of treatment. Diabetes, an example, is described on pages 715–723.

XEROSTOMIA

Saliva has many functions in the oral cavity relating to the maintenance of health of the teeth and soft tissues. It is protective in its functions of lubrication and cleansing. It contains immunoglobulins, electrolytes, and other substances that aid in resistance to disease (table 12–2).

Xerostomia means dryness of the mouth. It is caused by absence or diminished quantity of saliva. Lack of saliva and the resulting dry mouth are important contributing factors to oral discomfort and disease. It is a symptom, not a disease entity.

Table 12–2. Functions of Saliva

Lubrication of membranes, gingiva, teeth
Cleansing in self-cleansing mechanism
Tasting
Digestion: Food breakdown: Chewing
Food bolus formation
Swallowing
Protection Against Diseases
Antibacterial
Antifungal
Buffering: pH control
Remineralization
Protection against demineralization
Speech

I. Causes of Xerostomia

Xerostomia may be permanent or temporary. Temporary dry mouth occurs in diseases accompanied by high fever with dehydration or fluid loss; with control of certain diseases such as diabetes or hyperthyroidism, salivary flow returns to normal. Major causes of permanent xerostomia are as follows:

A. Radiation to Head and Neck for Cancer Therapy
Permanent damage to the salivary glands can result.

B. Surgical Removal of Glands
The glands may be removed because of neoplasm.

C. Sjögren's Syndrome
The syndrome is an autoimmune disorder of the salivary glands.

D. Pharmacologically-Induced Xerostomia
At least 400 drugs that are common prescription items produce dry mouth as a side effect.[14] When the drug prescription can be changed to a drug that does not have such a side effect, then this category can be called temporary.

II. Effects of Xerostomia

A. Symptoms
During patient examination and history preparation, questions and clinical observations can point to the existence of dry mouth even when a patient does not complain of the symptoms.
1. Feeling of oral dryness; tongue sticks to palate.
2. Difficulty with mastication, swallowing, or speech.
3. Impaired taste.
4. Thirst, with resultant increased use of fluids; licking of lips.
5. Smarting, burning, and soreness of mucosa and tongue.

B. Heavy bacterial plaque, materia alba, and debris accumulation can lead to increased severity of periodontal infection and dental caries.

C. Predisposition to dental caries, particularly root caries.

D. Problems of denture wearing.

E. Dietary changes because of discomfort during eating; may use large quantities of liquid to soften food for swallowing.

III. Treatment for Xerostomia

A. Prevention of Dental Caries
Severe, rampant dental caries related to radiation therapy is described on page 604. Even before the radiation treatments are started, oral hygiene and caries prevention instruction must start, and a fluoride program must be initiated.

B. Personal Care Program
1. Rigorous plaque control effort by the patient for bacterial plaque removal.
2. Multiple fluorides: use of dentifrice, rinse, and brush-on gel (or tray).
3. Avoid tobacco and alcohol use, and use foods that are noncariogenic.

C. Environmental Factors
Adjust air humidification in living quarters.

D. Use of a Saliva Substitute
A saliva substitute is a preparation with physical and chemical properties similar to real saliva. The ideal substitute should be able to coat the mucosa and teeth to keep them moist, reduce enamel solubility, and remineralize the surface, as well as help to prevent accumulation of bacterial plaque.

Saliva substitutes contain carboxymethylcellulose (CMC) and the minerals calcium and phosphorous, fluoride, and other ions typical of normal human saliva. A small amount is sprayed into the mouth and distributed over all surfaces with the tongue. Patients can use the preparation at will, as needed for comfort.

FACTORS TO TEACH THE PATIENT

I. What a pocket is and how it forms.
II. How a pocket is measured with a probe and that, until the sulci and pockets are probed, it is not possible to tell whether disease is present and how far it has progressed. Pockets and sulci must be checked regularly all around every tooth to be sure nothing is developing insidiously.
III. Treatment measures for xerostomia: diet, personal care, where to obtain and how to use a saliva substitute.
IV. Factors that contribute to disease development and progression: individual patient problems explained.

References

1. American Academy of Periodontology: *Current Procedural Terminology for Periodontics.* 5th ed. Chicago, American Academy of Periodontology, 1987, p. 1.
2. Listgarten, M.A., Mao, R., and Robinson, P.J.: Periodontal Probing and the Relationship of the Probe Tip to Periodontal Tissues, *J. Periodontol., 47,* 511, September, 1976.
3. Weinmann, J.P.: Progress of Gingival Inflammation into the Supporting Structures of the Teeth, *J. Periodontol., 12,* 71, July, 1941.
4. Armitage, G.C.: *Biologic Basis of Periodontal Maintenance Therapy.* Berkeley, California, Praxis Publishing Co., 1980, pp. 88–94.
5. Selvig, K.A.: Biologic Changes at the Tooth-Saliva Interface in Periodontal Disease, *J. Dent. Res., 48,* 846, September-October, 1969.
6. Bhaskar, S.N., ed.: *Orban's Oral Histology and Embryology,* 10th ed. St. Louis, The C.V. Mosby Co., 1986, p. 188.
7. Furseth, R. and Johansen, E.: A Microradiographic Comparison of Sound and Carious Human Dental Cementum, *Arch. Oral Biol., 13,* 1197, October, 1968.
8. Bhaskar: op. cit., p. 178.
9. Butler, R.T., Kalkwarf, K.L., and Kaldahl, W.B.: Drug-induced Gingival Hyperplasia: Phenytoin, Cyclosporine, and Nifedipine, *J. Am. Dent. Assoc., 114,* 56, January, 1987.

10. Rivera-Hidalgo, F.: Smoking and Periodontal Disease. A Review of the Literature, *J. Periodontol., 57,* 617, October, 1986.
11. Moriconi, M.B.: Effects of Smokeless Tobacco on Periodontal Tissue, *RDH, 4,* 14, May/June, 1984.
12. Johnson, R. and Herzog, A.: Oral Effects of Smokeless Tobacco Use, *Dent. Hyg., 61,* 354, August, 1987.
13. Grant, D.A., Stern, I.B., and Listgarten, M.A., eds.: *Periodontics,* 6th ed. St. Louis, The C.V. Mosby Co., 1988, p. 408.
14. Sreebny, L.M. and Valdini, A.: Xerostomia. A Neglected Symptom, *Arch. Intern. Med., 147,* 1333, July, 1987.

Suggested Readings

Addy, M., Dummer, P.M.H., Hunter, M.L., Kingdon, A., and Shaw, W.C.: A Study of the Association of Fraenal Attachment, Lip Coverage, and Vestibular Depth with Plaque and Gingivitis, *J. Periodontol., 58,* 752, November, 1987.

Adelson, L.J., Hanks, C.T., Ramfjord, S.P., and Caffesse, R.G.: *In Vitro* Cytotoxicity of Periodontally Diseased Root Surfaces, *J. Periodontol., 51,* 700, December, 1980.

Aleo, J.J. and Vandersall, D.C.: Cementum. Recent Concepts Related to Periodontal Disease Therapy, *Dent. Clin. North Am., 24,* 627, October, 1980.

Allen, D.L., McFall, W.T., and Jenzano, J.W.: *Periodontics for the Dental Hygienist,* 4th ed. Philadelphia, Lea & Febiger, 1987, pp. 79–92.

Armitage, G.C.: *Biologic Basis of Periodontal Maintenance Therapy.* Berkeley, California, Praxis Publishing Co., 1980, pp. 204–216.

Goldman, H.M. and Cohen, D.W.: *Periodontal Therapy,* 6th ed. St. Louis, The C.V. Mosby Co., 1980, pp. 105–146, 177–221.

Goldstein, A.R.: Enamel Pearls as a Contributing Factor in Periodontal Breakdown, *J. Am. Dent. Assoc., 99,* 210, August, 1979.

Ramfjord, S.P. and Ash, M.M.: *Periodontology and Periodontics.* Philadelphia, W.B. Saunders Co., 1979, pp. 112–137.

Ranney, R.R.: Pathogenesis of Periodontal Disease, in *International Conference on Research in the Biology of Periodontal Disease.* Chicago, College of Dentistry, University of Illinois, 1977, pp. 222–304.

Sabag, N., Saglie, R., and Mery, C.: Ultrastructure of the Normal Human Epithelial Attachment to the Cementum Root Surface, *J. Periodontol., 52,* 94, February, 1981.

Smukler, H. and Machtei, E.: Gingival Recession and Plaque Control, *Compend. Contin. Educ. Dent., 8,* 194, March, 1987.

Swartz, M.L. and Phillips, R.W.: Comparison of Bacterial Accumulations on Rough and Smooth Enamel Surfaces, *J. Periodontol., 28,* 304, October, 1957.

Watson, P.J.: Gingival Recession, *J. Dent., 12,* 29, March, 1984.

Tooth Position

Bakdash, M.B. and Jernberg, G.R.: Proximal Tooth Open Contacts and Periodontal Health: Evolution and Current Knowledge, *Northwest Dent., 65,* 15, November-December, 1986.

Behlfelt, K., Ericsson, L., Jacobson, L., and Linder-Aronson, S.: The Occurrence of Plaque and Gingivitis and Its Relationship to Tooth Alignment within the Dental Arches, *J. Clin. Periodontol., 8,* 329, August, 1981.

Buckley, L.A.: The Relationships Between Irregular Teeth, Plaque, Calculus and Gingival Disease, A Study of 300 Subjects, *Br. Dent. J., 148,* 67, February 5, 1980.

Buckley, L.A.: The Relationships Between Malocclusion, Gingival Inflammation, Plaque and Calculus, *J. Periodontol., 52,* 35, January, 1981.

Griffiths, G.S. and Addy, M.: Effects of Malalignment of Teeth in the Anterior Segments on Plaque Accumulation, *J. Clin. Periodontol., 8,* 481, December, 1981.

Kepic, T.J. and O'Leary, T.J.: Role of Marginal Ridge Relationships as an Etiologic Factor in Periodontal Disease, *J. Periodontol., 49,* 570, November, 1978.

Koral, S.M., Howell, T.H., and Jeffcoat, M.K.: Alveolar Bone Loss Due to Open Interproximal Contacts in Periodontal Disease, *J. Periodontol., 52,* 447, August, 1981.

Silness, J. and Røynstrand, T.: Effects of the Degree of Overbite and Overjet on Dental Health, *J. Clin. Periodontol., 12,* 389, May, 1985.

Silness, J. and Røynstrand, T.: Relationship Between Alignment Conditions of Teeth in Anterior Segments and Dental Health, *J. Clin. Periodontol., 12,* 312, April, 1985.

Silness, J. and Røynstrand, T.: Effects on Dental Health of Spacing of Teeth in Anterior Segments, *J. Clin. Periodontol., 11,* 387, July, 1984.

Waerhaug, J.: Eruption of Teeth into Crowded Position, Loss of Attachment and Downgrowth of Subgingival Plaque, *Am. J. Orthod., 78,* 453, October, 1980.

Restorations

Bazirgan, M.K. and Bates, J.F.: Effect of Clasp Design on Gingival Health, *J. Oral Rehabil., 14,* 271, May, 1987.

Block, P.L.: Restorative Margins and Periodontal Health: A New Look at an Old Perspective, *J. Prosthet. Dent., 57,* 683, June, 1987.

Chan, C. and Weber, H.: Plaque Retention on Teeth Restored with Full Ceramic Crowns: A Comparative Study, *J. Prosthet. Dent., 56,* 666, December, 1986.

Checchio, L.M., Gaskill, W.F., and Carrel, R.: The Relationship Between Periodontal Disease and Stainless Steel Crowns, *ASDC J. Dent. Child., 50,* 205, May-June, 1983.

Claman, L.J., Koidis, P.T., and Burch, J.G.: Proximal Tooth Surface Quality and Probing Depth, *J. Am. Dent. Assoc., 113,* 890, December, 1986.

Durr, D.P., Ashrafi, M.H., and Duncan, W.K.: A Study of Plaque Accumulation and Gingival Health Surrounding Stainless Steel Crowns, *ASDC J. Dent. Child., 49,* 343, September-October, 1982.

Eid, M.: Relationship Between Overhanging Amalgam Restorations and Periodontal Disease, *Quintessence Int., 18,* 775, November, 1987.

El Ghamrawy, E. and Runov, J.: Proximal Plaque Accumulation with Two Minor Connector Designs, *J. Oral Rehabil., 7,* 27, January, 1980.

Gardner, F.M.: Margins of Complete Crowns—Literature Review, *J. Prosthet. Dent., 48,* 396, October, 1982.

Hadavi, F., Caffesse, R.G., and Charbeneau, G.T.: A Study of the Gingival Response to Polished and Unpolished Amalgam Restorations, *Can. Dent. Assoc. J., 52,* 211, March, 1986.

Hakkarainen, K. and Ainamo, J.: Influence of Overhanging Posterior Tooth Restorations on Alveolar Bone Height in Adults, *J. Clin. Periodontol., 7,* 114, April, 1980.

Hancock, E.B., Mayo, C.V., Schwab, R.R., and Wirthlin, M.R.: Influence of Interdental Contacts on Periodontal Status, *J. Periodontol., 51,* 445, August, 1980.

Jacobson, T.E.: Periodontal Considerations in Removable Partial Denture Design, *Compend. Contin. Educ. Dent., 8,* 530, July/August, 1987.

Jameson, L.M. and Malone, W.F.P.: Crown Contours and Gingival Response, *J. Prosthet. Dent., 47,* 620, June, 1982.

Jernberg, G.R., Bakdash, M.B., and Keenan, K.M.: Relationship Between Proximal Tooth Open Contacts and Periodontal Disease, *J. Periodontol., 54,* 529, September, 1983.

Kodis, P.T., Burch, J.G., and Melfi, R.C.: Clinical Crown Contours: Contemporary View, *J. Am. Dent. Assoc., 114,* 792, June, 1987.

Koth, D.L.: Full Crown Restorations and Gingival Inflammation in a Controlled Population, *J. Prosthet. Dent., 48,* 681, December, 1982.

Lang, N.P., Kiel, R.A., and Anderhalden, K.: Clinical and Microbiological Effects of Subgingival Restorations with Overhanging or Clinically Perfect Margins, *J. Clin. Periodontol., 10,* 563, November, 1983.

Lekholm, U., Ericsson, I., Adell, R., and Slots, J.: The Condition of the Soft Tissues at Tooth and Fixture Abutments Supporting Fixed Bridges. A Microbiological and Histological Study, *J. Clin. Periodontol., 13,* 558, July, 1986.

List, G., Meister, F., Nery, E.B., and Mayer, J.C.: Gingival Crevicular Fluid Response to Subgingival Composite Resin Restoration, *Gen. Dent., 35,* 281, July-August, 1987.

Mihalow, D.M. and Tinanoff, N.: The Influence of Removable Partial Dentures on the Level of *Streptococcus mutans* in Saliva, *J. Prosthet. Dent., 59,* 49, January, 1988.

Orkin, D.A., Reddy, J., and Bradshaw, D.: The Relationship of the Position of Crown Margins to Gingival Health, *J. Prosthet. Dent., 57,* 421, April, 1987.

Sachs, R.I.: Restorative Dentistry and the Periodontium, *Dent. Clin. North Am., 29,* 261, April, 1985.

Silness, J., Gustavsen, F., and Mangersnes, K.: The Relationship Between Pontic Hygiene and Mucosal Inflammation in Fixed Bridge Recipients, *J. Periodont. Res., 17,* 434, July, 1982.

van Dijken, J.W.V., Sjöström, S., and Wing, K.: Development of Initial Gingivitis Around Different Types of Composite Resin, *J. Clin. Periodontol., 14,* 257, May, 1987.

Wunderlich, R.C. and Caffesse, R.G.: Periodontal Aspects of Porcelain Restorations, *Dent. Clin. North Am., 29,* 693, October, 1985.

Orthodontic Appliances

Årtun, J.: Caries and Periodontal Reactions Associated With Long-term Use of Different Types of Bonded Lingual Retainers, *Am. J. Orthod., 86,* 112, August, 1984.

Årtun, J., Spadafora, A.T., Shapiro, P.A., McNeill, R.W., and Chapko, M.K.: Hygiene Status Associated with Different Types of Bonded Orthodontic Canine-to-Canine Retainers, *J. Clin. Periodontol., 14,* 89, February, 1987.

Årtun, J. and Osterberg, S.K.: Periodontal Status of Secondary Crowded Mandibular Incisors. Long-term Results After Orthodontic Treatment, *J. Clin. Periodontol., 14,* 261, May, 1987.

Diamanti-Kipioti, A., Gusberti, F.A., and Lang, N.P.: Clinical and Microbiological Effects of Fixed Orthodontic Appliances, *J. Clin. Periodontol., 14,* 326, July, 1987.

Goultschin, J. and Zilberman, Y.: Gingival Response to Removable Orthodontic Appliances, *Am. J. Orthod., 81,* 147, February, 1982.

Mattingly, J.A., Sauer, G.J., Yancey, J.M., and Arnold, R.R.: Enhancement of *Streptococcus mutans* Colonization by Direct Bonded Orthodontic Appliances, *J. Dent. Res., 62,* 1209, December, 1983.

Scheie, A.A., Arneberg, P., and Krogstad, O.: Effect of Orthodontic Treatment on Prevalence of *Streptococcus mutans* in Plaque and Saliva, *Scand. J. Dent. Res., 92,* 211, June, 1984.

Drug-Induced Gingival Enlargement

Barak, S., Engelberg, I.S., and Hiss, J.: Gingival Hyperplasia Caused by Nifedipine. Histopathologic Findings, *J. Periodontol., 58,* 639, September, 1987.

Bennett, J.A. and Christian, J.M.: Cyclosporine-induced Gingival Hyperplasia: Case Report and Literature Review, *J. Am. Dent Assoc., 111,* 272, August, 1985.

Daley, T.D., Wysocki, G.P., and Day, C.: Clinical and Pharmacologic Correlations in Cyclosporin-induced Gingival Hyperplasia, *Oral Surg. Oral Med. Oral Pathol., 101,* 417, October, 1986.

Lucas, R.M., Howell, L.P., and Brian, A.W.: Nifedipine-induced Gingival Hyperplasia. A. Histochemical and Ultrastructural Study, *J. Periodontol., 56,* 211, April, 1985.

Rateitschak-Plüss, E.M., Hefti, A., Lörtscher, R., and Thiel, G.: Initial Observation that Cyclosporin-A Induces Gingival Enlargement in Man, *J. Clin. Periodontol., 10,* 237, May, 1983.

Rostock, M.H., Fry, H.R., and Turner, J.E.: Severe Gingival Overgrowth Associated with Cyclosporin Therapy, *J. Periodontol., 57,* 294, May, 1986.

Savage, N.W., Seymour, G.J., and Robinson, M.F.: Cyclosporin-A-Induced Gingival Enlargement. A Case Report, *J. Periodontol., 58,* 475, July, 1987.

Seymour, R.A., Smith, D.G., and Rogers, S.R.: The Comparative Effects of Azathioprine and Cyclosporin on Some Gingival Health Parameters of Renal Transplant Patients. A Longitudinal Study, *J. Clin. Periodontol., 14,* 610, November, 1987.

van der Wall, E.E., Tuinzing, D.B., and Hes, J.: Gingival Hyperplasia Induced by Nifedipine, an Arterial Vasodilating Drug, *Oral Surg. Oral Med. Oral Pathol., 60,* 38, July, 1985.

Wysocki, G.P., Gretzinger, H.A., Laupacis, A., Ulan, R.A., and Stiller, C.R.: Fibrous Hyperplasia of the Gingiva: A Side Effect of Cyclosporin A Therapy, *Oral Surg. Oral Med. Oral Pathol., 55,* 274, March, 1983.

Xerostomia

Atkinson, J.C. and Fox, P.C.: Clinical Pathology Conference: Xerostomia, *Gerodontics, 2,* 193, December, 1986.

Baum, B.J., Bodner, L., Fox, P.C., Izutsu, K.T., Pizzo, P.A., and Wright, W.E.: Therapy-induced Dysfunction of Salivary Glands: Implications for Oral Health, *Spec. Care Dentist., 5,* 274, November-December, 1985.

Epstein, J.B.: Clinical Trials of a Sialogogue in Humans: A Preliminary Report, *Spec. Care Dentist., 2,* 17, January-February, 1982.

Ettinger, R.L.: Xerostomia—A Complication of Ageing, *Aust. Dent. J., 26,* 365, December, 1981.

Fox, P.C., van der Ven, P.F., Baum, B.J., and Mandel, I.D.: Pilocarpine for the Treatment of Xerostomia Associated with Salivary Gland Dysfunction, *Oral Surg. Oral Med. Oral Pathol., 61,* 243, March, 1986.

Fox, P.C., van der Ven, P.F., Sonies, B.C., Weiffenbach, J.M., and Baum, B.J.: Xerostomia: Evaluation of a Symptom with Increasing Significance, *J. Am. Dent. Assoc., 110,* 519, April, 1985.

Fox, P.C., Busch, K.A., and Baum, B.J.: Subjective Reports of Xerostomia and Objective Measures of Salivary Gland Performance, *J. Am. Dent. Assoc., 115,* 581, October, 1987.

Gelhard, T.B., Fidler, V., 's-Gravenmade, E.J., and Vissink, A.: Remineralization of Softened Human Enamel in Mucin- or CMC-containing Artificial Salivas, *J. Oral Pathol., 12,* 336, October, 1983.

Glass, B.J., Van Dis, M.L., Langlais, R.P., and Miles, D.A.: Xerostomia: Diagnosis and Treatment Planning Considerations, *Oral Surg. Oral Med. Oral Pathol., 58,* 248, August, 1984.

Grad, H., Grushka, M., and Yanover, L.: Drug Induced Xerostomia. The Effects and Treatment, *Can. Dent. Assoc. J., 51,* 296, April, 1985.

Markitziu, A., Gedalia, I., Stabholz, A., and Shuval, J.: Prevention of Caries Progress in Xerostomic Patients by Topical Fluoride Applications: A Study *in vivo* and *in vitro, J. Dent., 10,* 248, September, 1982.

Miller, S.E. and Barkmeier, W.W.: Dental Management of the Patient with Xerostomia, *Dent. Hyg., 55,* 41, November, 1981.

Newbrun, E.: *Cariology,* 2nd ed. Baltimore, Williams & Wilkins, 1983, pp. 17–27.

Rhodus, N.L.: Detection and Management of the Dental Patient with Sjögren's Syndrome, *Compend. Cont. Educ. Dent., 8,* 578, September, 1987.

Slome, B.A.: Rampant Caries: A Side Effect of Tricyclic Antidepressant Therapy, *Gen. Dent., 32,* 494, November-December, 1984.

Toljanic, J.A. and Zucuskie, T.G.: Use of a Palatal Reservoir in Denture Patients with Xerostomia, *J. Prosthet. Dent., 52,* 540, October, 1984.

Vissink, A., 's-Gravenmade, E.J., Panders, A.K., Olthof, A., Vermey, A., Huisman, M.C., and Visch, L.L.: Artificial Saliva Reservoirs, *J. Prosthet. Dent., 52,* 710, November, 1984.

13 *Examination Procedures*

Parts of the gingival and dental examinations are made by direct *visual* observation, while other parts require *tactile* examination using a probe and an explorer. These two types of instruments, assisted by a mouth mirror, are key instruments in patient evaluation. Considerable skill is required for accurate and efficient probing and exploring.

General principles of instrumentation are described in Chapter 31, pages 429–438. Study that chapter for basic descriptions of instrument parts, grasp, finger rests, and stroke.

I. Precaution

A probe or an explorer should not be applied to the teeth and gingiva until an initial review of information from the patient history and oral examination has been made. The immediate application of information from the history was outlined on page 83. Of particular significance is knowledge of a patient's susceptibility to bacteremia. Patients at risk must receive prophylactic antibiotic premedication before instrumentation (pages 85 and 91).

II. Basic Set-up

All tray arrangements need a basic set-up composed of a mouth mirror, probe, explorer, and cotton pliers. Wrapping these together for sterilizing increases efficiency. The packet should be labeled "basic set-up."

THE MOUTH MIRROR

I. Description
A. Parts
The mirror has three parts: the handle, shank, and working end, which is the mounted mirror or mirror head. Instrument parts are described on pages 429–430.

B. Mirror Surfaces
1. *Plane (Flat).* May produce a double image.
2. *Concave.* Magnifying.
3. *Front Surface.* The reflecting surface is on the front of the lens rather than on the back as with plane or magnifying mirrors. The front surface eliminates "ghost" images.

C. Diameters
Diameters vary from ⅝ to 1¼ inches. In addition, special examination mirrors are available in 1½- to 2-inch diameters.

D. Attachments
Mirrors may be threaded plain stem or cone socket to be joined to a handle. Because mirrors tend to become scratched, replacement of the working end is possible without purchasing new handles.

E. Handles
1. Thicker handles contribute to a more comfortable grasp and greater control.
2. Wider mirror handles are especially useful for mobility determination (page 206).

F. Disposable Mirrors
1. Plastic in one piece or a handle with replaceable head for professional use; may have front surface.
2. Take-home mirrors for patient instruction. Patient may observe lingual and posterior aspects. One type of mirror has a light attachment.

II. Purposes and Uses
The mouth mirror is used to provide:

A. Indirect Vision
This is particularly needed for distal surfaces of posterior teeth and lingual surfaces of anterior teeth.

B. Indirect Illumination
Reflection of light from the dental overhead light to any area of the oral cavity is accomplished by adapting the mirror.

C. Transillumination
Reflection of light through the teeth.
1. Mirror is held to reflect light from the lingual while the teeth are examined from the facial.
2. Mirror is held for indirect vision on the lingual while light from the overhead dental light passes through the teeth. Translucency of enamel can be seen clearly, whereas dental caries or calculus deposits appear opaque.

D. Retraction
The mirror is used to protect or prevent interference by the cheeks, tongue, or lips.

III. Technique for Use
A. Grasp
Use modified pen grasp with finger rest on a tooth surface wherever possible to provide stability and control.

B. Retraction
1. Use petrolatum or other lubricant on dry or cracked lips and corners of mouth.
2. Adjust the mirror position so that the angles of the mouth are protected from undue pressure of shank of the mirror.
3. Insert and remove mirror carefully to avoid hitting the teeth, because this can be very disturbing to the patient.

C. Maintain Clear Vision
1. Warm mirror with water, rub along buccal mucosa to coat mirror with thin transparent film of saliva, and request patient to breathe through the nose to prevent condensation of moisture on mirror. Use a detergent or other means for keeping a clear surface.
2. Discard scratched mirrors.

IV. Care of Mirrors

A. Dismantle mirror and handle for sterilization.
B. Examine carefully after scrubbing with brush prior to sterilization to assure removal of debris around back, shank, and rim of reflecting surface.
C. Handle carefully during sterilization procedures to prevent other instruments from scratching the reflecting surface.
D. Consult manufacturer's specifications for sterilizing or disinfecting procedures that may cloud the mirror, particularly the front surface type.

INSTRUMENTS FOR APPLICATION OF AIR

I. Purposes and Uses

With appropriate, timely application of air to clear saliva and debris and/or dry the tooth surfaces, the following can be accomplished:

A. Improve and Facilitate Examination Procedures
1. Make a thorough, more accurate examination.
2. Dry supragingival calculus to facilitate exploring and scaling. Small deposits may be light in color and not visible until they are dried. Dried calculus appears chalky and presents a contrast to tooth color.
3. Deflect free gingival margin for observation into the subgingival area. Subgingival calculus usually appears dark.
4. Make identification of areas of demineralization and carious lesions easier.
5. Recognize location and condition of restorations, particularly tooth-color restorations.

B. Improve Visibility of the Field of Operation during Instrumentation
1. Dry area for finger rest to provide stability during instrumentation.
2. Facilitate positive scaling techniques.
3. Minimize appointment time.
4. Evaluate complete removal of calculus after instrumentation.

C. Prepare Teeth and/or Gingiva for Certain Procedures
1. Dry tooth surfaces for application of caries-preventive agents.
2. Make impression for study cast.
3. Apply topical anesthetic.

II. Compressed Air Syringe

A. Description
1. *Air Source.* Air compressor with tubing attachment to syringe.
2. *Air Tip.* Has angled working end that can be turned for maxillary or mandibular application. Tip is removable for sterilization.

B. Technique for Use
1. Use palm grasp about the handle of the syringe; place thumb on release lever or on button on handle.
2. Test the air flow so that the strength of flow can be controlled.
3. Make controlled, relatively short, gentle applications of air.
4. Supplement air drying with use of saliva ejector and folded gauze sponge placed in vestibule.

C. Precautions
1. Avoid sharp blasts of air on sensitive cervical areas of teeth or open carious lesions. Such areas may be dried by blotting with a gauze sponge or cotton roll to avoid causing discomfort.
2. Avoid applying air directly into a pocket. Subgingival plaque may be forced into the tissues and a bacteremia created.
3. Avoid forceful application of air which can direct saliva and debris out of the oral cavity, contaminate the working area and clinician, and create aerosols (pages 10–11). Air directed toward the posterior region of the patient's mouth may cause coughing.
4. Avoid silicate cement or other restorations that may be harmed by excessive drying.
5. Avoid startling the patient: forewarn when air is to be applied.

PROBE

Early in patient examination, the patient's periodontal disease status must be determined. Treatment planning will vary depending on whether the condition is gingivitis or whether it is periodontitis with periodontal pockets, bone loss, and root surface involvement.

The probe is used to make the initial assessment, followed by a detailed evaluation to determine the extent and degree of severity of disease and tissue destruction for specific treatment planning. During treatment, the probe is applied to assess progress. After treatment, use of the probe helps to determine completion of professional services as recognized by the health status of the tissues. At each maintenance appointment, a reevaluation with the probe is needed to assure continued self-care by the patient and to identify early disease changes that require additional professional treatment.

I. Purposes and Uses

A probe is used to

A. Assess the Periodontal Status for Preparation of a Treatment Plan

1. Classify the disease as gingivitis or periodontitis by determining whether bone loss has occurred and the pockets are gingival or periodontal (figure 12–1, page 181).
2. Determine the extent of inflammation in conjunction with the overall gingival examination. Bleeding on probing is an early sign of inflammation in the gingiva.

B. Make a Sulcus and Pocket Survey

1. Examine the shape, topography, and dimensions of sulci and pockets.
2. Measure and record probed pocket depths.
3. Evaluate tooth-surface pocket wall.
   a. Chart calculus location and severity.
   b. Record other root surface irregularities discerned by the probe.
4. Determine probed attachment level (page 198).

C. Make a Mucogingival Examination

1. Determine relationship of the gingival margin, attachment level, and the mucogingival junction.
2. Measure the width of the attached gingiva (figure 13–10, page 200).

D. Make Other Gingival Determinations

1. Evaluate gingival bleeding on probing and prepare a gingival bleeding index (page 271).
2. Measure the extent of apparent, visible gingival recession (figure 11–7, page 172).
3. Determine the consistency of the gingival tissue.

E. Guide to Treatment

1. Determine gingival characteristics, including pocket depth, bleeding, and consistency (all determined using a probe), to provide a basis for patient instruction as part of the total treatment.
2. Define depth of sulcus or pocket for application of instruments for scaling and root planing, and depth for use of an explorer for evaluation of these procedures.
3. Detect anatomic configuration of roots, subgingival deposits, and root irregularities that complicate instrumentation. For this, the probe is used in conjunction with the explorer.

F. Evaluate Success and Completeness of Treatment

1. Evaluate tissue response to professional treatment postoperatively on an immediate, short-term basis as well as at periodic maintenance examinations.
2. Evaluate patient's self-treatment through therapeutic disease control procedures.
3. Signs of health revealed by probing
   a. No bleeding: healthy tissue does not bleed.
   b. Reduced pocket depth: comparison of pre- and postoperative pocket depth.
   c. Tissue is firm as shown by application of the probe to the surface of the free gingiva.

II. Description

A probe is a slender instrument with a blunt end designed for examination of the depth and topography of an area. It has three parts: the handle, the angled shank, and the working end, which is the probe itself.

A. Characteristics

1. *Straight Working End*
   a. Tapered, round, flat, or rectangular in cross section with a smooth rounded end.
   b. Calibrated in millimeters at intervals specific for each kind of probe; some have color coding. Figure 13–1 shows a comparison of a few typical markings; table 13–1 lists probe markings with examples.
2. *Curved Working End.* Noncalibrated, curved, usually paired, smooth, furcation probes have rounded blunt end for investigation of the topography and anatomy around roots in a furca. Examples are the Nabers 1N and 2N probes.

B. Selection

The probe chosen for use by a dentist or a dental hygienist is frequently the instrument first used when a particular technique was learned, or one that provides comfort and ease of manipulation. Another reason for selection is that consistency in reading can be accomplished.

Analysis of a probe and comparison with other probes is recommended. Important features to be considered in probe selection are

1. *Adaptability.* The probe should be adaptable around the complete circumference of each tooth, both posterior and anterior, so that no millimeter of pocket depth can be neglected. Flat probes require more attention to adaptation and are useful primarily on facial and lingual surfaces.
2. *Markings.* Markings should be easy to read so that pocket depth can be readily identified and measured, and no disease area will be overlooked.

GUIDE TO PROBING

The information in Chapters 11 and 12 concerning the gingival examination, the normal tissues, and the development and types of pockets should be studied in conjunction with this outline of probing techniques.

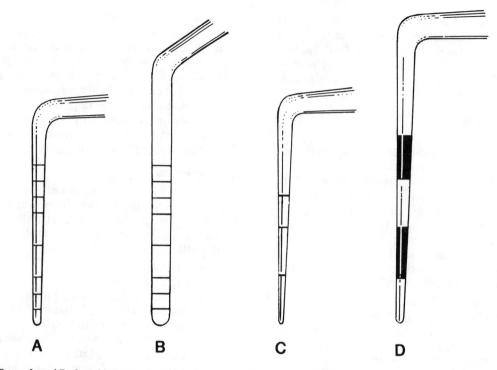

Figure 13–1. Examples of Probes. Names and calibrated markings shown are **A.** Williams (1-1-1-2-2-1-1-1), **B.** Goldman-Fox (1-1-1-2-2-1-1-1), **C.** Michigan O (3-3-2), and **D.** Hu-Friedy or Marquis Color-coded (3-3-3-3 or 3-3-2-3). See Table 13–1 for additional data on probes.

Table 13–1. Types of Probes

Probe Markings (mm)	Examples	Description
Marks at 1-2-3-5-7-8-9-10	Williams	Round, tapered (available with color-code)
	University of Michigan with Williams marks	Round, narrow diameter, fine
	Glickman	Round, with longer lower shank
	Merritt A and B	Round, single bend in shank
Marks at 3-3-2	University of Michigan O	Round, fine, tapered, narrow diameter
	Premier O	
	Marquis M-1	
Marks at 3-6-9-12 3-6-8-11 (and other variations)	Hu-Friedy QULIX	Round, tapered, fine
	Marquis	Color-coded
	Nordent	
Marks at 3.5-5.5-8.5-11.5	WHO Probe (World Health Organization)	Round, tapered, fine, with ball end
		Color-coded (figure 19–13, page 278)
No marks	Gilmore	Tapered, sharper than other probes
	Nabers 1N, 2N	Curved, with curved shank for furcation examination

A pocket is a diseased gingival sulcus. The use of a probe is the only accurate, dependable method to locate, assess, and measure sulci and pockets.

I. Pocket Characteristics

A. A pocket is measured from the base of the pocket (top of attached periodontal tissue) to the gingival margin. Figure 13–2 shows two pockets of different depths beneath gingival margins that are at the same level.

B. The pocket (or sulcus) is continuous around the entire tooth, and the entire pocket or sulcus must be measured. "Spot" probing is inadequate.

C. The depth varies around an individual tooth: a pocket rarely measures the same all around a tooth or even around one side of a tooth.
   1. The level of attached tissue assumes a varying position around the tooth.
   2. The gingival margin varies in its position on the tooth.

D. Proximal surface pockets must be examined by entering from both the facial and lingual surfaces of the tooth.
   1. Gingival and periodontal disease begin in the col area more frequently than in other areas (figure 11–5, page 169).
   2. Pocket may be deepest directly under the contact area because of crater formation in the alveolar bone (figure 13–3).

E. Anatomic features of the tooth-surface wall of the pocket influence the direction of probing. Examples are concave surfaces, anomalies, shape of cervical third, and position of furcations.

II. Evaluation of Tooth Surface

During the movement of the probe, calculus and tooth surface irregularities can be felt and evaluated.

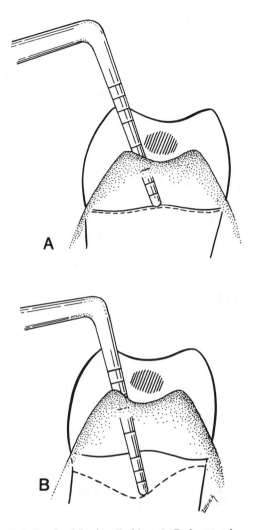

Figure 13–3. Proximal Surface Probing. A. Probe must be applied more than one-half way across from facial to overlap with probing from the lingual. **B.** Probe in area of crater formation. A pocket is usually deeper on the proximal under the contact area than on the facial or lingual.

The information obtained is used to plan the scaling and root planing appointments.

III. Factors That Affect Probe Determinations

The general objectives of probing are accuracy and consistency so that recordings are dependable for comparison with future probings. At the same time, patient discomfort and trauma to the tissues must be minimal. Probing is influenced by many factors, such as those that follow:

A. Severity and Extent of Periodontal Disease

With application of a light pressure, the probe passes along the tooth surface to the attached tissue level. Diseased tissue offers less resistance so that with increased severity of disease, the probe inserts to a deeper level.[1] Average levels show that the probe is stopped as follows:

1. *Normal Tissue.* The probe is at the base of the

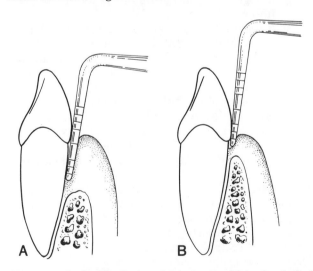

Figure 13–2. Pocket Depth. A pocket is measured from the gingival margin to the attached periodontal tissue. Shown is the contrast of probe measurements with gingival margins at the same level. **A.** Deep periodontal pocket (7 mm.) with apical migration of attachment. **B.** Shallow pocket (2 mm.) with the attachment near the cementoenamel junction.

sulcus or crevice, at the coronal end of the junctional epithelium.

2. *Gingivitis and Early Periodontitis.* The probe tip is within the junctional epithelium.

3. *Advanced Periodontitis.* Probe tip may penetrate through the junctional epithelium to reach attached connective tissue fibers.

B. The Probe Itself

1. *Calibration.* Must be accurately marked.

2. *Thickness.* A thinner probe slips through a narrow pocket more readily.

3. *Readability.* Aided by the markings and color-coding.

C. Technique

1. *Grasp.* Appropriate for maximum tactile sensitivity.

2. *Finger Rest.* Placed on non-mobile tooth with uniformity.

D. Placement Problems

1. *Anatomic Variations.* Tooth contours, furcations, contact areas, anomalies.

2. *Interferences.* Calculus, irregular margins of restorations, fixed dental appliances.

3. *Accessibility, Visibility.* Obstructed by tissue bleeding, limited opening by patient, macroglossia.

E. Application of Pressure

Consistent pressure is accomplished by consistent grasp and finger rest in addition to keen tactile sensitivity.

POCKET PROBING TECHNIQUE

I. Preparation for Probe Insertion

A. Grasp probe with modified pen grasp (page 431).

B. Establish finger rest on a neighboring tooth, preferably in the same dental arch.

C. Hold side of instrument tip flat against the tooth near the gingival margin with the probe approximately parallel with the long axis of the tooth for insertion. The cervical third of a primary tooth is more convex (figure 13–4).

D. Gently insert the tip under the gingival margin.

1. Healthy or firm fibrotic tissue: insertion is more difficult because of the close adaptation of the tissue to the tooth surface; underlying gingival fibers are strong and tight.

2. Spongy, soft tissue: gingival margin is loose and flabby because of the destruction of underlying gingival fibers. Probe will insert readily and bleeding can be expected on gentle probing.

II. Advance Probe to Base of Pocket

A. Hold side of probe tip flat against the tooth surface. Widespread roots of primary molars may make this probe position difficult unless the tis-

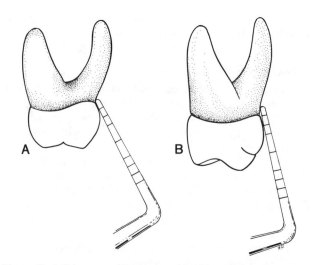

Figure 13–4. Primary and Permanent Maxillary Molars. A. Accentuated convexity of the cervical third and widespread roots of the primary molar complicate probe placement. Probe may encounter the root. **B.** Permanent tooth with less convexity of the cervical third and roots that are less widely spread.

sue is unduly distended by the probe (figure 13–4).

B. Slide the probe along the tooth surface vertically down to the base of the sulcus or pocket.

1. Maintain contact of the side of the tip of the probe with the tooth.

   a. Gingival pocket: side of probe is on enamel.

   b. Periodontal pocket: side of probe is on the cemental or dentinal surface when inserted to a level below the cementoenamel junction.

2. As the probe is passed down the side of the tooth, roughness may be felt. Evaluation of the topography and nature of the tooth surface is important to instrumentation.

3. If obstruction by hard bulky calculus deposit is encountered, lift the probe away from tooth and follow over the edge of the calculus until the probe can move vertically into the pocket again.

4. The base of the sulcus or pocket will feel soft and elastic (compared with the hard tooth surface and calculus deposits) and with slight pressure, the tension of the attached periodontal tissue at the base of the pocket can be felt.

C. Use only the pressure needed to detect by tactile means the level of the attached tissue, whether junctional epithelium or deep connective tissue fibers. A light pressure of 10 grams, or of no more than 20 grams, is ample.

D. Position probe for reading.

1. Bring the probe to position as nearly parallel with the long axis of the tooth as possible for reading the depth.

2. Interference of the contact area does not permit placing the probe parallel for the meas-

urement directly beneath the contact area. Hold the side of shank of the probe against the contact to minimize the angle (figure 13–3).

III. Read the Probe

A. Measurement of a pocket is made from the gingival margin to the attached periodontal tissue.

B. Count the millimeters that show on the probe above the gingival margin and subtract the number from the total number of millimeters marked on the particular probe being used. A comparison of pocket measurement using probes with different calibrations is shown in figure 13–5.

C. When the gingival margin appears at a level between probe marks, use the higher mark for the final reading.

D. Drying the area being probed improves visibility for specific reading.

IV. Circumferential Probing

A. Probe Stroke

Maintain the probe in the sulcus or pocket of each tooth as the probe is moved in a walking stroke.

1. It is not correct to remove the probe and reinsert it to make individual readings.

2. Repeated withdrawal and reinsertion cause unnecessary trauma to the gingival margin and hence increase postoperative discomfort.

B. Walking Stroke

1. Hold the side of the tip against the tooth at the base of the pocket.

2. Slide the probe up (coronally) about 1 to 2 mm. and back to the attachment in a "touch . . . touch . . . touch . . ." rhythm (figure 13–6).

3. Observe probe measurement at the gingival margin at each touch.

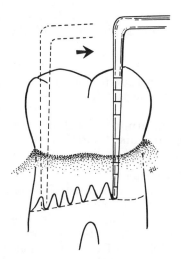

Figure 13–6. Probe Walking Stroke. The side of the tip of the probe is held in contact with the tooth. From the base of the pocket, the probe is moved up and down in 1- to 2-mm. strokes as it is advanced in 1-mm. steps. The attached periodontal tissue at the base of the pocket is contacted on each down stroke to identify pocket depth in each area.

4. Advance millimeter by millimeter along the facial and lingual surfaces into the proximal areas.

V. Adaptation of Probe for Individual Teeth

A. Molars and Premolars

1. Orient the probe at the distal line angle for both facial and lingual application.

2. Insert probe at the distal line angle and probe in a distal direction; adapt the probe around the line angle; probe across the distal surface until the side of the probe contacts the contact area, then slant the probe to continue under the contact area.

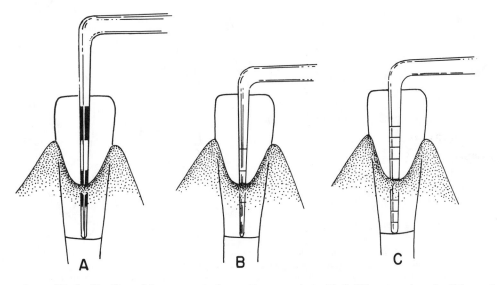

Figure 13–5. Comparison of Probe Readings. Measurement of same 5-mm. pocket with 3 different probes. **A.** Color-coded, **B.** Michigan O, **C.** Williams.

3. Reinsert the probe at the distal line angle and proceed in the mesial direction, around the mesial line angle and across the mesial surface.

B. Anterior Teeth

1. Initial insertion may be at the distal line angle or from the midline of the facial or lingual surfaces.
2. Proceed around the distal line angle and across the distal surface; reinsert and probe the other half of the tooth.

C. Proximal Surfaces

1. Continue the walking stroke around each line angle and onto the proximal surface.
2. Roll the instrument handle between the fingers to keep the side of the probe tip adapted to the tooth surface at line angles and as the tooth contour varies.
3. Continue stroke under the contact area. Overlap strokes from facial with strokes from lingual to assure full coverage (figure 13–3). Make sure that the col area under each contact has been thoroughly examined.

PROBED ATTACHMENT LEVEL

Attachment level refers to the position of the periodontal attached tissues at the base of a sulcus or pocket. It is measured from a fixed point to the attachment, whereas the probed pocket depth is measured from a changeable point (the crest of the free gingiva) to the attachment (figure 13–7A).

I. Rationale

A loss of attachment occurs in disease as the junctional epithelium migrates toward the apex. Stability of attachment is characteristic in health, and treatment procedures may be aimed to obtain a gain of attachment.

Evaluation can be made of the outcome of periodontal treatment and the stability of the attachment during maintenance examinations. When periodontal disease is active, pocket formation and migration of the attachment along the cemental surface will continue.

II. Procedure

A. Selection of a Fixed Point

1. Cementoenamel junction is usually used.
2. Margin of a permanent restoration.
3. For animal research, a notch may be made in the tooth; in human research studies, a template or splint may be made for each patient.

B. Measuring in the Presence of Visible Recession

1. Cementoenamel junction is visible directly.
2. Measure from the cementoenamel junction to the attachment (figure 13–7B).
3. The probed attachment level is greater than the probed pocket depth.

C. Measuring When the Cementoenamel Junction Is Covered by Gingiva

1. Slide the probe along the tooth surface, into the pocket, until the cementoenamel junction is felt (figure 13–7C).
2. Remove the calculus when it covers the cementoenamel junction.

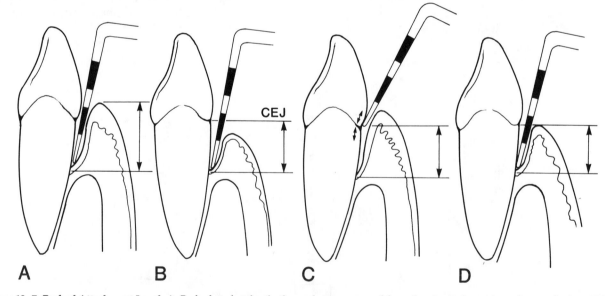

Figure 13–7. Probed Attachment Level. A. Probed pocket depth: the pocket is measured from the gingival margin to the attached periodontal tissue. **B.** Probed attachment level in the presence of gingival recession is measured directly from the cementoenamel junction (CEJ) to the attached tissue. **C.** Probed attachment level when the gingival margin covers the cementoenamel junction: first the cementoenamel junction is located as shown, and then the distance to the cementoenamel junction is measured and subtracted from the probed pocket depth. **D.** The probed attachment level is equal to the probed pocket depth when the gingival margin is at the level of the cementoenamel junction.

3. Measure from the gingival crest to the cementoenamel junction.
4. Subtract the millimeters from cementoenamel junction to gingival crest from the total pocket depth to the attachment.
5. Probed pocket depth is greater than the probed attachment level.

D. Measuring When the Free Gingival Margin Is Level with the Cementoenamel Junction
1. Apply the probe as has been described.
2. The probed pocket depth equals the probed attachment level (figure 13–7D).

FURCATIONS EXAMINATION

When a pocket extends into a furcation area, special adaptation of the probe must be made to determine the extent and topography of the furcation involvement. The classification of types of furcation involvement is shown on page 183.

I. Anatomic Features

A. Bifurcation (teeth with two roots)
1. *Mandibular Molars.* The furcation area is accessible for probing from the facial and lingual (figure 13–8).
2. *Maxillary First Premolars.* The furcation area is accessible from the mesial and distal, under the contact area.
3. *Primary Mandibular Molar.* Widespread roots.

B. Trifurcation (teeth with three roots)
1. *Maxillary Molars.* A palatal root and two buccal roots, the mesiobuccal and the distobuccal roots. Access for probing is from the mesial, buccal, and distal.
2. *Maxillary Primary Molars.* Widespread roots (figure 13–4, page 196).

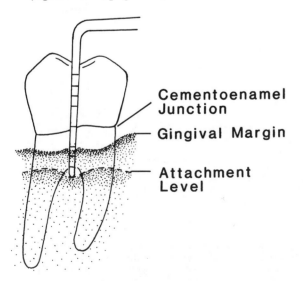

Cementoenamel Junction

Gingival Margin

Attachment Level

Figure 13–8. Furcation Examination. Probe inserted into bifurcation in area of gingival recession shows pocket of 3 mm. The probe is used to examine the topography of the furcation area.

II. Examination Methods

A. Early Furcation
1. Probe to measure pocket depth.
2. Inspect the area by adapting the probe closely to the tooth surface and moving the end of the probe over the anatomic curvatures of the roots. An example is shown in figure 33–2C, page 457.
3. Check radiograph for early signs of furcation involvement (figure 13–18, page 208).

B. Points of Access
Probe to measure pocket depths at points of access for each bifurcation or trifurcation area. Position of gingival margin will vary. Figure 13–8 shows apparent recession and 3-mm. pocket in bifurcation.

C. Probe Adaptation
Use probe in diagonal or horizontal position to examine between roots when there is gingival recession or a flexible, short, soft pocket wall that permits access.

D. Use of Curved Instrument
Use a curved instrument, such as a curved probe (Nabers 1N or 2N) or a curet, to examine advanced furcation.

E. Complications
Anatomic variations that complicate furcation examination: fused roots, anomalies, such as extra roots, or low or high furcations (figure 33–1, page 457).

MUCOGINGIVAL EXAMINATION

I. Tension Test[2]

A. Purposes
1. To detect adequacy of the width of the attached gingiva.
2. To locate frenal attachments and their proximity to the free gingiva.
3. To identify promptly the mucogingival junction.

B. Procedures
1. *Facial*
   a. Retract cheeks and lips laterally by grasping the lips with the thumbs and index fingers.
   b. Move the lips and cheeks up and down and across, creating tension at the mucogingival junction.
   c. Follow around from the molar areas on the right to molar areas on the left, both maxillary and mandibular.

2. *Lingual (Mandible)*

   a. Hold a mouth mirror to tense the mucosa of the floor of the mouth, gently retracting the side of the tongue, so that the mucogingival junction is clearly visible.

   b. Request patient to move the tongue to the left, to the right, and up to touch the palate.

C. Observations

1. Blanching at the mucogingival junction.
2. Frenal attachments.
3. Area(s) of apparent recession where there is very little keratinized gingiva and the base of the sulcus or pocket is near the mucogingival junction (figure 11–8, page 173).
4. Area where color, size, loss of stippling, smooth shininess, or other characteristic indicates the need for careful probing to determine the amount of attached gingiva.
5. Area where tension pulls the free gingiva away from the tooth, thereby indicating no attached gingiva.

II. Gingival Tissue Examination

When inflammation is present and a pocket extends to or through the mucogingival junction, a streak of color (red, bluish-red) that shows the inflammatory changes from the gingival margin to the mucogingival junction may be apparent. When such an area does not pull away during a tension test or does not permit passage of a probe through to the alveolar mucosa, the area should be noted in the record for examination after elimination of inflammation.

III. Probing

When a pocket extends to or beyond the mucogingival junction, the probe may pass through the pocket

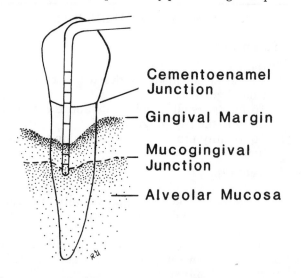

Figure 13–9. Mucogingival Examination. Probe in position for measuring pocket depth where attached gingiva is missing. Absence of attached gingiva permits the probe to pass through the mucogingival junction into the alveolar mucosa.

directly into the alveolar mucosa (figure 13–9). Mucogingival involvement was described on page 184.

IV. Measure the Amount of Attached Gingiva

A. Place the probe on the external surface of the gingiva and measure from the mucogingival junction to the gingival margin to determine the width of the total gingiva (figure 13–10A).
B. Insert the probe and measure pocket depth (figure 13–10B).
C. Subtract the pocket depth from the total gingival measurement to get the width of the attached gingiva.
D. Record findings.

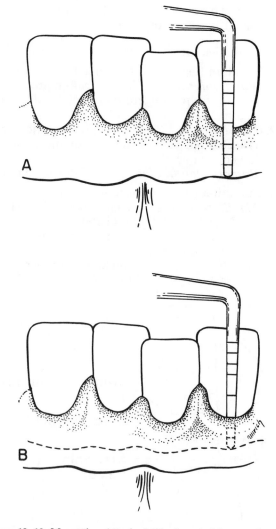

Figure 13–10. Measuring Attached Gingiva. A. Measure the total gingiva by laying the probe over the surface of the gingiva and measuring from the free margin to the mucogingival junction. **B.** Measure the pocket depth. Dotted line represents the base of the pocket. Subtract the pocket measurement (B) from the total gingiva (A) to obtain the width of attached gingiva. The area illustrated shows 2 mm. of attached gingiva.

PERIODONTAL CHARTING

Charting of findings while using the probe is a part of the complete periodontal record. The summary of periodontal observations and records may be found on pages 286 and 288.

The procedure described here assumes the use of a chart form with outline drawings of teeth with both facial and lingual root drawings. The exact procedure and format are entirely the choice of an individual dentist. A composite chart that includes dental as well as periodontal findings is frequently used.

In the preparation of the charting, contrasting colors should be used. For example, when red is used to chart dental caries on a composite charting, red would not be a good color selection for drawing the gingival margin because of possible interference with a drawing of a Class V carious lesion. One procedure for a relatively simple charting system is described here.

I. Teeth Identification

Mark missing, unerupted, or impacted teeth. Prepare these markings in advance of the patient's appointment by reviewing and comparing the radiographs and the study casts.

II. Draw Gingival Lines

A. Gingival Margin

1. Draw the outline of the position and contour of the gingival margin on the chart form as it appears in relation to the teeth both facial and lingual.
2. Prepare in advance of the patient's appointment when study casts are available.

B. Mucogingival Lines

1. *General Procedures*
   a. Use contrasting color to that used for drawing the gingival line.
   b. Draw on the facial for all quadrants; draw lingual only on mandibular.
2. *Three Methods.* For all, draw the gingival line first.

a. Draw the lines directly, estimating distances between the gingival margin and the mucogingival junction.
b. Measure with probe.
   i. Measure the total gingiva from gingival margin to mucogingival junction at the center of each tooth (facial and lingual). Write the millimeters on the tooth crown in light pencil to be erased later.
   ii. Place a dot on the tooth chart at the point of millimeters measured from the margin; connect the dots in a relatively straight line representing the mucogingival junction for the molars and premolars and in a scalloped line for the anterior teeth, in keeping with the actual appearance.
c. Study casts. When parts or all of the mucogingival lines show clearly on the casts, the drawing can be made in advance of the patient's appointment.

III. Record Pocket Measurements

A. Record all diseased pockets of any depth.
B. Record deepest millimeter measurement for each of the six areas around a tooth as shown in figure 13–11. Areas numbered 1, 3, 4, 6 extend from the line angle to under the contact area.
C. Supplement the six recordings with additional readings to show particular areas of unusually deep pockets, furcation involvement, or mucogingival involvement.
D. Record on the charting form. Figure 13–12 shows five possible methods for recording the millimeter depth.

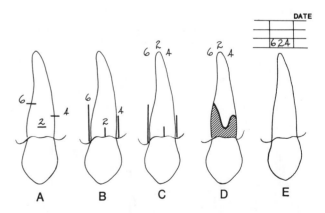

Figure 13–12. **Methods for Charting Pocket Measurements. A., B.** Chart forms with free-hand lines that designate relative depths. **C.** Numeric notations written at the apex of each tooth. **D.** A continuous line that defines the entire pocket and that can be shaded. **E.** Multiple spaces over the apex of each tooth, used to record the pocket depths. Each row can be dated, thus allowing comparisons of measurements at successive follow-up and maintenance examinations.

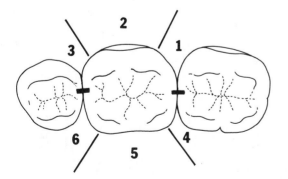

Figure 13–11. **Charting Pocket Measurements.** The pocket/sulcus is measured completely around each tooth. Record the deepest measurement for each of the six areas around the tooth. Areas 1, 3, 4, and 6 extend from the line angle to under the contact area.

IV. Record Special Disease Problems

Furcation involvement, mucogingival involvement, and frenal pull must be recorded either by a conspicuous symbol or by writing directly on the chart or in the record. See previous section for methods of examination for these conditions.

EXPLORERS

I. General Purposes and Uses

An explorer is used to
A. Detect, by tactile sense, the texture and character of the tooth surface.
B. Examine the supragingival tooth surfaces for calculus, demineralized and carious lesions, defects or irregularities in the surfaces and margins of restorations, and other irregularities that are not apparent to direct observation. An explorer is used to confirm direct observation.
C. Examine the subgingival tooth surfaces for calculus, demineralized and carious lesions, diseased altered cementum, and other cemental changes that can result from periodontal pocket formation.
D. Define the extent of instrumentation needed and guide techniques for
   1. Scaling and root planing.
   2. Finishing a restoration.
   3. Removing an overhanging filling.
E. Evaluate the completeness of treatment as shown by the smooth, glassy tooth surface or the smooth restoration.

II. Description

The basic parts of an instrument are described on pages 429–430.

A. Working End
   1. Slender, wire-like, metal *tip* that is approximately 1 to 2 mm. in length, is circular in cross section, and tapers to a fine sharp *point.*

   2. Design
      a. Single: a single instrument may be universal and adaptable to any tooth surface, or it may be designed for specific groups of surfaces. In figure 13–13, Numbers 2 through 7, 17, 18, 20, and 23 are single instruments.
      b. Paired: paired instruments are mirror images of each other, curved to provide access to contralateral tooth surfaces. In figure 13–13, Numbers 9 and 10, 11 and 12, 13 and 14, and 21 and 22 are paired.
      c. Design of a balanced instrument: middle of working end (tip of an explorer) should be centered over the long axis of the handle (figure 13–14).

B. Shank
   1. *Straight, Curved, or Angulated.* Whether a shank is straight, curved, or angulated depends on the use and adaptation for which the explorer was designed. In figure 13–13 compare the straight shanks of Numbers 2, 5, 6, 7, 13, and 14 with the others in the series, which are not straight. A curved shank may facilitate application of the instrument to proximal surfaces, particularly of posterior teeth.
   2. *Flexibility.* The slender, wire-like explorers have a degree of flexibility that contributes to increased sensitivity.

C. Handle
   1. *Weight.* For increased acute tactile sensitivity, a lightweight handle is more effective.
   2. *Diameter.* A wider diameter with serrations for friction while grasping can prevent finger cramping from too tight a grasp. With a lighter grasp, tactile sensitivity can be increased.

D. Construction
   1. *Single-ended.* A single-ended instrument has one working end on a separate handle.
   2. *Double-ended.* A double-ended instrument has two working ends, one on each end of a

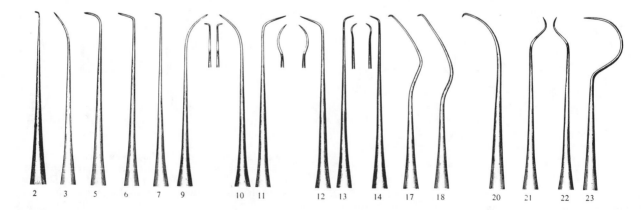

Figure 13–13. Explorers. This series from Numbers 2 through 23 shows standard shapes of explorer tips. Numbers 2 through 7, 17, 18, 20, and 23 are single instruments. Numbers 9 and 10, 11 and 12, 13 and 14, and 21 and 22 are paired instruments. (Courtesy of the S.S. White Company, Philadelphia, Pennsylvania.)

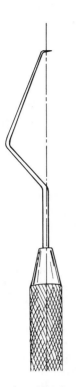

Figure 13–14. Balanced Explorer Design. With the middle of the tip centered over the long axis of the handle (shown by broken line from tip), the explorer can be positioned in a sulcus or pocket with ease and does not cause trauma to the gingival tissue. Shown is the balanced TU-17 explorer.

common handle. Most paired instruments are available double-ended. Other double-ended instruments combine two single instruments; for example, two unpaired explorers or an explorer with a probe.

III. Preparation of Explorers

Sharpen and retaper a dull explorer tip (page 453). With the explorer tip sharp and tapered, the following can be expected:

A. Increased tactile sensitivity with less pressure required.

B. Prevention of unnecessary trauma to the gingival tissue, because less pressure allows greater control.

C. Decreased operating time with increased patient comfort.

IV. Specific Explorers and Their Uses

A variety of explorers is available as shown by the examples in figure 13–13. The function of each type is related to its adaptability to specific surfaces of teeth at particular angulations. Certain explorers can be used effectively for detection of dental caries in pits and fissures, and others are designed to be adapted to examine proximal surfaces for calculus or dental caries. By other criteria, some can be used subgingivally, whereas others cannot be adapted subgingivally without inflicting damage to the sul-

cular epithelium. Therefore, such explorers are limited to supragingival adaptation only.

A. Subgingival Explorer (figure 13–14)

1. *Names and Numbers.* Orban Number 20, TU-17, pocket explorer.

2. *Shape.* The pocket explorer has an angulated shank with a short tip at a right-angle bend (figure 13–14). The tip should be measured to assure that it is less than 2 mm. A longer tip cannot be adapted to narrow roots, where a pocket narrows near the base.

3. *Use*

   a. Subgingival root examination.

   b. Features.

      i. Back of tip can be applied directly to the attached periodontal tissue at the base of the pocket without lacerating. When a straight or sickle explorer is directed toward the base of the pocket, the sharp tip can pass into the epithelium without resistance.

      ii. The short tip can be adapted to rounded tooth surfaces and line angles. Long tips of other explorers have tangential relationship with the tooth and cause distention and trauma to sulcular or pocket epithelium.

      iii. Narrow short tip can be adapted at the base where the pocket narrows without undue displacement of the pocket soft tissue wall.

   c. Supragingival use of Number TU-17. It may be adapted to all surfaces and is especially useful for proximal surface examination. It is not readily adaptable to pits and fissures.

B. Sickle or Shepherd's Hook (Number 23 in figure 13–13)

1. *Use.* Examining pits and fissures and supragingival smooth surfaces; examining surfaces and margins of restorations.

2. *Adaptability*

   a. Difficult to apply to proximal surfaces because the wide hook can contact an adjacent tooth and the straight long section of the tip can pass over a small proximal carious lesion.

   b. Not adaptable for deep subgingival exploration. When the point is directed to the base of a pocket, trauma to the attachment area can result. In the attempt to prevent such damage, the operator may not explore to the base of the pocket, thus providing incomplete service.

C. Pigtail or Cowhorn (Numbers 21 and 22 in figure 13–13)

1. *Use.* Proximal surfaces for calculus, dental caries, or margins of restorations.

2. *Adaptability.* As paired, curved tips, they are applied to opposite tooth surfaces.

D. Straight (Numbers 2, 6, 7 in figure 13–13)
1. *Use.* Supragingival, for pits and fissures, tooth irregularities of smooth surfaces, and surfaces and margins of restorations.
2. *Adaptability*
   a. For pit and fissure caries, the explorer tip is held parallel with the long axis of the tooth and applied straight into a pit.
   b. Not adaptable deep in subgingival area. Straight shanked instruments or those with long tips cannot be adapted readily in the apical portion of the pocket near the attached tissue or on line angles.

BASIC TECHNIQUES FOR USE OF EXPLORERS

Development of ability to use an explorer and a probe is achieved first by learning the anatomic features of each tooth surface and the types of irregularities that may be encountered on the surfaces. The second step is repeated practice of careful and deliberate techniques for application of the instruments.

The objective is to adapt the instruments in a routine manner that relays consistent comparative information about the nature of the tooth surface. Concentration, patience, attention to detail, and alertness to each irregularity, however small it may seem, are necessary.

I. Use of Sensory Stimuli

Both explorers and probes can transmit tactile stimuli from tooth surfaces to the fingers. A fine explorer usually gives a more acute reaction to small irregularities than does a thicker explorer. Probes vary in diameter; the narrower types may provide greater sensitivity.

A. Tooth Surface Irregularities

Three basic tactile sensations must be distinguished when probing or exploring. These may be grouped as normal tooth surface, irregularities created by excess or elevations in the surface, and irregularities caused by depressions in the tooth surface. Examples of these are listed here.
1. *Normal*
   a. Tooth structure: the smooth surface of enamel and root surface that has been planed; anatomic configurations such as cingula, furcations.
   b. Restored surfaces: smooth surfaces of metal (gold, amalgam) and the softer feeling of plastic; smooth margin of a restoration.
2. *Irregularities: Increases or Elevations in Tooth Surface*
   a. Deposits: calculus, and stain that is thick.
   b. Anomalies: enamel pearl; unusually pronounced cementoenamel junction.
   c. Restorations: overcontoured, irregular margins (overhang).

3. *Irregularities: Depressions, Grooves*
   a. Tooth surface: demineralized or carious lesion, abrasion, erosion, pits such as those caused by enamel hypoplasia, areas of cemental resorption on the root surface.
   b. Restorations: deficient margin, rough surface (figure 41–2, page 529).

B. Types of Stimuli

During exploring and probing, distinction of irregularities can be made through auditory and tactile means.
1. *Tactile.* Tactile sensations pass through the instrument to the fingers and hand and to the brain for registration and action. Tactile sensations, for example, may be the result of catching on an overcontoured restoration, dropping into a carious lesion, hooking the edge of a restoration or lesion, encountering an elevated deposit, or simply passing over a rough surface.
2. *Auditory.* As an explorer or probe moves over the surface of enamel, cementum, a metallic restoration, a plastic restoration, or any irregularity of tooth structure or restoration, a particular surface texture is apparent. With each contact, sound may be created. The clean smooth enamel is quiet; the rough cementum or calculus is scratchy or noisy. Sometimes a metallic restoration may "squeak" or have a metallic "ring." With experience, differentiations can be made.

II. Procedures: Supragingival

A. Use of Vision

Supragingival exploration for defects of the tooth surface differs from subgingival in that, when a surface is dried, much of the actual exploration is performed to confirm visual observation. The exceptions are the proximal areas near and around contact areas that cannot be directly observed.

Unnecessary exploring should be avoided. With adequate light and a source of air, proper retraction, and use of mouth mirror, dried supragingival calculus can generally be seen as either chalky white or brownish-yellow in contrast to tooth color. A minimum of exploration can confirm the finding.

B. Facial and Lingual Surfaces
1. Adapt the side of tip with the point always on the tooth surface.
2. Move the instrument in short walking strokes over the surface being examined, or direct the tip gently into a suspected carious lesion.
3. Avoid deliberate exploration of cervical third areas where there is recession or where the patient has previously exhibited sensitivity. If a sensitive area must be dried, avoid an air blast, and blot with a gauze sponge or a cotton

roll. Methods for desensitization are described on pages 499–500.

C. Proximal Surfaces

1. Lead with the tip onto the proximal surface, rolling the handle between the fingers to assure adaptation around the line angle.
2. Explore under the proximal contact area when there is recession of the papilla and the area is exposed. Overlap strokes from facial and lingual to assure full coverage.

III. Procedures: Subgingival

A. Essentials for Detection of Tooth Surface Irregularities

1. Definite but light grasp.
2. Consistent finger rest with light pressure.
3. Definite contact of the instrument with the tooth.
4. Light touch as the instrument is moved over the tooth surface.

B. Steps

1. With the tip in contact with the tooth supragingivally, hold the part of the shank that is next to the tip parallel with the long axis of the tooth. Gently slide the tip under the gingival margin into the sulcus or pocket.
2. Keep the point in contact with the tooth at all times to prevent unnecessary trauma to the pocket or sulcular epithelium. Adapt the tip closely to the tooth surface on the side of the point.
3. Slide the explorer tip over the tooth surface to the base of the pocket until, with the back of the tip, the resistance of the soft tissue of the attached periodontal tissue is felt (figure 13–15A). Calculus deposits may obstruct direct passage of the instrument to the base of the pocket. Lift the tip slightly away from the tooth surface and follow over the deposit to proceed to the base of the pocket.
4. Use a "walking" stroke, vertical or diagonal (oblique).
   a. Lead with the tip. Move it ahead as the instrument progresses (figure 13–15B).
   b. Length of stroke depends on the depth of a pocket.
      i. Shallow pocket: the stroke may extend the entire depth, from the base of the pocket to just beneath the gingival margin.
      ii. Deep pocket: controlled strokes 2- to 3-mm. long can provide more acute sensitivity to the surface and allow improved adaptation of the instrument. A deep pocket should be explored in sections. One should first explore the apical area next to the base of the pocket, then move up to a higher section, overlapping to assure full coverage.
   c. Do not remove the explorer from the pocket for each stroke on a particular surface because
      i. Trauma to the gingival margin caused by repeated withdrawal and reinsertion can cause the patient postoperative discomfort.
      ii. Concentration on the texture of the tooth surface is interrupted.
      iii. More time is consumed.
5. Proximal surface
   a. Lead with tip of instrument: do not "back into" an area.
   b. Continue the strokes around the line angle. Roll the instrument handle between the

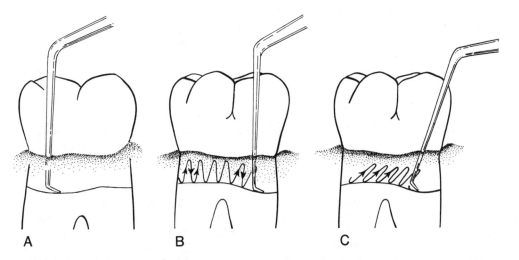

Figure 13–15. Use of Subgingival Explorer. A. The lower shank (next to tip) is held parallel with the long axis of the tooth. The explorer is passed into the pocket and lowered until the back of the working tip meets resistance from the attached periodontal tissue at the base of the pocket. **B.** Vertical walking stroke. With the side of the tip in contact with the tooth surface at all times, the explorer is moved over the surface. **C.** Diagonal walking stroke. Complete exploration of the surface is needed; therefore, groups of strokes are overlapped.

fingers to keep the tip closely adapted as the tooth contour changes.

   c. Continue strokes under the contact area. Overlap strokes from facial and lingual to assure full coverage.

IV. Record Findings

A. Supragingival Calculus

1. *Distribution.* Supragingival calculus is generally localized. It is most commonly confined to the lingual surfaces of the mandibular anterior teeth and the facial surfaces of the maxillary first and second molars, opposite the openings to the salivary ducts (page 247).
2. *Amount.* Slight, moderate, heavy.

B. Subgingival Calculus

1. *Distribution.* Subgingival calculus can be either localized or generalized.
2. *Amount.* Slight, moderate, heavy.

C. Other Irregularities of Tooth Surface

Note on the chart or in the record any other deviation from normal detected while using the explorer.

MOBILITY EXAMINATION

Because of the nature and function of the periodontal ligament, teeth have a slight normal mobility. Mobility can be considered abnormal or pathologic when it exceeds normal. Increased mobility can be an important clinical sign of disease.

I. Causes of Mobility

A. Inflammation

Inflammation in the periodontal ligament leads to degeneration or destruction of the fibers.

B. Loss of Support

Loss of sufficient support by alveolar bone and periodontal ligament (destroyed in periodontal disease) can increase the mobility.

C. Trauma from Occlusion

Injury to the periodontal tissues can result from occlusal forces (page 232–233).

II. Procedure for Determination of Mobility

A. Position the patient for clear visibility with maximum light and ready accessibility through convenient retraction.

B. Stabilize the head. Motion of the head, lips, or cheek can interfere with a true evaluation of tooth movement.

C. Use two single-ended metal instruments with wide blunt ends, held with a modified pen grasp. Use of wooden tongue depressors or plastic mirror handles is not recommended because of their flexibility. Testing with the fingers without the metal instruments can be misleading because the soft tissue of the finger tips can move and give an illusion of tooth movement.

D. Apply specific, firm finger rests (fulcrums). A standardized finger rest pressure contributes increased consistency to the determinations. The teeth may be dried with air or sponge to prevent slipping of the instruments or the finger on the finger rest.

E. Apply the blunt ends of the instruments to opposite sides of a tooth, and rock the tooth to test horizontal mobility. Keep both instrument ends on the tooth as pressure is applied first from one side and then the other.

F. Test vertical mobility (depression of the tooth into its socket) by applying, on the occlusal or incisal surface, pressure with one of the mirror handles.

G. Test each primary abutment tooth of a fixed partial denture.

H. Move from tooth to tooth in a systematic order.

III. Record Degree of Movement

A. Scale

N, 1, 2, 3 or I, II, III are frequently used, sometimes with a + to indicate mobility between numbers.

B. Recording

Although subjective, interpretation may be considered as follows:[3]

N = normal, physiologic

1 = slight mobility, greater than normal

2 = moderate mobility, greater than 1 mm. displacement

3 = severe mobility, may move in all directions, vertical as well as horizontal.

C. The Letter N Means *Normal* Mobility

All teeth that have a periodontal ligament have normal mobility. No tooth has zero mobility except in a condition, such as ankylosis, in which there is no periodontal ligament.

D. Chart Form

A chart form should provide for a place to record mobility. Preferably more than one place should be reserved so that comparative readings may be recorded at successive maintenance appointments.

FREMITUS

I. Definition

Fremitus means palpable vibration or movement. In dentistry it refers to the vibratory patterns of the teeth. A tooth with fremitus has excess contact, possibly related particularly to a premature contact. Usually, the tooth also demonstrates some degree of mobility because the excess contact forces the tooth to move. The test is used in conjunction with occlusal analysis and adjustment.

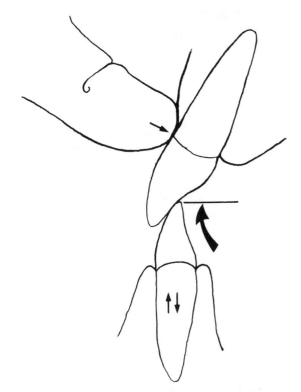

Figure 13–16. Fremitus. With the patient seated upright, an index finger is placed firmly over the cervical third of each maxillary tooth in succession starting with the most posterior tooth on one side and moving around the arch. The patient is requested to click the posterior teeth.

II. Procedure for Determination of Fremitus

A. Seat the patient upright.

B. Press an index finger on each maxillary tooth at about the cervical third (figure 13–16).

C. Request the patient to "click the back teeth" repeatedly.

D. Start with the most posterior maxillary tooth on one side and move the index finger tooth by tooth around the arch.

E. Record by tooth number the teeth where vibration is felt and the teeth where actual movement is noted. The degree recorded may be subjective, but the following range has been suggested:[4]

1. One-degree fremitus (+): when only slight movement can be felt.

2. Two-degree fremitus (+ +): when the tooth is clearly palpable but movement is barely visible.

3. Three-degree fremitus (+ + +): when movement is clearly observed visually.

RADIOGRAPHIC EXAMINATION

Radiographs provide essential information to aid and supplement clinical findings. During other phases of the examination, and especially during probing, the mounted radiographs should be on a viewbox for viewing in conjunction with examina-tion. When the radiographs have not been processed at the time of probing, areas for special confirmation can be marked on the record for review at the next appointment.

For observing evidence of periodontal involvement, periapical radiographs are needed. Bitewing radiographs do not show the complete periodontal tissues that extend around the roots. When bone loss is moderate to severe, the crest of the bone cannot usually be seen in a bitewing survey.

Principles for use of radiographs were described on pages 144–145. The need for mounted radiographs free from errors of technique and viewed on an adequately lighted viewbox cannot be overemphasized. A magnifying reading glass is of special assistance when studying periodontal findings.

I. Radiographic Changes in Periodontal Diseases

A. Bone Level

1. *Normal Bone Level.* The crest of the interdental bone appears from 1.0 to 1.5 mm. from the cementoenamel junction (figure 13–17).

2. *Bone Level in Periodontal Disease.* The height of the bone is lowered progressively as the inflammation is extended and bone is resorbed.

B. Shape of Remaining Bone

1. *Horizontal*

a. When the crest of the bone is parallel with a line between the cementoenamel junctions of two adjacent teeth, the term "horizontal bone loss" is used (figures 13–18 and 13–19).

b. When inflammation is the sole destructive factor, the bone loss usually appears horizontal.

c. When the amount of remaining bone is fairly evenly distributed throughout the dentition, the condition is described as *generalized* horizontal bone loss. It may be

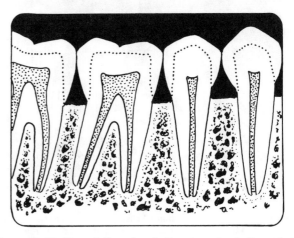

Figure 13–17. Normal Bone Level. Drawing of a radiograph to show normal bone level, 1 to 1.5 mm. from the cementoenamel junction.

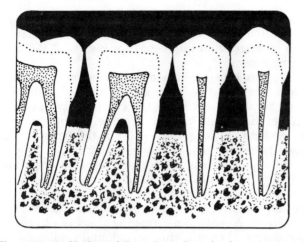

Figure 13–18. Horizontal Bone Loss. Bone level in periodontal disease is more than 1 to 1.5 mm. from the cementoenamel junction. When bone loss is horizontal, the crest of the alveolar bone is parallel with a line between the cementoenamel junctions of adjacent teeth. Note early furcation involvement in the second molar and moderate furcation involvement in the first molar.

designated either by millimeters from the position of the normal bone level or by percentage. When making estimates, referral to the table of average root lengths can be helpful (Appendix, tables A–3 and A–4).

    d. When bone loss is confined to specific areas, the condition is described as *localized* horizontal bone loss.

  2. *Angular or Vertical*

    a. Reduction in height of crestal bone that is irregular; the bone level is not parallel with a line joining the adjacent cementoenamel junctions (figure 13–20); and bone loss is greater on the proximal surface of one tooth than on the adjacent tooth.

    b. Angular bone loss is more commonly localized than generalized.

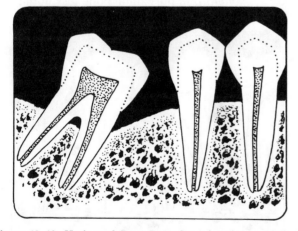

Figure 13–19. Horizontal Bone Loss. Second molar has drifted mesially into the space created when the first molar was removed. Note that the level of the crestal bone is parallel with a line between the cementoenamel junctions of the second premolar and the tipped second molar.

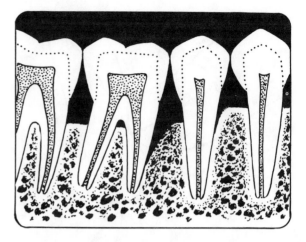

Figure 13–20. Angular or Vertical Bone Loss; Mesial of the First Molar. The level of the crestal bone between the second premolar and the first molar is not parallel with a line between the cementoenamel junctions of the same teeth.

    c. When inflammation and trauma from occlusion are combined in causing the destruction and irregular shape of the bone, the bone may appear with "angular defects" or with "vertical bone loss."

C. Crestal Lamina Dura

  1. *Normal.* White, radiopaque; continuous with and connects the lamina dura about the roots of two adjacent teeth; covers the interdental bone (figure 13–18).

  2. *Evidence of Disease.* The crestal lamina dura is indistinct, irregular, radiolucent, fuzzy.

D. Furcation Involvement

  1. *Normal.* Bone fills the area between the roots (figure 13–17).

  2. *Evidence of Disease.* Radiolucent area in the furcation.

    a. Early furcation involvement may appear as a small radiolucent black dot or as a slight thickening of the periodontal ligament space. It can be confirmed by probing. Early furcation involvement is shown in the second molar in figure 13–18.

    b. Furcation involvement of maxillary molars may become advanced before radiographic evidence can be seen. Superimposition of the palatal root may mask a small area of involvement. When the proximal bone level in the radiograph appears at the level where the furcation is normally located, furcation involvement should be suspected and probed for confirmation.

    c. Maxillary first premolar furcation involvement cannot be seen in a radiograph except at an unusual angulation or unusual position of the tooth. With correct vertical and horizontal angulation the roots are superimposed.

    d. Furcations may show at one angulation but

not at another; variations in technique can obscure a furcation involvement. All furcations must be carefully probed.

E. Periodontal Ligament Space

1. *Normal.* The periodontal ligament is connective tissue and, hence, appears radiolucent in a radiograph. It appears as a fine black radiolucent line next to the root surface. On its outer side is the lamina dura, the bone that lines the tooth socket and appears radiopaque (figure 13–21).

2. *Evidence of Disease.* Widening or thickening.
   a. Angular thickening or triangulation: the space is widened only near the coronal third, near the crest of the interdental bone.
   b. Complete periodontal ligament thickened along an entire side of a root to the apex, or around the root (figure 13–21): when viewed at different angulations (in the various radiographs of a complete survey), the ligament space may reveal varying thicknesses, thus showing that the disease involvement is not consistent around the entire root or that other structures are superimposed.

II. Early Periodontal Disease

The real preventive service a dental hygienist can perform is to recognize *early signs* of periodontal involvement so that treatment can be initiated to arrest the disease and prevent more severe involvement, which could lead to tooth loss. The recognition of severe bone loss, advanced furcation involvement, and marked thickening of the periodontal ligament space is not difficult after a basic understanding has been gained. The difficult part is to watch carefully for incipient, often isolated indications of early peri-

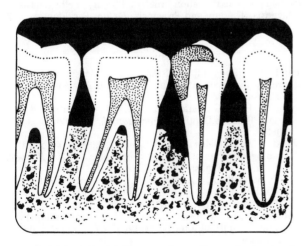

Figure 13–21. Periodontal Ligament Space. First and second molars have a normal periodontal ligament space which appears as a fine black line about the roots. The first premolar shows thickening of the ligament space about the entire root, and the second premolar has thickening about the mesial only.

odontal disease. These changes can be seen in all age groups, from young children to elderly patients.

A. Earliest Signs

The earliest signs of periodontal involvement are not evident in a radiograph. Only after the inflammation has extended from the soft tissue (gingivitis) to the supporting periodontal tissues and bone resorption has become sufficient does radiographic evidence appear.

B. Initial Bone Destruction

1. The usual interproximal pathway of inflammation from gingivitis to periodontitis is directly from the inflamed gingival connective tissue into the crest of the interdental bone (page 182).

2. Initial bone destruction takes place at the crest of the interdental bone in the crestal lamina dura.

C. Radiographic Evidence

1. Crestal lamina dura may appear slightly irregular, fuzzy, and radiolucent. At this stage it is best examined with a hand magnifying glass.

2. Angular thickening of the periodontal ligament space (triangulation) may also be apparent.

III. Other Radiographic Findings

Any other radiographic findings that may be directly or indirectly related to periodontal involvement and its contributing factors should be noted in the record for the attention of the dentist. Certain findings have a direct relation to dental hygiene care and instruction, particularly local factors that contribute to food impaction or plaque retention.

A. Calculus

Gross deposits, primarily those on proximal surfaces, may be seen in radiographs. Observing these may be helpful, but the probe and explorer are needed to define the exact location and extent.

The density and contrast of the radiograph influence whether or not calculus is seen. Because all deposits are not visible, the use of radiographs has limited value for specific calculus detection.

B. Overhanging Restorations

Some proximal overhanging margins may be seen in radiographs. The use of an explorer is necessary to detect irregular margins and to examine all proximal margins that do not reveal irregularities in the radiographs. Superimposition can mask an overhanging margin. Types of irregularities of restorations are described on pages 528–529.

C. Dental Caries

Clinical and radiographic identification of carious lesions is described on pages 218–220. Certain findings should be noted for their relationship to the periodontal tissues.

1. Large carious lesions may leave open contact areas that permit food impaction and hence damage to the periodontal tissues.
2. Carious lesions, either enamel or root caries, hold plaque and provide a rough surface for retention of food debris and materia alba.
3. Root caries and demineralization may interfere with techniques of root planing (page 183).

D. Relationship to Pockets

Radiographs do not show pockets; soft tissue does not show in a radiograph. Because a pocket is measured from the gingival margin to the base of the pocket, both of which are soft tissue, pockets cannot be seen in a radiograph. Probing is necessary to identify pockets.

TECHNICAL HINTS

I. Use topical anesthetic to help to alleviate discomfort while probing.
II. Avoid the most common errors in probing:
A. Not passing the probe to the full pocket depth.
B. Not holding the probe as parallel with the long axis of a tooth as possible, and therefore obtaining a false reading.
C. Not measuring around the entire tooth and therefore missing pockets. This error most commonly applies to proximal pockets. The probe must be passed more than halfway across from the facial to overlap with the probe used on the lingual, which should also be passed more than halfway across.
III. Check the markings on a new probe by measuring on a standard millimeter ruler.
IV. When bleeding is readily elicited on probing or exploring and tooth surfaces are obscured so that examination is complicated, initiate toothbrushing and other appropriate disease control methods. Explain the problem to the patient and outline a specific home care routine designed to reduce gingival inflammation. Postpone the complete examination for 1 week, after which the gingival condition should be improved.
V. Replace mirror heads frequently. Scratched mirrors obscure vision and delay procedures.
VI. Handle explorers and probes carefully. Because the tips are pliable and relatively fragile, precautions must be taken against breakage or bending (pages 43–44).

FACTORS TO TEACH THE PATIENT

I. The need for a careful, thorough examination if treatment is to be complete and effective.
II. Information about the instruments and techniques of examination and how their use makes the examination complete. Examples are the complete radiographic survey, probing 360 degrees around each tooth, and exploring each subgingival tooth surface.
III. Why bleeding can occur when probing. Healthy tissue does not bleed.
IV. Relation of pocket measurements to normal sulci.
V. Significance of mobility.
VI. Signs of periodontal disease in radiographs.

References

1. Listgarten, M.A.: Periodontal Probing: What Does It Mean? *J. Clin. Periodontol., 7,* 165, June, 1980.
2. Kopczyk, R.A. and Saxe, S.R.: Clinical Signs of Gingival Inadequacy: The Tension Test, *J. Dent. Child., 41,* 352, September-October, 1974.
3. Miller, S.C.: *Textbook of Periodontia,* 3rd ed. Philadelphia, The Blakiston Co., 1950, p. 125.
4. Goldman, H.M. and Cohen, D.W.: *Periodontal Therapy,* 6th ed. St. Louis, The C.V. Mosby Co., 1980, pp. 1092, 1107, 1110.

Suggested Readings

Bjorn, A.-L. and Hjort, P.: Bone Loss of Furcated Mandibular Molars, A Longitudinal Study, *J. Clin. Periodontol., 9,* 402, September, 1982.

Coatoam, G.W., Behrents, R.G., and Bissada, N.F.: The Width of Keratinized Gingiva During Orthodontic Treatment: Its Significance and Impact on Periodontal Status, *J. Periodontol., 52,* 307, June, 1981.

Croxson, L.J.: A Simplified Periodontal Screening Examination: The Community Periodontal Index of Treatment Needs (WHO) in General Practice, *Int. Dent. J., 34,* 28, March, 1984.

Eskow, R.N. and Kapin, S.H.: Furcation Invasions: Correlating a Classification System with Therapeutic Considerations. Part I. Examination, Diagnosis, and Classification, *Compend. Contin. Educ. Dent., 5,* 479, June, 1984.

Hug, H.U., van't Hof, M.A., Spanauf, A.J., and Renggli, H.H.: Validity of Clinical Assessments Related to the Cemento-enamel Junction, *J. Dent. Res., 62,* 825, July, 1983.

O'Hehir, T.: Periodontal Charting Magnifies Patient and Practice Benefits, *RDH, 7,* 28, May, 1987.

Pritchard, J.R. and Laws, A.J.: Gingival Crevice Depth. I. Predictability of Probing Deepest Points, *Aust. Dent. J., 29,* 404, December, 1984.

Waerhaug, J.: The Furcation Problem. Etiology, Pathogenesis, Diagnosis, Therapy and Prognosis, *J. Clin. Periodontol., 7,* 73, April, 1980.

Probing

Aeppli, D.M., Boen, J.R., and Bandt, C.L.: Measuring and Interpreting Increases in Probing Depth and Attachment Loss, *J. Periodontol., 56,* 262, May, 1985.

Agudio, G., Prato, G.P., and Bartolucci, E.G.: Computerized Charting of Probing Depths, *J. Periodontol., 56,* 766, December, 1985.

Badersten, A., Nilvéus, R., and Egelberg, J.: Reproducibility of Probing Attachment Level Measurements, *J. Clin. Periodontol., 11,* 475, August, 1984.

Birek, P., McCulloch, C.A.G., and Hardy, V.: Gingival Attachment Level Measurements with An Automated Periodontal Probe, *J. Clin. Periodontol., 14,* 472, September, 1987.

Borsboom, P.C.F., ten Bosch, J.J., Corba, N.H.C., and Tromp, J.A.H.: A Simple Constant-force Pocket Probe, *J. Periodontol., 52,* 390, July, 1981.

Caton, J., Greenstein, G., and Polson, A.M.: Depth of Periodontal Probe Penetration Related to Clinical and Histologic Signs of Gingival Inflammation, *J. Periodontol., 52,* 626, October, 1981.

Chamberlain, A.D.H., Renvert, S., Garrett, S., Nilvéus, R., and Egelberg, J.: Significance of Probing Force for Evaluation of Healing Following Periodontal Therapy, *J. Clin. Periodontol., 12,* 306, April, 1985.

Detsch, S.G.: A Periodontal Probe that Measures to One Tenth Millimeter, *J. Periodontol., 51,* 298, May, 1980.

Fowler, C., Garrett, S., Crigger, M., and Egelberg, J.: Histologic Probe Position in Treated and Untreated Human Periodontal Tissues, *J. Clin. Periodontol., 9,* 373, September, 1982.

Freed, H.K., Gapper, R.L., and Kalkwarf, K.L.: Evaluation of Periodontal Probing Forces, *J. Periodontol., 54,* 488, August, 1983.

Hancock, E.B. and Wirthlin, M.R.: The Location of the Periodontal Probe Tip in Health and Disease, *J. Periodontol., 52,* 124, March, 1981.

Jeffcoat, M.K., Jeffcoat, R.L., Jens, S.C., and Captain, K.: A New Periodontal Probe with Automated Cemento-enamel Junction Detection, *J. Clin. Periodontol., 13,* 276, April, 1986.

Kalkwarf, K.L., Kaldahl, W.B., and Patil, K.D.: Comparison of Manual and Pressure-controlled Periodontal Probing, *J. Periodontol., 57,* 467, August, 1986.

Listgarten, M.A., Mao, R., and Robinson, P.J.: Periodontal Probing and the Relationship of the Probe Tip to Periodontal Tissues, *J. Periodontol., 47,* 511, September, 1976.

McCulloch, C.A.G., Birek, P., and Hardy, V.: Comparison of Gingival Attachment Level Measurements with an Automated Periodontal Probe and a Pressure-sensitive Probe, *J. Periodont. Res., 22,* 348, September, 1987.

Mombelli, A. and Graf, H.: Depth-force-patterns in Periodontal Probing, *J. Clin. Periodontol., 13,* 126, February, 1986.

Pattison, G.L. and Pattison, A.M.: *Periodontal Instrumentation.* Reston, Virginia, Reston Publishing Co., 1979, pp. 19–98, 104–136.

Sanderink, R.B.A., Mörmann, W.H., and Barbakow, F.: Periodontal Pocket Measurements with a Modified Plast-o-Probe and a Metal Probe, *J. Clin. Periodontol., 10,* 11, January, 1983.

Tal, H.: A Probe for Measuring the Depth of Furcal Defects, *J. Clin. Periodontol., 9,* 393, September, 1982.

Van der Velden, U.: Location of Probe Tip in Bleeding and Nonbleeding Pockets With Minimal Gingival Inflammation, *J. Clin. Periodontol., 9,* 421, November, 1982.

Van der Velden, U., Abbas, F., and Winkel, G.: Probing Considerations in Relation to Periodontal Breakdown, *J. Clin. Periodontol., 13,* 894, November, 1986.

Watts T.: Constant Force Probing with and without a Stent in Untreated Periodontal Disease: the Clinical Reproducibility Problem and Possible Sources of Error, *J. Clin. Periodontol., 14,* 407, August, 1987.

Radiographs

Allen, D.L., McFall, W.T., and Jenzano, J.W.: *Periodontics for the Dental Hygienist,* 4th ed. Philadelphia, Lea & Febiger, 1987, pp. 118–124.

Buchanan, S.A., Jenderseck, R.S., Granet, M.A., Kircos, L.T., Chambers, D.W., and Robertson, P.B.: Radiographic Detection of Dental Calculus, *J. Periodontol., 58,* 747, November, 1987.

Carranza, F.A.: *Glickman's Clinical Periodontology,* 6th ed. Philadelphia, W.B. Saunders Co., 1984, pp. 513–523.

Hangorsky, U.: Radiographic Interpretation of Periodontal Disease, *Compend. Contin. Educ. Dent., 3,* 117, March/April, 1982.

Hirschmann, P.N.: Radiographic Interpretation of Chronic Periodontitis, *Int. Dent. J., 37,* 3, March, 1987.

Lang, N.P. and Hill, R.W.: Radiographs in Periodontics, *J. Clin. Periodontol., 4,* 16, February, 1977.

Mann, J., Pettigrew, J., Beideman, R., Green, P., and Ship, I.: Investigation of the Relationship Between Clinically Detected Loss of Attachment and Radiographic Changes in Early Periodontal Disease, *J. Clin. Periodontol., 12,* 247, March, 1985.

Pawlak, E.A. and Hoag, P.M.: *Essentials of Periodontics,* 3rd ed. St. Louis, The C.V. Mosby Co., 1984, pp. 127–130.

14 *The Teeth*

Clinical examination of the teeth is essential prior to treatment to provide guidelines for treatment planning, instrumentation, instruction, and follow-up evaluation. In general, patients tend to be more concerned about their teeth than about their gingiva. The reasons may be related to personal appearance, degree of information, which is usually greater about teeth than gingiva, and the sensitivity and pain associated with ailments of the teeth.

Background study of histology, dental anatomy, and oral pathology is important to this phase of clinical practice. *Suggested Readings* at the end of this chapter have been selected for additional information, reference, and review.

I. Objectives

With information from the patient's personal dental history (table 6–2, page 84) and a thorough clinical and radiographic examination, the dental hygienist can

A. Prepare a charting and provide a record of deviations from the normal teeth for the diagnostic work-up.

B. Identify the dental hygiene treatment and instruction needed in relation to the teeth for the particular patient.

C. Outline the patient's preventive dental program (page 297).

D. Utilize the specific data needed during treatment for instrument selection and adaptation.

II. Clinical Examination of the Teeth

Following is a list of major factors to observe when examining the teeth. Several of these are described in other chapters, for which page references are noted. Information about hypoplasia, attrition, erosion, abrasion, dental caries, and tooth vitality will be described in this chapter. Table 14–1 lists factors to observe during the examination of the teeth and suggests relationships to appointment procedures.

A. General Characteristics
1. Number of teeth; eruption pattern (Appendix, tables A–1 and A–2).
2. Anomalies of size, form, number.
3. Replacements such as restorations for individual teeth and groups of teeth (fixed and removable).

B. Deposits (table 16–1, page 236)
1. Calculus.
2. Bacterial Plaque.
3. Materia alba.

C. Color
1. Intrinsic stains (pages 257–258).
2. Extrinsic stains (pages 254–257).

D. Developmental Defects
1. Enamel hypoplasia.
2. Amelogenesis imperfecta; dentinogenesis imperfecta (page 257).

E. Regressive Changes
1. Attrition.
2. Erosion.
3. Abrasion.

F. Occlusion (pages 226–234)
1. Proximal contact relation: areas of food impaction.
2. Mobility (page 206).

G. Dental Caries and Demineralization

H. Vitality of Pulp

I. Tooth Fractures

ENAMEL HYPOPLASIA

I. Definition

Enamel hypoplasia is a defect that occurs as a result of a disturbance in the formation of the organic enamel matrix.

II. Types and Etiology

A. Hereditary
Enamel is partly or wholly missing; an anomaly.

B. Systemic (Environmental)
Factors that may contribute to enamel hypoplasia during tooth development include severe nutritional deficiency, particularly rickets; fever-producing diseases, such as measles, chickenpox, and scarlet fever; congenital syphilis; hypoparathyroidism; birth injury; prematurity; Rh hemolytic disease; idiopathic.

C. Local
A single tooth is affected; caused by trauma or periapical inflammation about a primary tooth;

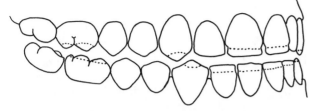

Figure 14–1. Enamel Hypoplasia. Chronologic hypoplasia, usually in the form of grooves or pits, appears in the enamel at a level corresponding with the stage of development of the teeth. For this patient, the disturbance in enamel development occurred at approximately 10 months of age.

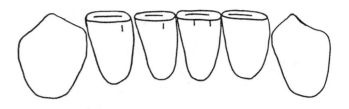

Figure 14–3. Attrition. Attrition of the incisal surfaces of mandibular anterior teeth has extended to expose the dentin. Dentin usually appears as a brown line or ring.

can injure the adjacent developing permanent tooth.

III. Appearance

A. Hereditary

May appear brown (page 257).

B. Systemic

Called also "chronologic hypoplasia" because the lesions are found in areas of those teeth where the enamel was formed during the systemic disturbance.

1. *Single Narrow Zone* (smooth or pitted). Disturbance lasted a short period of time (figure 14–1).
2. *Multiple.* Disturbance to the ameloblast occurred over a period of time, or several times.
3. *Teeth Most Frequently Affected.* First molars, incisors, canines, because the disturbances generally occur during the first year when those teeth are mineralizing. A table of tooth development is available for reference in Appendix, tables A–1 and A–2.

C. Hypoplasia of Congenital Syphilis[1]

Transmission of syphilis from mother to fetus after the sixteenth week of pregnancy may alter the development of the tooth germs. Figure 14–2 illustrates tooth forms that may result. The mesiodistal width may be reduced, and incisors are frequently narrowed at the incisal third.

Other conditions may also cause similar variations of tooth form.

D. Local

A single tooth with a yellow or brown intrinsic stain.

ATTRITION

I. Definition

Attrition is the wearing away of a tooth as a result of tooth-to-tooth contact (figure 14–3).

II. Occurrence

A. Location

May be found on occlusal, incisal, and proximal surfaces.

B. Age Factor

Increases with age, and more attrition is seen in men than women of comparable age.

III. Etiology

A. Bruxism

Predisposing factors may be psychologic, tension, or occlusal interferences.

B. Usage

Wear of surfaces on each other. Predisposing factors may be coarse foods, chewing tobacco, or

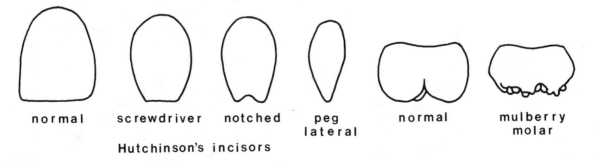

normal   screwdriver   notched   peg lateral   normal   mulberry molar

Hutchinson's incisors

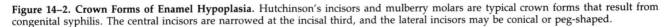

Figure 14–2. Crown Forms of Enamel Hypoplasia. Hutchinson's incisors and mulberry molars are typical crown forms that result from congenital syphilis. The central incisors are narrowed at the incisal third, and the lateral incisors may be conical or peg-shaped.

Table 14–1. Examination of the Teeth

Feature	To Observe	Suggested Relationship to Appointment Procedures
Morphology	Number of teeth (missing teeth verified by radiographic examination) Size, shape Arch form Position of individual teeth Injuries; fractures of the crown (root fractures observed in radiographs)	Selection and adaptation of instruments Areas prone to dental caries initiation, particularly the difficult-to-reach areas during plaque control Pulp test for vitality may be indicated
Development	Anomalies and developmental defects Pits and white spots	Distinguish hypoplasia and dental fluorosis from demineralization Identify pits for sealants
Eruption	Sequence of eruption: normal, irregular Unerupted teeth observed in radiographs	Care in using floss in the col area where the epithelium is usually less mature in young children Orthodontic needs Procedures for preservation of primary teeth

Deposits
Food debris
Plaque
Calculus
  Supragingival
  Subgingival
	Overall evaluation of self-care and plaque-control measures
	Relation of appearance of teeth to gingival health
	Extent and location of plaque, debris, and calculus
	Calculus and the tooth surface pocket wall
		Need for instruction and guidance
		
		Frequency of follow-up and maintenance appointments

Stains Extrinsic Intrinsic	Extrinsic: colors relate to causes Intrinsic: dark, grayish Tobacco stain	Need for test for pulp vitality Stain removal procedures; selection of polishing agent Dentifrice recommendation Plaque-control emphasis for plaque-related stains Provide information concerning the oral effects of tobacco use
Regressive Changes	Attrition: primary and permanent Abrasion: physical agents that may be a cause Erosion	Evaluate causes and treat or counsel for prevention Dietary analysis: for finding foods that may be related Selection of non-abrasive dentifrice Habit evaluation
Exposed Cementum	Relation to gingival recession, pocket formation Areas of narrow attached gingiva Hypersensitivity	Special care areas where only slight attached gingiva remains Non-abrasive dentifrice advised Measures to prevent root-surface caries Care during instrumentation Indication for application of desensitizing agent
Dental Caries	Areas of demineralization Carious lesions (proximal lesions observed in radiographs) Arrested caries Root caries	Charting Treatment plan Preventive program for caries control, fluoride, dietary factors Follow-up and frequency of maintenance

Table 14–1. Examination of the Teeth *Continued*

Feature	To Observe	Suggested Relationship to Appointment Procedures
Restorations	Contour of restorations, overhangs Proximal contact (see separate heading later in this table) Surface smoothness Staining	Chart and correct inadequate margins Selection of instruments and polishing agents Dentifrice selection to prevent discoloration
Factors Related to Occlusion Tooth Wear Proximal Contacts Mobility Classification Habits	Facets; worn-down cusp tips Health of supporting structures; observation of radiographs for signs of trauma from occlusion Use of floss to find open contact areas Areas of food retention Degree; comparison of chartings Possible causes Position of teeth Angle's classification Nail or object biting; lip or cheek biting Observe effects on lip, cheek, teeth Tongue thrust; reverse swallow	Need for study of bruxism and other parafunctional habits Chart inadequate contacts for corrective measures Use of floss by patient Need for reduction of inflammatory factors that may be related Dentist will identify and treat factors related to trauma from occlusion Relationship to orthodontic treatment needs Guidance for habit correction when indicated
Edentulous Areas	Radiographic evaluation for impacted, unerupted teeth, retained root tips, other deviations from normal	Supplemental fulcrum selection during instrumentation Applied plaque-control procedures for abutment teeth
Replacement for Missing Teeth Dentures Partial dentures	Teeth and tissue that support an appliance Cleanliness of an appliance Factors that contribute to food and debris retention	Preventive measures for harm to supporting teeth and soft tissues Instruction in personal care of fixed and removable dentures; use of floss under fixed partial denture; other appropriate care
Saliva	Amount and consistency Dryness of mouth	Relation to instruction for prevention of dental caries: more caries can be expected in a dry mouth. Use of saliva substitute; fluoride

abrasive dusts associated with certain occupations.

IV. Appearance

A. Initial Lesion
Small polished facet on a cusp tip or ridge, or slight flattening of an incisal edge.

B. Advanced
Gradual reduction in cusp height, flattening of occlusal plane (figure 14–3).

C. Staining of Exposed Dentin
May occur; stain usually is brown.

D. Radiographic
The pulp chamber and canals may be narrowed and sometimes obliterated as the result of formation of secondary dentin.

EROSION

I. Definition
Erosion is the loss of tooth substance by a chemical process that does not involve known bacterial action.

II. Occurrence

A. Location
Facial or lingual surfaces, depending on cause.

B. Usually Involves Several Teeth

III. Etiology

The lesions are caused by some form of chemical dissolution.

A. May Be Idiopathic (unknown).

B. Chronic Vomiting
Acid of chronic vomiting affects lingual surfaces, particularly anterior teeth.
1. Pregnancy.
2. Eating disorder, such as bulimia (pages 380–381).

C. Extrinsic
1. *Industrial.* Workers' teeth can be exposed to atmospheric acids.
2. *Dietary.* Facial surfaces most frequently affected.
   a. Carbonated beverages or lemon juice used frequently.
   b. Lemons or other citrus fruit sucked frequently.

IV. Appearance

A. Smooth, shallow, hard, shiny (in contrast to dental caries, in which appearance is soft and discolored).
B. Shape varies from shallow saucer-like depressions to deep wedge-shaped grooves; margins are not sharply demarcated.
C. May progress to involve the dentin and stimulate secondary dentin.
D. May occur in combination with dental caries, calculus, or dental restorations.[2]

ABRASION

I. Definition

Abrasion is the mechanical wearing away of tooth substance by forces other than mastication.

II. Occurrence

A. Location
Exposed root surfaces, generally.

B. Other Types
At incisal edge.

III. Etiology

The lesion originates from a mechanical abrasive activity. The action of microorganisms is not essential for the development of abrasion. Dental caries may occur in the abraded area as a secondary lesion.

A. Abrasive Agent
The most common cause is an abrasive dentifrice applied with vigorous horizontal toothbrushing (figure 14–4).

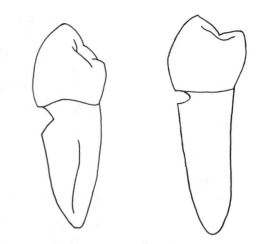

Figure 14–4. Abrasion. Profile view of the facial surface of mandibular premolars shows shape of abrasion on the cementum. Note that the area of abrasion undermines the enamel.

B. Other Types
Abrasion may occur at the incisal or occlusal surfaces.
1. Opening bobby pins may leave a small notch in one incisal edge. People with this habit usually utilize the same tooth each time.
2. Occupational: tacks held by carpenters, pins by dressmakers.
3. Pipe held between teeth; usually held in the same place over many years.

IV. Appearance

A. V- or wedge-shaped with hard, smooth, shiny surface and clearly defined margins.
B. Except for incisal biting habits, the lesions occur initially on exposed cementum, then extend into the dentin.

DENTAL CARIES

Dental caries is a disease of the mineralized structures of the teeth that is characterized by demineralization of the hard components and dissolution of the organic matrix. As defined by the World Health Organization, dental caries is a "localized, post-eruptive, pathological process of external origin involving softening of the hard tooth tissue and proceeding to the formation of a cavity."[3]

I. Development of Dental Caries

Requirements for the development of a carious lesion are microorganisms, carbohydrate, primarily sucrose, and a susceptible tooth surface. Bacterial plaque contains numerous types of acid-forming bacteria, and *Streptococcus mutans* has been specifically implicated. The role of plaque and the factors in the initiation of caries are described in Chapter 16, page 242.

A. Enamel Caries
1. *Steps in the Formation of a Cavity*
   a. Starts in pits or fissures or smooth surfaces that are not accessible for plaque removal.

b. Follows the general direction of the enamel rods.

c. Spreads at the dentinoenamel junction.

d. Continues along the dentinal tubules (figure 14–5).

2. *Types of Dental Caries* (described by location)

a. Pit and fissure. Caries begins in a minute fault in the enamel.

  i. Occurs where three or more lobes of the developing tooth join; closure of the enamel plates is imperfect. *Examples:* occlusal pits of molars and premolars.

  ii. Occurs at the endings of grooves of the teeth. *Example:* the buccal groove of a mandibular molar.

b. Smooth surface. Caries begins in smooth surfaces where there is no pit, groove, or other fault. It occurs in areas where bacterial plaque collects, such as proximal tooth surfaces, cervical thirds of teeth, and other difficult-to-clean areas.

B. Root Surface Caries

1. *Definition.* Root surface caries is a soft, progressive lesion of cementum and dentin that involves bacterial infection and invasion. It is also called cemental caries, cervical caries, or radicular caries.

2. *Steps in the Formation of a Cavity*

a. Gingival recession exposes the cemental surface. Caries does not form in the root surface while periodontal fibers are still attached.

b. Dental caries starts near cementoenamel junction. Cementum is very thin and is soon destroyed; dentin is invaded.

c. Enamel is not involved except by extension or when it is undermined. Root caries occurs in a mildly acidic environment. If the pH were lower, enamel would also become carious. The critical pH for enamel is about 5.0; for cementum 6.7.

d. *Actinomyces viscosus* has been found in cariogenic plaque of the root surfaces. Other organisms that may cause caries include *Actinomyces naeslundii, Lactobacillus,* and *Streptococcus mutans* (see table 16–3, page 242). A specific single organism has not been determined as being responsible for root caries.[4,5]

3. *Clinical Recognition*

a. Soft, shallow, ill-defined lesion.

b. Increases laterally to coalesce with other small lesions, and eventually may extend completely around the tooth with undermining of the enamel (figure 14–6).

c. Yellowish, light brown, dark brown to black.

d. Leathery in texture when explored (active lesion).

e. Arrested root caries displays cavitation and discoloration, but is hard to the touch of the explorer.[6]

4. Predisposing Factors

a. Root exposure. The incidence of root caries increases with age, but not because of age. Gingival recession is necessary for root caries, and gingival recession is related to periodontal conditions that lead to recession.

b. Lack of fluoride. Root caries incidence has been shown to be directly related to the fluoride concentration in the drinking water.[7] Lifelong residence in a community with near-optimum levels of fluoride in the water was shown to be associated with at least an average 30% decrease in the incidence of root caries compared with that associated with lifelong residence in a nonfluoridated community.[8]

c. Xerostomia[9]

  i. Medications with xerostomic effects. Many older patients use medications

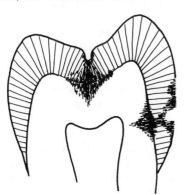

Figure 14–5. Dental Caries. Cones of dental caries in a pit and fissure and on a smooth tooth surface. Dental caries follows the general direction of the enamel rods, spreads at the dentinoenamel junction, and then continues along the dentinal tubules.

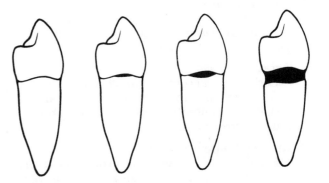

Figure 14–6. Root Surface Caries. A root surface lesion starts near the cementoenamel junction after gingival recession has exposed the root surface. The lesion is progressive, undermines the enamel, and may eventually surround the cervical third of the cementum. (Drawn after Banting, D.W. and Courtright, P.N.: Distribution and Natural History of Carious Lesions on the Roots of the Teeth, *Can. Dent. Assoc. J.,* 41, 45, January, 1975.)

or undergo therapies that reduce salivary flow.

    ii. Radiation therapy to the oral regions (pages 603–604).

  d. Inadequate personal daily plaque removal.

  e. Use of a cariogenic diet.[10]

II. Classification of Cavities

A. G.V. Black's Classification[11]

The standard method for classifying dental caries was developed by Dr. G.V. Black, a noted dental educator who divided the categories into classes according to surfaces of the teeth; each class is represented by a Roman numeral. These categories are customarily used for carious lesions, cavity preparations, and finished restorations. See table 14–2 for definitions and illustrations.

B. Nomenclature by Surfaces

1. *Simple Cavity.* Involves one tooth surface. *Example:* occlusal cavity.
2. *Compound Cavity.* Involves two tooth surfaces. *Example:* mesio-occlusal cavity, referred to as an "M-O" cavity.
3. *Complex Cavity.* Involves more than two tooth surfaces. *Example:* mesio-occlusal-distal, referred to as an "M-O-D" cavity.

III. Other Descriptive Terminology

A. Primary Dental Caries

On a surface not previously affected; sometimes called initial or incipient dental caries.

B. Secondary Caries

Adjacent to a previously restored area.

C. Recurrent Caries (generally referred to as secondary)

On tooth surface adjacent to a restoration when the lesion may be a continuation of the previous carious lesion.

D. Rampant Caries

Widespread formation of chalky areas and incipient cavities in numerous teeth over a comparatively short time lapse.

E. Arrested Caries

Caries that becomes stationary and does not show a tendency to progress further is called arrested. It frequently takes on a dark brown or reddish-brown color.

F. Nursing Bottle Caries

Nursing bottle caries is a form of rampant caries found in very young children who routinely have been given a nursing bottle at times when they were going to sleep or who have experienced prolonged at-will breast feeding. Other names for the same condition are nursing caries syndrome, nursing bottle mouth, baby bottle syndrome, baby bottle caries, and prolonged nursing habit.

1. *Etiology*
   a. Nursing bottle that contains sweetened milk or other fluid sweetened with sucrose.
   b. Pacifier dipped or filled with a sweet agent, such as honey.
   c. Prolonged at-will breast feeding.
2. *Effects.* Maxillary anterior teeth are the most severely affected. As the baby falls asleep, pools of sweet liquid can collect about the teeth. While the sucking is active, the liquid passes beyond the teeth. The nipple covers the mandibular anterior teeth; hence, they are rarely affected.
3. *Recognition.* Children should be seen for a dental examination no later than 12 months of age.[12] Demineralization may be noted along the cervical third of the maxillary anterior teeth. The source of the problem may be detected and preventive procedures initiated through parental counseling.

At a later stage the lesions appear dark brown. Eventually, the crowns may be destroyed to the gum line, abscesses may develop, and the child may suffer severe pain and discomfort.

RECOGNITION OF CARIOUS LESIONS

Both visual and exploratory means are used to recognize dental caries.

I. Preparation

Dry each tooth or group of teeth with compressed air and carefully inspect each surface, first visually, and then with an explorer as necessary to confirm visual findings.

II. Visual Examination: Enamel Caries

Characteristic changes in the color and translucency of tooth structure may be observed. Such changes either are definite signs of dental caries progress or may lead the examiner to suspect dental caries, which can then be inspected further with an explorer. Variations in color and translucency include the following:

A. Chalky white areas of demineralization.
B. Grayish-white discoloration of marginal ridges caused by dental caries of the proximal surface underneath.
C. Grayish-white color spreading from margins of restorations caused by lesions of secondary dental caries.
D. In relation to an amalgam restoration, dental caries appears translucent in outer portion and white and opaque adjacent to the amalgam.
E. Open carious lesions may vary in color from yellowish-brown to dark brown.
F. Less discoloration is generally present when dental caries progresses rapidly than when it progresses slowly.
G. Dull, flat white, opaque areas under direct light

Table 14–2. Dental Caries Charting: Classification of Cavities

Classification: Location	Appearance	Method of Examination
Class I. **Cavities in Pits or Fissures** a. Occlusal surfaces of premolars and molars b. Facial and lingual surfaces of molars c. Lingual surfaces of maxillary incisors		Direct or indirect visual Exploration Radiographs not useful
Class II. **Cavities in Proximal Surfaces of Premolars and Molars**		Early caries: by radiographs only Moderate caries not broken through from proximal to occlusal: (1) Visual by color changes in tooth and loss of translucency (2) Exploration from proximal Extensive caries involving occlusal: direct visual
Class III. **Cavities in Proximal Surfaces of Incisors and Canines That Do Not Involve the Incisal Angle**		Early caries: by radiographs or transillumination Moderate caries not broken through to lingual or facial: (1) Visual by tooth color change (2) Exploration (3) Radiograph Extensive caries; direct visual
Class IV. **Cavities in Proximal Surfaces of Incisors or Canines That Involve the Incisal Angle**		Visual Transillumination
Class V. **Cavities in the Cervical ⅓ of Facial or Lingual Surfaces** (not Pit or Fissure)		Direct visual: dry surface for vision Exploration to distinguish demineralization: whether rough or hard and unbroken Areas may be sensitive to touch
Class VI. **Cavities on Incisal Edges of Anterior Teeth and Cusp Tips of Posterior Teeth**		Direct visual May be discolored

show loss of translucency, particularly of the enamel.

H. Dark shadow on a proximal surface may be shown by transillumination. This type of observation is especially useful for anterior teeth and unrestored posterior teeth.

III. Exploratory Examination

A. Smooth Surface Caries

1. *Technique.* Adapt the side of the tip of the explorer closely to the tooth surface as described on page 205. Examine for hardness versus softness, roughness versus smoothness, and continuity of tooth surface versus breaks in continuity.
2. *Restorations.* Follow the margins of all restorations around with an explorer. Overhanging margins may or may not appear in the radiographs, depending on superimposition. Types of overhangs are described on pages 528–529. Chart all irregularities of existing restorations.

B. Pit and Fissure Caries

When a pit or fissure is discolored, one cannot determine visually whether dental caries is present except when a large obvious cavity can be seen. When a cavity is obvious, it should not be explored.

1. Direct the explorer tip so that it can pass straight into the pit or fissure. When the tip is not positioned correctly, caries in a small narrow pit can go undetected.
2. Explorer will catch when dental caries is present and there will be evidence of softening of tooth structure.

FRACTURES OF TEETH

Trauma to the face may involve fractured bones and teeth in addition to soft tissue injuries. Fractured jaws and methods of treatment are described in Chapter 48, pages 593–597.

I. Causes of Tooth Fractures

A. Automobile, bicycle, and diving accidents.
B. Contact sports when mouth protectors are not worn.
C. Blows incurred while fighting.
D. Iatrogenic, caused by dental treatments, such as certain endodontic or restorative procedures.

II. Description

A. Line of Fracture

1. Horizontal.
2. Diagonal.
3. Vertical.

B. Radiographic Signs of Recent Trauma[13]

1. Widened periodontal ligament space.
2. Radiolucent fracture line.

3. Radiopaque areas where fracture segments overlap.
4. Tooth displacement.

III. Classification: World Health Organization[14]

Classification provided by the World Health Organization is numbered as a special section of the International Classification of Diseases. Both primary and permanent dentitions are included. Figure 14–7 illustrates fractures of a central incisor.

873.60 Fracture of enamel of tooth only. Includes chipping and incomplete fractures (cracks).

873.61 Fracture of crown of tooth without pulpal involvement.

873.62 Fracture of crown with pulpal involvement.

873.63 Fracture of root of tooth.

873.64 Fracture of crown and root of tooth with or without pulpal involvement.

873.65 Fracture of tooth, unspecified.

873.66 Luxation (dislocation) of tooth. This category may involve concussion, subluxation, and luxation. A tooth with concussion is sensitive to percussion but is not loosened or displaced. Loosening without displacement is subluxation, and loosening with displacement is luxation.

873.66 Intrusion or extrusion of tooth. Intrusion into the alveolar bone is usually accompanied by fracture of the alveolar socket. Extrusion from the socket is a partial displacement.

873.68 Avulsion of tooth. Avulsion is the complete displacement of the tooth out of its socket. The emergency care for a tooth forcibly displaced may be found in table 60–1, page 754.

RADIOGRAPHIC EXAMINATION

During the clinical examination, information revealed by radiographs is utilized for supplementation and confirmation. Neither clinical nor radiographic examination is complete without the other. A few principal items to be seen in a radiographic examination of the teeth are

> Anomalies
> Impactions
> Fractures
> Internal and root resorption
> Dental caries
> Periapical radiolucencies

I. Technique Principles

Periapical radiographs usually provide sufficient information concerning the teeth, but panoramic, extraoral, or occlusal radiographs may be needed for detecting or defining anomalies and pathologic lesions outside the scope of periapical radiographs. Bitewing radiographs or periapical radiographs made

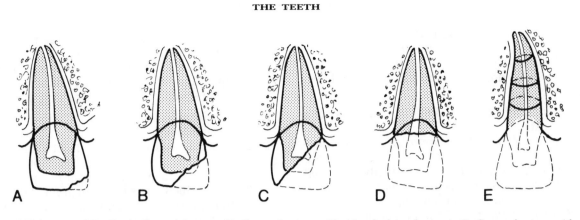

Figure 14–7. Fractures of Teeth. A. Enamel fracture. **B.** Crown fracture without pulpal involvement. **C.** Crown fracture with pulpal involvement. **D.** Fracture of crown and root near neck of tooth. **E.** Root fractures involving cementum, dentin, and the pulp may occur in the apical, middle, or coronal third of the root.

by a paralleling technique with no overlapping are most satisfactory for dental caries detection.

Principles for examination were described on pages 144–145. Mounted radiographs on an adequately lighted viewbox are a necessity during charting and treatment procedures. For the detection of early carious lesions a hand magnifying reading glass can be of invaluable assistance.

II. Detection of Dental Caries

Radiographs are not needed for facial, lingual, or occlusal carious lesions because they are accessible and best observed by exploration and direct vision. Because of superimposition of other parts of the tooth, facial, lingual, and occlusal carious lesions need to be fairly well advanced before they are definitely discernible in a radiograph.

A. Proximal Caries

Proximal surface lesions may be missed if radiographs are not used. Clinical skills for caries discernment need to be perfected, however, to prevent excess exposure of a patient to unnecessary radiation.

1. *Small Proximal Lesions.* Properly angulated radiographs with no overlapping are required for the detection of small lesions that involve the enamel or extend slightly into the dentin.
2. *Proximal Overhanging Restorations.* An overhanging filling or dental caries under that filling may be present, even if none can be seen in the radiograph because of superimposition. An explorer must be passed around the complete margin to confirm the condition.

B. Cemental Caries

1. *Location.* Most cemental carious lesions occur in the vicinity of and just beneath the cementoenamel junction.
2. *Appearance.* Cemental caries appears as a saucer-shaped lesion in a radiograph. It may appear to undermine the enamel or it may be located beneath an overhanging filling.

TESTING FOR PULPAL VITALITY

Any tooth suspected of being nonvital must be tested for pulpal vitality or degree of vitality. Such testing is particularly significant prior to treatment involving periodontal surgery, any restorative procedures, and orthodontic appliance placement. Diagnosis of vitality is made not only on the basis of a pulp test, but also on consideration of all data from the patient history and clinical and radiographic examinations.

A tooth may become nonvital from bacterial causes, particularly invasion of the pulp from dental caries or periodontal disease. Physical causes may be mechanical or thermal injuries. Examples of mechanical injuries are trauma, such as a blow, or iatrogenic dental procedures, such as cavity preparation or too-rapid orthodontic movement.

I. Observations That Suggest Loss of Vitality

A. Clinical

1. Discoloration of a tooth crown (intrinsic stains, page 257).
2. Fracture (part of the crown may be missing).
3. Large carious lesion or large restoration.
4. Fistula with opening into the oral cavity over the apical region of a tooth.

B. Radiographic

1. Apical radiolucency, which may indicate a granuloma, cyst, or abscess.
2. Bone loss with a widened periodontal ligament space extending to the apex.
3. Fractured root.
4. Large carious lesion or restoration that appears closely related to the pulp chamber.

II. Response to Pulp Testing

A. Rationale

Electrical pulp testing is based on the knowledge that an electrical stimulus can create pain to which a patient can react. The pulp tester, therefore, determines the conduction of stimuli to the sensory receptors. The vitality of the pulp depends on its blood supply and not on its nerve supply. For that reason, a positive or negative pulp test may not always show the true condition of the pulp.

B. Factors That Influence a Patient's Response to a Pulp Tester
1. *Degree of Pulpal Degeneration or Inflammation.* A necrotic pulp gives no response at all, whereas an acutely or chronically inflamed pulp responds at varying degrees between no response and full normal response.
2. *Pain Perception Threshold.* The lowest perceptible intensity of pain caused by a threshold stimulus. A threshold stimulus is the minimum stimulus necessary to induce patient response.
3. *Reaction to Pain.* May vary with a patient's attitude, age, sex, emotional security, fatigue, drugs used, as well as the size of the pulp and thickness of the dentin, particularly the amount of secondary dentin.
4. *Nerve Transmission Blocks.* Injuries or lesions of nerves, and anesthetics.
5. *Adjacent Metal.* Restorations or continuous bridgework.

III. Electrical Pulp Tester (Vitalometer)

Although thermal tests using hot or cold applications have been used, the electrical pulp testers are considered more consistent and reliable.

A. Types
1. *Battery-operated*
   a. Advantages. Hand held so a clinician can work alone; portable.
   b. Disadvantage. Battery can run down. Some types have a light to indicate current in circuit.
2. *Plug-in*
   a. Advantage. More dependable than battery-operated.
   b. Disadvantage. Not self-contained; requires house-current plug.

B. Precaution
   The application of an electrical current to a patient with a cardiac pacemaker or any electronic life-support device by the use of a pulp tester, ultrasonic scaler, desensitizing equipment, or electrosurgical instrument can interfere with the function of the life-support device and may constitute a serious health hazard.[15,16] A review of the patient history is necessary prior to application of a pulp tester.

C. Preparation and Use of Equipment
   Manufacturer's instructions are provided for each pulp tester and should be followed carefully. When the tester rheostat is separate from the applicator tip, an assistant is needed.

Consistency of procedures is essential to obtain consistent readings. The same pulp tester should be used for a particular patient at continuing comparative tests. Notes in a patient's record can indicate specific directions for that patient.

D. General Procedures
1. Assemble equipment.
2. Explain briefly to the patient what is to be done, but avoid detailed description, which could create anxiety or apprehension.
3. Dry the teeth to be tested to prevent the current from passing to the gingiva: isolate with cotton rolls and insert a saliva ejector, or use rubber dam.
4. Moisten the end of the tip of the tester with a small amount of toothpaste. Another electrolyte (conductor) may be used if its consistency allows it to remain where placed and prevents it from flowing over the tooth surface.
5. Instruct the patient to signal when a sensation is felt: suggest raising a hand or making a sound.
6. Apply tester tip. For certain types of pulp testers, the patient lightly holds the handle with the gloved clinician to complete the circuit.[17]
   a. Apply first to at least one tooth other than the one in question, preferably an adjacent tooth and the same tooth on the contralateral side. Such a procedure determines a normal response for the patient.
   b. Place *without pressure* but with definite contact on sound tooth structure in a consistent location on the middle or gingival third. The middle third of the crown of a single-rooted tooth and the middle third of each cusp of a multirooted tooth are frequently used (figure 14–8).

E. Readings
1. Avoid contact with gingival or other soft tissues. A low resistance circuit can be formed, thus allowing the circuit to by-pass the tooth.
2. Avoid contact with metallic restorations. The metal forms a more rapid conductor than does tooth structure. When approximal restorations are in contact, the circuit can be transmitted across to the adjacent tooth. The reading obtained would not pertain to the tooth in question (figure 14–9). A nonconductive clear plastic matrix strip may be inserted to separate the two metallic restorations.
3. Start with the rheostat at zero; advance slowly but steadily, stopping only momentarily after each number. Do not proceed with such regularity that the patient can count and anticipate.
4. Test each tooth at least twice. Average the readings.
5. Record on patient's record the lowest number (average number) at which a minimal stimulus

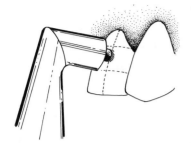

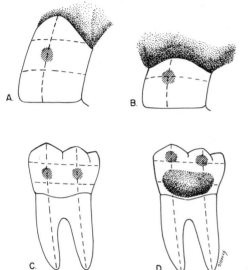

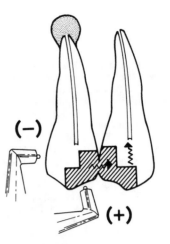

Figure 14–9. Use of Pulp Tester. False-positive response can result when the tester is placed on a metallic restoration. The current can be transmitted across a contact area to give a reading for the adjacent tooth rather than for the tooth in question. (Redrawn from Antel, J. and Christie, W.J.: Electrical Pulp Testing, *Can. Dent. Assoc. J. 45,* 597, November, 1979.)

Figure 14–8. Pulp Tester in Position. A. Correct contact point for tip of pulp tester is within the middle third of the crown. Avoid contact with gingiva or restorations. **B.** Adjustment of position of contact point because of gingival enlargement. **C.** Contact points on multirooted tooth. Place tip of pulp tester in the middle third over each root. **D.** Adjustment of position of contact points because of large Class V restoration.

induced a response. Record for all teeth tested, not only the tooth in question.

F. Reasons for False-negative Responses[18]

1. Patient premedicated with analgesics, tranquilizers, narcotics, or alcohol.
2. Recently traumatized tooth.
3. Pulp canal narrow and calcified.
4. Newly erupted tooth with incomplete closure at the apex; immature tooth.
5. Operational factors
   a. Inadequate contact with tooth causes insufficient conduction.
   b. Wearing surgical gloves changes the conduction so that the circuit is incomplete.[19] (See III., D., 6.)
   c. Tester not turned on; batteries weak or dead.

FACTORS TO TEACH THE PATIENT

I. The cause and process of enamel or root caries formation and development for the patients at risk.

II. A description of the hardness of the enamel and why a cavity is sometimes larger in the dentin before there is evidence from the external surface.

III. Why radiographs may be used to detect proximal incipient caries.

IV. Reasons for preservation of primary teeth.

V. Frequency of complete oral examination in relation to a continuing preventive program.

VI. Methods for prevention of dental caries: fluorides, plaque prevention and control, and control of cariogenic foods in the diet.

VII. Preventive measures for control and prevention of tooth abrasion: dentifrice selection and correction of brush selection and use.

VIII. Dietary factors related to erosion.

IX. When the patient asks specific questions about oral findings, explain why the dentist must observe and check before explanations can be made.

X. Methods for prevention of nursing bottle caries.[12] Explain that nothing but plain water should be used in bedtime or naptime nursing bottles. Discourage the use of a sweetener on a pacifier. Also teach the use of a cup for milk or juice by the baby's first birthday.

XI. Discuss accident prevention procedures, such as always wearing a mouthguard for contact sports and wearing seat belts.

References

1. Giunta, J.L.: *Oral Pathology,* 2nd ed. Baltimore, Williams & Wilkins, 1984, p. 40.

2. Sognnaes, R.F., Wolcott, R.B., and Xhonga, F.A.: Dental Erosion. I. Erosion-like Patterns Occurring in Association with Other Dental Conditions, *J. Am. Dent. Assoc., 84,* 571, March, 1972.

3. World Health Organization: *The Etiology and Prevention of Dental Caries.* WHO Technical Report Series, Number 494, Geneva, World Health Organization, 1972, 19 pp.

4. Sumney, D.L. and Jordan, H.V.: Characterization of Bacteria Isolated from Human Root Surface Carious Lesions, *J. Dent. Res., 53,* 343, March-April, 1974.

5. Syed, S.A., Loesche, W.J., Pape, H.L., and Grenier, E.: Predominant Cultivable Flora Isolated from Human Root Surface Caries Plaque, *Infect. Immun., 11,* 727, April, 1975.

6. Katz, R.V.: The Clinical Identification of Root Caries, *Gerodontology, 5,* 21, Spring, 1986.

7. Burt, B.A., Ismail, A.I., and Eklund, S.A.: Root Caries in an Optimally Fluoridated and a High-fluoride Community, *J. Dent. Res., 65,* 1154, September, 1986.

8. Stamm, J.W. and Banting, D.W.: Comparison of Root Caries Prevalence in Adults with Life-long Residence in Fluoridated and Non-fluoridated Communities, *J. Dent. Res., 59,* 405, Abstract 552, Special Issue A., March, 1980.

9. Kitamura, M., Kiyak, H.A., and Mulligan, K.: Predictors of Root Caries in the Elderly, *Community Dent. Oral Epidemiol., 14,* 34, February, 1986.

10. Ravald, N., Hamp, S.-E., and Birkhed, D.: Long-term Evaluation of Root Surface Caries in Periodontally Treated Patients, *J. Clin. Periodontol., 13,* 758, September, 1986.

11. Blackwell, R.E.: *G.V. Black's Operative Dentistry,* Volume II, 9th ed. Milwaukee, Medico-Dental Publishing Company, 1955, pp. 1–4.

12. American Academy of Pediatric Dentistry: Policy Statement on Infant Dental Care, May, 1986. American Academy of Pediatric Dentistry, 211 East Chicago Avenue, Chicago, Illinois, 60611.

13. Tyndall, D.A.: Seminar II. The Radiology of Trauma, *Dent. Radiog. Photog., 57,* 17, Numbers 1–4, 1985.

14. World Health Organization: Application of the International Classification of Diseases to Dentistry and Stomatology, ICD-DA, 2nd ed. Geneva, World Health Organization, 1978, pp. 88–89.

15. Woolley, L.H., Woodworth, J., and Dobbs, J.L.: A Preliminary Evaluation of the Effects of Electrical Pulp Testers on Dogs with Artificial Pacemakers, *J. Am. Dent. Assoc., 89,* 1099, November, 1974.

16. Ore, D.E. and Shriner, W.A.: Doctor: Don't Shut Off that Pacemaker, *Chicago Dent. Soc. Rev.,* pp. 22–23, August, 1974.

17. Kolbinson, D.A. and Teplitsky, P.E.: Electric Pulp Testing with Examination Gloves, *Oral Surg. Oral Med. Oral Pathol., 65,* 122, January, 1988.

18. Cohen, S. and Burns, R.C., eds.: *Pathways of the Pulp,* 4th ed. St. Louis, The C.V. Mosby Co., 1987, p. 21.

19. King, D.R. and King, A.C.: Use of the Vitalometer with Rubber Gloves, *Can. Dent. Assoc. J., 43,* 182, April, 1977.

Suggested Readings

Croll, T.P., Pascon, E.A., and Langeland, K.: Traumatically Injured Primary Incisors: A Clinical and Histological Study, *ASDC J. Dent. Child., 54,* 401, November-December, 1987.

Fitzgerald, L.R., Harris, E.F., Obermann, K., and McKnight, J.T.: Incisor Mamelon Morphology: Diagnostic Indicators of Abnormal Development, *J. Am. Dent. Assoc., 107,* 63, July, 1983.

Graves, R.C., Bohannan, H.M., Disney, J.A., Stamm, J.W., Bader, J.D., and Abernathy, J.R.: Recent Dental Caries and Treatment Patterns in US Children, *J. Public Health Dent., 46,* 23, Winter, 1986.

Koulourides, T. and Cameron, B.: Enamel Remineralization as a Factor in the Pathogenesis of Dental Caries, *J. Oral Pathol., 9,* 255, September, 1980.

Massler, M. and Schour, I.: *Atlas of the Mouth,* 2nd ed. Chicago, American Dental Association, Plates 7–16.

Miller, M.F.: Odontologic Diseases, in Lynch, M.A., ed.: *Burket's Oral Medicine,* 8th ed. Philadelphia, J.B. Lippincott Co., 1984, pp. 283–301.

Mitropoulos, C.M.: The Use of Fibre-optic Transillumination in the Diagnosis of Posterior Approximal Caries in Clinical Trials, *Caries Res., 19,* 379, July-August, 1985.

Rowe, N.H.: Dental Caries, in Steele, P.F., ed.: *Dimensions of Dental Hygiene,* 3rd ed. Philadelphia, Lea & Febiger, 1982, pp. 209–237.

Russell, R.R.B. and Johnson, N.W.: The Prospects for Vaccination Against Dental Caries, *Br. Dent. J., 162,* 29, January 10, 1987.

Sawada, K., Koike, M., Suda, H., and Sunada, I.: A New Device for Detecting Dental Caries, *Quintessence Int., 17,* 373, June, 1986.

Shaw, J.H.: Causes and Control of Dental Caries, *N. Engl. J. Med., 317,* 996, October 15, 1987.

Stephen, K.W., Russell, J.I., Creanor, S.L., and Burchell, C.K.: Comparison of Fibre Optic Transillumination with Clinical and Radiographic Caries Diagnosis, *Community Dent. Oral Epidemiol., 15,* 90, April, 1987.

Enamel Defects

Carlsson, G.E., Johansson, A., and Lundquist, S.: Occlusal Wear. A Follow-up Study of 18 Subjects with Extensively Worn Dentitions, *Acta Odontol. Scand., 43,* 83, Number 2, 1985.

Crawford, A.W. and de Bruin, H.J.: Concentration Changes in Surface Ca, P, F, Zn, Fe, and Sr During White Spot Formation, *J. Dent. Res., 62,* 964, September, 1983.

Johnson, G.K. and Sivers, J.E.: Attrition, Abrasion and Erosion: Diagnosis and Therapy, *Clin. Prevent. Dent., 9,* 12, September-October, 1987.

King, N.M. and Brook, A.H.: A Prevalence Study of Enamel Defects Among Young Adults in Hong Kong: Use of the FDI Index, *N.Z. Dent. J., 80,* 47, April, 1984.

Sarnat, H. and Moss, S.J.: Diagnosis of Enamel Defects, *N.Y.S. Dent. J., 51,* 103, February, 1985.

Smith, B.G.N. and Knight, J.K.: A Comparison of Patterns of Tooth Wear With Aetiological Factors, *Br. Dent. J., 157,* 16, July 7, 1984.

Root Caries

Banting, D.W., Ellen, R.P., and Fillery, E.D.: Prevalence of Root Surface Caries Among Institutionalized Older Persons, *Community Dent. Oral Epidemiol., 8,* 84, April, 1980.

Banting, D.W., Ellen, R.P., and Fillery, E.D.: A Longitudinal Study of Root Caries: Baseline and Incidence Data, *J. Dent. Res., 64,* 1141, September, 1985.

Banting, D.W. and Stamm, J.W.: Effects of Age and Length of Exposure to Fluoridated Water on Root Surface Fluoride Concentration, *Clin. Prevent. Dent., 4,* 3, July-August, 1982.

Billings, R.J., Brown, L.R., and Kaster, A.G.: Contemporary Treatment Strategies for Root Surface Dental Caries, *Gerodontics, 1,* 20, February, 1985.

Brustman, B.A.: Impact of Exposure to Fluoride-adequate Water on Root Surface Caries in Elderly, *Gerodontics, 2,* 203, December, 1986.

Ellen, R.P., Banting, D.W., and Fillery, E.D.: Streptococcus mutans and Lactobacillus Detection in the Assessment of Dental Root Surface Caries Risk, *J. Dent. Res., 64,* 1245, October, 1985.

Ellen, R.P., Banting, D.W., and Fillery, E.D.: Longitudinal Microbiological Investigation of a Hospitalized Population of Older Adults With a High Root Surface Caries Risk, *J. Dent. Res., 64,* 1377, December, 1985.

Feiglin, B.: Root Resorption, *Aust. Dent. J., 31,* 12, February, 1986.

Katz, R.V., Hazen, S.P., Chilton, N.W., and Mumma, R.D.: Prevalence and Intraoral Distribution of Root Caries in an Adult Population, *Caries Res., 16,* 265, Number 3, 1982.

Katz, S., Park, K.K., and Palenik, C.J.: In-vitro Root Surface Caries Studies, *J. Oral Med., 42,* 40, January-March, 1987.

Mitchell, T.L. and Forgay, M.G.E.: Root Surface Caries: Implications for Dental Hygienists, *Can. Dent. Hyg./Probe, 21,* 31, March, 1987.

Mount, G.J.: Root Surface Caries: A Recurrent Dilemma, *Aust. Dent. J., 31,* 288, August, 1986.

Newbrun, E.: *Cariology,* 2nd ed. Baltimore, Williams & Wilkins, 1983, pp. 52, 54–57, 251–253.

Newitter, D.A., Katz, R.V., and Clive, J.M.: Detection of Root Caries: Sensitivity and Specificity of a Modified Explorer, *Gerodontics, 1,* 65, April, 1985.

Nyvad, B. and Fejerskov, O.: Root Surface Caries: Clinical, Histopathological and Morphological Features and Clinical Implications, *Int. Dent. J., 32,* 312, December, 1982.

Nyvad, B. and Fejerskov, O.: Active Root Surface Caries Converted into Inactive Caries As a Response to Oral Hygiene, *Scand. J. Dent. Res., 94,* 281, June, 1986.

Ravald, N. and Hamp, S.-E.: Prediction of Root Surface Caries in Patients Treated for Advanced Periodontal Disease, *J. Clin. Periodontol., 8,* 400, October, 1981.

Seichter, U.: Root Surface Caries: A Critical Literature Review, *J. Am. Dent. Assoc., 115,* 305, August, 1987.

Vehkalahti, M.M.: Relationship Between Root Caries and Coronal Decay, *J. Dent. Res., 66,* 1608, October, 1987.

Vehkalahti, M.M., Rajala, M., Tuominen, R., and Paunio, I.: Prevalence of Root Caries in the Adult Finnish Population, *Community Dent. Oral Epidemiol., 11,* 188, June, 1983.

Nursing Bottle Caries

Berkowitz, R.J.: Streptococcus Mutans and Dental Caries in Infants, *Compend. Contin. Educ. Dent., 6,* 463, June, 1985.

Croll, T.P.: A Child's First Dental Visit: A Protocol, *Quintessence Int., 15,* 625, June, 1984.

Derkson, G.D. and Ponti, P.: Nursing Bottle Syndrome; Prevalence and Etiology in a Non-fluoridated City, *Can. Dent. Assoc. J., 48,* 389, June, 1982.

Dilley, G.J., Dilley, D.H., and Machen, J.B.: Prolonged Nursing Habit: A Profile of Patients and Their Families, *ASDC J. Dent. Child., 47,* 102, March-April, 1980.

Johnsen, D.C.: Dental Caries Patterns in Preschool Children, *Dent. Clin. North Am., 28,* 3, January, 1984.

Johnsen, D.C., Gerstenmaier, J.H., DiSantis, T.A., and Berkowitz, R.J.: Susceptibility of Nursing-caries Children to Future Approximal Molar Decay, *Pediatr. Dent., 8,* 168, June, 1986.

Kelly, M. and Bruerd, B.: The Prevalence of Baby Bottle Tooth Decay Among Two Native American Populations, *J. Public Health Dent., 47,* 94, Spring, 1987.

Milnes, A.R. and Bowden, G.H.W.: The Microflora Associated with Developing Lesions of Nursing Caries, *Caries Res., 19,* 289, July-August, 1985.

Roberts, G.J.: Is Breast Feeding a Possible Cause of Dental Caries? *J. Dent., 10,* 346, December, 1982.

Scanlan, D.: Nursing Bottle Caries—A Hospital Program, *Can. Dent. Hyg., 13,* 86, Winter, 1979.

Smith, A.J. and Shaw, L.: Baby Fruit Juices and Tooth Erosion, *Br. Dent. J., 162,* 65, January 24, 1987.

van Houte, J., Gibbs, G., and Butera, C.: Oral Flora of Children With "Nursing Bottle Caries," *J. Dent. Res., 61,* 382, February, 1982.

Walton, J.L. and Messer, L.B.: Dental Caries and Fluorosis in Breast-fed and Bottle-fed Children, *Caries Res., 15,* 124, Number 2, 1981.

Winter, G.B.: Problems Involved with the Use of Comforters, *Int. Dent. J., 30,* 29, March, 1980.

Tooth Fractures

American Dental Association, Bureau of Health Education and Audiovisual Services; Council on Dental Materials, Instruments, and Equipment: Mouth Protectors and Sports Team Dentists, *J. Am. Dent. Assoc., 109,* 84, July, 1984.

Bakland, L.K.: Traumatic Injuries, in Ingle, J.I. and Tainter, J.F.: *Endodontics,* 3rd ed. Philadelphia, Lea & Febiger, 1985, pp. 708–769.

Bender, I.B. and Freedland, J.B.: Clinical Considerations in the Diagnosis and Treatment of Intra-alveolar Root Fractures, *J. Am. Dent. Assoc., 107,* 595, October, 1983.

Bender, I.B. and Freedland, J.B.: Adult Root Fracture, *J. Am. Dent. Assoc., 107,* 413, September, 1983.

Gher, M.E., Dunlap, R.M., Anderson, M.H., and Kuhl, L.V.: Clinical Survey of Fractured Teeth, *J. Am. Dent. Assoc., 114,* 174, February, 1987.

Grossman, L.I., Oliet, S., and del Rio, C.E.: *Endodontic Practice,* 11th ed. Philadelphia, Lea & Febiger, 1988, pp. 23–25, 278–286.

Meister, F., Lommel, T.J., and Gerstein, H.: Diagnosis and Possible Causes of Vertical Root Fractures, *Oral Surg. Oral Med. Oral Pathol., 49,* 243, March, 1980.

Pulp Vitality

American Dental Association, Council on Dental Materials, Instruments, and Equipment: *Dentist's Desk Reference: Materials, Instruments, and Equipment,* 2nd ed. Chicago, American Dental Association, 1983, pp. 337–340.

Chambers, I.G.: The Role and Methods of Pulp Testing in Oral Diagnosis: A Review, *Int. Endod. J., 15,* 1, January, 1982.

Cooley, R.L., Stilley, J., and Lubow, R.M.: Evaluation of a Digital Pulp Tester, *Oral Surg. Oral Med. Oral Pathol., 58,* 437, October, 1984.

Dreven, L.J., Reader, A., Beck, F.M., Meyers, W.J., and Weaver, J.: An Evaluation of an Electric Pulp Tester as a Measure of Analgesia in Human Vital Teeth, *J. Endod., 13,* 233, May, 1987.

Dummer, P.M.H., Tanner, M., and McCarthy, J.P.: A Laboratory Study of Four Electric Pulp Testers, *Int. Endod. J., 19,* 161, July, 1986.

Dummer, P.M.H. and Tanner, M.: The Response of Caries-free, Unfilled Teeth to Electrical Excitation: A Comparison of Two New Pulp Testers, *Int. Endod. J., 19,* 172, July, 1986.

Fanibunda, K.B.: Diagnosis of Tooth Vitality by Crown Surface Temperature Measurement: A Clinical Evaluation, *J. Dent., 14,* 160, August, 1986.

Fuss, Z., Trowbridge, H., Bender, I.B., Rickoff, B., and Sorin, S.: Assessment of Reliability of Electrical and Thermal Pulp Testing Agents, *J. Endod., 12,* 301, July, 1986.

Grossman, L.I., Oliet, S., and del Rio, C.E.: *Endodontic Practice,* 11th ed. Philadelphia, Lea & Febiger, 1988, pp. 12–18.

Ingle, J.I. and Tainter, J.F: *Endodontics,* 3rd ed. Philadelphia, Lea & Febiger, 1985, pp. 456–460.

Kerr, D.A., Ash, M.M., and Millard, H.D.: *Oral Diagnosis,* 6th ed. St. Louis, The C.V. Mosby Co., 1983, pp. 302–309.

Kitamura, T., Takahashi, T., and Horiuchi, H.: Electrical Characteristics and Clinical Application of a New Automatic Pulp Tester, *Quintessence Int., 14,* 45, January, 1983.

Kleier, D.J., Sexton, J.R., and Averbach, R.E.: Electronic and Clinical Comparison of Pulp Testers, *J. Dent. Res., 61,* 1413, December, 1982.

Lado, E.A.: Use, Abuse, and Misuse of the Electric Pulp Tester, *Oper. Dent., 8,* 140, Autumn, 1983.

Rosenthal, A.B., Taintor, J.F., and Karp, G.: Human Pulp's Electrical Responsiveness in Hodgkin's Disease Patients Who Are Undergoing Chemotherapy, *J. Endod., 10,* 28, January, 1984.

Seltzer, S. and Bender, I.B.: *The Dental Pulp. Biologic Considerations in Dental Procedures,* 3rd ed. Philadelphia, J.B. Lippincott Co., 1984, pp. 377–380.

15 *The Occlusion*

The occlusion is examined and recorded as part of the oral examination. The dental hygienist, by studying the occlusion of each patient, can contribute significantly to the complete dental care and instruction. Recognition of malocclusion assists the dentist in the referral of patients to the orthodontist, gives many valuable points of reference for patient instruction, and determines necessary adaptations in techniques.

I. Objectives for Observing Occlusion

Recognizing a patient's occlusion and understanding the oral health problems of malocclusion can aid in accomplishing the following:
A. Provide information for the diagnostic work-up and planning dental hygiene care.
B. Plan personalized instruction in relation to such factors as oral habits, masticatory efficiency, personal oral care procedures, and predisposing factors to dental and periodontal infections.
C. Adapt techniques of instrumentation to malpositioned teeth or groups of teeth.
D. Plan the frequency of maintenance appointments for professional care on the basis of deposit retention areas, particularly those that are difficult to reach in routine personal care.
E. Assist by recording the general features of malocclusion for special consideration by the dentist, who may wish to refer the patient to an orthodontist.

II. Definitions*

A. Occlusion
The relationship of the teeth in the mandibular arch with those in the maxillary arch as they are brought together.

B. Static Occlusion
The relationships of the teeth when the jaws are closed in centric occlusion.

C. Centric Occlusion
The centric occlusion is the relation of opposing occlusal surfaces that provides the maximum contact and/or intercuspation.

*For additional definitions to those appearing in this chapter, the reader is referred to the *Orthodontic Glossary, 1987* (or the most recent edition) available from the American Association of Orthodontists, 460 N. Lindbergh Blvd., St. Louis, MO 63141–7883.

D. Functional Occlusion
Functional or dynamic occlusion refers to tooth contacts while the mandible is in action, such as during mastication and swallowing.

E. Centric Relation
Centric relation is the most unstrained, retruded anatomic and functional position of the heads of the condyles of the mandible in the glenoid fossae of the temporomandibular joints.

STATIC OCCLUSION

Static occlusion relationships may be efficiently observed in occluded study casts, although they can be seen directly in the oral cavity when the lips and cheeks are retracted. Classification of malocclusion and the variations that occur with each category are described here.

I. Normal (Ideal) Occlusion
The ideal mechanical relationship between the teeth of the maxillary arch and the teeth of the mandibular arch.
A. All teeth in maxillary arch in maximum contact with all teeth in mandibular arch in a definite pattern.
B. Maxillary teeth slightly overlapping the mandibular teeth on the facial surfaces.

II. Malocclusion
Any deviation from the physiologically acceptable relationship of the maxillary arch and/or teeth to the mandibular arch and/or teeth.

III. Types of Facial Profile (figure 15–1)
A. Mesognathic
Having slightly protruded jaws, which gives the facial outline a relatively flat appearance (straight profile).
B. Retrognathic
Having a prominent maxilla and a mandible posterior to its normal relationship (convex profile).
C. Prognathic
Having a prominent, protruded mandible and normal (usually) maxilla (concave profile).

IV. Malrelations of Groups of Teeth
A. Crossbites
1. *Anterior.* Maxillary incisors are lingual to the mandibular incisors (figure 15–10).

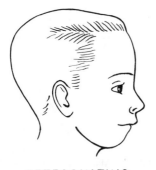 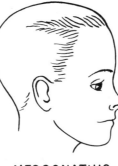 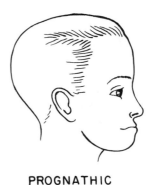

RETROGNATHIC MESOGNATHIC PROGNATHIC

Figure 15–1. Types of Facial Profiles.

2. *Posterior.* Maxillary or mandibular posterior teeth are either facial or lingual to their normal position. This condition may occur bilaterally or unilaterally (figure 15–2).

B. Edge-to-Edge Bite

Incisal surfaces of maxillary teeth occlude with incisal surfaces of mandibular teeth instead of overlapping as in normal occlusion (figure 15–3).

C. End-to-End Bite

Molars and premolars occlude cusp-to-cusp as viewed mesiodistally (figure 15–4).

D. Openbite

Lack of occlusal or incisal contact between certain maxillary and mandibular teeth because either or both have failed to reach the line of occlusion. The teeth cannot be brought together, and a space remains as a result of the arching of the line of occlusion (figure 15–5).

E. Overjet

The horizontal distance between the labioincisal surfaces of the mandibular incisors and the linguoincisal surfaces of the maxillary incisors (figure 15–6). One way to measure the amount of overjet is to place the tip of a probe on the labial surface of the mandibular incisor and, holding it horizontally against the incisal edge of the maxillary tooth, read the distance in millimeters.

F. Underjet (maxillary teeth are lingual to mandibular teeth)

The horizontal distance between the labioincisal surfaces of the maxillary incisors and the linguoincisal surfaces of the mandibular incisors (figure 15–7).

G. Overbite (vertical overlap)

Overbite is the vertical distance by which the maxillary incisors overlap the mandibular incisors.

1. *Normal Overbite.* An overbite is considered normal when the incisal edges of the maxillary teeth are within the incisal third of the mandibular teeth as shown in figure 15–8 in side view and in figure 15–11A in anterior view.

2. *Moderate Overbite.* An overbite is considered moderate when the incisal edges of the maxillary teeth appear within the middle third of the mandibular teeth (figure 15–11B).

3. *Deep (Severe) Overbite.* An overbite is considered deep (severe) when the incisal edges of the maxillary teeth are within the cervical third of the mandibular teeth (figure 15–11C). When in addition the incisal edges of the mandibular teeth are in contact with the maxillary lingual gingival tissue, the overbite is called very deep. A side view of very deep overbite is shown in figure 15–9.

4. *Anterior Crossbite.* The opposite situation occurs in anterior crossbite, in which the maxillary anterior teeth are lingual to the mandibular anterior teeth (figure 15–10).

5. *Clinical Examination of Overbite.* Normal, moderate, and severe anterior overbite are observed directly when the teeth are closed in occlusion. With the posterior teeth closed together, the lips can be retracted and the teeth observed as in figure 15–11. The degree of anterior overbite is judged by the position of the incisal edge of the maxillary teeth: normal (slight) within the incisal third of the man-

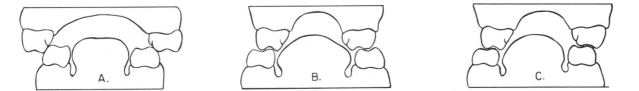

Figure 15–2. Posterior Crossbite. **A.** Mandibular teeth lingual to normal position. **B.** Mandibular teeth facial to normal position. **C.** Unilateral crossbite: right side, normal; left side, mandibular teeth facial to normal position.

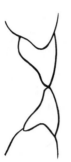

Figure 15–3. Edge-to-Edge Bite. Incisal surfaces occlude.

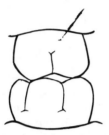

Figure 15–4. End-to-End Bite. Molars in cusp-to-cusp occlusion as viewed from the facial.

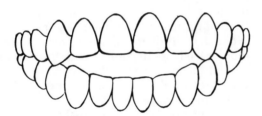

Figure 15–5. Openbite. Lack of incisal contact. Posterior teeth in normal occlusion.

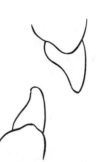

Figure 15–6. Overjet. Maxillary incisors are labial to the mandibular incisors. Measurable horizontal distance is evident between the incisal edge of the maxillary incisors and the incisal edge of the mandibular incisors. A periodontal probe can be used to measure for recording the distance.

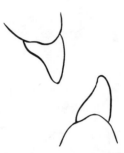

Figure 15–7. Underjet. Maxillary incisors are lingual to the mandibular incisors. Measurable horizontal distance is evident between the incisal edges of the maxillary incisors and the incisal edges of the mandibular incisors.

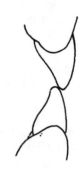

Figure 15–8. Normal Overbite. Profile view to show position of incisal edge of maxillary tooth within the incisal third of the facial surface of the mandibular incisor.

Figure 15–9. Deep (Severe) Anterior Overbite. Incisal edge of maxillary tooth is at the level of the cervical third of the facial surface of the mandibular anterior tooth. See the facial view in figure 15–11C.

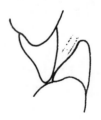

Figure 15–10. Anterior Crossbite. Maxillary anterior teeth are lingual to the mandibular anterior teeth. Anterior crossbite occurs in Angle's Class III malocclusion.

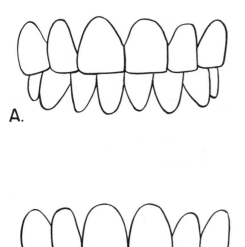

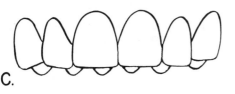

Figure 15–11. Overbite, Anterior View. A. Normal overbite: incisal edges of the maxillary teeth are within the incisal third of the facial surfaces of the mandibular teeth. **B.** Moderate overbite: incisal edges of maxillary teeth are within the middle third of the facial surfaces of the mandibular teeth. **C.** Severe overbite: the incisal edges of the maxillary teeth are within the cervical third of the facial of the mandibular teeth. When the incisal edges of the mandibular teeth are in contact with the maxillary lingual gingival tissue, the overbite is considered very severe. See the profile view in figure 15–9.

dibular incisors; moderate overbite within the middle third; and severe overbite within the cervical third. By placing a mouth mirror under the incisal edge of the maxillary teeth, one can sometimes see the mandibular teeth in contact with the maxillary lingual gingiva. When contact is not visible, an examination of the lingual gingiva may reveal teeth prints, or at least enlargement and redness from the contact.

V. Malpositions of Individual Teeth

A. Labioversion
A tooth that has assumed a position labial to normal.

B. Linguoversion
Position lingual to normal.

C. Buccoversion
Position buccal to normal.

D. Supraversion
Elongated above the line of occlusion.

E. Torsiversion
Turned or rotated.

F. Infraversion
Depressed below the line of occlusion. (Example: primary tooth that is submerged or ankylosed.)

DETERMINATION OF THE CLASSIFICATION OF MALOCCLUSION

The determination of the classification of occlusion is based upon the principles of Edward H. Angle, presented in the early 1900s. He defined normal occlusion as "the normal relations of the occlusal inclined planes of the teeth when the jaws are closed"[1] and based his system of classification upon the relationship of the first permanent molars.

Although authorities have since agreed that the maxillary first permanent molars do not occupy a fixed position in the dental arch, Angle's system serves to provide an acceptable basis for a useful classification. A more comprehensive picture of malocclusion is made by the orthodontist, who studies the relationships of the position of the teeth to the jaws, the face, and the skull.

Three general classes of malocclusion are described below. These are designated by Roman numerals. Because the mandible is movable and the maxilla is stationary, the classes describe the relationship of the mandible to the maxilla. For example, in Distoclusion (Class II) the mandible is distal, whereas in Mesioclusion (Class III) the mandible is mesial to the maxilla, as compared to the normal position.

I. Normal (Ideal) Occlusion (figure 15–12)

A. Facial Profile
Mesognathic (figure 15–1).

B. Molar Relation
The mesiobuccal cusp of the maxillary first permanent molar occludes with the buccal groove of the mandibular first permanent molar.

C. Canine Relation
The maxillary permanent canine occludes with the distal half of the mandibular canine and the mesial half of the mandibular first premolar.

II. Malocclusion

A. Class I or Neutroclusion (figure 15–12)
1. *Facial Profile.* Same as Normal Occlusion (I, A, above).
2. *Molar Relation.* Same as Normal Occlusion (I, B, above).

Figure 15–12. Normal Occlusion and Classification of Malocclusion.

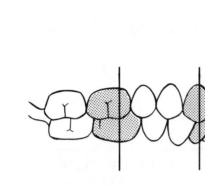

Normal (Ideal) Occlusion

Molar relationship: mesiobuccal cusp of maxillary first permanent molar occludes with the buccal groove of the mandibular first permanent molar.

Malocclusion

Class I: Neutroclusion. Molar relationship same as Normal, with malposition of individual teeth or groups of teeth.

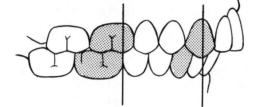

Class II: Distoclusion.

Molar relationship: buccal groove of the mandibular first permanent molar is distal to the mesiobuccal cusp of the maxillary first permanent molar by at least the width of a premolar.

Division 1: mandible is retruded and all maxillary incisors are protruded.

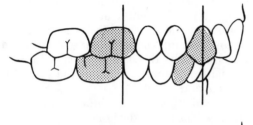

Division 2: mandible is retruded and one or more maxillary incisors are retruded.

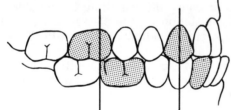

Class III: Mesioclusion.

Molar relationship: buccal groove of the mandibular first permanent molar is mesial to the mesiobuccal cusp of the maxillary first permanent molar by at least the width of a premolar.

3. *Canine Relation.* Same as Normal Occlusion (I, C, above).
4. *Malposition of Individual Teeth or Groups of Teeth.*
5. *General Types of Conditions That Frequently Occur in Class I.*
   a. Crowded maxillary or mandibular anterior teeth.
   b. Protruded or retruded maxillary incisors.
   c. Anterior crossbite.
   d. Posterior crossbite.
   e. Mesial drift of molars resulting from premature loss of teeth.

B. **Class II or Distoclusion** (figure 15–12)
   1. *Description.* Mandibular teeth posterior to normal position in their relation to the maxillary teeth.

2. *Facial Profile.* Retrognathic; maxilla protrudes; lower lip is full and often rests between the maxillary and mandibular incisors; the mandible appears retruded or weak (figure 15–1, Retrognathic).
3. *Molar Relation*
   a. The buccal groove of the mandibular first permanent molar is distal to the mesiobuccal cusp of the maxillary first permanent molar by at least the width of a premolar.
   b. When the distance is less than the width of a premolar the relation should be classified as "tendency toward Class II."
4. *Canine Relation*
   a. The distal surface of the mandibular canine is distal to the mesial surface of the max-

illary canine by at least the width of a premolar.

    b. When the distance is less than the width of a premolar the relation should be classified as "tendency toward Class II."

5. *Class II, Division 1*
    a. *Description:* The mandible is retruded and all maxillary incisors are protruded.
    b. *General types of conditions that frequently occur in Class II, Division 1 malocclusion:* deep overbite, excessive overjet, abnormal muscle function (lips), short mandible, or short upper lip.

6. *Class II, Division 2*
    a. *Description:* the mandible is retruded, and one or more maxillary incisors are retruded.
    b. *General types of conditions that frequently occur in Class II, Division 2 malocclusion:* maxillary lateral incisors protrude while both central incisors retrude, crowded maxillary anterior teeth, or deep overbite.

7. *Subdivision.* One side is Class I, the other side is Class II (may be Division 1 or 2).

C. Class III or Mesioclusion (figure 15–12)

1. *Description.* Mandibular teeth are anterior to normal position in relation to maxillary teeth.

2. *Facial Profile.* Prognathic; lower lip and mandible are prominent (figure 15–1).

3. *Molar Relation*
    a. The buccal groove of the mandibular first permanent molar is mesial to the mesiobuccal cusp of the maxillary first permanent molar by at least the width of a premolar.
    b. When the distance is less than the width of a premolar the relation should be classified as "tendency toward Class III."

4. *Canine Relation*
    a. The distal surface of the mandibular canine is mesial to the mesial surface of the maxillary canine by at least the width of a premolar.
    b. When the distance is less than the width of a premolar the relation should be classified as "tendency toward Class III."

5. *General Types of Conditions That Frequently Occur in Class III Malocclusion*
    a. True Class III: maxillary incisors are lingual to mandibular incisors in an anterior crossbite (figure 15–10).
    b. Maxillary and mandibular incisors are in edge-to-edge occlusion.
    c. Mandibular incisors are very crowded, but lingual to maxillary incisors.

OCCLUSION OF THE PRIMARY TEETH[2]

I. Normal (Ideal)

A. Canine Relation

Same as permanent dentition.

1. *With Primate Spaces* (page 770 for definition).

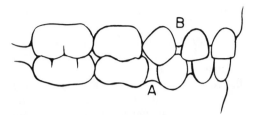

Figure 15–13. Primary Teeth With Primate Spaces. A. Mandibular primate space between canine and first molar. **B.** Maxillary primate space between the lateral incisor and the canine.

    a. Mandibular: between mandibular canine and first molar (figure 15–13A).
    b. Maxillary: between maxillary lateral incisor and canine (figure 15–13B).

2. *Without Primate Spaces.* Closed arches.

B. Second Molar Relation

The mesiobuccal cusp of the maxillary second primary molar occludes with the buccal groove of the mandibular second primary molar.

1. *Variations in Distal Surfaces Relationships.* Terminal step.
    a. The distal surface of the mandibular molar is mesial to that of the maxillary, thereby forming a mesial step (figure 15–14A).
    b. Morphologic variation in molar size: maxillary and mandibular molars have approximately the same mesiodistal width.

2. *Variation.* Terminal plane.
    a. The distal surfaces of the maxillary and mandibular molars are on same vertical plane (figure 15–14B).
    b. The maxillary molar is narrower mesiodistally than the mandibular molar (occurs in high percentage of patients).

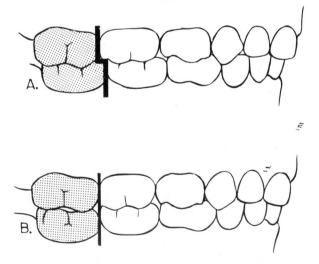

Figure 15–14. Eruption Patterns of the First Permanent Molars. A. Terminal step. The distal surface of mandibular second primary molar is mesial to the distal surface of the maxillary primary molar. **B.** Terminal plane. The distal surfaces of the mandibular and maxillary second primary molars are on the same vertical plane; permanent molars erupt in end-to-end occlusion.

3. *Effects on Occlusion of First Permanent Molars*
   a. Terminal step: first permanent molar erupts directly into proper occlusion (figure 15–14A).
   b. Terminal plane: first permanent molars erupt end-to-end. With mandibular primate space, early mesial shift of primary molars into the primate space occurs, and the permanent mandibular molar shifts into proper occlusion. Without primate spaces late mesial shift of permanent mandibular molar into proper occlusion occurs, following exfoliation of second primary molar (figure 15–14B).

II. Malocclusion of the Primary Teeth

Same as permanent dentition.

FUNCTIONAL OCCLUSION

In contrast to static occlusion, which pertains to the relationship of the teeth when the jaws are closed, functional occlusion consists of all contacts during chewing, swallowing, or other normal action. Functional occlusion is associated with performance.

The pressures or forces created by the muscles of mastication are transmitted from the teeth, after contact, to the periodontium. Such forces are necessary to maintain the occlusal relationship of the teeth and guide the teeth during eruption. The forces are also necessary to provide functional stimulation for the preservation of the health of the attachment apparatus, namely the periodontal ligament, the cementum, and the alveolar bone.

I. Types of Occlusal Contacts

A. Functional Contacts

Functional contacts are the normal contacts that are made between the maxillary teeth and the mandibular teeth during chewing and swallowing. Each contact is momentary, so the total contact time is only a few minutes each day.

B. Parafunctional Contacts

Parafunctional contacts are those made outside the normal range of function.
1. They result from occlusal habits and neuroses.
2. They are potentially injurious to the periodontal supporting structures, but only in the presence of bacterial plaque and inflammatory factors.
3. They create wear facets and attrition on the teeth. A facet is a shiny, flat, worn spot on the surface of a tooth, frequently on the side of a cusp.
4. They can be divided into the following:
   a. Tooth-to-tooth contacts: bruxism, clenching, tapping, doodling.
   b. Tooth-to-hard-object contacts: nail biting, occupational use of such objects as tacks or pins, smoking equipment such as a pipe stem or hard cigarette holder.
   c. Tooth-to-oral tissues contacts: lip or cheek biting.

II. Proximal Contacts

Proximal contacts serve to stabilize the position of teeth in the dental arches and to prevent food impaction between the teeth. Attrition or wear of the teeth occurs at the proximal contacts.

A. Drifting

When proximal contact is lost, teeth can drift into spaces created by unreplaced missing teeth. There is also a natural tendency for mesial migration of teeth toward the midline. In the absence of disease, the surrounding periodontal tissues adapt to repositioned teeth (figure 13–19, page 208).

B. Pathologic Migration

With destruction of the supporting structures of a tooth as a result of periodontal infection and with a force to move a tooth weakened by disease and bone loss, migration of the tooth can result. *Pathologic migration occurs when disease is present, in contrast to drifting, which is migration with a healthy periodontium.*

TRAUMA FROM OCCLUSION

Periodontal tissue injury caused by repeated occlusal forces that exceed the physiologic limits of tissue tolerance is called trauma from occlusion. Other names are periodontal traumatism, occlusal traumatism, and periodontal trauma.

I. Types of Trauma from Occlusion

A. Primary

When the excessive occlusal force is exerted on a tooth with normal bone support, *primary trauma from occlusion* results. An example is the effect of a new restoration placed above the line of occlusion.

B. Secondary

When the excessive occlusal force is exerted on a tooth with bone loss and inadequate alveolar bone support, and the ability of the tooth to withstand occlusal forces is impaired, *secondary trauma from occlusion* results. When a tooth has lost the support of the surrounding bone, even the pressures of what are usually considered normal occlusal forces may create lesions of trauma from occlusion.

II. Effects of Trauma from Occlusion

The attachment apparatus (periodontal ligament, cementum, and alveolar bone) has as its main purpose the maintenance of the tooth in the socket in a functional state. In a healthy situation, occlusal pressures and forces during chewing and swallowing are readily dispersed or absorbed and no unusual effects are produced.

A. Excess Forces

When the forces of occlusion are greater than can be taken care of by the attachment apparatus, damage can result. Circulatory disturbances, tissue destruction from crushing under pressure, bone resorption, and other pathologic processes are initiated.

B. Relation to Inflammatory Factors

1. *Trauma from occlusion does not cause gingivitis, periodontitis, or pocket formation.* The steps in the development of inflammatory disease and pockets were outlined on pages 181–182.
2. In the presence of inflammatory disease, the existing periodontal destruction may be aggravated or promoted by trauma from occlusion.

III. Methods of Application of Excess Pressure

To understand the nature of the occlusal forces that can cause periodontal trauma from occlusion, it is helpful to recognize types of tooth contacts that can overburden a tooth or group of teeth.[3]

A. Individual Teeth that Touch Before Full Closure

The contact is premature and may put excessive force on an individual tooth.

B. Two or Only a Few Teeth in Contact During Movement of the Jaw

The teeth involved receive a disproportionate amount of force.

C. Initial Contacts on Inclined Planes of Cusps

Following the initial contact, when the teeth are brought together in a closed position, there may be excess pressure on the teeth where initial contact was made.

D. Heavy Forces Not in a Vertical or Axial Direction

Normal occlusal relationships imply a direct cusp-to-fossa position during closure, with the force of occlusion in a vertical direction toward the tooth apex and parallel with the long axis. When pressures are exerted laterally or horizontally, excess force is placed on the periodontal attachment apparatus.

E. Increased Frequency, Intensity, and Duration of Contacts

In the presence of parafunctional habits, such as bruxism, clenching, tapping, or biting objects, many more than the usual number of tooth contacts are made each day, and the intensity and duration are altered.

IV. Recognition of Signs of Trauma from Occlusion

No one clinical or radiographic finding will clearly define the presence of trauma from occlusion. Diagnosis of the condition is complex. The possible observations listed as follows should be looked for specifically and recorded for evaluation and correlation with the patient history and all other clinical determinations.

A. Clinical Findings That May Occur in Trauma from Occlusion

1. Tooth mobility.
2. Fremitus.
3. Sensitivity of teeth to pressure and/or percussion.
4. Pathologic migration.
5. Wear facets or atypical occlusal wear.
6. Open contacts related to food impaction.
7. Neuromuscular disturbances in the muscles of mastication. In severe cases muscle spasm can occur.
8. Temporomandibular joint symptoms.

B. Radiographic Findings

Characteristics that may occur in trauma from occlusion include:

1. Widened periodontal ligament spaces, particularly angular thickening (triangulation). This finding frequently occurs in conjunction with tooth mobility.
2. Angular (vertical) bone loss in localized areas (figure 13–20, page 208).
3. Root resorption.
4. Furcation involvement.
5. Thickened lamina dura. Although related to occlusal forces, thickened lamina dura should not be considered a detrimental or destructive effect of trauma from occlusion. It may be a defense reaction to strengthen tooth support against occlusal forces. Thickened lamina dura is frequently associated with teeth that have undergone orthodontic treatment.

TECHNICAL HINTS

I. Observe the facial profile as the patient enters and is seated in the dental chair to estimate the classification of occlusion before examination of the teeth.
II. Avoid mention of a dentofacial deformity that would make the patient feel self-conscious.
III. Avoid suggesting to the patient or a parent the possible procedures the orthodontist may use in treatment because complications become known only after the complete diagnosis.
IV. Closing to centric relation can be performed most effectively by instructing the patient to curl the tongue and to try to hold the tip of the tongue as far back as possible while closing.
V. When a small child has difficulty in occluding, the clinician may firmly but gently press the cushions of the thumbs on the mucous membrane over the pterygomandibular raphe, holding the thumbs between the cheek and buccal surfaces of the teeth as the patient is requested to close.

VI. Study the occlusion of the patient with removable dentures with the dentures in place in the mouth.

FACTORS TO TEACH THE PATIENT

I. Interpretation of the *general* purposes of orthodontic care (function and esthetics) to patients whom the dentist has referred to an orthodontist.
   A. Dependence of masticatory efficiency on the occlusion of the teeth.
   B. Influence of masticatory efficiency on food selection in the diet.
   C. Influence of masticatory efficiency and diet on the nutritional status of the body and oral health.
II. Interpretation of the dentist's suggestions for the correction of oral habits.
III. The space-maintaining function of the primary teeth in prevention of malocclusion of permanent teeth.
IV. The role of malocclusion as a predisposing factor in the formation of dental caries and periodontal diseases.
V. Plaque removal methods for reducing dental calculus and soft deposit retention in areas where teeth are crowded, displaced, or otherwise not in normal occlusion.
VI. The relation of the occlusion and the position of the teeth to the patient's personal oral care procedures.
   A. Selection of the proper type of toothbrush.
   B. Application of thorough toothbrushing method or methods.
   C. Use of dental floss.
VII. Specific reasons for frequency of maintenance examinations when related to malocclusion.

References

1. Angle, E.H.: *Malocclusion of the Teeth,* 7th ed. Philadelphia, S.S. White, 1907.
2. Baume, L.J.: Physiological Tooth Migration and Its Significance for the Development of the Occlusion.
   I. The Biogenetic Course of the Deciduous Dentition, *J. Dent. Res., 29,* 123, April, 1950.
   II. The Biogenesis of the Accessional Dentition, *J. Dent. Res., 29,* 331, June, 1950.
   III. The Biogenesis of the Successional Dentition, *J. Dent. Res., 29,* 338, June, 1950.
   IV. The Biogenesis of Overbite, *J. Dent. Res., 29,* 440, August, 1950.
3. Allen, D.L., McFall, W.T., and Jenzano, J.W.: *Periodontics for the Dental Hygienist,* 4th ed. Philadelphia, Lea & Febiger, 1987, pp. 85–86.

Suggested Readings

Ash, M.M.: *Wheeler's Dental Anatomy, Physiology, and Occlusion,* 6th ed. Philadelphia, W.B. Saunders Co., 1984, pp. 378–438.

Barber, T.K. and Luke, L.S.: Preventive Orthodontics, in Stallard, R.E.: *A Textbook of Preventive Dentistry,* 2nd ed. Philadelphia, W.B. Saunders Co., 1982, pp. 347–386.

Currier, G.F.: Fundamentals of Orthodontics with Criteria for Referral, *Pediatr. Ann., 14,* 117, February, 1985.

Feliu, J.L.: Long-term Benefits of Orthodontic Treatment on Oral Hygiene, *Am. J. Orthod., 82,* 473, December, 1982.

Fox, R.N., Albino, J.E., Green, L.J., Farr, S.D., and Tedesco, L.A.: Development and Validation of a Measure of Attitudes Toward Malocclusion, *J. Dent. Res., 61,* 1039, September, 1982.

Ganssle, C.L. and Everett, M.S.: Dental Hygiene Utilization in Orthodontics, *Dent. Hyg., 57,* 17, November, 1983.

Jacobson, A.: Psychological Aspects of Dentofacial Esthetics and Orthognathic Surgery, *Angle Orthod., 54,* 18, January, 1984.

Kiyak, H.A., West, R.A., Hohl, T., and McNeill, R.W.: The Psychological Impact of Orthognathic Surgery: A 9-month Follow-up, *Am. J. Orthod., 81,* 404, May, 1982.

Margolis, F.S.: Ordinary versus Orthodontic Pacifiers, *Dent. Surv., 56,* 44, July, 1980.

Merow, W.W.: Orthodontics, in Steele, P.F., ed.: *Dental Specialties for the Dental Hygienist,* 2nd ed. Philadelphia, Lea & Febiger, 1978, pp. 199–237.

Proffit, W.R.: On the Aetiology of Malocclusion, *Br. J. Orthod., 13,* 1, January, 1986.

Rubel, I.: Avulsion of Central Incisors by Elastic Bands with Subsequent Orthodontic Treatment, *J. Am. Dent. Assoc., 100,* 211, February, 1980.

Shefter, G.J. and McFall, W.T.: Occlusal Relations and Periodontal Status in Human Adults, *J. Periodontol., 55,* 368, June, 1984.

Functional and Parafunctional

Carranza, F.A.: *Glickman's Clinical Periodontology,* 6th ed. Philadelphia, W.B. Saunders Co., 1984, pp. 266–282, 427–443.

Gallagher, S.J.: Diagnosis and Treatment of Bruxism: A Review of the Literature, *Gen. Dent., 28,* 62, March-April, 1980.

Grant, D.A., Stern, I.B., and Listgarten, M.A., eds.: *Periodontics,* 6th ed. St. Louis, The C.V. Mosby Co., 1988, pp. 479–509, 513–514, 977–979, 1017–1044.

Hanamura, H., Houston, F., Rylander, H., Carlsson, G.E., Haraldson, T., and Nyman, S.: Periodontal Status and Bruxism. A Comparative Study of Patients with Periodontal Disease and Occlusal Parafunctions, *J. Periodontol., 58,* 173, March, 1987.

Kerr, D.A., Ash, M.M., and Millard, H.D.: *Oral Diagnosis,* 6th ed. St. Louis, The C.V. Mosby Co., 1983, pp. 200–237.

Oliver, G.V.: Periodontics, in Steele, P.F., ed.: *Dimensions of Dental Hygiene,* 3rd ed. Philadelphia, Lea & Febiger, 1982, pp. 388–390, 415.

Habits

Martinez, N.P. and Hunckler, R.J.: Managing Digital Habits in Children, *Compend. Contin. Educ. Dent., 6,* 188, March, 1985.

Massler, M.: Oral Habits: Development and Management, *J. Pedod., 7,* 109, Winter, 1983.

Odenrick, L. and Brattström, V.: Nailbiting: Frequency and Association with Root Resorption During Orthodontic Treatment, *Br. J. Orthod., 12,* 78, April, 1985.

Villarosa, G.A. and Moss, R.A.: Oral Behavioral Patterns as Factors Contributing to the Development of Head and Facial Pain, *J. Prosthet. Dent., 54,* 427, September, 1985.

16 Bacterial Plaque and Other Soft Deposits

Dental caries and gingival and periodontal infections are caused by microorganisms in bacterial plaque. Disease-producing bacteria attach to the tooth surfaces and colonize. They bring about carious lesions of the enamel and root surfaces, in pits and fissures, and on smooth surfaces (pages 216–217). They also bring about inflammatory changes in the periodontium that can lead to destruction of tissues and loss of attachment.

During the clinical examination of the teeth and surrounding soft tissues, the soft and hard deposits that accumulate on the teeth and within the sulci or pockets must be recognized and assessed. From the findings, an initial treatment plan can be formulated based on the individual needs of the patient.

The soft deposits are acquired pellicle or cuticle, bacterial plaque, materia alba, and food debris, each of which is an entity, and the terms should not be interchanged. The hard, calcified deposit on teeth is dental calculus, which is described in Chapter 17. A classification with definitions of the dental deposits is presented in table 16–1.[1]

TERMINOLOGY

Acquired pellicle: an homogenous, organic, tenacious layer that forms over exposed oral surfaces. It is acellular, that is, free from microorganisms, until plaque begins to collect on it.

Bacterial plaque: organized masses of microorganisms held together by a gel-like intermicrobial matrix. Plaque forms on the acquired pellicle on the teeth, on other oral surfaces, and in the gingival sulcus and pockets. It is also called microbial plaque or bacterial dental plaque.

Materia alba: "white material" that is an informal collection of microorganisms and cellular debris. It forms a soft deposit over acquired pellicle and microbial plaque.

Microorganisms: minute living organisms, usually microscopic. They include bacteria, viruses, and fungi.

Bacteria: single-cell microorganisms. The several forms of bacteria are shown in figure 16–1.

Viruses: very small microorganisms that are incapable of growth or reproduction apart from living cells.

Fungi: plant-like organisms that occur as yeasts or molds. Yeasts are single-cell organisms.

Oral Flora: the various bacterial and other microscopic organisms that inhabit the oral cavity. The mouth has an indigenous flora, meaning

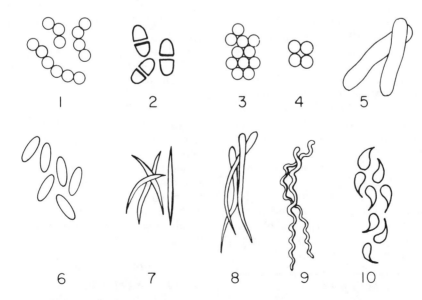

Figure 16–1. Morphologic Forms of Bacteria. 1. Streptococci, **2.** Diplococci, **3.** Staphylococci, **4.** Sarcina, **5.** Bacilli, **6.** Coccobacilli, **7.** Fusiform bacilli, **8.** Filamentous bacilli, **9.** Spirochetes, **10.** Vibrios. (From Hammond, B.: Bacterial structure and function, in Schuster, G.S., ed.: *Oral Microbiology and Infectious Disease*, 2nd Student edition. Toronto, B.C. Decker, 1988, p. 23.)

Table 16–1. Tooth Deposits

Category	Tooth Deposit	Description	Derivation
Nonmineralized	Acquired Pellicle	Translucent, homogenous, thin, unstructured film covering and adherent to the surfaces of the teeth, restorations, calculus, and other surfaces in the oral cavity	Supragingival: saliva Subgingival: gingival sulcus fluid
	Bacterial Plaques	Dense, organized bacterial systems embedded in an intermicrobial matrix that adhere closely to the teeth, calculus, and other surfaces in the oral cavity Water irrigation removes only the outer layer of loose organisms	Colonization of oral microorganisms
	Materia Alba	Loosely adherent, unstructured, white or grayish-white mass of oral debris and bacteria that lies over bacterial plaque Vigorous rinsing and water irrigation can remove materia alba	Incidental accumulation
	Food Debris	Unstructured, loosely attached particulate matter Self-cleansing activity of tongue and saliva and rinsing vigorously will remove debris	Food retention following eating
Mineralized	Calculus	Calcified bacterial plaque; hard, tenacious mass that forms on the clinical crowns of the natural teeth and on dentures and other appliances	Plaque mineralization
	a. Supragingival	Occurs coronal to the margin of the gingiva; is covered with bacterial plaque	Supragingival: source of minerals is saliva
	b. Subgingival	Occurs apical to the margin of the gingiva; is covered with bacterial plaque	Subgingival: source of minerals is gingival sulcus fluid

(Adapted from Schroeder, H.E.: *Formation and Inhibition of Dental Calculus.* Vienna, Hans Huber, 1969, pp. 14–15.)

those organisms that are native to the area. Certain organisms specifically reside in certain parts, for example, on the tongue, on the mucosa, or in the gingival sulcus.

Aerobe: a microorganism that can live and grow in the presence of oxygen. An *obligate* aerobe lives or grows only in the presence of oxygen.

Anaerobe: a microorganism that thrives best, or only, in the absence of oxygen. A *facultative* organism is able to grow in the presence or absence of oxygen; an *obligate* anaerobe grows only in the absence of oxygen.

Leukocytes: white blood cells. They are body defense cells and collect in the tissues and pockets during periodontal and gingival infections. For a description of the various types of white blood cells, see page 701 and figure 57–1.

ACQUIRED PELLICLE

The acquired pellicle is an amorphous, organic, tenacious membranous layer that forms over exposed tooth surfaces, as well as over restorations and dental calculus. Its thickness, which varies from 0.1 to 0.8 μm, usually is thicker near the gingiva. Pellicles are acellular, that is, they are free from bacteria or other cell forms.

I. Formation

Within minutes after all external material has been removed by polishing the tooth surfaces with an abrasive, the acquired pellicle begins to form. It is composed primarily of glycoproteins from the saliva that are selectively adsorbed by the hydroxyapatite of the tooth surface. The adsorbed material becomes a highly insoluble coating over the teeth, calculus deposits, restorations, and complete and partial dentures.

II. Types of Pellicles[2]

A. Surface Pellicle, Unstained

The unstained pellicle is clear, translucent, insoluble, and not readily visible until a disclosing agent has been applied. When stained with a disclosing agent, it appears thin, with a pale staining that contrasts with the thicker, darker staining of bacterial plaque.

B. Surface Pellicle, Stained
Unstained pellicle can take on extrinsic stain and become brown, grayish, or other colors as described on page 256.

C. Subsurface Pellicle
Surface pellicle is continuous with pellicle that is embedded in tooth structure, particularly where the tooth surface is partially demineralized.[3]

III. Significance of Pellicle

A. Protective
Pellicle appears to provide a barrier against acids; thus it may aid in reducing dental caries attack.[3]

B. Nidus for Bacteria
Pellicle participates in plaque formation by aiding the adherence of microorganisms.

C. Attachment of Calculus
One mode of calculus attachment is by the acquired pellicle (page 250).

BACTERIAL PLAQUE

Bacterial plaque is a dense, nonmineralized, complex mass of bacterial colonies in a gel-like intermicrobial matrix. It adheres firmly to the acquired pellicle and hence to the teeth, calculus, and fixed and removable restorations.

Characteristics of supragingival and subgingival plaques are shown in table 16–2.

I. Steps in the Formation of Plaque

Plaque is formed in three basic steps, namely, pellicle formation, bacterial colonization, and plaque maturation (figure 16–2). Plaque formation does not occur randomly but involves a series of complex interactions.

A. Formation of a Pellicle
The pellicle forms on the tooth surface by selective adsorption of protein components from the saliva.

B. Bacteria Attach to the Pellicle
Initial attachment of bacteria to the pellicle is by selective adherence of specific bacteria from the oral environment. Innate characteristics of the bacteria and the pellicle determine the adhesive interactions that make a particular organism adhere to a particular pellicle.

C. Bacterial Multiplication
Microcolonies form in layers as the bacteria multiply and grow. With increased size of colonies, they meet and coalesce to form a continuous bacterial mass.

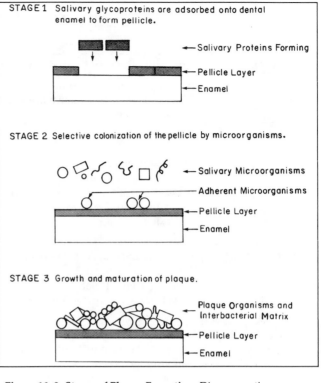

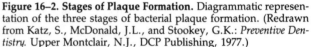

Figure 16–2. Stages of Plaque Formation. Diagrammatic representation of the three stages of bacterial plaque formation. (Redrawn from Katz, S., McDonald, J.L., and Stookey, G.K.: *Preventive Dentistry.* Upper Montclair, N.J., DCP Publishing, 1977.)

D. Plaque Growth and Maturation
The increase in the mass and thickness of plaque results from
1. Continued bacterial multiplication.
2. Continuous adherence of bacteria to the plaque surface.

E. Matrix Formation
The intermicrobial substance is derived mainly from saliva for supragingival plaque and from gingival sulcus fluid and exudate for subgingival plaque. Other components of the intermicrobial substance are the polysaccharides, glucans, and fructans or levans produced by certain bacteria from dietary sucrose. The polysaccharides are sticky and contribute to the adhesion of the plaque to the teeth.

II. Changes in Plaque Microorganisms

Bacterial plaque consists of a complex mixture of microorganisms that occur primarily as microcolonies. The population density is very high and increases as plaque ages. The probability of the development of dental caries and/or gingivitis increases as the number of microorganisms increases.

Changes in the types of organisms occur within plaque as the plaque matures. When oral hygiene practices are discontinued, the numbers of bacteria increase rapidly. The changes in oral flora follow a

Table 16–2. Characteristics of Supragingival and Subgingival Plaque

Characteristic	Supragingival Plaque	Subgingival Plaque
Location	Coronal to the margin of the free gingiva	Apical to the margin of the free gingiva
Origin	Salivary glycoprotein forms pellicle Microorganisms from saliva are selectively attracted to pellicle	Downgrowth of bacteria from supragingival plaque

Distribution	Starts on proximal surfaces and other protected areas
	Heaviest collection on
	  Areas not cleaned daily by patient
	  Cervical third, especially facial
	  Lingual mandibular molars
	  Proximal surfaces
	  Pit and fissure plaque
		Shallow pocket: similar to supragingival plaque
		Undisturbed; held by pocket wall
		Attached plaque covers calculus
		Unattached plaque extends to the periodontal attachment

Adhesion	Firmly attached to acquired pellicle, other bacteria, and tooth surfaces Surface bacteria (unattached): loose, washed away by saliva or swallowed	Adheres to tooth surface, subgingival pellicle, and calculus Subgingival flora: loose, floating, motile organisms in deep pocket do not adhere; they are between adherent plaque on tooth and the pocket epithelium
Retention	Rough surfaces of teeth or restorations Malpositioned teeth Carious lesions (See Chapter 12 for other factors)	Pocket holds plaque against tooth Overhanging margins of fillings that extend into pockets

Shape and Size	Friction of tongue, cheeks, lips limits shape and size
	Thickness: thicker at the cervical third and on proximal surfaces
	  Healthy gingiva: thin plaque, 15 to 20 cells thick
	  Chronic gingivitis: thick plaque, 100 to 300 cells thick
		Molded by pocket wall to shape of the tooth surface
		Follows form created by subgingival calculus
		May become thicker as the diseased pocket wall becomes less tight

Structure	Adherent, densely packed microbial layer over pellicle on tooth surface Intermicrobial matrix Onset: small isolated colonies 2 to 5 days: colonies merge to form a covering of plaque	Three layers (see figure 34–1, page 476) 1. Tooth-surface-attached plaque: many gram-positive rods and cocci 2. Unattached plaque in middle: many gram-negative, motile forms; spirochetes; leukocytes 3. Epithelium-attached plaque: gram-negative, motile forms predominate; many leukocytes migrate through epithelium
Microorganisms	Early plaque: primarily gram-positive cocci Older plaque (3 to 4 days): increased numbers of filaments and fusiforms 4 to 9 days undisturbed: more complex flora with rods, filamentous forms 7 to 14 days: vibrios, spirochetes, more gram-negative organisms	Environment conducive to growth of anaerobic population Diseased pocket: primarily gram-negative, motile, spirochetes, rods See table 16–4
Sources of Nutrients for Bacterial Proliferation	Saliva Ingested food	Tissue fluid (gingival sulcus fluid) Exudate Leukocytes

Significance	Etiology of
	  Gingivitis
	  Supragingival calculus
	  Dental caries (figure 16–5)
		Etiology of
		  Gingivitis
		  Periodontal infections
		  Subgingival calculus

pattern such as shown in figure 16–4, page 240. The changes can be described as follows:[4]

A. Days 1 to 2

Early plaque consists primarily of cocci. Streptococci, which dominate the bacterial population, include *Streptococcus mutans* and *Streptococcus sanguis.*

B. Days 2 to 4

The cocci still dominate, and increasing numbers of filamentous forms and slender rods may be seen on the surface of the cocci colonies. Gradually, the filamentous forms grow into the cocci layer and replace many of the cocci. Slow plaque formers continue to form plaque comprised primarily of cocci for a longer time than do fast plaque formers.

C. Days 4 to 7

Filaments increase in numbers, and a more mixed flora begins to appear with rods, filamentous forms, and fusobacteria. Plaque near the gingival margin is thicker and develops a more mature flora earlier, with spirochetes and vibrios. As plaque spreads coronally, the new plaque has the characteristic coccal forms.

D. Days 7 to 14

Vibrios and spirochetes appear, and the number of white blood cells increases. As plaque matures and thickens, more gram-negative and anaerobic organisms appear. During this period, signs of inflammation are beginning to be observable in the gingiva.

E. Days 14 to 21

Older plaque. Vibrios and spirochetes are prevalent, along with cocci and filamentous forms. The densely packed filamentous microorganisms arrange themselves perpendicular to the tooth surface in a palisade. Gingivitis is evident clinically.

III. Distribution of Plaque

A. By Location

1. *Supragingival Plaque.* Plaque is coronal to the gingival margin.
2. *Subgingival Plaque.* Plaque is located between the periodontal attachment and the gingival margin, within the sulcus or pocket.
3. *Fissure Plaque.* Plaque also develops in pits and fissures and is referred to as *fissure* plaque.
4. *Gingival Plaque.* Plaque forms on the external surfaces of the oral epithelium and attached gingiva.

B. By Surfaces

1. *During Formation.* Supragingival plaque formation begins at the gingival margin, particularly on proximal surfaces, and increases rapidly when left undisturbed. It spreads over the gingival third and on towards the middle third of the crown.

2. *Tooth Surfaces Involved*
   a. Plaque occurs most frequently on proximal surfaces and around the gingival third, associated with protected areas (figure 16–3).
   b. Least amounts occur on the palatal surfaces of maxillary teeth because of the activity of the tongue.

C. Factors Influencing Plaque Accumulation

In Chapter 12 (pages 185–188) many factors that influence deposit accumulation and disease development were outlined. A review of those factors can be helpful in conjunction with the material in this section.

1. Figure 16–3 illustrates the accumulation of bacterial plaque around crowded mandibular anterior teeth. Research has shown that, when personal plaque removal efforts are made conscientiously, plaque accumulation around crowded teeth is not greater than that around teeth in good alignment.[5]
2. More rapid collection occurs on rough surfaces of teeth, restorations, and calculus.
3. Thick, dense deposits usually collect in difficult-to-clean areas, such as under overhanging margins of crowns or fillings, under ledges of calculus, and in areas associated with carious lesions.
4. Deposits may extend over an entire crown of a tooth that is unopposed, out of occlusion, or not used during mastication.

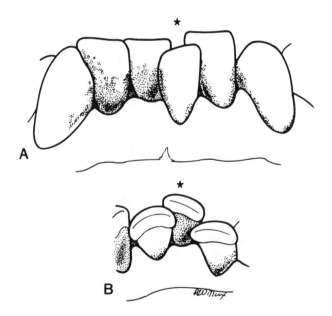

Figure 16–3. Plaque Accumulation in Protected Areas. Crowded mandibular anterior teeth demonstrate bacterial plaque after use of a disclosing agent. The thickest plaque is on the proximal surfaces and at the cervical thirds of the teeth. Note the central incisors in facial view (**A**) and lingual view (**B**), with thick extensive plaque on the less accessible protected surfaces.

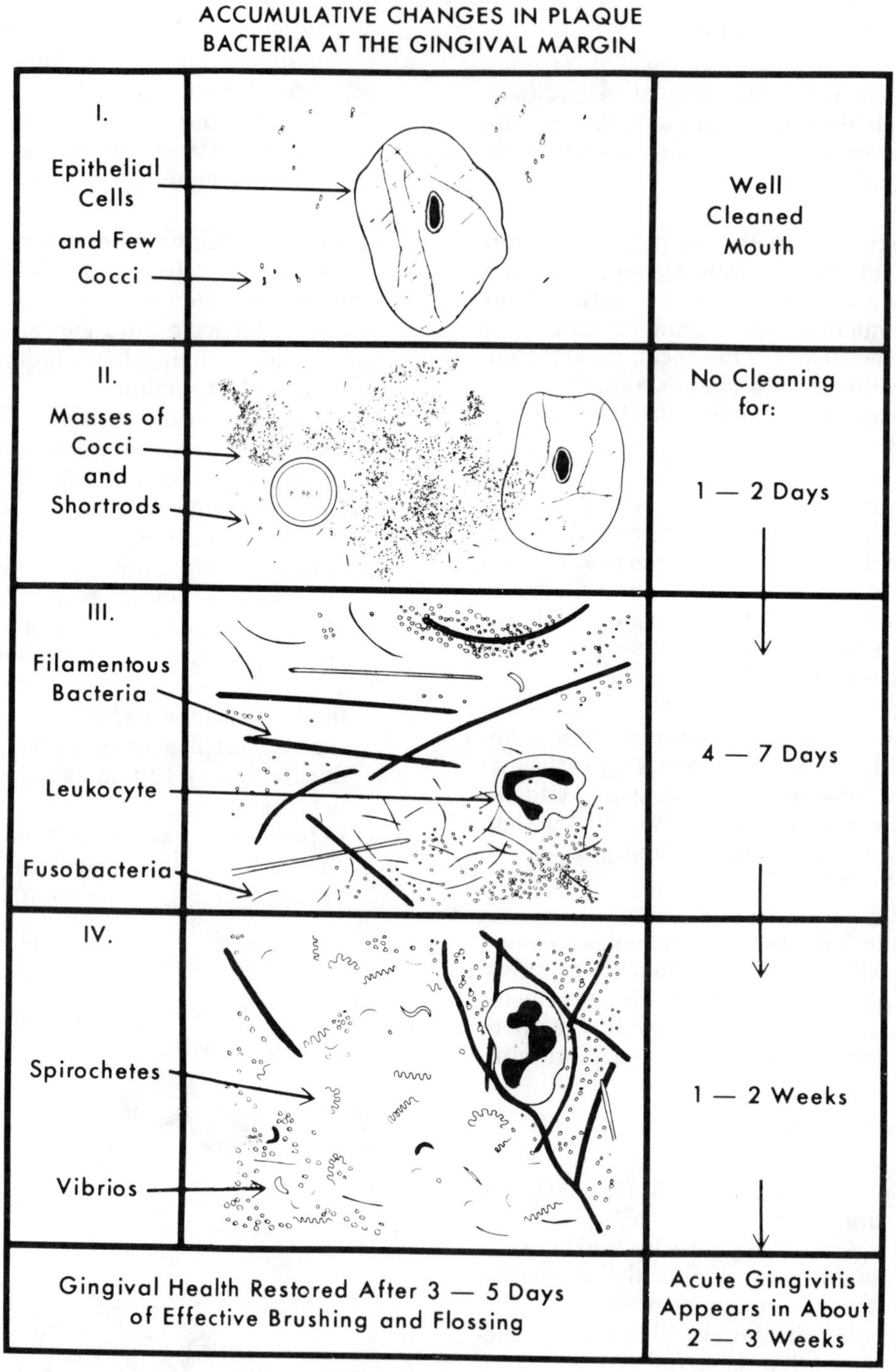

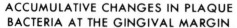

ACCUMULATIVE CHANGES IN PLAQUE BACTERIA AT THE GINGIVAL MARGIN

I. Epithelial Cells and Few Cocci		Well Cleaned Mouth
II. Masses of Cocci and Shortrods		No Cleaning for: 1 — 2 Days
III. Filamentous Bacteria Leukocyte Fusobacteria		4 — 7 Days
IV. Spirochetes Vibrios		1 — 2 Weeks
Gingival Health Restored After 3 — 5 Days of Effective Brushing and Flossing		Acute Gingivitis Appears in About 2 — 3 Weeks

Figure 16–4. Plaque Microorganisms. On the right are the time intervals from 1 day to 3 weeks. On the left are the changes in the plaque content that take place as plaque ages. As the numbers of microorganisms increase, the numbers of defense cells (leukocytes) also increase. (From Crawford, J.J.: Microbiology, in Barton, R.E., Matteson, S.R., and Richardson, R.E.: The Dental Assistant, 6th ed. Philadelphia, Lea & Febiger, 1988.)

IV. Composition

Plaque is composed of microorganisms and intermicrobial matrix. Organic and inorganic solids constitute approximately 20 percent, and water accounts for 80 percent. Microorganisms make up at least 70 to 80 percent of the solid matter, which is higher in subgingival plaque than in supragingival.

Composition differs between individuals and between different tooth surfaces of an individual. As plaque ages, it changes.

A. Inorganic Elements[6,7]

1. *Calcium and Phosphorus.* The concentration of calcium, phosphorus, magnesium, and fluoride is higher in plaque than in saliva, thus illustrating the ability of plaque to concentrate inorganic elements.

   Plaque on the lingual surfaces of the mandibular anterior teeth contains a higher concentration of calcium and phosphate than does plaque on the other teeth, and the amount is even higher on those same surfaces in heavy calculus formers.

2. *Fluoride.* The concentration of fluoride in plaque is higher when fluoridated water is used, and is increased following professional topical applications of fluoride, and the use of fluoride-containing dentifrices and mouthrinses.

B. Organic Components

The organic intermicrobial substance surrounds the microorganisms of plaque and contains primarily carbohydrates and proteins, with small amounts of lipids.

1. *Carbohydrates.* Carbohydrates, which are produced by several types of bacteria, include glucans and fructans or levans made from dietary sucrose. Dextran is a type of glucan. These carbohydrates contribute to the following:
   a. Adherence of the microorganisms to each other and the tooth. An example is *Streptococcus mutans,* which may be linked to glucans.
   b. Energy storage of carbohydrate for reserve use by plaque bacteria.
2. *Proteins*
   a. Supragingival plaque contains proteins derived from saliva.
   b. Subgingival plaque contains proteins from gingival exudate and sulcus fluid.
3. *Lipids.* The lipid content may include lipopolysaccharide endotoxins from gram-negative bacteria.

V. Detection

A. Direct Vision

1. *Thin Plaque.* May be translucent and therefore not visible.
2. *Stained Plaque.* May acquire extrinsic stains that make it visible; for example, yellow, green, tobacco, as described on pages 254–256.
3. *Thick Plaque.* The tooth may appear dull, dingy, with a matted fur-like surface. Materia alba or food debris may collect over the plaque.

B. Use of Explorer or Probe

1. *Tactile Examination.* When calcification has started, plaque may feel slightly rough; otherwise the surface may feel only somewhat slippery because of the coating of soft, slimy plaque.
2. *Removal of Plaque.* When no plaque is visible, an explorer can be passed over the tooth surface. If present, plaque will adhere to the explorer tip. This technique is used when evaluating for a Plaque Index (page 262).

C. Use of Disclosing Agent

When a disclosing agent is applied, plaque takes on the color and becomes readily visible (figure 26–1, page 367). Disclosing agent should not be applied until the evaluation of the oral mucosa and gingival color has been recorded.

D. Clinical Record

1. Record plaque by location and extent (slight, moderate, or heavy). An index or plaque score may be used (figures 19–1, 19–2, pages 264, 265).
2. Plaque recordings and indices are kept for comparison in conjunction with the instructional plan for plaque control by the patient, both current and for maintenance appointments.
3. Plaque evaluation records are included with the complete charting and oral examination.

SIGNIFICANCE OF BACTERIAL PLAQUE

The role of plaque in the initiation and perpetuation of both dental caries and periodontal infections has led to a realization that all bacterial plaque is not the same, but that the content and effects vary. Two hypotheses have been used to describe plaque differences.

The "Non-specific Plaque Hypothesis" suggests that dental caries and periodontal infections result from the bacterial products of the entire plaque flora. The level or threshold of disease activity would be determined by the quantity of microorganisms and the response by host defense.

The "Specific Plaque Hypothesis," on the other hand, is based on the realization that the principal differences between plaques are brought about by specific pathogenic microorganisms. By this system, particular microorganisms must always be present in association with specific infections. Prevention or treatment procedures would then be directed at the specific plaque microorganisms.

On the basis of their pathogenic effects, the three main categories of plaques are as follows:

1. *Cariogenic Plaque.* Associated with the initiation of dental caries. A high sucrose diet favors the cariogenic flora.
2. *Periodontal-Disease-Producing Plaque.* Directly involved in promoting the inflammatory responses demonstrated by gingivitis, periodontitis, and other periodontal infections.
3. *Calculus Plaque or Calculogenic Plaque.* Invites mineralization of the plaque, leading to calculus formation.

DENTAL CARIES

Dental caries is a disease of the dental calcified structures (enamel, dentin, and cementum) that is characterized by demineralization of the mineral components and dissolution of the organic matrix. Clinical characteristics and types of cavities were described in Chapter 14.

I. Essentials for Dental Caries

The sequence of events leading to demineralization and dental caries is shown in figure 16–5.

A. Susceptible Tooth Surface

A tooth with optimum fluoride content resists the process of dental caries.

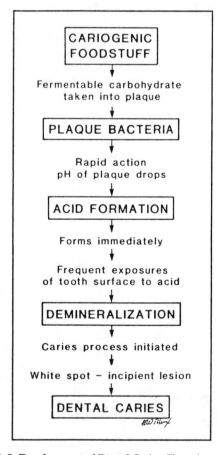

Figure 16–5. Development of Dental Caries. Flow chart shows the step-by-step action within the microbial plaque on the tooth surface.

B. Specific Microorganisms[8]

Bacterial plaque contains many acidogenic microorganisms, especially streptococci, which have been shown to be involved in the etiology of dental caries. *Streptococcus mutans* has particular cariogenic potential in the development of enamel caries. Table 16–3 shows the significant microorganisms in dental caries.

C. Cariogenic Foodstuff Source

1. Cariogenic foodstuff, particularly sucrose, enters the microbial plaque.
2. Acid-forming bacteria break down the sugar to an acid.
3. Acid on the tooth surface causes demineralization.
4. Frequent exposures to acid produce a carious lesion.

II. Contributing Factors

A. Time

Acid formation begins *immediately* when the sucrose from food is taken into the plaque.

B. The pH of the Plaque

The pH of the plaque is lowered promptly, and 1 to 2 hours are required for the pH to return to a normal level, assuming the plaque is left undisturbed.

1. Plaque pH before eating ranges from 6.2 to 7.0; it is lower in the caries susceptible person and higher in the caries-resistant person.
2. Immediately following sucrose intake into plaque, a rapid drop in the pH of the plaque occurs.[9,10]
3. Critical pH for enamel demineralization averages between 5.2 to 5.5, below which the enamel demineralizes.
4. The amount of demineralization depends on the length of time and the frequency with which the acid with a pH of 5.2 or below the critical pH is in contact with the tooth surface.

Table 16–3.   Significant Microorganisms in Dental Caries

Type of Caries	Etiologic Microorganism
Pit and fissure	*Streptococcus mutans* Lactobacillus
Smooth surface	*Streptococcus mutans*
Root surface	*Streptococcus mutans* *Actinomyces viscosus* *Actinomyces naeslundii* Other filamentous rods
Deep dentinal caries	Lactobacillus *Actinomyces naeslundii* Other filamentous rods
(From Newbrun, E.: *Cariology*, 3rd ed. Chicago, Quintessence, 1989.)	

C. Frequency of Carbohydrate Intake

With each meal or snack that contains sucrose, the pH of the plaque is lowered, provided the specific streptococci are present. Large amounts of sucrose eaten at mealtimes can be expected to be less cariogenic than small amounts eaten at frequent intervals during the day.[11] These and other related facts can be presented to the patient when the diet is discussed as a part of the basic instruction or as part of a total dental caries control program with dietary analysis (pages 382–389).

PERIODONTAL INFECTIONS

Bacterial plaque is unquestionably the single most important etiologic factor in most periodontal infections. The variations in clinical manifestations in different individuals can be accounted for by the differences in the bacterial activity within the plaque, as well as by the tissue response and resistance to the microorganisms and their products.

Table 16–4 lists significant microorganisms present in the bacterial plaque of the various periodontal infections. Total counts of microorganisms in diseased periodontal pockets are extremely high. Several hundreds of types exist. Morphologic varieties include cocci, rods, fusiforms, filaments, spirilla, and spirochetes (figure 16–1, page 235).

I. Initiation of Gingival Disease

Microorganisms of the bacterial plaque at the gingival margin multiply and extend beneath the margin. A high concentration of microorganisms is in contact with the sulcular epithelium. The irritation from the bacteria and their products leads to degeneration of the sulcular epithelium. Inflammation in the adjacent connective tissue results. The steps in the development of gingivitis and pocket formation are described on pages 181–182.

II. Experimental Gingivitis[4]

Gingivitis develops in 2 to 3 weeks when plaque is left undisturbed on the tooth surfaces. The microbiologic changes were outlined on page 239. Acute gingivitis is reversible, and when the gingiva are treated by plaque removal procedures, the gingiva returns to health within a few days.

An experimental gingivitis program to demon-

Table 16–4. Significant Microorganisms in Periodontal Health and Disease

Periodontal Condition	Bacterial and Immunologic Features	Bacterial Species
Periodontal Health	Gram-positive coccal and rod forms Few motile forms, few spirochetes	Streptococcus spp. Actinomyces spp.
Gingivitis	Gram-positive and gram-negative bacteria Few motile rods and spirochetes Total numbers 10 to 20 times those in healthy gingiva	Streptococcus spp. Actinomyces spp. Bacteroides spp. Fusobacterium spp. Veillonella spp. Treponema spp.
Necrotizing Ulcerative Gingivitis	Spirochetes invading tissue Gram-negative bacteria primarily	Treponema spp. Fusobacterium spp. *Bacteroides intermedius*
Juvenile Periodontitis	Subgingival: gram-negative, anaerobic bacteria Soft tissue invasion of gram-negative organisms in pocket wall Depressed neutrophil function (chemotaxis and phagocytosis)	*Actinobacillus actinomycetemcomitans* Capnocytophaga spp.
Rapidly Progressive Periodontitis	Gram-negative, anaerobic bacteria Depressed neutrophil function	*Actinobacillus actinomycetemcomitans* Bacteroides spp. Capnocytophaga spp.

Adult Periodontitis	Subgingival plaque: gram-negative, anaerobic, motile bacteria
	
	Complex flora: coccoid, spiral, and rod forms
		Bacteroides spp.:
		  B. gingivalis
		  B. intermedius
		Treponema spp.
		Actinomyces spp.
		Streptococcus spp.
		Fusobacterium nucleatum
		Eikenella corrodens
		Wolinella recta

strate the effect of plaque can be conducted as follows:

A. Observe and record characteristics of the healthy gingiva at the outset. Record a gingival index, a plaque index, and a bleeding index.

B. Withhold all plaque control procedures for a period of 3 weeks.

C. Repeat clinical observations of tissues and record indices at least weekly during the test period. Note initial evidence of gingivitis.

D. Reinstate plaque removal measures after 3 weeks. Make daily observations relative to gingival bleeding and indications that healing is taking place. In 1 week, repeat gingival and plaque indices.

III. Calculus Formation

Bacterial plaque forms a matrix for calculus formation (page 248). The significance of calculus in periodontal infections is described on page 251.

EFFECT OF DIET ON PLAQUE

I. Cariogenic Foods

A. Dental Caries

The relationship of the cariogenic food content of the diet and its frequency of use to the development of dental caries is well defined in research and clinical application. Dental caries initiation is outlined in figure 16–5.

B. Effect of Sucrose on Amount and pH of Plaque

When a cariogenic diet is used, plaque forms and grows more profusely.[12] Patients fed sucrose by stomach tube had a less acidogenic plaque than did patients who were fed sucrose by mouth.[13]

II. Food Intake

Food particles are not needed in the mouth for plaque to form. In one study, neither varying the number of meals nor feeding by stomach tube affected the development of plaque.[14] In another study, less plaque developed in a group of stomach-fed patients when compared with those fed by mouth.[13]

III. Texture of Diet

A. Mechanical Removal of Plaque

The friction of mastication has been shown to affect only the occlusal and incisal thirds of the crowns of teeth. Plaque on the gingival third collected in spite of a normal diet that included coarse bread and fresh fruit,[4] or chewing raw carrots 3 times daily as the only methods for personal care.[15] Chewing apples did not affect moderate amounts of plaque, but did tend to remove food debris in a group of 12-year-olds.[16]

B. Soft Diet

A soft diet tends to favor plaque accumulation. Although not well documented in the literature,

clinical experience has shown that the soft diet, especially one with excess fermentable carbohydrates, leads to excess plaque formation. In one experiment using dogs, more plaque developed when a soft diet was used.[17]

MATERIA ALBA

Materia alba is a loosely adherent mass of bacteria and cellular debris that frequently occurs on top of bacterial plaque.

Materia alba ("white material") distinguishes itself clinically as a bulky, soft deposit that is clearly visible without application of a disclosing agent. It is white, or grayish-white, and characteristically may resemble cottage cheese.

Materia alba forms over bacterial plaque. It is a product of informal accumulation of living and dead bacteria, desquamated epithelial cells, disintegrating leukocytes, salivary proteins, and particles of food debris.

Surface bacteria in contact with the gingiva contribute to gingival inflammation. Tooth surface demineralization and dental caries are seen frequently under materia alba.

Clinical distinction between materia alba, food debris, and bacterial plaque is necessary, but patient instruction for the removal of all three involves the same basic plaque control procedures. Materia alba can be removed with a water spray or oral irrigator, whereas bacterial plaque cannot.

FOOD DEBRIS

Loose food particles collect about the cervical third and proximal embrasures of the teeth.

When there are open contact areas, mobility of teeth, or irregularities of occlusion, such as plunger cusps, food may be forced between the teeth during mastication and vertical food impaction results. Horizontal or lateral food impaction occurs in facial and lingual embrasures, particularly when the interdental papillae are reduced or missing.

Food debris adds to a general unsanitary condition of the mouth. Cariogenic foods contribute to dental caries because liquified carbohydrate diffuses rapidly into the plaque and hence to the acid-forming bacteria.

Some self-cleansing through the action of the tongue, lips, saliva, and related factors takes place. Debris removal by toothbrushing, flossing, and other aids constitutes a total plaque control program. Cleansing of debris from about fixed prosthetic and orthodontic appliances is important to the plan for oral sanitation.

TECHNICAL HINTS

I. Check all surfaces of restorations and prosthetic appliances and remove rough areas and overhanging margins. Soft deposits accumulate on rough or irregular surfaces more rapidly and in greater quantity than on smooth surfaces.

II. Withhold the use of a disclosing agent until the intraoral mucosal and gingival examinations have been made. Coloring agents can disguise soft tissue changes and deviations from normal.

FACTORS TO TEACH THE PATIENT

I. Location, composition, and properties of bacterial plaque with emphasis on its role in dental caries and periodontal infections.

II. The cause and prevention of dental caries.

III. Effects of personal oral care procedures in the prevention of bacterial plaque and materia alba.

IV. Plaque control procedures with special adaptations for individual needs.

V. Sources of cariogenic foodstuff in the diet with suggestions for control.

VI. Relationship of frequency of eating cariogenic foods to dental caries.

References

1. Schroeder, H.E.: *Formation and Inhibition of Dental Calculus.* Vienna, Hans Huber, 1969, pp. 14–15.
2. Meckel, A.H.: Formation and Properties of Organic Films on Teeth, *Arch. Oral Biol., 10,* 585, July-August, 1965.
3. Meckel, A.H.: The Nature and Importance of Organic Deposits on Dental Enamel, *Caries Res., 2,* 104, Number 2, 1968.
4. Löe, H., Theilade, E., and Jensen, S.B.: Experimental Gingivitis in Man, *J. Periodontol., 36,* 177, May-June, 1965.
5. Årtun, J. and Osterberg, S.K.: Periodontal Status of Secondary Crowded Mandibular Incisors. Long-term Results After Orthodontic Treatment, *J. Clin. Periodontol., 14,* 261, May, 1987.
6. Mandel, I.D.: Relation of Saliva and Plaque to Caries, *J. Dent. Res., 53,* 246, March-April, 1974, Supplement.
7. Grøn, P., Yao, K., and Spinelli, M.: A Study of Inorganic Constituents in Dental Plaque, *J. Dent. Res., 48,* 799, September-October, 1969.
8. Newbrun, E.: *Cariology,* 3rd ed. Chicago, Quintessence, 1989.
9. Stephan, R.M.: Intra-oral Hydrogen-Ion Concentrations Associated with Dental Caries Activity, *J. Dent. Res., 23,* 257, August, 1944.
10. Rosen, S. and Weisenstein, P.R.: The Effect of Sugar Solutions on pH of Dental Plaques from Caries-Susceptible and Caries-free Individuals, *J. Dent. Res., 44,* 845, September-October, 1965.
11. Gustafsson, B.E., Quensel, C.E., Lanke, L.S., Lundquist, C., Grahnén, H., Bonow, B.E., and Krasse, B.: The Vipeholm Dental Caries Study. The Effect of Different Levels of Carbohydrate Intake on Caries Activity in 436 Individuals Observed for Five Years, *Acta Odontol. Scand., 11,* 232, Number 3–4, 1954.
12. Carlsson, J. and Egelberg, J.: Effect of Diet on Early Plaque Formation in Man, *Odont. Revy, 16,* 112, Number 1, 1965.
13. Littleton, N.W., Carter, C.H., and Kelley, R.T.: Studies of Oral Health in Persons Nourished by Stomach Tube. I. Changes in pH of Plaque Material after the Addition of Sucrose, *J. Am. Dent. Assoc., 74,* 119, January, 1967.
14. Egelberg, J.: Local Effect of Diet on Plaque Formation and Development of Gingivitis in Dogs. III. Effect of Frequency of Meals and Tube Feeding, *Odont. Revy, 16,* 50, Number 1, 1965.
15. Lindhe, J. and Wicén, P-O.: The Effects on the Gingivae of Chewing Fibrous Foods, *J. Periodont. Res., 4,* 193, Number 3, 1969.
16. Birkeland, J.M. and Jorkjend, L.: The Effect of Chewing Apples on Dental Plaque and Food Debris, *Community Dent. Oral Epidemiol., 2,* 161, Number 4, 1974.
17. Egelberg, J.: Local Effect of Diet on Plaque Formation and Development of Gingivitis in Dogs. I. Effect of Hard and Soft Diets, *Odont. Revy, 16,* 31, Number 1, 1965.

Suggested Readings

Abbas, D.K., Skjørland, K.K., Gjermo, P., and Sønyu, T.: Chemical and Morphological Studies of the Acquired Pellicle Formed Subgingivally on Dentin *in vivo, Acta Odontol. Scand., 43,* 31, March, 1985.

Alaluusua, S. and Renkonen, O.-V.: *Streptococcus mutans* Establishment and Dental Caries Experience in Children from 2 to 4 Years Old, *Scand. J. Dent. Res., 91,* 453, December, 1983.

Beltrami, M., Bickel, M., and Baehni, P.C.: The Effect of Supragingival Plaque Control on the Composition of the Subgingival Microflora in Human Periodontitis, *J. Clin. Periodontol., 14,* 161, March, 1987.

Brecx, M., Theilade, J., and Attström, R.: Influence of Optimal and Excluded Oral Hygiene on Early Formation of Dental Plaque on Plastic Films. A Quantitative and Descriptive Light and Electron Microscopic Study, *J. Clin. Periodontol., 7,* 361, October, 1980.

Carranza, F.A.: *Glickman's Clinical Periodontology,* 6th ed. Philadelphia, W.B. Saunders Co., 1984, pp. 361–390.

Emilson, C.-G. and Krasse, B.: Support for and Implications of the Specific Plaque Hypothesis, *Scand. J. Dent. Res., 93,* 96, April, 1985.

Fure, S., Romaniec, M., Emilson, C.G., and Krasse, B.: Proportions of *Streptococcus mutans,* Lactobacilli and Actinomyces spp. in Root Surface Plaque, *Scand. J. Dent. Res., 95,* 119, April, 1987.

Gibbons, R.J. and van Houte, J.: On the Formation of Dental Plaques, *J. Periodontol., 44,* 347, June, 1973.

Goh, C.J.W., Waite, I.M., Groves, B.J., and Cornick, D.E.R.: The Influence of Gingival Inflammation and Pocketing on the Rate of Plaque Formation During Non-surgical Periodontal Treatment, *Br. Dent. J., 161,* 165, September 6, 1986.

Grant, D.A., Stern, I.B., and Listgarten, M.A., eds.: *Periodontics,* 6th ed. St. Louis, The C.V. Mosby Co., 1988, pp. 150–197.

Greenlee, J.S.: Microbiology and Prevention of Disease Transmission, in Darby, M.L. and Bushee, E.J., eds.: *Mosby's Comprehensive Review of Dental Hygiene.* St. Louis, The C.V. Mosby Co., 1986, pp. 269–276.

Greenstein, G. and Polson, A.: Microscopic Monitoring of Pathogens Associated With Periodontal Diseases. A Review, *J. Periodontol., 56,* 740, December, 1985.

Harris, N.O.: The Life Cycle of the Dental Plaque: From Acquired Pellicle to Dental Plaque, to Calculus Formation, in Harris, N.O. and Christen, A.G.: *Primary Preventive Dentistry,* 2nd ed. Norwalk, Connecticut, Appleton & Lange, 1987, pp. 19–35.

Hayes, M.L., Carter, E.C., and Griffiths, S.J.: The Acidogenic Microbial Composition of Dental Plaque from Caries-free and Caries-prone People, *Arch. Oral Biol., 28,* 381, Number 5, 1983.

Holm-Pedersen, P., Folke, L.E.A., and Gawronski, T.H.: Composition and Metabolic Activity of Dental Plaque From Healthy Young and Elderly Individuals, *J. Dent. Res., 59,* 771, May, 1980.

Kornman, K.: The Microbiologic Etiology of Periodontal Disease, *Compend. Contin. Educ. Dent.,* Supplement 7, S173, 1986.

Liakoni, H., Barber, P.M., and Newman, H.N.: Bacterial Penetration of the Pocket Tissues in Juvenile/Postjuvenile Periodontitis After the Presurgical Oral Hygiene Phase, *J. Periodontol., 58,* 847, December, 1987.

Listgarten, M.A. and Levin, S.: Positive Correlation Between the Proportions of Subgingival Spirochetes and Motile Bacteria and Susceptibility of Human Subjects to Periodontal Deterioration, *J. Clin. Periodontol., 8,* 122, April, 1981.

Loesche, W.J., Syed, S.A., Schmidt, E., and Morrison, E.C.: Bacterial Profiles of Subgingival Plaques in Periodontitis, *J. Periodontol., 56,* 447, August, 1985.

Maetani, T., Miyoshi, R., Nahara, Y., Kawazoe, Y., and Hamada,

T.: Plaque Accumulation on Teflon-coated Metal, *J. Prosthet. Dent., 51,* 353, March, 1984.

Matsson, L. and Goldberg, P.: Gingival Inflammatory Reaction in Children at Different Ages, *J. Clin. Periodontol., 12,* 98, February, 1985.

Müller, H.-P. and Flores de Jacoby, L.: Distribution of Morphologically Different Micro-organisms Associated with Active Periodontal Lesions, *J. Clin. Periodontol., 14,* 110, February, 1987.

Newman, H.N.: Update on Plaque and Periodontal Disease, *J. Clin. Periodontol., 7,* 251, August, 1980.

Saglie, F.R., Pertuiset, J.H., Rezende, M.T., Sabet, M.S., Raoufi, D., and Carranza, F.A.: Bacterial Invasion in Experimental Gingivitis in Man, *J. Periodontol., 58,* 837, December, 1987.

Savitt, E.D. and Socransky, S.S.: Distribution of Certain Subgingival Microbial Species in Selected Periodontal Conditions, *J. Periodont. Res., 19,* 111, March, 1984.

Schachtele, C.F. and Jensen, M.E.: Comparison of Methods for Monitoring Changes in the pH of Human Dental Plaque, *J. Dent. Res., 61,* 1117, October, 1982.

Slots, J. and Dahlén, G.: Subgingival Microorganisms and Bacterial Virulence Factors in Periodontitis, *Scand. J. Dent. Res., 93,* 120, April, 1985.

Smith, Q.T.: Acquired Pellicle: A Mediator of Enamel Demineralization and Remineralization, *Northwest Dent., 59,* 152, May-June, 1980.

Tabita, P.V., Bissada, N.F., and Maybury, J.E.: Effectiveness of Supragingival Plaque Control on the Development of Subgingival Plaque and Gingival Inflammation in Patients with Moderate Pocket Depth, *J. Periodontol., 52,* 88, February, 1981.

Takazoe, I., Nakamura, T., and Okuda, K.: Colonization of the Subgingival Area by *Bacteroides gingivalis, J. Dent. Res., 63,* 422, March, 1984.

Theilade, E. and Theilade, J.: Formation and Ecology of Plaque at Different Locations in the Mouth, *Scand. J. Dent. Res., 93,* 90, April, 1985.

van Houte, J.: Bacterial Specificity in the Etiology of Dental Caries, *Int. Dent. J., 30,* 305, December, 1980.

van Houte, J., Aasenden, R., and Peebles, T.C.: Lactobacilli in Human Dental Plaque and Saliva, *J. Dent. Res., 60,* 2, January, 1981.

van Palenstein Helderman, W.H.: Microbial Etiology of Periodontal Disease. *J. Clin. Periodontol., 8,* 261, August, 1981.

Waerhaug, J.: Effect of Toothbrushing on Subgingival Plaque Formation, *J. Periodontol., 52,* 30, January, 1981.

Walker, C.B., Gordon, J.M., and Socransky, S.S.: Antibiotic Susceptibility Testing of Subgingival Plaque Samples, *J. Clin. Periodontol., 10,* 422, July, 1983.

Wikner, S.: Short Term Effect of Mechanical Plaque Control on Salivary Concentration of *S. mutans* and Lactobacilli, *Scand. J. Dent. Res., 94,* 320, August, 1986.

Wilson, R.F., Woods, A., and Ashley, F.P.: Dark-field Microscopy of Dental Plaque. A Clinical and Laboratory Evaluation, *Br. Dent. J., 159,* 114, August 24, 1985.

Winkel, E.G., Abbas, F., van der Velden, U., Vroom, T.M., Scholte, G., and Hart, A.A.M.: Experimental Gingivitis in Relation to Age in Individuals Not Susceptible to Periodontal Destruction, *J. Clin. Periodont., 14,* 499, October, 1987.

Wojeicki, C.J., Harper, D.S., and Robinson, P.J.: Differences in Periodontal Disease-associated Microorganisms of Subgingival Plaque in Prepubertal, Pubertal, and Postpubertal Children, *J. Periodontol., 58,* 219, April, 1987.

17 *Dental Calculus*

Dental calculus, which is mineralized bacterial plaque, is a hard, tenacious mass that forms on the clinical crowns of the natural teeth and on dentures and other dental appliances. It forms as a *result* of periodontal infection and is covered with a layer of bacterial plaque.

Calculus is significant in the progression of inflammatory periodontal disease. The rough surface of the calculus holds the disease-producing bacteria close to the gingival tissue and perpetuates the inflamed state.

The control of plaque deposits by the patient, supplemented by complete calculus removal, can reduce or eliminate gingival inflammation. A relationship exists between the amount of plaque and calculus on the teeth and the severity of most gingival and periodontal infections.

Comprehensive understanding of the characteristics, origin, development, and methods of prevention of calculus is essential to patient examination, evaluation, treatment, and instruction. For successful treatment and prevention, the patient needs to know the interrelationship between plaque, calculus, and oral health, the need for complete removal of calculus, and the reasons for the painstaking manner in which scaling procedures must be carried out.

I. Classification and Distribution

Dental calculus is classified by its location on a tooth surface as related to the adjacent free gingival margin, that is, supragingival and subgingival (figure 17–1).

A. Supragingival Calculus
1. *Location.* On the clinical crown above the margin of the gingiva.
2. *Distribution*
   a. Most frequent sites: on the lingual surfaces of mandibular anterior teeth and the facial surfaces of maxillary first and second molars, opposite the openings of the ducts of the salivary glands.
   b. Crowns of teeth out of occlusion; nonfunctioning teeth; or teeth that are neglected during daily plaque removal (toothbrushing, flossing, or other personal care).
   c. Surfaces of dentures and dental appliances.
3. *Other Names for Supragingival Calculus*

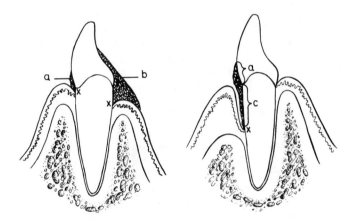

Figure 17–1. Dental Calculus. a. Supragingival calculus on cervical third of a mandibular anterior tooth. **b.** Supragingival calculus over crown, exposed root surface, and the margin of the gingiva. **c.** Subgingival calculus along root to the bottom of a periodontal pocket. **x.** Bottom of pocket.

   a. Supramarginal*
   b. Extragingival
   c. Coronal: indicating that the calculus is on the anatomic crown.
   d. Salivary: a term that indicates that the source of the minerals is the saliva.

B. Subgingival Calculus
1. *Location.* On the clinical crown beneath the margin of the gingiva. It extends nearly to the bottom of the pocket. As the pocket is deepened by disease, calculus forms on the exposed root surface.
2. *Distribution*
   a. May be generalized or localized on single teeth or a group of teeth.
   b. Proximal surfaces have heaviest deposits.
3. *Other Names for Subgingival Calculus*
   a. Submarginal
   b. Serumal: term that indicates the source of the minerals is the blood serum.

II. Occurrence

A. Age
Calculus occurs at any age and on both permanent and primary teeth. Incidence increases

---

*The terms supra- and subgingival are at present probably the most widely used. Supra- and submarginal are more specific in their definition because the margin of the free gingiva is the dividing line between the two categories. The gingiva includes free and attached.

with age, and in some populations, 100 percent of the people over 30 have calculus, usually because of continuing accumulation, not an increased tendency to form new deposits as age advances.

B. Calculus in Children

In a survey of children ages 9 to 14, 56 to 85 percent had supragingival and 30 to 67 percent had subgingival calculus in the various age, sex, and racial–ethnic groups measured.[1] In another study in normal children, 9 percent of ages 4 to 6, 18 percent of ages 7 to 9, and 43 percent of ages 10 to 15 had calculus. In a group of children ages 10 to 15 with cystic fibrosis, 90 percent had calculus, and in a group of the same age with asthma, 100 percent had calculus.[2]

III. Clinical Characteristics

A. Appearance and Consistency

Identification of calculus prior to removal depends on knowledge of its appearance, consistency, and distribution. Appointment planning, selection of instruments, and techniques depend on understanding the texture, morphology, and mode of attachment of calculus. Table 17–1 provides a summary of clinical characteristics.

B. Supragingival Examination

1. *Direct Examination.* Supragingival deposits may be seen directly or indirectly, using a mouth mirror.
2. *Use of Compressed Air.* Small amounts of calculus that have not been stained are frequently invisible when they are wet with saliva. With a combination of retraction, light, and drying with air, small deposits usually can be seen. An explorer may be used when visual examination is not definite (page 204).

C. Subgingival Examination

1. *Visual Examination.* Of calculus within a pocket
   a. Dark edge of calculus may be seen at or just beneath the margin.
   b. Diseased gingival margin does not adapt closely to a tooth surface, thus permitting a view into the pocket where calculus can be seen.
   c. Gentle air blast can deflect the margin from the tooth for observation into the pocket.
   d. Transillumination: when light shines through anterior teeth, a dark opaque shadow-like area seen on a proximal tooth surface could be subgingival calculus. Supragingival calculus may also be found by this method. Without calculus, stain, or thick, soft deposit, the enamel is translucent.
2. *Gingival Tissue Color Change.* Dark calculus may reflect through a thin margin and suggest the presence of subgingival calculus.

3. *Tactile Examination*
   a. Probe. While probing for sulcus/pocket characteristics, a rough subgingival tooth surface can be felt when calculus is present. Although there are other causes for roughness, subgingival calculus is the most common (page 183).
   b. Explorer. A fine subgingival explorer is needed that can be adapted close to the root surface all the way to the bottom of a pocket. Each subgingival area must be examined carefully to the bottom of the pocket, completely around each tooth.

D. Clinical Record

Calculus deposits are described in the examination record. The location of supra- and subgingival deposits and their extent (slight, moderate, or heavy) must be designated. A calculus index may be useful for patient evaluation and counseling at continuing maintenance appointments (page 277).

The calculus record is included with the complete charting and oral examination, page 286.

CALCULUS FORMATION[4]

Subgingival calculus does not develop by direct extension from supragingival calculus. First, subgingival bacterial plaque forms by extension of supragingival plaque. Each plaque mineralizes separately.

Calculus results from the deposition of minerals into a plaque organic matrix. Calculus formation occurs in three basic steps: *pellicle formation, plaque formation,* and *mineralization.* Mineralization of supra- and subgingival calculus is essentially the same, although the source of the elements for mineralization is not the same.

I. Pellicle Formation

The formation and characteristics of pellicle were described on page 236. The pellicle, or cuticle, is composed of mucoproteins from the saliva and is an acellular material. Its thickness and contour vary on the tooth surface. It begins to form within minutes after all deposits have been removed from the tooth surface.

II. Plaque Maturation

A. Microorganisms settle in the pellicle layer.
B. Colonies are formed. Originally, the colonies consist primarily of cocci and rod-shaped organisms. By the fifth day, the plaque is mostly made up of filamentous organisms.
C. The colonies grow together to form a cohesive plaque layer (figure 16–2, page 237).

III. Mineralization

A. Mineralization Foci (Centers) Form

Within 24 to 72 hours, more and more mineralization centers develop close to the under-

Table 17–1. Clinical Characteristics of Dental Calculus

Characteristic	Supragingival Calculus	Subgingival Calculus
Color	White, creamy-yellow, or gray May be stained by tobacco, food, or other pigments Slight deposits may be invisible until dried with compressed air	Light to dark brown, dark green, or black Stains derived from blood pigments from diseased pocket
Shape	Amorphous, bulky Gross deposits may (1) Form interproximal bridge between adjacent teeth (2) Extend over the margin of the gingiva Shape of calculus mass is determined by the anatomy of the teeth, contour of gingival margin, and pressure of the tongue, lips, cheeks	Flattened to conform with pressure from the pocket wall Combinations of the following calculus formations occur:[3] (1) Crusty, spiny, or nodular (2) Ledge or ring-like formations (3) Thin, smooth veneers (4) Finger- and fern-like formations (5) Individual calculus islands
Consistency and Texture	Moderately hard Newer deposits less dense and hard Porous Surface covered with non-mineralized plaque	Brittle, flint-like Harder and more dense than supragingival calculus Newest deposits near bottom of pocket are less dense and hard Surface covered with plaque
Size and Quantity	Quantity has direct relationship to (1) Personal oral care procedures and plaque control measures (2) Physical character of diet (3) Individual tendencies (4) Function and use Increased amount in tobacco smokers	Related to pocket depth Increased amount with age because of accumulation Quantity is related to personal care, diet, and individual tendency as it is with supragingival. Subgingival is primarily related to the development and progression of periodontal disease
Distribution on Individual Tooth	Above margin of gingiva May cover a large portion of the visible clinical crown, or may form fine thin line near gingival margin	Below margin of gingiva Extends to bottom of the pocket and follows contour of soft tissue attachment With gingival recession, subgingival calculus may become supragingival and become covered with typical supragingival calculus
Distribution on Teeth	Symmetrical arrangement on teeth except when influenced by (1) Malpositioned teeth (2) Unilateral hypofunction (3) Inconsistent personal care (4) Abrasion from food Occurs with or without associated subgingival deposits Location related to openings of the salivary gland ducts: (1) Facial of maxillary molars (2) Lingual mandibular anterior teeth	May be generalized or localized on a few teeth Heaviest on proximal surfaces, lightest on facial surfaces Occurs with or without associated supragingival deposits

lying tooth surface. Eventually, the centers grow large enough to touch and unite.

B. Organic Matrix

Mineralization first occurs within the inter-microbial matrix. The filamentous microorganisms provide the matrix for the deposition of minerals.

A calculus-like deposit has been observed on the teeth of germ-free animals that have no bacterial plaque.[5,6,7] It may indicate that other organic substances such as the pellicle may mineralize.

C. Sources of Minerals

1. *Supragingival Calculus.* The source of elements for supragingival calculus is the saliva.
2. *Subgingival Calculus.* The gingival sulcus fluid and the inflammatory exudate supply the minerals for the subgingival deposits. Gingival sulcus fluid was described on page 168. Because the amount of sulcus fluid and exudate increases with increases in inflammation, more minerals are available for mineralization of subgingival plaque.

D. Crystal Formation

Mineralization consists of crystal formation, namely, hydroxyapatite, octocalcium phosphate, whitlockite, and brushite, each with a characteristic developmental pattern. The crystals form in the intercellular matrix and on the surface of bacteria, and finally within the bacteria.[8,9,10]

E. Mechanism of Mineralization

The mineralization process is considered the same for both supra- and subgingival calculus.

The process by which minerals, mainly calcium and phosphate, become incorporated from the saliva or gingival sulcus fluid into the plaque matrix is still not completely understood.

Current research studies point to the probability that calcification of calculus may involve the same phenomena as other ectopic calcifications (such as urinary or renal calculi) and with similarities to normal calcification of bone, cartilage, enamel, or dentin. For those wishing to read about this complex subject, a list of references is provided in the *Suggested Readings* at the end of this chapter.

IV. Formation Time

Formation time means the average number of days required for the primary soft deposit to change to the mature mineralized stage. The average time is about 12 days, with a range from 10 days for rapid calculus formers to 20 days for slow calculus formers.[11] Mineralization can begin as early as 24 to 48 hours.

Formation time depends on individual tendency, but it is strongly influenced by the roughness of the tooth surface, and the care and character of personal plaque control measures. Determination of the ap-proximate formation time for an individual is important to instruction and counseling, as well as treatment planning for professional care and frequency of maintenance appointments.

V. Structure of Calculus

A. Layers

Calculus forms in layers that are more or less parallel with the tooth surface. The layers are separated by a line that appears to be a pellicle that was deposited over the previously formed calculus, and, as mineralization progressed, the pellicle became imbedded.

The lines between the layers of calculus can be called incremental lines. They form around the tooth in supragingival calculus, but irregularly from crown to apex on the root surface in subgingival calculus. The lines are evidence that calculus grows or increases by apposition of new layers.

B. Surface

The surface of a calculus mass is rough and can be detected by use of an explorer. As observed by electron microscope, the surface roughness appears as peaks, valleys, and pits.

C. Outer Layer

The outer layer is partly calcified. On the surface is a thick, mat-like soft layer of plaque and/or materia alba. It is the outer surface of the plaque on the subgingival calculus that is in contact with the diseased pocket epithelium.

VI. Attachment of Calculus

Calculus is more readily removed from some tooth surfaces than from others. The ease or difficulty of removal can be related to the manner of attachment of the calculus to the tooth surface.

Several modes of attachment have been observed by conventional histologic techniques and by electron microscopy. On any one tooth and in any one area, more than one mode of attachment may be found.

When studying the attachment types, the character of the hard, smooth enamel surface, and the rough, porous, cemental surface should be considered. Three general modes of attachment can be identified.[12]

A. Attachment by Means of an Acquired Pellicle or Cuticle

1. The pellicle is a thin, acellular, homogeneous layer positioned between the calculus and the tooth surface.
2. Calculus attachment is superficial because no interlocking or penetration occurs.
3. Pellicle attachment occurs most frequently on enamel and newly scaled and planed root surfaces.
4. Calculus may be removed readily because of the smooth attachment.

B. Attachment to Minute Irregularities in the Tooth Surface by Mechanical Locking into Undercuts
1. Enamel irregularities include cracks, lamellae, and carious defects.
2. Cemental irregularities include tiny spaces left at previous locations of Sharpey's fibers, resorption lacunae, scaling grooves, cemental tears or fragmentation.
3. Difficult to be certain all calculus is removed when it is attached by this method.

C. Attachment by Direct Contact Between Calcified Intercellular Matrix and the Tooth Surface
1. Interlocking of inorganic crystals of the tooth with the mineralizing bacterial plaque.
2. Distinction between calculus and cementum is difficult during root planing.

VII. Composition

Calculus is made up of inorganic and organic components and water. Although the percentage varies depending on the age and hardness of a deposit and the location from which the sample for analysis is taken, mature calculus usually contains between 75 and 85 percent inorganic components; the rest is organic components and water. The chemical content of supra- and subgingival calculus is similar.[13,14,15]

A. Inorganic
1. *Inorganic Components.* The components are mainly salts of calcium, primarily calcium phosphate, with small amounts of magnesium phosphate and calcium carbonate.
2. *Trace Elements.* Various trace elements have been identified, including sodium (Na), chlorine (Cl), zinc (Zn), strontium (Sr), bromine (Br), copper (Cu), manganese (Mn), tungsten (W), gold (Au), aluminum (Al), silicon (Si), iron (Fe), and fluorine (Fl).[16]
3. *Fluoride in Calculus*
   a. Concentration. The concentration of fluoride in calculus varies and is influenced by the amount of fluoride received from fluoride in the drinking water, topical application,[17] dentifrices,[18,19] or any form that is received by contact with the external surface of the calculus.
   b. Uptake. The surface of the cementum, which is more permeable, has a much higher content of fluoride than the enamel surface.

      Supragingival calculus has a much higher fluoride concentration than subgingival calculus, and supragingival calculus can have a higher fluoride content than the enamel surface,[20] because the calculus would be more porous than the enamel.
4. *Crystals.* At least two thirds of the inorganic matter of calculus is crystalline, principally apatite. Predominating is hydroxyapatite, which is the same crystal present in enamel,

dentin, cementum, and bone. Calculus also contains varying amounts of brushite, whitlockite, and octocalcium phosphate.[21]
5. *Calculus Compared with Teeth and Bone.* Dental enamel is the most highly calcified tissue in the body and contains 96 percent inorganic salts as compared with dentin, 65 percent, and cementum and bone at 45 to 50 percent.[22] Mature calculus has approximately 75 to 85 percent inorganic content. A comparison of calculus with the tooth parts provides insight into the effects of instrumentation, the difficulty of distinguishing calculus from cementum or dentin when scaling subgingivally, and the modes of attachment of calculus to the tooth surface.

B. Organic

The organic portion of calculus consists of various types of nonvital microorganisms, desquamated epithelial cells, leukocytes, and mucin from the saliva. Substances identified in the organic matrix include cholesterol, cholesterol esters, phospholipids, and fatty acids in the lipid fraction; reducing sugars and carbohydrate-protein complexes in the carbohydrate fraction; and keratins, nucleoproteins, and amino acids in the protein portion.[23,24]

The microorganisms are predominantly filamentous. In early calculus, during the first 5 days, cocci are found with some rods.[23,25] Most of the organisms within calculus are considered nonviable. The plaque on the calculus surface contains viable organisms.

SIGNIFICANCE OF DENTAL CALCULUS

Calculus has long been considered to have an important role in the development, promotion, and recurrence of gingival and periodontal infections.

Significant to the rationale for calculus removal and the production of a smooth tooth surface are the points listed here concerning the relationship of calculus to periodontal and gingival diseases.

I. Relation to Plaque

A. Calculus is mineralized plaque. Therefore, calculus prevention depends on plaque prevention.
B. Calculus has a rough surface and provides a haven for plaque collection on its surface.

II. Relation to Pocket

A. Subgingival calculus is always covered by active plaque that is in direct contact with the pocket epithelium. Plaque bacteria initiate gingivitis and periodontitis.
B. Subgingival calculus forms as a result of the calcification of the plaque on the subgingival tooth surface. Therefore, subgingival calculus is secondary to plaque, and its formation is secondary

to pocket formation. Subgingival calculus is a *result* of pocket formation, not a cause.

C. With the perpetuation of inflammation in the pocket wall by the plaque on the calculus surface, the secretion of gingival sulcus fluid is promoted and increased. With more fluid come more minerals for calculus formation.

III. Relation to Disease Control Techniques and Scaling

A. Plaque over a rough calculus surface is much more difficult to remove by toothbrushing, flossing, or other disease control procedures than from a smooth surface. The proximal surface calculus may tear and shred dental floss as it is passed over and under the deposit.

B. Removal and prevention of calculus provides a smooth tooth surface that is easier for the patient to keep clean by toothbrushing and flossing, and that is resistant to plaque retention.

IV. Permeability of Calculus

With its rough surface and permeable structure, calculus can act as a reservoir for toxic microbial and tissue breakdown products. In a pocket, calculus holds the toxic products adjacent to the pocket lining, and inflammation can persist.

V. Drainage from Diseased Pocket

Calculus can reduce drainage from the pocket by helping to trap bacteria and debris. Healing is prevented and the advancement of disease is encouraged. Gingival abscess formation may result (pages 485–486).

FACTORS TO TEACH THE PATIENT

I. What calculus is and how it forms from bacterial plaque.

II. The effect of calculus on the health of the periodontal tissues and, therefore, on the general health of the oral cavity.

III. Properties of calculus that explain the need for detailed, meticulous scaling procedures.

IV. Reasons for producing a smooth tooth surface during scaling and planing.

V. Plaque control measures that the patient may carry out to minimize calculus deposits.

References

1. Suomi, J.D., Smith, L.W., McClendon, B.J., Spolsky, V.W., and Horowitz, H.S.: Oral Calculus in Children, *J. Periodontol., 42,* 341, June, 1971.

2. Wotman, S., Mercadante, J., Mandel, I.D., Goldman, R.S., and Denning, C.: The Occurrence of Calculus in Normal Children, Children with Cystic Fibrosis, and Children with Asthma, *J. Periodontol., 44,* 278, May, 1973.

3. Everett, F.G. and Potter, G.R.: Morphology of Submarginal Calculus, *J. Periodontol., 30,* 27, January, 1959.

4. Mandel, I.D.: Calculus Formation and Prevention: An Overview, *Compend. Contin. Educ. Dent., 8,* S235, Supplement Number 8, 1987.

5. Fitzgerald, R.J. and McDaniel, E.G.: Dental Calculus in the Germ-free Rat, *Arch. Oral Biol., 2,* 239, August, 1960.

6. Gustafsson, B.E. and Krasse, B.: Dental Calculus in Germfree Rats, *Acta Odontol. Scand., 20,* 135, Number 2, 1962.

7. Theilade, J., Fitzgerald, R.J., Scott, D.B., and Nylen, M.U.: Electron Microscopic Observations of Dental Calculus in Germfree and Conventional Rats, *Arch. Oral Biol., 9,* 97, January-February, 1964.

8. Gonzales, F. and Sognnaes, R.F.: Electron Microscopy of Dental Calculus, *Science, 131,* 156, January 15, 1960.

9. Zander, H.A., Hazen, S.P., and Scott, D.B.: Mineralization of Dental Calculus, *Proc. Soc. Exp. Biol. and Med., 103,* 257, February, 1960.

10. McMillan, L., Hutchinson, A.C.W., and Fosdick, L.S.: Electron Microscopic Study of Dental Calculus, *Dental Prog., 1,* 188, April, 1961.

11. Schroeder, H.E.: *Formation and Inhibition of Dental Calculus.* Vienna, Hans Huber Publishers, 1969, pp. 73–74.

12. Canis, M.F., Kramer, G.M., and Pameijer, C.M.: Calculus Attachment. Review of the Literature and New Findings, *J. Periodontol., 50,* 406, August, 1979.

13. Mandel, I.D.: Biochemical Aspects of Calculus Formation, *J. Periodont. Res., 9,* 10, Number 1, 1974.

14. Glock, G.E. and Murray, M.M.: Chemical Investigation of Salivary Calculus, *J. Dent. Res., 17,* 257, August, 1938.

15. Mandel, I.D. and Levy, B.M.: Studies on Salivary Calculus. I. Histochemical and Chemical Investigations of Supra- and Subgingival Calculus, *Oral Surg., 10,* 874, August, 1957.

16. Mukherjee, S.: Formation and Prevention of Supra-Gingival Calculus, *J. Periodont. Res.,* Supplementum 2, 1968, pp. 1–35.

17. Schait, A. and Mühlemann, H.R.: Fluoride Uptake by Calculus Following Topical Application of Fluorides, *Helv. Odont. Acta, 15,* 132, October, 1971.

18. Kinoshita, S., Schait, A., Schroeder, H.E., and Mühlemann, H.R.: Origin of Fluoride in Early Dental Calculus, *Helv. Odont. Acta, 9,* 141, October, 1965.

19. Mühlemann, H.R., Schait, A., and Schroeder, H.E.: Salivary Origin of Fluorine in Calcified Dental Plaques, *Helv. Odont. Acta, 8,* 128, October, 1964.

20. Yardeni, J., Gedalia, I., and Kohn, M.: Fluoride Concentration of Dental Calculus, Surface Enamel, and Cementum, *Arch. Oral Biol., 8,* 697, November-December, 1963.

21. Grøn, P., van Campen, G.J., and Lindstrom, I.: Human Dental Calculus. Inorganic Chemical and Crystallographic Composition, *Arch. Oral Biol., 12,* 829, July, 1967.

22. Bhaskar, S.N., ed.: *Orban's Oral Histology and Embryology,* 10th ed. St. Louis, The C.V. Mosby Co., 1986, pp. 46, 101, 175.

23. Mandel, I.D., Levy, B.M., and Wasserman, B.H.: Histochemistry of Calculus Formation, *J. Periodontol., 28,* 132, April, 1957.

24. Mandel, I.D.: Histochemical and Biochemical Aspects of Calculus Formation, *Periodontics, 1,* 43, March-April, 1963.

25. Turesky, S., Renstrup, G., and Glickman, I.: Histologic and Histochemical Observations Regarding Early Calculus Formation in Children and Adults, *J. Periodontol., 32,* 7, January, 1961.

Suggested Readings

Epstein, S.R., Mandel, I., and Scopp, I.W.: Salivary Composition and Calculus Formation in Patients Undergoing Hemodialysis, *J. Periodontol., 51,* 336, June, 1980.

Friskopp, J.: Ultrastructure of Nondecalcified Supragingival Calculus, *J. Periodontol., 54,* 542, September, 1983.

Friskopp, J. and Hammarström, L.: A Comparative, Scanning Electron Microscopic Study of Supragingival and Subgingival Calculus, *J. Periodontol., 51,* 553, October, 1980.

Friskopp, J. and Isacsson, G.: A Quantitative Microradiographic Study of Mineral Content of Supragingival and Subgingival Dental Calculus, *Scand. J. Dent. Res., 92,* 25, February, 1984.

Mandel, I.D. and Gaffar, A.: Calculus Revisited. A Review, *J. Clin. Periodontol., 13,* 249, April, 1986.

Calculus Formation and Mineralization

Allen, D.L., McFall, W.T., and Jenzano, J.W.: *Periodontics for the Dental Hygienist,* 4th ed. Philadelphia, Lea & Febiger, 1987, pp. 42–44.

Carranza, F.A.: *Glickman's Clinical Periodontology,* 6th ed. Philadelphia, W.B. Saunders Co., 1984, pp. 402–404.

Grant, D.A., Stern, I.B., and Listgarten, M.A., eds.: *Periodontics,* 6th ed. St. Louis, The C.V. Mosby Co., 1988, pp. 198–215.

Jenkins, G.N.: *The Physiology and Biochemistry of the Mouth,* 4th ed. Philadelphia, J.B. Lippincott Co., 1978, pp. 403–409.

Leung, S.W.: Calculus Formation. Salivary Factors, *Dent. Clin. North Am.,* p. 723, November, 1960.

Lindhe, J.: *Textbook of Clinical Periodontology.* Philadelphia, W.B. Saunders Co., 1985, pp. 110–117.

Mandel, I.D.: Calculus Formation and Prevention: An Overview, *Compend. Contin. Educ. Dent., 8,* S235, Supplement Number 8, 1987.

Mukherjee, S.: Formation and Prevention of Supra-gingival Calculus, *J. Periodont. Res.,* Supplementum 2, 1968, pp. 14–21.

Ramfjord, S.P. and Ash, M.M.: *Periodontology and Periodontics.* Philadelphia, W.B. Saunders Co., 1979, pp. 156–161.

Schroeder, H.E.: *Formation and Inhibition of Dental Calculus.* Vienna, Hans Huber Publishers, 1969, pp. 37–44, 94–108.

Calculus Attachment

Jones, S.J.: Morphology of Calculus Formation on the Human Tooth Surface, *Proc. R. Soc. Med., 65,* 903, October, 1972.

Kopczyk, R.A. and Conroy, C.W.: The Attachment of Calculus to Root Planed Surfaces, *Periodontics, 6,* 78, April, 1968.

Moskow, B.S.: Calculus Attachment in Cemental Separations, *J. Periodontol., 40,* 125, March, 1969.

Selvig, K.A.: Attachment of Plaque and Calculus to Tooth Surfaces, *J. Periodont. Res., 5,* 8, Number 1, 1970.

Shroff, F.R.: An Observation on the Attachment of Calculus, *Oral Surg., 8,* 154, February, 1955.

Theilade, J.: Electron Microscopic Study of Calculus Attachment to Smooth Surfaces, *Acta Odontol. Scand., 22,* 379, Number 3, 1964.

Voreadis, E.G. and Zander, H.A.: Cuticular Calculus Attachment, *Oral Surg., 11,* 1120, October, 1958.

Zander, H.A.: Attachment of Calculus to Root Surfaces, *J. Periodontol., 24,* 16, January, 1953.

18 Dental Stains and Discolorations

Discolorations of the teeth and restorations occur in three general ways: (1) stain adhering directly to the surfaces, (2) stain contained within calculus and soft deposits, and (3) stain incorporated within the tooth structure or the restorative material. Instructional and clinical techniques apply to all three. The first two may be removed by scaling or polishing. Certain stains may be prevented by the patient's routine personal care.

The significance of stains is primarily the appearance or cosmetic effect. In general, any detrimental effect on the teeth or gingival tissues is related to the soft deposit or calculus in which the stain occurs. Thick deposits of stain conceivably can provide a rough surface on which bacterial plaque can collect and irritate the adjacent gingiva. Certain stains provide a means of evaluating oral cleanliness and the patient's habits of personal care.

I. Classification of Stains

A. Classified by Location
1. *Extrinsic.* Extrinsic stains occur on the external surface of the tooth and may be removed by techniques of toothbrushing, scaling, and/or polishing.
2. *Intrinsic.* Intrinsic stains occur within the tooth substance and cannot be removed by techniques of scaling or polishing.

B. Classified by Source
1. *Exogenous.* Exogenous stains develop or originate from sources outside the tooth. Exogenous stains may be extrinsic and stay on the outer surface of the tooth or intrinsic and become incorporated within the tooth structure.
2. *Endogenous.* Endogenous stains develop or originate from within the tooth. Endogenous stains are always intrinsic and usually are discolorations of the dentin reflected through the enamel.

II. Recognition and Identification

Accurately prepared medical and dental histories can provide information to supplement clinical observations when the need arises to identify a certain stain.

A food diary may aid in identifying certain contributing factors. The history of personal plaque removal with the type and frequency of use of toothbrush, floss, and other supplemental materials and devices may help to explain the presence of certain stains. The state of oral hygiene and oral cleanliness is significant to the occurrence of dental stains.

More than one type of stain may occur and more than one etiologic factor may cause the stains of an individual's dentition. Making a differential diagnosis may seem complicated.

III. Application of Techniques for Stain Removal

A. Stains Occurring Directly on the Tooth Surface
1. Stains that are directly associated with the plaque or pellicle on the surface of the enamel or exposed cementum are removed as much as possible during toothbrushing by the patient. Some stains are removed by scaling, whereas others will require polishing.
2. When stains are tenacious, excessive polishing should be avoided. Precautions should be taken to prevent (1) abrasion of the tooth surface or gingival margin, (2) removal of a layer of fluoride-rich tooth surface, or (3) overheating with a power-driven polisher.

B. Stains Incorporated within Tooth Deposits
When stain is included within the substance of a soft deposit or calculus, it is removed with the deposit.

EXTRINSIC STAINS

The most frequently observed stains, yellow, green, black line, and tobacco will be described first; descriptions of the less common orange, red, and metallic stains will follow.

I. Yellow Stain

A. Clinical Appearance
Dull, yellowish discoloration of bacterial plaque appears.

B. Distribution on Tooth Surfaces
Yellow stain is associated with presence of bacterial plaque. (Note distribution of bacterial plaque, table 16–2, page 238.)

C. Occurrence
1. Common to all ages.
2. More evident when personal oral care procedures are neglected.

D. Etiology
Usually food pigments.

II. Green Stain

A. Clinical Appearance

1. Light or yellowish green to very dark green.
2. Embedded in bacterial plaque.
3. Shape: occurs in three general forms.
   a. Small curved line following contour of facial gingival crest.
   b. Smeared irregularly, may even cover entire facial surface.
   c. Streaked, following grooves or lines in enamel.
4. The stain is frequently superimposed by soft yellow or gray debris (materia alba and food debris).
5. Dark green occasionally becomes embedded in surface enamel and may be observed as an exogenous intrinsic stain when superficial layers of deposit are removed.
6. Enamel under stain is sometimes demineralized as a result of cariogenic plaque or materia alba. The rough demineralized surface encourages plaque retention, demineralization, and recurrence of green stain.

B. Distribution on Tooth Surfaces

1. Primarily facial; may extend to proximal.
2. Most frequently facial cervical third of maxillary anterior teeth.

C. Composition

1. Chromogenic bacteria and fungi.
2. Decomposed hemoglobin.
3. Inorganic elements include calcium, potassium, sodium, silicon, magnesium, phosphorus, and others in small amounts.[1]

D. Occurrence

1. May occur at any age; primarily found in childhood.
2. Collects on both permanent and primary teeth.

E. Recurrence

Recurrence depends on fastidiousness of personal care procedures.

F. Etiology

Green stain results from oral uncleanliness, chromogenic bacteria, and gingival hemorrhage.
1. Chromogenic bacteria or fungi are retained and nourished in bacterial plaque where the green stain is produced.
2. Blood pigments from hemoglobin are decomposed by bacteria.
3. Predisposing factors are the presence of means for retention and proliferation of chromogenic bacteria: bacterial plaque, materia alba, and food debris.

G. Clinical Approach

1. Do not scale the area. Often, an area of demineralized tooth structure underlies the stain and soft deposits.
2. Have the patient remove the soft deposits during a disease control lesson. Initiate a daily fluoride remineralization program.
3. Polish the area gently, preferably with a porte polisher, until the area has shown evidence of remineralization.

H. Other Green Stains

In addition to the clinical entity "Green Stain" described above, bacterial plaque and acquired pellicle may become stained by a variety of substances. Differential distinction may be determined by questioning the patient or from items in the medical or dental histories. Green discoloration may result from the following:
1. Chlorophyll preparations.
2. Metallic dusts of industry.
3. Certain drugs. The stain from smoking marijuana may appear grayish green.

III. Black Line Stain

Black line stain is a highly retentive black or dark brown calculus-like stain that forms along the gingival third near the gingival margin. It may occur on primary or permanent teeth.

A. Other Names

Mesenteric line, pigmented dental plaque, brown stain, black stain.

B. Clinical Features

1. Continuous or interrupted fine line, 1 mm. wide (average), no appreciable thickness.
2. May be a wider band or even occupy entire gingival third in severe cases (rare).
3. Follows contour of gingival crest about 1 mm. above crest.
4. Usually demarcated from gingival crest by clear white line of unstained enamel.
5. Appears black at bases of pits and fissures.
6. Heavy deposits slightly elevated from the tooth surface may be detected with an explorer.
7. Gingiva is firm, with little or no tendency to bleed.
8. Teeth are frequently clean and shiny, with a tendency to lower incidence of dental caries.

C. Distribution on Tooth Surfaces

1. Facial and lingual; follows contour of gingival crest onto proximal surfaces.
2. Rarely on facial of maxillary anterior.
3. Most frequently: lingual and proximal surfaces of maxillary posterior teeth.

D. Composition and Formation[2,3]

1. Black line stain is like calculus in that it is composed of microorganisms embedded in an intermicrobial substance.
2. The microorganisms are primarily gram-positive rods with other bacteria, including cocci, in smaller percentages.

The composition of black line stain is different from the composition of supragingival calculus, in which cocci predominate. Attachment to the tooth of black line stain is by a pellicle-like structure.[4]

Oral disease does not result from the presence of black line stain. In contrast, gingivitis is related to the formation of supragingival plaque, and in the presence of a cariogenic substrate, dental caries develops.

3. Mineralization in black line stain is similar to the formation of calculus.

E. Occurrence
1. All ages; more common in childhood.
2. More common in females.
3. Frequently found in clean mouths.

F. Recurrence
Black line stain tends to form again despite regular personal care, but quantity may be less when plaque control procedures are meticulous.

G. Predisposing Factors
None apparent, except a natural tendency.

IV. Tobacco Stain

A. Clinical Appearance
1. Light brown to dark leathery brown or black.
2. Shape
   a. Diffuse staining of bacterial plaque.
   b. Narrow band that follows contour of gingival crest, slightly above the crest.
   c. Wide, firm, tar-like band may cover cervical third and extend to central third of crown.
3. May be incorporated in calculus deposit.
4. Heavy deposits (particularly from smokeless tobacco) may penetrate the enamel and become exogenous intrinsic.

B. Distribution on Tooth Surfaces
1. Cervical third, primarily.
2. Any surface, as well as pits and fissures.
3. Most frequently on lingual surfaces.

C. Composition
1. Tar products of combustion.
2. Brown pigment from smokeless tobacco.

D. Predisposing Factors
1. Natural tendencies. The quantity of stain is not proportional to the amount of tobacco used.
2. Personal oral care procedures; increased deposits occur with neglect.
3. Extent of bacterial plaque and calculus available for adherence.

V. Other Brown Stains

A. Brown Pellicle
The acquired pellicle is smooth and structureless and recurs readily after removal.[5] The pellicle can take on stains of various colors that result from chemical alteration of the pellicle.[6]

B. Stannous Fluoride[7,8,9]
Light brown, sometimes yellowish, stain forms on the teeth in the pellicle after repeated use of a stannous fluoride dentifrice or other product, or having a topical fluoride application. The brown stain results from the formation of stannous sulfide or brown tin oxide from the reaction of the tin ion in the fluoride compound.

C. Foodstuffs
Tea, coffee, and soy sauce are often implicated in the formation of a brownish-stained pellicle. As with other brown pellicle stains, there is less when the personal oral hygiene and plaque control are excellent.

D. Anti-plaque Agents[10,11]
Chlorhexidine and alexidine are used in mouthrinse, gel, and dentifrice and shown effective against plaque formation (page 330). A brownish stain of the tooth surfaces results, usually more pronounced on proximal and other surfaces less accessible to routine plaque control procedures. The stain also tends to form more rapidly on exposed roots than on enamel. Tooth staining has been considered a significant side effect.

E. Betel Leaf[12]
Betel leaf chewing is common among people of all ages in eastern countries. Betel has a caries-inhibiting effect.

The discoloration imparted to the teeth is a dark mahogany brown, sometimes almost black. It may become thick and hard, with partly smooth and partly rough surfaces.

Microscopically, the black deposit consists of microorganisms and mineralized material with a laminated pattern characteristic of subgingival calculus. It should be removed by scaling.

VI. Orange and Red Stains

A. Clinical Appearance
Orange or red stains appear at the cervical third.

B. Distribution on Tooth Surfaces
1. More frequently on anterior than on posterior teeth.
2. Both facial and lingual of anterior teeth.

C. Occurrence
Rare (red more rare than orange).

D. Etiology
Chromogenic bacteria.

VII. Metallic Stains

A. Metals or Metallic Salts from Metal-containing Dust of Industry
1. *Clinical Appearance.* Examples of colors on teeth
   a. Copper or brass: green or bluish-green.
   b. Iron: brown to greenish-brown.
   c. Nickel: green.
   d. Cadmium: yellow or golden brown.
2. *Distribution on Tooth Surfaces*
   a. Primarily anterior; may occur on any teeth.

    b. Cervical third more commonly.
  3. *Manner of Formation*
    a. Industrial worker inhales dust through mouth, bringing metallic substance in contact with teeth.
    b. Metal imparts color to bacterial plaque.
    c. Occasionally, stain may penetrate tooth substance and become exogenous intrinsic stain.

B. Metallic Substances Contained in Drugs

  1. *Clinical Appearance.* Examples of colors on teeth.
    a. Iron: black (iron sulfide) or brown.
    b. Manganese (from potassium permanganate): black.
  2. *Distribution on Tooth Surfaces.* General, may occur on all.
  3. *Manner of Formation*
    a. Drug enters plaque substance, imparts color to plaque and calculus.
    b. Pigment from drug may attach directly to tooth substance.
  4. *Prevention.* Use a medication through a straw or in tablet or capsule form to prevent direct contact with the teeth.

ENDOGENOUS INTRINSIC STAINS

Stains incorporated within the tooth structure may be related to the period of tooth development or may be acquired after eruption. Occasionally, a patient, desiring an improvement in the appearance of the anterior teeth, may request removal of a discoloration. The dentist may employ one of two alternatives in the treatment of these teeth. Improvement in tooth color can be produced by bleaching in certain instances. In other cases, a jacket crown is indicated to cover the discoloration.

I. Pulpless Teeth

Not all pulpless teeth discolor. Improved endodontic procedures have contributed to the prevention of many discolorations formerly associated with that cause.

A. Clinical Appearance

A wide range of colors exists; stains may be light yellow-brown, slate gray, reddish-brown, dark brown, bluish-black, or black. Others have an orange or greenish tinge.

B. Manner of Formation

  1. Blood and other pulp tissue elements may be made available for breakdown as a result of hemorrhages in the pulp chamber, root canal operations, or necrosis and decomposition of the pulp tissue.
  2. Pigments from the decomposed hemoglobin and pulp tissue penetrate the dentinal tubules.

II. Tetracyclines[13]

A. Tetracycline antibiotics, used widely for combatting many types of infections, have an affinity for mineralized tissues and are absorbed by the bones and teeth. They can be transferred through the placenta and enter fetal circulation.

B. Discoloration of the teeth of a child can result when the drug is administered to the mother during the third trimester of pregnancy or to the child in infancy and early childhood.

C. Color of teeth may be light green to dark yellow, or a gray-brown. The discoloration depends on the dosage, length of time the drug was used, and the type of tetracycline.

D. Discoloration may be generalized or limited to specific parts of individual teeth that were developing at the time of administration of the antibiotic. Reference to the Table of Tooth Development can assist in determining the patient's age at the time the drug was administered, and the patient's medical history at that age may reveal the probable cause of the intrinsic stain (Appendix, tables A–1 and A–2).

III. Imperfect Tooth Development

Defective tooth development may result from factors of genetic abnormality or environmental influences during tooth development.

A. Hereditary: Genetic[14]

  1. *Amelogenesis Imperfecta.* The enamel is partially or completely missing because of a generalized disturbance of the ameloblasts. Teeth are yellowish-brown or gray-brown.
  2. *Dentinogenesis Imperfecta ("Opalescent Dentin").* The dentin is abnormal as a result of disturbances in the odontoblastic layer during development. The teeth appear translucent or opalescent, and vary in color from gray to bluish-brown.

B. Enamel Hypoplasia[14]

  1. *Systemic Hypoplasia* (chronologic hypoplasia resulting from ameloblastic disturbance of short duration). Teeth erupt with white spots or with pits. Over a long period of time, the white spots may become discolored from food pigments or other substances taken into the mouth. Figure 14–1 (page 213) shows an example of chronologic hypoplasia.
  2. *Local Hypoplasia* (affects single tooth). White spots may become stained as in systemic hypoplasia.

C. Dental Fluorosis

Dental fluorosis was originally called "brown stain." Later, Dr. Frederick S. McKay, who studied the condition and described it in the dental literature, named it "mottled enamel" (page 397).

  1. *Manner of Formation*
    a. Enamel hypomineralization results from

ingestion of excessive fluoride ion in drinking water (more than 2 parts per million) during the period of mineralization. The enamel alterations are a result of toxic damage to the ameloblasts.

b. When the teeth erupt, they have white spots or areas that later become discolored from oral pigments and appear light or dark brown.

c. Severe effects of excess fluoride during development may produce cracks or pitting; the discoloration concentrates in these. It was that condition and appearance that led to the name mottled enamel.

2. *Classification*[15,16]

Grade of Fluorosis	Description of Fluorosis
Normal	No irregularities present
Questionable	A few white flecks or white spots
Very Mild	Small opaque, paper-white areas involving less than 25 percent of the surface
Mild	White opacities are more extensive, but do not involve more than 50 percent of the surface
Moderate	Distinct brown stain; all enamel surfaces affected
Severe	Besides brown staining, the tooth is worn and hypoplastic. All enamel surfaces are affected and discrete or confluent pitting is present

IV. Other Systemic Causes

Several types of tooth discolorations may result from blood-borne pigments.

Pigments circulating in the blood are transmitted to the dentin from the capillaries of the pulp. *Example:* prolonged jaundice early in life can impart yellow or greenish discoloration to the teeth.

Erythroblastosis fetalis (Rh incompatibility) may leave a green, brown, or blue hue to the teeth.

EXOGENOUS INTRINSIC STAINS

When intrinsic stains come from an outside source, not from within the tooth, the stain is called exogenous intrinsic. Extrinsic stains can provide stain that becomes intrinsic. Tobacco and green stains are examples of this.

I. Restorative Materials

A. Silver Amalgam

1. Silver amalgam can impart a gray to black discoloration to the tooth structure around a restoration.

2. Metallic ions migrate from the amalgam restoration into the enamel and dentin.

3. Silver, tin, and mercury ions eventually contact debris at the junction of the tooth and the restoration and form sulfides, which are products of corrosion.

B. Copper Amalgam

Copper amalgam used for filling primary teeth may impart a bluish-green color.

II. Endodontic Therapy and Restorative Materials

A. Silver nitrate: bluish-black.
B. Volatile oils: yellowish-brown.
C. Strong iodine: brown.
D. Aureomycin: yellow.
E. Silver-containing root canal sealer: black.

III. Drugs

A. Stannous Fluoride Topical Application[7]

1. Light to dark brown staining from the formation of tin sulfide.

2. Located most frequently in occlusal pits and grooves of posterior teeth and cervical third facial surfaces of anterior teeth; in carious and pre-carious lesions; and margins of tooth color and amalgam restorations.

3. Staining may accompany dental caries arrestment.

B. Ammoniacal Silver Nitrate

Used in treatment of sensitive areas such as exposed cementum or for inhibition of demineralization in dental caries prevention, imparts a dark brown to black discoloration.

IV. Stain in Dentin

Example: discoloration resulting from a carious lesion.

TECHNICAL HINTS

I. Record color, type, extent, and location of stains with the patient's examination.

II. Make additions to the dental history as information is gained concerning the origin of stains such as those related to tooth development, systemic disease, occupations, or medications.

III. Avoid making patient feel self-conscious by overemphasizing the appearance of stains, particularly those that may occur in spite of conscientious toothbrushing habits.

IV. Use tact when questioning patients with brown stain, because nonsmokers do not appreciate having an assumption made concerning the cause of a stain on the teeth.

V. Refer patient's questions concerning the removal of intrinsic stains to the dentist. Avoid expressing an opinion in terms of diagnosis or prognosis of treatment until the dentist has recommended a procedure.

FACTORS TO TEACH THE PATIENT

I. Predisposing factors that contribute to stain accumulation.

II. Personal care procedures that can aid in the prevention or reduction of stains.

III. Reasons for not using an abrasive dentifrice with vigorous brushing strokes to lessen or remove stain accumulation.

IV. The need to avoid tobacco, coffee, tea, and other beverages or foodstuffs that can stain, to prevent discoloration of new restorations.

V. Reasons for the difficulty of removing certain extrinsic stains during scaling and polishing.

VI. Effect of tetracyclines on developing teeth. Need to avoid use during pregnancy and by children to age 12.

References

1. Shay, D.E., Haddox, J.H., and Richmond, J.L.: An Inorganic Qualitative and Quantitative Analysis of Green Stain, *J. Am. Dent. Assoc., 50,* 156, February, 1955.

2. Theilade, J., Slots, J., and Fejerskov, O.: The Ultrastructure of Black Stain on Human Primary Teeth, *Scand. J. Dent. Res., 81,* 528, Number 7, 1973.

3. Slots, J.: The Microflora of Black Stain on Human Primary Teeth, *Scand. J. Dent. Res., 82,* 484, Number 7, 1974.

4. Theilade, J.: Development of Bacterial Plaque in the Oral Cavity, *J. Clin. Periodontol., 4,* 1, December, 1977.

5. Meckel, A.H.: The Formation and Properties of Organic Films on Teeth, *Arch. Oral Biol., 10,* 585, July-August, 1965.

6. Eriksen, H.M. and Nordbø, H.: Extrinsic Discoloration of Teeth, *J. Clin. Periodontol., 5,* 229, November, 1978.

7. Horowitz, H.S. and Chamberlin, S.R.: Pigmentation of Teeth following Topical Applications of Stannous Fluoride in a Nonfluoridated Area, *J. Public Health Dent., 31,* 32, Winter, 1971.

8. Shannon, I.L.: Stannous Fluoride: Does It Stain Teeth? How Does It React with Tooth Surfaces? A Review, *Gen. Dent., 26,* 64, September-October, 1978.

9. Leverett, D.H., McHugh, W.D., and Jensen, Ø.E.: Dental Caries and Staining after Twenty-eight Months of Rinsing with Stannous Fluoride or Sodium Fluoride, *J. Dent. Res., 65,* 424, March, 1986.

10. Flötra, L., Gjermo, P., Rölla, G., and Waerhaug, J.: Side Effects of Chlorhexidine Mouthwashes, *Scand. J. Dent. Res., 79,* 119, April, 1971.

11. Formicola, A.J., Deasy, M.J., Johnson, D.H., and Howe, E.E.: Tooth Staining Effects of an Alexidine Mouthwash, *J. Periodontol., 50,* 207, April, 1979.

12. Reichart, P.A., Lenz, H., König, H., Becker, J., and Mohr, U.: The Black Layer on the Teeth of Betel Chewers: A Light Microscopic, Microradiographic, and Electronmicroscopic Study, *J. Oral Path., 14,* 466, July, 1985.

13. American Dental Association, Council on Dental Therapeutics: *Accepted Dental Therapeutics,* 40th ed. Chicago, American Dental Association, 1984, pp. 288–290.

14. Ash, M.M. and Ward, M.L.: *Kerr and Ash's Oral Pathology,* 5th ed. Philadelphia, Lea & Febiger, 1986, pp. 54–56.

15. Dean, H.T.: Investigation of Physiological Effects by Epidemiological Method, in Moulton, F.R., ed.: *Fluorine and Dental Health.* Washington, American Association for the Advancement of Science, Number 19, 1942.

16. Newbrun, E., ed.: *Fluorides and Dental Caries,* 3rd ed. Springfield, Illinois, Charles C Thomas, 1986, p. 5.

17. Ash and Ward: op. cit., pp. 270–271.

Suggested Readings

Burke, S.W.: Oral Physiology and Oral Physiotherapy, in Steele, P.F., ed.: *Dimensions of Dental Hygiene,* 3rd ed. Philadelphia, Lea & Febiger, 1982, pp. 97–100.

Ceen, R.F. and Gwinnett, A.J.: Indelible Iatrogenic Staining of Enamel following Debonding. A Case Report, *J. Clin. Orthod., 14,* 713, October, 1980.

Chan, K.C., Fuller, J.L., and Hormati, A.A.: The Ability of Foods to Stain Two Composite Resins, *J. Prosthet. Dent., 43,* 542, May, 1980.

Chan, K.C., Hormati, A.A., and Kerber, P.E.: Staining Calcified Dental Tissues with Food, *J. Prosthet. Dent., 46,* 175, August, 1981.

Cooley, R.L. and Berkmeier, W.W.: Staining of Composite and Microfilled Resin with Stannous Fluoride, *J. Prosthet. Dent., 49,* 346, March, 1983.

Dayan, D., Heifferman, A., Gorski, M., and Begleiter, A.: Tooth Discoloration—Extrinsic and Intrinsic Factors, *Quintessence Int., 14,* 195, February, 1983.

Dummett, C.O., Sakumura, J.S., and Barens, G.: The Relationship of Facial Skin Complexion to Oral Mucosa Pigmentation and Tooth Color, *J. Prosthet. Dent., 43,* 392, April, 1980.

Eriksen, H.M., Nordbø, H., Kantanen, H., and Ellingsen, J.E.: Chemical Plaque Control and Extrinsic Tooth Discoloration. A Review of Possible Mechanisms, *J. Clin. Periodontol., 12,* 345, May, 1985.

Massler, M. and Schour, I.: *Atlas of the Mouth.* Chicago, American Dental Association, Plate 12.

Schuurs, A.H.B., Abraham-Inpijn, L., van Straalen, J.P., and Sastrowijoto, S.H.: An Unusual Case of Black Teeth, *Oral Surg. Oral Med. Oral Pathol., 64,* 427, October, 1987.

Solheim, H., Eriksen, H.M., and Nordbø, H.: Chemical Plaque Control and Extrinsic Discoloration of Teeth, *Acta Odontol. Scand., 38,* 303, Number 5, 1980.

Developmental Defects

Atkinson, D.: Tetracycline and Its Effect on Teeth, *Dent. Assist., 47,* 36, November/December, 1978.

DeSort, K.D.: Amelogenesis Imperfecta: The Genetics, Classification, and Treatment, *J. Prosthet. Dent., 49,* 786, June, 1983.

Fleming, P., Witkop, C.J., and Kuhlmann, W.H.: Staining and Hypoplasia of Enamel Caused by Tetracycline: Case Report, *Pediatr. Dent., 9,* 245, September, 1987.

Gertzman, G.B.R., Gaston, G., and Quinn, I.: Amelogenesis Imperfecta: Local Hypoplastic Type with Pulpal Calcification, *J. Am. Dent. Assoc., 99,* 637, October, 1979.

Giansanti, J.S. and Budnick, S.D.: Six Generations of Hereditary Opalescent Dentin: Report of Case, *J. Am. Dent. Assoc., 90,* 439, February, 1975.

Guggenheimer, J.: Tetracyclines and the Human Dentition, *Compend. Contin. Educ. Dent., 5,* 245, March, 1984.

Thylstrup, A. and Fejerskov, O.: Clinical Appearance of Dental Fluorosis in Permanent Teeth in Relation to Histologic Changes, *Community Dent. Oral Epidemiol., 6,* 315, December, 1978.

Winter, G.B. and Brook, A.H.: Enamel Hypoplasia and Anomalies of the Enamel, *Dent. Clin. North Am., 19,* 3, January, 1975.

Witkop, C.J.: Hereditary Defects of Dentin, *Dent. Clin. North Am., 19,* 25, January, 1975.

Chlorhexidine Stains

Addy, M. and Moran, J.: Extrinsic Tooth Discoloration by Metals and Chlorhexidine. II. Clinical Staining Produced by Chlorhexidine, Iron and Tea, *Br. Dent. J., 159,* 331, November 23, 1985.

Addy, M. and Prayitno, S.W.: Light Microscopic and Color Television Image Analysis of the Development of Staining on Chlorhexidine-treated Surfaces, *J. Periodontol., 51,* 39, January, 1980.

Addy, M. and Roberts, W.R.: Comparison of the Bisbiguanide Antiseptics Alexidine and Chlorhexidine. II. Clinical and *in vitro* Staining Properties, *J. Clin. Periodontol., 8,* 220, June, 1981.

Addy, M., Moran, J., Davies, R.M., Beak, A., and Lewis, A.: The Effect of Single Morning and Evening Rinses of Chlorhexidine on the Development of Tooth Staining and Plaque Accumulation. A Blind Cross-over Trial, *J. Clin. Periodontol., 9,* 134, March, 1982.

Addy, M., Moran, J., Griffiths, A.A., and Wills-Wood, N.J.: Extrinsic Tooth Discoloration by Metals and Chlorhexidine. I. Surface Protein Denaturation or Dietary Precipitation? *Br. Dent. J., 159,* 281, November 9, 1985.

Addy, M., Prayitno, S., Taylor, L., and Cadogan, S.: An *in vitro* Study of the Role of Dietary Factors in the Aetiology of Tooth Staining Associated with the Use of Chlorhexidine, *J. Periodont. Res., 14,* 403, September, 1979.

Dolles, O.K., Eriksen, H.M., and Gjermo, P.: Tooth Stain During 2 Years' Use of Chlorhexidine—and Fluoride-containing Dentifrices, *Scand. J. Dent. Res., 87,* 268, August, 1979.

Nordbö, H., Attramadal, A., and Eriksen, H.M.: Iron Discoloration of Acrylic Resin Exposed to Chlorhexidine or Tannic Acid: A Model Study, *J. Prosthet. Dent., 49,* 126, January, 1983.

Prayitno, S. and Addy, M.: An *in vitro* Study of Factors Affecting the Development of Staining Associated with the Use of Chlorhexidine, *J. Periodont. Res., 14,* 397, November, 1979.

Prayitno, S., Taylor, L., Cadogan, S., and Addy, M.: An *in vivo* Study of Dietary Factors in the Aetiology of Tooth Staining Associated with the Use of Chlorhexidine, *J. Periodont. Res., 14,* 411, September 1979.

19 *Indices and Scoring Methods*

An index is an expression of clinical observations in numeric values. It is used to describe the status of the individual or group with respect to a condition being measured. The use of a numeric scale and a standardized method for interpreting observations of a condition results in an index score that is more consistent and less subjective than a word description of that condition.

Indices using various criteria have been developed to compare the extent and severity of disease. For example, dental caries is indexed by the number of teeth or surfaces with carious lesions and restorations. An index for dental fluorosis identifies very mild, mild, moderate, or severe involvement of the enamel, ranging respectively from white spots visible only when a tooth is dry to marked brown stains with pitting.[1]

Various factors associated with gingivitis and periodontal infections have been used in the development of indices. Measurement criteria include recession, bone loss, pocket formation, mobility of teeth, gingival inflammation, gingival bleeding, and the amount and distribution of plaque and calculus.

Several indices will be described in this chapter. Those included have been selected because they are well known and widely used in the assessment of oral health status. The *Suggested Readings* at the end of the chapter contain references to other indices. Familiarity with the various types of indices may prove helpful when different evaluation criteria are needed.

I. Purposes and Uses of an Index

A distinction must be made between an individual oral health assessment score, a clinical trial, and a community health epidemiologic survey.

A. Individual Clinical Score
1. *Purpose.* In clinical practice, an index, plaque record, or scoring system for an individual patient can be used for education, motivation, and evaluation. The effects of personal disease control efforts, the progress of healing during professional treatments, and the maintenance of health over time can be monitored. An example is the plaque-free score described on page 264 in which a patient is able to measure the effects of personal daily care efforts by the changes in the scores. This system may prove to be a valuable motivating device.

2. *Uses*
   a. Provides individual assessment to help a patient recognize an oral problem.
   b. Reveals the degree of effectiveness of present oral hygiene practices.
   c. Motivates the person in preventive and professional care for the elimination and control of oral disease.
   d. Evaluates the success of individual and professional treatment over a period of time by comparing index scores.

B. Clinical Trial
1. *Purpose.* A clinical trial is planned for the determination of the effect of an agent or procedure on the progression, control, or prevention of a disease. The trial is conducted by comparing an experimental group with a control group that is similar to the experimental group in every way except for the variable being studied.

   Examples of indices used for clinical trials are the Plaque Index (Pl I) of Silness and Löe[2] and the Patient Hygiene Performance (PHP) of Podshadley and Haley.[3] These and other indices are described in this chapter.

2. *Uses*
   a. Determines baseline data before experimental factors are introduced.
   b. Measures the effectiveness of specific agents for the prevention, control, or treatment of oral conditions.
   c. Measures the effectiveness of mechanical devices for personal care, such as toothbrushes, interdental cleaning devices, or water irrigators.

C. Epidemiologic Survey
1. *Purpose.* The word epidemiology denotes the study of disease characteristics of populations. An example of an index designed for a survey of population groups is the DMF (Decayed, Missing, and Filled Teeth) Index. It has been used with populations around the world to determine the extent of dental caries. Such a survey was not designed for evaluation of an individual patient.

2. *Uses*
   a. Shows the prevalence and incidence of a particular condition occurring within a given population.

b. Provides baseline data to show existing dental health practices.
c. Assesses the needs of a community.
d. Compares the effects of a community program and evaluates the results.

II. Characteristics of an Index

A. Descriptive Categories of Indices
1. *General Categories*
   a. Simple index. One that measures the presence or absence of a condition. An example is an index that measures the presence of bacterial plaque without evaluating its effect on the gingiva.
   b. Cumulative index. One that measures all the evidence of a condition, past and present. An example is the DMF Index for dental caries.
2. *Types of Simple and Cumulative Indices*
   a. Irreversible. One that measures conditions that will not change. An example is an index that measures dental caries.
   b. Reversible. One that measures conditions that can be changed. Examples are indices that measure bacterial plaque.
3. *Other Definitions*
   a. Incidence. The number of new cases of a specific disease or condition within a defined population over a period of time.
   b. Prevalence. The number of specific cases or lesions within a defined population at a single point in time or during a stated period of time.[4]

B. Selection Criteria
A useful and effective index will
1. Be simple to use and calculate.
2. Require minimal equipment and expense.
3. Require a minimal amount of time to complete.
4. Not cause patient discomfort or otherwise be unacceptable to a patient.
5. Have clear-cut criteria that are readily understandable.
6. Be as free as possible from subjective interpretation.
7. Be reproducible by the same examiner or different examiners.
8. Be amenable to statistical analysis; have validity and reliability.

III. Indices Described in This Chapter

The sequence of indices included follows a general outline for the descriptions of bacterial plaque; plaque, debris, and calculus; gingival bleeding; gingivitis; and periodontal diseases. Dental caries indices for permanent and primary teeth are then outlined.

One should realize that plaque indices are applicable for preventive instruction related to bacterial plaque control for dental caries, as well as for gingival and periodontal diseases.

A. Bacterial Plaque
1. Plaque Index (Pl I) (page 262).
2. Plaque Control Record (page 263).
3. Plaque-free Score (page 264).

B. Plaque, Debris, Calculus
1. Patient Hygiene Performance (PHP) (page 265).
2. Oral Hygiene Index (OHI) (page 267).
3. Simplified Oral Hygiene Index (OHI-S) (page 269).

C. Gingival Bleeding
1. Sulcus Bleeding Index (SBI) (page 271).
2. Gingival Bleeding Index (GBI) (page 271).

D. Gingival Changes/Gingivitis
1. Papillary-Marginal-Attached Index (P-M-A) (page 271).
2. Gingival Index (GI) (page 273).

E. Periodontal Diseases
1. Periodontal Index (PI) (page 274).
2. Periodontal Disease Index (PDI) (page 274).
3. Community Periodontal Index of Treatment Needs (CPITN) (page 277).

F. Dental Caries
1. Decayed, Missing, and Filled Permanent Teeth (DMFT) (page 279).
2. Decayed, Missing, and Filled Permanent Tooth Surfaces (DMFS) (page 280).
3. Primary teeth indices (page 281).

PLAQUE INDEX (Pl I)
(Silness and Löe[2,5])

I. Purpose
To assess the thickness of plaque at the gingival area.

II. Selection of Teeth
The entire dentition or selected teeth can be evaluated.

A. Areas Examined
Four gingival areas (distal, facial, mesial, lingual) are examined systematically for each tooth.

B. Modified Procedures
Examine only the facial, mesial, and lingual. Assign double score to the mesial reading, and divide the total by 4.

III. Procedure
A. Dry the teeth and examine visually using adequate light, mouth mirror, and probe or explorer.
B. Evaluate bacterial plaque on the cervical third; pay no attention to plaque that has extended to the middle or incisal thirds.
C. Probe to test the surface when no plaque is visible. Pass the probe or explorer across the tooth

surface in the cervical third and near the entrance to the sulcus. When no plaque adheres to the probe tip, the area is scored 0. When plaque adheres, a score of 1 is assigned.

D. Use a disclosing agent, if necessary, to assist evaluation for the 0 to 1 scores. When the Pl I is used in conjunction with the Gingival Index (GI, page 273), the GI must be completed first because the disclosing agent masks the gingival characteristics.

E. Include plaque on the surface of calculus and on dental restorations in the cervical third in the evaluation.

F. Criteria

0 = No plaque.

1 = A film of plaque adhering to the free gingival margin and adjacent area of the tooth. The plaque may be recognized only after application of disclosing agent or by running the explorer across the tooth surface.

2 = Moderate accumulation of soft deposits within the gingival pocket that can be seen with the naked eye or on the tooth and gingival margin.

3 = Abundance of soft matter within the gingival pocket and/or on the tooth and gingival margin.

IV. Scoring

A. Pl I for Area

Each area (distal, facial, mesial, lingual or palatal) is assigned a score from 0 to 3.

B. Pl I for a Tooth

Scores for each area are totalled and divided by 4.

C. Pl I for Groups of Teeth

Scores for individual teeth may be grouped and totalled and divided by the number of teeth. For instance, a Plaque Index may be determined for specific teeth or groups of teeth. The right side may be compared with the left.

D. Pl I for the Individual

Add the scores for each tooth and divide by the number of teeth examined. The Pl I ranges from 0 to 3.

E. Suggested Nominal Scale for Patient Reference

Rating	Scores
Excellent	0
Good	0.1–0.9
Fair	1.0–1.9
Poor	2.0–3.0

F. Pl I for a Group

Add the scores for each member of a group and divide by the number of individuals.

PLAQUE CONTROL RECORD
(O'Leary, Drake, and Naylor[6])

I. Purpose

To record the presence of bacterial plaque on individual tooth surfaces to permit the patient to visualize progress while learning plaque control.

II. Selection of Teeth and Surfaces

A. All teeth are included. Missing teeth are identified on the record form by a single thick horizontal line.

B. Four surfaces are recorded: facial, lingual, mesial, and distal.

C. Six areas may be recorded. The mesial and distal segments of the diagram may be divided to provide space to record proximal surfaces from the facial separately from the lingual or palatal (figure 19–1).[7]

III. Procedure

A. Apply disclosing agent or give a chewable tablet. Instruct patient to swish and rub the solution over the tooth surfaces with the tongue before rinsing.

B. Examine each tooth surface for bacterial plaque at the gingival margin. No attempt is made to differentiate quantity of plaque.

C. Record by making a dash or coloring in the appropriate spaces on the diagram (figure 19–1) to indicate plaque on facial, lingual, palatal, mesial, and/or distal surfaces.

IV. Scoring

A. Total the number of teeth present; multiply by 4 (or 6 if modification is used) to obtain the number of available surfaces. Count the number of surfaces with plaque.

B. Multiply the number of plaque-stained surfaces by 100 and divide by the total number of available surfaces to derive the percent of surfaces.

C. Compare over subsequent appointments as the patient learns and practices plaque control. Ten percent or fewer plaque-stained surfaces can be considered a good goal, but if the plaque is regularly left in the same areas, special instruction is indicated to prevent pocket formation.

D. Calculation example for plaque control record:

Individual findings: 26 teeth scored
8 surfaces with plaque

1. Multiply the number of teeth by 4:
26 × 4 = 104 surfaces

2. Percent with plaque =

$$\frac{\text{Number of surfaces with plaque} \times 100}{\text{Number of available tooth surfaces}}$$

$$= \frac{8 \times 100}{104} = \frac{800}{104} = 7.6$$

Interpretation: Although 0 percent is ideal, fewer than 10 percent plaque-stained surfaces has been suggested as a guideline in periodontal therapy. After initial therapy and when the patient has reached a 10 percent level of plaque control or better, necessary additional periodontal and restorative procedures may be initiated.[6] In comparison, a similar evaluation using a plaque-free score would mean that a goal

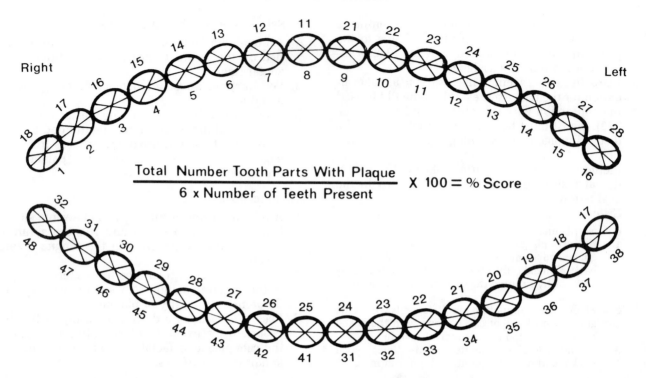

$$\frac{\text{Total Number Tooth Parts With Plaque}}{6 \times \text{Number of Teeth Present}} \times 100 = \% \text{ Score}$$

Figure 19–1. Plaque Control Record. Diagrammatic representation of the teeth includes spaces to record plaque on six areas of each tooth. The facial surfaces are on the outer and the lingual and palatal surfaces on the inner portion of the arches. Teeth are numbered by the ADA System on the inside and by the FDI System on the outside. (Modified from Ramfjord, S.P. and Ash, M.M.: *Periodontology and Periodontics.* Philadelphia, W.B. Saunders Co., 1979, page 273; and from O'Leary, T.J., Drake, R.B., and Naylor, J.E.: *J. Periodontol.*, 43, 38, 1972.)

of over 90 percent or better plaque-free surfaces would have to be reached before the surgical phase of treatment could be undertaken.

PLAQUE-FREE SCORE
(Grant, Stern, Everett[8])

I. Purpose

To determine the location, number, and percent of plaque-free surfaces for individual motivation and instruction. Interdental bleeding can also be documented.

II. Selection of Teeth and Surfaces

A. All erupted teeth are included. Missing teeth are identified on the record form by a single thick horizontal line through the box in the chart form.
B. Four surfaces are recorded for each tooth: facial, lingual or palatal, mesial, and distal.

III. Procedure

A. Plaque-free Score

1. Apply disclosing agent or give chewable tablet. Instruct patient to swish and rub the solution over the tooth surfaces with the tongue before rinsing.
2. Examine each tooth surface for evidence of plaque. Use adequate light and a mouth mirror

for visualizing all surfaces. In patient instruction, the patient needs a hand mirror to see the location of the plaque that has been missed during personal hygiene techniques.

3. Record in red the surfaces showing plaque. Use an appropriate tooth chart form or a diagrammatic form, such as that shown in figure 19–2. The use of red ink for recording the plaque is suggested when a red disclosing agent is used to help the patient associate the location of the plaque in the mouth with the recording.

B. Papillary Bleeding on Probing

1. The small circles between the diagrammatic tooth blocks in figure 19–2 are used to record proximal bleeding on probing.
2. Improvement in the gingival tissue health will be demonstrated over a period of time as fewer bleeding areas are noted.

IV. Scoring

A. Plaque-free Score

1. Total the number of teeth present.
2. Total the number of surfaces with plaque that appear in red on the tooth diagram.
3. Consult table 19–1.
   a. Read across the top or bottom to locate the number of teeth and total surfaces.

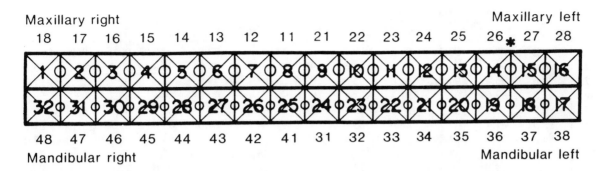

Maxillary right
18 17 16 15 14 13 12 11 21 22 23 24 25 26 * 27 28

48 47 46 45 44 43 42 41 31 32 33 34 35 36 37 38
Mandibular right   Mandibular left

b. Read down the side to locate the number of surfaces with plaque.

c. Find the intersection of the top and side numbers; this number is the plaque-free score in percent.

4. To calculate without table 19–1 for reference
   a. Multiply the number of teeth by 4 to determine the number of available surfaces.
   b. Subtract the number of surfaces with plaque from the total available surfaces to find the number of plaque-free surfaces.
   c. Plaque-free score =

$$\frac{\text{Number of plaque-free surfaces} \times 100}{\text{Number of available surfaces}}$$

= Percent plaque-free surfaces

5. Evaluate plaque-free score. Ideally, 100 percent is the goal. When a patient maintains a percent under 85, check individual surfaces to determine whether plaque is usually left in the same areas. To prevent the development of specific areas of periodontal infection, remedial instruction in the areas usually missed is indicated.

B. Papillary Bleeding on Probing

1. Total the number of small circles marked for bleeding. A person with 32 teeth has 30 interdental areas. The mesial or distal of a tooth adjacent to an edentulous area is probed and counted.

2. Evaluate total interdental bleeding. In health, bleeding on probing does not occur.

C. Calculation Example for Plaque-free Score

Individual findings: 24 teeth scored
37 surfaces with plaque

1. With table 19–1
   a. Locate the number of teeth across the top of table 19–1 (24–96): there are 96 total surfaces.
   b. Locate the number of surfaces with plaque down the side (37); find the intersection.
   c. The percent of plaque-free surfaces is 61.5.

2. Without reference table 19–1
   a. Multiply the number of teeth by 4:
      24 × 4 = 96 available surfaces

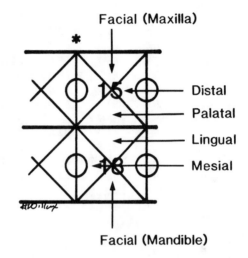

Facial (Maxilla)

Distal
Palatal
Lingual
Mesial

Facial (Mandible)

Figure 19–2. Plaque-free Score. Diagrammatic representation of the teeth used to record plaque and papillary bleeding. Enlargement of teeth (*) shows tooth surfaces. Teeth are numbered by the ADA System inside each block and by the FDI System outside each block. (Adapted from Grant, D.A., Stern, I.B., and Listgarten, M.A.: *Periodontics*, 6th ed. St. Louis, The C.V. Mosby Co., 1988, page 613.)

b. Subtract the number of surfaces with plaque from total available surfaces:
   96 − 37 = 59 plaque-free surfaces
c. Percent plaque-free surfaces =

$$\frac{59 \times 100}{96} = 61.5$$

Interpretation: On the basis of the ideal 100 percent, 61.5 percent is poor. More instruction is indicated.

PATIENT HYGIENE PERFORMANCE (PHP)
(Podshadley and Haley[3])

I. Purpose

To assess the extent of plaque and debris over a tooth surface. Debris is defined for the PHP as the soft foreign material consisting of bacterial plaque,

Table 19–1. Plaque-Free Score

Number of Tooth Surfaces

Number of Tooth Surfaces with Plaque	32–128	31–124	30–120	29–116	28–112	27–108	26–104	25–100	24–96	23–92	22–88	21–84	
1	99.2	99.2	99.2	99.2	99.2	99.1	99.1	99.0	99.0	99.0	98.9	98.9	
4	96.9	96.8	96.7	97.6	96.5	96.3	96.2	96.0	95.9	95.7	95.5	95.3	
7	94.6	95.4	94.2	94.0	93.8	93.6	93.3	93.0	92.8	92.4	92.1	91.7	
10	92.2	92.0	91.7	91.4	91.1	90.8	90.4	90.0	89.6	89.2	88.7	88.1	
13	89.9	89.6	89.2	88.8	88.4	88.0	87.5	87.0	86.5	85.9	85.3	84.5	
16	87.5	87.1	86.7	86.3	85.8	85.2	84.7	84.0	83.4	82.7	81.9	81.0	
19	85.2	84.7	84.2	83.7	83.1	82.5	81.8	81.0	80.3	79.4	78.5	77.4	
22	83.9	82.3	81.7	81.1	80.4	79.7	78.9	78.0	77.1	76.1	75.0	73.9	
25	80.4	79.9	79.2	78.5	77.7	76.9	76.0	75.0	74.0	72.9	71.6	70.3	
28	78.2	77.5	76.7	75.9	75.0	74.1	73.1	72.0	70.9	69.6	68.2	66.4	
31	75.8	75.0	74.2	73.3	72.4	71.3	70.2	69.0	67.8	66.4	64.8	63.1	
34	73.5	72.6	71.7	70.7	69.7	68.6	67.4	66.0	64.6	63.1	61.4	59.6	
37	71.1	70.2	69.2	68.2	67.0	65.8	64.5	63.0	61.5	59.8	58.0	56.0	
40	68.8	67.8	66.7	65.6	64.3	63.0	61.6	60.0	58.4	56.6	54.6	52.4	
43	66.5	65.4	64.2	63.0	61.7	60.2	58.7	57.0	55.3	53.3	51.2	48.9	
46	64.1	63.0	61.7	60.4	59.0	57.5	55.8	54.0	52.1	50.0	47.8	45.3	
49	61.8	60.5	59.2	57.8	56.3	54.7	52.9	51.0	49.0	46.8	44.4	41.7	
52	59.4	58.1	56.7	55.2	53.6	51.9	50.0	48.0	45.9	43.5	41.0	38.1	
55	57.1	55.7	54.2	52.6	50.9	49.1	47.2	45.0	42.8	40.3	37.5	34.6	
58	54.7	53.3	51.7	50.0	48.3	46.3	44.3	42.0	39.6	37.0	34.1	31.0	
61	52.4	50.9	49.2	47.5	45.6	43.6	41.4	39.0	36.4	33.7	30.7	27.4	
64	50.0	48.4	46.7	44.9	42.9	40.8	38.5	36.0	33.4	30.5	27.3	23.9	
67	47.7	46.0	44.2	42.3	40.2	38.0	35.6	33.0	30.3	27.2	23.9	20.3	
70	45.4	43.6	41.7	39.7	37.5	35.2	32.7	30.0	27.1	24.0	20.5	16.7	
73	43.0	41.2	39.2	37.1	34.9	32.5	29.9	27.0	24.0	20.7	17.1	13.1	
76	40.7	38.8	36.7	34.5	32.2	29.7	27.0	24.0	20.9	17.4	13.7	9.6	
79	38.3	36.3	34.2	31.9	29.5	26.9	24.1	21.0	17.8	14.2	10.3	6.0	
82	36.0	33.9	31.7	29.4	26.8	24.1	21.2	18.0	14.6	10.9	6.9	2.4	
85	33.6	31.5	29.2	26.8	24.2	21.3	18.3	15.0	11.5	7.7	3.3	—	
88	31.3	29.1	26.7	24.2	21.5	18.6	15.4	12.0	8.4	4.4	0.0	—	
91	29.0	26.7	24.2	21.6	18.8	15.8	12.5	9.0	5.3	1.1	—	1.3	79
94	27.6	24.2	21.7	19.0	16.1	13.0	9.7	6.0	2.1	—	0.0	5.0	78
97	24.3	21.8	19.2	16.4	13.4	10.2	6.8	3.0	—	—	4.0	8.8	73
100	21.9	19.4	16.7	13.8	10.8	7.5	3.9	0.0	—	2.8	7.9	12.5	70
103	19.9	17.0	14.2	11.3	8.1	4.7	1.0	—	1.5	7.0	11.9	16.3	67
106	17.2	14.6	11.7	8.7	5.4	1.9	—	0.0	5.9	11.2	15.8	20.0	64
109	14.9	12.1	9.2	6.1	2.7	—	—	4.7	10.3	15.3	19.8	23.8	61
112	12.5	9.7	6.7	3.5	0.0	—	3.4	9.4	14.8	19.5	23.7	27.5	58
115	11.2	7.3	4.2	.9	—	1.8	8.4	14.1	19.2	23.7	27.7	31.3	55
118	7.9	4.9	1.7	—	0.0	7.2	13.4	18.8	23.6	27.8	31.6	35.0	52
121	5.5	2.5	—	—	5.8	12.5	18.4	23.5	28.0	32.0	35.6	38.8	49
124	3.2	0.0	—	4.2	11.6	17.9	23.4	28.2	32.4	36.2	39.5	42.5	46
128	0.0	—	2.3	10.5	17.4	23.3	28.4	32.9	36.8	40.3	43.5	46.3	43
	—	0.0	9.1	16.7	23.1	28.6	33.4	37.5	41.2	44.5	47.4	50.0	40
	—	7.5	16.0	23.0	28.9	34.0	38.4	42.2	45.6	48.7	51.4	53.8	37
	5.6	15.0	22.8	29.2	34.7	39.3	43.4	46.9	50.0	52.8	55.3	57.5	34
	13.9	22.5	29.6	35.5	40.4	44.7	48.4	51.6	54.5	57.0	59.3	61.3	31
	22.3	30.0	36.4	41.7	46.2	50.0	53.4	56.3	58.9	61.2	63.2	65.0	28
	30.6	37.5	43.2	48.0	52.0	55.4	58.4	61.0	63.3	65.3	67.2	68.8	25
	38.9	45.0	50.0	54.2	57.7	60.8	63.4	65.7	67.7	69.5	71.1	72.5	22
	47.3	52.5	56.9	60.5	63.5	66.1	68.4	70.4	72.1	73.7	75.0	76.3	19
	55.6	60.0	63.7	66.7	69.3	71.5	73.4	75.0	76.5	78.8	79.0	80.0	16
	63.9	67.5	70.5	73.0	75.0	76.8	78.4	79.7	80.9	82.0	82.9	83.8	13
	72.3	75.0	77.3	79.2	80.8	82.2	83.4	84.4	85.3	86.2	86.9	87.5	10
	80.6	82.5	84.1	85.5	86.6	87.5	88.4	89.1	89.8	90.3	90.8	91.3	7
	88.9	90.0	91.0	91.7	92.4	92.9	93.4	93.8	94.2	94.5	94.8	95.0	4
	97.3	97.5	97.8	98.0	98.1	98.3	98.4	98.5	98.6	98.7	98.7	98.8	1
	9–36	10–40	11–44	12–48	13–52	14–56	15–60	16–64	17–68	18–72	19–76	20–80	

(From Grant, D.A., Stern, I.B., and Everett, F.G.: *Periodontics*, 5th ed. The C.V. Mosby Co., 1979.)

materia alba, and food debris that is loosely attached to tooth surfaces.

II. Selection of Teeth and Surfaces

A. Teeth Examined

(FDI System tooth numbers are in parentheses.)

Maxillary	Mandibular
No. 3 (16) Right first molar	No. 19 (36) Left first molar
No. 8 (11) Right central incisor	No. 24 (31) Left central incisor
No. 14 (26) Left first molar	No. 30 (46) Right first molar

B. Substitutions

When a first molar is missing, is less than three-fourths erupted, has a full crown, or is broken down, the second molar is used. The third molar is used when the second is missing. The adjacent central incisor is used for a missing incisor.

C. Surfaces

The facial surfaces of incisors and maxillary molars and the lingual of mandibular molars are examined. These surfaces are the same as those used for the Simplified Oral Hygiene Index (figure 19–6, page 270).

III. Procedure

A. Apply disclosing agent. Instruct the patient to swish for 30 seconds and expectorate but not rinse.
B. Examination is made using a mouth mirror.
C. Each tooth surface to be evaluated is subdivided (mentally) into five sections (figure 19–3) as follows:
   1. Vertically: three divisions, mesial, middle, and distal.
   2. Horizontally: the middle third is subdivided into gingival, middle, and occlusal or incisal thirds.
D. Each of the five subdivisions is scored for the presence of stained debris as follows:

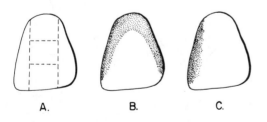

    A.   B.   C.

Figure 19–3. Patient Hygiene Performance (PHP). A. Oral debris is assessed by dividing a tooth into five subdivisions, each of which is scored 1 when debris is shown to be present after use of a disclosing agent. **B.** Example of Debris Score of 3. Shaded portion represents debris stained by disclosing agent. **C.** Example of Debris Score of 1. (Podshadley and Haley, Public Health Reports, *83*, 259, 1968.)

0 = No debris (or questionable).
1 = Debris definitely present.
Identify by *M* when all three molars or both incisors are missing.
Identify by *S* when a substitute tooth is used.

IV. Scoring

A. Debris Score for Individual Tooth

Add the scores for each of the five subdivisions. The scores range from 0 to 5.

B. PHP for the Individual

Total the scores for the individual teeth and divide by the number of teeth examined. The PHP ranges from 0 to 5.

C. Suggested Nominal Scale for Evaluation of Scores

Rating	Scores
Excellent	0– (no debris)
Good	0.1–1.7
Fair	1.8–3.4
Poor	3.5–5.0

D. Calculation Example for an Individual

Tooth	Debris Score
No. 3 (16)	5
No. 8 (11)	3
No. 14 (26)	4
No. 19 (36)	5
No. 24 (31)	2
No. 30 (46)	3
Total	22

$$PHP = \frac{\text{Total Debris Score}}{\text{Number of Teeth Scored}} = \frac{22}{6} = 3.66$$

Interpretation: According to the suggested nominal scale, this person with a PHP of 3.66 would be classified as exhibiting poor hygiene performance.

E. PHP for a Group

To obtain the average PHP score for a group or population, total the individual scores and divide by the number of people examined.

ORAL HYGIENE INDEX (OHI)
(Greene and Vermillion,[9] Waggener[10])

I. Purpose

To measure existing debris and calculus as an indication of oral cleanliness. The OHI has two components, the *Debris Index* and the *Calculus Index*. Each is based on 12 numerical determinations that designate the amount of debris or calculus found on selected tooth surfaces. The two scores may be used singly or may be combined for an OHI.

II. Selection of Teeth and Surfaces

A. Divide the dentition into sextants. Posterior sextants begin distal to the canines.

1. Score only fully erupted permanent teeth. A tooth is considered fully erupted when it has reached the occlusal plane.
2. Exclude third molars, teeth with full crown restorations, and teeth reduced in height because of severe dental caries or trauma.

B. Select the 12 tooth surfaces, 1 facial and 1 lingual or palatal in each sextant, that are covered with the greatest amount of debris, plaque, or calculus.
  1. Facial and lingual or palatal surfaces in each sextant may be taken from different teeth.
  2. Include proximal surfaces to the contact area. A score represents half the circumference of the selected tooth.

III. Procedure

A. Evaluation

Evaluate each sextant to record first the debris and then the calculus.

B. Sequence

Proceed in routine order from maxillary right, anterior, and left sextants to mandibular left, anterior, and right sextants.

C. Record 12 Debris Scores

1. *Definition of Oral Debris.* Oral debris is the soft foreign matter on the surfaces of the teeth that consists of bacterial plaque, materia alba, and food debris.
2. *Examination.* Run the side of the tip of a probe or explorer across the tooth surface to assist in estimating the surface area covered by debris.
3. *Criteria* (figure 19–4)

   0 = No debris or stain present.
   1 = Soft debris covering not more than one third of the tooth surface being examined, or the presence of extrinsic stains without debris, regardless of surface area covered.
   2 = Soft debris covering more than one third but not more than two thirds of the exposed tooth surface.
   3 = Soft debris covering more than two thirds of the exposed tooth surface.

D. Record 12 Calculus Scores

1. *Definition of Calculus.* Dental calculus is a hard deposit of inorganic salts composed primarily of calcium carbonate and phosphate

mixed with debris, microorganisms, and desquamated epithelial cells.
2. *Examination.* Use an explorer to supplement visual examination for supragingival calculus deposits. Identify subgingival deposits by exploring and/or probing. Record only definite deposits of hard calculus.
3. *Criteria* (figure 19–5)

   0 = No calculus present
   1 = Supragingival calculus covering not more than one third of the exposed tooth surface being examined.
   2 = Supragingival calculus covering more than one third but not more than two thirds of the exposed tooth surface, or the presence of individual flecks of subgingival calculus around the cervical portion of the tooth.
   3 = Supragingival calculus covering more than two thirds of the exposed tooth surface or a continuous heavy band of subgingival calculus around the cervical portion of the tooth.

IV. Scoring

A. OHI for an Individual

1. Determine Debris Index (DI) and Calculus Index (CI)
   a. Divide total scores by number of sextants.
      i. Each selected surface has a severity score of 0 to 3 (see Criteria, above).
      ii. The total score for debris or calculus ranges from 0 to 36 (12 scores multiplied by maximum severity of 3).
   b. Debris Index (DI) or Calculus Index (CI) ranges from 0 to 6.
2. Oral Hygiene Index (OHI) = DI + CI
   a. Combine the Debris Index and the Calculus Index.
   b. The OHI ranges from 0 to 12.

B. Suggested Nominal Scale

1. DI and CI

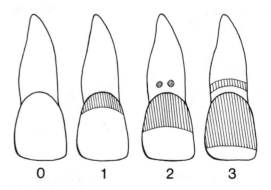

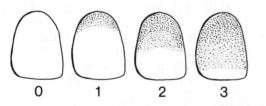

Figure 19–4. Oral Hygiene Index. For the Debris Index, 12 surfaces are scored, 2 in each sextant. Scoring of 0 to 3 is based on tooth surfaces covered by debris as shown.

Figure 19–5. Oral Hygiene Index. For the Calculus Index, 12 surfaces are scored, 2 in each sextant. Scoring of 0 to 3 is based on location and tooth surface area with calculus as shown. Note slight subgingival calculus recorded as 2 and more extensive subgingival calculus by 3.

Rating	Scores
Excellent	0
Good	0.1–1.2
Fair	1.3–3.0
Poor	3.1–6.0

2. OHI

Rating	Scores
Excellent	0
Good	0.1–2.4
Fair	2.5–6.0
Poor	6.1–12.0

C. Calculation Example for Individual OHI

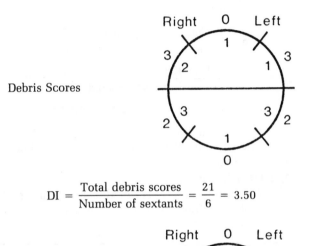

Debris Scores

$$DI = \frac{Total\ debris\ scores}{Number\ of\ sextants} = \frac{21}{6} = 3.50$$

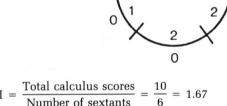

Calculus scores

$$CI = \frac{Total\ calculus\ scores}{Number\ of\ sextants} = \frac{10}{6} = 1.67$$

$$OHI = DI + CI = 3.50 + 1.67 = 5.17$$

Interpretation: According to the suggested nominal scale, the score for this individual OHI score (5.17) indicates a fair oral hygiene status.

D. OHI for a Group

1. *Group Debris Index.* Divide total DI scores by number of individuals.
2. *Group Calculus Index.* Divide total CI scores by number of individuals.
3. *Mean Oral Hygiene Index (OHI).* Divide total DI and CI scores for all individuals by the number of individuals.

SIMPLIFIED ORAL HYGIENE INDEX (OHI-S)
(Greene and Vermillion[11,12])

I. Purpose

To assess oral cleanliness by estimating the tooth surface covered with debris and/or calculus.

A. Components

The OHI-S has two components, the Simplified Debris Index (DI-S) and the Simplified Calculus Index (CI-S). The two scores may be used separately or may be combined for the OHI-S.

B. Comparison with OHI (page 267)

After experience with the Oral Hygiene Index (OHI), the need for simplification was recognized because of the length of time required to evaluate debris and calculus, as well as to make subjective decisions on tooth selection.

1. *Tooth Selection.* In the OHI the examiner has to select the tooth with the most debris or calculus in each sextant. The OHI-S assesses 6 specific teeth, 1 in each sextant.
2. *Number of Surfaces.* In the OHI, 12 surfaces are evaluated; only 6 surfaces are used in the OHI-S.
3. *Scoring.* The OHI ranges from 0 to 12; the OHI-S ranges from 0 to 6.

II. Selection of Teeth and Surfaces

A. Identify the 6 Specific Teeth (figure 19–6)

1. *Posterior.* The first fully erupted tooth distal to each second premolar is examined. The facial surfaces of the maxillary molars and the lingual surfaces of the mandibular molars are used. Although usually the first molars, the second or third molars may be used.
2. *Anterior.* The facial surfaces of the maxillary right and the mandibular left central incisors are used. When either is missing, the opposite central incisor is scored.

B. Extent

A score represents half the circumference of the selected tooth; includes proximal surfaces to the contact areas.

III. Procedure

A. Qualification

At least two of the six possible surfaces must have been examined for an individual score to be expressed.

B. Record Six Debris Scores and Six Calculus Scores

Follow the routine and use the same criteria as for the OHI described on page 268. Figures 19–4 (debris) and 19–5 (calculus) illustrate the extent of deposits for each score from 0 to 3.

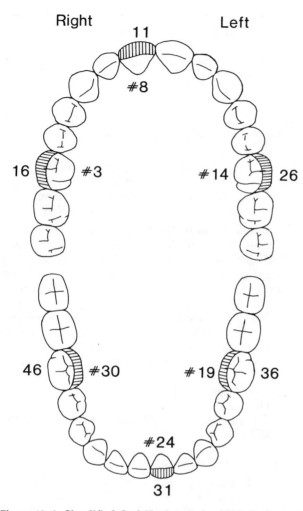

Right   Left

Figure 19–6. Simplified Oral Hygiene Index (OHI-S). Six tooth surfaces are scored as follows: facial surfaces of maxillary molars and of the maxillary right and mandibular left central incisors, and the lingual surfaces of mandibular molars. Teeth are numbered by the ADA System on the lingual and by the FDI System on the facial.

IV. Scoring

A. OHI-S for an Individual
  1. *Determine Simplified Debris Index (DI-S) and Simplified Calculus Index (CI-S)*
    a. Divide total scores by number of sextants.
    b. DI-S and CI-S values range from 0 to 3.
  2. *Simplified Oral Hygiene Index (OHI-S)*
    a. Combine the DI-S and CI-S.
    b. OHI-S value ranges from 0 to 6.

B. Suggested Nominal Scale[12]

DI-S and CI-S

Rating	Scores
Excellent	0
Good	0.1–0.6
Fair	0.7–1.8
Poor	1.9–3.0

OHI-S

Excellent	0
Good	0.1–1.2
Fair	1.3–3.0
Poor	3.1–6.0

C. Calculation Example for an Individual

Tooth	Individual Scores	
	DI-S	CI-S
No. 3 (16)	2	2
No. 8 (11)	1	0
No. 14 (26)	3	2
No. 19 (36)	3	2
No. 24 (31)	2	1
No. 30 (46)	2	2
Total	13	9

$$\text{DI-S} = \frac{\text{Total Debris Scores}}{\text{Number of Teeth Scored}} = \frac{13}{6} = 2.17$$

$$\text{CI-S} = \frac{\text{Total Calculus Scores}}{\text{Number of Teeth Scored}} = \frac{9}{6} = 1.50$$

$$\text{OHI-S} = \text{DI-S} + \text{CI-S} = 2.17 + 1.50 = 3.67$$

Interpretation: According to the suggested nominal scale, the score for this individual (3.67) indicates a poor oral hygiene status.

D. OHI-S Group Score
  Compute the average of the individual scores by totalling the scores and dividing by the number of individuals.

BLEEDING INDICES

Bleeding on gentle probing or flossing is an early sign of gingival inflammation and precedes color changes and enlargement of the gingival tissues.[13,14] Based on the principle that healthy tissue does not bleed, testing for bleeding has become a significant procedure for evaluation prior to treatment planning, after therapy to show the effects of treatment aimed to eliminate inflammation, and at maintenance appointments.

For patient instruction and motivation, a variety of bleeding indices and scoring methods has been developed. The Gingival Index (GI) described on page 273 includes an estimate of bleeding on probing along with other clinical observations to arrive at a score to designate the severity of gingivitis. The GI has been used extensively in research, as well as for patient instruction and motivation.

Another example is the record of bleeding following interdental probing, which may accompany a plaque-free score as described on page 264. The form illustrated in figure 19–2 has small circles that can be colored in to illustrate interproximal bleeding. A series of diagrams made over several weeks can show the patient's progress toward health, as less and less bleeding is charted.

Two of the well-known bleeding indices will be

described below. They are the Sulcus Bleeding Index developed by Mühlemann and the Gingival Bleeding Index of Carter and Barnes.

SULCUS BLEEDING INDEX (SBI)
(Mühlemann[13])

I. Purpose

To locate areas of gingival sulcus bleeding upon gentle probing and thus recognize and record the presence of early (initial) inflammatory gingival disease.

II. Areas Examined

Four gingival units are scored systematically for each tooth: the marginal gingiva, labial and lingual (M units), and the papillary gingiva, mesial and distal (P units).

III. Procedure

A. Use standardized lighting while probing each of the four areas.
B. Hold the probe parallel with the long axis of the tooth for M units, and direct the probe toward the col area for P units.
C. Wait 30 seconds after probing before scoring apparently healthy gingival units.
D. Dry the gingiva gently if necessary to observe color changes clearly.
E. Criteria

   0 = Healthy appearance of P and M, no bleeding on sulcus probing.
   1 = Apparently healthy P and M showing no change in color and no swelling, but bleeding from sulcus on probing.
   2 = Bleeding on probing *and* change of color caused by inflammation. No swelling or macroscopic edema.
   3 = Bleeding on probing *and* change in color and slight edematous swelling.
   4 = (1) Bleeding on probing *and* change in color *and* obvious swelling.
       (2) Bleeding on probing and obvious swelling.
   5 = Bleeding on probing and spontaneous bleeding *and* change in color, marked swelling with or without ulceration.

IV. Scoring

A. SBI for Area

Each of the 4 gingival units (M and P) is scored 0 to 5.

B. SBI for Tooth

Scores for the 4 units are totalled and divided by 4.

C. SBI for Individual

By totalling scores for individual teeth and dividing by the number of teeth, the SBI is determined. Indices range from 0 to 6.

GINGIVAL BLEEDING INDEX (GBI)
(Carter and Barnes[15])

I. Purpose

To record the presence or absence of gingival inflammation as determined by bleeding from interproximal gingival sulci.

II. Areas Examined

Each interproximal area has two sulci, which are scored as one interdental unit, or may be scored individually. Certain areas may be excluded from scoring because of accessibility, tooth position, diastemas, or other factors, and if exclusions are made, a consistent procedure should be followed for an individual and for a group if a study is to be made.

A full complement of teeth has 28 proximal areas. In the original studies, third molars were excluded, and 26 units were recorded.[15]

III. Procedure
A. Instrument

Unwaxed dental floss is used. The use of floss has the advantages of being readily available, disposable, and usable by the instructed patient.

B. Steps

1. Pass the floss interproximally first on one side of the papilla and then on the other.
2. Curve the floss around the adjacent tooth (figure 23–1 E and F, page 319), and bring the floss to the bottom of the sulcus.
3. Move the floss up and down for one stroke, with care not to lacerate the gingiva. Adapt finger rests to provide controlled, consistent pressure.
4. Use a new length of clean floss for each area.
5. Retract for visibility of bleeding from both facial and lingual.
6. Allow 30 seconds for reinspection of an area that does not show blood immediately either in the area or on the floss.

C. Criteria

Bleeding indicates the presence of disease. No attempt is made to quantify the severity of bleeding because the important factor is no bleeding at all in health.

IV. Scoring

The number of bleeding areas and the number of scorable units are recorded. Patient motivation can result when the patient participates in observing and recording over a series of appointments.

PAPILLARY-MARGINAL-ATTACHED GINGIVAL INDEX (P-M-A)
(Schour and Massler[16,17])

I. Purpose

To assess the extent of gingival changes in large groups for epidemiologic studies.

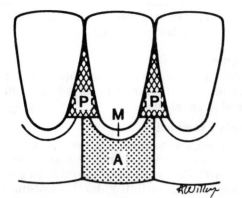

Figure 19–7. Papillary-Marginal-Attached Gingival Index (P-M-A). Each of the 3 parts of the gingiva is scored from 0 (healthy) to 5 (marked disease characteristics). Units are scored and recorded separately to show P (Papillary), M (Marginal), and A (Attached) conditions.

II. Selection of Teeth and Areas

Three gingival units are examined for each tooth (figure 19–7)

P = *Papillary* portion between the teeth
  1. Number each papilla by the tooth just distal. No papilla is present when teeth are separated by a diastema or edentulous area.
  2. Mild gingivitis is associated with papillary changes. Inflammation usually begins within the papilla at the col area.

M = *Marginal* collar around the tooth
  1. Located between papillae, attached by junctional epithelium, and demarcated from attached gingiva by the free gingival groove (page 167).
  2. Moderate gingivitis is associated with papillary and marginal gingival inflammation.

A = *Attached* gingiva overlying the alveolar bone
  1. Stippled gingiva between the free gingival groove and the mucogingival junction.
  2. Severe gingivitis is associated with spread of inflammation from papillary and marginal gingivitis into the attached gingiva.

III. Procedure

A. Instruments and Equipment
  1. Adequate lighting; headrest for stabilization.
  2. Mouth mirror.
  3. Probe for pressing on gingiva. In the original studies, a blunt explorer was used.

B. Examine Facial Surfaces Only
  1. Proceed in a routine order from left maxillary second molar around to right second molar; then mandibular right second molar around to left.
  2. Third molars are not included.

C. Criteria

Gingival Area	Score	Criteria
Papillary	P	0 = Normal; no inflammation.
		1 + = Mild papillary engorgement; slight increase in size.
		2 + = Obvious increase in size of gingival papilla; bleeding on pressure.
		3 + = Excessive increase in size with spontaneous bleeding.
		4 + = Necrotic papilla.
		5 + = Atrophy and loss of papilla (through inflammation).
Marginal	M	0 = Normal; no inflammation visible.
		1 + = Engorgement; slight increase in size; no bleeding.
		2 + = Obvious engorgement; bleeding upon pressure.
		3 + = Swollen collar; spontaneous bleeding; beginning infiltration into attached gingiva.
		4 + = Necrotic gingivitis.
		5 + = Recession of the free marginal gingiva below the CEJ as a result of inflammatory changes.
Attached	A	0 = Normal; pale rose; stippled.
		1 + = Slight engorgement with loss of stippling; change in color may or may not be present.
		2 + = Obvious engorgement of attached gingiva with marked increase in redness. Pocket formation present.
		3 + = Advanced periodontitis. Deep pockets evident.

IV. Scoring

A. P-M-A for an Individual
  1. Count the number of Papillary, Marginal, and Attached units scored and record separately as follows:

$$\text{P-M-A} = 10\text{-}5\text{-}0$$

  2. Keep totals separate. If added together the sum would reflect different meanings and would not represent the areas of the gingiva where the inflammation occurred.

B. Suggested Nominal Scale for the P-M-A[16]

Mild gingivitis	1 to 4 papillae 0 to 2 margins
Moderate gingivitis	4 to 8 papillae 2 to 4 margins
Severe gingivitis	more than 8 papillae more than 4 margins

C. P-M-A for a Group

Compute the average of the P, M, and A by totalling each for all individuals and then dividing each by the number of individuals examined.

GINGIVAL INDEX (GI)
(Löe and Silness[5,18])

I. Purpose

To assess the severity of gingivitis based on color, consistency, and bleeding on probing.

II. Selection of Teeth and Gingival Areas

A gingival index may be determined for selected teeth or for the entire dentition.

A. Areas Examined

Four gingival areas (distal, facial, mesial, lingual) are examined systematically for each tooth.

B. Modified Procedure

Omit the distal examination for each tooth. The score for the mesial is doubled, and the total score for each tooth is divided by 4.

III. Procedure

A. The teeth and gingiva are dried, and under adequate light, a mouth mirror and probe are used.
B. The probe is used to press on the gingiva to determine the degree of firmness.
C. The probe is used to run along the soft tissue wall near the entrance to the gingival sulcus to evaluate bleeding (figure 19–8).
D. Criteria

   0 = Normal gingiva.
   1 = Mild inflammation—slight change in color, slight edema. *No bleeding on probing.*
   2 = Moderate inflammation—redness, edema, and glazing. *Bleeding on probing.*
   3 = Severe inflammation—marked redness and edema. Ulceration. *Tendency to spontaneous bleeding.*

IV. Scoring

A. GI for Area

Each of the 4 gingival surfaces (distal, facial, mesial, lingual) is given a score of 0 to 3.

B. GI for a Tooth

Scores for each area are totalled and divided by 4.

C. GI for Groups of Teeth

Scores for individual teeth may be grouped and totalled, and divided by the number of teeth. A Gingival Index may be determined for specific teeth, group of teeth, quadrant, or side of mouth.

D. GI for the Individual

By totalling scores and dividing by the number of teeth examined, the Gingival Index is determined. Indices range from 0 to 3.

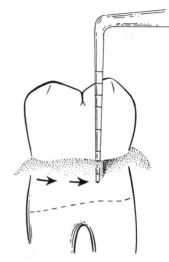

Figure 19–8. Gingival Index (GI). Probe stroke for bleeding evaluation. The broken line represents the level of attachment of the periodontal tissues. The probe is inserted a few millimeters and moved along the soft tissue pocket wall with light pressure in a circumferential direction. The stroke shown here is in contrast with the walking stroke used for pocket evaluation and measurement as described on page 197.

E. Suggested Nominal Scale for Patient Reference

Rating	Scores
Excellent (healthy tissue)	0
Good	0.1–0.9
Fair	1.0–1.9
Poor	2.0–3.0

F. Calculation Example for an Individual
(using 6 teeth for an example of screening; see figure 19–9)

		Gingival Area		
	M	F	D	L
3 (16)	3	1	3	1
9 (21)	1	0	1	1
12 (24)	2	1	2	0
19 (36)	3	1	3	3
25 (41)	1	1	1	1
28 (44)	2	1	2	0
Total	12 +	5 +	12 +	6 = 35

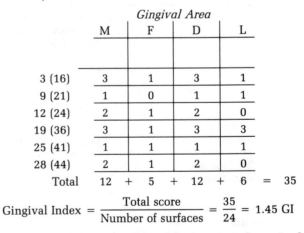

$$\text{Gingival Index} = \frac{\text{Total score}}{\text{Number of surfaces}} = \frac{35}{24} = 1.45 \text{ GI}$$

Interpretation: According to the suggested nominal scale, the score for this individual (1.45) indicates only fair gingival health (moderate inflammation). The ratings for each gingival area or surface can be used to help the patient compare gingival changes toward health at each appointment.

G. GI for a Group

Add the individual GI scores and divide by the number of individuals examined.

THE PERIODONTAL INDEX (PI)
(Russell[19,20])

I. Purpose

To assess and score the periodontal disease status of populations in epidemiologic studies.

II. Procedure

A. Instruments

Each tooth present is examined using a mouth mirror and explorer with adequate illumination. In the original examinations,[19] a Jacquette scaler and chip blower were used to define the presence of periodontal pockets. At present, a periodontal probe is the preferred instrument.

B. Criteria

0 = Negative		There is neither overt inflammation in the investing tissues nor loss of function caused by destruction of supporting tissue.
1 = Mild Gingivitis		There is an overt area of inflammation in the free gingiva that does not circumscribe the tooth.
2 = Gingivitis		Inflammation completely circumscribes the tooth, but there is no apparent break in the epithelial attachment.
6 = Gingivitis with Pocket Formation		The epithelial attachment has been broken and there is a pocket (not merely a deepened gingival crevice caused by swelling in the free gingiva). There is no interference with normal masticatory function; the tooth is firm in its socket and has not drifted.
8 = Advanced Destruction with Loss of Masticatory Function		The tooth may be loose; may have drifted; may sound dull on percussion with a metallic instrument; may be depressible in its socket.

III. Scoring

A. Each tooth is assigned a score from 0 (no disease) to 8 (severe disease with loss of function).
B. Add the scores for each tooth and divide by the number of teeth present and examined to obtain the individual's score.
C. PI group score: total the individuals' scores and divide by the number of individuals examined. The average ranges from 0 to 8.
D. Suggested Nominal Scale for Patient Reference[20]

Condition	Scores
Clinically normal supportive tissues	0–0.2
Simple gingivitis	0.3–0.9
Beginning destructive periodontal disease	0.7–1.9
Established destructive periodontal disease	1.6–5.0
Terminal disease	3.8–8.0

E. Breakdown of scores: In a population group, scores may be averaged by specific age groups, such as ages 1 to 9, 10 to 19, 20 to 29, and so forth. Scores may be calculated for each sex or for each sex within the various age groups. Data may also be used to calculate disease in relation to economic factors or educational background of the individuals.

THE PERIODONTAL DISEASE INDEX (PDI)
(Ramfjord[21,22])

I. Purpose

To assess the prevalence and severity of gingivitis and periodontitis and to show the periodontal status of an individual or a group.

The Periodontal Disease Index (PDI) combines the evaluation of gingival status with the probed attachment level (crevice depth measured from the cementoenamel junction).

Although not part of the PDI, a Calculus Index (CI) and Plaque Index (PI) have usually been included when making a survey and will be described after the PDI.

II. Selection of Teeth and Surfaces

A. Six teeth are used to represent the six segments of the dentition (figure 19–9).

(FDI System tooth numbers are in parentheses.)

Maxillary	Mandibular
No. 3 (16) right first molar	No. 19 (36) left first molar
No. 9 (21) left central incisor	No. 25 (41) right central incisor
No. 12 (24) left first premolar	No. 28 (44) right first premolar

B. Only fully erupted teeth are used.
C. Substitutions are not made for missing teeth; scores are derived from the teeth present.

III. Procedure

A. Determine Gingival Status

1. Under consistent standardized light, dry the gingiva with cotton to observe color and form.
2. Apply gentle pressure with the probe to determine consistency (density). When the color

Right   Left

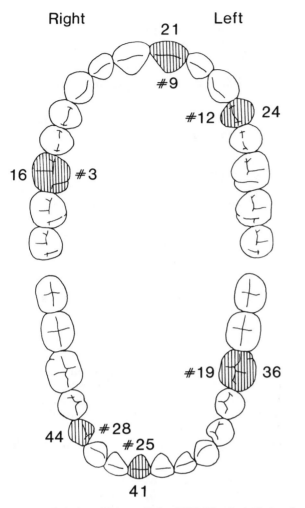

Figure 19–9. Periodontal Disease Index (PDI). The six shaded teeth are scored. Teeth are numbered by the ADA System on the lingual and the FDI System on the facial.

change definitely indicates the presence of inflammation, the consistency is not checked.

3. Criteria for gingival status

   0 = Absence of signs of inflammation.
   1 = Mild to moderate inflammatory gingival changes, not extending around the tooth.
   2 = Mild to moderately severe gingivitis extending all around the tooth.
   3 = Severe gingivitis characterized by marked redness, swelling, tendency to bleed, and ulceration, not necessarily extending around the tooth.

4. Summary for an individual
   a. Individual teeth. Add the scores for each area and divide by the number of areas examined.
   b. Score for individual. Add the scores for all the examined teeth and divide by the total number of teeth examined. The range is from 0 to 3.

B. Determine Crevice Depth from Cementoenamel Junction (CEJ)

1. *Technique Objective.* To measure the crevice or sulcus depth from the CEJ to the bottom of the gingival crevice or pocket. This technique measures the probed attachment level and is described in detail on page 198.
2. *Instrument.* To obtain consistent readings, a probe is needed that has been calibrated for shape, thickness, angulation, and the placement and definition of reference marks. When the index was first used, a Michigan probe No. 0 was used (figure 13–1–C, page 194).
3. *Locations of Measurements*
   a. Two measurements. When two measurements are made, they are at the middle of the facial surface and at the facial aspect of the mesial contact area, with the side of the probe held touching both teeth (figure 19–10).
   b. Original PDI. Four measurements were made for each tooth, on the facial, mesial, distal, and lingual. It was later found that no significant loss in accuracy resulted from using only two measurements. Four measurements are still used for certain types of research evaluations.
4. *Measurements*
   a. When the CEJ is covered by gingiva, determine the location of the CEJ by sliding the probe subgingivally (figure 19–11A), and measure the distance to the CEJ from the margin. Scale to remove calculus when deposits cover the CEJ (figure 19–11B). Measure from the gingival margin to determine the probed pocket depth (figure 19–11C) and subtract the measured distance from the gingival margin to the CEJ to determine the probed attachment level.
   b. When the CEJ is visible because of gingival recession, the crevice depth can be measured directly from the CEJ (figure 19–11D).
   c. When the gingival margin is level with the CEJ, the probed pocket depth and the

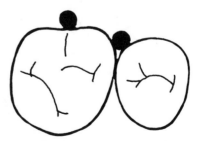

Figure 19–10. Periodontal Disease Index (PDI). Probe positions for measuring crevice depth are shown by the black dots. One measurement is made at the middle of the facial surface and the other at the facial aspect of the mesial contact area. The side of the probe is held touching both teeth.

probed attachment level are equal (figure 13–7D, page 198).

5. Criteria for PDI

0 to 3 (Gingivitis Index)	= When the gingival crevice or pocket in none of the measured areas extends apical to the cementoenamel junction.
4	= When the crevices (pockets) of any 2 (or 4) recorded areas extend apically to the cementoenamel junction not more than, but including, 3 mm. (The gingivitis score is then disregarded.)
5	= When the crevices (pockets) of any of the 2 (or 4) recorded areas extend apically to the cementoenamel junction from 3 mm. to 6 mm inclusive. (The gingivitis score is disregarded.)
6	= When the crevices (pockets) extend more than 6 mm. apically to the cementoenamel junction in any of the 2 (or 4) measured areas. (The gingivitis score is disregarded.)

IV. Scoring

A. PDI for an Individual

Add scores for individual teeth and divide by the number of teeth examined. The PDI ranges from 0 to 6.

B. Suggested Nominal Scale for Evaluation of Scores

1. *Gingivitis.* Numbers 0 to 3 indicate gingival involvement only, with increasing severity from 0 (no disease) through 3.9 (severe gingivitis).
2. *Periodontitis.* Numbers 4 through 6 indicate periodontal involvement with migration of the junctional epithelium and bone loss of increasing degree of severity from 4 (early disease) through 6 (advanced disease).

C. Calculation Example for an Individual

Tooth	Periodontal Disease Score
No. 3 (16)	4
No. 9 (21)	0
No. 12 (24)	5
No. 19 (36)	6
No. 25 (41)	4
No. 28 (44)	2
Total	21

$$PDI = \frac{Total\ scores}{Number\ of\ teeth} = \frac{21}{6} = 3.5$$

Interpretation: For epidemiologic purposes, using the average (mean) group score of 3.5 can be acceptable for showing overall characteristics of a large population. In the example above, however, the 3.5 PDI, which by the nominal score represents "severe gingivitis," would be misleading when reporting the condition of this individual. The scores for each tooth clearly show that 4 of the 6 teeth examined have measurements that show loss of attachment and loss of bone typical of periodontitis. Care must be taken when interpreting the PDI on an individual basis.

D. PDI Group Score

Total the individual PDI scores and divide by the number of individuals examined. The average ranges from 0 to 6.

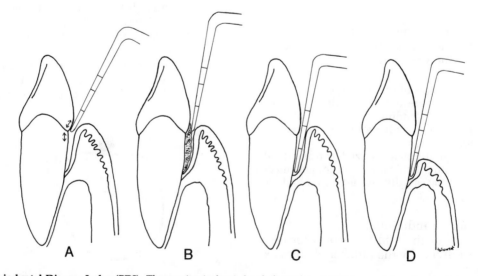

Figure 19–11. Periodontal Disease Index (PDI). The crevice (sulcus) depth from the cementoenamel junction is determined as follows. **A.** Locate the cementoenamel junction with the probe tip and measure the distance from the gingival margin. **B.** When calculus interferes with efforts to locate the cementoenamel junction, scaling is performed. **C.** Apply probe to measure the pocket depth from gingival margin to attached periodontal tissue, and subtract the distance to the cementoenamel junction. **D.** When there is apparent recession, the direct reading from the cementoenamel junction can be measured. Note use of Michigan 0 probe.

CALCULUS SCORE (Used with PDI)
(Ramfjord[22])

I. Purpose

To evaluate the presence and extent of calculus. This index is not an integral part of the PDI but was developed and used in conjunction with the PDI.

Because calculus may have to be removed to determine the location of the cementoenamel junction for crevice and pocket measurements in the PDI, calculus should be scored first, before its removal.

II. Surfaces Examined

For each of the 6 teeth (figure 19–9), 4 surfaces (facial, lingual (or palatal), mesial, and distal) are scored from 0 to 3.

III. Procedure
A. Instruments

A subgingival explorer (for example, the No. TU-17, figure 13–14, page 203) may be used to locate subgingival calculus and determine its extent. The probe (such as the Michigan 0) used for crevice and pocket determinations may provide sufficient sensitivity for calculus evaluation.

B. Criteria

0 = No calculus
1 = Supragingival calculus extending only slightly below the free gingival margin (not more than 1 mm.).
2 = Moderate amount of supra- and subgingival calculus, or subgingival calculus only.
3 = Abundance of supra- and subgingival calculus.

IV. Scoring
A. Individual Teeth

Add scores for each surface and divide by the number of surfaces (4).

B. Calculus Score for an Individual

Add the scores for the individual teeth and divide by the number of teeth. The calculus score ranges from 0 to 3.

DENTAL PLAQUE SCORE (Used with PDI)
(Ramfjord[22])

I. Purpose

To evaluate the extent of plaque on the basis of tooth surface coverage.

II. Selection of Teeth and Surfaces

For each of the 6 teeth (figure 19–9), 4 surfaces (facial, lingual, mesial, and distal) are scored from 0 to 3.

III. Procedure

A. Apply disclosing agent, using two saturated pellets, one for the maxillary and one for the mandibular teeth.
B. Request patient to expectorate, then rinse with water.
C. Use direct or indirect (mirror) vision to observe specific surfaces with disclosed plaque.
D. Criteria

0 = No plaque
1 = Plaque present on some but not all interproximal, facial, and lingual surfaces of the tooth.
2 = Plaque present on all interproximal, facial, and lingual surfaces, but covering less than one half of these surfaces.
3 = Plaque extending over all interproximal, facial, and lingual surfaces, and covering more than one half of these surfaces.

E. The original criteria listed above serve adequately for epidemiologic purposes. Criteria were developed later to refine the scoring for small differences in the distribution of bacterial plaque.[23] By the modified system, scores are recorded for the gingival half of the facial and lingual surfaces as shown in figure 19–12, and recorded as follows:

0 = No plaque on the gingival half.
1 = Plaque covering less than one third of the gingival half.
2 = Plaque covering one third or less than two thirds of the gingival half.
3 = Plaque covering two thirds or more of the facial or lingual of the gingival half.

IV. Scoring

Add the plaque scores for each tooth and divide by the number of teeth examined.

COMMUNITY PERIODONTAL INDEX OF TREATMENT NEEDS (CPITN)
(Fédération Dentaire Internationale,[24] Ainamo[25])

I. Purpose

To screen and monitor individual or group periodontal treatment needs.

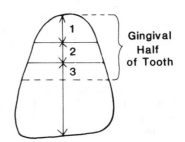

Figure 19–12. Ramfjord Dental Plaque Index. In the criteria modification, scores are recorded for the gingival half of the facial and lingual surfaces. Scores are recorded from 0 (no plaque present) to 3.

II. Selection of Teeth

A. Adults (20 years and older)
1. Divide the dentition into sextants. Evaluate all teeth.
   a. Posterior sextants begin distal to canines.
   b. A sextant must have two or more functional teeth. A functional tooth is one that is not indicated for extraction. When only one functional tooth is present, it is assessed with the adjacent sextant. The sextant with no teeth or one tooth is recorded as missing and marked X on the record form.
2. Third molars are included only when they function in place of second molars.

B. Children and Adolescents (7 to 19 years of age)
1. Divide the dentition into sextants.
2. Evaluate one tooth per sextant: the first molars in posterior; right central incisor in maxilla; left central incisor in mandibular anterior.[24]
3. When a designated tooth is missing, the sextant is recorded as missing and marked with an X.

III. Procedure

A. Instrument: WHO Periodontal Probe (figure 19–13)
1. *Markings.* At intervals from tip: 3.5, 2.0, 3.0, and 3.0 mm. (total 11.5 mm.).
2. *Working Tip.* A ball 0.5 mm. in diameter. The functions of the ball tip are
   a. To aid in detection of calculus and other tooth surface roughness.
   b. To facilitate assessment of the base of the pocket and reduce the risk of overmeasurement.
3. *Color-Coding.* Color-coded between 3.5 and 5.5 mm.

B. Probe Application
1. Objectives are to determine pocket depth, bleeding response, and presence of calculus.
2. Insert probe into sulcus/pocket gently. Keep light contact with tooth surface to detect calculus; use a force no greater than 15 to 25 grams to reveal disease without causing patient discomfort.
3. Observe color-coded area for prompt identification of pocket depth below 3.5 mm., between 3.5 and 5.5 mm. (within the color-coded zone), and above the 5.5-mm. level to facilitate classification.

C. Criteria
Five codes are used. Each includes conditions identified with the preceding codes, for example, Code 3 with 4- or 5-mm. pockets includes calculus and bleeding, typical of Codes 1 and 2.

Code 0 = Healthy periodontal tissues.
Code 1 = Bleeding after gentle probing.
Code 2 = Supra- or subgingival calculus or defective margin of filling or crown.

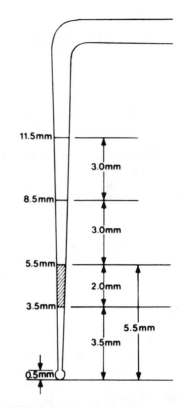

Figure 19–13. WHO Periodontal Probe. The probe, with markings as shown, is used to make determinations for the Community Periodontal Index of Treatment Needs (CPITN). (From FDI A Simplified Periodontal Examination for Dental Practices. Fédération Dentaire Internationale, 64 Wimpole Street, London W1M 8AL.)

Code 3 = 4- or 5-mm. pocket.
Code 4 = 6-mm. or deeper pathologic pocket.

D. Recording
1. Use a simple box chart for recording as shown in figure 19–14. The chart can be made into peel-off stick-on labels or a rubber stamp to facilitate the recording procedure on any examination form or individual patient record.
2. Place X for missing sextant.
3. Mark one score to represent each sextant. Record only the highest code that corresponds with the most severe condition.
4. Do not examine remaining teeth in a sextant after a Code 4 has been recorded.
5. The use of only Codes 0, 1, and 2 for patients aged 7 to 11 years may be advisable because of frequent occurrence of gingival ("false") pockets without attachment loss. The possibility of periodontal disease with attachment loss, however, should not be overlooked in young patients, nor should the need for treatment of deep chronic gingival pockets.

IV. Scoring

A. Periodontal Treatment Needs Scale
Patients are classified (0, I, II, III) into treatment needs according to the highest coded score recorded during the examination.

0 = No need for treatment (Code 0).
I = Oral hygiene instruction (Code 1).
II = Oral hygiene instruction plus scaling and root planing, including elimination of plaque retentive margins of fillings and crowns (Codes 2 and 3).
III = I + II + complex periodontal therapy that may include surgical intervention and/or deep scaling and root planing with local anesthesia (Code 4).

B. CPITN for an Individual

1. Example for adult patient (figure 19–14)
   Interpretation: Two sextants are marked for missing (X). Codes 2, 3, and 4 indicate need for thorough periodontal examination, charting, and detailed treatment plan.
2. Example for young patient (figure 19–15)
   Interpretation: Code 1 indicates need for improved oral hygiene. Code 3 indicates need for scaling and root planing after a complete periodontal examination and charting. The possibility of juvenile periodontitis should be considered.

C. CPITN for Groups

The recordings for a group may be presented in a variety of ways, such as the following:[25]
1. Treatment needs can be reported as the number or percent of subjects in each treatment need category.
2. Mean number of sextants with bleeding, calculus, and moderate or deep pockets for each age group can be shown.
3. To identify high and low priorities for treatment in a community, calculations of the number and percent of individuals with the following can be made:
   a. No sextant scoring each code.
   b. 1 to 2 sextants scoring Code 1, 2, 3, or 4.
   c. 3 to 4 sextants scoring Code 1, 2, 3, or 4.
   d. 5 to 6 sextants scoring Code 1, 2, 3, or 4.

DENTAL CARIES INDICES

The most widely used indices are the DMFT (Decayed, Missing, Filled Teeth) and DMFS (Decayed,

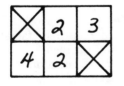

Figure 19–14.

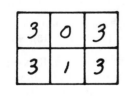

Figure 19–15.

Missing, Filled Surfaces) for permanent teeth.[26] Their counterparts deft (decayed, extracted, filled teeth) and defs (decayed, extracted, filled surfaces) are used for the primary teeth.[27] For a mixed dentition, two separate indices are indicated, one for the permanent teeth and one for the primary teeth.

From the indices, information can be derived to show the number of persons affected by dental caries, the number of teeth that need treatment, the proportion of teeth that have been treated, and other statistical data useful in organizing and evaluating dental health program efforts.

When a survey is made, specific procedures must be carefully defined to fulfill the objectives of a specific study. The basic descriptions included in this section can be adapted in most situations.

DECAYED MISSING AND FILLED PERMANENT TEETH (DMFT)[26]

I. Purpose

To determine total dental caries experience, past and present.

II. Selection of Teeth

A. DMFT is Based on 28 Teeth

B. Teeth Not Counted

1. Third molars.
2. Unerupted teeth. A tooth is considered erupted when any part projects through the gingiva. Certain types of research may require differentiation between clinical emergence, partial eruption, and full eruption.
3. Congenitally missing and supernumerary teeth.
4. Teeth removed for reasons other than dental caries, such as for an impaction or during orthodontic treatment.
5. Teeth restored for reasons other than dental caries, such as trauma (fracture), cosmetic purposes, or for use as a bridge abutment.
6. Primary tooth retained with the permanent successor erupted. The permanent tooth is evaluated because a primary tooth is never included in this index.

III. Procedures

A. Instruments

Each tooth is examined in a systematic sequence, using a mouth mirror and adequate light. Explorers of the same design and with standardized dimensions of the working ends are needed throughout a given survey.

B. Examination

1. *Use of Explorer.* Teeth should be observed by visual means as much as possible. Unnecessary discomfort for the patient can be avoided by exploring only questionable small lesions.

2. *Criteria for Identification of Dental Caries.* A detailed description for clinical recognition of dental caries appears on page 218, and a review of that material is suggested. In brief, for a dental caries index, a tooth can be considered carious when
   a. The lesion is clinically visible and obvious.
   b. The explorer tip can penetrate into soft yielding material.
   c. Discoloration or loss of translucency typical of undermined or demineralized enamel is apparent.
   d. The explorer tip in a pit or fissure catches or resists removal after moderate to firm pressure on insertion, and when softness occurs at the base of the area.

C. Criteria for Recording
1. *Each Tooth is Recorded Once.*
2. *"D" Recordings*
   a. When both dental caries and a restoration are present, the tooth is listed as D.
   b. When a crown is broken down as a result of dental caries, it may be recorded as D.
3. *"M" Recordings.* A tooth is considered missing
   a. When it has been extracted because of dental caries.
   b. When it is carious, nonrestorable, and indicated for extraction.
4. *"F" Recordings*
   a. Permanent and temporary fillings are recorded as F.
   b. A tooth with a defective filling but without evidence of dental caries is recorded as F.

IV. Scoring

A. Individual DMFT
1. Total each component separately.
2. Total D + M + F = DMF

   Example:
   a. D = 3, M = 2, F = 5
      DMF = 3 + 2 + 5 = 10
   b. A DMF of 10 may have different derivations. An individual who had regular dental care may have a distribution: $D = 0, M = 0, F = 10$.

B. Group Average
1. Total the DMFs for each individual examined.
2. Divide the total DMFs by the number of individuals in the group.

   Example:
   30 individuals with a total DMF of 210.
   $$\frac{210}{30} = 7.0 \text{ average DMF for the group.}$$

3. This DMF average represents accumulated dental caries experience. It can be presented by age groups.

C. Specific Treatment Needs of a Group
1. To calculate the percent of DMF teeth needing restorations, divide the total D component by the total DMFT.

   Example: D = 175, M = 55, F = 18
   Total DMFT = 248
   $$\frac{D}{DMF} = \frac{175}{248} = .70 \text{ or } 70\% \text{ of the teeth need restorations.}$$

2. Tooth mortality in a group of 20 individuals.
   a. To calculate the percent of teeth lost by extraction, divide the total M component by the total DMFT.

      Example: D = 175, M = 55, F = 18
      Total DMFT = 248
      $$\frac{M}{DMF} = \frac{55}{248} = .22 \text{ or } 22\% \text{ of the DMF teeth are accounted for by extraction.}$$

   b. To calculate the percent of *all* teeth lost by extraction because of dental caries: Twenty individuals have 28 × 20 = 560 permanent teeth.
      $$\frac{M}{\text{total teeth}} = \frac{55}{560} = .09 \text{ or } 9\% \text{ of all of their teeth lost because of dental caries.}$$

3. The same type of calculation can be used to determine the percent of filled teeth.

DECAYED MISSING AND FILLED PERMANENT TOOTH SURFACES (DMFS)

I. Purpose

To determine total dental caries experience, past and present, by recording tooth surfaces involved instead of teeth, as in the DMFT previously described.

II. Selection of Teeth and Surfaces

A. Teeth not Counted
The same as listed for the DMFT (page 279).

B. Surfaces
1. *Posterior Teeth.* Each tooth has five surfaces examined and recorded: facial, lingual, mesial, distal, and occlusal.
2. *Anterior Teeth.* Each tooth has four surfaces for evaluation: facial, lingual, mesial, and distal.
3. *Total Surface Count for a DMFS.* 128 surfaces.

   Of 28 teeth, 16 are posterior (16 × 5 = 80) and 12 are anterior (12 × 4 = 48).

4. *Missing Posterior Teeth.* Recorded as five surfaces. The number of surfaces that were carious before extraction usually cannot be determined.

III. Procedures

The same criteria for instruments and examination apply as listed previously for DMFT. In all surveys, specific criteria must be predetermined.

IV. Scoring

A. Individual DMFS

Teeth present = 24 (4 teeth have not yet erupted)
D (surfaces) = 3, M = 0, F (surfaces) = 8
DMFS = D + M + F = 3 + 0 + 8 = 11

B. Group DMFS

A group of 20 individuals 15 to 18 years old lives in a community with fluoridated water. All have lived there continuously except 3 who moved there from a nonfluoridated town after reaching 12 years of age. The following data show the distribution of DMFS:

	Total DMFS
10 individuals (each with 0 DMFS)	0
7 individuals (DMFS = 2,2,3,3,3,3,4)	20
3 individuals who had not lived continuously in the area (DMFS = 9,12,12)	33
Total DMFS	53

Average DMFS for the group $= \dfrac{53}{20} = 2.65$

Interpretation: The differences between those who had not lived with fluoridation are notable. The two groups should be presented separately because of the wide difference. The group average DMFS is 2.65, whereas the DMFS for those who lived in the fluoridated area all their lives is 1.18, and the DMFS for the other 3 is 11.0.

DECAYED, INDICATED FOR EXTRACTION, FILLED TEETH OR SURFACES
(dft and dfs) (deft and defs)[27]

I. Purpose

To determine the dental caries experience as shown for the primary teeth present in the oral cavity by evaluating teeth or surfaces.

II. Selection of Teeth or Surfaces

A. deft or dft
20 teeth evaluated.

B. defs or dfs
88 surfaces evaluated.
1. *Posterior Teeth.* Each has 5 surfaces: facial, lingual or palatal, mesial, distal, and occlusal. (8 teeth × 5 surfaces = 40 surfaces.)
2. *Anterior Teeth.* Each has 4 surfaces: facial, lingual or palatal, mesial, and distal. (12 teeth × 4 surfaces = 48 surfaces.)

C. Teeth Not Counted
1. Missing teeth, including unerupted and congenitally missing.
2. Supernumerary teeth.
3. Teeth restored for reasons other than dental caries are not counted as f.

III. Procedure

A. Instruments and Examination
Same as for DMFT (page 279).

B. Criteria for Identification of Dental Caries
Same as for DMFT (page 280).

C. Criteria for def

d = number of primary teeth or surfaces with dental caries but not restored.

e = number of teeth indicated for extraction because of dental caries.

f = number of filled primary teeth on surfaces that do not have dental caries (each surface is scored once only, "d" has first score).

D. Difference Between deft/defs and dft/dfs
In the deft and defs, both "d" and "e" are used to describe teeth with dental caries. Thus, d and e are sometimes combined, and the index becomes the "dft" or "dfs."

IV. Scoring

A. Individual dft

A 2½-year-old child with nursing bottle caries (page 218) has 18 teeth. Teeth A (55) and J (65) are unerupted. There is no sign of dental caries in teeth M (73), N (72), 0 (71), P (81), Q (82), and R (83). All other teeth have 2 carious surfaces each except B (54), which is broken down to the gumline.

Summary: Total teeth = 18
Caries-free = 6
"d" teeth = 12
"f" teeth = 0
dft = d + f = 12 + 0 = 12

Interpretation: 12 of 18 teeth with carious lesions indicates a serious need for dental treatment for the child.

B. Individual dfs
Using the same 2½-year-old child to calculate dfs:

Total number of carious surfaces: 11 × 2 = 22
Tooth B: 1 × 5 = 5
Total 27 dfs

Interpretation: The child has 48 anterior surfaces (12 teeth × 4 surfaces) and 30 posterior surfaces (6 teeth × 5 surfaces) to total 78 surfaces.

$$\frac{dfs}{number\ of\ surfaces} = \frac{27}{78} = .34 \text{ or } 34\% \text{ of the surfaces in need of dental treatment.}$$

C. Mixed Dentition
A DMFT or DMFS and a deft or defs are never added together. Each child is given a separate

index for permanent teeth and another for primary teeth. The index for the permanent teeth is usually determined first, and then the index for the primary teeth separately.

DECAYED, MISSING, AND FILLED
(dmft or dmfs)

I. Purpose

To determine dental caries experience past and present for children older than 7 and up to 11 or 12 years of age.

II. Selection of Teeth or Surfaces

A. dmft: 12 teeth evaluated (8 primary molars; 4 primary canines).
B. dmfs: 56 surfaces evaluated.
  1. Primary molars: 8 × 5 surfaces each = 40.
  2. Primary canines: 4 × 4 surfaces each = 16.
C. A primary molar or canine is presumed missing because of dental caries when it has been lost before the normal exfoliation time.

III. Procedure

A. Instruments and examination: same as for DMFT or DMFS (pages 279, 280).
B. Criteria for dmft or dmfs

  d   = number of primary molars and canines or number of surfaces that are carious (*decayed*).
  m   = number of primary molars and canines *missing*.
  f   = number of *filled* primary molars and canines without caries (teeth or surfaces).

C. Each tooth is counted only once. When both dental caries and a restoration are present, the tooth or surface is listed as *d,* dental caries.

IV. Scoring

A. Individual dmf

A 10-year-old boy has all primary molars and canines present.
Examination reveals d = 2, m = 0, f = 1

dmf = d + m + f = 2 + 0 + 1 = 3 dmf

B. Mixed Dentition

Permanent and primary teeth are evaluated separately. A DMFT or DMFS and a dmft and a dmfs are never added together.

TECHNICAL HINTS

  I. Select an index or scoring method that best fits the needs of the situation or patient.
 II. Calibrate criteria for each index used.
III. Implement an index at the beginning of an appointment series.
IV. Permit the patient to graph or chart the plaque or gingival index used and correlate the numeric values with the oral findings that may be seen.

V. Keep a continuing record, graph, or chart for index recording in the patient's permanent file for observation and review at each maintenance appointment.

FACTORS TO TEACH THE PATIENT

  I. How an index is used and calculated and what the scores mean.
 II. Correlation of index scores with current oral health practices and procedures.
III. Procedures to follow to improve index scores and bring the oral tissues to health.

References

 1. Horowitz, H.S.: Indexes for Measuring Dental Fluorosis, *J. Public Health Dent., 46,* 179, Fall, 1986.
 2. Silness, J. and Löe, H.: Periodontal Disease in Pregnancy. II. Correlation between Oral Hygiene and Periodontal Condition, *Acta Odontol. Scand., 22,* 121, Number 1, 1964.
 3. Podshadley, A.G. and Haley, J.V.: A Method for Evaluating Oral Hygiene Performance, *Public Health Rep., 83,* 259, March, 1968.
 4. Darby, M.L. and Bowen, D.M.: *Research Methods for Oral Health Professionals.* St. Louis, The C.V. Mosby Co., 1980, p. 11.
 5. Löe, H.: The Gingival Index, the Plaque Index and the Retention Index Systems, *J. Periodontol., 38,* 610, November-December, 1967 (Part II).
 6. O'Leary, T.J., Drake, R.B., and Naylor, J.E.: The Plaque Control Record, *J. Periodontol., 43,* 38, January, 1972.
 7. Ramfjord, S.P. and Ash, M.M.: *Periodontology and Periodontics.* Philadelphia, W.B. Saunders Co., 1979, p. 273.
 8. Grant, D.A., Stern, I.B., and Everett, F.G.: *Periodontics,* 5th ed. St. Louis, The C.V. Mosby Co., 1979, pp. 529–531.
 9. Greene, J.C. and Vermillion, J.R.: Oral Hygiene Index: A Method for Classifying Oral Hygiene Status, *J. Am. Dent. Assoc., 61,* 172, August, 1960.
10. Waggener, E.W.: Community Dentistry, in Steele, P.F., ed.: *Dimensions of Dental Hygiene,* 2nd ed. Philadelphia, Lea & Febiger, 1975, pp. 13–16.
11. Greene, J.C. and Vermillion, J.R.: The Simplified Oral Hygiene Index, *J. Am. Dent. Assoc., 68,* 7, January, 1964.
12. Greene, J.C.: The Oral Hygiene Index—Development and Uses, *J. Periodontol., 38,* 625, November-December, 1967 (Part II).
13. Mühlemann, H.R. and Son, S.: Gingival Sulcus Bleeding—A Leading Symptom in Initial Gingivitis, *Helv. Odontol. Acta, 15,* 107, October, 1971.
14. Meitner, S.W., Zander, H.A., Iker, H.P., and Polson, A.M.: Identification of Inflamed Gingival Surfaces, *J. Clin. Periodontol., 6,* 93, April, 1979.
15. Carter, H.G. and Barnes, G.P.: The Gingival Bleeding Index, *J. Periodontol., 45,* 801, November, 1974.
16. Schour, I. and Massler, M.: Prevalence of Gingivitis in Young Adults, *J. Dent. Res., 27,* 733, Abstract Number 33, December, 1948.
17. Massler, M.: The P-M-A Index for the Assessment of Gingivitis, *J. Periodontol., 38,* 592, November-December, 1967 (Part II).
18. Löe, H. and Silness, J.: Periodontal Disease in Pregnancy. I. Prevalence and Severity, *Acta Odontol. Scand., 21,* 533, Number 6, 1963.
19. Russell, A.L.: A System of Classification and Scoring for Prevalence Surveys of Periodontal Disease, *J. Dent. Res., 35,* 350, June, 1956.
20. Russell, A.L.: The Periodontal Index, *J. Periodontol., 38,* 585, November-December, 1967 (Part II).

21. Ramfjord, S.P.: Indices for Prevalence and Incidence of Periodontal Disease, *J. Periodontol., 30,* 51, January, 1959.

22. Ramfjord, S.P.: The Periodontal Disease Index (PDI), *J. Periodontol., 38,* 602, November-December, 1967 (Part II).

23. Shick, R.A. and Ash, M.M.: Evaluation of the Vertical Method of Toothbrushing, *J. Periodontol., 32,* 346, October, 1961.

24. Fedération Dentaire Internationale: A Simplified Periodontal Examination for Dental Practices, FDI WG6 and Joint FDI/WHO WG1, Fedération Dentaire Internationale, 64 Wimpole Street, London, WIM 8AL.

25. Ainamo, J., Barmes, D., Beagrie, G., Cutress, T., Martin, J., and Sardo-Infirri, J.: Development of the World Health Organization (WHO) Community Periodontal Index of Treatment Needs (CPITN), *Int. Dent. J., 32,* 281, September, 1982.

26. Klein, H. and Palmer, C.E.: Studies on Dental Caries. I. Dental Status and Dental Needs of Elementary School Children, *Public Health Rep., 53,* 751, May 13, 1938.

27. Gruebbel, A.O.: A Measurement of Dental Caries Prevalence and Treatment Service for Deciduous Teeth, *J. Dent. Res., 23,* 163, June, 1944.

Suggested Readings

Ainamo, J., Parviainen, K., and Murtomaa, H.: Reliability of the CPITN in the Epidemiological Assessment of Periodontal Treatment Needs at 13–15 Years of Age, *Int. Dent. J., 34,* 214, September, 1984.

Ainamo, J., Nordblad, A., and Kallio, P.: Use of the CPITN in Populations Under 20 Years of Age, *Int. Dent. J., 34,* 285, December, 1984.

Armitage, G.C.: *Biologic Basis of Periodontal Maintenance Therapy.* Berkeley, California, Praxis Publishing Co., 1980, pp. 8–20.

Barnes, G.P., Parker, W.A., Lyon, T.C., and Fultz, R.P.: Indices Used to Evaluate Signs, Symptoms and Etiologic Factors Associated with Diseases of the Periodontium, *J. Periodontol., 57,* 643, October, 1986.

Barmes, D.E. and Leous, P.A.: Assessment of Periodontal Status by CPITN and Its Applicability to the Development of Long-term Goals on Periodontal Health of the Population, *Int. Dent. J., 36,* 177, September, 1986.

Bloem, T.J., Razzoog, M.E., Chamberlain, B.B., and Lang, B.: Efficacy of Tissue Brushing as Measured by the Prosthodontic Tissue Index, *Spec. Care Dentist., 4,* 70, March-April, 1984.

Blount, R.L. and Stokes, T.F.: A Comparison of the OHI-S and the PHP in an Oral Hygiene Program, *ASDC J. Dent. Child., 53,* 53, January-February, 1986.

Bollmer, B.W., Sturzenberger, O.P., Lehnhoff, R.W., Bosma, M.L., Lang, N.P., Mallatt, M.E., and Meckel, A.H.: A Comparison of 3 Clinical Indices for Measuring Gingivitis, *J. Clin. Periodontol., 13,* 392, May, 1986.

Burger, P., Cleaton-Jones, P., du Plessis, J., and de Vries, J.: Comparison of Two Fluorosis Indices in the Primary Dentition of Tswana Children, *Community Dent. Oral Epidemiol., 15,* 95, April, 1985.

Burt, B.A.: Methods for Assessing the Distribution of Oral Diseases, in Striffler, D.F., Young, W.O., and Burt, B.A.: *Dentistry, Dental Practice and the Community,* 3rd ed. Philadelphia, W.B. Saunders Co., 1983, pp. 75–114.

Ciancio, S.G.: Current Status of Indices of Gingivitis, *J. Clin. Periodontol., 13,* 375, May, 1986.

Croxson, L.J.: A Simplified Periodontal Screening Examination: the Community Periodontal Index of Treatment Needs (WHO) in General Practice, *Int. Dent. J., 34,* 28, March, 1984.

Cutress, T.W., Hunter, P.B.V., and Hoskins, D.I.H.: Comparison of the Periodontal Index (P.I.) and Community Periodontal Index of Treatment Needs (CPITN), *Community Dent. Oral Epidemiol., 14,* 39, February, 1986.

Emslie, R.D.: The 621 Periodontal Probe, *Int. Dent. J., 30,* 287, December, 1980.

Engelberger, T., Hefti, A., Kallenberger, A., and Rateitschak, K.-H.: Correlations Among Papilla Bleeding Index, Other Clinical Indices and Histologically Determined Inflammation of Gingival Papilla, *J. Clin. Periodontol., 10,* 579, November, 1983.

Fischman, S.L.: Current Status of Indices of Plaque, *J. Clin. Periodontol., 13,* 371, May, 1986.

Fleiss, J.L., Park, M.H., Chilton, N.W., Alman, J.E., Feldman, R.S., and Chauncey, H.H.: Representativeness of the "Ramfjord Teeth" for Epidemiologic Studies of Gingivitis and Periodontitis, *Community Dent. Oral Epidemiol., 15,* 221, August, 1987.

Gettinger, G., Patters, M.R., Testa, M.A., Löe, H., Anerud, A., Boysen, H., and Robertson, P.B.: The Use of Six Selected Teeth in Population Measures of Periodontal Status, *J. Periodontol., 54,* 155, March, 1983.

Hunt, R.J.: The Efficiency of Half-mouth Examinations in Estimating the Prevalence of Periodontal Disease, *J. Dent. Res., 66,* 1044, May, 1987.

Mander, C.I. and Mainwaring, P.J.: Assessment of the Validity of Two Plaque Indices, *Community Dent. Oral Epidemiol., 8,* 139, June, 1980.

Massler, M. and Schour, I.: The P-M-A Index of Gingivitis, *J. Dent. Res., 28,* 634, Abstract Number 7, December, 1949.

Massler, M., Schour, I., and Chopra, B.: Occurrence of Gingivitis in Suburban Chicago School Children, *J. Periodontol., 21,* 146, July, 1950.

Sturzenberger, O.P., Lehnhoff, R.W., and Bollmer, B.W.: A Clinical Procedure for Determining the Proficiency of Gingivitis Examiners, *J. Clin. Periodontol., 12,* 756, October, 1985.

Tervonen, T. and Ainamo, J.: Relative Influence of Calculus and Overhangs of Fillings on the Frequency of Score 2 of the CPITN, *Community Dent. Oral Epidemiol., 14,* 136, June, 1986.

Tsamtsouris, A., White, G.E., and Clark, R.E.: A Comparison Between the Plaque Indices of Silness-Löe and Greene-Vermillion, *J. Pedod., 5,* 51, Fall, 1980.

van der Velden, U., Winkel, E.G., and Abbas, F.: Bleeding/Plaque Ratio. A Possible Prognostic Indicator for Periodontal Breakdown, *J. Clin. Periodontol., 12,* 861, November, 1985.

Wei, S.H.Y. and Lang, N.P.: Periodontal Epidemiological Indices for Children and Adolescents: I. Gingival and Periodontal Health Assessments, *Pediatr. Dent., 3,* 353, December, 1981; II. Evaluation of Oral Hygiene; III. Clinical Applications, *Pediatr. Dent., 4,* 64, March, 1982.

World Health Organization: *Epidemiology, Etiology and Prevention of Periodontal Diseases,* WHO Technical Report Series, Number 621, Geneva, WHO, 1978.

Zarkowski, P.: Community Oral Health Planning and Practice, in Darby, M.L. and Bushee, E.J., eds.: *Comprehensive Review of Dental Hygiene.* St. Louis, The C.V. Mosby Co., 1986, pp. 584–592.

Other Indices

Adams, R.A. and Nystrom, G.P.: A Periodontitis Severity Index, *J. Periodontol., 57,* 176, March, 1986.

Caton, J.G. and Polson, A.M.: The Interdental Bleeding Index: A Simplified Procedure for Monitoring Gingival Health, *Compend. Contin. Educ. Dent., 6,* 88, February, 1985.

Chosack, A.: A Dental Caries Severity Index for Primary Teeth, *Community Dent. Oral Epidemiol., 14,* 86, April, 1986.

Fischman, S., Cancro, L.P., Pretara-Spanedda, P., and Jacobs, D.: Distal Mesial Plaque Index. A Technique for Assessing Dental Plaque About the Gingiva, *Dent. Hyg., 61,* 404, September, 1987.

Gourdon, A.M., Buyle-Bodin, Y., Woda, A., and Faraj, M.: Development of an Abrasion Index, *J. Prosthet. Dent., 57,* 358, March, 1987.

Granath, L., Widenheim, J., and Birkhed, D.: Diagnosis of Mild Enamel Fluorosis in Permanent Maxillary Incisors Using Two Scoring Systems, *Community Dent. Oral Epidemiol., 13,* 273, October, 1985.

Horowitz, H.S., Driscoll, W.S., Meyers, R.J., Heifetz, S.B., and Kingman, A.: A New Method for Assessing the Prevalence of Dental Fluorosis—the Tooth Surface Index of Fluorosis, *J. Am. Dent. Assoc., 109,* 37, July, 1984.

Katz, R.V.: Assessing Root Caries in Populations: The Evolution of the Root Caries Index, *J. Public Health Dent., 40,* 7, Winter, 1980.

Katz, R.V.: Development of an Index for the Prevalence of Root Caries, *J. Dent. Res., 63,* Special Issue, 814, May, 1984.

Koch, A.L., Gershen, J.A., and Marcus, M.: A Children's Oral Health Status Index Based on Dentists' Judgment, *J. Am. Dent. Assoc., 110,* 36, January, 1985.

Lobene, R.R., Weatherford, T., Ross, N.M., Lamn, R.A., and Menaker, L.: A Modified Gingival Index for Use in Clinical Trials, *Clin. Prevent. Dent., 8,* 3, January-February, 1986.

Marcus, M., Koch, A.L., and Gershen, J.A.: A Proposed Index of Oral Health Status: A Practical Application, *J. Am. Dent. Assoc., 107,* 729, November, 1983.

Niederman, R. and Sullivan, T.M.: Oral Hygiene Skill Achievement Index I, *J. Periodontol., 52,* 143, March, 1981.

Niederman, R., Sullivan, T.M., Weiss, D., Morhart, R., Robbins, W., and Maier, D.: Oral Hygiene Skill Achievement Index II, *J. Periodontol., 52,* 150, March, 1981.

Nowicki, D., Vogel, R.I., Melcer, S., and Deasy, M.J.: The Gingival Bleeding Time Index, *J. Periodontol., 52,* 260, May, 1981.

Øilo, G., Dahl, B.L., Hatle, G., and Gad, A.-L.: An Index for Evaluating Wear of Teeth, *Acta Odontol. Scand., 45,* 361, Number 5, 1987.

Quigley, G.A. and Hein, J.W.: Comparative Cleansing Efficiency of Manual and Power Brushing, *J. Am. Dent. Assoc., 65,* 26, July, 1962.

Shaw, L. and Murray, J.J.: A New Index for Measuring Extrinsic Stain in Clinical Trials, *Community Dent. Oral Epidemiol., 5,* 116, May, 1977.

Smith, B.G.N. and Knight, J.K.: An Index for Measuring the Wear of Teeth, *Br. Dent. J., 156,* 435, June 23, 1984.

20 Records and Charting

Complete and accurate examinations with proper documentation by records and chartings are basic to all patient care. All findings of the diagnostic work-up are recorded. Some systems of recording involve the completion of forms with topics and spaces to check or fill in the information, whereas others call for a prose-style summary.

Radiographs, study casts, photographs, and all other materials collected during the initial examination and during continuing patient appointments are official parts of the permanent records. A filing system that makes these records readily accessible is needed. Every part must be dated.

I. Purposes for Charting

The purpose of each type of charting is defined by its title: the dental charting includes diagrammatic representation of existing conditions of the teeth, whereas the periodontal charting indicates clinical features of the periodontium. Separate types of chart forms may be used to record the special features of each, or the two may be combined on one chart. Neatness in the markings of symbols, drawings, and labels goes hand in hand with the accuracy of the examination itself.

A sense of responsibility to the patient and an earnest desire to be of the greatest possible assistance to the dentist are prerequisite. The dental hygienist does not diagnose. When the charting is prepared, a picture or diagram of observations is recorded. The charting is not described specifically to a patient unless the dentist requests that certain aspects of the diagnosis and treatment plan be presented to the patient.

An accurate, detailed, and carefully recorded charting is used as follows:

A. For Treatment Planning
The charting is a graphic representation of the existing condition of the patient's teeth and periodontium from which needed treatment procedures can be organized into a treatment plan.

B. For Treatment
During dental and dental hygiene appointments, the charting is useful for guiding specific techniques.

C. For Evaluation
The outcome and degree of lasting effects of treatment are determined by comparing the findings of the initially recorded examination with periodic follow-up examinations.

D. For Protection
In the event of misunderstanding by a patient, or if legal questions should arise, the records and chartings are realistic evidence.

E. For Identification
In the event of emergency, accident, or disaster, a patient may be identified by the teeth for which a record has been maintained.

II. Materials for Charting

A. Instruments
1. Probe.
2. Sharp explorers.
3. Mouth mirror: clear and unscratched.
4. Dental floss.
5. Gauze sponges.
6. Airtip and saliva ejector.
7. Topical anesthetic if probing proves discomforting to the patient.

B. Study Casts

C. Radiographs
1. Advanced preparation of the radiographic survey facilitates coordination between clinical and radiographic examinations. The completely processed and mounted radiographs provide greater assurance of a thorough analysis.
2. A bitewing survey may be sufficient for the charting of dental caries, but a periapical survey is essential for periodontal evaluation.

D. Chart Form
Many variations of chart forms are in current use, some available commercially, some designed by the dentist to meet particular needs. Specifications for an adequate form include ample space to chart neatly, accurately, and completely; to label as needed for clarity; and to record in a manner that will be interpretable by all who use it. Three types of forms are described here.
1. *Anatomic Tooth Drawings of the Complete Teeth.* Such a chart form lends itself to combined dental and periodontal charting. Figure 20–2 is an example of this type of chart form (page 288).
2. *Anatomic Drawings of the Crowns of Teeth*

Only. Difficult to chart adequately the periodontal findings; designed primarily for charting dental caries.

3. *Geometric.* A diagrammatic representation for each tooth with space for each surface; generally does not include the roots. This type of chart includes two circles. The inner circle represents the occlusal surface, and the outer circle, divided into four parts, represents the mesial, facial, distal, and lingual. The individual tooth diagrams may be arranged in a linear format (figure 20–1A) or in arches to simulate the oral cavity (figure 20–1B).

E. Marking Pencils

1. Pens and pencils of various colors in keeping with the system of charting selected by the dentist are needed.
2. Sanitize pencils or pens to be used by rubbing vigorously with gauze sponge moistened in a chemical disinfectant.
3. When charting without an assistant, particular care must be exercised to keep sterile dental instruments apart from materials that cannot be sterilized. Transmission of oral microorganisms to chart form, pencils, eraser, or radiographs presents a real problem in the maintenance of a clinically clean environment.

III. Clinic Procedures

A. Patient Position

Position for optimum visibility of and accessibility to the field of operation.

B. Illumination

Maximum illumination is important. Use direct or indirect (mirror) light or transillumination.

C. Sequence for Charting

The use of a set routine is prerequisite to accomplishing a complete and accurate charting not only for the tooth surface-to-surface pattern, but also for the parts of the charting itself.

Charting of all of one kind of item for the entire mouth, rather than complete chartings of one tooth, helps to obtain accuracy because only one train of thought is required at a time. For example, in the dental charting, record all the restorations first. Then start again at the first tooth and chart all the deviations from normal. Charting all restorations and deviations for each tooth separately is a less efficient method.

PERIODONTAL RECORDS AND CHARTING

The patient's permanent records include the itemized findings of all the clinical and radiographic examinations. Material for the periodontal charting has been described on pages 201–202. Entries should be clear and easily understood by all who will read them and use them in continuing treatment.

Additions to the records are made to show the progress of treatment and comparative observations throughout the series of treatment appointments. After the mouth has been brought to a state of health the patient can maintain, a maintenance plan is outlined. At each succeeding appointment, new and comparative records and chartings are made.

Basic periodontal recordings are listed here. The dentist may prefer to perform some parts of the examination and assign other parts to the dental hygienist.

I. Clinical Observations of the Gingiva

A. Describe gingiva: color, size, position, shape, consistency, and surface texture; extent of bleeding when probed; and areas where exudate can be pressed from the pockets (pages 171–173 and table 11–1, pages 174–175).
B. Describe distribution of gingival changes: localized or generalized; specify the areas of severest disease involvement. Use tooth numbers to identify adjacent gingival tissue. Tooth numbering systems are described on pages 73–75.
C. Describe degree of severity of disease: slight, moderate, severe.

II. Items to Be Charted

A. Chart missing teeth.
B. Gingival line (margin) and mucogingival lines (junction).
C. Pocket measurements.
D. Areas of suspected mucogingival involvement.
E. Furcation involvement.
F. Abnormal frenal attachments.
G. Mobility and fremitus of teeth.

III. Deposits

A. Stains

1. *Extrinsic.* Record type of stain, color, distribution, specific location by tooth number, whether slight, moderate, or heavy.
2. *Intrinsic.* Record separately from extrinsic and identify by type when known.

B. Calculus

Record distribution and amount of supragingival and subgingival calculus separately for treatment planning purposes.

C. Soft Deposits

1. *Materia Alba and Food Debris.* Distribution and amount. Record location by teeth when the plaque control instruction will require special emphasis on a particular area.
2. *Bacterial Plaque*
   a. Record direct observations with or without

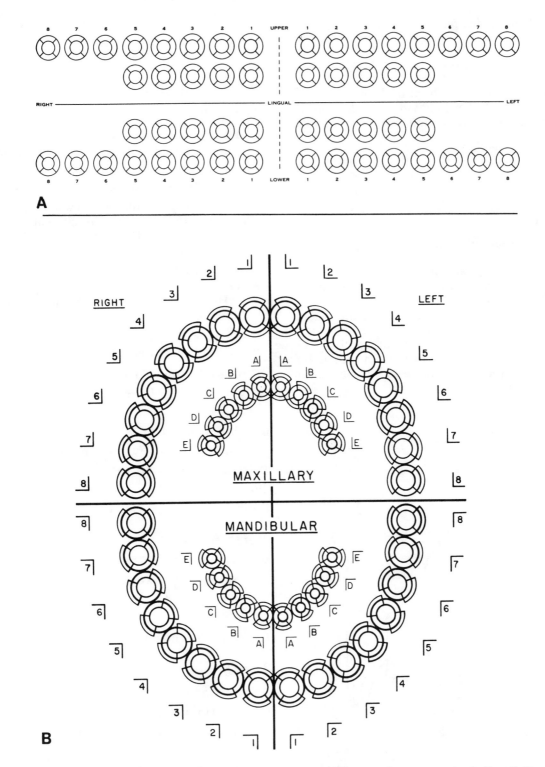

Figure 20–1. Geometric Charting Form. Type A. Linear format with primary teeth between the permanent teeth. **Type B.** Permanent teeth in arch form with primary teeth inside. Teeth are numbered by quadrant numbers 1 through 8 (page 74).

disclosing agent: distribution and degree or amount.

   b. Plaque index recorded.

IV. Factors Related to Occlusion

Clinical signs of trauma from occlusion were described on page 233. The following list is for consideration with other records for the treatment planning.

A. Mobility of Teeth

Record degree for each tooth (page 206). In figure 20–2, an example of a method for recording mobility is shown. The small box associated with each root apex and tooth number is used to record mobility.

B. Fremitus (pages 206–207)

C. Possible Food Impaction Areas

1. Inquire of patient where fibrous foods usually catch between the teeth.
2. Use dental floss to identify inadequate contact areas that may contribute to food impaction. An example of one method for recording an open contact is shown by the vertical parallel lines between teeth numbered 21 and 22 in figure 20–2.

D. Occlusion-related Habits

1. Observe for evidence of, and question patient concerning, parafunctional habits, such as bruxism or clenching.
2. Note wear patterns and facets on study cast.
3. Note attrition.

E. Tooth Migration (page 232)

F. Sensitivity to Percussion (page 73)

G. Radiographic Evidences

Related to trauma from occlusion (page 233).

V. Radiographic Findings

Specific notes should be made to correlate the radiographic findings with the clinical observations just listed. Details of radiographic findings in periodontal disease were described on pages 207–210. The following should be noted in particular:

A. Bone Level

Height of bone as related to the cementoenamel junction.

B. Shape of Remaining Bone

Horizontal or angular.

C. Crestal Lamina Dura

Intact, broken, or missing.

Missing Tooth I or X

Unerupted or impacted; Encircle tooth

Drift and Migration ⌇⌇

Open Contact ‖

Food Impaction ↓ (at occlusal)

Periodontal

Gingival Margin: Black line

Mucogingival Junction: Dashed line

Furca involved ● (in furcation)

Probed pocket depths (mm) P–1

Probed attachment level (mm) At–1

Teeth

Dental Caries: red

Restoration: blue

Defective Restoration: circle with red

Overhang ▼ (at occlusal)

Mobility M–1 (N, 1, 2, 3)

Fremitus F–1 (recorded on maxillary only)

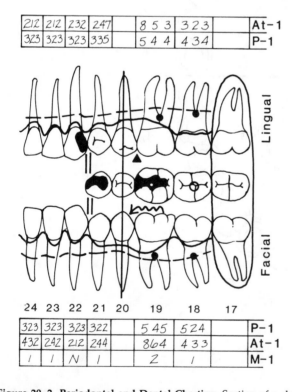

2 1 2	2 1 2	2 3 2	2 4 7		8 5 3	3 2 3		At–1
3 2 3	3 2 3	3 2 3	3 3 5		5 4 4	4 3 4		P–1

| | 24 | 23 | 22 | 21 | 20 | 19 | 18 | 17 |

3 2 3	3 2 3	3 2 3	3 2 2		5 4 5	5 2 4		P–1
4 3 2	2 4 2	2 1 2	2 4 4		8 6 4	4 3 3		At–1
1	1	N	1		2	1		M–1

Figure 20–2. Periodontal and Dental Charting. Section of a charting (mandibular left quadrant) shows combined dental and periodontal charting. Dental caries and restorations are usually marked with colored pencils, such as blue for restorations and red for dental caries, on the anatomic crowns or roots. The gingival margin is clearly drawn to show areas of recession. Boxes at the apices of each tooth provide spaces for pocket and attachment level recordings, as well as for mobility notations.

D. **Furcation Involvement**

E. **Widening of Periodontal Ligament Space**

F. **Overhanging Fillings and Large Carious Lesions**
Bacterial plaque-retention factors.

DENTAL RECORDS AND CHARTING

The patient's permanent records include the itemized findings of the clinical and radiographic examinations along with subjective symptoms reported by the patient. Material for the dental records has been included in Chapter 14 and for occlusion in Chapter 15. Mobility of teeth has been charted with the periodontal examination because the causes of mobility are periodontally oriented. The outline here is for summary in anticipation of treatment planning.

After initial entries into the record, additions are made to show the progress of treatment. At each periodic maintenance visit, new and comparative records and chartings must be prepared.

The need for meticulous examination and recording cannot be overemphasized. Finding and recording a carious lesion may mean saving a tooth for the patient's lifetime; inadvertent neglect of a tooth may lead eventually to a need for endodontic therapy or even extraction.

I. Before Patient Appointment

Radiographs and study casts prepared at an initial appointment before clinical examination for charting help to conserve patient chair time.

A. Radiographic Charting

The following may be charted without the presence of the patient: missing, unerupted, impacted teeth, endodontic restorations, overhanging margins of existing restorations, proximal surface carious lesions, and any other deviation from normal evident from the radiographs.

Supplemental and confirmational observations and checks are made during the clinical examination with the patient. For example, when an overhanging restoration is noted but dental caries is not visible in the radiograph, examination by exploration is required because the restoration may be superimposed over the carious lesion.

B. Study Casts

Record the classification of occlusion (pages 229–231).

II. Patient Appointment

Figure 20–2 is an example of a quadrant of dental charting using anatomic tooth drawings. Dental findings can also be charted on a geometric form, such as is shown in figure 20–1.

A. Chart missing teeth.

B. Chart existing restorations, including fixed and removable prostheses and sealants.

C. Chart apparent carious lesions and other deviations from normal.

D. Coordinate clinical and radiographic findings.

E. Use dental floss. Chart inadequate contact areas and observe proximal surface roughness. Fraying of dental floss as it is passed over a rough proximal surface may mean the defective margin of a restoration, a sharp cavity margin, or dental calculus.

F. Chart pulp vitality. Record numbers in the permanent record. Chart forms sometimes include a specific place for the recording of such data. Procedures were described on pages 221–223.

G. Chart tooth sensitivity. The patient may report hypersensitive areas, or they may be discovered during instrumentation. Record the tooth number and surface for reference during the treatment phase.

TECHNICAL HINTS

I. Use a record form with adequate space for recording details.

II. Prepare permanent records in ink.

III. Use abbreviations and symbols only when their meaning will be clear to all who read them.

IV. Check that all records are complete, accurate, clearly stated, readable, and neat.

V. Plan appointments, when possible, in order that radiographs and study casts will be available prior to and at the time of clinical charting. When the medical and dental history and the extraoral and intraoral examinations can be completed in advance, time can be saved. Necessary consultations with a patient's physician, preparation with premedication when indicated for the patient susceptible to bacteremia, or other special adaptation can be made.

VI. Explain to a patient who asks specific questions about the charting or other recordings why the dentist must observe and check such records before explanations can be made.

FACTORS TO TEACH THE PATIENT

I. The importance of making a complete study of the patient's oral problems before beginning treatment.

II. Advantages of cooperation and patience in furnishing information that will help dental personnel to interpret observations accurately so that the correct diagnosis and appropriate treatment plan can be made.

III. All information received is completely confidential, and the records are locked when the office is closed.

Suggested Readings

Allen, D.L., McFall, W.T., and Jenzano, J.W.: *Periodontics for the Dental Hygienist,* 4th ed. Philadelphia, Lea & Febiger, 1987, pp. 99–135.

Carranza, F.A.: *Glickman's Clinical Periodontology,* 6th ed. Philadelphia, W.B. Saunders Co., 1984, pp. 500–523.

Castano, F.A. and Alden, B.A., eds.: *Handbook of Expanded Den-*

tal Auxiliary Practice, 2nd ed. Philadelphia, J.B. Lippincott Co., 1980, pp. 5–25.

Grant, D.A., Stern, I.B., and Listgarten, M.A., eds.: *Periodontics,* 6th ed. St. Louis, The C.V. Mosby Co., 1988, pp. 537–559.

Helburn, R.L.: The Computer-assisted Periodontal Chart: A Tool to Aid in the Control of Periodontal Disease, *Compend. Contin. Educ. Dent., 5,* 80, January, 1984.

Murrell, C.: Record Keeping. Its Role in Malpractice Avoidance and Defense, Part 1, *Dent. Hyg., 60,* 324, July, 1986.

O'Reilly, P.: An Overview of Forensic Dentistry, *Clin. Prevent. Dent., 8,* 16, January-February, 1986.

21 *The Dental Hygiene Treatment Plan*

All the information about the patient, collected as parts of the diagnostic work-up, is organized for evaluation. From the evaluation, the dentist makes the diagnosis and the treatment plan is prepared before treatment is started.

The *total treatment plan* is a sequential outline of the essential services and procedures that must be carried out by the dentist, the dental hygienist, and the patient to eliminate disease and restore the oral cavity to health and normal function. The *dental hygiene treatment plan,* which consists of those services to be performed by the dental hygienist with the patient, is formulated within the framework of the total treatment plan and is an integral part of it.

I. Objectives

The objectives of a treatment sequence are:

A. To Eliminate and Control Etiologic and Predisposing Disease Factors

The principal etiologic agents in both dental caries and periodontal and gingival diseases are the microorganisms of bacterial plaque. The goal should be to control the etiologic agent and, thus, to prevent future recurrences of the same conditions.

B. To Eliminate the Signs and Symptoms of Disease

Treatment planning includes measures to eliminate signs of disease, such as carious lesions, inflammation, and pockets.

C. To Restore Normal Function

This includes occlusal adjustment, restoration of teeth, replacement of missing teeth, orthodontic tooth movement, and recontouring of gingival form (gingivoplasty).

D. To Maintain Health and Prevent the Recurrence of Disease

Methods used are counseling and supervision of the patient in daily self-care and provision of regular follow-up professional supervision and care.

II. Preparation for the Treatment Plan

A. Diagnostic Work-up

The parts of a diagnostic work-up were listed on page 71 and described in Chapters 6 through 20. The histories, dental and periodontal chartings, radiographs, study casts, recorded information from the extraoral and intraoral examinations, indices, and all other available information are studied by the dentist. The key pertinent findings that point to the disease problems are selected and the diagnosis is made.

B. Diagnosis

The *diagnosis* is the identification of the disease condition by recognition of characteristic signs and symptoms. A *differential diagnosis* distinguishes the disease from other diseases that have similar manifestations.

Patients frequently have more than one disease condition. For example, dental caries and periodontal or gingival diseases commonly occur simultaneously. When the treatment plan is made, the treatment for each disease condition is outlined, and a coordinated treatment sequence is determined.

III. Parts of a Total Treatment Plan

A total treatment plan usually involves several interdependent areas of oral care based on an individual patient's diagnosis and disease symptoms. Divisions for a treatment plan are listed below with examples of services included in each.

A. Priority Treatment
1. Emergency care for pain or other acute condition.
2. Procedures such as biopsy of a lesion found during the extraoral and intraoral examinations, or a laboratory test for a suspected systemic condition.

B. Preventive Phase
1. Procedures for the patient's daily self-care, including plaque control.
2. Introduction to self-applied fluoride.

C. Preparatory Phase
1. Initial (Phase 1) periodontal therapy includes disease control procedures performed by the patient, and professional complete scaling and root planing.
2. Dental caries is treated initially by excavation of large carious lesions; placement of sedative temporary fillings; pulp treatment as indicated.
3. Endodontic therapy.
4. Preparation for oral surgery includes plaque control and scaling to reduce the bacterial count and inflammation.

5. Removal of hopeless teeth that cannot be successfully treated.

D. Treatment Phase
1. Gingival and periodontal treatment, including elimination of inflammation and pockets; surgical procedures; occlusal adjustment.
2. Restorative treatment.
3. Prosthetic treatment.
4. Orthodontic treatment.
5. Tissue maintenance during therapy (page 293).

E. Maintenance Phase
1. Patient is instructed in specific daily plaque control and other preventive measures.
2. Professional appointments at designated intervals.
   a. Complete re-evaluation and updating of records and all parts of the diagnostic work-up.
   b. Maintenance treatment plan may include any service as a continuation, supplement, or addition to previous preventive, educational, or therapeutic measures. The maintenance appointment is described on pages 540–541.

PLANNING THE DENTAL HYGIENE TREATMENT PLAN

The dental hygienist's objective is to prepare a flexible, realistic, dental hygiene plan and sequence of procedures based on the plan for total care of the patient. As described on page 3, a dental hygienist's services may be divided into preventive, educational, and therapeutic, all of which are applicable at various levels in the total treatment plan. Services to be performed depend on state or area practice acts, and any examples cited here are not intended to represent a specific location.

An objective in planning dental hygiene care is to ensure the best possible sequence of procedures that will contribute to the restoration of the patient's oral health in the shortest possible time and will pave the way to the long-range preventive program that will continue throughout the patient's lifetime. To achieve the goals of planned care, the dental hygienist must see the dental hygiene aspects within the total plan for the patient and contribute to the overall continuity of the corrective and maintenance phases.

I. Characteristics of a Well-planned Treatment Plan
An effective plan will be
A. Adapted to the needs of the patient's oral condition.
B. Orderly in sequence to allow for thoroughness in each procedure and to prevent duplication or repetition of efforts.
C. Composed of purposefully selected procedures that are

1. Planned with a reasonable degree of predictability of outcome.
2. Expected to resolve the condition and reach an optimum result in a minimum of time.
3. Projected toward a state of health the patient can maintain with self-care procedures.

II. Record and Explain
The treatment plan is recorded in the patient's record. The patient or parent of a young or mentally disabled patient must understand the treatment plan and be aware of the expected outcome of each appointment, as well as of the total series. The role of the patient in treatment through self-care on a daily basis must be written into the treatment plan and explained to the patient.

STEPS IN PLANNING

I. Objectives
A. Review the patient's oral problems as described in the diagnosis and total treatment plan.
B. Identify objectives that may be attained.
1. Overall objectives of the total treatment and anticipated state of oral health after treatment.
2. Dental hygiene goals, both short-term and long-term.

II. Services
Preventive, educational, preparatory, and treatment procedures are selected that can be expected to meet the objectives. The services to be performed for each phase of the total treatment plan are listed in sequence for the appointment series, and time requirements for each phase are estimated and recorded.

Examples are given here for each phase of the treatment plan.

A. Preventive
A typical program includes plaque control measures, self-applied and professionally applied fluorides, diet counseling, and pit and fissure sealants.

B. Preparatory
Complete scaling and root planing may be the major services to prepare a patient for periodontal surgery. *Preparatory* treatment is in contrast to *definitive* treatment, which means the complete treatment needed by a patient to bring the oral tissues to a state of health at that time.

C. Treatment
1. *Periodontal.* Scaling, root planing, and selective gingival curettage that are preparatory for one patient may be the definitive and curative treatment for another patient.
2. *Periodontal Post-surgical Procedures.* Suture removal, removal and replacement of periodontal dressings, and other postoperative care

and instruction are parts of the patient's treatment plan that may be performed by the dental hygienist.

3. *Restorative.* Finishing and polishing of restorations may best be scheduled in conjunction with topical fluoride application. After polishing restorations, a topical fluoride application should be made to protect the enamel that has been highly polished adjacent to the restoration.

D. Tissue Maintenance During Long-term Therapy

When restorative, prosthetic, orthodontic, or other treatment continues over a long period, appointments are needed for gingival evaluation, supervision of plaque control measures, calculus removal, topical fluoride applications, and other procedures specific for the patient.

III. Criteria for Determination of Sequence

Sequence planning involves first an outline of a series of appointments with the services to be performed. Secondly, sequence refers to the order in which the parts of an individual appointment are carried out. The sequence is influenced by numerous factors, including urgency of treatment, need for treating etiologic factors first, the severity and extent of the condition, and certain special patient requirements. These factors are described here with examples.

A. Urgency

When discomfort or pain is present, the area involved requires first attention. In the dental hygiene treatment plan, this could apply to an area of the gingiva where the patient has particular difficulty, and either specially adapted plaque control instruction or scaling may be needed.

B. Etiologic Factors Should Be Treated First

The factors that caused or contributed to the development of the existing disease must be arrested and controlled. In patients with gingival or periodontal infections, the continued success of treatment depends on the removal of bacterial plaque.

Disease will recur when daily control measures for the removal of the etiologic agent, plaque, are not carried out. New dental caries also can develop unless continued attention is paid to preventive measures.

Pellicle forms within minutes after a tooth surface has been completely cleaned, and disclosable plaque will be present within 24 hours or less. Therefore, plaque control measures must be introduced in the treatment plan before scaling or root planing.

C. Special Patient Requirements (Items from the Patient History)

1. *Antibiotic Premedication.* A list of conditions that require antibiotic premedication may be found on pages 85 and 91. For patients who need antibiotics, all instrumentation, including the examination procedures when instruments are used (probing, exploring), as well as tooth movement for mobility determination, must be done under antibiotic coverage.

Bacteremias have been demonstrated during brushing, flossing, and other disease control measures. Instruction and practice of the plaque-removing procedures must be carried out while the patient is premedicated.

Appointments must be planned and conducted efficiently to prevent the need for unnecessary premedication. When a patient's physical health and strength do not contraindicate, appointments that are longer than customary may be reserved so that more can be accomplished.

2. *Systemic Diseases.* Chronic disease or physical disability may influence the content or length of appointments.

3. *Infectious Diseases.* Disease transmission problems for patients with a history of a communicable disease may require postponement of all except urgent needs.

D. Severity and Extent of the Condition

Findings that indicate the severity of gingival or periodontal infection include changes in color, size, shape, consistency, and bleeding of the gingiva, pocket measurements, mobility of teeth, and radiographic signs. To determine the length of appointments and sequence of procedures, consideration is given necessarily to the depth of pockets in relation to the distribution and hardness of dental calculus. The number of appointments and the length of appointments increase with severity.

A suggested division of conditions graded by the severity of infection follows.

1. *Moderate to Severe Periodontal Disease.* For the patient who requires complicated periodontal, restorative, and prosthetic treatment, the dental hygiene treatment plan includes preventive and preparatory procedures as well as maintenance during therapy, postsurgical care, and follow-up.

2. *Moderate or Slight Periodontal Disease.* The dental hygiene treatment plan includes the preventive phase, complete scaling, planing, and gingival curettage as indicated. This treatment may be definitive, or the follow-up evaluation may show the need for surgical or other additional treatment.

3. *Gingivitis with Supra- and Subgingival Calculus.* The preventive phase and complete scaling are indicated, and gingival pockets may require curettage. The treatment may be definitive, or upon re-evaluation, gingivoplasty or other treatment may be needed.

4. *Gingivitis with Slight Supragingival Calculus or No Calculus.* Dental hygiene services usually constitute the definitive treatment. To eliminate gingival inflammation, plaque control measures may be the total treatment, which is supplemented by scaling when there is calculus or only polishing when stain is unsightly.

INDIVIDUAL APPOINTMENT SEQUENCE

I. Evaluation

Each appointment starts with an evaluation of the gingival tissues.

A. Previously Treated Area

The area is examined for progress toward health, the signs of inflammation that may still be present, and indications for additional treatment that is needed.

B. Effects of Plaque Control Measures

The self-treatment by the patient is evaluated. After the color, size, shape, consistency, and other characteristics of the gingiva are observed, a disclosing agent is used to evaluate the degree of plaque present on the teeth. This evaluates the patient's techniques and thoroughness in plaque removal.

II. Instruction for Disease Control

Instruction begins when evaluation starts, and continues throughout. Specific techniques for the use of plaque removal devices, such as toothbrush, floss, or other aid, are presented before instrumentation or other professional clinical services are performed. The reasons for this sequence are presented on page 371.

III. Tissue Conditioning

Preparation or conditioning of the gingival tissue for scaling can be of particular importance when there is spongy, soft tissue that bleeds on slight provocation, and when the area is generally septic from plaque, materia alba, and debris accumulation.

Tissue conditioning is accomplished by initiating plaque control procedures and prescribing a concentrated daily program of plaque removal and hot salt water rinsing. A quadrant that needs tissue conditioning is not selected for scaling until gingival healing and patient cooperation have been demonstrated.

Objectives of such a program include:

A. Gingival Healing

The tissue becomes less edematous, bleeding is minimized, and scaling procedures are facilitated.

B. General Oral Cleanliness with Lowered Bacterial Accumulation

There is less likelihood that bacteremias will be produced during scaling, and there is less contamination in aerosols produced.

C. Learning by the Patient

The patient can practice and see benefits of plaque removal.

IV. Clinical Services

The questions of which area or quadrant should be scaled first and in which order the other areas and quadrants should follow can be answered for most patients by considering the following order of choices:

A. Patient Selection

When the patient indicates an area of discomfort, that area may be taken first.

B. Apprehensive Patient

To make the first scaling less complicated and to help orient the patient to the procedures to be followed, either the quadrant with the fewest teeth or the quadrant with the least deep periodontal disease can be selected.

C. When Two Quadrants Are To Be Treated at the Same Appointment

Select a maxillary and mandibular of the same side.

SAMPLE DENTAL HYGIENE TREATMENT PLAN

It would be impossible to present sample treatment plans for each of the wide variety of patient problems or combinations of problems encountered in practice. Each patient must be handled individually.

Examples of treatment sequences and plans are found in special areas of this book. An outline for maintenance appointment can be found on pages 540–541, and a treatment sequence for a patient with necrotizing ulcerative gingivitis is found on pages 483–484.

For the patient whose dental hygiene treatment plan is sketched below, the diagnostic work-up was completed by the dental hygienist. The dentist indicated a diagnosis of generalized moderate periodontal disease. The preliminary total treatment plan includes occlusal adjustment, restorative procedures, and the prosthetic replacement of two missing teeth. No emergency measures are required. None of the periodontal surgery or dental treatment will be started until the dental hygiene preventive and preparatory appointments have been completed and the patient's mouth has been re-evaluated.

The examinations revealed slight localized supragingival calculus and generalized moderate-to-heavy subgingival calculus. Because the patient has enlarged, spongy marginal gingiva with generalized bleeding on probing and plaque on the cervical thirds of most teeth, scaling is not started on the first appointment. The importance of tissue conditioning is described in the previous section and the rationale for introducing plaque control before scaling is described on page 371.

More detail is included in the treatment plan recorded below than probably would be written in practice. Abbreviations would be used that could be recognized by all personnel involved in using the patient's record. For example, "Plaque I," "Plaque II," "Plaque III" might be sufficient notation for the plaque control instruction series.

APPOINTMENT I

1. Record plaque or bleeding scores (pages 262–265, 271).
2. Give disease control instruction: *First Lesson*, pages 372–373.
3. Introduce self-applied fluoride program.
   a. Discuss dentifrice recommendation.
   b. Explain the need for frequent brushing to gain most benefit from fluoride in dentifrice.
   c. Demonstrate use of fluoride mouthrinse.

APPOINTMENT II

1. Evaluate disease control with the patient.
   a. Assess gingival tissue (table 11–1, pages 174–175).
   b. Record indices.
2. Instruction: *Second Lesson,* page 373.
3. Perform scaling
   a. First quadrant scaling and root planing with anesthesia.
   b. Curettage as indicated; dressing placed when needed.
   c. Postoperative instructions.

APPOINTMENT III

1. Remove dressing.
2. Evaluation
   a. Assess gingival tissue; record bleeding index.
   b. Examine first quadrant scaled: note healing. Explore to check for residual calculus.
   c. Evaluate plaque. Disclose for Plaque Index.
3. Instruction: *Third Lesson,* pages 373–374.
4. Perform scaling and root planing
   a. Complete first quadrant when residual calculus is found.
   b. Second quadrant scaling with anesthesia.
   c. Gingival curettage as directed; dressing when needed.

APPOINTMENT IV

1. Remove dressing.
2. Evaluation
   a. Assess gingival tissue.
   b. Record bleeding or other indices.
   c. Examine previously scaled quadrants; explore for residual calculus.
   d. Evaluate plaque.
3. Instruction: continue as needed.
4. Perform scaling and root planing.
   a. Complete first and second quadrants.
   b. Third quadrant scaling with anesthesia.
   c. Gingival curettage as directed; dressing when needed.

APPOINTMENT V

The same basic structure is followed as outlined for Appointments III and IV. Each time the previously treated quadrants must be checked and completed. Each time the instruction is continued if the patient is still not accomplishing disease control. The fourth quadrant is scaled under anesthesia and curettage performed as needed.

APPOINTMENT VI

1. Evaluation of four quadrants; additional scaling when indicated.
2. Evaluate need for stain removal. Scaling, planing, and the patient's daily therapeutic plaque removal often remove stains so that stain removal will be highly selective.
3. Re-evaluation by the dentist; planning for the next phase of appointments when patient is ready as shown by the health of the gingival tissue.

APPOINTMENT VII: Maintenance During Therapy

When the restorative and prosthetic treatment extends over a period of time, periodic appointments are needed for monitoring the continued success of the patient's self-care. A gingival tissue evaluation, checks with a probe to determine bleeding, plaque checks with disclosing agents, additional instruction, particularly for the care of newly fixed or removable prosthetic appliances, and motivational encouragement are essential.

APPOINTMENT VIII: Maintenance

The maintenance appointment frequency is determined. Components of the maintenance appointment are described on pages 540–541.

INFORMED CONSENT

Informed consent simply means that the patient has been informed about the nature of the oral condition and the treatment needed, and that the patient has consented to follow the recommendations made. In other words, informed consent is the permission granted by the patient, or the patient's parent or guardian, for the professional person to proceed. Each state has its own law on this subject.

Suggested forms are available, and each dental office or clinic needs printed forms with the official name and address heading.[1,2] The forms are used with duplicate or triplicate copies so that the file, the patient, and any other required specialist can maintain a copy.

Prior to obtaining the signature on the form, the patient should receive information about the following:

   I. The health problem and its need for treatment.
   II. The diagnosis and a description of the severity, extent, and what can occur if the treatment is not carried out.
   III. The recommended treatment and any risks involved.
   IV. The responsibilities of the patient relative to supplementary personal care and follow-up.
   V. Expected outcomes.
   VI. Appointments needed and financial arrangements.

TECHNICAL HINTS

I. Treatment plans for minors or mentally disabled patients should be discussed with the parent or guardian. Permission should be obtained by signature, particularly when anesthesia will be used or prescriptions issued.

II. Complete records are essential. Misunderstandings can lead to legal involvements.

FACTORS TO TEACH THE PATIENT

I. Why a treatment plan is made.

II. Explanation of unclear parts of the total treatment plan.

III. Parts of the treatment plan carried out by the patient. Interrelation of roles of patient and members of the dental team in eliminating the patient's oral disease.

IV. The long-term effects of comprehensive continuing care.

V. Why disease control measures must be learned before scaling and planing are done.

VI. Significance of the indices as guides for evaluating the health of the gingiva.

VII. What presurgical preparation means, what it consists of, and what its expected advantages are.

References

1. Robbins, K.S.: Medical-legal Considerations, in Malamed, S.F.: *Handbook of Medical Emergencies in the Dental Office*, 3rd ed. St. Louis, The C.V. Mosby Co., 1987, pp. 73–83.
2. Bailey, B.L.: Informed Consent in Dentistry, *J. Am. Dent. Assoc., 110,* 709, May, 1985.

Suggested Readings

Carranza, F.A.: *Glickman's Clinical Periodontology*, 6th ed. Philadelphia, W.B. Saunders Co., 1984, pp. 542–544.

Darby, M.L.: Viewpoint. The Dental Hygiene Process—A Step Toward Professionalism, *Dent. Hyg., 55,* 8, September, 1981.

Friedlander, A.H. and Frederick, C.J.: Interpretation of the Psychiatric Diagnostic Scheme: An Aid to Dental Treatment Planning, *Spec. Care Dentist., 7,* 165, July-August, 1987.

Goldman, H.M. and Cohen, D.W.: *Periodontal Therapy*, 6th ed. St. Louis, The C.V. Mosby Co., 1980, pp. 412–438.

Grant, D.A., Stern, I.B., and Listgarten, M.A., eds.: *Periodontics*, 6th ed. St. Louis, The C.V. Mosby Co., 1988, pp. 592–608.

Kerr, D.A., Ash, M.M., and Millard, H.D.: *Oral Diagnosis*, 6th ed. St. Louis, The C.V. Mosby Co., 1983, pp. 343–367.

Miller, P.L.: Treatment Planning for the Periodontal Patient, *Dent. Hyg., 54,* 331, July, 1980.

Miller, S.S.: Dental Hygiene Diagnosis, *RDH, 2,* 46, July-August, 1982.

Nielsen, N.J.: Decision Making Associated with Dental Hygiene Practice, *Dent. Hyg., 57,* 24, December, 1983.

O'Hehir, T.: Planning Treatment . . . From Px to Tx, *RDH, 4,* 18, July/August, 1984.

Pattison, G.L. and Pattison, A.M.: *Periodontal Instrumentation*. Reston, Virginia, Reston, 1979, pp. 337–344.

IV

Prevention

INTRODUCTION

This section, *Prevention,* includes procedures for bacterial disease control, use of fluorides, application of pit and fissure sealants, diet counseling, and all related preventive measures. In planning the sequence of treatment for the patient, initiation of preventive measures precedes dental and dental hygiene clinical services except in an emergency.

Dental caries and periodontal infections are caused by microorganisms of bacterial plaque. The long-range success of professional treatment is limited unless the causes of the condition, namely the microorganisms, are eliminated or brought to a controllable level.

Primary prevention, involving measures to prevent disease completely, is basic to continuing benefits of dental and dental hygiene treatment. The fluoridation of water supplies, bacterial plaque control, and limitation of cariogenic food substances for the prevention of dental caries are examples of primary preventive activities.

Secondary preventive measures are those related to the early recognition and treatment of incipient disease before extensive lesions develop. The restoration of small carious lesions and the recognition and biopsy of a suspected lesion of the mucous membrane are examples of secondary prevention. The relationship of primary and secondary prevention to dental hygiene practice was introduced on page 3.

Tertiary preventive measures are represented in more complex and involved dental and periodontal therapy, even to the extent of the replacement of missing teeth. Prevention is still involved as long as complete breakdown and loss of function are prevented.

Preventive dentistry is the sum total of the efforts to promote, restore, and maintain the oral health of the individual. A *program for prevention* is composed of the cooperative steps taken by the patient and members of the dental team to preserve the natural dentition and the supporting structures by preventing the onset, progress, and recurrence of oral diseases and other destructive or disfiguring conditions.

STEPS IN A PREVENTIVE PROGRAM

Each patient needs a *preventive treatment plan.* Planning and carrying out the preventive program may be divided into the six basic steps that are discussed in this section. Details to describe each step either were part of the diagnostic work-up described in previous chapters or will be parts of the chapters to follow.

I. Assess Patient's Needs

A. Review all information from the diagnostic work-up: history, examinations, radiographs, chartings.
B. Identify the presence and severity of disease and predisposing factors.
C. Utilize indices to rate the extent of the needs and provide a baseline for continuing comparisons.

II. Select Applicable Preventive Methods

A. Apply information about the patient: educational level, occupation, socioeconomic background, and attitudes toward oral health.
B. Recognize the influence of physical or mental disabilities.
C. Determine the current personal oral care procedures carried out by the patient, and their frequency.
D. Outline the instruction recommended and the goals to be attained by the patient.

III. Provide Instruction for Self-care

A. Provide motivating demonstration and supervision for specific daily bacterial plaque removal, self-applied fluoride, and other applicable preventive measures.

B. Show methods for self-evaluation.

IV. Perform Clinical Preventive Services

A. Complete scaling and root planing.

B. Apply caries-preventive agents.

V. Evaluate Changes in the Patient's Oral Health

A. Evaluate gingival tissue, bleeding, plaque, and techniques performed by the patient.

B. Use successive indices to compare progress.

C. Provide preventive counseling for corrective action when initial goals are not met.

VI. Plan Long-term Maintenance

A. Re-evaluate periodically to monitor continuance of preventive practices.

B. Provide additional preventive measures when indicated, particularly following placement of new restorations or prosthetic devices.

PATIENT INSTRUCTION

Instruction is an essential part of the preventive program if goals for attaining a patient's oral health are to be reached. Personalized patient instruction contributes first to the knowledge, attitudes, and practices of the individual and then, through the individual, to the family and the community.

The outmoded concept that all teeth eventually must be removed has been replaced by a new concept of preservation based on current research findings. It is now known that periodontal infections and dental caries can be prevented or controlled, and therefore, teeth can be preserved throughout the lifetime of the individual.

Dental health education is the provision of oral health information to people in such a way that they can apply it in everyday living.[1] Knowledge of and belief in health facts are not enough; benefits result only when knowledge is put into action. Learning occurs when an individual changes behavior and when changes are incorporated as a part of everyday living.

I. Motivation

Instruction is tailored to individual needs and motivations. An individual is motivated to practice behavior that leads to achievement of goals that are valued. Dental health instruction can be effective if the patient considers oral health a valuable asset or goal.

Stimulation of behavior, or motivation, stems from basic physiologic and social needs. Peer group approval and the need to conform to group standards, as well as the fear of disapproval or rejection when appearance of the teeth or odor of the breath is unacceptable, are frequently much stronger motivating factors than is a health reason, such as freedom from infection or the ability to chew food for body cell maintenance.

The need for relief from pain can bring a patient to seek immediate dental care; however, additional motivation will be needed to help the patient to realize that, through a preventive care program, future pain can be avoided.

Motivation and what the patient will learn and practice are proportional to the sincerity and concern of the dental team members. A motivated dental professional develops patient-centered systems of instruction that are meaningful to the patient.

II. Patient-centered Instruction

For most patients, major emphasis must be placed on control of dental caries or periodontal infections. Attention should also be paid to prevention of oral accidents, particularly those related to mouth protectors for contact sports, safety belts for automobiles, and children's accidents that lead to fractured anterior teeth.

Whereas patient instruction of the past connoted teaching a patient how and when to use a toothbrush, usually by means of a model and in one short session, patient instruction now envelops a wide range of essential areas of learning aimed at developing a patient's knowledge, attitudes, and practices for continuing oral health. The ability to interpret and apply current dental research findings requires continuing review through reading and other educational efforts.

DISEASE CONTROL

Bacterial plaque is the most important etiologic factor in the development of dental caries and inflammatory periodontal infection.

Disease control in the individual is directly related to the measures employed for removing bacterial plaque from the teeth on a regular daily basis. The most effective means for plaque removal available at present are mechanical, that is, toothbrushing for tooth surfaces that can be reached with the brush, and dental floss or other devices for proximal surfaces.

Pellicle begins to form immediately, and microbial plaque forms again within a few to 24 hours following its removal. Self-care measures for control clearly are necessary on a day-to-day basis.

Personal measures for disease control need supplementation by professional care. The removal of dental calculus, overhanging fillings, and other local plaque retainers is essential to create an environment that can be maintained effectively by the individual.

Continuing personal and professional care are mutually interdependent in a successful patient-centered plaque control program. Plaque control in combination with periodic scaling and root planing has been shown to arrest the progress of periodontal disease.

Oral physical therapy is accomplished by the use

of physical agents in the prevention, management, and control of oral diseases. In physical medicine, physical therapy includes the use of various agents, particularly light, heat, water, electricity, and exercise. A few of the same agents are used in oral care, and many mechanical devices have been developed for specific application to the teeth and gingiva. The satisfactory use of an oral physical therapy device depends on the patient's understanding of the goals to be attained. Objectives may need reconsideration from time to time depending on new research findings relative to the cause and prevention of oral diseases.

FACTORS TO TEACH THE PATIENT

I. The relationship between preventive measures and clinical services.
II. Why particular preventive measures were selected for the particular patient.
III. Self-evaluation methods for determining health of gingiva.
IV. Objectives for bacterial plaque disease control.

Reference

1. Young, W.O. and Striffler, D.F.: *The Dentist, His Practice, and His Community,* 2nd ed. Philadelphia, W.B. Saunders Co., 1969, p. 296.

22 Oral Disease Control: Toothbrushes and Toothbrushing

The toothbrush is the principal instrument in general use for accomplishing bacterial plaque removal as a necessary part of disease control. Many different designs of toothbrushes and supplementary devices have been manufactured and promoted.

Patients who have not previously received professional advice concerning the best brush for their particular oral conditions very likely have used brushes selected on the basis of cost, availability, advertising claims, family tradition, or habit. Because of the variety in shapes, sizes, textures, and other characteristics, dental professionals must become familiar with the many available products to advise patients appropriately.

DEVELOPMENT OF TOOTHBRUSHES[1-4]

Crudely contrived toothpicks, presumably used for relief from food impaction, are believed to be the earliest implements devised for the care of the teeth. Excavations in Mesopotamia uncovered elaborate gold toothpicks used by the Sumerians about 3000 B.C.

The earliest record of the "chewstick," which has been considered the primitive toothbrush, dates back in the Chinese literature to about 1600 B.C. The care of the mouth was associated with religious training and ritual: the Buddhists had a "toothstick," and the Mohammedans used the "miswak" or "siwak." Chewsticks, made from various types of tasty woods by crushing an end and spreading the fibers in a brush-like manner, are still used by many Asiatic and African people.

The Ebers Papyrus, compiled about 1500 B.C. and dating probably at about 4000 B.C., contained reference to conditions similar to periodontal diseases and preparations used as mouthwashes and dentifrices. The writings of Hippocrates (about 300 B.C.) include descriptions of diseased gums related to calculus and of complex preparations for the treatment of unhealthy mouths.

It is believed that the first brush made of hog's bristles, was mentioned in the early Chinese literature. Pierre Fauchard in 1728 in *Le Chirurgien Dentiste* described many aspects of oral health. He condemned the toothbrush made of horse's hair because it was rough and destructive to the teeth and advised the use of sponges or herb roots. Fauchard recommended scaling of teeth and developed instruments and splints for loose teeth, as well as dentifrices and mouthwashes.

One of the earlier toothbrushes made in England was produced by William Addis about 1780. By the early nineteenth century, craftsmen in various European countries constructed handles of gold, ivory, or ebony, in which replaceable brush heads could be fitted. The first patent for a toothbrush in the United States was issued to H.N. Wadsworth in the middle of the nineteenth century.

Many new varieties of toothbrushes were developed around 1900, when celluloid was available for the manufacture of toothbrush handles. In 1919, the American Academy of Periodontology defined specifications for toothbrush design and brushing methods in an attempt to standardize professional recommendations.[5]

Nylon came into use in toothbrush construction in 1938. World War II complications prevented Chinese export of wild boar bristles, and synthetic materials were substituted for natural bristles. Since then, synthetic materials have been improved and manufacturer's specifications standardized. Many current toothbrushes are made exclusively of synthetic materials. Powered toothbrushes, although developed earlier, were not actively promoted until about 1960.

MANUAL TOOTHBRUSHES

Although the American Dental Association does not evaluate and classify manual toothbrushes, certain recommendations have been made.[6] Desirable characteristics of a brush designed primarily to promote oral cleanliness are that it

1. Conform to individual patient requirements in size, shape, and texture.
2. Be easily and efficiently manipulated.
3. Be readily cleaned and aerated; impervious to moisture.
4. Be durable and inexpensive.
5. Have prime functional properties of flexibility, softness, and diameter of the bristles or filaments; and strength, rigidity, and lightness of the handle.
6. Be designed for utility, efficiency, and cleanliness.

I. General Description

A. Parts (figure 22–1)

1. *Handle.* The part grasped in the hand during toothbrushing.
2. *Head.* The working end; consists of tufts of bristles or filaments and the stock where the tufts are secured.
3. *Shank.* The section that connects the head and the handle.

B. Dimensions

1. *Total Brush Length.* About 15–19 cm. (6–7.5 inches); junior and child sizes may be shorter.
2. *Head.* Should be only large enough to accommodate the tufts.
   a. Length of brushing plane: 25.4 to 31.8 mm. (1 to 1¼ inches); width: 7.9 to 9.5 mm. (⁵⁄₁₆ to ⅜ inch).
   b. Bristle or filament height: 11 mm. (⁷⁄₁₆ inch).

II. Handle

A. Composition

Nearly all current brush handles are plastics, which combine durability, imperviousness to moisture, pleasing appearance, low cost, sufficient rigidity, and smooth texture.

B. Shape

1. *Preferred Characteristics*
   a. Handle aligned on same plane as the head.
   b. Easy to grasp.
   c. Will not slip or rotate during use.
   d. No sharp corners or projections.
   e. Light weight, consistent with strength.
2. *Variations.* A twist, curve, offset, or angle in the shank with or without thumb rests may frequently be related to new ideas for advertising appeal or for adaptation to difficult-to-reach areas. Slight deviations may not complicate manipulation or affect control of the brush placement and pressure.

Bent or thickened handles can be helpful for use by patients with certain types of disability (pages 622–623).

III. Head

A. Stock

The stock is the extension of the handle where the tufts are attached in rows.

B. Tufts

A tuft is a cluster of bristles or filaments secured together in one hole in the stock.

C. Design (figure 22–2)

1. *Tufted.* Five or six tufts long and two or three rows wide, spaced for easy cleaning of the brush.
2. *Multitufted.* Ten or twelve tufts long and three or four rows wide, spaced closely to provide a smooth brushing plane and to allow the filaments to support each other for longer durability.

D. Brushing Plane (profile)

Brushes are available with variously shaped filament profiles. They may range from brushes with filaments all of equal lengths (flat planes, figure 22–2) to those with variable lengths such as dome-shaped, bi-level, or rippled. All filaments should be soft and end-rounded for safety to oral soft tissues and tooth structure. When used properly, the variable length profiles can be more efficient for cleaning the hard-to-reach areas such as extension onto proximal surfaces, malpositioned teeth, or exposed root surfaces.

IV. Bristles and Filaments

Most current toothbrushes have nylon filaments. Natural bristles are relatively unsanitary, and their physical qualifications cannot be standardized.

The stiffness (described commercially for the patient as soft, medium, or hard) depends on the diameter and length of the filament.

A. Factors Influencing Stiffness

1. *Diameter.* Thinner filaments are softer and more resilient.
2. *Length.* Shorter filaments are stiffer and have less flexibility.
3. *Number of Filaments in a Tuft.* Each filament

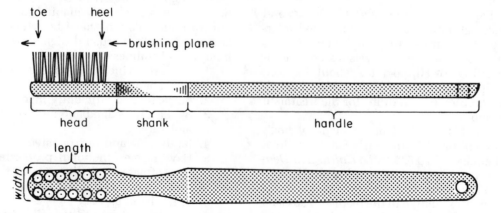

Figure 22–1. Parts of a Toothbrush.

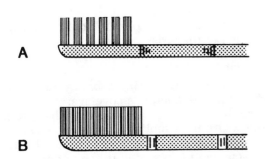

Figure 22–2. Toothbrush Design. A. Tufted brush with 5 or 6 spaced tufts in 2 or 3 rows. Filaments or bristles may have equal lengths to form a smooth trim as shown, or the brushing plane may have tapered tufts. **B.** Multitufted brush 10 or 12 tufts long and 3 or 4 tufts wide. Tufts are spaced closely to provide a smooth brushing plane.

gives support to the adjacent filaments; each tuft gives support to adjacent tufts.

B. Natural Bristles

1. *Source.* Historically, bristles have been obtained from the hair of the hog or wild boar.
2. *Uniformity.* Bristles are not consistent in texture or wearing properties. Their inherent resiliency varies with the breed of animal, as well as with the geographic location and season when the bristles were taken.
3. *Diameter.* They vary in size from 0.087 mm. (.0035 inch) to 0.475 mm. (.019 inch) depending on the portion of the bristle and the age and life of the animal.
4. *Shape.* Bristles have deficient, irregular, frequently open ends.
5. *Disadvantages.*[7] Toothbrushes with natural bristles are not recommended because the bristles
   a. Cannot be standardized.
   b. Wear more rapidly and irregularly.
   c. Are hollow, thereby allowing microorganisms and debris to collect inside.
   d. Are water absorbent (water softens the bristle).

C. Filaments

1. *Composition.* Synthetic, plastic materials, primarily nylon.
2. *Uniformity.* Controlled.
3. *Diameter*
   a. Filaments may range from extra soft to hard. Diameters range from 0.15 mm (.006 inch) to 0.3 mm (.012 inch).
   b. Small interdental brushes are made with filaments of 0.075 mm. (.003 inch) (page 323).
4. *Shape.* End-rounded filaments cause the least trauma to the tissues.
5. *Advantages of Filaments Over Natural Bristles*
   a. Rinse clean and dry rapidly when left in open.
   b. More durable and maintain their form longer.
   c. Ends, rounded and closed, repel water and debris.
   d. More resistant to accumulation of bacteria and fungi than are natural bristles.

V. Toothbrush Selection for the Patient

A. Influencing Factors (see also pages 370–371)

Factors that influence the selection of the proper toothbrush for an individual patient include the following:

1. *Patient*
   a. Ability of the patient to use the brush and remove plaque from all tooth surfaces without damage to the soft tissue or tooth structure.
   b. Manual dexterity of patient.
   c. Motivation, ability, and willingness to follow the prescribed procedures.
2. *Gingiva*
   a. Status of gingival or periodontal health.
   b. Anatomic configurations of the gingiva.
3. *Position of Teeth.* Displaced teeth require variations in brush placement.
4. *Personal Preferences*
   a. Professional personnel may prefer to instruct certain methods and with certain brushes.
   b. Patient may have preferences and may resist change.
5. *Technique Selected.* Method of brushing to be recommended and instructed.

B. Toothbrush Size and Shape

The brush selected must be able to reach all facial, lingual, palatal, and occlusal surfaces for bacterial plaque removal.

C. Soft Nylon Brush: Tufted or Multitufted

Tufted medium or hard brushes were formerly used to a greater extent than currently. They are generally contraindicated because of potential damage to gingiva and teeth while removing plaque from the cervical thirds of the teeth, particularly if an abrasive dentifrice is used. The following are suggested as advantages for the use of a soft brush with rounded ends:

1. More effective in cleaning the cervical areas, both proximal and marginal.
2. Less traumatic to the gingival tissue; therefore patients can brush at the cervical areas without fear of pain or lacerating the tissues.
3. Can be directed into the sulcus for sulcular brushing and into interproximal areas.
4. Applicable around fixed orthodontic appliances or fixation appliances used to treat a fractured jaw.
5. Tooth abrasion and/or gingival recession is prevented or less severe in an over-vigorous brusher.

6. More effective use for sensitive gingiva in such conditions as necrotizing ulcerative gingivitis or desquamative gingivitis, or during healing stages following scaling and curettage or periodontal surgery.

7. Small size is ideal for a young child as a first brush on primary teeth.

TOOTHBRUSHING PROCEDURES

Complete toothbrushing instruction for a patient involves teaching many details related to why, what, when, where, and how. In addition to descriptions of specific toothbrushing methods, the succeeding sections will consider the grasp of the brush, the sequence and amount of brushing, the areas of limited access, supplementary brushing for the occlusal surfaces and the tongue, the possible detrimental effects from improper toothbrushing as well as contraindications, and the care of toothbrushes.

I. Grasp of Brush

A. Objectives

Manipulation of the brush for successful plaque removal can be related to the manner in which the brush is held. Patients may need specific instruction in how to hold and place the brush. When they start to brush to remove the bacterial plaque that has been colored with a disclosing agent, the tenaciousness of the plaque and the need for controlled pressure are realized. With a firm, comfortable grasp, the following can be expected:

1. Control of the brush during all movements.

2. Effective positioning at the beginning of each brushing stroke, follow-through during the complete stroke, and repositioning for the next stroke.

3. Sensitivity to the amount of pressure applied. Pressure is necessary for removal of the bacterial plaque. Too much pressure, however, bends the filaments and curves them away from the gingival sulcus where brushing is indicated.

B. Procedure

1. Grasp toothbrush handle in the palm of the hand with thumb against the shank.
   a. Near enough to the head of the brush so that it can be controlled effectively.
   b. Not so close to the head of the brush that manipulation of the brush is hindered or that fingers can touch the anterior teeth when reaching the brush head to molar regions.

2. Direct filaments in the direction needed for placement on the teeth; direction depends on the brushing method to be used.

3. Adapt grasp for the various positions of the brush head on the teeth throughout the procedure; adjust to permit unrestricted movement of the wrist and arm.

II. Sequence

A. The procedure in brushing, for any method used, should assure complete coverage.

B. Omission of an area is prevented when brushing follows from the molar region of one arch around to the opposite side, then back around the lingual or facial, and is repeated in the opposing arch.

C. Each brush placement must overlap the previous one for thorough coverage (figure 22–3).

D. Encourage the patient to begin by brushing one of the areas that most meets the individual needs.
   1. Areas that are most frequently missed.
   2. Areas that are most difficult for brush placement and/or manipulation, such as the right side for the right-handed brusher or the left side for the left-handed brusher.

E. Suggest that the sequence be changed at least once each day so that the same areas are not always brushed last when time may be limited and plaque removal may be less complete.

III. Amount of Brushing

A. The Count System

To ensure thorough coverage with an even distribution of amount of brushing and to help the patient concentrate on the performance, a system of counting is useful.

1. Count six strokes in each area (or five or ten, whichever is most appropriate for the particular patient) for modified Stillman or other method in which a stroke is used.

2. Count slowly to ten for each brush position

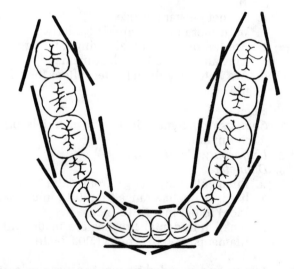

Figure 22–3. Brushing Positions. Each brush position, as represented by a black line, should overlap the previous position. Note placement at canines, where the distal of the canine is brushed with the premolars and the mesial aspect is brushed with the incisors. Short lines on lingual anterior indicate brush placed the long narrow way. The maxillary teeth require a similar number of brushing positions.

while brush is vibrated and filament ends are held in position for the Bass, Charters, or other vibratory method.

B. The Clock System

Some patients brush thoroughly while watching a clock or an egg timer for 3 or 4 minutes. Timed procedures cannot assure thorough coverage, because single areas that are most accessible may get more brushing time.

C. Combination

For many patients, use of the "count" system in combination with the "clock" system produces the most complete removal of bacterial plaque.

IV. Frequency of Brushing

Because of individual variations, one set rule for frequency cannot be applied. The emphasis in patient education should be placed on complete plaque removal rather than on number of brushings.

For the control of bacterial plaque, and for oral sanitation and halitosis prevention, at least two brushings, one of which includes thorough flossing, are recommended for each day.

Going to sleep with a clean mouth should be encouraged. Patients who use a chewable fluoride tablet, mouthrinse, or gel application before going to bed should complete plaque removal before fluoride application.

V. Methods

Most toothbrushing methods can be classified into one of eight groups based on the motion and position of the brush. Noted below beside certain categories are names of methods that utilize the designated motion as part or all of their particular procedure. Some of these methods are recorded for descriptive, comparative, or historic purposes only, and are not currently recommended. A few even have been proved detrimental.

A. **Sulcular:** Bass.
B. **Roll:** Rolling stroke, modified Stillman.
C. **Vibratory:** Stillman, Charters.
D. **Circular:** Fones.
E. **Vertical:** Leonard.
F. **Horizontal.**
G. **Physiologic:** Smith.
H. **Scrub-brush.**

THE BASS METHOD: SULCULAR BRUSHING

The Bass technique is widely accepted as the most effective method for bacterial plaque removal adjacent to and directly beneath the gingival margin. This area around the tooth is the most significant in the control of gingival and periodontal disease.

I. Purposes and Indications

A. For all patients for bacterial plaque removal adjacent to and directly beneath the gingival margin.
B. Particularly for open interproximal areas, cervical areas beneath the height of contour of the enamel, and exposed root surfaces.
C. For the patient who has had periodontal surgery.

II. Brush Selection

Because of potential damage to the gingival tissue, only a soft nylon brush with end-rounded filaments is indicated.

III. Technique[8]

A. Grasp Brush Handle

Direct the filaments apically (up for maxillary, down for mandibular teeth). Even though the brush placement calls for directing the filaments at a 45-degree angle, it is usually easier and safer for the patient to first place the brush parallel with the long axis of the tooth. From that position the brush can be turned slightly and brought to the gingival margin to the 45-degree angle (figure 22–4).

B. Angle the Filaments

Place the brush with the filament tips directed straight into the gingival sulcus. The filaments will be directed at approximately 45 degrees to

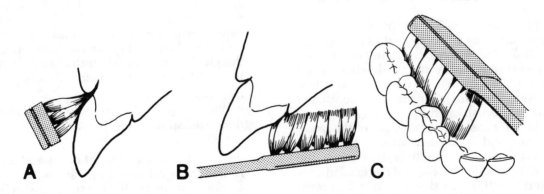

Figure 22–4. Sulcular Brushing. A. Filament tips are directed into the gingival sulcus at approximately 45 degrees to the long axis of the tooth. **B.** Position for lingual surface of maxillary anterior teeth. **C.** Brush in position for mandibular posterior teeth, lingual surfaces.

the long axis of the tooth, as shown in figure 22–4A.

C. Press Lightly Without Flexing

Press lightly so the filament tips enter the gingival sulci and embrasures and cover the gingival margin. Do not bend the filaments.

D. Vibrate the Brush

Vibrate the brush back and forth with very short strokes without disengaging the tips of the filaments from the sulci. Count at least 10 vibrations.

E. Reposition the Brush

Apply the brush to the next group of two or three teeth. Take care to overlap placement, as shown in figure 22–3.

F. Repeat Stroke

The entire stroke (Parts A. through D., above) is repeated at each position around the maxillary and mandibular arches, both facially and lingually.

G. Position Brush for Lingual and Palatal Anterior Surfaces (figure 22–4B)

Hold the brush the long narrow way for the anterior components as described for the rolling stroke technique. The filaments are kept straight and directed into the sulci.

IV. Problems

A. An over-eager brusher may convert the "very short strokes" (note III., D., above) into a scrub-brush technique and cause injury to the gingival margin.

B. Dexterity requirement may be too high for certain patients.

C. Rolling stroke procedure may precede the sulcular brushing when a patient believes it helps to clean the teeth. The two techniques should be performed separately rather than trying to combine them in what has been referred to as a "modified Bass."

The procedure of rolling the brush down over the crown after the vibratory part of the sulcular brush stroke has several disadvantages: (1) too often the brush is hastily and carelessly replaced into the sulcus position, or the opposite is true and considerable time is consumed in the attempt to replace the brush carefully; (2) gingival margin injury by the constant replacement of the brush is common; and (3) concentration is not on the important objective, which is to remove the plaque at and under the gingival margin. Patients may tend to roll the brush down over the crown prematurely, thereby accomplishing very little sulcular brushing.

THE ROLL or ROLLING STROKE METHOD

I. Purposes and Indications

A. Cleaning gingiva and removal of plaque, materia alba, and food debris from the teeth without emphasis on gingival sulcus.
 1. For children with relatively healthy gingiva and normal tissue contour when a sulcular technique may seem difficult for the patient to master.
 2. For general cleaning in conjunction with the use of a vibratory technique (Charters, Stillman).

B. Useful for preparatory instruction (first lesson) for modified Stillman technique because the initial brush placement is the same. This can be particularly helpful when there is a question as to how complicated a technique the patient can master and practice.

II. Technique[5,9]

A. Grasp Brush Handle

Direct filaments apically (up for maxillary, down for mandibular teeth).

B. Place Side of Brush on the Attached Gingiva

The filaments are directed apically. When the plastic portion of the brush head is level with the occlusal or incisal plane, generally the brush will be at the proper height, as shown in figure 22–5A.

C. Press to Flex the Filaments

The sides of the filaments are pressed against the gingiva. The gingiva will blanch.

D. Roll the Brush Slowly Over the Teeth

As the brush is rolled, the wrist is turned slightly. The filaments remain flexed and follow the contours of the teeth, thereby permitting cleaning of the cervical areas. Some filaments may reach interdentally.

E. Replace and Repeat Five Times or More

The entire stroke (Parts A through D, above) is repeated at least five times for each tooth or group of teeth. When the brush is removed and repositioned, the wrist is rotated, the brush is moved away from the teeth, and the cheek is stretched facially with the back of the plastic portion. Care must be taken not to drag the filament tips over the gingival margin when the brush is returned to the initial position (figure 22–5A).

F. Overlap Strokes

When moving the brush to an adjacent position, overlap the brush position, as shown in figure 22–3.

G. Position Brush for Lingual or Palatal Surfaces

1. Use the brush the long, narrow way.
2. Hook the heel of the brush on the incisal edge (figure 22–5D).
3. Press down for maxillary (up for mandibular)

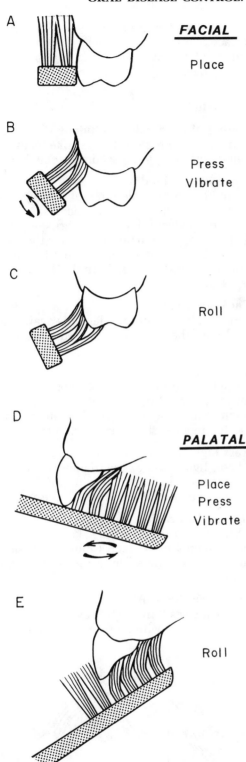

FACIAL

Place

Press
Vibrate

Roll

PALATAL

Place
Press
Vibrate

Roll

Figure 22–5. Modified Stillman Method of Brushing. A. Initial brush placement with sides of bristles or filaments against the attached gingiva. **B.** The brush is pressed and angled, then vibrated. **C.** Vibrating is continued as the brush is rolled slowly over the crown. **D.** Maxillary anterior lingual placement with the brush applied the long way. **E.** Vibrating continues as the brush is rolled over the crown and interdental areas. Placement is similar for the lingual of the mandibular anterior. The roll or rolling stroke brushing method has the same brush positions.

until the filaments lie flat against the teeth and gingiva.
4. Press and roll (curve up for mandibular, down for maxillary teeth).
5. Replace and repeat five times for each brush width. (Brush placement across the anterior lingual can be compared with the hands of a clock or spokes of a wheel.)

III. Problems
A. Brushing too high during initial placement can lacerate the alveolar mucosa.
B. Tendency to use quick, sweeping strokes results in no brushing for the cervical third of the tooth because the brush tips pass over rather than into the area; likewise for the interproximal areas.
C. Replacing brush with filament tips directed into the gingiva can produce punctate lesions (page 313).

THE MODIFIED STILLMAN METHOD

This method as originally described by Stillman[10] was designed for massage and stimulation, as well as for cleaning the cervical areas. The brush ends were placed partly on the gingiva and partly on the cervical areas of the tooth and were directed slightly apically. Pressure was applied to effect a blanching. The handle was given a slight rotary motion, and the brush ends were maintained in position on the tooth surface. After several applications, the brush was moved to the adjacent tooth.

A modified Stillman, which incorporates a rolling stroke after the vibratory (rotary) phase, generally is used at present. The modifications minimize the possibility of gingival trauma and increase the plaque removal effects.[11]

I. Purposes and Indications
A. Bacterial plaque removal from cervical areas below the height of contour of the crown and from exposed proximal surfaces.
B. General application for cleaning tooth surfaces and massage of the gingiva.

II. Technique (figure 22–5)
A. Grasp Brush Handle
Direct filaments apically (up for maxillary, down for mandibular teeth).

B. Place Side of Brush on the Attached Gingiva
The filaments are directly apically. When the plastic portion of the brush head is level with the occlusal or incisal plane, generally the brush will be at the proper height, as shown in figure 22–5A.

C. Press to Flex the Filaments
The sides of the filaments are pressed lightly against the gingiva. The gingiva will blanch.

D. Angle the Filaments
Turn the handle by rotating the wrist so that the filaments are directed at an angle of approximately 45 degrees with the long axis of the tooth.

E. Vibrate the Brush

Vibrate gently but firmly. Maintain light pressure on the filaments, and keep the tips of the filaments in position with constant contact. Count to ten slowly as the brush is vibrated by a rotary motion of the handle.

F. Roll and Vibrate the Brush

Turn the wrist and work the vibrating brush slowly down over the gingiva and tooth. Make some of the filaments reach interdentally.

G. Replace Brush for Repeat Stroke

Reposition the brush by rotating the wrist. Avoid dragging the filaments back over the free gingival margin by holding the brush out, slightly away from the tooth.

H. Repeat Stroke Five Times or More

The entire stroke (Parts A through F, above) is repeated at least five times for each tooth or group of teeth. When moving the brush to an adjacent position, overlap the brush position, as shown in figure 22–3.

I. Position Brush for Lingual and Palatal Surfaces

1. Position the brush the long, narrow way for the anterior components, as described for the rolling stroke technique and shown in figure 22–5 D and E.
2. Press and vibrate, roll, and repeat.

III. Problems

A. Without careful brush placement, tissue laceration can result when a hard brush is used. A soft brush used with lighter pressure is needed.
B. Patient may try to move the brush into the rolling stroke too quickly, and the vibratory aspect may be ineffective for plaque removal at the gingival margin.

THE CHARTERS METHOD

The original intent, as described by Charters,[12] was to use the toothbrush in a manner that would stimulate the gingival margin "all around each tooth, especially in the inter-dental spaces." The method is generally not used when interdental papillae are normal because other methods may be easier to teach.

I. Purposes and Indications

A. Loosening of debris and bacterial plaque.
B. Massage and stimulation for marginal and interdental gingiva.
C. Indicated to aid in plaque removal from proximal tooth surfaces when interproximal tissue is missing, for example, following periodontal surgery.
D. Adaptable to cervical areas below the height of contour of the crown and to exposed root surfaces.
E. Useful for removing bacterial plaque from abutment teeth and under the gingival border of a fixed partial denture (bridge) or from the undersurface of a sanitary bridge.
F. Aids in cleansing orthodontic appliances (figure 24–2C, page 338).

II. Technique[13]

A. Apply Rolling Stroke Technique

Instruct in a basic rolling stroke technique for general cleaning to be accomplished first.

B. Grasp Brush Handle

Hold brush (outside the oral cavity) with filaments directed toward the occlusal or incisal plane of the teeth that will be brushed. The tips are pointed down for application to the maxillary and pointed up for application to the mandibular arch. Insert the brush held in the direction it will be used.

C. Place the Brush

Place the sides of the filaments against the enamel with the brush tips toward the occlusal or incisal plane.

D. Angle the Filaments

Angle at approximately 45 degrees to the occlusal or incisal plane. Slide the brush to a position at the junction of the free gingival margin and the tooth surface (figure 22–6B).

E. Press Lightly

Press lightly to flex the filaments and force the tips between the teeth. The sides of the filaments are pressed against the gingival margin.

F. Vibrate the Brush

Vibrate gently but firmly, keeping the tips of the filaments in contact. Count to 10 slowly as the brush is vibrated by a rotary motion of the handle.

G. Reposition the Brush and Repeat

Repeat Parts B through F, as described, several times in each position around the dental arches.

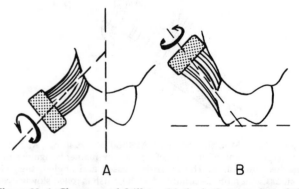

Figure 22–6. Charters and Stillman Methods Compared. A. Stillman. The brush is angled at approximately 45 degrees to the long axis of the tooth. B. Charters. The brush is angled at approximately 45 degrees to the occlusal plane, with brush tips directed toward the occlusal or incisal.

H. Overlap Strokes

When moving the brush to an adjacent position, overlap the brush position, as shown in figure 22–3.

I. Position Brush for Lingual and Palatal Surfaces

Since Charters brush position is difficult to accomplish on the lingual, a modified Stillman technique is frequently advised. When Charters method is preferred, the positions are as follows:

1. *Posterior*
   a. With brush tips pointed toward the occlusal, extend the brush handle across the incisal of the canine of the side opposite that to be brushed.
   b. Place the sides of the toe-end filaments against the distal of the most posterior tooth and subsequently at each embrasure.
   c. Press and vibrate.

2. *Anterior*
   a. With brush handle parallel with the long axis of the tooth, place the sides of the toe-end filaments over the interproximal embrasure.
   b. Press and vibrate.

J. Application of Brush for Fixed Partial Denture

When placing the brush, check that the filament tips are directed under the gingival border of the pontic.

III. Problems

A. Brush ends do not engage the gingival sulcus to remove subgingival bacterial accumulations.

B. In some areas, the correct brush placement is limited or impossible; therefore, modifications become necessary, consequently adding to the complexity of the procedure.

C. Requirements in digital dexterity are high.

OTHER TOOTHBRUSHING METHODS

The rolling stroke, modified Stillman, and Bass are probably the methods most used for patient instruction by dentists and dental hygienists. Other methods are and have been used, and a few of the well-known methods are included here. The technique and intent of some of the methods overlap. Evaluation prior to special instruction generally reveals that a mixture of techniques may be in use by a patient.

I. Circular: The Fones Method

Many patients, especially school children, probably received instruction in this method because it was advocated by Fones, who founded the first course for dental hygienists. He described the technique in the first dental hygiene text that was used for many years by dental hygiene students throughout the United States.

Although now considered possibly detrimental for adults, particularly when used by a vigorous brusher, this method may be recommended as an easy-to-learn first technique for young children. A soft brush with .006- to .008-inch filament diameter is selected. In abbreviated form, the technique described by Dr. Fones includes the following:[14]

A. With the teeth closed, place the brush inside the cheek with the brush tips lightly contacting the gingiva over the last maxillary molar.

B. Use a fast, wide, circular motion that sweeps from the maxillary gingiva to the mandibular gingiva with very little pressure (figure 22–7).

C. Bring anterior teeth in end-to-end contact, and hold lip out when necessary to make the continuous circular strokes.

D. Lingual and palatal tooth surfaces require an in-and-out stroke. Brush sweeps across palate on maxillary and back and forth to the molars on the mandibular.

II. Vertical: Leonard Method

As described by Hirschfeld,[15] the up-and-down stroke was employed when teeth were cleaned with a primitive crude twig toothbrush. The true vertical stroke passes from the gingiva over the maxillary teeth to the gingiva over the mandibular teeth, with a vigorous sweeping motion.

Leonard described and advocated a vertical stroke in which maxillary and mandibular teeth were brushed separately. Paraphrased, he described his method as follows:[16]

A. With the teeth edge-to-edge, place the brush with the filaments against the teeth at right angles to the long axes of the teeth.

B. Brush vigorously, without great pressure, with a stroke that is mostly up and down on the tooth

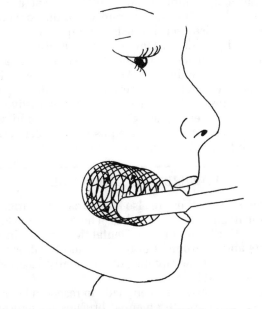

Figure 22–7. Fones Method of Brushing. With the teeth closed, a circular motion extends from the maxillary gingiva to the mandibular gingiva using a light pressure.

surfaces, with just a slight rotation or circular movement after striking the gingival margin with force.

C. Use enough pressure to force the filaments into the embrasures, but not enough to damage the brush.

D. The upper and lower teeth are not brushed in the same series of strokes. The teeth are placed edge-to-edge to keep the brush from slipping over the occlusal or incisal.

III. Horizontal

Horizontal or crosswise brushing is generally accepted as detrimental. An unlimited sweep with a horizontal scrubbing motion bears pressure on teeth that are most facially inclined or prominent. With the use of an abrasive dentifrice, such brushing may produce tooth abrasion. Because the interdental areas are not touched by this method, various gingival and periodontal problems may ensue.

IV. Physiologic: Smith's Method

The physiologic method was described by Smith[17] and advocated later by Bell.[18] It was based on the principle that the toothbrush should follow the same physiologic pathway that food follows when it traverses over the tissues in a "natural" masticating act.

A soft brush with "small tufts of fine bristles arranged in four parallel rows and trimmed to an even length" was used in a brushing stroke directed down over the lower teeth onto the gingiva and upward over the teeth for the maxillary. Smith also suggested a few gentle horizontal strokes to clean the portion of the sulci directly over the bifurcations of the roots.

V. Scrub-Brush

Vigorously combined horizontal, vertical, and circular strokes, with some vibratory motions for certain areas, comprise a scrub-brush technique. A soft brush with end-rounded filaments, such as that recommended in particular for the Bass technique, can be used with a very short-stroked scrub-brush technique for plaque removal in the cervical area following periodontal surgery. Without caution, however, vigorous scrubbing can encourage gingival recession and, with a dentifrice of sufficient abrasiveness, can create areas of tooth abrasion.

POWERED TOOTHBRUSHES

Powered brushes are also known as automatic, mechanical, and electric brushes. The American Dental Association Council on Dental Materials, Instruments and Equipment evaluates and classifies powered brushes as acceptable, provisionally acceptable, or unacceptable.[19]

Comparisons have been made in research between the powered and the manual brushes to determine the ability of each type to remove plaque, prevent calculus development, and reduce the incidence of gingivitis. Both types have been shown effective when used correctly.

I. Description

A. Head

The head, connected to the shank, is detachable from the handle and replaceable. In general, powered brush heads are smaller than manual brush heads. They range in size from approximately 6 to 12 mm. (¼ to ½ inch) wide by 15 to 18 mm. (¾ inch) long.

B. Motion

The action on different models may be one of the following:

1. *Reciprocating.* Moves back and forth in a line.
2. *Arcuate.* Filament ends follow an arc as they move up and down.
3. *Orbital.* Circular.
4. *Vibratory.*
5. *Elliptical.* Oval.
6. *Dual Motion.* More than one of the previously listed motions.

C. Power Source

1. *Direct.* Cord from electrical outlet connects directly to the toothbrush handle.
2. *Replaceable Batteries.* Disadvantage in the nuisance and cost of repeatedly replacing or recharging batteries; also, as the batteries lose their power, the brush is slowed. Corrosion may be a problem if water gets into the case.
3. *Rechargeable.* The instrument is placed into a stand that contains the recharger and is connected to the electrical outlet. A few models have a recharger built into the handle.
4. *Switches.* A few models require that the push button be held down during operation. This requirement may present difficulties for some patients, such as small children or persons with certain types of disabilities.

D. Speeds

Speeds vary from low to high among the different models. Some have the speed coordinated with the filament texture, for example, a soft small brush with a fast vigorous action, or a larger, harder brush with a slower, more gentle motion. The number of strokes per minute varies from, for example, as low as 1000 cycles per minute for a replaceable battery type, to about 3600 oscillations per minute for an arcuate model. The rechargeable battery types operate at approximately 2000 complete strokes per minute.

II. Purposes and Indications

A. General Application

For all patients for the removal of bacterial plaque, materia alba, and food debris. All of the general objectives that apply to plaque control measures and to manual brushes apply to powered brushes.

B. Patients with Disabilities

Powered brushes with their thick handles have been shown to be easily handled and manipulated by patients with certain disabilities, especially when grasping is difficult to accomplish (pages 622–624).

C. Patients Unable to Brush

A powered brush may be readily handled by a parent, attendant, or other person who cares for the patient.

III. Instruction

With a manual brush, an individual must learn to apply the brush tips in certain ways in order that each surface of each tooth can be reached, slight pressure can be applied for a thorough brushing effect, and the stroke can be repeated a number of times. With a powered brush, the action is built in. The only muscle training required is turning the handle to apply the brush to each surface of each tooth and holding it on each surface for a reasonable length of time in a correct position.

IV. Methods for Use

The general suggestions presented here are basic and, as with all brushing techniques, need adaptations for an individual mouth. Familiarity with the instructions provided by the manufacturers of the various powered brushes is a prerequisite.

A. Select brush with extra-soft filaments. The tips included with a newly purchased brush handle are not usually extra-soft.

B. Select dentifrice with minimum abrasivity. The extra strokes made by a powered brush increase the effects of abrasion to the tooth surface.

C. Place a small amount of dentifrice on the brush and spread the dentifrice over the teeth to prevent splashing when the power is turned on.

D. Any of the brushing techniques previously described in this chapter can be applied for use with a powered brush.

E. Vary the brush position for each tooth surface. Brush each tooth separately.
   1. Apply the brush for sulcular brushing to the distal, facial, and mesial surfaces of each tooth as the brush is moved from the most posterior teeth toward the anterior, quadrant by quadrant.
   2. Hold the brush in one location. Then turn it or move it to reach adjacent areas while keeping the power on.
   3. Angulate for access to surfaces of rotated, crowded, or otherwise displaced teeth.
   4. Retract lip with fingers of other hand to give access to and visibility of anterior facial surfaces, particularly including prominent canines.
   5. Modify brush positions for application to proximal surfaces when interdental papillae

are missing. Brush head may be positioned parallel with the long axis and inserted proximally.

F. Make strokes slowly, with a slight steady pressure. Pressure should not be great enough at any time to bend the filaments.

G. Precautions
   1. Acrylic restorations should be avoided or treated without pressure because they can wear down under repeated application of the fast-moving filaments with dentifrice.
   2. Avoid pressure with abrasive dentifrice over exposed cementum or dentin.

SUPPLEMENTAL BRUSHING

I. Problem Areas

Each surface of each tooth must be brushed. Initial instruction necessarily may be limited to a basic procedure, particularly when it varies from the patient's present procedures.

At succeeding lessons, the special hard-to-get areas are shown to the patient. Suggestions are made and demonstrated for brush adaptation for areas that were missed. Methods for cleaning the interdental areas and fixed and removable appliances are described in Chapters 23 and 24.

Attention in teaching should be given to the following:

A. Facially displaced teeth, especially canines and premolars, where the zone of attached gingiva may be minimal and where toothbrush abrasion frequently occurs.

B. Surfaces of teeth next to edentulous areas.

C. Inclined teeth, for example, lingual surfaces of mandibular molars that are inclined lingually.

D. Exposed root surfaces; cemental and dentinal surfaces may become abraded by extended application of an abrasive dentifrice.

E. Exposed furcation areas.

F. Right canine and lateral incisor, both maxillary and mandibular, are commonly missed by right-handed brushers; the opposite is true for left-handed brushers.

G. Distal surfaces of most posterior teeth (figure 22–8). At best, the brush may reach only the distal line angles. Supplementation with dental floss, yarn, or tufted dental floss is needed for the distal surface (pages 319–321).

II. Occlusal Brushing

A. Objectives

   1. To loosen plaque microorganisms packed in pits and fissures.
   2. To remove plaque deposits from occlusal surfaces of teeth out of occlusion or not used during mastication.
   3. To remove plaque from the margins of restorations.
   4. To apply fluoride from fluoride dentifrice.

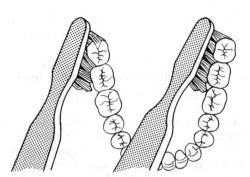

Figure 22–8. Brushing Problems. Brush placement to remove plaque from the distal surfaces of the most posterior teeth. The distobuccal is approached by stretching the cheek; the distolingual is approached by directing the brush across from the canine of the opposite side.

B. Technique
1. Place brush on occlusal of molar teeth with filament tips pointed into the occlusal pits at a right angle. The handle should be parallel with the occlusal surface. The toe of the brush should cover the distal grooves of the most posterior tooth.
2. Two acceptable strokes are suggested.
   a. Vibrate the brush in a slight circular movement while maintaining the filament tips on the occlusal surface throughout a count of ten. Press moderately so filaments do not bend but go straight into the pits and fissures (figure 22–9).
   b. Force the filaments against the occlusal surface with sharp, quick strokes; lift the brush off each time to dislodge debris; repeat about ten times.
3. Move brush to premolar area, overlapping previous brush position.

C. Precaution
Long scrubbing strokes from anterior to posterior on an occlusal surface may contact only the prominent parts of the cusps (figure 22–9B and 9C).

III. Tongue Brushing
Total mouth cleanliness includes tongue brushing.

A. Microorganisms of the Tongue
1. Main foci for oral microorganisms
   a. Dorsum of tongue.
   b. Gingival sulci and pockets.
   c. Bacterial plaque on all teeth.
2. Microorganisms in saliva are principally from the tongue.
3. Tongue organisms influence the flora of the entire oral cavity.

B. Effects of Cleaning the Tongue
1. Reduction of oral debris.
2. Retardation of bacterial plaque formation and total plaque accumulation.
3. Reduction of number of microorganisms.

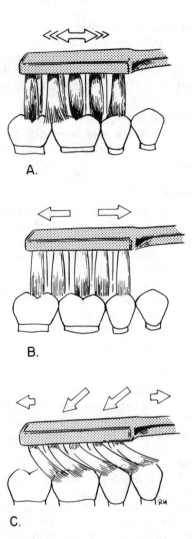

Figure 22–9. Occlusal Brushing. A. Vibrating brush with light pressure while maintaining filament tips on the occlusal surface permits tips to work their way into pits and fissures. **B.** Long horizontal strokes contact only the cusp tips. **C.** Excess pressure curves the filaments so that tips cannot get into the pits and fissures.

When brushing of the tongue is discontinued, the number of organisms increases.
4. Contribution to overall cleanliness.

C. Anatomic Features of Tongue Conducive to Debris Retention
1. *Surface Papillae.* Numerous filiform papillae extend as minute projections, whereas fungiform papillae are not as high and create elevations and depressions that entrap debris and microorganisms.
2. *Fissured Tongue.* Fissures may be several millimeters deep and retain debris.

D. Brushing Procedure
1. Hold the brush handle at a right angle to the midline of the tongue and direct the brush tips toward the throat.
2. With the tongue extruded, the sides of the filaments are placed on the posterior part of the surface.

3. With light pressure draw the brush forward and over the tip of the tongue. Repeat three or four times. Do not scrub the papillae.

DETRIMENTAL EFFECTS FROM TOOTHBRUSHING

I. Toothbrush Trauma: The Gingiva

Trauma to the gingiva occurs most frequently on the facial surfaces over teeth prominent in the dental arch. The lesions frequently are found over canines and premolars.

Lesions are especially apt to occur after initial instruction in use of a new method of brushing. The patient may have been over-zealous or may have misunderstood correct brush placement. Examination of a patient's gingiva within a few days to a week after instruction can be important.

A. Acute Alterations

Acute lesions are usually lacerations or ulcerations. The severity of the lesion may depend on the frequency and extent of brushing, as well as on the stiffness of the filaments and the force applied.

1. *Appearance*
   a. Scuffed epithelial surface with denuded underlying connective tissue.
   b. Punctate lesions that appear as red, pinpoint spots.
   c. Diffuse redness and denuded attached gingiva.
2. *Precipitating Factors*
   a. Horizontal or vertical scrub toothbrushing method.
   b. Excess pressure applied using firm palm grasp of handle.[20]
   c. Abrasive dentifrice used.[21]
   d. Overvigorous placement and application of the toothbrush.
   e. Penetration of gingiva by filament ends.
   f. Use of toothbrush with frayed, broken bristles or filaments.
   g. Application of filaments beyond attached gingiva.

B. Chronic Alterations

1. *Location*
   a. Usually appear only on the facial gingiva, because of the vigor with which toothbrush is used.
   b. Frequently, inversely related to the right- or left-handedness of the patient.
   c. Areas most often involved are around canines or teeth in labioversion or buccoversion.
2. *Recession*
   a. Margin of gingiva has receded toward the apex, and the cementum is exposed.
   b. Predisposing anatomic factors include a narrow band of attached gingiva and thin facial bone over teeth malposed in labioversion. Vigorous, pressured brushing, particularly when horizontal strokes are used, contributes to recession.
3. *Changes in Gingival Contour*
   a. Rolled, bulbous, hard, firm marginal gingiva, in "piled up" or festoon shape (pages 172, 176 and figure 11–9D).
   b. Gingival cleft, which is a narrow groove or slit that extends from the crest of the gingiva to the attached gingiva ("Stillman's Cleft," figure 11–10, pages 172 and 176).
4. *Precipitating Factors*
   a. Repeated use of a vigorous rotary, vertical, or horizontal toothbrushing method with an abrasive dentifrice.
   b. Use of a long, brisk stroke with excessive pressure, over a long period of time.
   c. Habitual prolonged brushing in one area.
   d. Excessive pressure applied with a worn, nonresilient brush.

C. Suggested Corrective Measures

1. Recommend use of a soft toothbrush with end-rounded filaments.
2. Correct the patient's toothbrushing technique; demonstrate a toothbrushing method better suited to the oral condition.
3. Temporary cessation of brushing the traumatized area may be needed. An antiplaque rinse may assist in the healing process.

II. Abrasion of the Teeth

Abrasion is the loss of tooth substance produced by mechanical wear other than that caused by mastication. Abrasion also may be defined as the pathologic wearing away of tooth substance through some abnormal mechanical process, in contrast with erosion that generally involves a chemical process.

A. Contributing Factors

1. Hard toothbrush with abrasive agent in the dentifrice.
2. Horizontal brushing.
3. Excessive pressure during brushing.
4. Prominence of the tooth surface labially or buccally.

B. Location of Abraded Areas

1. Primarily on facial surfaces, especially of canines, premolars, and sometimes first molars, or on any tooth in buccoversion or labioversion, those most available to the pressure of the toothbrush. The canines are susceptible because of their prominence on the curvature of the dental arches.
2. Most abraded areas are on the cervical areas of exposed root surfaces, but occasionally may occur on the enamel. When adjacent teeth are involved, the lesions appear in line with each other.

C. Appearance

Wedge-shaped indentations with smooth, shiny surfaces (figure 14–4, page 216).

D. Corrective Measures

1. Explain the problem to the patient to assure full cooperation.
2. Advise a specific brush with soft-textured filaments.
3. Change or correct the toothbrushing technique.
4. Recommend a less abrasive dentifrice.
5. Use a smaller amount of dentifrice.
   a. Start brushing in the area of the dentition where the most plaque and calculus are noted at a maintenance appointment.
   b. Avoid applying the dentifrice vigorously to the same tooth surfaces.[22]

CONTRAINDICATIONS FOR TOOTHBRUSHING

Even when an unusual oral condition develops, a patient must be encouraged to brush whenever possible to reduce the possibility of infection by decreasing the oral bacterial count. Prolonged omission of techniques of plaque removal is never indicated. Examples of conditions that may indicate a temporary departure from personal care routines follow.

I. Acute Oral Inflammatory or Traumatic Lesions

When an acute oral condition precludes normal brushing, the patient should be instructed to brush all areas of the mouth that are not affected and to resume regular plaque control measures on the affected area as soon as possible. When not otherwise contraindicated by instructions from the dentist, rinsing with a warm, mild saline solution can encourage healing and debris removal.

II. Following Periodontal Surgery

Patients must receive specific instructions concerning brushing temporarily while sutures and/or dressing are in place. Because direct, vigorous brushing of a periodontal dressing could cause its displacement, brushing of the occlusal surfaces and light strokes over the dressing may be advised. Other teeth and gingiva should be brushed as usual. Additional instructions appear in table 36–1, on pages 492–493.

III. Acute Stage of Necrotizing Ulcerative Gingivitis

A major contributing factor in the development of this disease is a lack of oral cleanliness. During the acute stage, the oral tissues are sensitive to any touch, and toothbrushing will be neglected. Instructions for these patients are on pages 484 and 485. A very soft brush is indicated along with careful brush placement to avoid trauma.

IV. Following Dental Extraction

Instructions may be found on page 592 and include brushing all teeth and gingiva except the surgical wound area. Teeth adjacent to the extraction site need cleaning as soon as possible to reduce bacterial collections and decrease the possibility of oral infection.

V. Following Dental Restorations

Patients tend to avoid brushing a new crown, newly placed fixed partial denture, or other appliance. Specific instructions should be given at the time of insertion.

CARE OF TOOTHBRUSHES

When discussing the type and features of the brush selected for an individual patient, the number of brushes needed and the frequency of replacement should be included. Perhaps the ideal time to teach cleaning and daily care of brushes would be after a practice session when the brush has to be washed and cleaned for storage at the dental office.

The condition of a brush depends on many factors, including the amount and manner of use, the type of care, and the quality of the brush at the start.

I. Supply of Brushes

A. Advise at least two brushes for home use and a third in a portable container for use at work, school, or travel.
B. Purchase of brushes should be staggered so that all brushes are not new at the same time and, more important, so that they are all not old at the same time, thereby resulting in less than optimum maintenance of the gingival condition.
C. Replace brushes before bristles or filaments become splayed, frayed, or lose resiliency. Worn brushes remove significantly less plaque than do new brushes.
D. No time limit can be specified for brush replacement. Duration of a brush depends on many factors, including frequency, method, and forces used.[7]

II. Cleaning Toothbrushes

A. Clean thoroughly after each use.
B. Hold brush head under strong stream of warm water from faucet to force particles, dentifrice, and bacteria from between the bristles.
C. Tap the handle on edge of sink to remove remaining particles.
D. Use another toothbrush to clean a brush: bristles or filaments can be worked between those of the other brush to remove resistant debris.
E. Rinse completely and tap out excess water.

III. Brush Storage

A. Keep brush in open air with head in an upright position, apart from contact with other brushes, particularly those of another person.

B. Portable brush container should have sufficient holes to give air temporarily until the brush can be completely exposed for drying. A closed container encourages bacterial growth.

References

1. Hirschfeld, I.: *The Toothbrush: Its Use and Abuse.* Brooklyn, N.Y., Dental Items of Interest Publishing Co., 1939, pp. 1–27.
2. Kimery, M.J. and Stallard, R.E.: The Evolutionary Development and Contemporary Utilization of Various Oral Hygiene Procedures, *Periodont. Abstr., 16,* 90, September, 1968.
3. McCauley, H.B.: Toothbrushes, Toothbrush Materials and Design, *J. Am. Dent. Assoc., 33,* 283, March 1, 1946.
4. Weinberger, B.W.: *An Introduction to the History of Dentistry.* St. Louis, The C.V. Mosby Co., 1948, pp. 43, 140–144.
5. American Academy of Periodontology, Committee Report: The Tooth Brush and Methods of Cleaning the Teeth, *Dent. Items Int., 42,* 193, March, 1920.
6. American Dental Association, Council on Dental Therapeutics: *Accepted Dental Therapeutics,* 40th ed. Chicago, American Dental Association, 1984, pp. 386–387.
7. Massassati, A. and Frank, R.M.: Scanning Electron Microscopy of Unused and Used Manual Toothbrushes, *J. Clin. Periodontol., 9,* 148, March, 1982.
8. Bass, C.C.: An Effective Method of Personal Oral Hygiene, *J. Louisiana State Med. Soc., 106,* 100, March, 1954.
9. Hard, D.: Oral Prophylaxis, in Bunting, R.W.: *Oral Hygiene,* 3rd ed. Philadelphia, Lea & Febiger, 1957, pp. 280–283.
10. Stillman, P.R.: A Philosophy of the Treatment of Periodontal Disease, *Dent. Dig., 38,* 315, September, 1932.
11. Hirschfeld: op. cit., p. 380.
12. Charters, W.J.: Immunizing Both Hard and Soft Mouth Tissue to Infection by Correct Stimulation with the Toothbrush, *J. Am. Dent. Assoc., 15,* 87, January, 1928.
13. Charters, W.J.: Home Care of the Mouth. I. Proper Home Care of the Mouth, *J. Periodontol., 19,* 136, October, 1948.
14. Fones, A.C., ed.: *Mouth Hygiene,* 4th ed. Philadelphia, Lea & Febiger, 1934, pp. 299–306.
15. Hirschfeld: op. cit., pp. 369–371.
16. Leonard, H.J.: Conservative Treatment of Periodontoclasia, *J. Am. Dent. Assoc., 26,* 1308, August, 1939.
17. Smith, T.S.: Anatomic and Physiologic Conditions Governing the Use of the Toothbrush, *J. Am. Dent. Assoc., 27,* 874, June, 1940.
18. Bell, D.G.: Home Care of the Mouth. III. Teaching Home Care to the Patient, *J. Periodontol., 19,* 140, October, 1948.
19. American Dental Association, Council on Dental Materials, Instruments, and Equipment: *Dentist's Desk Reference: Materials, Instruments and Equipment,* 2nd ed. Chicago, American Dental Association, 1983, pp. 14, 418.
20. Niemi, M.-L., Ainamo, J., and Etemadzadeh, H.: The Effect of Toothbrush Grip on Gingival Abrasion and Plaque Removal During Toothbrushing, *J. Clin. Periodontol., 14,* 19, January, 1987.
21. Niemi, M.-L., Sandholm, L., and Ainamo, J.: Frequency of Gingival Lesions After Standardized Brushing as Related to Stiffness of Toothbrush and Abrasiveness of Dentifrice, *J. Clin. Periodontol., 11,* 254, April, 1984.
22. Moore, W.F.: Oral Hygiene (Letter to Editor), *J. Am. Dent. Assoc., 101,* 896, December, 1980.

Suggested Readings

Ainamo, J.: Relative Roles of Toothbrushing, Sucrose Consumption and Fluorides in the Maintenance of Oral Health in Children, *Int. Dent. J., 30,* 54, March, 1980.

Bastiaan, R.J.: The Cleaning Efficiency of Different Toothbrushes in Children, *J. Clin. Periodontol., 13,* 837, October, 1986.

Bastiaan, R.J.: Comparison of the Clinical Effectiveness of a Single and a Double Headed Toothbrush, *J. Clin. Periodontol., 11,* 331, May, 1984.

Bergenholtz, A., Gustafsson, L.B., Segerlund, N., Hagberg, C., and

Östby, P.N.: Role of Brushing Technique and Toothbrush Design in Plaque Removal, *Scand. J. Dent. Res., 92,* 344, August, 1984.

Chong, M.P. and Beech, D.R.: Characteristics of Toothbrushes, *Aust. Dent. J., 28,* 202, August, 1983.

Frandsen, A.: Mechanical Oral Hygiene Practices. State-of-the-Science Review, in Löe, H. and Kleinman, D.V.: *Dental Plaque Control Measures and Oral Hygiene Practices.* Washington, D.C., IRL Press, 1986, pp. 93–97.

Glass, R.T. and Lare, M.M.: Toothbrush Contamination: A Potential Health Risk? *Quintessence Int., 17,* 39, January, 1986.

Glaze, P.M. and Wade, A.B.: Toothbrush Age and Wear As It Relates to Plaque Control, *J. Clin. Periodontol., 13,* 52, January, 1986.

Golding, P.S.: The Development of the Toothbrush. A Short History of Tooth Cleansing, Part 1. *Dent. Health (London), 21,* 25, Number 4, 1982.

Hawkins, B.F., Kohout, F.J., Lainson, P.A., and Heckert, A.: Duration of Toothbrushing for Effective Plaque Control, *Quintessence Int., 17,* 361, June, 1986.

Hills, J.M.: Evolution of the Omnii Cleaner, *Clin. Prevent. Dent., 5,* 8, January-February, 1983.

Honkala, E., Nyyssönen, V., Knuuttila, M., and Markkanen, H.: Effectiveness of Children's Habitual Toothbrushing, *J. Clin. Periodontol., 13,* 81, January, 1986.

Hyde, R.J., Feller, R.P., and Sharon, I.M.: Tongue Brushing, Dentifrice, and Age Effects on Taste and Smell, *J. Dent. Res., 60,* 1730, October, 1981.

Khoory, T.: The Use of Chewing Sticks in Preventive Oral Hygiene, *Clin. Prevent. Dent., 5,* 11, July-August, 1983.

Kreifeldt, J.G., Hill, P.H., and Calisti, L.J.P.: A Systematic Study of the Plaque Removal Efficiency of Worn Toothbrushes, *J. Dent. Res., 59,* 2047, December, 1980.

Lavstedt, S., Modeer, T., and Welander, E.: Plaque and Gingivitis in a Group of Swedish Schoolchildren with Special Reference to Toothbrushing Habits, *Acta Odontol. Scand., 40,* 307, Number 5, 1982.

MacGregor, I.D.M.: Toothbrushing Efficiency in Smokers and Nonsmokers, *J. Clin. Periodontol., 11,* 313, May, 1984.

Mueller, L.J., Darby, M.L., Allen, D.S., and Tolle, S.L.: Rotary Electric Toothbrushing. Clinical Effects on the Presence of Gingivitis and Supragingival Plaque, *Dent. Hyg., 61,* 546, December, 1987.

Nygaard-Østby, P., Edvardsen, S., and Spydevold, B.: Access to Interproximal Tooth Surfaces by Different Bristle Designs and Stiffnesses of Toothbrushes, *Scand. J. Dent. Res., 87,* 424, December, 1979.

Nyyssönen, V. and Honkala, E.: Toothbrushing Frequency in 4 Consecutive Studies of Finnish Adolescents, *J. Clin. Periodontol., 11,* 682, November, 1984.

Nyyssönen, V. and Honkala, E.: Oral Hygiene Status and Habitual Toothbrushing in Children, *ASDC J. Dent. Child., 51,* 285, July-August, 1984.

Park, K.K., Matis, B.A., and Christen, A.G.: Choosing an Effective Toothbrush. A Risky Venture, *Clin. Prevent. Dent., 7,* 5, July-August, 1985.

Schifter, C.C., Emling, R.C., Seibert, J.S., and Yankell, S.L.: A Comparison of Plaque Removal Effectiveness of an Electric Versus a Manual Toothbrush, *Clin. Prevent. Dent., 5,* 15, September-October, 1983.

Shory, N.L., Mitchell, G.E., and Jamison, H.C.: A Study of the Effectiveness of Two Types of Toothbrushes for Removal of Oral Accumulations, *J. Am. Dent. Assoc., 115,* 717, November, 1987.

Stean, H. and Forward, G.C.: Measurement of Plaque Growth Following Toothbrushing, *Community Dent. Oral Epidemiol., 8,* 420, December, 1980.

Van der Velden, U., Van Winkelhoff, A.J., Abbas, F., and DeGraaff, J.: The Habitat of Periodontopathic Micro-organisms, *J. Clin. Periodontol., 13,* 243, March, 1986.

Vogel, R.I., Alfano, M.J., and Manhold, J.H.: The Effect of Intrasulcular Brushing on Sulcular Epithelial Permeability, *J. Periodontol., 52,* 244, May, 1981.

Waerhaug, J.: Effect of Toothbrushing on Subgingival Plaque Formation, *J. Periodontol., 52,* 30, January, 1981.

Walsh, T.F. and Glenwright, H.D.: Relative Effectiveness of a Rotary and Conventional Toothbrush in Plaque Removal, *Community Dent. Oral Epidemiol., 12,* 160, June, 1984.

Wasserman, B.H.: A New Deep-grooved Design Toothbrush. A Clinical Evaluation, *Clin. Prevent. Dent., 7,* 7, March-April, 1985.

Zier, B.A. and Pimlott, J.F.L.: Mechanical Plaque Control: Are Concepts Changing? *Can. Dent. Hyg./Probe, 21,* 123, September, 1987.

Toothbrush and Restorations

Aker, D.A., Aker, J.R., and Sorensen, S.E.: Toothbrush Abrasion of Color-corrective Porcelain Stains Applied to Porcelain-fused-to-metal Restorations, *J. Prosthet. Dent., 44,* 161, August, 1980.

Aker, J.R.: New Composite Resins: Comparison of Their Resistance to Toothbrush Abrasion and Characteristics of Abraded Surfaces, *J. Am. Dent. Assoc., 105,* 633, October, 1982.

Bativala, F., Weiner, S., Berendsen, P., Vincent, G.R., Ianzano, J., and Harris, W.T.: The Microscopic Appearance and Effect of Toothbrushing on Extrinsically Stained Metal-Ceramic Restorations, *J. Prosthet. Dent., 57,* 47, January, 1987.

Van Dijken, J.W.V., Stadigh, J., and Meurman, J.H.: Appearance of Finished and Unfinished Composite Surfaces After Toothbrushing. A Scanning Electron Microscopy Study, *Acta Odontol. Scand., 41,* 377, Number 6, 1983.

Detrimental Effects

Axéll, T. and Koch, G.: Traumatic Ulcerative Gingival Lesion, *J. Clin. Periodontol., 9,* 178, May, 1982.

Blasberg, B., Jordon-Knox, A., and Conklin, R.J.: Gingival Ulceration Due to Improper Toothbrushing, *Can. Dent. Assoc. J., 47,* 462, July, 1981.

Carranza, F.A.: *Glickman's Clinical Periodontology,* 6th ed. Philadelphia, W.B. Saunders Co., 1984, pp. 422–423.

Gillette, W.B. and Van House, R.L.: Ill Effects of Improper Oral Hygiene Procedures, *J. Am. Dent. Assoc., 101,* 476, September, 1980.

Niemi, M.-L.: Gingival Abrasion and Plaque Removal After Toothbrushing With an Electric and a Manual Toothbrush, *Acta Odontol. Scand., 45,* 367, Number 5, 1987.

Niemi, M.-L., Ainamo, J., and Etemadzadeh, H.: Gingival Abrasion and Plaque Removal With Manual Versus Electric Toothbrushing, *J. Clin. Periodontol., 13,* 709, August, 1986.

Nordbø, H. and Skogedal, O.: The Rate of Cervical Abrasion in Dental Students, *Acta Odontol. Scand., 40,* 45, Number 1, 1982.

Sandholm, L., Niemi, M.-L., and Ainamo, J.: Identification of Soft Tissue Brushing Lesions. A Clinical and Scanning Electron Microscopic Study, *J. Clin. Periodontol., 9,* 397, September, 1982.

Smukler, H. and Landsberg, J.: The Toothbrush and Gingival Traumatic Injury, *J. Periodontol., 55,* 713, December, 1984.

23 *Auxiliary Plaque Control Measures*

Auxiliary measures are selected to complement toothbrushing. Because plaque on proximal tooth surfaces is not accessible to usual brushing, a means for proximal plaque removal is necessary for complete preventive care. Other objectives and uses are outlined as each auxiliary aid is described in this chapter. Following in Chapter 24, particular applications are given for care of teeth and tissues related to dental appliances. In Chapter 25, necessary adaptations are described for a mouth with complete rehabilitation and for dental implants.

When the bacterial plaque control and oral physical therapy regimen is outlined for an individual patient, the first consideration is given to the specific oral condition and how it can be improved or maintained in health. Next, one must consider which goals of oral health can be reached by the use of particular implements. For example, certain devices can be expected to remove plaque, whereas others do not remove plaque, but are efficient at removing debris, materia alba, and superficial layers of less tenaciously attached microorganisms over the surface of the plaque.

After matching the available devices with the goals for health of the individual's oral condition, teaching, learning, and time must be considered. The simplest possible procedures are selected for the patient's convenience and ease of learning, as well as for keeping the daily oral care regimen at a realistic level with respect to the time the patient is able and willing to spend.

INTERDENTAL PLAQUE CONTROL

Normally, the interdental gingiva fills the gingival embrasure between two teeth and beneath their contact area. Between posterior teeth are two papillae, one facial and one lingual, connected by a col, which is a depressed concave area (figure 11–5, page 169). Between anterior teeth in contact, is a single papilla with a pyramidal shape. The epithelium covering the col is thin and less resistant to disease. When inflammation is present in the papilla, the size of the papilla is enlarged and the col becomes deeper.

The interdental col area is generally inaccessible for toothbrushing. It is a protected area when the teeth are in normal position. Because of its shape, it harbors microorganisms. Most gingival disease starts in the interdental areas, and the incidence of gingivitis is highest in the interdental col gingiva.

When interdental papillae are reduced in height or are missing, the proximal tooth surfaces are exposed and the gingiva takes on a different shape, sometimes craterlike. Bacterial plaque collects on the tooth surfaces and retention of debris in the interproximal area can occur. Irregularities of tooth position, such as rotation or alterations related to malocclusion or tooth loss, contribute to alterations in the shape of the gingival embrasure and further complicate the plan for plaque control.

I. Objectives of Interdental Care

The interdental papillae may be missing or reduced in height because of (1) disease such as necrotizing ulcerative gingivitis, (2) surgical procedures essential in the treatment of periodontal infection, or (3) habitual pressure atrophy caused by the use of interdental tips or other devices that are contraindicated when interdental gingiva fill the embrasure. As a result of the exposure of the tooth surfaces, the changes in shape of the interdental tissue, and the general trapping of debris in the unnatural spaces, specific care is needed.

With the judicious use of the various methods and devices available, disease control of the interdental area can be accomplished by a motivated patient.

II. Role of Toothbrushing

Interproximal vibratory and sulcular brushing, such as the Charters, Stillman, and Bass techniques using a soft brush, can be successful to some degree in removing dental plaque from the proximal surfaces of the teeth. All the proximal plaque, however, cannot be removed by toothbrushing because the col and the tooth surface around the contact area are not accessible to the toothbrush.

For complete plaque and debris removal from proximal tooth surfaces, more than the toothbrush is needed. Various materials and devices are described in the sections following.

Removal of all calculus and smoothing of the tooth surface by root planing increase the effectiveness of devices. Rough tooth surfaces retain bacterial plaque, which initiates inflammation. Large deposits of calculus and overhanging restorations interfere with the use of devices; for example, dental floss catches and shreds when applied to overhanging margins of restorations or calculus deposits.

DENTAL FLOSS AND TAPE

When dental floss or tape is applied with firm pressure to a flat or convex proximal tooth surface, plaque can be removed. A concave tooth surface escapes contact with the floss. Figure 23–8A (page 322) illustrates this problem for the mesial of a maxillary first premolar.

When contact is inadequate and the patient indicates that floss or toothpicks are required to relieve pressure from impacted food, dental attention may be needed. The area should be charted or otherwise brought to the attention of the dentist.

I. Types of Floss

Research has shown no difference in the effectiveness of waxed or unwaxed floss for the removal of bacterial plaque.[1,2,3]

A. Unwaxed

Unwaxed floss is frequently recommended because it is thinner and slips through close contacts with ease.

B. Waxed

Waxed floss may be indicated, especially during the initial period of patient care before restorative work is completed and tooth surfaces are completely scaled and root planed, because the unwaxed floss shreds and tears more easily. The tearing may aggravate the patient and discourage continued use.

II. Procedure

For most patients dental floss is best used before toothbrushing to assure that caries-susceptible proximal surfaces will be de-plaqued and that the fluoride from the dentifrice used during brushing will be able to reach the proximal surfaces for caries prevention.

A. Floss Preparation

1. Hold a 12- to 15-inch length of floss with the thumb and index finger of each hand: grasp firmly with ½ inch of floss between the finger tips. The ends of the floss may be tucked into the palm and held by the ring and little finger, or the floss may be wrapped around the middle fingers (figure 23–1A, B, and C).
2. A circle of floss may be made by tying the ends together; the circle may be rotated as the floss is used (figure 23–2).

B. Application

1. *Maxillary Teeth.* Direct the floss up by holding the floss over two thumbs or a thumb and an index finger as shown in figure 23–1A and B. Rest a side of a finger on teeth of opposite side of the maxillary arch to provide balance and a fulcrum.
2. *Mandibular Teeth.* Direct the floss down by holding the two index fingers on top of the strand. One index finger holds the floss on the lingual and the other on the facial (figure 23–1C). The side of the finger on the lingual is held on the teeth of the opposite side of the mouth to serve as a fulcrum or rest.

C. Insertion

1. Hold floss in a diagonal or oblique position (figure 23–3).
2. Ease the floss past each contact area with a gentle sawing motion.
3. Control floss to prevent snapping through the contact area onto the gingival tissue.

D. Cleaning Stroke

1. Clean adjacent teeth separately: for the distal aspect curve the floss mesially, and for the mesial aspect curve the floss distally, around the tooth (figure 23–1E and F).
2. Pass the floss below the gingival margin, press to adapt the floss around the tooth, and slide up the tooth surface. Repeat.
3. Loop the floss over the distal of the most posterior teeth in each quadrant and the teeth next to edentulous areas (figure 23–1G). Hold firmly against the tooth and move the floss in both an up-and-down motion and a "shoeshine" stroke.

E. Additional Suggestions

1. When a dentifrice is used, dental tape may retain the dentifrice against the tooth better than floss.
2. Slide the floss to a new, unused portion for succeeding proximal tooth surfaces.
3. Floss may be doubled to provide a wider rubbing surface.

III. Precautions

A. Pressure in Col Area

The col area is not keratinized and is vulnerable to disease. Plaque control of the area is of great importance because most gingival and periodontal disease begins in the col area.

Too great a pressure with floss one or more times daily, particularly very fine floss that tends to cut more easily than thicker floss, can be destructive to the attachment. Excess pressure of the floss against the attachment is particularly significant in children, while teeth are in the process of eruption and the junctional epithelium is less firmly attached.

B. Prevention of Floss Cuts and Floss Clefts

1. *Location.* Floss cuts or clefts occur primarily on facial or lingual surfaces directly beside or in the middle of an interdental papilla. They appear as straight line cuts from the gingival margin toward the mucogingival junction (pages 172–173).
2. *Causes*
   a. Using too long a piece of floss between the fingers when held for insertion.

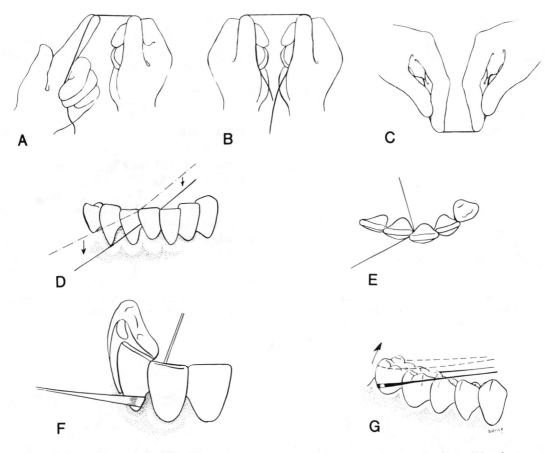

Figure 23–1. Use of Dental Floss. For maxillary insertion hold the floss between the thumb and index finger **(A)** or between thumbs **(B)**. Grasp the floss firmly. Allow ½- to 1-inch length between fingers. **C.** For the mandibular teeth, direct the floss down, guided by the index fingers. **D.** Work the floss slowly between the teeth in a short sawing motion. Avoid snapping through the contact area. **E.** Curve the floss around the tooth in a C-shape. Hold the floss toward the mesial for cleaning the distal surfaces and toward the distal for cleaning the mesial surfaces. **F.** Press the floss firmly against the tooth. Move gently beneath the gingiva until tissue resistance is felt. Slide the floss horizontally and vertically with pressure to remove bacterial plaque. **G.** Begin flossing with the distal of the most posterior tooth, and work systematically around the arch.

b. Snapping the floss through the contact area.

c. Not curving the floss about the teeth; floss held straight across the papilla.

d. Not using a rest to prevent undue pressure.

C. Aid for Flossing

A floss holder can be helpful for a person with a handicap or for a parent or attendant serving a child or patient. Floss holders are described on page 624.

TUFTED DENTAL FLOSS

I. Description

Tufted dental floss is also called a floss/yarn combination. Regular dental floss is alternated with a thickened tufted portion. Two variations are available commercially.

A. Single, Pre-cut Lengths

"Super Floss" is available in a 2-foot length composed of a 5-inch tufted portion adjacent to a 3-inch stiffened end for inserting under a fixed appliance or orthodontic attachment (figure 23–4A).

B. Roll

"NUFloss" is available in a roll that is similar to that of regular floss and has a cutting device to allow selection of a preferred length. The tufted portions (about 1 inch long) alternate with the plain floss (about 1½ inches long) (figure 23–4B).

II. Indications for Use

A. Plaque removal from tooth surfaces adjacent to wide embrasures where interdental papillae have been lost.

B. Plaque removal from mesial and distal abutments and under pontic of a fixed partial denture or orthodontic appliance. The stiff end of "Super Floss" is inserted; "NUFloss" is threaded using a floss threader (figure 24–10, page 342).

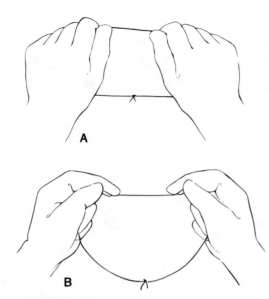

Figure 23–2. **Circle of Floss.** The ends of the floss are tied together for convenient holding. A child may be able to manage floss better with this technique. **A.** Floss held for maxillary teeth. **B.** Floss held for mandibular teeth.

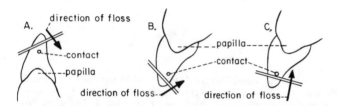

Figure 23–3. **Insertion of Floss.** Hold floss in a diagonal or oblique position over the teeth where the floss will be inserted. Arrows indicate the direction of movement of the floss. **A.** Floss held for mandibular insertion. **B.** Floss held for maxillary insertion. **C.** Floss held incorrectly. When floss is held horizontally, the possibility for damage to the papilla is greater.

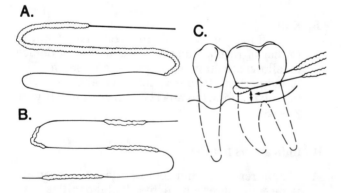

Figure 23–4. **Tufted Dental Floss.** The floss/yarn combination may be "Super Floss" **(A)** in a pre-cut length with a tufted portion and a 3-inch stiffened end for insertion under a fixed appliance, or "NUFloss" **(B)** with tufted portions alternated with plain floss. A preferred length of "NUFloss" is obtained from the container. **C.** "NUFloss" applied to the proximal surface of a molar. It may be used in an up-and-down and a shoe-shine stroke.

III. Technique

Curve floss and/or tufted portion around the tooth in a "C" to clean individual surfaces and remove bacterial plaque (figure 23–4C).

KNITTING YARN

I. Indications for Use

A. For tooth surfaces adjacent to wide proximal spaces, dental floss is too narrow and does not remove plaque efficiently.
B. For mesial and distal abutments of fixed partial dentures and under pontics, use a floss threader (pages 342–343).
C. For isolated teeth, teeth separated by a diastema, and distal surfaces of most posterior teeth.

II. Technique

A. Fold yarn double. Use about 8 inches of 3- or 4-ply smooth synthetic yarn. Loop through about

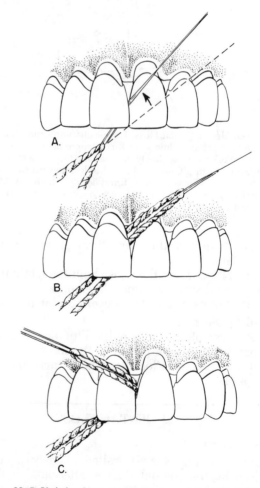

Figure 23–5. **Knitting Yarn. A.** Yarn is looped through dental floss, and the floss is drawn through the contact area in the usual manner, shown by the arrow. **B.** Yarn is drawn through the embrasure. **C.** Yarn is positioned against the surface of the tooth for plaque removal. When tooth contact is missing and space permits, the yarn is used without floss.

8 inches of dental floss; tie floss with 1 overhand knot.

B. Insert floss through the contact area. Draw the yarn into the embrasure (figure 23–5).
C. Clean adjacent teeth separately with a facial-lingual back-and-forth stroke. Hold the ends of the yarn distally and then around mesially.
D. For specific areas where a papilla may be high or access is not otherwise sufficient for the wide yarn, use the dental floss end of the combination.
E. Use dentifrice if desired.
F. For closed contacts, use a floss threader (figure 24–10, page 342).

GAUZE STRIP

I. Indications for Use

A. For proximal surfaces of widely spaced teeth. Gauze is too thick to pass through contact areas.
B. For surfaces of teeth next to edentulous areas.
C. For distal and mesial surfaces of abutment teeth.
D. For areas under posterior cantilevered section of a fixed appliance, such as the distal portion of a denture supported by implants (page 362).

II. Technique

A. Cut 1-inch gauze bandage into a 6- to 8-inch length and fold in thirds or down the center.
B. Position the fold of the gauze on the cervical area next to the gingival crest and work back and forth several times; hold ends toward distal to clean a mesial surface, and toward mesial to clean a distal surface (figure 23–6).

PIPE CLEANER

I. Indications for Use

A. For proximal surfaces when interdental gingiva is missing.
B. For furcation areas.

II. Technique

A. Use one third of a regular length pipe cleaner at a time. Check wire end to prevent damage to the gingiva or scratching of the cemental surface.
B. Carefully work the end of the cleaner through the space. Take care not to press wire end into the gingiva.
C. Work back and forth pressing toward one surface and then the other.
D. Slide pipe cleaner between exposed roots of a furcation. Work back and forth (figure 23–7).

TOOTHPICK IN HOLDER

I. Description

A round toothpick is inserted into a plastic handle with contra-angled ends for adaptation to the facial, lingual, or palatal surfaces.

II. Indications for Use

A. Patient with Periodontitis

For plaque removal at and just under the gingival margin, for interdental cleaning, particularly for concave proximal tooth surfaces (figure 23–8), and for exposed furcation area.

B. Orthodontic Patient

For plaque removal at gingival margin above appliance and for cleaning around fixed appliances (figure 24–3, page 339).

III. Technique

A. Prepare Instrument

1. Insert round tapered toothpick into the end of the holder. One type of holder has angulated ends for use in various positions.

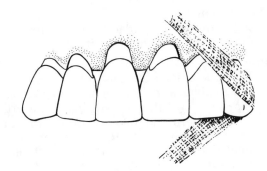

Figure 23–6. Gauze Strip. A 6- or 8-inch length of 1-inch bandage is folded in thirds and placed around a tooth adjacent to an edentulous area, a tooth with interdental spacing, or the distal of the most posterior tooth. A shoe-shine stroke is used to clean the bacterial plaque from the surface.

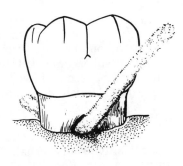

Figure 23–7. Pipe Cleaner. An exposed furcation area may be cleaned by inserting a pipe cleaner and moving it back and forth.

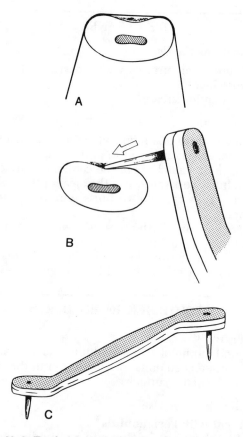

Figure 23–8. Toothpick in Holder. Cross section of the maxillary first premolar at the cementoenamel junction shows concave surface. **A.** Note inability of dental floss to remove bacterial plaque from the concavity. **B.** Toothpick in holder can be applied for plaque removal from facial and from lingual. **C.** Holder or handle for toothpick is angulated to accommodate toothpick directed from facial on the one end and from lingual on the other end.

2. Twist the toothpick firmly into place. Break off the long end cleanly so that sharp edges cannot scratch the inner cheek or the tongue during use.

B. Application

1. Apply toothpick at the gingival margin. At a right-angle application, with moderate pressure, trace the gingival margin around each tooth.
2. To remove plaque just below the gingival margin, apply the end at less than 45 degrees, maintain the tip on the tooth surface, and follow around the sulcus or pocket (figure 23–9).
3. Use a tip that has become frayed from use as a small cleaning "brush" to rub on tooth surfaces where plaque has collected. It should be checked for loose bits of wood that could become deposited in the sulcus or gingiva.
4. For hypersensitive spots, usually at the cervical third of a tooth, the patient can use the tip daily to massage dentifrice for densensitization (pages 499–500).

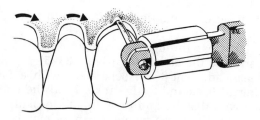

Figure 23–9. Toothpick in Holder for Bacterial Plaque at Gingival Margin. The tip is placed at or just below the gingival margin. Trace the margin around each tooth.

WOOD INTERDENTAL CLEANER

I. Description

The wood cleaner is a 2-inch-long device made of bass wood or birchwood. It is triangular in cross section as shown in figure 23–10.

II. Indications for Use

A. Application

For cleaning proximal tooth surfaces where the tooth surfaces are exposed and interdental gingiva missing. Space must be adequate; otherwise the gingival tissue can be traumatized.

B. Limitation

As with most interdental devices, the wood cleaner is advised only for the patient who will follow instructions carefully. A fresh cleaner may be advised for each arch or quadrant because the wood may become splayed.

III. Technique

A. Fulcrum (Rest)

First teach the patient to use a rest by placing the hand on the cheek or chin, or by placing a finger on the gingiva convenient to the place where the tip will be applied. This precaution will help to prevent inserting the wedge with too much pressure.

B. Preparation

Soften the wood by placing the pointed end in the mouth and moistening with saliva.

C. Procedure

1. Hold the base of the triangular wedge toward the gingival border of the interdental area and insert with the tip pointed slightly toward the occlusal or incisal to follow the contour of the embrasure (figure 23–10). When the wedge is held horizontally, the interdental tissue can be flattened.
2. Clean the tooth surfaces by moving the wedge in and out while applying a burnishing stroke with moderate pressure first to one side of the embrasure and then the other, about 4 strokes each.

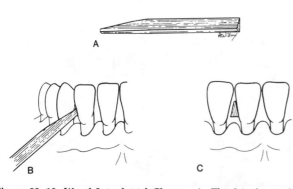

Figure 23–10. Wood Interdental Cleaner. A. The 2-inch wooden triangular cleaner. **B.** Application on proximal surface of a tooth with missing interdental papilla. The base of the triangle is on the gingival side. **C.** The side of the triangle is rubbed in and out against the proximal surface to remove bacterial plaque.

   3. Discard the cleaner as soon as the first signs of splaying are evident.

INTERDENTAL BRUSHES

I. Types

A. Small Insert Brushes with Reusable Handle
   1. Soft nylon filaments are twisted into a fine stainless steel wire for insertion into a handle with an angulated shank (figure 23–11D).
   2. The small tapered or cylindric brush heads are of varying sizes approximately 12 to 15 mm. (½ inch) in length, with a diameter of 3 to 5 mm. (⅛ to ¼ inch).

B. Brush with Wire Handle
   1. Soft nylon filaments are twisted into a fine stainless steel wire. The wire is continuous with the handle, which is approximately 35 to 45 mm. (1½ to 1¾ inches) in length (figure 23–11C).
   2. The filaments form a narrow brush approximately 30 to 35 mm. (1¼ to 1½ inches) in length and 5 to 8 mm. (¼ to ⁵⁄₁₆ inches) in diameter.

II. Indications for Use

A. For open interdental areas.
B. For exposed bifurcations or trifurcations.
C. For plaque removal to supplement toothbrushing.

III. Technique

A. Select brush of appropriate diameter.
B. Moisten the brush and insert into interdental area or furcation at an angle in keeping with gingival form; brush in and out.

IV. Care of Brushes

A. Clean brush during use to remove debris and plaque by holding under actively running water.
B. Clean thoroughly after use and dry in open air.

C. Discard when filaments become loose or deformed.

SINGLE-TUFT BRUSH (END-TUFT, UNITUFT)

I. Description

   The single tuft, or group of small tufts, may be from 3 to 6 mm. in diameter and may be flat or tapered (figure 23–11A and B). The handle may be straight or contra-angled.

II. Indications for Use

A. For Open Interproximal Areas

B. For Fixed Dental Appliances
   The single-tuft brush may be adaptable around and under a fixed partial denture, pontic, orthodontic appliance, precision attachment, and implant abutment.

C. For Difficult-to-Reach Areas
   The lingual surfaces of the mandibular molars, abutment teeth, the distals of the most posterior teeth, and teeth that are crowded are examples of areas where an end-tuft brush may prove of value. The shank may be bent for easy adaptation to lingual surfaces (figure 24–8, page 341).

III. Technique

A. Direct the end of the tuft into the interproximal area along the gingival margin.
B. Combine a rotating motion with intermittent pressure.
C. Use a sulcular brushing stroke.

INTERDENTAL TIP

I. Composition and Design

   Conical or pyramidal flexible rubber or plastic tip is attached to the end of the handle of a toothbrush, or is on a special plastic handle. The soft, pliable rubber tip is preferred because it can be adapted to the interdental area more easily than can the hard, more rigid plastic tip.

II. Indications for Use

A. For cleaning debris and materia alba from the interdental area and for removal of bacterial plaque by rubbing the exposed tooth surfaces.
B. For adaptation to areas where toothbrushing is difficult, for example, exposed furcation areas, mesial of mesially inclined teeth, or concave surfaces, such as shown in figure 23–8.
C. Contraindicated for clinically healthy gingiva with intact interdental papillae.

III. Technique

A. Trace along the gingival margin with the tip positioned just beneath the margin. The adaptation is similar to the toothpick in holder (figure 23–9).

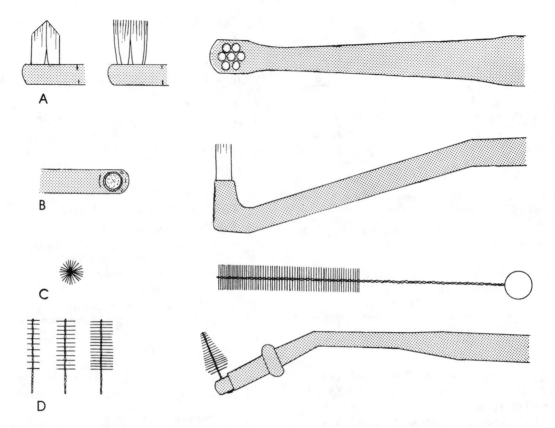

Figure 23–11. Single-tuft and Interdental Brushes. A. Single-tuft brush with tapered and flat groups of filaments. **B.** Single-tuft brush on handle with angulated shank. **C.** Interdental brush with filaments twisted into a fine wire that ends in a handle. **D.** Insert brushes for a reusable handle with an angulated shank.

B. For additional cleaning of the proximal surfaces of the teeth, rub the tip against the teeth as it is moved in and out of an embrasure and under a contact area.

C. Rinse the tip as indicated during use to remove debris, and wash thoroughly at the finish.

ORAL IRRIGATION

The use of a forced intermittent or steady stream of water in oral physical therapy is sometimes called hydrotherapy. The use of oral irrigation (a form of hydrotherapy) has proved to be a useful adjunct to toothbrushing but must not be considered a substitute for brushing or other plaque removal devices because it is not effective in the complete removal of bacterial plaque.

Oral irrigating devices are evaluated by the American Dental Association, Council on Dental Materials, Instruments and Equipment. They are classified as acceptable, provisionally acceptable, or unacceptable (page 331 and figure 23–15).[4]

I. Objectives

A water irrigation device has been shown to be a useful adjunct for maintaining the health and cleanliness of the oral cavity. Benefits that may be derived from the use of irrigation include the following:

A. Removal of Debris

Effective removal of unattached debris from about the teeth and interdental areas for oral sanitation. Attached deposits (bacterial plaque or calculus) are not removed.

B. Removal of Bacteria

Reduction in numbers of microorganisms.

C. Reduction of Unattached Plaque

Reduction in plaque accumulation as the result of removal of loosely adherent supragingival plaque.[5,6]

D. Delivery of Chemical Plaque Control Agents

When a dilute antiplaque agent used in place of water in an irrigator is to be recommended for daily use by a patient, specific instructions for proper dilution, frequency of use, and position of the delivery tip will be needed. Usually, minimal water pressure is indicated.

1. *Penetration into Pocket.* A chemical agent must contact the microorganisms directly to be effective. Supragingival irrigation has limited clinical effect on the subgingival microorganisms. Studies have shown that supragingival irrigation can deliver an aqueous solution into pockets, but the depth of penetration varies.[7,8]

Aiming the solution at a 45-degree angle toward the sulcus did not improve penetration over the recommended angulation perpendicular to the long axis of the tooth.[8] When a blunted hypodermic needle was used to apply the irrigating solution below the gingival margin, disclosing agent showed that the penetration to the apex was more frequent.[7,9]

2. *Agents Used.* Chemicals that have been researched for use in an irrigator include weak solutions of stannous fluoride,[10] chlorhexidine gluconate,[11,12,13,14] metronidazole,[13,14] and sanguinaria.[15,16]

A specially designed tip for the home-use irrigator has been studied for daily subgingival insertion by a patient.[17,18] Carefully supervised instruction is needed.

II. Types and Description of Irrigators

A. Sources of Action

1. *Power-driven.* Power-driven pump unit that generates an intermittent or pulsating jet of water.
    a. Adjustable dial to regulate water pressure and a reservoir to maintain a steady flow.
    b. Hand-held, interchangeable, adjustable tip that can be turned a complete 360 degrees for application at various angulations.
2. *Water Faucet Attachment.* Single-line type that attaches directly to the water faucet.
    a. Delivers a continuous stream of water that is adjustable by varying the line pressure.
    b. Hand-held interchangeable tip that rotates a complete 360 degrees for application to all areas.

B. Delivery Tips (figure 23–12)

1. Monojet (single stream)
2. Fractionated Microjet (7 streams)

III. Technique and Operational Factors

A. Instruction of Patient

1. Debris can be removed by irrigation, thus leaving tooth surfaces available for plaque removal and for exposure to fluoride from the dentifrice.
2. Precaution: Because water irrigation tends to impart a feeling of oral cleanliness, the patient may not realize the need for complete plaque removal and may neglect toothbrushing or other necessary procedures.

B. Procedure

The user turns on and adjusts the water jet stream, leans over the washbowl, and directs the tip toward an interproximal area in a horizontal direction perpendicular to the long axis of the tooth. The stream should not be directed into the sulcus or pocket (figure 23–13).

C. Operational Factors

1. *Limit Water Pressure.* Pressure need only be great enough to flush out interdental areas. Avoid high pressures.

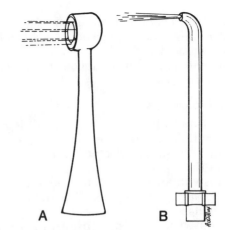

Figure 23–12. Irrigator Delivery Tips. A. Fractionated microjet tip with seven streams. **B.** Monojet tip (single stream).

2. *Undesirable Effects.* Application to a single area should be limited in duration to prevent adverse effects. Periodontal abscess formation from water forced below the attachment level is possible. Particles and bacteria from the sulcus and pocket may be forced into the subepithelial tissue.[19]

IV. Indications

Use of daily irrigation with an antiplaque agent may prove especially helpful in controlling bacterial infection in periodontal pockets for such patients as those unable to receive conventional therapy and those with periodontal conditions not satisfactorily controlled by routine nonsurgical periodontal therapy. As an adjunct to treatment, benefit can be realized during the maintenance phase, especially for patients with refractory periodontal disease.

Without an antiplaque agent, the cleansing effects of water irrigation can be beneficial for patients with conditions that increase the potential for retention of debris and bacteria, including the following:

A. Missing or reduced interdental papillae.
B. Fixed orthodontic appliances.

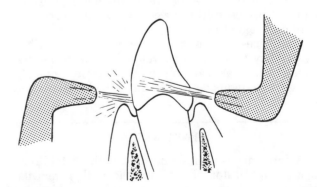

Figure 23–13. Water Irrigator. Monojet delivery tip used in horizontal direction through interproximal area. When tip is directed toward a pocket or sulcus, only low pressures must be used. High irrigation pressure may force microorganisms into the gingival tissues, thus creating bacteremias.

C. Restorative rehabilitative appliances: fixed partial dentures, splints, precision attachments, implant abutments.

D. Intermaxillary fixation for reconstructive surgery or fractured jaws.[20]

V. Contraindications

A. Patients at risk for infective endocarditis who require antibiotic premedication (pages 85, 91) should not use an irrigator because bacteremia can result.[21,22]

B. Patients with deep periodontal pockets or tissue flaps covering unerupted or partially erupted third molars.

C. Patients with acute conditions, for example, necrotizing ulcerative gingivitis or periodontal abscess.

D. Patients with clinically healthy gingiva, with minimum or normal sulcus depths and no bleeding on probing, and who are capable of doing satisfactory plaque removal and cleaning with a toothbrush and dental floss. The patient who does not need an irrigating device for a particular reason should not be encouraged to purchase and use one. Constant pressure of the water stream over an interdental papilla and col area may reduce the height of the papilla.

CHEMICAL PLAQUE REMOVAL

The first part of this chapter described various methods to supplement toothbrushing in the *mechanical* removal of bacterial plaque. The objective in mechanical removal is the physical clearing away of microorganisms and their pathogenic products to prevent or treat dental and periodontal infections.

Chemical plaque removal agents are intended to eliminate, reduce, or alter plaque so that it is no longer pathogenic to the teeth or soft tissues. Most chemical agents for patient use have been made available through dentifrice or mouthrinse. The irrigator, described in the previous section of this chapter, is a mechanical device, but because chemical agents can be applied during irrigation, it may serve as a combined agent in disease control.

Dentifrices and mouthrinses will be described next. They have purposes related to cleansing and tissue healing after treatment, and they may contain active ingredients for dental and periodontal disease control.

DENTIFRICES

A dentifrice is a substance used with a toothbrush or other applicator for removing bacterial plaque, materia alba, and debris from the gingiva and teeth for cosmetic and sanitary purposes, and for applying specific agents to the tooth surfaces for preventive and/or therapeutic purposes. As a result of research, the dentist and dental hygienist can apply current knowledge to aid the patient in the selection of an appropriate dentifrice that will benefit the teeth and gingiva and help to maintain them in a healthy state.

I. Basic Components[23,24]

Powder dentifrices contain abrasives, detergents, flavoring, and sweetener. Paste dentifrices contain the same ingredients plus binders, humectants, preservative, and water. Either may have a coloring agent. The range of content of the various ingredients in commercially available dentifrices is as follows:

Detergent	1–2%
Cleaning and Polish Agents	25–60%
Binder (thickener)	1–2%
Humectant	20–40%
Flavoring	1–1.5%
Water	15–50%
Therapeutic Agent	1–2%
Preservative, Sweetener, and Coloring Agent	2–3%

A therapeutic dentifrice has a drug or chemical agent added for a specific preventive or treatment action. In manufacturing products, a major problem is to combine agents that are compatible with each other.

A. Detergents (Foaming Agents or Surfactants)

1. *Purposes.* To lower surface tension, penetrate and loosen surface deposits and stains, emulsify debris for easy removal by the toothbrush, and contribute to the foaming action, which many people like.

2. *Criteria for Use.* Nontoxic, neutral in reaction, active in acid or alkaline media, stable, compatible with other dentifrice ingredients, no distinctive flavor, and foaming characteristics.

3. *Substances Used.* Synthetic detergents

   Sodium lauryl sulfate USP
   Sodium n-lauryl sarcosinate
   Sodium cocomonoglyceride sulfonate

B. Cleaning and Polishing Agents

A dentifrice may have a combination of agents in an *abrasive system* to accommodate both cleaning and polishing objectives.

1. *Purposes.* An abrasive to clean, and a polishing agent to produce a smooth, shiny tooth surface that will resist discoloration and bacterial accumulation and retention.

2. *Criteria for Use.* The ideal abrasive cleans well with no damage to the tooth surface and provides a high polish that can prevent or delay the reaccumulation of stains and deposits.

3. *Abrasives Used*

   Calcium carbonate
   Calcium pyrophosphate
   Dicalcium phosphate, dihydrate
   Dicalcium phosphate, anhydrous
   Insoluble sodium metaphosphate (IMP)
   Hydrated aluminum oxide
   Silica, silicates, and dehydrated silica gels

For gel dentifrices:[23]
    Synthetic amorphous silica zerogel
    Synthetic amorphous complex aluminosilicate salt

C. Binders (Thickeners)

1. *Purpose.* To prevent separation of the solid and liquid ingredients during storage.
2. *Criteria.* Stable, nontoxic, compatible with other ingredients.
3. *Types Used.* Organic hydrophilic colloids

    Alginates
    Synthetic derivatives of cellulose

Organic colloids require a preservative to prevent microbial growth.

D. Humectants

1. *Purposes.* To retain moisture and prevent hardening on exposure to air.
2. *Criteria.* Stable, nontoxic.
3. *Substances Used*

    Glycerin
    Sorbitol
    Propylene glycol

These agents require a preservative to prevent microbial growth.

E. Preservatives

1. *Purpose.* To prevent bacterial growth.
2. *Criterion.* Compatible with other ingredients.
3. *Substances Used*

    Alcohols
    Benzoates
    Formaldehyde
    Dichlorinated phenols

F. Sweetening Agents

1. *Purpose.* To impart a pleasant flavor.
2. *Criterion.* Must be nonfermentable sugar.
3. *Substances Used*

    Artificial non-cariogenic sweetener
    Sorbitol and glycerin, used as humectants, contribute to sweet flavor

G. Flavoring Agents

1. *Purposes.* To make the dentifrice desirable; to mask other ingredients that may have a less pleasant flavor.
2. *Criteria.* Remain unchanged during manufacturing and storage; compatible with other ingredients.
3. *Substances Used*

    Essential oils (peppermint, cinnamon, wintergreen, clove)
    Menthol
    Artificial non-cariogenic sweetener

H. Coloring Agents

1. *Purpose.* Attractiveness.
2. *Criteria.* Does not stain teeth or discolor other oral tissues.
3. *Types.* Vegetable dyes.

II. Prophylactic or Therapeutic Dentifrices

The American Dental Association, Council on Dental Therapeutics evaluates only those dentifrices that claim therapeutic value. Categories of acceptance are described on page 331.

Over the years, research on chlorophyll dentifrices, ammoniated dentifrices, dentifrices containing such enzyme inhibitors as sodium n-lauryl sarcosinate and sodium dehydroacetate, and antibiotics, such as penicillin and tyrothricin, contributed to the search for a major break into dental caries prevention. Research has shown that fluoride dentifrices contribute the greatest benefits at the present time.

Problems with dentifrice formulation have been related to finding compatible constituents to be combined with the active ingredient in the dentifrice formula.

III. Dentifrice Selection

The dentifrice that has been used by a patient should be recorded with other information about self-care habits when the dental history is prepared. Later the dentifrice must be evaluated and a change recommended when necessary in accord with the individual oral condition and treatment objectives.

There are specific reasons for recommending the use of particular dentifrices and for discouraging the use of others. The patient looks to the dentist and dental hygienist for professional advice in keeping with current research. The factors described below should be considered in dentifrice selection.

A. Dental Caries Control; Remineralization

The use of a fluoride-containing dentifrice is generally recommended for all age groups and is mandatory for children and caries-prone adults. Fluoride for prevention of root caries is necessary after gingival recession and root exposure after periodontal therapy.

Fluoride dentifrices are described on page 409.

B. Gingival Health

The health of the gingival tissue and the prevention of periodontal infections are prime objectives when using a toothbrush and auxiliary aids for bacterial plaque removal from proximal tooth surfaces. A dentifrice can assist in plaque removal. With the addition of a chemotherapeutic agent, the dentifrice can provide the medium for application of the agent to the teeth and gingiva. Agents that may destroy or inhibit the growth of microorganisms in plaque have been researched extensively. Selected references are provided in the *Suggested Readings* at the end of the chapter.

C. Abrasiveness

The degree of abrasiveness of a dentifrice is influenced by several factors, including dentifrice concentration, hardness of toothbrush used, and brushing force or pressure. The greater the dilution of the abrasive agent, the less abrasive the preparation. The harder the toothbrush, the more abrasion of tooth structure. The more force used with a brush, the greater abrasiveness of the agent. Even the temperature can alter the abrasive effect because the toothbrush filaments are softer in a warmer environment. Ranking of dentifrices by their abrasiveness should be relative and subject to several variables.[25,26]

Reference tables for the comparative abrasiveness of commercial dentifrices to dentin and enamel are available.[23,27,28] Dentifrice abrasion is described on page 313.

A patient with exposed cementum or dentin must be advised to use an exceptionally mild abrasive dentifrice.

D. Desensitization

Dentifrices designated specifically for desensitization are within the scope of the acceptance program of the Council on Dental Therapeutics. Potassium nitrate, strontium chloride, and sodium citrate have been shown to be effective agents. Desensitizing effects of fluoride preparations also have been demonstrated (page 500).

Because most tooth sensitivity is related to areas of exposed dentin and cementum, careful attention must be paid to the abrasiveness of a dentifrice with desensitizing claims.

MOUTHRINSES

Mouthrinses may be classified as cosmetic or therapeutic. When claims for therapeutic value have not been scientifically substantiated, the repeated use of a product may be harmful.

Mouthrinses that claim no therapeutic or disease preventive value are not included in the acceptance program of the American Dental Association, Council on Dental Therapeutics. At present, the routine unsupervised use of medicated mouthrinses by the public cannot be considered appropriate. Several fluoride solutions have been accepted as effective agents for use as mouthrinses for reducing the incidence of dental caries.[29]

When recording information about the oral health practices of a patient as part of the medical and dental history, one should determine whether a particular mouthrinse is used, the frequency of use, and what the patient believes to be the benefit from its use. If any detrimental effects are suspected after the oral examination, or if adverse effects are known to be possible, the patient can be informed and alternate procedures for rinsing can be recommended.

I. Purposes and Uses

A. Dental Office or Clinic

1. Preoperative rinse to reduce microorganisms, thereby providing a more septic working field.[30–32]
2. Preoperative rinse to reduce aerosol contamination during use of handpiece and ultrasonic scaler (pages 56, 467).
3. To facilitate impression procedures (page 152).
4. To rinse and refresh the mouth during film placement for radiography and following a dental or dental hygiene procedure.

B. Patient at Home

1. *Mouth Cleaning.* Vigorous rinsing to dislodge food debris contributes to general oral cleanliness. Rinsing with clear water after meals and after snacks, particularly sweet snacks, has been suggested when toothbrushing and interdental cleaning are not possible.

   The limitations of rinsing for cleansing should be understood: although rinsing aids in the removal of gross debris and unattached surface microorganisms, attached plaque is not disturbed.
2. *Postsurgical Care*
   a. After oral surgery as directed (page 592).
   b. After periodontal surgery (page 493).
   c. Antiplaque rinse to promote healing when tissues are not ready for routine brushing. Chlorhexidine use is described on pages 330–331.
3. *After Nonsurgical Periodontal Therapy* (page 538). A saline rinse can promote healing of the gingival tissues, and a fluoride rinse can benefit the exposed root planed surfaces for dental caries prevention.
4. *Treatment.* During pathologic conditions, for example, necrotizing ulcerative gingivitis, to remove debris, encourage healing, and soothe tender gingiva (page 484).
5. *Dental Caries Prevention.* The use of fluoride mouthrinses for dental caries control is included in the chapter on fluoride application (pages 408–409).
6. *Cosmetic Purposes.* Advertising claims can be misleading, and patients need assistance in interpreting what they read and hear. Without advice, people may select a mouthrinse on the basis of advertising promises or flavor. Purposes and effects that may be expected from the use of a cosmetic mouthrinse are:
   a. Removes loose debris when rinsing is vigorous.
   b. Gives temporary benefit through mechanical reduction in numbers of oral microorganisms.
   c. Imparts a pleasant taste, odor, and stimulating sensation to the oral cavity.
   d. Contributes to a temporary suppression of halitosis when causes are local.

II. Procedure for Rinsing

Many patients, particularly children, should be shown very specifically how to rinse, and the method should be practiced under supervision. Uninstructed patients may hold water in their mouths and bow the head from side to side, or perform some other action that cannot force the water about and between the teeth.

A. A small amount of fluid is taken into the mouth; lips are closed.

B. With the teeth kept slightly apart, the fluid is forced through the interdental areas with as much pressure as possible to loosen debris.

C. A combination of lip, tongue, and cheek action is used as the fluid is forced back and forth between the teeth while the cheeks are ballooned and sucked in alternately.

D. The mouth is divided into three sections, and the rinsing should be concentrated on first the anterior, then on one side followed by the other.

E. Expectorate or swallow.

III. Self-prepared Mouthrinses

Plain water, saline solutions, or solutions of bicarbonate of soda may be considered the most practical mouthrinses from the point of view of availability, cost, and effectiveness for debris removal and general oral cleanliness. Frequently prescribed or recommended by dentists, they may be helpful in postoperative care following dental and dental hygiene procedures.

When a salt solution is of greater strength than the physiologic salt solution concentration of body cells, fluid is drawn out of the cells by osmotic force to balance the pressure. This action may produce a reduction of edema and related benefits. The patient history must be checked, as a patient on a low-salt or sodium-free diet should not use a saline rinse.

A. Water

B. Isotonic Sodium Chloride Solution

1. Isotonic is normal or physiologic salt solution, which is 0.9% aqueous solution; same concentration as cellular fluids.

2. Preparation (household measurements): level ½ teaspoonful salt added to 1 cup (8 ounces) of warm water.

C. Hypertonic Sodium Chloride Solution

1. A salt solution that has an osmotic pressure greater than that of physiologic salt solution is hypertonic.

2. Preparation (household measurements): ½ teaspoonful salt added to ½ cup (4 ounces) of warm water.

D. Sodium Bicarbonate Solution

Level ½ teaspoonful "soda" added to 1 cup (8 ounces) of warm water.

E. Sodium Chloride—Sodium Bicarbonate Solution (flavored)

Sodium chloride	2.0 g. (½ teaspoonful)
Sodium bicarbonate	1.0 g. (¼ teaspoonful)
Amaranth solution	2.0 ml. (½ teaspoonful)
Peppermint water to make	240.0 ml. (8-ounce glass)

IV. Commercial Mouthrinse Ingredients[23]

Basic ingredients for both cosmetic and therapeutic oral rinses include water, alcohol, flavoring oils, and coloring materials.

A. Water

Makes up the largest percent by volume.

B. Alcohol

Ethyl alcohol is used to increase the solubility of the essential oils. The concentration may be as much as 15 to 30 percent. Alcohol lowers surface tension and is mildly astringent.

C. Flavoring

Essential oils and their derivatives (eucalyptus oil, oil of wintergreen) or aromatic waters (peppermint, spearmint, wintergreen, or others).

D. Coloring

Must not discolor oral tissues.

E. Sweetening Agent

Artificial non-cariogenic sweetener.

V. Active Ingredients

Commercial mouthrinses generally contain more than one active ingredient and, therefore, may advertise more than one claim for usefulness. Several factors influence how effective an agent may be, including the dilution by the saliva, the length of time the agent may be in contact with the tissue or bacteria, and the effect that contact with the organic matter of the mouth may have in changing the action. Agents and products listed below are for information only and should not be considered recommendations.

A. Antimicrobial Agents

1. *Purposes*
   a. Reduce the oral microbacterial count.
   b. Inhibit bacterial activity.

2. *Limitations of Agents to Use.* Many have disagreeable flavors or high cost, or their activity decreases when contact is made with organic matter in the mouth.

3. *Active Ingredients*

   Povidone-iodine
   Phenolic compounds
   Hexylresorcinol, thymol, and other phenol derivatives
   Quaternary ammonium compounds
      Benzethonium chloride
      Cetylpyridinium chloride
   Boric and benzoic acid

Chlorine-liberating compounds
Hexetidine

B. Oxygenating Agents[33,34]

1. *Purposes*
   a. Cleansing: The effervescence makes these agents effective in debridement.
   b. Antimicrobial: Action is limited; the agent is effective only as long as oxygen is being released.
2. *Uses.* Particularly in the treatment of necrotizing ulcerative gingivitis.
3. *Active Ingredients*

   Hydrogen peroxide (hydrogen peroxide USP diluted with water)
   Sodium perborate
   Urea peroxide

4. *Precaution.* Continued use of hydrogen peroxide solution, as well as of most other oxygen-liberating drugs after the treatment of a disease, can lead to sponginess of the gingiva, formation of black hairy tongue, hypersensitivity of exposed root surfaces, and, because an acid is produced when water is added, demineralization of tooth surfaces.

C. Astringents

1. *Purpose.* Shrink tissues.
2. *Use.* During impression making.
3. *Active Ingredients*

   Zinc chloride
   Zinc acetate
   Alum
   Tannic, acetic, and citric acids

4. *Precaution.* The agents are acid in water solution and can cause tooth demineralization and tissue irritation with repeated use.

D. Anodynes

1. *Purposes.* Alleviate pain, soothe sore spots.
2. *Uses.* Temporary pain relief for lesions of mucous membranes; during radiographic film exposure; aid in impression making.
3. *Active Ingredients*

   Phenol derivatives
   Essential oils

E. Buffering Agents

1. *Purpose and Uses.* Reduce oral acidity created by the fermentation of food debris; dissolve mucinous films; give relief for soreness of soft tissues.
2. *Active Ingredients*

   Sodium borate solution NF
   Sodium perborate NF
   Sodium bicarbonate USP

F. Deodorizing Agents

1. *Purpose.* Neutralize odors from decomposed oral debris.

2. *Use.* Lessen possibility of halitosis from local causes.
3. *Active Ingredients*

   Chlorophyll and other deodorizing agents

VI. Preventive and Therapeutic Agents

A. Fluorides

Fluoride rinses are described in Chapter 29, pages 408–409. Sodium fluoride is effective in the prevention of dental caries when used daily at 0.05% solution or weekly at 0.2% solution.

B. Plaque and Gingivitis Prevention

Suggested requirements for an effective chemotherapeutic agent include at least the following:[35]

1. *Nontoxic.* The agent should not damage oral tissues or create systemic disturbances.
2. *No or Limited Absorption.* The agent should not be absorbed through the membranes of the gastrointestinal tract. The action should be confined to bacterial plaque.
3. *Substantivity.* Substantivity means the ability of an agent to be bound to the pellicle and tooth surface and to be released over an extended period of time with retention of potency. With time, the bacterial succession and, ultimately, disease are altered.
4. *Bacterial Specificity.* The agent may have a broad antimicrobial spectrum, but it should have specificity for the organisms most pathogenic for a given infection. The agent may act directly on the organism, may interfere with bacterial attachment, may act on the plaque matrix, or may alter the tooth surface.
5. *Low Induced Drug Resistance.* Long-range effectiveness is lost when a drug induces resistance of microorganisms.

C. Chlorhexidine

Chlorhexidine has been tested extensively and has been shown to be the most effective antiplaque and antigingivitis chemotherapeutic agent available.

1. *Preparations*
   a. 0.2% Chlorhexidine gluconate: Early studies showed that twice-daily use of 0.2% rinse prevented bacterial plaque accumulation and gingivitis.[36] The 0.2% solution has been used extensively throughout the world except in the United States.
   b. 0.12% Chlorhexidine gluconate: The 0.12% solution has approval in the United States. Research has shown that the clinical effects of 0.12% mouthrinse compare favorably with those of the 0.2% mouthrinse.[37]
2. *Mechanism of Action*
   a. Bactericidal: Chlorhexidine is active against a wide range of gram-positive and gram-negative organisms and fungi.

b. Substantivity: Chlorhexidine is rapidly adsorbed to teeth and pellicle and is released slowly, thus prolonging the bactericidal effect.

3. *Clinical Uses.* No chemotherapeutic agent is intended to substitute for mechanical plaque removal on a daily basis as the most effective disease-preventive method.

    a. Decrease supragingival bacterial plaque formation and inhibit development of gingivitis.

    b. Use for short-term adjunctive therapy following surgical treatment that limits the amount of mechanical plaque removal because of healing tissue, dressings, or accessibility.

    c. Use for selected patients to control inflammation in necrotizing ulcerative gingivitis and to encourage and motivate when oral hygiene has been neglected for a period of time.

    d. Suppress *Streptococcus mutans;* prevent smooth surface dental caries.[38]

4. *Side Effects.* Brown staining of teeth has been the most generalized side effect. Certain patients, however, also manifest one or more of the following conditions.

    a. Temporary loss of taste.

    b. Discomfort from the bitter taste of the mouthrinse. Masking with a flavoring agent has been customary with more recent commercial products.

    c. Burning sensations of the mucosa.

    d. Dryness and soreness of the mucosa.

    e. Epithelial desquamation.

    f. Discoloration of the teeth, tongue, and restorations.

    g. Slight increase in supragingival calculus formation related to the dead bacteria that remain as a result of the bactericidal action of the chlorhexidine. The dead bacteria are trapped in the usual calculus formation process.

AMERICAN DENTAL ASSOCIATION EVALUATION PROGRAMS

The purposes of the programs for approval of products are to determine the safety and effectiveness of a product or device, to review advertising claims, and to inform the profession and the public about the safety and efficacy of the agent or device. The approval of the American Dental Association is shown by the use of official seals (figures 23–14 and 23–15).

Guidelines are set up and specific requirements must be fulfilled before the product or device can be recognized. Periodic reviews are required. The Councils publish a list of all accepted products and devices.[29] The depth and importance of the programs are recognized internationally.

Figure 23–14. Seal of Acceptance. The American Dental Association, Council on Dental Therapeutics official stamp for drugs and chemicals that meet specific standards for use in diagnosis, treatment, and prevention of oral disease.

I. Council on Dental Therapeutics[39]

Within the responsibilities of the Council on Dental Therapeutics (CDT) are all drugs and chemicals used in diagnosis, treatment, and prevention of oral disease. The products of a therapeutic nature that are used by patients are also surveyed, including dentifrices and mouthrinses.

The CDT uses *Accepted, Provisionally Accepted,* and *Unaccepted* for classification. In general, commercial products are examined upon request of the manufacturer, and research is submitted to show the effectiveness of the product. After study by the Council, the seal of acceptance may be placed on the product when the evidence for its safety and effectiveness is adequate (figure 23–14).

The Council prepares and publishes guidelines, such as those now available for acceptance of fluoride-containing dentifrices[40] and for the acceptance of chemotherapeutic products for the control of supragingival bacterial plaque and gingivitis.[41]

II. Council on Dental Materials, Instruments, and Equipment[42]

The Council on Dental Materials, Instruments, and Equipment (CDMIE) has a *certification* program for dental materials and instruments that meet official specifications. A special seal can be used (figure 23–15).

Also, an *acceptance* program identifies safety and effectiveness of appropriate items. After review, the items are classified as *Acceptable, Provisionally Acceptable,* or *Unacceptable.* Acceptable products can use the seal (figure 23–15).

When an existing certification or acceptance program is not applicable, a product may be evaluated for a stamp of *Professionally Recognized* (figure 23–15).

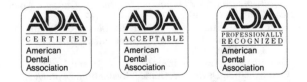

Figure 23–15. Seals for Certification, Acceptance, and Professional Recognition. The American Dental Association, Council on Dental Materials, Instruments, and Equipment permits the use of an official seal when criteria are met.

TECHNICAL HINTS

I. While preparing the patient's dental history, inquire about and record specific devices, dentifrices, mouthrinses, or other auxiliary aids used, in anticipation of evaluation for professional advice needed.

II. Request that a patient bring for demonstration a plaque control device being used, to assure that no harm is being done that, although not producing symptoms currently, could cause problems after long-term use.

III. Take care that preparations containing alcohol are not recommended for use by alcoholic patients, recovering alcoholic patients, or young people that may have a sensitivity to alcoholism.

IV. Check patient history for risk of bacteremia and need for antibiotic premedication while teaching the use of new plaque removal devices. Those who floss only every 2 to 3 days are subject to bacteremia.[43]

FACTORS TO TEACH THE PATIENT

I. Significance of American Dental Association product approval stamp. How to select approved products.

II. Ask dental hygienist and dentist about new products and whether they are appropriate to use.

III. How to use each supplementary aid for bacterial plaque removal. Bring implements to the office for approval of how each is being used.

IV. Avoid prolonged use of commercial mouthrinses.

V. How to prepare saline rinse for use after a scaling and root planing appointment.

References

1. Hill, H.C., Levi, P.A., and Glickman, I.: The Effects of Waxed and Unwaxed Dental Floss on Interdental Plaque Accumulation and Interdental Gingival Health, *J. Periodontol., 44,* 411, July, 1973.

2. Finkelstein, P. and Grossman, E.: The Effectiveness of Dental Floss in Reducing Gingival Inflammation, *J. Dent. Res., 58,* 1034, March, 1979.

3. Lamberts, D.M., Wunderlich, R.C., and Caffesse, R.G.: The Effect of Waxed and Unwaxed Dental Floss on Gingival Health. Part I. Plaque Removal and Gingival Response, *J. Periodontol., 53,* 393, June, 1982.

4. American Dental Association, Council on Dental Materials, Instruments, and Equipment: *Dentist's Desk Reference: Materials, Instruments and Equipment,* 2nd ed. Chicago, American Dental Association, 1983, pp. 421–422.

5. Hugoson, A.: Effect of the Water Pik Device on Plaque Accumulation and Development of Gingivitis, *J. Clin. Periodontol., 5,* 95, May, 1978.

6. Oshrain, R.L., Fiorello, L.A., Harper, D.S., and Lamster, I.B.: Oral Irrigation Devices. A Clinical Evaluation, *Dent. Hyg., 61,* 551, December, 1987.

7. Hardy, J.H., Newman, H.N., and Strahan, J.D.: Direct Irrigation and Subgingival Plaque, *J. Clin. Periodontol., 9,* 57, January, 1982.

8. Eakle, W.S., Ford, C., and Boyd, R.L.: Depth of Penetration in Periodontal Pockets With Oral Irrigation, *J. Clin. Periodontol., 13,* 39, January, 1986.

9. Pitcher, G.R., Newman, H.N., and Strahan, J.D.: Access to Subgingival Plaque by Disclosing Agents Using Mouthrinsing and Direct Irrigation, *J. Clin. Periodontol., 7,* 300, August, 1980.

10. Boyd, R.L., Leggott, P., Quinn, R., Buchanan, S., Eakle, W., and Chambers, D.: Effect of Self-administered Daily Irrigation with 0.02% SnF$_2$ on Periodontal Disease Activity, *J. Clin. Periodontol., 12,* 420, July, 1985.

11. Lang, N.P. and Räber, K.: Use of Oral Irrigators as Vehicle for the Application of Antimicrobial Agents in Chemical Plaque Control, *J. Clin. Periodontol., 8,* 177, June, 1981.

12. Lang, N.P. and Ramseier-Grossman, K.: Optimal Dosage of Chlorhexidine Digluconate in Chemical Plaque Control When Applied by the Oral Irrigator, *J. Clin. Periodontol., 8,* 189, June, 1981.

13. Aziz-Gandour, I.A. and Newman, H.N.: The Effects of a Simplified Oral Hygiene Regime Plus Supragingival Irrigation with Chlorhexidine or Metronidazole on Chronic Inflammatory Periodontal Disease, *J. Clin. Periodontol., 13,* 228, March, 1986.

14. Sanders, P.C., Linden, G.J., and Newman, H.N.: The Effects of a Simplified Mechanical Oral Hygiene Regime Plus Supragingival Irrigation with Chlorhexidine or Metronidazole on Subgingival Plaque, *J. Clin. Periodontol., 13,* 237, March, 1986.

15. Southard, G.L., Parsons, L.G., Thomas, L.G., Woodall, I.R., and Jones, B.J.B.: Effect of Sanguinaria Extract on Development of Plaque and Gingivitis When Supragingivally Delivered as a Manual Rinse or Under Pressure in an Oral Irrigator, *J. Clin. Periodontol., 14,* 377, August, 1987.

16. Parsons, L.G., Thomas, L.G., Southard, G.L., Woodall, I.R., and Jones, B.J.B.: Effect of Sanguinaria Extract on Established Plaque and Gingivitis When Supragingivally Delivered As a Manual Rinse or Under Pressure in an Oral Irrigator, *J. Clin. Periodontol., 14,* 381, August, 1987.

17. Macaulay, W.J.R. and Newman, H.N.: The Effect on the Composition of Subgingival Plaque of a Simplified Oral Hygiene System Including Pulsating Jet Subgingival Irrigation, *J. Periodont. Res., 21,* 375, July, 1986.

18. Watts, E.A. and Newman, H.N.: Clinical Effects on Chronic Periodontitis of a Simplified System of Oral Hygiene Including Subgingival Pulsated Jet Irrigation With Chlorhexidine, *J. Clin. Periodontol., 13,* 666, August, 1986.

19. O'Leary, T.J., Shafer, W.G., Swenson, H.M., Nesler, D.C., and Van Dorn, P.R.: Possible Penetration of Crevicular Tissue from Oral Hygiene Procedures: I. Use of Oral Irrigating Devices, *J. Periodontol., 41,* 158, March, 1970.

20. Phelps-Sandall, B.A. and Oxford, S.J.: Effectiveness of Oral Hygiene Techniques on Plaque and Gingivitis in Patients Placed in Intermaxillary Fixation, *Oral Surg. Oral Med. Oral Pathol., 56,* 487, November, 1983.

21. Romans, A.R. and App, G.R.: Bacteremia, a Result from Oral Irrigation in Subjects with Gingivitis, *J. Periodontol., 42,* 757, December, 1971.

22. Felix, J.E., Rosen, S., and App, G.R.: Detection of Bacteremia After the Use of an Oral Irrigation Device in Subjects with Periodontitis, *J. Periodontol., 42,* 785, December, 1971.

23. Volpe, A.R.: Dentifrices and Mouth Rinses, in Stallard, R.E., ed.: *A Textbook of Preventive Dentistry,* 2nd ed. Philadelphia, W.B. Saunders Co., 1982, pp. 170–216.

24. Harris, N.O.: Dentifrices, Mouthrinses, and Oral Irrigators, in Harris, N.O. and Christen, A.G.: *Primary Preventive Dentistry,* 2nd ed. Norwalk, Connecticut, Appleton & Lange, 1987, pp. 137–151.

25. Harte, D.B. and Manly, R.S.: Effect of Toothbrush Variables on Wear of Dentin Produced by Four Abrasives, *J. Dent. Res., 54,* 993, September-October, 1975.

26. Harte, D.B. and Manly, R.S.: Four Variables Affecting Mag-

nitude of Dentifrice Abrasiveness, *J. Dent. Res.,* *55,* 322, May-June, 1976.

27. Ciancio, S.G. and Bourgeault, P.C.: *Clinical Pharmacology for Dental Professionals.* New York, McGraw-Hill, 1980, pp. 141–146.

28. Hembree, M.E. and Hembree, J.H.: Relative Abrasiveness of Dentifrices, *Dent. Hyg.,* *51,* 253, June, 1977.

29. American Dental Association: *Products for Your Practice.* ADA Council-Evaluated Products. Chicago, American Dental Association, current year.

30. Scopp, I.W. and Orvieto, L.D.: Gingival Degerming by Povidone-iodine Irrigation: Bacteremia Reduction in Extraction Procedures, *J. Am. Dent. Assoc.,* *83,* 1294, December, 1971.

31. Brenman, H.S. and Randall, E.: Local Degerming with Povidone-iodine. II. Prior to Gingivectomy, *J. Periodontol.,* *45,* 870, December, 1974.

32. Bender, I.B., Naidorf, I.J., and Garvey, G.J.: Bacterial Endocarditis: A Consideration for Physician and Dentist, *J. Am. Dent. Assoc.,* *109,* 415, September, 1984.

33. American Dental Association, Council on Dental Therapeutics: *Accepted Dental Therapeutics,* 40th ed. Chicago, American Dental Association, 1984, pp. 322–323.

34. Weitzman, S.A., Weitberg, A.B., Niederman, R., and Stossel, T.P.: Chronic Treatment With Hydrogen Peroxide. Is It Safe? *J. Periodontol.,* *55,* 510, September, 1984.

35. Newbrun, E.: Chemical and Mechanical Removal of Plaque, *Compend. Contin. Educ. Dent.,* *6,* S110, Supplement Number 6, 1985.

36. Löe, H. and Schiøtt, C.R.: The Effect of Mouthrinses and Topical Application of Chlorhexidine on the Development of Dental Plaque and Gingivitis in Man, *J. Periodont. Res.,* *5,* 79, Number 2, 1970.

37. Segreto, V.A., Collins, E.M., Beiswanger, B.B., de la Rosa, M., Isaacs, R.L., Lang, N.P., Mallatt, M.E., and Meckel, A.H.: A Comparison of Mouthrinses Containing Two Concentrations of Chlorhexidine, *J. Periodont. Res.,* *21,* 23, Supplement Number 16, 1986.

38. Gisselsson, H., Birkhed, D., and Björn, A.-L.: Effect of Professional Flossing with Chlorhexidine Gel on Approximal Caries in 12- to 15-year-old Schoolchildren, *Caries Res.,* *22,* 187, May-June, 1988.

39. Jakush, J.: ADA Evaluation Programs: A Proud History of Service to the Profession and the Public, *J. Am. Dent. Assoc.,* *114,* 446, April, 1987.

40. American Dental Association, Council on Dental Therapeutics: Guidelines for the Acceptance of Fluoride-containing Dentifrices, *J. Am. Dent. Assoc.,* *110,* 545, April, 1985.

41. American Dental Association, Council on Dental Therapeutics: Guidelines for Acceptance of Chemotherapeutic Products for the Control of Supragingival Dental Plaque and Gingivitis, *J. Am. Dent. Assoc.,* *112,* 529, April, 1986.

42. American Dental Association, Council on Dental Materials, Instruments, and Equipment: op. cit., pp. 10–18.

43. Carroll, G.C. and Sebor, R.J.: Dental Flossing and Its Relationship to Transient Bacteremia, *J. Periodontol.,* *51,* 691, December, 1980.

Suggested Readings

Bassiouny, M.A. and Grant, A.A.: Oral Hygiene for the Partially Edentulous, *J. Periodontol.,* *52,* 214, April, 1981.

Ciancio, S.C.: Chemotherapeutic Agents and Periodontal Therapy. Their Impact on Clinical Practice, *J. Periodontol.,* *57,* 108, February, 1986.

Fédération Dentaire Internationale, Core Working Group: Topical and Systemic Antimicrobial Agents in the Treatment of Chronic Gingivitis and Periodontitis, Fédération Dentaire Internationale Technical Report No. 26, *Int. Dent. J.,* *37,* 52, March, 1987.

Kornman, K.S.: Antimicrobial Agents. State-of-the-Science Review, in Löe, H. and Kleinman, D.V., eds.: *Dental Plaque Control Measures and Oral Hygiene Practices.* Washington, D.C., IRL Press, 1986, pp. 121–142.

Kornman, K.S.: The Role of Supragingival Plaque in the Prevention

and Treatment of Periodontal Diseases, *J. Periodont. Res.,* *21,* 5–22, Supplement Number 16, 1986.

Loesche, W.J.: Chemotherapy of Dental Plaque Infections, *Oral Sciences Reviews,* *9,* 65, Munksgaard, 1976.

Newman, H.N.: Modes of Application of Anti-plaque Chemicals, *J. Clin. Periodontol.,* *13,* 965, November, 1986.

Scheirton, L.S.: Personal Oral Hygiene: Auxiliary Measures to Complement Toothbrushing, in Harris, N.O. and Christen, A.G.: *Primary Preventive Dentistry,* 2nd ed. Norwalk, Connecticut, Appleton & Lange, 1987, pp. 107–135.

Socransky, S.S.: Microbiology of Plaque, *Compend. Contin. Educ. Dent.,* *5,* S53, Supplement Number 5, 1984.

Takei, H.H.: The Interdental Space, *Dent. Clin. North Am.,* *24,* 169, April, 1980.

Zier, B.A. and Pimlott, J.F.L.: Mechanical Plaque Control: Are Concepts Changing? *Can. Dent. Hyg. (Probe),* *21,* 123, September, 1987.

Dental Floss

Abelson, D.C., Barton, J.E., Maietti, G.M., and Cowherd, M.G.: Evaluation of Interproximal Cleaning by Two Types of Dental Floss, *Clin. Prevent. Dent.,* *3,* 19, July-August, 1981.

Barton, R.F. and Diamond, B.: Evaluation and Patient Acceptance of a Mechanical Dental Flossing Device Compared to Hand-held Floss, *Clin. Prevent. Dent.,* *2,* 10, May-June, 1980.

Bass, C.C.: The Optimum Characteristics of Dental Floss for Personal Oral Hygiene, *Dent. Items Int.,* *70,* 921, September, 1948.

Boyer, E.M. and Field, H.M.: Tissue Response to Initial Performance of Flossing and Sulcular Toothbrushing, *Dent. Hyg.,* *54,* 370, August, 1980.

Jerman, A.C. and Christen, A.G.: Floss Holders: What Do Periodontists Think of Them? *Clin. Prevent. Dent.,* *3,* 5, January-February, 1981.

Lobene, R.R., Soparkar, P.M., and Newman, M.B.: Use of Dental Floss. Effect on Plaque and Gingivitis, *Clin. Prevent. Dent.,* *4,* 5, January-February, 1982.

Murtomaa, H., Turtola, L., and Rytomaa, I.: Use of Dental Floss by Finnish Students, *J. Clin. Periodontol.,* *11,* 443, August, 1984.

Perry, D.A. and Pattison, G.: An Investigation of Wax Residue on Tooth Surfaces After Use of Waxed Dental Floss, *Dent. Hyg.,* *60,* 16, January, 1986.

Reitman, W.R., Whiteley, R.T., and Robertson, P.B.: Proximal Surface Cleaning by Dental Floss, *Clin. Prevent. Dent.,* *2,* 7, May-June, 1980.

Samant, A., Martin, J.O., and Cinotti, W.R.: The Role of Dental Floss in Restorative Dentistry, *J. Prosthet. Dent.,* *53,* 597, April, 1985.

Smith, B.A., Collier, C.M., and Caffesse, R.G.: *In vitro* Effectiveness of Dental Floss in Plaque Removal, *J. Clin. Periodontol.,* *13,* 211, March, 1986.

Stevens, A.W.: A Comparison of the Effectiveness of Variable Diameter vs. Unwaxed Floss, *J. Periodontol.,* *51,* 666, November, 1980.

Vercaigne, M.A. and Gelskey, S.C.: The Efficacy of Professional Flossing in the Control of Gingival Health, *Can. Dent. Hyg.,* *16,* 16, Spring, 1982.

Waerhaug, J.: Healing of the Dento-epithelial Junction Following the Use of Dental Floss, *J. Clin. Periodontol.,* *8,* 144, April, 1981.

Walsh, M.M. and Heckman, B.L.: Interproximal Subgingival Cleaning by Dental Floss and the Toothpick, *Dent. Hyg.,* *59,* 464, October, 1985.

Wong, C.H. and Wade, A.B.: A Comparative Study of Effectiveness in Plaque Removal by Super Floss and Waxed Dental Floss, *J. Clin. Periodontol.,* *12,* 788, October, 1985.

Wunderlich, R.C., Lamberts, D.M., and Caffesse, R.G.: The Effect of Waxed and Unwaxed Dental Floss on Gingival Health. Part II. Crevicular Fluid Flow and Gingival Bleeding, *J. Periodontol.,* *53,* 397, June, 1982.

Interdental Aids

Bergenholtz, A., Bjorne, A., Glantz, P.-O., and Vikstrom, B.: Plaque Removal by Various Triangular Toothpicks, *J. Clin. Periodontol., 7,* 121, April, 1980.

Bergenholtz, A. and Brithon, J.: Plaque Removal by Dental Floss or Toothpicks, An Intra-individual Comparative Study, *J. Clin. Periodontol., 7,* 516, December, 1980.

Bergenholtz, A. and Olsson, A.: Efficacy of Plaque-removal Using Interdental Brushes and Waxed Dental Floss, *Scand. J. Dent. Res., 92,* 198, June, 1984.

El Ghamrawy, E.: A Tooth-brush Designed for Proximal Surfaces Adjacent to Toothless Spaces in the Partially Edentulous Patient, *J. Oral Rehabil., 6,* 323, October, 1979.

Naylor, W.P. and Stewart, D.M.: The End-tuft Toothbrush for the Partially Edentulous Patient, *J. Prosthet. Dent., 52,* 311, August, 1984.

Smith, B.A., Shanbour, G.S., Caffesse, R.G., Morrison, E.C., and Dennison, J.D.: *In vitro* Polishing Effectiveness of Interdental Aids on Root Surfaces, *J. Clin. Periodontol., 13,* 597, July, 1986.

Waerhaug, J.: The Interdental Brush and Its Place in Operative and Crown and Bridge Dentistry, *J. Oral Rehabil., 3,* 107, April, 1976.

Irrigation

Braatz, L., Garrett, S., Claffey, N., and Egelberg, J.: Antimicrobial Irrigation of Deep Pockets to Supplement Non-surgical Periodontal Therapy. II. Daily Irrigation, *J. Clin. Periodontol., 12,* 630, September, 1985.

Drisko, C.L., White, C.L., Killoy, W.J., and Mayberry, W.E.: Comparison of Dark-field Microscopy and a Flagella Stain for Monitoring the Effect of a Water Pik on Bacterial Motility, *J. Periodontol., 58,* 381, June, 1987.

Greenstein, G.: Effects of Subgingival Irrigation on Periodontal Status, *J. Periodontol., 58,* 827, December, 1987.

Kelly, A., Resteghini, R., Williams, B., and Dolby, A.E.: Pressures Recorded During Periodontal Pocket Irrigation, *J. Periodontol., 56,* 297, May, 1985.

Mazza, J.E., Newman, M.G., and Sims, T.N.: Clinical and Antimicrobial Effect of Stannous Fluoride on Periodontitis, *J. Clin. Periodontol., 8,* 203, June, 1981.

Ross, C.H. and Beeson, M.D.: Oral Irrigation . . . A New Clinical Horizon, *RDH, 5,* 26, October, 1985.

Schmid, E., Kornman, K.S., and Tinanoff, N.: Changes of Subgingival Total Colony Forming Units and Black Pigmented Bacteroides After a Single Irrigation of Periodontal Pockets with 1.64% SnF_2, *J. Periodontol., 56,* 330, June, 1985.

Soh, L.L., Newman, H.N., and Strahan, J.D.: Effects of Subgingival Chlorhexidine Irrigation on Periodontal Inflammation, *J. Clin. Periodontol., 9,* 66, January, 1982.

Wunderlich, R.C.: Subgingival Penetration of an Applied Solution, *Int. J. Periodontics Restorative Dent., 4,* 64, Number 5, 1984.

Local Drug Delivery

Addy, M., Langeroudi, M., and Hassan, H.: The Development and Clinical Use of Acrylic Strips Containing Anti-microbial Agents in the Management of Chronic Periodontitis, *Int. Dent. J., 35,* 124, June, 1985.

Coventry, J. and Newman, H.N.: Experimental Use of a Slow Release Device Employing Chlorhexidine Gluconate in Areas of Acute Periodontal Inflammation, *J. Clin. Periodontol., 9,* 129, March, 1982.

Goodson, J.M., Hogan, P.E., and Dunham, S.L.: Clinical Responses Following Periodontal Treatment by Local Drug Delivery, *J. Periodontol., 56,* 81, Supplement, 1985.

Goodson, J.M., Offenbacher, S., Farr, D.H., and Hogan, P.E.: Periodontal Disease Treatment by Local Drug Delivery, *J. Periodontol., 56,* 265, May, 1985.

Newman, H.N., Yeung, F.I.S., Wan Yusof, W.Z.A.B., and Addy, M.: Slow Release Metronidazole and a Simplified Mechanical Oral Hygiene Regimen in the Control of Chronic Periodontitis, *J. Clin. Periodontol., 11,* 576, October, 1984.

Wan Yusof, W.Z.A., Newman, H.N., Strahan, J.D., and Coventry, J.F.: Subgingival Metronidazole in Dialysis Tubing and Subgingival Chlorhexidine Irrigation in the Control of Chronic Inflammatory Periodontal Disease, *J. Clin. Periodontol., 11,* 166, March, 1984.

Dentifrices

Allen, C.E. and Nunez, L.J.: A Look at Toothpaste Ingredients, *Gen. Dent., 33,* 58, January-February, 1985.

American Dental Association, Council on Dental Therapeutics: *Accepted Dental Therapeutics,* 40th ed. Chicago, American Dental Association, 1984, pp. 421–428.

American Dental Association Health Foundation Research Institute: Clinical Methods for Determining Dentifrice-cleaning Ability, *J. Am. Dent. Assoc., 109,* 759, November, 1984.

Baxter, P.M., Davis, W.B., and Jackson, J.: Toothpaste Abrasive Requirements to Control Naturally Stained Pellicle, *J. Oral Rehabil., 8,* 19, January, 1981.

Bay, I. and Rølla, G.: Plaque Inhibition and Improved Gingival Condition by Use of a Stannous Fluoride Toothpaste, *Scand. J. Dent. Res., 88,* 313, August, 1980.

Boackle, R.J., Draughn, R.A., and Vesely, J.: Disruption of Complement-mediated Reactions by Insoluble Dentifrice Ingredients, *J. Periodontol., 52,* 621, October, 1981.

De Boer, P., Duinkerke, A.S.H., and Arends, J.: Influence of Tooth Paste Particle Size and Tooth Brush Stiffness on Dentine Abrasion *in vitro, Caries Res., 19,* 232, May-June, 1985.

Dowell, T.B.: The Use of Toothpaste in Infancy, *Br. Dent. J., 150,* 247, May 5, 1981.

Duke, S.A.: Effect of a Chalk-based Toothpaste on pH Changes in Dental Plaque *in vivo, Caries Res., 20,* 278, May-June, 1986.

Duke, S.A. and Forward, G.C.: The Conditions Occurring *in vivo* When Brushing with Toothpastes, *Br. Dent. J., 152,* 52, January 19, 1982.

Etemadzadeh, H., Ainamo, J., and Heikki, M.: Plaque Growth-inhibiting Effects of an Abrasive Fluoride-Chlorhexidine Toothpaste and a Fluoride Toothpaste Containing Oxidative Enzymes, *J. Clin. Periodontol., 12,* 607, August, 1985.

Jones, P.A., Fisher, S.E., and Wilson, H.J.: Abrasivity of Dentifrices on Anterior Restorative Materials, *Br. Dent. J., 158,* 130, February 23, 1985.

Joyston-Bechal, S., Smales, F.C., and Duckworth, R.: Effect of Metronidazole on Chronic Periodontal Disease in Subjects Using a Topically Applied Chlorhexidine Gel, *J. Clin. Periodontol., 11,* 53, January, 1984.

Kleber, C.J., Putt, M.S., and Muhler, J.C.: Dental Plaque Scores of Children Brushing with a Gel or Paste-dentifrice, *ASDC J. Dent. Child., 49,* 288, July-August, 1982.

Lamb, D.J., Howell, R.A., and Constable, G.: Removal of Plaque and Stain from Natural Teeth by a Low Abrasivity Toothpaste, *Br. Dent. J., 157,* 125, August 25, 1984.

Lobene, R.R.: Clinical Studies of the Cleaning Functions of Dentifrices, *J. Am. Dent. Assoc., 105,* 798, November, 1982.

Makinen, K.K., Soderling, E., Hurttia, H., Lehtonen, O.-P., and Luukkala, E.: Biochemical, Microbiologic, and Clinical Comparisons Between Two Dentifrices That Contain Different Mixtures of Sugar Alcohols, *J. Am. Dent. Assoc., 111,* 745, November, 1985.

Moran, J. and Addy, M.: The Antibacterial Properties of Some Commercially Available Toothpastes *in vitro, Br. Dent. J., 156,* 175, March 10, 1984.

Naylor, M.N. and Pindborg, J.J., eds.: The Contribution of Dentifrices to Oral Health, *Community Dent. Oral Epidemiol., 8,* 217–285, Extra Issue, 1980.

O'Connor, B.S.: Consumer-oriented Aspects of Dentifrices, *Dent. Hyg., 54,* 121, March, 1980.

Saxton, C.A. and Cowell, C.R.: Clinical Investigation of the Effects of Dentifrices on Dentin Wear at the Cementoenamel Junction, *J. Am. Dent. Assoc., 102,* 38, January, 1981.

Sherrill, C.A. and Krouse, M.: A Critical Look at Recent Dentifrice Claims, *Dent. Hyg., 60,* 410, September, 1986.

Svinnseth, P.N., Gjerdet, N.R., and Lie, T.: Abrasivity of Toothpastes. An *in vitro* Study of Toothpastes Marketed in Norway, *Acta Odontol. Scand., 45,* 195, Number 3, 1987.

Toothpastes, *Consumer Reports, 51,* 144, March, 1986.

Zier, B.A. and Pimlott, J.F.L.: Dentifrice Dimensions, *Can. Dent. Hyg./Probe, 21,* 169, December, 1987.

Anticalculus Dentifrice

Lobene, R.R., Soparkar, P.M., Newman, M.B., and Kohut, B.E.: Reduced Formation of Supragingival Calculus with Use of Fluoride-Zinc Chloride Dentifrice, *J. Am. Dent. Assoc., 114,* 350, March, 1987.

Lobene, R.R.: A Clinical Comparison of the Anticalculus Effect of Two Commercially-available Dentifrices, *Clin. Prevent. Dent., 9,* 3, July-August, 1987.

Lu, K.H., Yen, D.J.C., Zacherl, W.A., Ruhlman, C.D., Sturzenberger, O.P., and Lehnhoff, R.W.: The Effect of a Fluoride Dentifrice Containing an Anticalculus Agent on Dental Caries in Children, *ASDC J. Dent. Child., 52,* 449, November-December, 1985.

Rustogi, K.N., Volpe, A.R., and Petrone, M.E.: A Clinical Comparison of Two Anticalculus Dentifrices, *Compend. Contin. Educ. Dent., 9,* 78, January, 1988.

Schiff, T.G.: The Effect of a Dentifrice Containing Soluble Pyrophosphate and Sodium Fluoride on Calculus Deposits. A 6-month Clinical Study, *Clin. Prevent. Dent., 9,* 13, March-April, 1987.

Zacherl, W.A., Pfeiffer, H.J., and Swancar, J.R.: The Effect of Soluble Pyrophosphates on Dental Calculus in Adults, *J. Am. Dent. Assoc., 110,* 737, May, 1985.

Zacherl, W.A. and Albrecht, E.B.: Soluble Pyrophosphate As a Calculus Inhibitor, *RDH, 6,* 51, May/June, 1986.

Mouthrinses

Axelsson, P. and Lindhe, J.: Efficacy of Mouthrinses in Inhibiting Dental Plaque and Gingivitis in Man, *J. Clin. Periodontol., 14,* 205, April, 1987.

Dahlén, G.: Effect of Antimicrobial Mouthrinses on Salivary Microflora in Healthy Subjects, *Scand. J. Dent. Res., 92,* 38, February, 1984.

Emling, R.C. and Yankell, S.L.: First Clinical Studies of a New Prebrushing Mouthrinse, *Compend. Contin. Educ. Dent., 6,* 636, October, 1985.

Grenby, T.H. and Saldanha, M.G.: The Antimicrobial Activity of Modern Mouthwashes, *Br. Dent. J., 157,* 239, October 6, 1984.

Gross, K.B.W., Overman, P.R., Clark, B.R., Eberhart, A., and Love, J.: Sanguinarine and Essential Oil Mouthrinses. Effects on Plaque and Gingivitis, *Dent. Hyg., 61,* 62, February, 1987.

Helldén, L., Camosci, D., Hock, J., and Tinanoff, N.: Clinical Study to Compare the Effect of Stannous Fluoride and Chlorhexidine Mouthrinses on Plaque Formation, *J. Clin. Periodontol., 8,* 12, February, 1981.

Mankodi, S., Ross, N.M., and Mostler, K.: Clinical Efficacy of Listerine in Inhibiting and Reducing Plaque and Experimental Gingivitis, *J. Clin. Periodontol., 14,* 285, May, 1987.

Mueller, H.J.: Some Considerations Regarding the Degradational Interactions Between Mouth Rinses and Silver-soldered Joints, *Am. J. Orthod., 81,* 140, February, 1982.

Oppermann, R.V. and Gjermo, P.: *In vivo* Effect of Four Antibacterial Agents Upon the Acidogenicity of Dental Plaque, *Scand. J. Dent. Res., 88,* 34, February, 1980.

Schaeken, M.J.M., de Jong, M.H., Franken, H.C.M., and van der Hoeven, J.S.: Effects of Highly Concentrated Stannous Fluoride and Chlorhexidine Regimes on Human Dental Plaque Flora, *J. Dent. Res., 65,* 57, January, 1986.

Selbst, S.M., De Maio, J.G., and Boenning, D.: Mouthwash Poisoning. Report of a Fatal Case, *Clin. Pediatr. (Phila), 24,* 162, March, 1985.

Chlorhexidine

Addy, M.: Chlorhexidine Compared with Other Locally Delivered Antimicrobials. A Short Review, *J. Clin. Periodontol., 13,* 957, November, 1986.

Brown, A.T., Largent, B.A., Ferretti, G.A., and Lillich, T.T.: Chemical Control of Plaque-dependent Oral Diseases: The Use of

Chlorhexidine, *Compend. Contin. Educ. Dent., 7,* 719, November/December, 1986.

Fardal, O. and Turnbull, R.S.: A Review of the Literature on Use of Chlorhexidine in Dentistry, *J. Am. Dent. Assoc., 112,* 863, June, 1986.

Flötra, L., Gjermo, G., Rölla, G., and Waerhaug, J.: Side Effects of Chlorhexidine Mouth Washes, *Scand. J. Dent. Res., 79,* 119, April, 1971.

Greenstein, G., Berman, C., and Jaffin, R.: Chlorhexidine. An Adjunct to Periodontal Therapy, *J. Periodontol., 57,* 370, June, 1986.

Hepsø, H.U., Bjornland, T., and Skoglund, L.A.: Side-effects and Patient Acceptance of 0.2% versus 0.1% Chlorhexidine Used as Postoperative Prophylactic Mouthwash, *Int. J. Oral Maxillofac. Surg., 17,* 17, February, 1988.

Lie, T. and Enersen, M.: Effects of Chlorhexidine Gel in a Group of Maintenance Care Patients with Poor Oral Hygiene, *J. Periodontol., 57,* 364, June, 1986.

Tonelli, P.M., Hume, W.R., and Kenney, E.B.: Chlorhexidine: A Review of the Literature, *J. West. Soc. Periodont. Periodont. Abstr., 31,* 5, Number 1, 1983.

Westfelt, E., Nyman, S., Lindhe, J., and Socransky, S.: Use of Chlorhexidine as a Plaque Control Measure Following Surgical Treatment of Periodontal Disease, *J. Clin. Periodontol., 10,* 22, January, 1983.

Westling, M. and Tynelius-Bratthall, G.: Microbiological and Clinical Short-term Effects of Repeated Intracrevicular Chlorhexidine Rinsings, *J. Periodont. Res., 19,* 202, March, 1984.

Sanguinaria

Etemadzadeh, H. and Ainamo, J.: Lacking Anti-plaque Efficacy of 2 Sanguinarine Mouth Rinses, *J. Clin. Periodontol., 14,* 176, March, 1987.

Greenfield, W. and Cuchel, S.J.: The Use of an Oral Rinse and Dentifrice as a System for Reducing Dental Plaque, *Compend. Contin. Educ. Dent., 5,* S82, Supplement Number 5, 1984.

Schonfeld, S.E., Farnoush, A., and Wilson, S.G.: *In vivo* Antiplaque Activity of a Sanguinarine-containing Dentifrice: Comparison with Conventional Toothpastes, *J. Periodont. Res., 21,* 298, May, 1986.

Southard, G.L., Parsons, L.G., Thomas, L.G., Boulware, R.T., Woodall, I.R., and Jones, B.J.B.: The Relationship of Sanguinaria Extract Concentration and Zinc Ion to Plaque and Gingivitis, *J. Clin. Periodontol., 14,* 315, July, 1987.

Southard, G.L., Boulware, R.T., Walborn, D.R., Groznick, W.J., Thorne, E.E., and Yankell, S.L.: Sanguinarine, A New Antiplaque Agent: Retention and Plaque Specificity, *J. Am. Dent. Assoc., 108,* 338, March, 1984.

Wennström, J. and Lindhe, J.: Some Effects of a Sanguinarine-containing Mouthrinse on Developing Plaque and Gingivitis, *J. Clin. Periodontol., 12,* 867, November, 1985.

Peroxide and Bicarbonate

Amigoni, N.A., Johnson, G.K., and Kalkwarf, K.L.: The Use of Sodium Bicarbonate and Hydrogen Peroxide in Periodontal Therapy: A Review, *J. Am. Dent. Assoc., 114,* 217, February, 1987.

Bakdash, M.B., Wolff, L.F., Pihlstrom, B.L., Aeppli, D.M., and Bandt, C.L.: Salt and Peroxide Compared with Conventional Oral Hygiene, *J. Periodontol., 58,* 308, May, 1987.

Cerra, M.B. and Killoy, W.J.: The Effect of Sodium Bicarbonate and Hydrogen Peroxide on the Microbial Flora of Periodontal Pockets. A Preliminary Report, *J. Periodontol., 53,* 599, October, 1982.

Gold, S.I.: Early Origins of Hydrogen Peroxide Use in Oral Hygiene, *J. Periodontol., 54,* 247, April, 1983.

Gomes, B.C., Shakun, M.L., and Ripa, L.W.: Effect of Rinsing with a 1.5% Hydrogen Peroxide Solution (Peroxyl®) on Gingivitis and Plaque in Handicapped and Nonhandicapped Subjects, *Clin. Prevent. Dent., 6,* 21, May-June, 1984.

Greenstein, G. and Rethman, M.: Hydrogen Peroxide and Salt Solutions: Are They Effective Antiplaque Agents? *Compend. Contin. Educ. Dent., 8,* 348, May, 1987.

Herrin, J.R., Rubright, W.C., Squier, C.A., Lawton, W.J., Osborn, M.O., Stumbo, P.J., and Grigsby, W.R.: Local and Systemic Effects of Orally Applied Sodium Salts, *J. Am. Dent. Assoc., 113,* 607, October, 1986.

Kaminsky, S.B., Gillette, W.B., and O'Leary, T.J.: Sodium Absorption Associated with Oral Hygiene Procedures, *J. Am. Dent. Assoc., 114,* 644, May, 1987.

Lehne, R.K.: Abrasivity of Sodium Bicarbonate, *Clin. Prevent. Dent., 5,* 17, January-February, 1983.

Lyne, S.M., Glasscock, N.D., and Allen, D.S.: Clinical Effectiveness of Hydrogen Peroxide-Sodium Bicarbonate Paste on Periodontitis Treated with and without Scaling and Root Planing, *Dent. Hyg., 60,* 450, October, 1986.

Miyasaki, K.T., Genco, R.J., and Wilson, M.E.: Antimicrobial Properties of Hydrogen Peroxide and Sodium Bicarbonate Individually and in Combination Against Selected Oral, Gram-negative, Facultative Bacteria, *J. Dent. Res., 65,* 1142, September, 1986.

Newbrun, E., Hoover, C.I., and Ryder, M.I.: Bactericidal Action of Bicarbonate Ion on Selected Periodontal Pathogenic Microorganisms, *J. Periodontol., 55,* 658, November, 1984.

Pihlstrom, B.L., Wolff, L.F., Bakdash, M.B., Schaffer, E.M., Jensen, J.R., Aeppli, D.M., and Bandt, C.L.: Salt and Peroxide Compared with Conventional Oral Hygiene. I. Clinical Results, *J. Periodontol., 58,* 291, May, 1987.

Rees, T.D. and Orth, C.F.: Oral Ulcerations with Use of Hydrogen Peroxide, *J. Periodontol., 57,* 689, November, 1986.

Walsh, M.M. and Kaufman, N.: Subgingival Application of a Hydrogen Peroxide/Baking Soda Mixture with a Toothpick, *Clin. Prevent. Dent., 7,* 21, March-April, 1985.

Weitzman, S.A., Weitberg, A.B., Stossel, T.P., Schwartz, J., and Shklar, G.: Effects of Hydrogen Peroxide on Oral Carcinogenesis in Hamsters, *J. Periodontol., 57,* 685, November, 1986.

West, T.L. and King, W.J.: Toothbrushing with Hydrogen Peroxide-Sodium Bicarbonate Compared to Toothpowder and Water in Reducing Periodontal Pocket Suppuration and Darkfield Bacterial Counts, *J. Periodontol., 54,* 339, June, 1983.

Wolff, L.F., Pihlstrom, B.L., Bakdash, M.B., Schaffer, E.M., Jensen, J.R., Aeppli, D.M., and Bandt, C.L.: Salt and Peroxide Compared with Conventional Oral Hygiene. II. Microbial Results, *J. Periodontol., 58,* 301, May, 1987.

24 Care of Dental Appliances

Total cleanliness of the oral cavity for the health of the teeth and supporting structures involves specific procedures for the care of the natural teeth and all appliances, both fixed and removable. A dental *appliance* is a device used for therapy and to provide function. A *prosthesis* is an appliance for the artificial replacement of a missing part of the body.

The fit and function of a dental appliance depend to a large degree on the cooperation of the patient in daily cleaning of the appliance and bacterial plaque control for the remaining natural teeth. Likewise, orthodontic appliances must be kept clean and periodontal health maintained if the treatment is to have long-term success.

The patient's cooperation depends on the motivation, information, and sense of appreciation and concern imparted by the members of the dental team. For the natural teeth involved, instruction begins early, before construction of the partial denture or placement of orthodontic appliances. Instruction is supplemented when an appliance is inserted to demonstrate specific techniques for daily care. Continuing supervision and review of procedures at succeeding appointments and maintenance appointments are required.

Fixed appliances include fixed partial dentures, space maintainers, periodontal splints, orthodontic appliances, and fixed complete and partial dentures with implant attached abutments. Examples of removable types are complete dentures, overdentures, and partial dentures, space maintainers, and orthodontic appliances, as well as obturators for closure of palatal defects.

A patient may have more than one prosthesis. For example, a complete maxillary denture may be accompanied by both fixed and removable partial dentures in the mandibular arch. For this patient, the regimen for personal care involves the natural teeth as well as the fixed and removable dentures. A program of instruction must be worked out for each patient, depending on individual needs.

ORTHODONTIC APPLIANCES

Without a strong and persistent preventive care program before, during, and following completion of orthodontic treatment, a high dental caries rate has been associated with orthodontic treatment. Gingival and periodontal infections during and following treatment are not unusual. An individualized preventive program that includes a specific plan of instruction, motivation, and supervision is essential for the patient with orthodontic appliances. The patient must understand that much more effort is required while in treatment than was required before the appliances were placed.

The dental hygienist who works with an orthodontist is in a position to perform a highly specialized service. Because the patient will be under care with regular appointments for a long period, frequently over a few years, periodic communication between the patient's referring dentist and dental hygienist is necessary to coordinate instruction along with other necessary dental and dental hygiene care.

I. Complicating Factors

A. Age Group
Many orthodontic patients are preteens and teen-agers, periods when the incidence of gingivitis is high. The incidence of periodontal infection increases from early childhood to late teenage years.

B. Gingivitis
Bacterial plaque retention by orthodontic appliances leads to gingivitis. The degree can vary from slight to severe with gingival enlargement particularly of the interdental papillae. The tissue may greatly enlarge and cover the fixed appliance. The enlarged tissue with pockets provides additional plaque-retentive areas.

C. Position of Teeth
Teeth that are irregularly positioned are naturally more susceptible to the retention of bacterial deposits and are more difficult to clean. With the severe malocclusions presented by orthodontic patients at the outset, this factor becomes even more significant.

D. Problems with Appliances
1. Orthodontic appliances retain plaque and debris.
2. Accidents may cause wires to bend adversely and become imbedded in the gingiva. A loosened band may be forced under the gingiva.
3. Removable appliances or their clasps may press excessively against the gingiva.
4. Rubber bands used during therapy may slip under the gingiva and detach the junctional epithelium.

E. Self-care Is Difficult

Even the patient who tries to maintain oral cleanliness has difficulty because the appliances are in the way and interfere with the application of the toothbrush and other devices used for plaque control.

II. Disease Control

A rigid program for dental caries and periodontal disease control is needed. The selection of plaque control procedures for an individual patient is determined by the anatomic features of the gingiva, the position of the teeth, and the type and position of the orthodontic appliance.

Many types of appliances are utilized for orthodontic treatment. Fixed orthodontic appliances may consist of brackets bonded directly to the tooth surfaces after an acid etch procedure, as shown in figure 40–1 (page 521). Other appliances are bands cemented around each tooth with brackets attached to the bands to support an arch wire. Figures 24–2 and 24–3 show teeth with complete bands.

A. General Instructions

1. Give instructions before appliances are placed. Every attempt must be made to have the oral tissues in health and the patient motivated to perform thorough daily plaque removal.
2. Perform brushing before a mirror so that brush application is accurate and brushing is thorough.
3. Use a disclosing solution rinse to assist in self-evaluation. Orthodontic patients may experience difficulty in chewing disclosing wafers without discomfort or pain.
4. Recommend an approved fluoride dentifrice to aid in dental caries control.

5. Place emphasis in brushing on sulcular brushing and cleaning the area between the orthodontic bands and brackets and the gingiva.

B. Toothbrushing

1. *Brush Selection*
   a. A soft brush with end-rounded filaments generally is recommended.
   b. A special orthodontic brush designed with two spaced rows of soft nylon filaments and with a third middle row that is shorter can be applied directly over the fixed appliance and used with a short horizontal stroke (figure 24–1).
2. *Brushing Procedure*
   a. A sulcular method is needed by most patients for cleaning the appliances and maintaining the gingiva.
   b. Special adaptation is required for facial surfaces. Place the brush in the Charters position for over the wire and bracket (or under for mandibular); place in Stillman position for the opposite side (figure 24–2).
   c. To assure cleanliness, one should brush the appliances in any way that the filaments can be manipulated. Insert the brush from below, over, and above the arch wire; rotate and vibrate to remove plaque and debris.
   d. Lingual approach to brushing is similar to the basic strokes used on the facial surfaces.

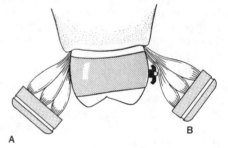

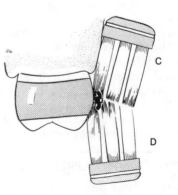

Figure 24–2. Toothbrushing for Orthodontic Appliance. A. Sulcular brushing for periodontal tissues. B. Facial over bracket. C. Cleaning the bracket using brush in Charters brushing position for the gingival side. D. Brush in Stillman position for occlusal side of the bracket and arch wire.

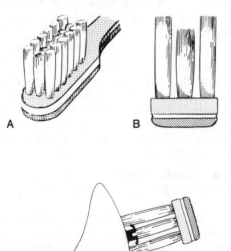

Figure 24–1. Orthodontic Toothbrush. A. Middle row of filaments trimmed shorter to fit over a fixed appliance. B. Cross section. C. Brush held over a bracket.

C. Additional Measures

1. *Interdental Aids*

The previously described applications for the interdental tip and toothpick in holder (pages 321–323) also apply for care of the orthodontic patient (figure 24–3). A floss threader is needed for plaque removal from proximal tooth surfaces when the appliance prevents passage of floss from the occlusal. Tufted dental floss or yarn used in the floss threader can remove plaque more efficiently than can regular dental floss.

An interdental brush and a single-tuft brush can be particularly beneficial around individual teeth. The entire system should be kept as simple as possible.

2. *Oral Irrigation*[1]

Most orthodontic patients can benefit from the regular use of an irrigator for removal of food particles.

III. Care of Removable Appliance or Hawley Retainer (figure 24–4)

A. Clean the appliance after each meal and before retiring. Instructions for cleaning procedures and agents for removable appliances are described with the care of the removable denture (pages 344–345).

B. Brush and rinse teeth and gingival tissue under the appliance each time the appliance is removed. Unless necessary as directed by the orthodontist, the health of the underlying tissues is best maintained when the appliance is not kept in the mouth continuously.

C. Brush the mucosa under the appliance. Methods are described on page 349.

D. Keep appliance in a container with water when it is out of the mouth.

IV. Self-applied Fluoride

A patient with an orthodontic appliance has an increased risk of enamel demineralization and dental caries because of bacterial plaque retention. A daily

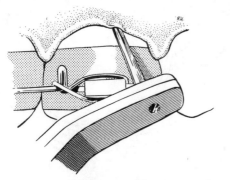

Figure 24–3. Toothpick Holder for Orthodontic Patient. Moistened toothpick in holder can be applied for cleaning about appliances and in the subgingival area of the sulcus. Directions for use of the device are on pages 321–322.

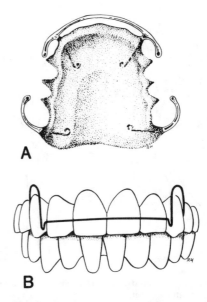

Figure 24–4. Hawley Retainer. A. Removable acrylic retainer with labial retaining wire and clasps of type worn by an orthodontic patient after removal of a fixed appliance. **B.** Anterior view of patient shows a Hawley appliance in position. The method for cleaning the appliance is similar to that for cleaning a removable denture (pages 344–345).

fluoride program is mandatory to supplement mechanical daily plaque removal and periodic professional topical applications of fluoride solution or gel.

Self-applied fluorides are described on pages 407–410. A fluoride dentifrice is recommended, along with a daily mouthrinse, gel tray, or brush-on gel. Encouragement, repetition, reinforcement, and motivation are needed to achieve continuing interest and cooperation of an orthodontic patient in both the plaque control and the self-applied fluoride programs.

SPACE MAINTAINERS

When teeth are lost, the surrounding teeth tend to move toward the space. The loss of a permanent tooth is illustrated in figure 24–5. With the extraction of the mandibular first molar, the second and third molars inclined mesially, and the maxillary first molar supererupted into the space. Prevention of such disruption of occlusion and function is a primary reason for the use of fixed or removable dental appliances described in the next sections (pages 341–345).

The premature loss of one or more primary molars disrupts the eruption pattern of the developing permanent teeth. The loss of a second primary molar creates a serious situation because the permanent molars begin to migrate mesially. The permanent premolars may be closed in and prevented from eruption, as shown in figure 24–6.

Many malocclusions result from early loss or prolonged retention of primary teeth. *Preventive orthodontics* refers to the elimination of factors that may lead to malocclusion in an otherwise normally developing dentition. When a primary tooth cannot be

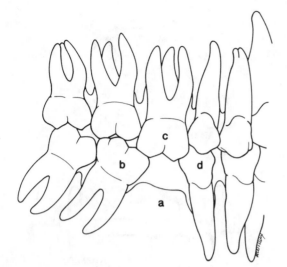

Figure 24–5. Loss of Mandibular First Permanent Molar. Mandibular second (b) and third molars incline into the space from which the first molar was removed (a). Second premolar (d) drifts to the distal. Maxillary first molar (c) supererupts into the space. Occlusion and mastication are disabled, and predisposition to periodontal involvement around the irregularly positioned teeth is greatly increased.

saved through treatment and restoration, the space then must be held.

I. Types of Space Maintainers

A space maintainer is a prosthetic replacement for prematurely lost primary teeth that is intended to prevent closure of the space before eruption of the permanent successors.*

The two general types of space maintainers are *fixed* and *removable.* An advantage of a fixed appliance is that the patient cannot lose or forget to wear the appliance. Some space maintainers may be designed for function during mastication, and others may have orthodontic attachments to move teeth.

II. Fixed Space Maintainer

A. Description

A fixed appliance is made of orthodontic arch wire soldered to a band or bands placed around natural teeth, usually around molars. A bilateral lingual appliance is shown in figure 24–7.

B. Personal Care Procedures

Bacterial plaque control can be accomplished by using many of the methods described for orthodontic appliances (pages 338–339). Adaptation of techniques is needed for cleaning the lingual arch wire and the lingual aspect of the molar bands for an appliance such as that shown in figure 24–7. A single-tuft brush with a bent shank may prove helpful (figure 24–8). Prevention of

---

*Definitions in this chapter that pertain to orthodontic appliances are taken from or adapted from the *Orthodontic Glossary*, 1987 edition, American Society of Orthodontists, 460 N. Lindbergh Blvd., St. Louis, Missouri 63141-7883.

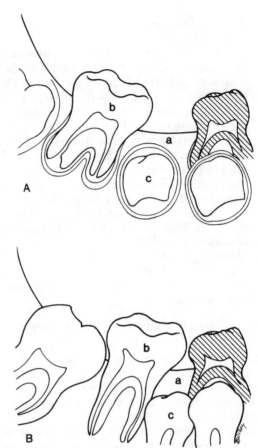

Figure 24–6. Premature Loss of Second Primary Molar. A. Developing first permanent molar (b) inclines and drifts to the mesial into the space (a) from which the second primary molar was removed. Developing second premolar (c) is crowded. **B.** Space from which molar was removed (a) is nearly closed by the mesial drift and eruption of the first permanent molar (b). Developing second premolar (c) is closed in and prevented from eruption. Note that the second permanent molar has impacted against the first molar.

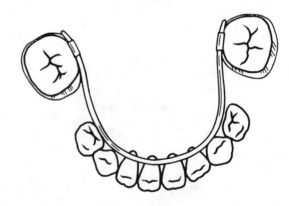

Figure 24–7. Space Maintainer. Bilateral lingual mandibular space maintainer with orthodontic bands cemented around the permanent molars to hold the lingual arch wire. Space from which primary molar was removed is being maintained for eruption of premolar.

dental caries and gingivitis can be especially important during the ages of mixed dentition.

III. Removable Space Maintainer

A. Description

The removable appliance is constructed with an acrylic base and stainless steel wire formed into clasps. A lingual bar of stainless steel may be used for a mandibular appliance.

B. Personal Care Procedures

The removable space maintainer is similar to a removable partial denture, and the methods for denture hygiene described on page 344 apply. Care of natural teeth, the abutments, and clasped teeth requires continuing demonstration and motivation for the young patient.

FIXED PARTIAL DENTURES

A partial denture replaces one or more, but less than all, of the natural teeth.* The fixed partial denture, otherwise called a fixed bridge, cannot be removed, but is permanently attached to natural teeth, roots, or dental implant, which furnish support to the appliance.

I. Components of a Fixed Partial Denture (figure 24–9)

A. Abutment

A tooth or portion of an implant used for the support or anchorage of a prosthesis is called an abutment.

B. Retainer

An inlay, onlay, or crown that restores an abutment tooth and is used for fixation and support of the fixed partial denture is called a retainer.

C. Pontic

A pontic is an artificial tooth that replaces a lost natural tooth, restores its function, and usually occupies the space previously occupied by the natural crown.

D. Connector

A connector unites the retainer to the pontic or joins two individual pontics. In a fixed partial denture, the connector may be a solder joint, or when the entire bridge is cast as a single unit,

*All definitions in this chapter that pertain to prosthetic appliances are taken from or adapted from and are in accord with the *Glossary of Prosthetic Terms*, 5th ed. *J. Prosthet. Dent., 58*, 717, December, 1987.

the connector may be continuous with the retainer.

E. Surfaces

1. *Occlusal.* The surface that occludes with opposing teeth.
2. *Gingival.* The portion or side of the pontic that is adjacent to the edentulous gingiva beneath it.

II. Characteristics

A. Types of Fixed Partial Dentures

1. *Natural Teeth Supported*
   a. Bilateral: Supported by one or more natural teeth at each end (figure 24–9A).
   b. Cantilever: Supported by one or more teeth at one end only (figure 24–9B).
   c. Resin-bonded cast metal bridge: Uses resin-bonded retainer attached to etched enamel; characterized by little or no removal of tooth structure.
2. *Implant Supported.* Blade, cylinder, and screw types of implants used for abutments are shown in figure 25–7 (page 360).

B. Criteria for Fixed Partial Denture[2]

1. Harmonious with the teeth and surrounding periodontium.
2. All parts accessible for cleaning by the patient and the professional.
3. Must not interfere with the cleaning regimen for the remaining natural dentition.
4. Must not traumatize oral tissues.

III. Care Procedures

A. Debris Removal

When suggesting a procedure to follow for cleaning the oral cavity when a fixed partial denture is present, debris removal with an oral irrigator may be recommended as a first step. By removing food and debris, access of the toothbrush and other aids for plaque removal is facilitated. The patient must understand the function of the irrigator and be aware that the bacterial plaque has not been removed. Procedure for use of an oral irrigator is described on pages 324–326.

B. Plaque Removal from Abutment Teeth

Nearly all the methods proposed for bacterial plaque control in the two previous chapters may be applicable to abutment teeth. The proximal surface and gingiva of an abutment tooth adjacent to a pontic usually require special attention.

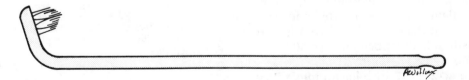

Figure 24–8. Single-tuft Brush with Bent Shank. Adaptation of brush permits easier access to the lingual and palatal aspects of natural teeth as well as to orthodontic or prosthetic appliances.

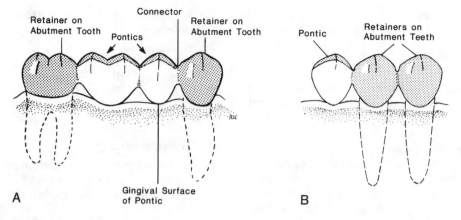

Figure 24–9. Fixed Partial Dentures. A. Characteristic parts of mandibular four-unit fixed partial denture. Cast gold crowns on the abutment teeth serve as the retainers for this bridge. **B.** Cantilever bridge supported by double abutment.

1. *Toothbrushing.* Sulcular brushing is generally indicated. The area of the tooth surface adjacent to and beneath the gingival margin must be kept meticulously free of bacterial plaque.

2. *Dentifrice Selection.* A nonabrasive dentifrice is indicated to prevent the possibility of abrasion when pontic or crown facings are made of acrylic, when the gold of the partial denture is highly polished and could be scratched, and when there are areas of root exposure on abutment teeth.

    A fluoride-containing dentifrice is important for protection of remaining tooth surfaces, particularly exposed cementum.

3. *Additional Interdental Care.* An interdental plaque removal method is indicated. This method is selected on the basis of the individual patient or the appliance. The interdental cleaning device is adapted specifically to the distal of the mesial abutment and the mesial of the distal abutment, and from both facial and lingual. The same interdental cleaning procedure can usually be applied to the gingival surface of the fixed partial denture. Interdental cleaning methods and devices are described on pages 317–324.

C. The Appliance

1. *Areas Requiring Emphasis.* The gingival surfaces of the pontics and beneath the connectors are particularly prone to plaque retention.

2. *Toothbrushing.* A toothbrush in the Charters position may be helpful for cleaning the gingival surface of the pontic from the facial aspect. The filaments can be directed under the pontic to clean the gingival surface. Charters brush position is described on page 308.

3. *Dental Floss*
    a. Thread a 12- to 15-inch length into a floss threader. Several types are available (figure 24–10).

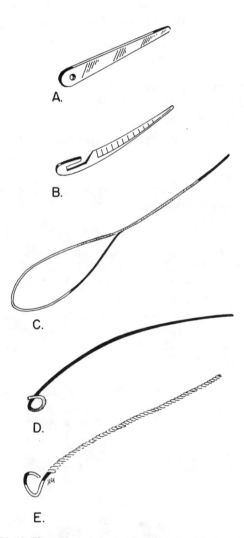

Figure 24–10. Floss Threaders. A. Clear plastic with closed eye. **B.** Tinted plastic with open eye. **C.** Soft plastic loop. **D.** Flexible wire. **E.** Twisted wire.

b. Apply threader between an abutment and pontic.

c. Draw the floss through, and using single or double thickness, remove loose debris (figure 24–11).

d. Apply dentifrice and a new section of the floss with moderate pressure to the undersurface (gingival surface) of the pontic and then to the proximal surfaces of each abutment tooth to remove bacterial plaque. Remove floss.

4. *Knitting Yarn.* Put length of yarn or tufted floss in floss threader and pull through under the appliance for a cleaning device that is thicker than floss alone (pages 320–321).

5. *Other Interdental Devices.* A pipe cleaner, interdental brush, a single-tuft brush, or an interdental tip should be recommended and demonstrated as indicated by the needs of the individual appliance. These devices usually fit mesial and distal to the pontic, but not over the gingival surface of the pontic. Yarn or tufted floss with threader is essential.

REMOVABLE PARTIAL DENTURES

The removable partial denture replaces one or more, but less than all, of the natural teeth and associated structures, and can be removed from the mouth and replaced at will. Depending on the location and number of remaining natural teeth, a partial denture may receive all its support from the teeth, or it may be partly toothborne and partly tissueborne.

Self-care procedures for the patient with a removable appliance involve much more than cleaning the appliance. The abutment teeth, the gingival tissue, and the mucosa of edentulous areas require regular attention. Gingival health is unfavorably affected by removable partial dentures because bacterial plaque tends to accumulate more readily and in greater quantities. Plaque control is a major factor in the long-term effectiveness of a removable partial denture.

Procedures suggested here for care of the removable partial denture apply also to various other removable appliances. Examples of these are removable space maintainers, appliances for orthodontic purposes, such as a Hawley biteplate or retainer (figure 24–4), obturators for closure of palatal openings, such as for cleft palate (page 585) or for replacement of tissue removed in the treatment of oral cancer.

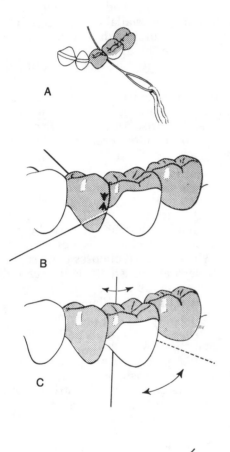

Figure 24–11. Use of Floss Threader. A. Use floss threader to draw the floss (or yarn or tufted floss) between abutment and a pontic. **B.** Apply floss to the distal surface of the mesial abutment; pull through 1 or 2 inches. **C.** Slide floss under pontic. Move back and forth several times, as shown by the arrows, to remove bacterial plaque from the gingival surface of the pontic. **D.** Apply new section of floss to the mesial surface of the distal abutment.

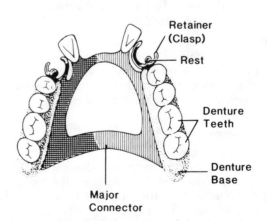
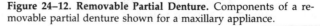

Figure 24–12. Removable Partial Denture. Components of a removable partial denture shown for a maxillary appliance.

I. Components of a Removable Partial Denture
(figure 24–12)

The selection of cleansing agents and the procedures for cleaning are complicated by the intricacy of the metallic parts and their relation to the natural teeth, as well as by the dental materials used in construction.

A. Abutment
An abutment is a natural tooth or portion of an implant used for the support or anchorage of an appliance.

B. Denture Base
The denture base is the part of the partial denture that rests on the oral mucosa and carries the artificial teeth. The base may be made of plastic resin or alloys of gold or chrome.

C. Denture Teeth
The teeth of a partial denture may be made of porcelain, plastic resin, or metal.

D. Major Connectors
Connectors are bars of rigid metal that unite the parts of a partial denture. In the maxillary arch, there can be one or two *palatal bars* or full palatal coverage. The mandibular arch contains a *lingual bar.*

Minor connectors may be placed between the major connectors and other units, such as clasps and occlusal rests.

E. Retainer
Any type of clasp, attachment, or device used for the fixation or stabilization of an appliance is called a retainer.

F. Precision Attachment
A precision attachment is a type of retainer that consists of a metal receptacle and a close-fitting part. The metal receptacle is usually included within the restoration of an abutment tooth, and the close-fitting part is attached to a pontic or denture framework. The precision attachments are used for removable partial dentures and occasionally for fixed partial and overdentures. A wide variety of attachments is available.[3]

G. Rest
A rigid, stabilizing extension of a fixed or removable partial denture that contacts a remaining tooth or teeth for the dissipation of vertical or horizontal forces is known as a rest.

II. Objectives

A. The Appliance
Because natural teeth are adjacent to the appliance, objectives for cleaning the appliance take on added significance. The basic objectives are to remove irritants to the oral tissues (primarily bacterial plaque), prevent mouth odors, and improve appearance.

B. The Natural Teeth
The objective is to control plaque for the prevention of dental caries and periodontal infection.

III. Cleaning a Removable Appliance

Rinsing, immersion, and brushing methods, as well as the cleansing agents described for the complete denture on pages 346–349, apply alike to the partial appliance, with the few additions noted below.

A. Rinsing
After each meal, the denture and the natural teeth should be brushed. When regular cleaning facilities are not available, rinsing is important for both the natural teeth and the removable appliance. While the appliance is out, the tongue can be used to rub the sides of abutment teeth.

B. Immersion
Before immersion, the denture must be cleaned by rinsing and brushing to remove all bacterial plaque and debris. An agent known to discolor metal can be avoided. Procedures for immersion cleaning are described on pages 347–348.

C. Brushing
1. *Recommended Brushes*
   a. Toothbrush: One or more should be reserved for the natural teeth. The use of a regular toothbrush for partial care of a removable appliance is not recommended. When a patient chooses to do so, however, a separate brush is definitely indicated. Brushing the clasps and other metal parts can deform the filaments and make the brush ineffective for use on natural teeth.
   b. Powered brush: A powered toothbrush is sometimes appropriate for the natural teeth of the patient with a partial denture. The powered brush, however, should not be used in and about the intricate clasps and other parts of a removable appliance because of the danger of catching the brush and damaging the appliance.
   c. Clasp brush: A specially designed narrow, tapered, cylindrical brush about 2 to 3 inches long that can be adapted to the inner surfaces of clasps is recommended (figure 24–13). Clasps and their connectors are closely adapted to the supporting teeth, and the protected internal surfaces are prone to plaque accumulation. These difficult-to-clean areas require special care.
   d. Denture brush: A denture brush is shown in figure 24–15 and described on page 348. It is an excellent brush for cleaning all the smooth surfaces and the metal bars of the partial denture.
2. *Precautions During Brushing.* Too tight a grasp of a partial appliance can result in bending or fracture of clasps or bars. Filaments of a brush

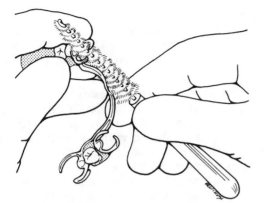

Figure 24–13. Clasp Brush. A brush specially designed to remove bacterial plaque from the inside surfaces of clasps is available. The denture must be held carefully to avoid accidents.

can inadvertently catch the appliance and cause it to drop. Partial filling of the sink with water or lining of the sink with a face cloth or towel is necessary to prevent accidents that cause breakage (page 348).

IV. The Natural Teeth

A. Plaque Control

Toothbrushing and interdental cleaning methods selected for the particular needs of the patient must be followed meticulously. The longevity of the removable appliance depends on the health of the supporting teeth, and in turn, the health of the natural teeth depends on the cleanliness of the appliance.

B. Dental Caries Control

The topical application of fluoride, the use of a fluoride dentifrice and other self-applied fluoride measures, such as a daily mouthrinse or application of a gel, and the control of refined sugars in the diet must be definite parts of the complete program of oral care for the patient with a removable appliance.

The patient must be constantly alert to the control of plaque retention by the appliance and to the need for rinsing immediately after eating when brushing is not possible. For the patient who has been caries-susceptible, and whose teeth are missing because of dental caries, a dietary analysis and specific dental caries control program may increase a patient's motivation.

COMPLETE DENTURES

One should not assume that the patient who is new to the dental office and is wearing dentures or a denture knows the proper techniques for caring for the appliances. During questioning for the patient history, information about the method and frequency of denture care is recorded. Later, the dentures are examined and the current method of care is reviewed.

Alternate cleansing agents, devices, or procedures are recommended and demonstrated as indicated.

Instruction may be given to the patient receiving a maxillary and mandibular denture for the first time, to the patient whose dentures have been remade or relined, or to the patient with a single denture that opposes natural teeth. Another patient may be receiving an immediate denture, that is, a denture inserted immediately following removal of natural teeth. Types of dentures and characteristics of the edentulous mouth are described on pages 573–574.

I. Components of a Complete Denture (figure 24–14)

In an effort to understand the effects of various cleansing agents and devices, information about the structure and material of the parts of a denture is pertinent.

A. Denture Base

The part of a denture that rests on the oral mucosa and to which the teeth are attached is the denture base. Most denture bases are made of plastic resin. Others may be metal, for example, chrome-cobalt or gold in combination with a plastic resin.

B. Surfaces

1. *Impression Surface.* Also called the tissue or inner surface, the impression surface is the part that lies adjacent to the mucous membrane of the alveolar ridge and immediately associated parts; in the maxillary, the tissue surface is adjacent to the hard palate.
2. *Polished Surface.* The external or outer surface is highly polished. The occlusal surface is not polished.
3. *Occlusal Surface.* The portion of the surface of a denture that makes contact or near contact with the corresponding surface of the oppos-

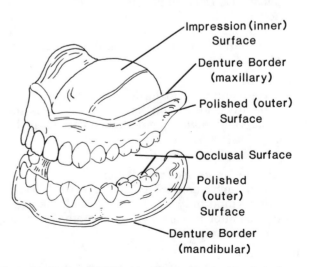

Figure 24–14. Complete Denture. The surfaces and borders of maxillary and mandibular dentures.

ing denture or natural teeth is the occlusal surface.

C. Teeth

The denture teeth may be made of plastic resin or porcelain. Some posterior teeth have metal occlusal inserts. Anterior porcelain teeth have metal pins for retention.

II. Purposes for Cleaning

Inadequate oral tissue care and denture hygiene practices are major causes of oral lesions under dentures.

A. Prevent Irritation to the Oral Tissues

1. *Mechanical Irritants.* Rough deposits of plaque, calculus, thick stains.
2. *Chemical Irritants.* Products of putrefaction of food debris and bacterial metabolic products.

B. Control Infection

Reactions to bacterial denture plaque and/or secondary infections by way of traumatic lesions may occur.

C. Prevent Mouth Odors

D. Maintain Appearance

III. Denture Deposits

Accumulation of stains and deposits on dentures varies between individuals in a manner similar to that on natural teeth. The phases of deposit formation may be divided as follows:

A. Mucin and Food Debris on the Denture Surface

Readily removed by rinsing or brushing.

B. Denture Pellicle and Bacterial Plaque

Denture pellicle forms readily after a denture is cleaned. Denture plaque is composed predominantly of gram-positive cocci, rods, and filamentous forms of bacteria in an intermicrobial substance. Denture plaque also includes varying accumulations of *Candida albicans.*

Plaque serves as a matrix for calculus formation and stain accumulation when the denture is not cleaned.

C. Calculus

Hard and fixed to the denture surface, calculus generally is located on the buccal of the maxillary molars and lingual of mandibular anterior region.

IV. Methods for Cleaning

A. Rinsing under Running Water

Although a denture that could be kept clean by this method only would be unusual, the use of rinsing after meals when other methods are not possible is necessary.

B. Brushing

Brush with water, soap, or other mild cleansing agent. Coarse abrasives produce scratches.

C. Immersion

The denture is soaked in a solvent or detergent in which chemical action removes or loosens stains and deposits that can then be rinsed or brushed away.

D. Mechanical Denture Cleansers[4]

Commercially available devices include ultrasonic, sonic, magnetic, and agitating mechanisms that can be combined with an immersion agent. The action of the mechanical cleansing device seems to make the solution more efficient than a solution used alone. Ultrasonic cleaning during a professional appointment is described on page 514.

V. Denture Cleansers[4–8]

A. Requirements for a Denture Cleanser[8]

1. Easy for a patient to use.
2. Reasonably priced.
3. Effective removal of denture deposits (organic and inorganic) without abrasion of the denture surface.
4. Bactericidal and fungicidal action.
5. Nontoxic.
6. Harmless to the dental materials used for partial or complete dentures.

B. Chemical Solution Cleansers (Immersion)

1. *Alkaline Hypochlorite*
   a. Active ingredient: Dilute sodium hypochlorite with bleaching properties.
   b. Action: Loosen debris and light stains; bleaching; dissolve mucin; dissolve plaque matrix.
   c. Example: Household bleach.
   d. Disadvantages: Odor; tarnish; surface pitting; bleaching effect on soft lining materials and denture materials containing fibers.[4]
2. *Alkaline Peroxide*
   a. Active ingredient: Alkaline detergent with an oxygen-liberating agent (sodium perborate or percarbonate).
   b. Action: Loosen debris and light stains by an oxygen-liberating mechanism. A preventive cleanser should be used regularly from the day a denture has been cleaned professionally to prevent accumulation of heavy deposits.
   c. Examples: Most proprietary cleansers are in the form of a powder or tablet that is dropped into water to create the alkaline solution of hydrogen peroxide.
   d. Disadvantage: Will not remove heavy stains or calculus.
3. *Dilute Acids*
   a. Active ingredient: Inorganic acids.
   b. Action: Dissolve inorganic components of denture deposits.
   c. Examples: 3% to 5% hydrochloric acid

alone or with phosphoric acid; commercially prepared ultrasonic solutions. The strong acids (although in dilute form) are not recommended for home use by the patient. Acetic acid (vinegar) has been used with some success if deposits are not old and hard.

    d. Disadvantage: Corrosion of metal parts of a denture.

  4. *Enzymes.* The enzymes act to break down plaque proteins and polysaccharides. Enzyme agents have been incorporated into various immersion-type cleansers.

  5. *Disinfectants.* A sanitary denture is necessary for the prevention of inflammation in the oral mucosa under the denture. Types of denture-induced lesions are described on pages 576–577.

    Effective methods for minimizing bacterial plaque accumulation are described in Section VI. Regular daily maintenance procedures must be carried out.

    Disinfection of dentures to prevent cross-contamination between patients and dental health care personnel can be accomplished by using a hypochlorite solution. Full-strength commercially available sodium hypochlorite has been shown to be an antimicrobial agent and can accomplish sterilization of a denture by immersion for 5 minutes.[9]

C. Abrasive Cleansers (Brushing)

  1. *Denture Pastes and Powders, Toothpastes and Powders*

    a. Active ingredient: An abrasive, such as calcium carbonate (see Dentifrices, page 326).

    b. Action: Mechanical removal of bacterial plaque and stains by brushing.

    c. Examples: Various commercial products.

    d. Disadvantage: Can abrade the plastic resin denture base and acrylic teeth. A paste with low abrasiveness should be selected.

  2. *Household Agents*

    a. Active ingredient: Detergent and/or abrasive agent.

    b. Examples: Salt and bicarbonate of soda are mildly abrasive; hand soap is cleansing and not particularly abrasive. Scouring powders or other excessively abrasive cleansers should not be used.

VI. General Cleaning Procedures

A. When to Clean

  1. Regularly after each meal and before retiring.

  2. Chemical immersion daily or twice weekly, depending on the rate of formation of calculus and stain and the type of solution used.

    a. May be at one of the daily cleanings.

    b. Suggested while bathing.

    c. Overnight when denture is removed as instructed by the dentist.

B. Selection of Procedure for Cleaning

    Immersion, followed by brushing, is recommended. When unable to clean, rinsing after eating is advised.

C. Preparation for Cleaning

  1. Rinse the denture thoroughly when it is taken from the mouth to remove saliva and loose debris.*

  2. Remove denture-adherent material

    a. Definition: A denture adherent is a commercially available paste or powder preparation.[4] A patient may use it under the direction of the dentist for temporary stabilization. An occasional patient may use an adherent indefinitely in an attempt to get along with ill-fitting dentures that should be adjusted or rebased.

    b. Method: Use a brush to remove the adherent with care.

    c. Denture-bearing mucosa: Rinse and clean with a brush twice or more times daily (page 349).

VII. Cleaning by Immersion

A. Advantages

  1. The solution reaches all areas of the denture for a complete cleaning.

  2. Minimizes danger of dropping the appliance. Prevents need for handling, which is required during brushing.

  3. Offers safe storage when dentures are out of the mouth.

  4. Aids persons with limited ability to manage a brush.

  5. When cleaning is distasteful, immersion involves the least handling and observation. This advantage is particularly attractive to an attendant or nurse who must clean the denture of a helpless patient.

B. Procedure

  1. Place denture in a plastic container with fitted cover that is maintained specifically for this purpose.

  2. Use only warm water for rinsing and for mixing the solution. Warm water promotes the action of the cleanser. Hot water should never be used because it can distort plastic resin.

  3. Follow manufacturer's specifications to assure correct dilution of cleanser.

  4. Check that the denture is completely submerged in the solution; cover the container.

  5. When the denture is removed, rinse under running water and remove loosened debris and chemicals before proceeding to clean by brushing.

  6. Empty and clean container daily. Mix fresh

---

*Procedure for removal of a denture for a patient is described on page 513.

solution to prevent contamination and growth of microorganisms.[10]

C. Solutions

1. *Proprietary.* Available in powder or tablet form.
   a. Preparation: Add measured warm water as directed by the manufacturer.
   b. Length of immersion: Usually 10 to 15 minutes or as suggested by the manufacturer. Because the action depends on the mechanical bubbling effect of released oxygen, the solution has little value after the available oxygen has been released.
   c. Effect: The solutions are only effective against loose debris; denture cleanliness depends on regular daily immersion supplemented by brushing.

2. *Hypochlorite Solution.* Household bleach (5% sodium hypochlorite) and Calgone. Calgone acts to improve the penetrating and detaching power of the bleach.
   a. Proportions

   > 1 tablespoon (15 ml.) sodium hypochlorite (household bleach)
   > 2 teaspoons (8 ml.) Calgone
   > 4 ounces (114 ml.) water

   b. Length of immersion: Usually 10 to 15 minutes. When stains or calculus form, the patient should be instructed to soak the denture overnight provided there are no metal parts that can become corroded.

3. *White Household Vinegar*
   a. Indication for use: Only when calculus is observed on the denture; not routinely.
   b. Proportion: 1 or 2 teaspoonfuls in 1 cup of warm water.
   c. Length of immersion: The denture may be immersed overnight when necessary for complete cleaning. Two or three soakings may be needed to loosen hard calculus.

VIII. Cleaning by Brushing

A. Type of Brush

1. *Denture Brush.* A good-quality denture brush with end-rounded filaments is recommended. The styles of denture brushes vary. One type shown in figure 24–15 is designed with two arrangements of filaments. One group in a large round arrangement of tufts permits access to the inner, curved impression surface of the denture. The second group of tufts is arranged to form a rectangular brush for convenient adaptation to the polished and occlusal denture surfaces. Another design is shown in figure 50–8, page 625.

2. *Other Brushes.* A few patients prefer not to have a denture brush for personal reasons. A hand brush can be used, provided the filaments are long enough to reach into the deeper

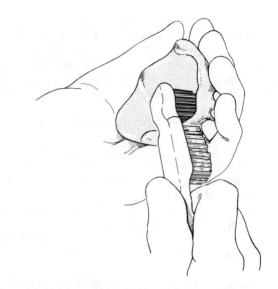

Figure 24–15. Denture Brush. The denture is held securely, but without squeezing, in the palm of the nonworking hand. Place a face cloth in the bottom of the sink and partially fill with water. The specially designed brush is preferred because one group of tufts is arranged to provide access to the inner impression surface of the denture, as shown.

portions of the impression surfaces. Prerequisite is that each area of each surface of the denture must be reached by the brush if bacterial plaque formation is to be controlled.

If a patient prefers to use an ordinary toothbrush, a multitufted soft nylon brush with end-rounded filaments should be acceptable if access to all the inner curvatures is possible without applying undue pressure on certain parts in the attempt to clean others. The patient who wears a single denture should keep separate brushes for the natural teeth and the denture to maintain the brush for the natural teeth in the best condition possible.

B. Procedure

1. Grasp denture in palm of hand securely, but without a squeezing pressure because dentures can be broken (figure 24–15).
2. Hold the denture low in a sink in which a towel, wash cloth, or rubber mat has been spread over the bottom to serve as a cushion should the denture be dropped. The sink should be partially filled with water.
3. Apply warm water, nonabrasive cleanser, and brush to all areas of the denture. Particular attention should be paid the impression surfaces where configurations of the surface correspond with those of the oral topography. The anterior areas of the inner surfaces of both the maxillary and mandibular dentures require special adaptations of the brush.
4. Rinse denture and brush under running water. Use the brush to remove denture cleanser that may be retained in the grooves.

5. Visually check each area carefully for bacterial plaque. Teach the patient to run a finger over the surfaces to find "slippery" plaque areas.

C. Precautions Related to Brushing
1. Overzealous brushing with an abrasive cleansing agent on the impression surface could alter the fit of the denture.
2. Plastic resin can be abraded. Scratches make a rough surface; the denture may become more subject to the collection of debris and calculus.
3. Possibility of incomplete coverage during cleaning, particularly in the more inaccessible areas.
4. Possibility of cleaning with uneven pressure when the brush is applied more vigorously to accessible areas.
5. Danger of dropping and breaking the denture is increased when it is wet and, therefore, slippery.
6. Patient who requires eyeglasses should be advised to wear them when brushing to watch the procedure and to observe the cleanliness of the denture after brushing.

IX. Additional Instructions

A. Care of Plastic Resin
An appliance made with plastic resin should be immersed in water or cleansing solution when it is not in the mouth.

B. Prevention of Denture Deposits
When the denture is kept clean by regular procedures from the time of insertion, accumulation of heavy stains and calculus can be prevented.

C. Professional Maintenance
A denture should never be scraped by the patient with a sharp instrument in the attempt to remove calculus deposits. When the cleaning methods recommended in this chapter do not remove deposits, the denture should be taken to the dental hygienist and dentist for professional cleaning. A regular maintenance plan is arranged.

D. Paste Cleaners
Paste cleansers (dentifrices or denture pastes) may cling and be difficult to rinse from the denture. Residual chemical agents, such as essential oils, may cause inflammatory or allergic reactions of the oral mucosa, and phenolic agents can have deleterious effects on plastic resin.

E. Soft Lining Materials
Temporary soft conditioning lining material may be sensitive to proprietary cleansers. Washing with cold water and a soft cloth, cotton, or soft brush (gently) can be suggested. The denture plaque should be removed several times each day. Outer, polished surfaces should be thoroughly brushed in the usual manner. When the denture is placed in water overnight, the teeth should be placed down so that the soft material at the denture border cannot become deformed.[11]

X. The Underlying Mucosa

A. Rinsing
Each time the denture is removed, the mouth should be rinsed thoroughly with warm water or a mild salt solution (pages 329). The patient can learn to clean the mucosa by rubbing over the edentulous areas with the tongue.

B. Cleaning
The edentulous mucosa should be brushed at least once daily. A soft brush with end-rounded filaments is applied in long, straight strokes from posterior to anterior.

C. Massage
For stimulation of circulation and increased resistance to trauma, frequent massage is recommended. Methods for massage that may be suggested to the patient are:
1. *Digital.* Place thumb and index finger over the ridge and apply massage with a press-and-release stroke. The palate may be rubbed with the ball of the thumb.
2. *Multitufted Soft Toothbrush.* Apply sides of filaments and vibratory motion to each area. Prevent trauma to the tissue by placing the brush carefully and avoiding scrubbing with undue pressure.
3. *Powered Brush.* Apply to each area with smooth, even strokes.

COMPLETE OVERDENTURE

An overdenture is a complete denture supported by both retained natural teeth or implants and the soft tissue of the residual alveolar ridge. It also has been known as an overlay denture, coping denture, and tooth-mucosa-supported denture.

I. Purposes
The advantages of an overdenture when compared with a denture in a completely edentulous mouth are that the natural teeth
A. Help to preserve bone.
B. Allow the remaining teeth to bear occlusal pressures, thereby reducing the pressures placed on edentulous areas.
C. Improve stability and retention of the denture.
D. Improve the patient's tactile and proprioceptive senses by having the periodontal ligament present.
E. Increase the patient's psychologic acceptance of the denture. The patient does not feel that all natural teeth have been lost.

II. Criteria
The overdenture should be considered for any patient whose treatment plan calls for extraction of all teeth. Teeth to be preserved must meet certain standards of health.

A. Periodontal Condition

Because wearing the overdenture brings stress to the periodontium, the tissues must have, or be treatable to obtain, the following:

1. Healthy sulci. There must be no bleeding or other signs of inflammation; minimal sulci depth; and all requirements of health (table 11–1, pages 174–175).
2. A band of attached gingiva (page 169).

B. Bone Support

The bone level following tooth preparation must be adequate to withstand occlusal forces.

C. Teeth

Teeth must have minimal mobility. Teeth selected are frequently the mandibular canines and premolars, and maxillary canines.

III. Preparation of the Teeth

A. Endodontics

Most preserved teeth need endodontic therapy because the crown will be reduced.

B. Periodontics

Treatment procedures depend on clinical findings, but may include measures to eliminate inflammation and pockets, to increase the zone of attached gingiva, or to reshape the architecture of the bone or gingival tissue.

C. Restorative

1. Tooth crowns are reduced to short rounded preparations or, for some patients, to the level and contour of the gingival margin.
2. An amalgam or composite restoration may cover the root canals, or the teeth may be protected by a gold coping (figure 24–16). A coping is a cast thin metal covering or cap.
3. The gold coping may be used as a retainer for a retentive attachment.

IV. Dental Hygiene Care and Instruction

The patient must be well informed concerning the problems of care of the retained teeth and gingiva. A high degree of motivation to want to save the remaining teeth is needed.

A. Denture Care

The impression surface of the denture must be kept meticulously free from plaque accumulation. Denture care is outlined on pages 347–349.

B. Gingival Tissue and Natural Teeth

1. Complete daily bacterial plaque removal using a soft brush with end-rounded filaments or a powered toothbrush is needed.
2. Interdental tip or a toothpick in holder should be used daily to trace around each natural tooth to clean subgingivally (pages 321, 323).
3. Massage of the edentulous mucosa should be demonstrated (page 349).

C. Fluoride

A specific fluoride application plan must be included. The requirements depend partly on the

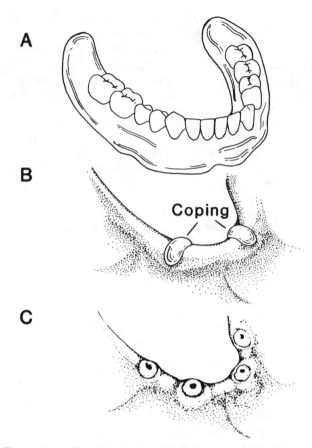

Figure 24–16. Overdenture. A. Mandibular complete denture. **B.** Support provided by gold cap copings. **C.** Natural teeth with amalgam restoration in the coronal portion of the root canal opening.

past history of dental caries. When the teeth have been extracted because of dental caries, caries control measures take on special significance, particularly if dietary habits remain the same. Current dietary habits must be checked by asking the patient to keep a daily food diary (pages 382–386). Limitations on sucrose intake can be recommended accordingly.

1. *Fluoride Self-application.* All patients must use a fluoride dentifrice. In addition, either a mouthrinse or a gel-tray can be recommended. After cleaning, the patient's denture can be used for a custom tray, and the gel drops can be placed inside at the locations of the natural teeth. Pressure of the denture as it is seated will force the gel about the teeth.
2. *Professional Topical Applications.* When daily mouthrinse or gel-tray is not carried out by the patient or when additional fluoride is indicated, professional topical applications are made. Because frequent maintenance appointments are needed to check the health of the gingival tissues, an application can be made at each such appointment. Benefit is derived from the fluoride in direct proportion to the frequency of application: the more fre-

quent the application of fluoride, the greater the benefit derived.

D. Maintenance Appointments

Supervision by frequent maintenance appointments for scaling and planing, topical fluoride applications, and motivation and instruction for plaque control is essential.

TECHNICAL HINTS

I. Review instructions for each patient with a fixed or removable prosthesis. Do not assume that, because a denture has been in use for a long time, the patient knows how to clean it properly or how to care for the adjacent soft tissue.

II. Prevent cross-contamination when receiving a denture from a patient by:
   A. Wearing protective gloves.
   B. Offering a container or disposable napkin in which the patient can place the denture.
   C. Scrubbing the denture with disinfectant soap using a disposable scrub brush or a brush that can be resterilized.
   D. Wearing gloves and a mask while cleaning the appliance and directing scrub strokes away from oneself and into the sink to prevent contamination of clothes.

III. Acrylic restorations, crowns and pontics are subject to toothbrush dentifrice abrasion. Select soft brush and nonabrasive cleansing material.

IV. Provide printed instructions for each patient. Personalize the instructions with notations related to particular problem areas of the patient.

V. Source of educational materials:

   American Dental Association
   Order Department
   211 East Chicago Avenue
   Chicago, Illinois 60611.

   Request current catalog. Samples of the following booklets are available on request:

   Orthodontics: Questions and Answers
   Removable Partial Dentures
   Fixed Bridges and Crowns
   Dentures: What You Don't Know Can Hurt You

References

1. Attarzadeh, F.: Water Irrigating Devices for the Orthodontic Patient, *Int. J. Orthod., 24,* 15, Spring, 1986.
2. Obreschkow, C.: Oral Hygiene and Periodontal Considerations in Restorative Treatment with Prefabricated Attachments and Precision-milled Prosthetic Devices, *Int. J. Periodont. Rest. Dent., 4,* 73, Number 1, 1985.
3. American Dental Association, Council on Dental Materials, Instruments, and Equipment: *Dentist's Desk Reference: Materials, Instruments and Equipment,* 2nd ed. Chicago, American Dental Association, 1983, pp. 137–166.
4. Ibid., pp. 422–426.
5. Budtz-Jorgensen, E.: Materials and Methods for Cleaning Dentures, *J. Prosthet. Dent., 42,* 619, December, 1979.
6. Gallagher, J.B., Jr.: *Handbook For Complete Dentures.* Boston, Tufts University School of Dental Medicine, 1981.
7. American Dental Association, Council on Dental Materials, Instruments, and Equipment: Denture Cleansers, *J. Am. Dent. Assoc., 106,* 77, January, 1983.
8. Abelson, D.C.: Denture Plaque and Denture Cleansers: Review of the Literature, *Gerodontics, 1,* 202, October, 1985.
9. Rudd, R.W., Senia, E.S., McCleskey, F.K., and Adams, E.D.: Sterilization of Complete Dentures with Sodium Hypochlorite, *J. Prosthet. Dent., 51,* 318, March, 1984.
10. DePaola, L.G. and Minah, G.E.: Isolation of Pathogenic Microorganisms from Dentures and Denture-soaking Containers of Myelosuppressed Cancer Patients, *J. Prosthet. Dent., 49,* 20, January, 1983.
11. Ortman, L.F.: Patient Education and Complete Denture Maintenance, in Winkler, S.: *Essentials of Complete Denture Prosthodontics.* Philadelphia, W.B. Saunders Co., 1979, p. 477.

Suggested Readings

Bloem, T.J., Razzoog, M.E., Chamberlain, B.B., and Lang, B.: Efficacy of Tissue Brushing as Measured By the Prosthodontic Tissue Index, *Spec. Care Dentist., 4,* 70, March-April, 1984.
Holt, R.A.: Instructions for Patients Who Receive Immediate Dentures, *J. Am. Dent. Assoc., 112,* 645, May, 1986.
Leivesley, W.D.: Guiding the Developing Mixed Dentition, *Aust. Dent. J., 29,* 154, June, 1984.
Tautin, F.S.: The Beneficial Effects of Tissue Massage for the Edentulous Patient, *J. Prosthet. Dent., 48,* 653, December, 1982.

Orthodontic Appliances

Bounoure, G.M. and Vezin, J.C.: Orthodontic Fluoride Protection, *J. Clin. Orthod., 14,* 321, May, 1980.
Boyd, R.L.: Longitudinal Evaluation of a System for Self-monitoring Plaque Control Effectiveness in Orthodontic Patients, *J. Clin. Periodontol., 10,* 380, July, 1983.
Carranza, F.A.: *Glickman's Clinical Periodontology,* 6th ed. Philadelphia, W.B. Saunders Co., 1984, pp. 409–411, 746–754.
Chung, A., Kudlick, E.M., Gregory, J.E., Royal, G.C., and Reindorf, C.A.: Toothbrushing and Transient Bacteremia in Patients Undergoing Orthodontic Treatment, *Am. J. Orthod. Dentofac. Orthop., 90,* 181, September, 1986.
Cohen, A.M., Moss, J.P., and Williams, D.W.: Oral Hygiene Instruction Prior to Orthodontic Treatment, A Preliminary Study, *Br. Dent. J., 155,* 277, October 22, 1983.
Corbett, J.A., Brown, L.R., Keene, H.J., and Horton, I.M.: Comparison of *Streptococcus mutans* Concentrations in Non-banded and Banded Orthodontic Patients, *J. Dent. Res., 60,* 1936, December, 1981.
Dyer, J.R. and Shannon, I.L.: MFP Versus Stannous Fluoride Mouthrinses for Prevention of Decalcification in Orthodontic Patients, *ASDC J. Dent. Child., 49,* 19, January-February, 1982.
Feliu, J.L.: Long-term Benefits of Orthodontic Treatment on Oral Hygiene, *Am. J. Orthod., 82,* 473, December, 1982.
Gaidry, D., Kudlick, E.M., Hutton, J.G., and Russell, D.M.: A Survey to Evaluate the Management of Orthodontic Patients with a History of Rheumatic Fever or Congenital Heart Disease, *Am. J. Orthod., 87,* 338, April, 1985.
Hamp, S.E., Lundström, F., and Nyman, S.: Periodontal Conditions in Adolescents Subjected to Multiband Orthodontic Treatment with Controlled Oral Hygiene, *Eur. J. Orthod., 4,* 77, May, 1982.
Hickory, W. and Nanda, R.: Nutritional Considerations in Orthodontics, *Dent. Clin. North Am., 25,* 195, January, 1981.
Huber, S.J., Vernino, A.R., and Nanda, R.S.: Professional Prophylaxis and Its Effect on the Periodontium of Full-banded Orthodontic Patients, *Am. J. Orthod. Dentofac. Orthop., 91,* 321, April, 1987.
Kvam, E., Gjerdet, N.R., and Bondevik, O.: Traumatic Ulcers and Pain During Orthodontic Treatment, *Community Dent. Oral Epidemiol., 15,* 104, April, 1987.
Lundström, F., Hamp, S.E., and Nyman, S.: Systematic Plaque Control in Children Undergoing Long-term Orthodontic Treatment, *Eur. J. Orthod., 2,* 27, Number 1, 1980.

Mattingly, J.A., Sauer, G.J., Yancey, J.M., and Arnold, R.R.: Enhancement of *Streptococcus mutans* Colonization by Direct Bonded Orthodontic Appliances, *J. Dent. Res., 62,* 1209, December, 1983.

Pender, N.: Aspects of Oral Health in Orthodontic Patients, *Br. J. Orthod., 13,* 95, April, 1986.

Polson, A.M. and Reed, B.E.: Long-term Effect of Orthodontic Treatment on Crestal Alveolar Bone Levels, *J. Periodontol., 55,* 28, January, 1984.

Rivera Circuns, A.L. and Tullock, J.F.C.: Gingival Invagination in Extraction Sites of Orthodontic Patients: Their Incidence, Effects on Periodontal Health, and Orthodontic Treatment, *Am. J. Orthod., 83,* 469, June, 1983.

Sadowsky, C. and BeGole, E.A.: Long-term Effects of Orthodontic Treatment on Periodontal Health, *Am. J. Orthod., 80,* 156, August, 1981.

Shaw, W.C., Addy, M., and Ray, C.: Dental and Social Effects of Malocclusion and Effectiveness of Orthodontic Treatment: A Review, *Community Dent. Oral Epidemiol., 8,* 36, February, 1980.

Stirrups, D.R., Laws, E.A., and Honigman, J.L.: The Effect of a Chlorhexidine Gluconate Mouthrinse on Oral Health During Fixed Appliance Orthodontic Treatment, *Br. Dent. J., 151,* 84, August 4, 1981.

Van Venrooy, J.R. and Proffit, W.R.: Orthodontic Care for Medically Compromised Patients: Possibilities and Limitations, *J. Am. Dent. Assoc., 111,* 262, August, 1985.

White, L.: Toothbrush Pressures of Orthodontic Patients, *Am. J. Orthod., 83,* 109, February, 1983.

Williams, S., Melsen, B., Agerbaek, N., and Asboe, V.: The Orthodontic Treatment of Malocclusion in Patients with Previous Periodontal Disease, *Br. J. Orthod., 9,* 178, October, 1982.

Partial Dentures

Bassiouny, M.A. and Grant, A.A.: Oral Hygiene for the Partially Edentulous, *J. Periodontol., 52,* 214, April, 1981.

Bergman, B., Hugoson, A., and Olsson, C.-O.: Caries, Periodontal and Prosthetic Findings in Patients with Removable Partial Dentures: A Ten-year Longitudinal Study, *J. Prosthet. Dent., 48,* 506, November, 1982.

Chandler, J.A. and Brudvik, J.S.: Clinical Evaluation of Patients Eight to Nine Years After Placement of Removable Partial Dentures, *J. Prosthet. Dent., 51,* 736, June, 1984.

Gomes, B.C., Renner, R.P., and Baer, P.N.: Periodontal Considerations in Removable Partial Dentures, *J. Am. Dent. Assoc., 101,* 496, September, 1980.

Gunne, H.-S.J.: The Effect of Removable Partial Dentures on Mastication and Dietary Intake, *Acta Odontol. Scand., 43,* 269, Number 5, 1985.

Markkanen, H., Lappalainen, R., Honkala, E., and Tuominen, R.: Periodontal Conditions with Removable Complete and Partial Dentures in the Adult Population Aged 30 Years and Over, *J. Oral Rehabil., 14,* 355, July, 1987.

Müller, H.-P.: The Effect of Artificial Crown Margins at the Gingival Margin on the Periodontal Conditions in a Group of Periodontally Supervised Patients Treated with Fixed Bridges, *J. Clin. Periodontol., 13,* 97, February, 1986.

Naylor, W.P. and Stewart, D.M.: The End-tuft Toothbrush for the Partially Edentulous Patient, *J. Prosthet. Dent., 52,* 311, August, 1984.

Rissin, L., Feldman, R.S., Kapur, K.K., and Chauncey, H.H.: Six-year Report of the Periodontal Health of Fixed and Removable Partial Denture Abutment Teeth, *J. Prosthet. Dent., 54,* 461, October, 1985.

Silness, J., Gustavsen, F., and Mangersnes, K.: The Relationship Between Pontic Hygiene and Mucosal Inflammation in Fixed Bridge Recipients, *J. Periodont. Res., 17,* 434, July, 1982.

Theilade, E., Budtz-Jorgensen, E., and Theilade, J.: Predominant Cultivable Microflora of Plaque on Removable Dentures in Patients with Healthy Oral Mucosa, *Arch. Oral Biol., 28,* 675, Number 8, 1983.

Wright, W.E.: Success with the Cantilever Fixed Partial Denture, *J. Prosthet. Dent., 55,* 537, May, 1986.

Denture Cleansing

Abelson, D.C.: Denture Plaque and Denture Cleansers, *J. Prosthet. Dent., 45,* 376, April, 1981.

American Dental Association, Council on Dental Materials, Instruments and Equipment: Denture Cleansers, *J. Am. Dent. Assoc., 106,* 77, January, 1983.

Augsburger, R.H. and Elahi, J.M.: Evaluation of Seven Proprietary Denture Cleansers, *J. Prosthet. Dent., 47,* 356, April, 1982.

Budtz-Jorgensen, E., Kelstrup, J., and Poulsen, S.: Reduction of Formation of Denture Plaque by a Protease (Alcalase), *Acta Odontol. Scand., 41,* 93, Number 2, 1983.

Catalan, A., Herrera, R., and Martinez, A.: Denture Plaque and Palatal Mucosa in Denture Stomatitis: Scanning Electron Microscopic and Microbiologic Study, *J. Prosthet. Dent., 57,* 581, May, 1987.

Davenport, J.C., Wilson, H.J., and Spence, D.: The Compatibility of Soft Lining Materials and Denture Cleansers, *Br. Dent. J., 161,* 13, July 5, 1986.

DePaola, L.G., Minah, G.E., and Elias, S.A.: Growth and Potential Pathogens in Denture-soaking Solution of Myelosuppressed Cancer Patients, *J. Prosthet. Dent., 51,* 554, April, 1984.

Frank, R.M. and Steuer, P.: Transmission Electron Microscopy of Plaque Accumulations in Denture Stomatitis, *J. Prosthet. Dent., 53,* 115, January, 1985.

Ghalichebaf, M., Graser, G.N., and Zander, H.A.: The Efficacy of Denture-cleansing Agents, *J. Prosthet. Dent., 48,* 515, November, 1982.

Goll, G., Smith, D.E., and Plein, J.B.: The Effect of Denture Cleansers on Temporary Soft Liners, *J. Prosthet. Dent., 50,* 466, October, 1983.

Gwinnett, A.J. and Caputo, L.: The Effectiveness of Ultrasonic Denture Cleaning: A Scanning Electron Microscope Study, *J. Prosthet. Dent., 50,* 20, July, 1983.

Heath, J.R., Davenport, J.C., and Jones, P.A.: The Abrasion of Acrylic Resin by Cleaning Pastes, *J. Oral Rehabil., 10,* 159, March, 1983.

Kastner, C., Svare, C.W., Scandrett, F.R., Kerber, P.E., Taylor, T.D., and Semler, H.E.: Effects of Chemical Denture Cleaners on the Flexibility of Cast Clasps, *J. Prosthet. Dent., 50,* 473, October, 1983.

Kempler, D., Myer, M., Kahl, E.A., and Martin, D.W.: The Efficacy of Sodium Hypochlorite as a Denture Cleanser, *Spec. Care Dentist., 2,* 112, May-June, 1982.

Lambert, J.P. and Kolstad, R.: Effect of a Benzoic Acid-detergent Germicide on Denture-borne *Candida albicans, J. Prosthet. Dent., 55,* 699, June, 1986.

Moore, T.C., Smith, D.E., and Kenny, G.E.: Sanitization of Dentures by Several Denture Hygiene Methods, *J. Prosthet. Dent., 52,* 158, August, 1984.

Mueller, H.J. and Greener, E.H.: Characterization of Some Denture Cleansers, *J. Prosthet. Dent., 43,* 491, May, 1980.

Mueller, H.J., Stanford, J.W., and Fan, P.L.: Silver Solders Exposed to Cleansers, *J. Am. Dent. Assoc., 106,* 43, January, 1983.

Murray, I.D., McCabe, J.F., and Storer, R.: Abrasivity of Denture Cleaning Pastes *in vitro* and *in situ, Br. Dent. J., 161,* 137, August 23, 1986.

Murray, I.D., McCabe, J.F., and Storer, R.: The Relationship Between the Abrasivity and Cleaning Power of the Dentifrice-type Denture Cleaners, *Br. Dent. J., 161,* 205, September 20, 1986.

Palenik, C.J. and Miller, C.H.: *In vitro* Testing of Three Denture-cleaning Systems, *J. Prosthet. Dent., 51,* 751, June, 1984.

Polyzois, G.L.: The Wearing of Complete Dentures: Guidance to Patients, *J. Oral Rehabil., 10,* 229, May, 1983.

Polyzois, G.L.: Denture Cleansing Habits. A Survey, *Aust. Dent. J., 28,* 171, June, 1983.

Robinson, J.G.: The Whitening of Acrylic Dentures: The Role of Denture Cleansers, *Br. Dent. J., 159,* 247, October 19, 1985.

Sharp, E.W., Biol, M.I., and Verran, J.: Denture Cleansers and *in vitro* Plaque, *J. Prosthet. Dent., 53,* 584, April, 1985.

Tamamoto, M., Hamada, T., Miyake, Y., and Suginaka, H.: Ability of Enzymes to Remove Candida, *J. Prosthet. Dent., 53,* 214, February, 1985.

Tarbet, W.J., Axelrod, S., Minkoff, S., and Fratarcangelo, P.A.: Denture Cleansing: A Comparison of Two Methods, *J Prosthet. Dent., 51,* 322, March, 1984.

Tarbet, W.J.: Denture Plaque: Quiet Destroyer, *J. Prosthet. Dent., 48,* 647, December, 1982.

Overdentures

Derkson, G.D. and MacEntee, M.M.: Effect of 0.4% Stannous Fluoride Gel on the Gingival Health of Overdenture Abutments, *J. Prosthet. Dent., 48,* 23, July, 1982.

Graser, G.N. and Caton, J.G.: Influence of Overdenture Abutment Tooth Contour on the Periodontium: A Preliminary Report, *J. Prosthet. Dent., 49,* 173, February, 1983.

Johnson, G.K. and Sivers, J.E.: Periodontal Considerations for Overdentures, *J. Am. Dent. Assoc., 114,* 468, April, 1987.

Johnson, L.: Overdentures Using Attachments and Inserts, *J. Am. Dent. Assoc., 106,* 352, March, 1983.

Keltjens, H.M.A.M., Schaeken, M.J.M., and van der Hoeven, J.S.: Microbial Aspects of Preventive Regimes in Patients with Overdentures, *J. Dent. Res., 66,* 1579, October, 1987.

Key, M.C.: Topical Fluoride Treatment of Overdenture Abutments, *Gen. Dent., 28,* 58, May-June, 1980.

Renner, R.P., Gomes, B.C., Shakun, M.L., Baer, P.N., Davis, R.K., and Camp, P.: Four-year Longitudinal Study of the Periodontal Health Status of Overdenture Patients, *J. Prosthet. Dent., 51,* 593, May, 1984.

Robbins, J.W.: Periodontal Considerations in the Overdenture Patient, *J. Prosthet. Dent., 46,* 596, December, 1981.

Toolson, L.B., Smith, D.E., and Phillips, C.: A 2-year Longitudinal Study of Overdenture Patients. Part II: Assessment of the Periodontal Health of Overdenture Abutments, *J. Prosthet. Dent., 47,* 4, January, 1982.

25 *The Patient with Oral Rehabilitation and Implants*

Complete oral rehabilitation refers to the combined treatment of the teeth and periodontium to restore health, function, and physical form. As generally used, *oral rehabilitation* applies to involved extensive restorative procedures in a mouth that cannot be treated with routine dental care. It is also known as *mouth rehabilitation, occlusal rehabilitation, occluso-rehabilitation, complete reconstruction,* or *periodontal prosthesis.*

The term *periodontal prosthesis* is used to designate restorative and prosthetic treatment that is necessary for the treatment of advanced periodontal disease. The prosthesis used may be a splint for immobilization or stabilization of a group of teeth or an entire arch, maxillary or mandibular.

Periodontal, restorative, and prosthetic treatments are interdependent. The function and duration of all restorative and prosthetic treatments depend directly on the health of the periodontium, which provides the attachment and support necessary for the restored tooth. Periodontal health, in turn, is influenced by restorative and prosthetic treatment. Many predisposing factors that contribute to the initiation, development, and progress of periodontal disease are a direct result of untreated dental caries, incomplete or inadequate restorations, unreplaced missing teeth, and inadequate occlusal relationships built into restorations or prostheses.

I. Objectives of Complete Rehabilitation

Objectives for complete rehabilitation involve the same principles as for all oral care and include the need to
A. Restore optimal functional occlusion.
B. Maintain the health of the periodontium.
C. Produce biologically contoured restorations in harmony with normal oral physiology.
D. Replace missing teeth.
E. Provide support to teeth with advanced bone loss and marked mobility.
F. Provide desirable esthetics.
G. Establish acceptable phonetics.

II. Components of Treatment

Complete oral reconstruction means total mouth involvement, which brings in many phases of dentistry, often accomplished by individual specialists. The overall treatment plan may include some or all of the following:

A. Extensive periodontal therapy involving various surgical procedures.
B. Occlusal adjustment.
C. Endodontic therapy.
D. Correction of oral habits.
E. Orthodontic tooth movement.
F. Splinting of teeth temporarily or permanently.
G. Restorations involving individual teeth: crowns, inlays, onlays.
H. Replacement of teeth by fixed and/or removable prostheses.
I. Dental implant.

III. Accomplishment of Treatment

Treatment may be long and involved for the patient who undergoes complete oral rehabilitation. It requires patience, persistence, and dedication of the patient, the dental hygienist, and the dentist.

The dental hygiene treatment plan overlaps every phase of the total treatment, beginning with the initial preparation of the patient's mouth. Maintenance and supervision of the patient's self-care program is essential throughout restorative and prosthetic therapy and continuing into the maintenance phase.

Specific measures for self-care in terms of plaque removal and dental caries prevention must be selected and supervised. The patient is shown how to self-evaluate, so that minor deviations from normal can be recognized and called to the attention of the dentist.

CHARACTERISTICS OF THE REHABILITATED MOUTH

To select the appropriate methods for plaque control and caries prevention, one must identify existing conditions, such as contour and position of the gingiva, contour of restorations, and problem areas adjacent to fixed prostheses. When these are known, the variety of possible techniques and devices for plaque removal can be reviewed and a plan for care outlined.

A patient who has undergone extensive periodontal therapy and restorative and prosthetic rehabilitation may have some or all of the characteristics listed here. Each condition may require specially selected or adapted plaque control measures. Fixed and removable appliances can provide many areas for plaque and debris retention.

I. Periodontal Findings

A. Gingival recession.

B. Exposed root surfaces.

C. Exposed furcation areas.

D. Alterations of gingival contour: the gingival margins may be rolled or rounded.

E. Changes in size and shape of the gingival embrasures.

   1. Missing interdental papillae: wide embrasures with gingival recession and increased root exposure (figure 25–1).

   2. Narrowed embrasures: created by overcontoured restorations or variously shaped pontics (figure 25–2).

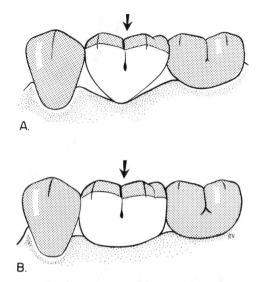

A.

B.

Figure 25–2. Shape of Pontics. Mandibular three-unit fixed partial denture: **A.** "Bullet"-shaped pontic with wide embrasures for access for bacterial plaque removal. **B.** Improperly shaped pontic with closed embrasures and wide gingival surface for plaque retention. Arrows indicate pontics.

II. Single Tooth Restorations

A. The gingival margin around a crown restoration may appear bluish or bluish-red when the crown margin is below the gingival margin.

B. Various restorations.

III. Fixed Prosthesis

The parts of a fixed prosthesis are described on page 341 and in figure 24–9.

   A patient may have

A. Fixed splinting around long segments of, or an entire, arch (figure 25–3).

B. Natural abutment teeth with difficult access areas adjacent to a pontic.

C. Implant abutment surfaces.

D. Closed contacts between teeth involved in a multitooth prosthesis.

E. Gingival surfaces of pontics.

F. Embrasures created by pontics may be wide and triangular, or narrow, unnatural, non-self-cleansing areas created by improperly shaped pontics (figure 25–2B).

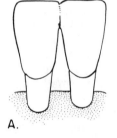

A.

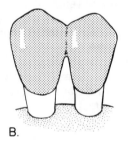

B.

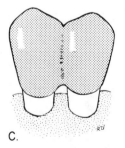

C.

Figure 25–1. Gingival Embrasures. **A.** Wide embrasure between two central incisors with missing interdental papilla and gingival recession. **B.** Double abutment with closed contact area with open embrasure provides access for plaque removal. **C.** Overcontoured crowns of a double abutment with a narrowed embrasure that provides limited access for bacterial plaque removal and cleaning of debris.

IV. Removable Prostheses

A. Complete denture may be used in one dental arch opposing natural teeth and partial dentures, fixed or removable.

B. Partial denture

   1. Creation of potential areas of plaque and debris retention.

      a. Alteration of tooth form by clasp, rest, or precision attachment (page 344).

      b. Improperly contoured edge of the partial denture at the junction of the partial and the abutment tooth.

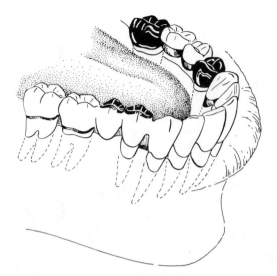

Figure 25–3. Complete-Arch Fixed Splint. A continuous therapeutic fixed appliance stabilizes periodontally involved teeth and replaces missing components to provide appropriate occlusal relationships. Numerous problem areas for bacterial-plaque removal exist.

2. Partial denture may impinge on the gingiva surrounding the abutment tooth.
3. Double abutment (two natural teeth with crowns that are soldered or cast together) has a closed contact requiring lateral (from facial or lingual) access to the gingival embrasure (figure 25–1B and C).
4. The mucosa under the partial denture needs special care.

SELF-CARE FOR THE REHABILITATED MOUTH

These special patients require greater than average attention, patience, and teaching skill to obtain a favorable result that will assure continuing health of the patient's periodontal tissues. Total commitment on the part of the patient is necessary if the selected plan is to meet the requirements for daily care.

I. Planning the Disease Control Program

The control program should be planned as a concentrated effort to maintain gingival tissue, the exposed tooth structure, and hence, the underlying supporting periodontium, as well as the restorations and prostheses. The instructions have three parts: first, before the surgical, restorative, and prosthetic treatment; second, during therapy; and third, after reconstruction.

A. Part 1

Basic plaque control measures are learned and practiced by the patient during the preparatory phase. The same treatment plan outlined on page 295 is typical of the procedure that can be used in conjunction with scaling appointments. During these lessons, principles for self-evaluation can be presented.

B. Part 2

During therapy, adaptations will be needed for applying techniques to temporary restorations. When the treatment extends over a long period, regular dental hygiene appointments for careful monitoring of the gingival health are essential.

C. Part 3

After therapy is completed, another set of self-care procedures is required in order to meet the needs of the rehabilitated mouth. Special devices and techniques are selected and tried until the most efficient and thorough procedures are determined.

II. Plaque Control: Selection of Methods[1]

Any of the methods and techniques described in Chapters 22, 23, and 24 may be needed in the care of the oral soft tissues, tooth surfaces, restorations, and fixed and removable prostheses. Methods selected must allow the patient to accomplish complete daily plaque removal from each area around every tooth or replacement. A summary of devices and methods is provided in table 25–1.

Most patients need a method for each of the following:
A. Debris removal, particularly from interproximal areas and around fixed prostheses.
B. Sulcular brushing.
C. Interdental plaque removal
   1. Proximal surfaces of natural and restored teeth, including exposed roots where access exists from the incisal or occlusal surfaces.
   2. Proximal surfaces of abutment teeth under closed contact areas (figure 25–4).
   3. Mesial and/or distal surfaces of teeth without proximal contact.

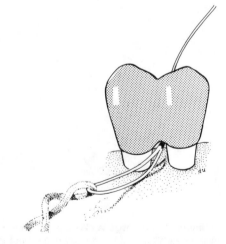

Figure 25–4. Bacterial Plaque Removal from Embrasure. A floss threader is used with yarn or tufted floss to clean under a double abutment embrasure. Narrowed embrasure from overcontoured crown increases plaque and debris retention and makes cleaning difficult.

Table 25–1.   Care of the Rehabilitated Mouth

Problem	Device/Method	Special Adaptations
Debris Removal	Water irrigation Toothbrush	Wide embrasures Under fixed partial dentures

Sulcular Brushing	Toothbrush with soft end-rounded
	  filaments
		Facial and lingual surfaces
		Distals of most-posterior teeth,
		  particularly terminal abutment

Proximal Surfaces Plaque removal	Floss Floss with threader Yarn with floss and/or threader Toothpick holder Pipe cleaner Interdental brush Single-tuft brush	Abutment teeth Proximal root surfaces Pontic surfaces Narrowed embrasures

Proximal Surfaces
  Without contact with
  an adjacent tooth
	Gauze strip
	Yarn
		Terminal abutment of removable partial
		  denture
		Distals of most-posterior teeth in the
		  dental arch

Exposed Furcation Molars	Pipe cleaner Floss/yarn in threader Interdental brush Interdental rubber tip	Rotated tooth
Exposed Furcation Maxillary first premolar	Interdental brush Interdental rubber tip	Fused root with groove
Exposed Root Surfaces	Dentifrice, containing desensitizing agent Nonabrasive fluoride dentifrice	Desensitization Prevent abrasion of cementum or dentin
Fixed Partial Denture	Toothbrush (soft nylon) Floss threader with floss/yarn Any other proximal surface procedures as applicable	Gingival surfaces of pontics Proximal surfaces of pontics and retainers

Edentulous Gingiva
  Under removable
  denture
	Toothbrush (soft nylon) (manual or
	  powered)
		Stimulation and plaque removal

Tongue Brushing	Toothbrush (soft nylon)	Deep fissures
Removable Denture	Denture brush Clasp brush Chemical cleanser for immersion	Clasps

D. Removal of bacterial plaque around a fixed partial denture must include the gingival and proximal surfaces of pontics.

E. Cleaning the removable prosthesis and care of the supporting tissues.

III. Fluorides

A. Selection of Fluorides

For the patient with porcelain or composite resin restorations, an acidulated fluoride preparation must be avoided. Porcelain and composite resin restorations become pitted and rough with repeated applications of a fluoride solution with an acid pH.[2,3,4,5,6]

Neutral fluoride products with low viscosity and low fluoride concentration can be advised.

B. Personal Daily Program

Fluoride dentifrice along with daily mouthrinse or brush-on gel is recommended to prevent root caries. For certain patients in the root caries risk groups and those with multiple sensitive teeth, a custom-tray application should be used daily.

C. Professional Topical Applications

When the patient does not use self-treatment methods on a regular basis or when additional fluoride is deemed beneficial, professional applications are recommended for each maintenance appointment.

IV. Dietary Survey

Whether the need for the rehabilitation was related to extensive dental caries or to a periodontal disease, dietary counseling is indicated. Every possible means must be taken to prevent carious lesions of the exposed root surfaces about the restorations. Overall dietary factors should be checked to assure support from a nutritional standpoint. Procedures for obtaining the Food Diary and conducting the counseling session are described on pages 383–389.

V. Procedure

No fixed procedure can be stated that will apply to every patient. A personalized sequence must be worked out, often by trial and error.
A. Outline a possible sequence.
1. Select methods and devices that can meet the requirements of the individual oral characteristics.
2. Demonstrate the use of the methods and have the patient practice under supervision. Avoid presenting too many procedures in one lesson, which can confuse and discourage the patient.
3. Provide step-by-step written directions for home reference.
B. Recheck successes within a few days and at least by 1 week.
1. Evaluate gingival tissue (table 11–1, pages 174–175).
2. Evaluate plaque. Use a disclosing agent to provide the patient with an evaluation of areas that need additional attention.
3. Evaluate technique performance.
a. Observe patient's dexterity in managing the techniques.
b. Note relationship of techniques to areas where disclosing agent revealed plaque retention.
4. Make necessary adjustments to simplify, clarify, and assure that all areas are completely deplaqued daily.
C. Reevaluate weekly or as frequently as needed to maintain the patient's motivation, to follow the health of the gingival tissues, and to recognize a need for changes in the procedures used.

VI. Sample Procedure

The patient described below has a complete maxillary fixed partial denture (splint), which has several natural teeth as abutments and four areas of double pontics; a mandibular removable partial denture with double abutments connecting mandibular canines and first premolars on each side; and wide embrasures between mandibular incisors caused by previous periodontal disease, which has since been treated with periodontal surgery.

The patient might use a procedure such as the following:

A. Morning After Eating
1. Complete brushing with powered brush (containing softest filaments available), applying the brush to proximal surfaces.
2. Brush partial removable denture and rinse thoroughly.

B. Noon After Eating (Away From Home)
1. Rinse partial denture under running water.
2. Use manual toothbrush, covering all surfaces as thoroughly as possible.
3. Rinse carefully, forcing the water under fixed partial denture areas.

C. Evening, After All Eating
1. Remove partial denture, rinse under running water, and place in cleansing solution. (Complete procedure for partial removable denture is described on page 344).
2. Use water irrigator to remove debris from all parts of fixed splint and from all proximal surfaces of mandibular teeth.
3. Use toothbrush for facial and lingual sulcular brushing, applying the brush interdentally as much as possible. Use fluoride dentifrice.
4. Brush tongue and edentulous gingiva under removable denture.
5. Use dental floss and/or yarn to proximal surfaces accessible from incisal.
6. Clean all gingival and proximal surfaces of fixed partial denture. Use floss and yarn with floss threader for all proximal and gingival surfaces not accessible from incisal or occlusal. Interdental brush may be needed for certain wide embrasures.
7. Use yarn or gauze strip for distal surfaces of the abutment teeth for the mandibular removable denture (mandibular premolars).
8. Use toothpick holder with dentifrice containing a desensitizing agent to massage hypersensitive areas of exposed roots.
9. Rinse with fluoride mouthrinse, vigorously forcing the solution between the teeth and under fixed appliances.
10. Clean partial denture, using denture brush and clasp brush, and rinse the denture thoroughly.

VII. Maintenance

Continuing supervision of the patient with oral rehabilitation is an absolute essential. The well-informed and conscientious patient who devotes up to an hour each day on personal care procedures expects a maintenance appointment that thoroughly evaluates the gingival tissue, the rehabilitation appliances, and the completeness of plaque control efforts.

Everything listed on pages 540–541 for inclusion in the maintenance examination applies with special meaning and emphasis to the rehabilitated patient. What could seem like a minute area of gingival bleeding on probing, whether the pocket is shallow or has started to deepen, should be a warning signal that an area may not be covered by present self-care procedures and needs some form of treatment. *Each millimeter of gingival sulcus must be probed carefully to detect incipient changes.*

DENTAL IMPLANTS

An *implant* is an alloplastic material grafted or inserted into intact tissues for prosthetic, therapeutic, diagnostic, or experimental purposes.[7] A *dental implant* is usually placed within or on mandibular or maxillary bone either to replace teeth or provide a stable and retentive base for support of a fixed or removable prosthesis. The various plates and screws used in the treatment of fractures are also implants.

New research has led to an increased use of implants in dental practice. Techniques for clinical applications have been refined. Factors that contribute to implant failure have been studied and defined, and criteria for implant success have been proposed.[8,9]

The success of an implant can be dependent on many factors, including especially patient understanding and skills for direct daily care of the prosthesis and the surrounding soft tissues. Frequent maintenance appointments for careful supervision and patient motivation are necessary.

I. Types of Dental Implants

The three general categories of dental implants are described here. They are subperiosteal, transosteal, and endosteal.

A. Subperiosteal

1. *Location.* The implant is placed over the bone, under the periosteum.
2. *Example.* A cast framework rests over the bone of the mandible or maxilla; it may be the complete arch or unilateral (figure 25–5).
3. *Material.* Cobalt-chromium-molybdenum (Vitallium) or titanium are used.
4. *Description*[10,11]
   a. Two-step. In the first step, a surgical flap is used to reflect mucosal tissues and to expose the underlying bone. An impression is made of the bony ridge. The metallic unit is cast and then placed in a second surgical step. Usually, four posts protrude into the oral cavity to hold the complete denture.
   b. One-step. Computer-assisted design and manufacturing have been applied, using a reformatted computed tomography scan from which approximate casts of the maxilla or mandible can be made. The implant is designed on this replica and is placed in one surgical procedure.[12]

B. Transosteal (Transosseous)

1. *Location.* The implant is placed through the bone.
2. *Example.* The mandibular-staple bone plate (figure 25–6).
3. *Material.* Titanium, aluminum, and vanadium alloy.
4. *Description.*[13,14] A metal plate, fitted to the

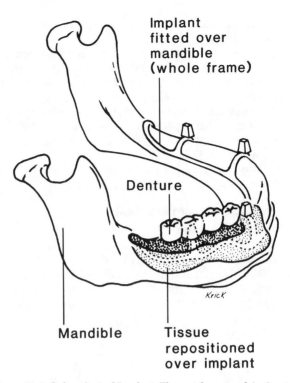

Figure 25–5. Subperiosteal Implant. The cast framework is situated on the left side of the mandible; on the right side, the cast framework is shown by dotted lines under the denture.

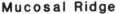
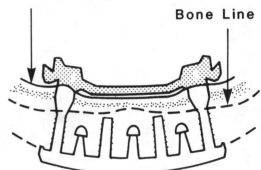

Figure 25–6. Transosteal Implant. Mandibular staple bone plate in the anterior region shows metal plate at the lower border of the mandible, with pins extending toward the occlusal surface. Terminal pins protrude into the oral cavity to hold the overdenture.

inferior border of the mandible, has five to seven pins extending toward the occlusal surface. Usually, two terminal pins protrude into the oral cavity to hold the overdenture. The pins are connected by a crossbar. The transosteal implant can be used when the patient has an atrophic edentulous mandible or a congenital or traumatic deformity of the mandible.

C. Endosteal (Endosseous)

1. *Location.* The implant is placed within the bone.

2. *Examples.* Blade, screw, and cylinder types are used (figure 25–7).
3. *Material.* Titanium (pure or alloy) and ceramic have been used. A layer of titanium oxide is created on the surface of the titanium during the manufacturing process.
4. *Description.*[8] The support, body, or fixture is placed during the first surgical step and left covered by mucosal tissue for several months while implant and bone bond. The abutment, post, or neck for the prosthesis is then added at a second-stage operation.

II. Preparation and Placement

A. Patient Selection

Careful screening is essential for patients with generally acceptable physical health and a real desire to go through the required treatment. Diagnosis and treatment planning are based on a risk-benefit analysis and follow a detailed medical, dental, and behavioral history along with an oral and radiographic examination. Sometimes a psychologic examination is used.

1. *Systemic Health*
   a. Medical history. The patient must be free of systemic conditions that can interfere with healing or acceptance of the implant. Biocompatibility of the implant with body tissues is essential.
   b. Contraindications. Examples of conditions that would make a patient a poor risk would be recent radiation therapy to the affected part, uncontrolled diabetes mellitus, alcoholism or heavy alcohol intake, substance abuse, an immunosuppressive disease or medication, anticoagulant medication, psychosis or paranoia.
2. *Oral Examination*
   a. Radiographic and clinical findings.
   b. The presence of an active oral disease such as periodontitis contraindicates implant placement until the disease is treated.
3. *Oral Hygiene.* The patient must demonstrate consistent and effective personal oral care.

B. Information for the Patient
1. Explain procedures to be performed and the time schedule.
2. Explain possible complications.
3. Emphasize the role of personal oral care and the need for daily bacterial plaque control.
4. Obtain an informed consent statement and agreement of understanding.

C. Surgical Steps

Acceptable bone integration has occurred with certain single-stage endosseous implants, but the more acceptable modality is a two-stage procedure. The entire implant usually cannot be inserted in one step because forces of occlusion (chewing, biting) cause mobility and prevent bone healing. When the implant is first placed it must be stabilized. Movement of the implant may cause the formation of a fibrous tissue layer instead of osseointegration.

1. *Instrumentation.* The surgical procedure requires atraumatic placement of the implant into the bone. High-speed handpiece or other heat-producing methods cannot be used because they cause bone damage. With certain implants, special titanium, plastic, or teflon coated instruments are required.
2. *Sterile Procedures.* Whenever microorganisms are introduced during a surgical procedure, healing can be impaired. Manufacturers prepare implants in sterile packages, or implants are sterilized by autoclave before placement.

D. Prosthetic Steps[15,16]

Attention to ideal requirements for acceptable prostheses is necessary. Margins, embrasure

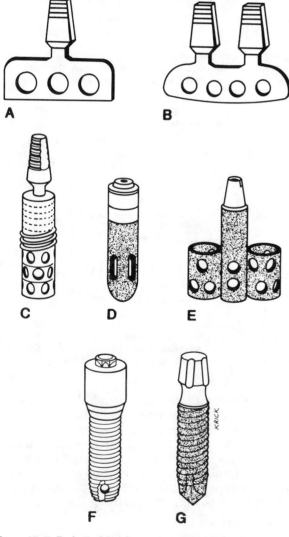

Figure 25–7. Endosteal Implants. A. and **B.** Blade types. **C., D., E.** Cylinder types. **F.** and **G.** Screw types.

shapes, crown contours, contact areas, and occlusal harmony must be designed to prevent bacterial plaque collection and permit thorough disease-control procedures by the patient.

III. Implant Interfaces

An implant has an inner interface with the *bone* and a *soft-tissue* interface where the terminal pin, abutment, post, or other protruding portion of the implant is surrounded by the mucosal or gingival tissue.

A. Implant Bone Interface

Osseointegration or direct implant-bone integration is the most effective mechanism; however, some implants have functioned for long periods with a fibrous tissue encapsulation.

1. *Osseointegration (Osteointegration).* This refers to direct structural and functional union between the implant and healthy living bone. There is no discernible connective tissue between the bone and the implant. Pure titanium has been shown effective for osseointegration when kept stable during the healing phase.[17]

2. *Fibro-osseous Integration.*[18] Fibro-osseous or fibrous integration means that dense collagenous tissue is interposed between implant and bone. Problems of mobility and inflammation within the connective tissue may limit the long-term expectation of success with this type of interface.

B. Implant/Soft Tissue Interface

The external environment of an implant is the oral cavity, with saliva, bacterial plaque, and debris.

1. *Biologic Seal (Permucosal Seal).*[19,20] Between the implant or post and the soft tissue, a biologic seal must exist to prevent microorganisms and inflammation-producing agents from entering the tissues.

2. *Soft-Tissue Connection.* Sulcular epithelium is in contact with the implant surface. The attachment appears similar to the epithelial attachment of the junctional epithelium of a natural tooth. Hemidesmosomes and basal lamina have been identified.[21,22,23,24] The epithelium resembles a long junctional epithelium.

IV. Peri-Implant Hygiene

A key requirement for implant success is the disease-control program for the tissue surrounding the implant. Meticulous hygiene is a necessity for which repeated instruction may be needed.

A. Bacterial Plaque (Implant Plaque)

Plaque microorganisms around implants with healthy permucosal tissue have been shown to be like the flora around natural teeth. Gram-positive, nonmotile coccoid and other forms predominate.[25,26,27]

The tissues around implant posts or abutments react to microorganisms and their toxic products in a manner similar to the gingiva surrounding natural teeth. When inflammation and pocket depths increase, the total numbers of microorganisms and numbers of spirochetes and motile rods increase also.[28,29,30]

B. Planning the Disease Control Program

1. *Relation to Treatment.* Supervision of a patient's oral hygiene must begin prior to the surgical phase for implant placement and carry on throughout the treatment phases.

2. *Types of Prostheses.* Implant-supported prostheses may be partial, complete, fixed, removable or single-tooth replacements. Prostheses may be supported by natural teeth and/or implants. An individual may have a variety of areas and prostheses to care for.

C. Selection of Plaque-Removal Methods[31]

Any of the methods for plaque removal described in Chapters 22, 23, and 24 may be required in various combinations. Each patient will need an individually planned program so that each type of abutment and appliance will be maintained in a plaque-free environment.

1. *Conventional Prostheses.* Removable or fixed, partial or complete dentures made of conventional dental materials are to be cleaned by the usual methods described earlier. Suggestions provided here pertain primarily to the posts, abutments, or other protruding portions of implants.

2. *Precautions*
   a. Prevent damage to implant materials. Care must be taken to use implements, dentifrices, or other cleaning agents that will not scratch or abrade the titanium or other material. Only smooth plastic or wooden implements or soft materials (yarn, gauze, or floss) should be used.
   b. Examples. The wire twisted to hold a pipe cleaner or the filaments of an interdental brush, may extrude and scratch the abutment or abrade the soft tissue. Each device should be checked before use.

   Toothbrush filaments must be smooth, soft, end-rounded, and usually used with warm water, to prevent damage to the peri-implant tissue.

3. *Subperiosteal Implant.* The posts and surrounding tissue need to be cleaned completely around the circumference. Yarn or gauze strip can be used with a floss threader to position the material under the crossbar.

4. *Endosteal Implant*
   a. Abutments or posts. A floss threader can be used to position yarn or a gauze bandage strip around an abutment and under a fixed prosthesis. Tufted dental floss is also

highly effective. Interdental brushes and single end-tuft brushes are adaptable. The end-tuft brush bent at the neck is particularly useful on lingual and palatal surfaces (figure 24–8, page 341).

A specially designed cleaning instrument made of hard plastic that cannot damage a titanium surface has been developed.[31] As shown in figure 25–8, one end has a crescent blade and the other a semicircular hook that can be rotated around the abutment cylinder.

b. Undersurface of fixed prosthesis with cantilever. Several endosteal implants may be placed anterior to the mental foramen, and the complete overdenture may have a cantilevered portion distal to the terminal implant. Cleaning plaque from under the cantilever may be accomplished by using gauze strips.

D. Rinsing and Irrigation

1. *General Cleaning.* Use of an irrigator can remove debris before specific cleaning with toothbrush and auxiliary aids.

2. *Chemotherapy.* Irrigation with an approved antimicrobial can be advised for selected patients. Specific directions for preparation of the agent, and for the use of the irrigator should be given.

3. *Fluoride Measures for Dental Caries Control.* For the patient with natural teeth, fluoride self-application daily should be incorporated into the regime (pages 407–410).

V. Maintenance

The patient's daily oral plaque removal and regular supervision and monitoring through maintenance appointments directly influence the long-term success of an implant. When teeth were lost originally because of lack of daily disease control by the patient, a more intense program of education and practice may be needed. Neglect may have been caused by lack of knowledge about, or appreciation for, preventive measures.

A. Frequency of Appointments

Each patient must have a personalized appointment interval, depending on individual needs. The first series of appointments following placement of the implant(s) should start within a week and be scheduled weekly until healing is com-

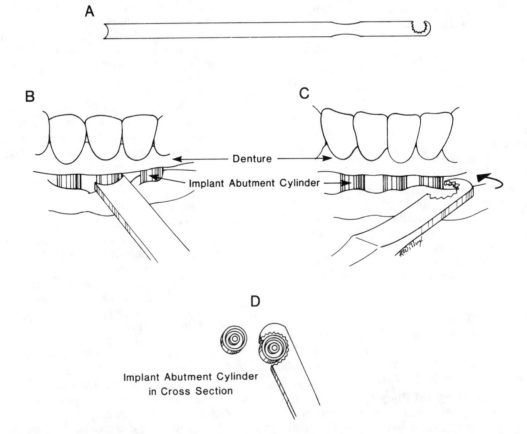

Figure 25–8. Plastic Cleaning Instrument. A. Specially designed plastic instrument for cleaning titanium abutment cylinders. One end is a semicircular hook and the other end a crescent blade. **B.** Application of crescent blade. **C.** Application of semicircular hook. **D.** Implant cylinder in cross-section with semicircular hook in position. (Adapted from: Balshi, T.J.: Hygiene Maintenance Procedures for Patients Treated with the Tissue Integrated Prosthesis, (Osseointegration), *Quintessence Int. 17*, 95, February, 1986)

pleted and the patient has demonstrated the ability to control the bacterial plaque.

Maintenance appointments during the first year may be at 1- or 2-month intervals.

B. The Maintenance Appointment

Factors outlined for a maintenance appointment (pages 540–541) apply to a patient with an implant. Health history, vital signs, intraoral/extraoral examination, and other appropriate reviews, are all a part of the total plan. At each maintenance appointment the dentist evaluates and records the condition of each implant.

1. *Basic Criteria for Implant Success*[8]
   a. Mobility: no mobility can be demonstrated clinically.
   b. Radiograph: no evidence of peri-implant radiolucency.
   c. Bone loss: less than 0.2 mm. annually after the first year.
   d. Clinical symptoms: no pain, infections, or paresthesia.
   e. Longevity: the rate of success overall for a particular type of implant: 85 percent after 5 years; 80 percent after 10 years.
2. *Examination*
   a. Peri-implant tissue. Visual examination should show no signs of inflammation as evidenced by the usual criteria of changes in color, size, shape, and consistency.
   b. Probing. Probing gently, primarily to determine bleeding tendency, may be a routine part of an examination for tissue health. The dentist will specify exactly what should be done, because probing may not be indicated for certain implants. A plastic probe is available.[32]
   c. Deposits. Bacterial plaque can be tested with a disclosing agent. The gingival surfaces of fixed appliances should be checked carefully.

      Calculus is usually not extensive, hard, or firmly attached to implant abutments or other protruding parts, provided the patient has been faithful with daily procedures and professional maintenance appointments.
3. *Review of Personal Disease Control Procedures.* The patient demonstrates, and the clinician provides recommendations for improvements.
4. *Instrumentation.* Each type of implant requires attention to certain features. Manufacturer's instructions should be followed. Care must be taken not to scratch or alter in any way the surfaces of titanium and other materials making up the implant superstructures.
   a. Calculus removal. Plastic or wooden instruments are indicated for titanium. A porte polisher with wood point may be appropriate. If a standard curet is used, it should be dull, applied carefully, and placed only where calculus is visible. Routine scaling procedures can be applied to the appliances, prostheses, and natural teeth present.

      Certain implants have a permucosal titanium ring that can be removed by the dentist. The implant part can then be cleaned in an ultrasonic solution and replaced into the fixture.
   b. Stain removal. Unless necessary for esthetics, polishing is not included routinely. When selective stain removal is indicated, only a nonabrasive agent should be used.

FACTORS TO TEACH THE PATIENT

I. Importance of Daily Care

The health of the periodontal tissues and the duration of the restorations and prostheses depend on daily self-care by the patient.

II. Need for Concentration

More thought and concentration are required to maintain the mouth with advanced restorative dentistry, periodontal prosthesis, or implants than are needed for an average mouth.

III. Time Requirement

Cleaning a mouth with complex restorations takes longer. Time must be allotted in the daily schedule for complete cleaning and plaque removal once each day, supplemented by cleaning at least three times each day, or after each meal.

IV. Diligence and Thoroughness

Do not go easy with the brush and other devices in the attempt to protect the restorations from breakage. *Protection* is for the gingival tissues and the preservation of the periodontium and is accomplished only by thorough bacterial plaque removal around every tooth.

V. Importance of Maintenance

Frequent, regular appointments for professional supervision and cooperative care are necessary.

References

1. Bradbury, E., Harvard University, School of Dental Medicine, Boston, personal communication.
2. Yaffe, A. and Zalkind, M.: The Effect of Topical Application of Fluoride on Composite Resin Restorations, *J. Prosthet. Dent., 45,* 59, January, 1981.
3. Kula, K., Nelson, S., Kula, T., and Thompson, V.: In Vitro Effect of Acidulated Phosphate Fluoride Gel on the Surface of Composites with Different Filler Particles, *J. Prosthet. Dent., 56,* 161, August, 1986.
4. Copps, D.P., Lacy, A.M., Curtis, T., and Carman, J.E.: Effects of Topical Fluorides on Five Low-fusing Dental Porcelains, *J. Prosthet. Dent., 52,* 340, September, 1984.

5. Wunderlich, R.C. and Yaman, P.: In Vitro Effect of Topical Fluoride on Dental Porcelain, *J. Prosthet. Dent., 55,* 385, March, 1986.

6. Sposetti, V.J., Shen, C., and Levin, A.C.: The Effect of Topical Fluoride Application on Porcelain Restorations, *J. Prosthet. Dent., 55,* 677, June, 1986.

7. Jablonski, S.: *Illustrated Dictionary of Dentistry.* Philadelphia, W.B. Saunders Co., 1982, p. 410.

8. Albrektsson, T., Zarb, G., Worthington, P., and Eriksson, A.R.: The Long-term Efficacy of Currently Used Dental Implants: A Review and Proposed Criteria of Success, *Int. J. Oral Maxillofac. Implants, 1,* 11, Number 1, 1986.

9. Schnitman, P.A. and Shulman, L.B., eds.: *Dental Implants: Benefit and Risk.* An NIH–Harvard Concensus Development Conference, United States Department of Health and Human Services, National Institutes of Health, Publication No. 81-1531, Bethesda, Maryland, December, 1980.

10. Goldberg, N.I.: Risk of Subperiosteal Implants, in Schnitman, P.A. and Shulman, L.B., eds.: *Dental Implants: Benefit and Risk.* An NIH–Harvard Concensus Development Conference, United States Department of Health and Human Services, National Institutes of Health, Publication No. 81-1531, Bethesda, Maryland, December, 1980, p. 89.

11. Cranin, A.N.: Surgical Aspects of the Subperiosteal Implant, in Clark, J.W., ed.: *Clinical Dentistry,* Volume 5, Chapter 50. Philadelphia, J.B. Lippincott Co., 1987, pp. 1–12.

12. Boyne, P.J. and James, R.A.: Advances in Subperiosteal Implant Reconstruction, *Dent. Clin. North Am., 30,* 259, April, 1986.

13. Small, I.A.: The Mandibular Staple Bone Plate. Its Use and Advantages in Reconstructive Surgery, *Dent. Clin. North Am., 30,* 175, April, 1986.

14. Cranin, A.N., Sher, J., and Schilb, T.P.: The Transosteal Implant: A 17-year Review and Report, *J. Prosthet. Dent., 55,* 709, June, 1986.

15. Finger, I.M. and Guerra, L.R.: Prosthetic Considerations in Reconstructive Implantology, *Dent. Clin. North Am., 30,* 69, January, 1986.

16. Stines, A.V.: Prosthodontic Reconstruction with the Mandibular Staple Bone Plate, *Dent. Clin. North Am., 30,* 189, April, 1986.

17. Hansson, H.-A., Albrektsson, T., and Brånemark, P.-I.: Structural Aspects of the Interface Between Tissue and Titanium Implants, *J. Prosthet. Dent., 50,* 108, July, 1983.

18. Weiss, C.M.: Tissue Integration of Dental Endosseous Implants: Description and Comparative Analysis of the Fibroosseous Integration and Osseous Integration Systems, *J. Oral Implantol., 12,* 169, Number 2, 1986.

19. McKinney, R.V., Steflik, D.E., and Koth, D.L.: Per, Peri, or Trans? A Concept for Improved Dental Implant Terminology, *J. Prosthet. Dent., 52,* 267, August, 1984.

20. McKinney, R.V., Steflik, D.E., and Koth, D.L.: Evidence for a Junctional Epithelial Attachment to Ceramic Dental Implants. A Transmission Electron Microscopic Study, *J. Periodontol., 56,* 579, October, 1985.

21. James, R.A. and Schultz, R.L.: Hemidesmosomes and the Adhesions of Junctional Epithelial Cells to Metal Implants: A Preliminary Report, *J. Oral Implantol., 4,* 294, Winter, 1974.

22. Swope, E.M. and James, R.A.: A Longitudinal Study on Hemidesmosome Formation at the Dental Implant–Tissue Interface, *J. Oral Implantol., 9,* 412, Number 3, 1981.

23. Gould, T.R.L., Westbury, L., and Brunette, D.M.: Ultrastructural Study of the Attachment of Human Gingiva to Titanium *in vivo, J. Prosthet. Dent., 52,* 418, September, 1984.

24. Jansen, J.A., de Wijn, J.R., Wolters-Lutgerhorst, J.M.L., and van Mullem, P.J.: Ultrastructural Study of Epithelial Cell Attachment to Implant Materials, *J. Dent. Res., 64,* 891, June, 1985.

25. Lekholm, U., Ericsson, I., Adell, R., and Slots, J.: The Condition of the Soft Tissues at Tooth and Fixture Abutments Supporting Fixed Bridges. A Microbiological and Histological Study, *J. Clin. Periodontol., 13,* 558, July, 1986.

26. Rams, T.E., Roberts, T.W., Tatum, H., and Keyes, P.H.: The Subgingival Microbial Flora Associated with Human Dental Implants, *J. Prosthet. Dent., 51,* 529, April, 1984.

27. Adell, R., Lekholm, U., Rockler, B., Brånemark, P.-I., Lindhe, J., Eriksson, B., and Sbordone, L.: Marginal Tissue Reactions at Osseointegrated Titanium Fixtures. I. A 3-year Longitudinal Prospective Study, *Int. J. Oral Maxillofac. Surg., 15,* 39, February, 1986.

28. Rams, T.E. and Link, C.C.: Microbiology of Failing Dental Implants in Humans: Electron Microscopic Observations, *J. Oral Implantol., 11,* 93, Number 1, 1983.

29. Holt, R., Newman, M.G., Kratochvil, F., Jeswani, S., Bugler, M., Khorsandi, S., and Sanz, M.: The Clinical and Microbial Characterization of the Peri-implant Environment, *J. Dent. Res., 65,* 247, Abstract 703, Special Issue, 1986.

30. Lekholm, U., Adell, R., Lindhe, J., Brånemark, P.-I., Eriksson, B., Rockler, B., Lindvall, A.-M., and Yoneyama, T.: Marginal Tissue Reactions at Osseointegrated Titanium Fixtures. II. A Cross-sectional Retrospective Study, *Int. J. Oral Maxillofac. Surg., 15,* 53, February, 1986.

31. Balshi, T.J.: Hygiene Maintenance Procedures for Patients Treated with the Tissue Integrated Prosthesis, (Osseointegration), *Quintessence Int., 17,* 95, February, 1986.

32. *Perio-Test.* Bernard Loewenthal, D.D.S., 278 Lafayette Road, Portsmouth, New Hampshire 03801.

Suggested Readings

Balshi, T.J. and Mingledorff, E.B.: Maintenance Procedures for Patients after Complete Fixed Prosthodontics, *J. Prosthet. Dent., 37,* 420, April, 1977.

Becker, C.M. and Kaldahl, W.B.: Using Removable Partial Dentures to Stabilize Teeth with Secondary Occlusal Traumatism, *J. Prosthet. Dent., 47,* 587, June, 1982.

Bergman, B.: Periodontal Reactions Related to Removable Partial Dentures: A Literature Review, *J. Prosthet. Dent., 58,* 454, October, 1987.

Block, P.L.: Restorative Margins and Periodontal Health: A New Look At An Old Perspective, *J. Prosthet. Dent., 57,* 683, June, 1987.

Carr, E.H.: Laminate Veneers. Restoration Alternative Means Special Care, *RDH, 2,* 11, July-August, 1982.

Conny, D.J., Tedesco, L.A., Brewer, J.D., and Albino, J.E.: Changes of Attitude in Fixed Prosthodontic Patients, *J. Prosthet. Dent., 53,* 451, April, 1985.

Goldman, H.M. and Cohen, D.W.: *Periodontal Therapy,* 6th ed. St. Louis, The C.V. Mosby Co., 1980, pp. 1112–1154.

Grant, D.A., Stern, I.B., and Listgarten, M.A., eds.: *Periodontics,* 6th ed. St. Louis, The C.V. Mosby Co., 1988, pp. 1045–1055.

Jones, J.D. and Snyder, N.C.: Role of the Dental Hygienist in the Prosthodontic Practice, *J. Prosthet. Dent., 52,* 885, December, 1984.

Kenney, E.B.: Restorative-Periodontal Interrelationships, in Carranza, F.A.: *Glickman's Clinical Periodontology,* 6th ed. Philadelphia, W.B. Saunders Co., 1984, pp. 906–945.

Nyman, S. and Ericsson, I.: The Capacity of Reduced Periodontal Tissues to Support Fixed Bridgework, *J. Clin. Periodontol., 9,* 409, September, 1982.

Dental Implants

Adell, R.: Tissue Integrated Prosthesis in Clinical Dentistry, *Int. Dent. J., 35,* 259, December, 1985.

Albrektsson, T. and Jacobsson, M.: Bone-metal Interface in Osseointegration, *J. Prosthet. Dent., 57,* 597, May, 1987.

Albrektsson, T., Jansson, T., and Lekholm, U.: Osseointegrated Dental Implants, *Dent. Clin. North Am., 30,* 151, January, 1986.

Babbush, C.A.: Endosteal Blade-vent Implants, *Dent. Clin. North Am., 30,* 97, January, 1986.

Babbush, C.A.: Titanium Plasma Spray Screw Implant System for Reconstruction of the Edentulous Mandible, *Dent. Clin. North Am., 30,* 117, January, 1986.

Babbush, C.A.: ITI Endosteal Hollow Cylinder Implant Systems, *Dent. Clin. North Am., 30,* 133, January, 1986.

Brånemark, P.-I.: Osseointegration and Its Experimental Background, *J. Prosthet. Dent., 50,* 399, September, 1983.

Ericsson, I., Lekholm, U., Brånemark, P.-I., Lindhe, J., Glantz, P.-O., and Nyman, S.: A Clinical Evaluation of Fixed-bridge Restorations Supported by the Combination of Teeth and Osseointegrated Titanium Implants, *J. Clin. Periodontol., 13,* 307, April, 1986.

Heimdahl, A., Kondell, P.-A., Nord, C.E., and Nordenram, A.: Effect of Insertion of Osseo-integrated Prosthesis on the Oral Microflora, *Swed. Dent. J., 7,* 199, Number 5, 1983.

Hobkirk, J.A.: Progress in Implant Research, *Int. Dent. J., 33,* 341, December, 1983.

Holt, R.: Dental Implants, *J. West. Soc. Periodont. Periodont. Abstr., 34,* 49, Number 2, 1986.

Kawahara, H.: Cellular Responses to Implant Materials: Biological, Physical, and Chemical Factors, *Int. Dent. J., 33,* 350, December, 1983.

Kent, J.N., Misiek, D.J., Silverman, H., and Rotskoff, K.: A Multicenter Retrospective Review of the Mandibular Staple Bone Plate, *J. Oral Maxillofac. Surg., 42,* 421, July, 1984.

Manski, R.J.: A Synopsis of Recent Literature Concerning the Dental Implant, *J. Oral Implantol., 10,* 275, Number 2, 1982.

McKinney, R.V., Steflik, D.E., and Koth, D.L.: The Biologic Response to the Single-crystal Sapphire Endosteal Dental Implant: Scanning Electron Microscopic Observations, *J. Prosthet. Dent., 51,* 372, March, 1984.

McKinstry, R.E. and Aramany, M.A.: Clinical Evaluation of the Mandibular Staple Bone Plate, *J. Prosthet. Dent., 50,* 374, September, 1983.

Meffert, R.M.: Endosseous Dental Implantology from the Periodontist's Viewpoint, *J. Periodontol., 57,* 531, September 1986.

Niznick, G.A.: Implant Prosthodontics Using the Core-vent System, *J. Oral Implantol., 12,* 45, Number 1, 1985.

O'Malley, J.P. and Gordon, A.B.: The Mandibular Orthopedic Bone Staple in the Treatment of the Atrophic Mandible, *J. Prosthet. Dent., 48,* 432, October, 1982.

Parr, G.R., Gardner, L.K., and Toth, R.W.: Titanium: The Mystery Metal of Implant Dentistry, *J. Prosthet. Dent., 54,* 410, September, 1985.

Shulman, L.B., Rogoff, G.S., Savitt, E.D., and Kent, R.L.: Evaluation in Reconstructive Implantology, *Dent. Clin. North Am., 30,* 327, April, 1986.

Small, I.A. and Misiek, D.: A Sixteen-year Evaluation of the Mandibular Staple Bone Plate, *J. Oral Maxillofac. Surg., 44,* 60, January, 1986.

Smithloff, M. and Fritz, M.E.: The Use of Blade Implants in a Selected Population of Partially Edentulous Adults. A Ten-year Report, *J. Periodontol., 53,* 413, July, 1982.

Toth, R.W., Parr, G.R., and Gardner, L.K.: Soft Tissue Response to Endosseous Titanium Oral Implants, *J. Prosthet. Dent., 54,* 564, October, 1985.

Walker, C., Aufdemorte, T.B., McAnear, J.T., and Key, M.C.: The Mandibular Staple Bone Plate: A 5½-year Follow up, *J. Am. Dent. Assoc., 114,* 189, February, 1987.

Young, L., Michel, J.D., and Moore, D.J.: A Twenty-year Evaluation of Subperiosteal Implants, *J. Prosthet. Dent., 49,* 690, May, 1983.

26 *Disclosing Agents*

A disclosing agent is a preparation in liquid, tablet, or lozenge form that contains a dye or other coloring agent. In dentistry, a disclosing agent is used to identify bacterial plaque deposits for instruction, evaluation, and research.

Bacterial plaque is nearly colorless unless stained by foods, beverages, or tobacco. After use of a disclosing agent, the soft deposits pick up the color of the agent, whereas the dye can be rinsed off readily from plaque-free surfaces (figure 26–1). After staining, the deposits that can be seen distinctly provide a valuable visual aid in patient instruction. Such a procedure can demonstrate dramatically to the patient the presence of deposits and the areas that need special attention during personal oral care.

I. Purposes

A disclosing agent clearly demarcates soft deposits that might otherwise be invisible, and therefore facilitates

A. Personalized patient instruction in the location of soft deposits and the techniques for removal.
B. Self-evaluation by the patient on a daily basis during initial instruction and periodic checks thereafter.
C. Continuing evaluation of the effectiveness of the instruction for the patient
   1. To determine the need for revisions of the plaque-control procedures.
   2. To study the long-term effects over successive maintenance appointments.
D. Preparation of plaque indices (pages 262–265).
E. Research studies to gain new information about the incidence and formation of deposits on the teeth, the effectiveness of specific devices for plaque control, antiplaque agents, and to evaluate clinical and instructional group health programs.

II. Properties of an Acceptable Disclosing Agent

A. Intensity of Color

A distinct staining of deposits should be evident. The color should contrast with normal colors of the oral cavity.

B. Duration of Intensity

The color should not rinse off immediately with ordinary rinsing methods, or be removable by the saliva for the period of time required to complete the instruction or clinical service. It is desirable for the color to be removed from the gingival tissue and lips by the completion of the appointment, as the patient may have a personal reaction to color retained for a long period of time.

C. Taste

The patient should not be made uncomfortable by an unpleasant or highly flavored substance. The main reason for using the disclosant is to motivate the patient; therefore the use of the agent should be pleasant and encourage cooperation.

D. Irritation to the Mucous Membrane

The patient should be questioned concerning the possibility of an idiosyncrasy to an ingredient. When this information is obtained, it should be entered on the patient's permanent history record. Because of the possibility of allergy, more than one type of disclosing agent should be available for use.

E. Diffusibility

A solution should be thin enough so it can be applied readily to the exposed surfaces of the teeth, yet thick enough to impart an intense color to bacterial plaque.

F. Astringent and Antiseptic Properties

These properties may be highly desirable in that the disclosing agent may contribute other factors to the treatment procedures. The application of an antiseptic before scaling is frequently recommended, and if an antiseptic disclosing agent is used, one solution serves a dual purpose.

A disclosant may inhibit the growth of microorganisms. In quantitative plaque research studies, therefore, disclosing agents without antibacterial properties should be used.

III. Formulae

A wide variety of disclosing agents has been used. Skinner's Iodine Solution was formerly the most classic and widely used. In general, iodine solutions are less desirable because of their unpleasant flavor.

Aniline dyes have been shown to have carcinogenic potential. Therefore, the use of basic fuchsin and beta rose (flavored basic fuchsin) has been discouraged.

The formulae of a few disclosing agents are included in this chapter. Other well-known ones are Buckley's, Berwick's, Talbot's Iodo-glycerol, and Metaphen solutions.

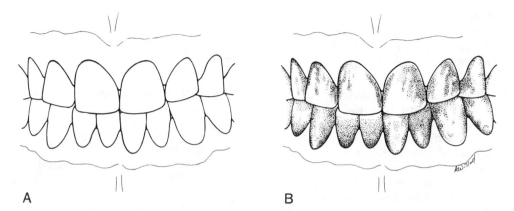

A   B

Figure 26–1. Use of Disclosing Agent. A. Appearance of the teeth before application of a disclosing agent. Bacterial plaque and pellicle are usually invisible. **B.** After use of a disclosing agent on the same teeth as those shown in **A.** Bacterial plaque and pellicle take on the color of the dye used in the disclosing agent. As noted, soft deposits are extensive, and are especially thick on the proximal surfaces.

A. Iodine Preparations

1. Skinner's Solution
Iodine crystals	3.3 g.
Potassium iodide	1.0 g.
Zinc iodide	1.0 g.
Water (distilled)	16.0 ml.
Glycerin	16.0 ml.
2. Diluted Tincture of Iodine
Tincture of iodine	21.0 ml.
Water (distilled)	15.0 ml.

B. Mercurochrome Preparations

1. Mercurochrome Solution (5%)
Mercurochrome	1.5 g.
Water (distilled) to make	30.0 ml.
2. Flavored Mercurochrome Disclosing Solution
Mercurochrome	13.5 g.
Water (distilled)	3.0 L.
Oil of peppermint	3 drops
Artificial noncariogenic sweetener	

C. Bismarck Brown (Easlick's Disclosing Solution)

Bismarck Brown	3.0 g.
Ethyl alcohol	10.0 ml.
Glycerin	120.0 ml.
Anise (flavoring)	1 drop

D. Merbromin

Merbromin, N.F.	450.0 mg.
Oil of peppermint	1 drop
Distilled water to make	100.0 ml.

E. Erythrosin

1. Concentrate for Application by Rinsing
F.D.&C. Red No. 3 or No. 28	6.0 g.
Water to make	100.0 ml.
2. For Direct Topical Application
Erythrosin	0.8 g.
Water (distilled)	100.0 ml.
Alcohol (95%)	10.0 ml.
Oil of peppermint	2 drops

3. Tablet[1]
F.D.&C. Red No. 3	15.0 mg.
Sodium chloride	.747%
Sodium sucaryl	.747%
Calcium stearate	.995%
Soluble saccharin	.186%
White oil	.124%
Flavoring	2.239%
Sorbitol to make a 7 grain tablet	

F. Fast Green

F.D.&C. Green No. 3	5% or 2.5%

G. Fluorescein[2]

F.D.&C. Yellow No. 8 (used with a special ultraviolet light source to make the agent visible)

H. Two-tone[3]

F.D.&C. Green No. 3
F.D.&C. Red No. 3
Thicker (older) plaque stains blue; thinner (newer) plaque stains red.

IV. Methods for Application

Make gingival tissue evaluation before application because disclosing agent will mask tissue colors.

A. Solution for Direct Application
1. Dry the teeth with compressed air, retracting cheek or tongue.
2. Use swab or small cotton pellet with cotton pliers to carry the solution to the teeth.
3. Apply solution to the crowns of the teeth only.
4. Direct the patient to spread the agent over all surfaces of the teeth with the tongue.
5. Examine the distribution of agent and request the patient to rinse if indicated.

B. Rinsing
A few drops of a concentrated preparation are placed in a paper cup and water is added for the appropriate dilution. Instruct the patient to rinse and swish the solution over all tooth surfaces.

C. Tablet or Wafer

The patient chews the wafer (one half may be sufficient for some patients), swishes it around for 30 to 60 seconds, and rinses.

D. Effect

Clean tooth surfaces do not absorb the coloring agent; when pellicle and bacterial plaque are present, they absorb the agent and are disclosed. Pellicle stains as a thin, relatively clear covering, whereas bacterial plaque appears darker, thicker, and more opaque.

The oral mucous membrane and lips may retain the color from certain disclosing agents. Application of petrolatum or other coating substance may prevent absorption of the color by the lips.

V. Patient Instruction

Since plaque and pellicle are frequently invisible to a patient, a disclosing agent can provide a method for patient instruction.

A. Explain Bacterial Plaque

The patient needs to be informed about the composition and effect of plaque in the production of gingival and periodontal infections, with particular reference to the individual mouth.

B. Show Location and Distribution of Plaque

With a hand mirror, the patient can observe the teeth and the disclosed bacterial plaque. A small mouth mirror is needed to show the lingual surfaces and posterior facial areas.

Show the special areas of concern. Relate these to the health of the gingiva.

C. Demonstrate Methods for Daily Plaque Removal

A plan of instruction is outlined in Chapter 27 (page 371). The techniques for toothbrushing and associated procedures were described in Chapters 22 and 23.

TECHNICAL HINTS

I. Avoid using disclosing or antiseptic solutions on teeth that have tooth color restorations because these materials may be stained by coloring agents.

II. Purchase solutions in small quantities. Do not keep solutions containing alcohol longer than 2 or 3 months because the alcohol will evaporate and render the solution too highly concentrated.

III. Use small bottles with dropper caps for solutions. Transfer solution to a dappen dish for use. Do not contaminate the solution by dipping cotton pliers with pellet directly into the container bottle.

IV. Use only small, unsaturated cotton pellets or swab with adequate retraction of cheeks and tongue to control staining of the tongue and alveolar mucosa.

V. Maintain a list of methods for spot removal in case the dye-containing solutions are inadvertently spilled.[4]

VI. Request local druggist to stock disclosing tablets for patients to purchase. Advise patients of the stores where the agents may be purchased.

FACTORS TO TEACH THE PATIENT

I. Purposes for use of disclosing agents: the appearance of stained bacterial plaque and the methods of daily care necessary to keep plaque controlled.

II. Self-evaluation of plaque control methods by using a disclosing agent.

III. For the parent: method of application of a disclosing agent to a small child's teeth to evaluate the presence of plaque.

References

1. Arnim, S.S.: Use of Disclosing Agents for Measuring Tooth Cleanliness, *J. Periodontol., 34,* 227, May, 1963.
2. Lang, N.P., Østergaard, E., and Löe, H.: A Fluorescent Plaque Disclosing Agent, *J. Periodont. Res., 7,* 59, Number 1, 1972.
3. Block, P.L., Lobene, R.R., and Derdivanis, J.P.: A Two-tone Dye Test for Dental Plaque, *J. Periodontol., 43,* 423, July, 1972.
4. Hunt, D.R. and Makinson, O.F.: Removal of Plaque Disclosing Stains from Clothing, *Aust. Dent. J., 29,* 5, February, 1984.

Suggested Readings

American Dental Association, Council on Dental Materials, Instruments, and Equipment: *Dentist's Desk Reference: Materials, Instruments and Equipment,* 2nd ed. Chicago, American Dental Association, 1983, pp. 417–418.

American Dental Association, Council on Dental Therapeutics: *Accepted Dental Therapeutics,* 40th ed. Chicago, American Dental Association, 1984, p. 388.

Baab, D.A., Broadwell, A.H., and Williams, B.L.: A Comparison of Antimicrobial Activity of Four Disclosant Dyes, *J. Dent. Res., 62,* 837, July, 1983.

Barton, J.E.: Disclosants: Their Role in Dentistry, *Dent. Hyg., 55,* 31, January, 1981.

Gallagher, I.H.C., Fussell, S.J., and Cutress, T.W.: Mechanism of Action of a Two-tone Plaque Disclosing Agent, *J. Periodontol., 48,* 395, July, 1977.

Gillings, B.R.D.: Recent Developments in Dental Plaque Disclosants, *Aust. Dent. J., 22,* 260, August, 1977.

Kieser, J.B. and Wade, A.B.: Use of Food Colourants as Plaque Disclosing Agents, *J. Clin. Periodontol., 3,* 200, November, 1976.

Kipioti, A., Tsamis, A., and Mitsis, F.: Disclosing Agents in Plaque Control. Evaluation of Their Role During Periodontal Treatment, *Clin. Prevent. Dent., 6,* 9, November-December, 1984.

Lim, L.P., Tay, F.B.K., Waite, I.M., and Cornick, D.E.R.: A Comparison of 4 Techniques for Clinical Detection of Early Plaque Formed During Different Dietary Regimes, *J. Clin. Periodontol., 13,* 658, August, 1986.

O'Brien, W.J. and Fanian, F.: Use of a Dual Filter-Mirror Device with a Fluorescent Plaque Disclosant, *Clin. Prevent. Dent., 6,* 13, May-June, 1984.

Pitcher, G.R., Newman, H.N., and Strahan, J.D.: Access to Subgingival Plaque by Disclosing Agents Using Mouthrinsing and Direct Irrigation, *J. Clin. Periodontol., 7,* 300, August, 1980.

Tan, A.E.S.: Disclosing Agents in Plaque Control: A Review, *J. West. Soc. Periodont. Periodont. Abstr., 29,* 81, Number 3, 1981.

Tan, A.E.S. and Wade, A.B.: The Role of Visual Feedback by a Disclosing Agent in Plaque Control, *J. Clin. Periodontol., 7,* 140, April, 1980.

27 Disease Control: Helping Patients Learn

People will learn and adhere to the principles and details of methods for the prevention and control of dental caries and periodontal diseases in proportion to the concern and professional enthusiasm shown for their future oral health by members of the dental team. Specialized knowledge of dental and periodontal infections and skill in teaching foster confidence, but of greatest importance is *conviction* that careful treatment and teaching for the particular patient is worthwhile.

An effective teaching program provides both detailed information and principles to guide and motivate the patient to cooperate in optimal personal management. The overall teaching objective is to assist the patient to acquire knowledge, attitudes, and practices that will aid in attaining and maintaining oral health.

I. Planned Patient Learning

Instruction must be planned if it is to stay directed toward goals, utilize available time efficiently, and help the patient to learn sequentially, from the simpler to the more complex. The design of instruction may be divided into certain basic steps.

A. Objectives
What knowledge and skills can be expected of the learner-patient if oral health is to be obtained and maintained?

B. Preparation
What is the patient's background and experience? How can the patient become aware of personal oral health status?

C. Presentation
What knowledge-content must be included? How will the patient be oriented to the overall requirements for reaching the goals? Which instructional methods can be most helpful? What teaching aids are the most efficient?

D. Demonstration/Motivation
What mode of demonstration will be most meaningful to this patient? What is the sequence of steps in the procedures to be learned? How can the steps be shown for sequential learning?

E. Practice
How will the procedures be practiced? How much practice will be needed? How can knowledge and skill-practice be integrated?

F. Evaluation
Can the patient demonstrate the procedures for self-care? Do the teeth and gingiva show the benefits of learning? Does the patient show basic understanding and motivation for continuing care?

The suggested procedure for patient instruction outlined in this chapter follows these six steps. The modes of presentation, demonstration, motivation, and practice are numerous.

Effective patient-centered systems of instruction can be developed that are in accord with the policies and beliefs of the dentist. The important considerations for the methods used are that they are based on current, sound, scientific knowledge, and that they are applied efficiently so that the patient acquires the skill and know-how for adequate daily self-care.

II. Principles of Learning[1]

A. Learning is more effective when an individual is physiologically and psychologically ready to learn.

B. Individual differences must be considered if effective learning is to take place.

C. Motivation is essential for learning.

D. What an individual learns in a given situation depends on what is recognized and understood.

E. Transfer of learning is facilitated by recognition of similarities and dissimilarities between past experiences and the present situation.

F. An individual learns what is actually used.

G. Learning takes place more effectively in situations from which the individual derives feelings of satisfaction.

H. Evaluation of the results of instruction is essential to determine whether learning is taking place.

III. The Learning Ladder[2]

Figure 27–1 illustrates the six steps from learner unawareness to habit formation. When beginning to help a patient learn about oral health and what the individual's needs are, one must determine where the patient stands on the ladder, and start from there. Briefly, the ladder steps are as follows:

A. Unawareness
Many patients have little concept of the new information about dental and periodontal infections and how these are prevented or controlled.

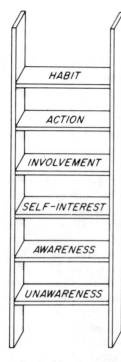

Figure 27–1. The Learning Ladder. Learning takes place in a series of steps from unawareness through interest and involvement to habit-forming. See the text for the description of each step on the ladder. (From Harris, N.O. and Christen, A.G.: *Primary Preventive Dentistry,* 2nd ed. Norwalk, Connecticut, Appleton & Lange, 1987.)

B. Awareness

Patients may have a good knowledge of the scientific facts, but do not apply the facts to personal action.

C. Self-interest

Realization of the application of facts/knowledge to the well-being of the individual is an initial motivation.

D. Involvement

With awareness and application to self, the response to action is forthcoming when attitude is influenced.

E. Action

Testing new knowledge and beginning of change in behavior may lead to an increased awareness that a real health goal is possible to attain.

F. Habit

Self-satisfaction in the comfort and value of sound teeth and healthy periodontal tissues helps to make certain practices become part of a daily routine. Ultimate motivation is finally reached.

INDIVIDUAL PATIENT PLANNING

Each patient has personal requirements for self-care, and objectives to fulfill these requirements must be related realistically to individual needs, interests,

and ability level. If the patient is to participate effectively in the learning process, active involvement in setting goals is necessary.

The general objectives for disease control are for a reduced incidence of new dental carious lesions and for the elimination, control, and prevention of gingival and periodontal infections. The objectives for patient learning are selected with the patient to accomplish these objectives.

I. Selection of Objectives

From the patient history, oral examination, radiographs, study casts, all other data collected during the initial evaluation, and the diagnosis, details of the self-care program are evolved.

The items listed below summarize factors that must be considered.

A. The Gingiva

1. *Current Status of Gingival Health.* As evidenced by the color, size, contour, consistency, surface texture, tendency to bleed, probing depths, and severity of the periodontal condition.
2. *Treatment Plan.* Whether scaling and root planing will complete the professional treatment, or whether the condition will require more complicated periodontal therapy.
3. *Specific Anatomic Features*
   a. Open interdental areas or intact interdental gingiva.
   b. Recession with root exposure.
   c. Width of attached gingiva.

B. The Teeth

1. *Position*
   a. Malrelations, such as crowding, overbite, crossbite; malpositions of individual teeth; normal alignment.
   b. Teeth adjacent to edentulous areas.
2. *Abutment Teeth.*
3. *Dental Appliances.* Fixed, removable, orthodontic.

C. General Health

1. *Chronic Disease.* Any systemic condition that may limit the ability to perform certain tasks or that may cause an exaggerated response of the gingiva to local irritants and require more intensive care.
2. *Capacity of Patient for Self-care.* Physical and mental handicaps that require that another person perform plaque-control procedures.

D. Age

1. Young children require parental assistance.
2. Motivation varies with age.

E. Dexterity

1. Occupation that requires manual or digital dexterity may contribute to increased facility in the manipulation of oral care devices.
2. For most patients, unless a physical handicap

is apparent, dexterity cannot be detected until after instruction has begun.

F. Motivational Factors

1. *Immediate Evaluation.* Previous oral health habits can reveal attitudes and motivation; but frequently, a lack of oral cleanliness can be attributed to a lack of knowledge. Many people have had little or no instruction in how to care for their mouths.
2. *Long-range Motivation.* Prejudging a patient's motivation and willingness to carry out prescribed procedures is rarely possible. Some people show tremendous enthusiasm that may be short-lived; others reveal little interest at first, but prove to be highly conscientious.
3. *Motivation Related to Attitude.* Motivation can be directly related to the concern and enthusiasm of the members of the dental health team.

II. Program Outline

A. Program Planning

All of the aforementioned factors that apply to an individual patient are matched with the available plaque removal and oral physical therapy procedures. These include the selection of a toothbrush, toothbrushing method, interdental care devices and methods, dentifrice, and applied techniques for fixed and removable dental appliances.

With a clear definition of the needs of a patient, a recommended regimen or program can be outlined. The patient is shown the oral condition, changes and benefits that can be expected are explained, and cooperation is solicited. In this framework, the patient helps to formulate the goals that must be accomplished.

B. Immediate and Long-range Planning

Immediate and long-range programs are usually indicated. The immediate program is related to the treatment phase, whereas the long-range program is related to the maintenance phase of care.

The immediate program may be more complicated and intensified than the long-range program. It may seem more complicated to the patient because of the anxieties generally associated with learning new procedures and changing former habits.

The new habits and attitudes acquired during the immediate program phase may aid the transition to the long-range program. With continuing reinforcement of instruction and encouragement, plaque-control measures become a part of the daily routine, and the health of the oral cavity can be maintained.

C. When to Teach

The initial instruction is best given *first*, before any clinical treatment. Reasons related to the educational aspects are as follows:

1. *Emphasis on Importance of Self-care.* Clinical professional services have only short-term effectiveness if the patient does not maintain tissue health through daily plaque removal. If considered first, and first in succeeding appointments, the degree of importance placed on self-care procedures by the dental team will become apparent to the patient.
2. *Teaching Is More Effective.* If instruction is delayed until after the clinical procedures in an appointment,
   a. Time may be limited.
   b. The gingival margin may be sensitive from instrumentation.
   c. Blood clots forming after scaling and root planing should not be disturbed.
   d. Patient may be tired, anxious to leave, and less receptive to instruction.
3. *Plaque on Patient's Teeth.* With removal of tooth deposits during scaling, the opportunity to utilize the patient's existing plaque for demonstration is lost. With the use of a disclosing agent, a method of instruction is available that can clearly and dramatically show the patient what is to be accomplished. Bacterial plaque is not visible on most teeth without staining. Words fail to impress upon the patient that bacterial colonies exist on the teeth and these multitudes of microorganisms are the responsible agents for dental and periodontal infections.

D. The Setting

Because of the need for the light and rinsing facilities during the demonstration, instruction may be given best at the dental chair. Without an extensive display of instruments and other equipment to distract the patient, and with the dental hygienist seated beside the dental chair at the patient's eye level, an atmosphere conducive to learning can be created.

A specific area may be set aside and furnished for plaque-control instruction in a dental office or clinic. Such an area should be planned with mirrors for the patient to use to observe the stained plaque on posterior teeth and distal surfaces. The patient should also be able to see placement of the toothbrush and floss in all areas of the mouth. Requirements for such a facility for a patient in a wheel chair are described on page 614 and in figure 50–2.

PRESENTATION, DEMONSTRATION, PRACTICE

A suggested outline for conducting the plaque-control program follows. Various adaptations will be needed to tailor the plan to individual patients.

Each of the "lessons" described in the following is meant to represent the opening few minutes of each of the treatment appointments. A plaque index or score (pages 262–266) and/or a bleeding index (page 271) is made at the start. The index or score is shown to the patient and new and review instruction is provided as indicated. The scaling and root planing planned for that time are then started.

I. First Lesson

A. Objective
Orientation to bacterial plaque removal.

B. Description
Describe the formation and composition of bacterial plaque, its relationship to oral disease, and specifically its relationship to the patient's present condition. Present an overview of the plaque-control program, what it can accomplish, and its purposes in relation to professional treatment.

C. Illustration
Sketch on a pad of paper or use prepared materials. Show a tooth and gingiva and point out where the bacterial masses collect to form plaque. Explain how inflammation develops in the gingiva. The complete description should be divided over more than one instruction period. Too long a "lecture" with too many facts and details at one time may mean the patient cannot absorb any of them.

1. *Patient with Gingivitis.* Show and explain the formation of dental calculus and how periodontal disease can develop if gingivitis is left untreated.
2. *Patient with Periodontitis.* Introduce pocket formation and the reasons for pocket elimination.
3. *Patient Whose Most Severe Problem is Dental Caries.* When a dietary survey is to be made, orientation to the preparation of the survey precludes discussion of plaque, sucrose, and dental caries, until the dietary record is obtained (page 383).

D. Demonstration
1. While the patient observes in a hand mirror, a healthy area of gingiva and an inflamed area can be compared.
2. A probe is used to show a gingival sulcus and/or increased pocket depth related to periodontal involvement. Bleeding on probing is an important indicator of disease and should be recorded.
3. Remove a sample of plaque with a curet to demonstrate the thickness and consistency of plaque, to use in a test for acid formation (methyl red spot plate test, or Snyder test, pages 389–390) and to use for a phase microscope demonstration.

E. Application of a Disclosing Agent
1. *Explain Its Purpose.* Discoloration of plaque shows where the masses of bacteria accumulate.

2. *Apply Disclosing Agent.* Use a topical application, provide diluted concentrate for a rinse, or request the patient to chew a tablet, swish for approximately 1 minute, and rinse (pages 367–368).
3. *Examine the Teeth with the Patient.* Point out the stained plaque and explain how these areas (generally the proximal surfaces and cervical third of the teeth) are adjacent to the gingiva, and therefore the bacteria must be removed to control inflammation.
4. *Record Plaque Score or Index* (pages 262–266). Explain the score to the patient and use it to compare at future evaluations.
5. *Observe Location.* Observation of the location of disclosed plaque will guide the instruction for plaque removal.

F. Instruction
1. *Keep Instruction Simple.* It may be better not to teach both flossing and brushing during the first control lesson depending on the patient's background and experience.
2. *Floss First*
   a. Review objective.
   b. Show manner of holding the floss, inserting proximally, pressing around the tooth, and activating for plaque removal (figure 23–1, page 319).
   c. Examine in mirror to observe proximal areas where plaque has been removed.
3. *Brush.* Give a soft brush and ask the patient to remove the stained plaque. No specific brushing instructions should be given at this time so that the patient can concentrate on the single objective related to plaque removal.
4. *After Brushing, Examine the Teeth with the Patient.* The patient will see where accessible plaque was removed.
5. *Explain.* The use of a toothbrush is the most effective means of plaque control for facial and lingual surfaces, as is the use of floss for proximal surfaces.

G. Summary of Lesson I
1. Review the basic objectives: to learn about plaque composition, occurrence, and relationship to oral disease; to learn about the use of a disclosing agent to aid in plaque detection and removal.
2. At the first lesson, a specific toothbrushing method is not necessarily presented. The basic objectives should not be obscured by inclusion of excess information or diversion of the patient's thinking by concentration on details of brush position. There are exceptions; for example:
   a. The patient who demonstrates an acceptable brushing technique, whose mouth has been kept reasonably clean and shows no signs of detrimental brushing, may only

need to be shown a few special adaptations for the difficult-to-reach areas or other improvements.

   b. The patient who demonstrates a brushing method that is detrimental such as a vigorous horizontal stroke or a haphazard scrub-brush method, and whose teeth and/or gingiva show the effects of harmful brushing, will need an introduction to a less destructive method.

H. Continuation of Appointment

Instruction and practice in plaque removal can occupy the first appointment. Clinical services may not be started until the gingival inflammatory clinical signs have been lessened and the patient shows good progress in learning self-care.

When calculus removal is initiated, the relation of clinical procedures to plaque control should be made clear to the patient. The satisfactory long-range outcome of scaling and other professional treatment is dependent on complete daily plaque removal.

I. Instruction at End of Appointment

1. Use of disclosing agent at home: provide patient with tablets or instructions for purchasing. Suggest using a tablet for daily plaque checks.
2. Emphasize the need for cleaning regularly for complete daily plaque removal. Discuss carrying a toothbrush and dental floss for use when not at home.
3. When extra brushes cannot be supplied, explain that the toothbrush that has been used that day will be kept in the office for use during future appointments. Write down the specific name (number) of the brush for the patient to purchase for home use.

J. Patient Records

Methods, procedures, and patient progress and problems should be recorded following each appointment. The documented record can be reviewed before each appointment as a guide to continuing instruction.

II. Second Lesson

A. Objectives

To evaluate patient's success to date and to review and expand the knowledge-content of the previous lesson.

B. Evaluation

1. *Examine the Gingival Tissue with the Patient.* Evaluate and compare with notes recorded from previous examination. Changes in color, size, and bleeding on probing should be noted and recorded.
2. *Apply the Disclosing Agent.* Evaluate the plaque as the patient self-evaluates, using a hand mirror. Chart plaque index or other record and compare, with the patient, with previous scores or indices.

C. Review and Extension of Knowledge

1. Invite questions from patient concerning plaque formation and gingival and periodontal infections to determine how clearly information from the previous lesson was understood and retained.
2. Discuss dentifrice recommendation when information from the dental history and the oral examination indicates the need for a change.
3. Explain why the patient needs a more scientific brushing method (or how a few alterations in the previous method can improve the oral condition).
4. Relate brushing to the treatment phase of oral care.

D. Demonstration

When not done previously, demonstrate the brushing technique of choice for this particular patient.

1. Show the basic stroke on the anterior teeth where the patient can observe brush position and activation. Explain each step. Demonstrate brush position for each quadrant.
2. Instruction is divided appropriately to permit the patient to learn at a comfortable pace. When a patient has a power-driven brush, it is recommended that initial instruction be given with the manual brush so that proficiency can be attained with both. The patient should be asked to bring the power-driven brush to the next appointment for demonstration and instruction.

E. Practice

1. Each position around each arch must be practiced because of the variations in grasp of brush and hand positions, the difficulty of access, and the individual tooth positions, particularly malpositions.
2. A recommended sequence for brushing that will include all areas and the tongue is discussed with the patient.

F. Instructions for Home Procedures

Use disclosing agent after flossing and brushing to test completeness of plaque removal. A mouth mirror for the patient to use at home can be helpful. Inexpensive plastic mirrors are available specifically for this purpose.

III. Third Lesson

A. Objectives

1. Patients with reasonable mastery of the flossing and brushing methods, who need auxiliary plaque control and oral physical therapy measures (interdental, dental appliances, or other), begin the third phase of their instruction.

2. When a patient is not ready and the plaque score or index still shows a lack of reasonable skill and motivation, introduction of new material may be postponed and previous instruction reviewed and practiced.

3. Many dentists will postpone therapy until the patient shows that an effective plaque control program can be carried out and an acceptable level of oral cleanliness can be maintained.

B. Evaluation and Review

1. *Evaluate Gingiva.* Inspect with the patient for color, size, bleeding, and other characteristics of disease. Review the features of normal gingiva and commend improvements. Quadrants that have been scaled and root planed can be compared with other quadrants so that the effect of healing can be shown.

   Question the patient about changes observed during the past week or since the previous appointment, such as less bleeding when brushing, better taste, and an overall feeling of cleanliness. Emphasize the role of self-care in accomplishing the improvements rather than the effects of professional treatment.

2. *Evaluate Plaque.* Apply disclosing agent and inspect for areas that need additional instruction. Relate areas of persistent gingival redness to areas inadequately flossed and brushed.

3. *Evaluate Brushing.* Patient demonstrates with emphasis on the areas missed as revealed by gingival and disclosing agent examinations. Help the patient to evaluate and make corrections. Supplement as needed with demonstration.

C. Introduction of New Material

Demonstrate auxiliary interdental or other methods; explain the purposes and procedures for each method selected for this patient.

D. Practice

Most interdental methods require continued instruction. A specific appointment to check the method of use is particularly important by at least the end of the first week, because incorrect habits may become permanent if allowed to persist.

IV. Continuous Instruction

A. Number of Lessons

It is not possible to predict in advance the number of specific teaching sessions a patient will need to demonstrate mastery of the recommended procedures and to show by the appearance of the teeth and health of the gingiva that the practices have been carried out daily. When additional supervision is indicated after professional treatment has been completed, short appointments may be scheduled in conjunction with dental appointments.

One teaching-learning experience is rarely ad-

equate. When a patient has been able to maintain relatively clean teeth and clinically healthy gingiva and can demonstrate an acceptable toothbrushing method, a review of difficult-to-reach areas can be made and reevaluated at a follow-up appointment.

B. Relationship to Gingival Health

When areas of gingival marginal redness and sponginess persist, tooth surfaces are checked carefully for residual calculus, and scaling and planing are completed as indicated. When the patient consistently fails to remove dental plaque in certain areas, a reevaluation of the program is made. Perhaps the selected procedures are too difficult for the patient to accomplish or perhaps supplementary measures are needed.

C. Maintenance

After the initial instruction series, a follow-up is best scheduled after a shorter interval than may be used for succeeding maintenance appointments. One must evaluate the patient's ability to continue adequate self-care and determine whether true learning has resulted and new habits have been adopted. Learning means that a change in behavior has occurred.

At each maintenance appointment, a plaque score or index is recorded, and the patient can evaluate the progress made. The complete procedures for the appointment are described on pages 540–541.

V. Instruction Adaptability

The methods for presentation, demonstration, practice, and evaluation described in the previous pages can be adapted readily to various age levels. Awareness of the changing motivation and interests from the young to the elderly, and adaptations of terminology with respect for the patient's level of understanding, ease the transition from patient to patient.

Others for whom instruction is provided are the nurses or family members who attend patients who are unable to care for themselves. In Section VI, the various chapters that pertain to patients with disabilities include suggestions for patient care. Aids and devices are described on pages 621–625.

THE PRESCHOOL CHILD

The establishment of positive health habits and attitudes in the adult has its beginnings in childhood. Even before birth and during the first year after birth, the parent's education for prevention of dental caries and gingival infection should begin.

After birth, regular daily systemic fluoride in the absence of fluoridation, as well as attention to the control of dietary sucrose, can mean a great deal to the future oral health of the child. Nursing bottle caries was described on page 218. Information about plaque control for gingival health can be applied while the child's primary teeth are erupting.

I. Early Plaque Control

Conditioning a child to associate cleaning of the oral cavity with total body cleanliness can begin when the first teeth erupt. A small, soft toothbrush may be used or, at first, the parent can rub the teeth and gingiva with a cloth wrapped over a finger.

As time goes on, the child will want to use the brush, particularly if given the opportunity to watch the parents brush their teeth. At first, a tiny child may only chew on the brush, but eventually may try to imitate the parents. Gradually, an actual brushing procedure can be encouraged.

For several years the parents will have the responsibility for brushing the child's teeth after meals and flossing and brushing before the child retires. The age varies with the individual child relative to when the child can take on the responsibility. It has been suggested that when a child attends to bathing, personal toothbrushing may also be done. Parental supervision and encouragement must continue for a few more years for most children.

II. Professional Instruction

A. The First Dental Appointment

Early visits to the dental office for orientation and getting acquainted are to be encouraged. If the child has not had a dental emergency and therefore visited the dental office earlier, oral examination and necessary treatment are indicated no later than 12 months of age.[3] Instruction in plaque control for child and parent should be introduced at the first appointment along with other preventive measures.

B. Effect of Age

Each year brings marked differences in the behavior of preschool children. The child at 2 years of age may be cooperative and well-behaved; at about 2½, contrary and difficult; by 3, amiable and in good control, yet at 4 be difficult and dogmatic. The general suggestions made below should be applied to the individual child, and are presented only as a basis from which instruction can be planned.

C. Instruction for the Child

1. *Toothbrush Selection.* A child-sized, soft nylon brush is recommended. When possible, let the child select the brush from assorted colors.
2. *Method.* Control of bacterial plaque at the gingival margin and on proximal tooth surfaces requires the same emphasis for the very young as at other ages. Although the very young child will have a short interest span for specific instruction, the mother can be coached to assist with supplementary home instruction. Many dentists favor instruction in a scrub-brush method for preschool children (page 310).

III. Instruction for the Parent

The parent who is a patient in the same dental practice may be familiar already with the teaching methods used and well-oriented to the importance of bacterial plaque control. Transfer of knowledge and skills to care of the child can be relatively easy. When the child is a patient in a pedodontic specialty practice or the parent is a patient elsewhere, orientation will be needed in accord with the parent's present knowledge.

A. Disclosing Agent

1. The use of tablets is preferable, for those older preschool children who will chew them, so that tablets can be used at home for the parent to evaluate plaque control. One-half tablet is sufficient. When a young child cannot understand about chewing the tablet, disclosing solution can be applied.
2. Examination: the child is given a mirror to "watch" the teeth. The plaque deposits are pointed out and discussed with the parent, and a little plaque removed with a probe to illustrate.

B. Demonstration

The brushing method of choice is shown to the parent while the child is in the dental chair under the light.

C. Procedure and Practice

1. *Provide Natural Setting.* Procedures are demonstrated to both the child and parent, to simulate the home setting. Several positions for parent and child are effective and are shown in figure 50–9 on page 627.
2. *Demonstrate Head Support.* Show the parent how, if the child's teeth are brushed from the front, the child's head falls back, unsupported, and seeing into the mouth is difficult.
3. *Suggested Standing Position.* Child stands in front of parent and leans back against the parent. Parent cradles the child's head with the nondominant arm and brings the hand around to hold the chin in the palm of the hand and to retract the lips and cheek with the fingers.
4. *Brush Mandibular Teeth.* Retract lip for anterior and cheek for posterior teeth. The back of the brush head will retract the tongue.
5. *Maxillary Teeth.* Child is asked to tip the head back so that the parent can look in the mouth while fingers retract the upper lip for anterior and the cheek for posterior teeth.
6. *Dental Floss.* With the child's head supported as described above for brushing, the parent can be shown how finger and hand rests (fulcrums) can be maintained while floss is applied. When primary teeth are widely spaced, brushing may be adapted to remove plaque from all surfaces without a need for flossing. If more efficient, the parent can use nylon yarn

for proximal surfaces. Flossing may not be recommended for all children (page 318).

7. *Dentifrice Recommendation.* A fluoride dentifrice is preferred, even when fluoride is in the drinking water. The amount of fluoride dentifrice that should be used is illustrated in figure 29–8 (page 410).

When a child has a dental caries problem, additional measures may be recommended. As the child matures and develops the ability to rinse, a daily fluoride rinse can be used.

D. Summary

Instructions include brushing after each meal and using the disclosing test before one of the brushings. In a nonfluoridated area, the most beneficial procedure is to use a fluoride supplement (mouthrinse and swallow, or chewable tablet, page 400) at bedtime after thorough plaque removal by toothbrushing and flossing.

E. Second Appointment

Procedure follows that for an adult. The gingiva are examined, and bleeding on probing is evaluated; plaque is disclosed and neglected areas are discovered; the child demonstrates brushing, and then the parent. Suggestions for improvement are offered.

As needed, calculus and dental stain are removed professionally. Brushing demonstration precedes each succeeding restorative appointment until proficiency is demonstrated.

IV. Maintenance

Instruction continues with each 4 to 6 months' maintenance appointment.

THE TEACHING SYSTEM

A simple, direct approach, such as has been described, with specific content and unembellished with excess distracting material focuses the attention of the patient-learner on the central theme: disease control. The more practical, realistic, and goal-centered the components of instruction can be, the more effective the outcomes will be in terms of treatment and prevention of recurrence of disease. An *informed,* knowledgeable patient will have reasons for *practicing* appropriate, scientifically based, self-care measures.

A teaching system must be reevaluated from time to time, particularly as new research reveals new aspects of prevention and treatment. New devices for plaque removal and gingival care may become available, and these must be studied before recommendations to patients can be made.

The teaching system presented in this chapter has a built-in-evaluation of patient learning. The outcomes of learning are shown by examination and demonstration: examination for the gingival characteristics consistent with health; demonstration of

disclosable plaque, and the demonstration of the patient's ability to use floss and brush for plaque removal without harm to the oral tissues.

Because the ultimate objective of plaque control is to prevent dental caries and periodontal infections, the oral health history of the patient over several years can be used to document a true evaluation. The teaching system must involve development of the patient's attitudes relative to continuing professional supervision and regular appointments for examination and treatment.

EVALUATION OF TEACHING AIDS

I. General Characteristics

Evaluation of teaching aids involves consideration of the following:

A. Simplicity

Ease of management, ready obtainability, ease of understanding by the patient.

B. Content

Practical, scientifically sound, meaningful.

C. Level of Orientation

Appropriate to the individual patient.

D. Durability

If reusable, the teaching aids must maintain their cleanliness and freshness. Washable materials can be selected when appropriate.

E. Cost

Reasonable. Cost relates to their essential value in reaching goals.

F. Objectives

1. Objective of a teaching aid must be clear and readily understood by the patient.
2. In teaching, activities should be reality-centered not fantasy-centered. A well-intentioned visual aid may provide entertainment rather than education and have no transfer value, in terms of the actual oral health lesson, to the behavioral pattern of the patient.

II. Reading Material for the Patient

Effectively presented, informational books and leaflets can supplement and reinforce individually presented instruction. Selected with a purpose, a booklet or other printed material may be presented to the patient to read while at the dental office or it may be given for "homework." The booklet's contents must be reviewed with the patient; particular sections may be marked to personalize the instruction and encourage reading. Indiscriminate distribution of printed materials is pointless.

Obtaining copies and reviewing newly available materials are essential parts of a dental hygienist's work, even as a teacher reviews new textbooks and materials for possible use in a classroom.

Instruction sheets and leaflets can be custom-made

by the dental hygienist with the cooperation and recommendations of the dentist. It is especially helpful to have postoperative instructions, plaque control, and oral physical therapy procedures outlined so that the patient will have a reference for home use. Materials can be personalized by writing on them the patient's name and special procedures or reminders.

III. Use of Models

A. Patient's Study Cast

The cast can be useful to explain oral conditions or restorations such as the need to replace missing teeth. With certain patients, aspects of plaque control and oral physical therapy can be demonstrated, provided the patient is properly oriented to associate the cast with the teeth in the mouth.

B. Commercially Available Models

Although plastic models (dentoforms) have been used extensively for teaching toothbrushing methods, their meaningfulness to the patient has not been demonstrated. When a toothbrush is to be available for the patient to practice brushing in his mouth, the usefulness of the time spent to demonstrate on a model first may be questioned. When teaching is by means of the model and brush only, and particularly when the oversized model will be used, the patient's learning should be carefully evaluated. All three of the patient evaluation methods described in this chapter (gingival status, disclosed plaque, and ability of patient to brush) should be utilized.

The model and the large toothbrush probably do not represent a problem to the patient, and most patients can imitate the motions of the toothbrush on the model accurately when asked. The difficulty comes in transferring the motions to the mouth and relating such motions to the bacterial collections on the teeth. The more complex the technique, the greater the difficulty of transfer.

References

1. Sand, O.: *Curriculum Study in Basic Nursing Education.* New York, Putnam, 1955, pp. 53–60.
2. Christen, A.G.: Understanding Human Motivation, in Harris, N.O. and Christen, A.G.: *Primary Preventive Dentistry,* 2nd ed. Norwalk, Connecticut, Appleton & Lange, 1987, pp. 390–393.
3. American Academy of Pediatric Dentistry: Oral Health Policies for Children. VIII. Policy Statement on Infant Dental Care, American Academy of Pediatric Dentistry, 211 East Chicago Avenue, Chicago, Illinois, May, 1986, p. 34.
4. Routh, D.K.: The Preschool Child, in Gabel, S. and Erickson, M.T., eds.: *Child Development and Developmental Disabilities.* Boston, Little, Brown and Company, 1980, pp. 21–42.

Suggested Readings

Arnim, S.S. and Williams, Q.E.: How to Educate Patients in Oral Hygiene, *Dent. Radiogr. Photogr., 32,* 61, Number 4, 1959.

Baab, D. and Weinstein, P.: Longitudinal Evaluation of a Self-inspection Plaque Index in Periodontal Recall Patients, *J. Clin. Periodontol., 13,* 313, April, 1986.

Baab, D.A. and Weinstein, P.: Oral Hygiene Instruction Using a Self Inspection Plaque Index, *Community Dent. Oral Epidemiol., 11,* 174, June, 1983.

Bakdash, M.B.: A Clinical Model for Monitoring Patients' Oral Hygiene Performance, *Northwest Dent., 60,* 77, March-April, 1981.

Bowen, D.M. and Darby, M.L.: Effectiveness of the Phase Contrast Microscope, *Dent. Hyg., 55,* 26, February, 1981.

Boyer, E.M.: Compliance and Dental Hygiene Self-care, *Dent. Hyg., 62,* 30, January, 1988.

Boyer, E.M. and Nikias, M.K.: Self-reported Compliance with a Preventive Dental Regimen, *Clin. Prevent. Dent., 5,* 3, January-February, 1983.

Brown, J.C.: Patient Noncompliance: A Neglected Topic in Dentistry, *J. Am. Dent. Assoc., 103,* 567, October, 1981.

Conte, T.G.: Realistic Dental Care in Jails and Prisons: Summary of Proceedings, *J. Am. Dent. Assoc., 102,* 343, March, 1981.

Corn, H., Marks, M.H., and Corn, B.M.: Educating the Patient in Effective Plaque Control, in Clark, J.W., ed.: *Clinical Dentistry,* Volume 2, Chapter 4, Philadelphia, J.B. Lippincott Co., 1985, pp. 1–64.

Emler, B.F., Windchy, A.M., Zaino, S.W., Feldman, S.M., and Scheetz, J.P.: The Value of Repetition and Reinforcement in Improving Oral Hygiene Performance, *J. Periodontol., 51,* 228, April, 1980.

Glavind, L.: The Result of Periodontal Treatment in Relationship to Various Background Factors, *J. Clin. Periodontol., 13,* 789, September, 1986.

Glavind, L. and Zeuner, E.: Evaluation of a Television-tape Demonstration for the Reinforcement of Oral Hygiene Instruction, *J. Clin. Periodontol., 13,* 201, March, 1986.

Glavind, L., Christensen, H., Pedersen, H., Rosendahl, H., and Attström, R.: Oral Hygiene Instruction in General Dental Practice by Means of Self-teaching Manuals, *J. Clin. Periodonto!., 12,* 27, January, 1985.

Glavind, L., Zeuner, E., and Attström, R.: Evaluation of Various Feedback Mechanisms in Relation to Compliance by Adult Patients with Oral Home Care Instructions, *J. Clin. Periodontol., 10,* 57, January, 1983.

Glavind, L., Zeuner, E., and Attström, R.: Oral Cleanliness and Gingival Health Following Oral Hygiene Instruction by Self-educational Programs, *J. Clin. Periodontol., 11,* 262, April, 1984.

Glavind, L., Zeuner, E., and Attström, R.: Oral Hygiene Instruction of Adults by Means of a Self-instructional Manual, *J. Clin. Periodontol., 8,* 165, June, 1981.

Hamp, S.-E., Johansson, L.-Å., and Karlsson, R.: Clinical Effects of Preventive Regimens for Young People in Their Early and Middle Teens in Relation to Previous Experience with Dental Prevention, *Acta Odontol. Scand., 42,* 99, Number 2, 1984.

Hoogstraten, J. and Moltzer, G.: Effects of Dental Health Care Instruction on Knowledge, Attitude, Behavior and Fear, *Community Dent. Oral Epidemiol., 11,* 278, October, 1983.

Huntley, D.E.: Andragogy in Plaque Control Instruction, *Dent. Hyg., 61,* 24, January, 1987.

Levine, R.S.: The Scientific Basis of Dental Health Education. A Health Education Council Policy Document. Part I. A General Guide for Those Involved in Dental Health Education, *Br. Dent. J., 158,* 223, March 23, 1985.

Martin, B.J. and Mauldin, B.B.: The Role of the Dental Hygienist in Patient Motivation, *J. Am. Dent. Assoc., 106,* 613, May, 1983.

McCaul, K.D., Glasgow, R.E., and Gustafson, C.: Predicting Levels of Preventive Dental Behaviors, *J. Am. Dent. Assoc., 111,* 601, October, 1985.

Miller, S.S.: Strategies and Techniques for Oral Health Maintenance and Disease Control, in Darby, M.L. and Bushee, E.J., eds.: *Mosby's Comprehensive Review of Dental Hygiene.* St. Louis, The C.V. Mosby Co., 1986, pp. 467–470.

Nestarick, D.J. and Shute, R.E.: Improving the Oral Hygiene Practices of Dental Hygienists, *Dent. Hyg., 57,* 26, April, 1983.

Odman, P.A., Lange, A.L., and Bakdash, M.B.: Utilization of Locus of Control in the Prediction of Patients' Oral Hygiene Performance, *J. Clin. Periodontol., 11,* 367, July, 1984.

Petersen, M.: Treating Adult Patients as Partners in Dental Health Education, *Dent. Hyg., 60,* 346, August, 1986.

Schou, L.: Active-involvement Principle in Dental Health Education, *Community Dent. Oral Epidemiol., 13,* 128, June, 1985.

Walsh, M.M.: Effects of School-based Dental Health Education on Knowledge, Attitudes and Behavior of Adolescents in San Francisco, *Community Dent. Oral Epidemiol., 13,* 143, June, 1985.

Walsh, M.M., Heckman, B.H., and Moreau-Diettinger, R.: Use of Gingival Bleeding for Reinforcement of Oral Home Care Behavior, *Community Dent. Oral Epidemiol., 13,* 133, June, 1985.

Weinstein, P., Getz, T., and Milgrom, P.: Oral Self-care: A Promising Alternative Behavior Model, *J. Am. Dent. Assoc., 107,* 67, July, 1983.

Children

Albino, J.E., Tedesco, L.A., and Lee, C.Z.: Peer Leadership and Health Status: Factors Moderating Response to a Children's Dental Health Program, *Clin. Prevent. Dent., 2,* 18, January-February, 1980.

Blinkhorn, A.S.: Factors Influencing the Transmission of the Toothbrushing Routine by Mothers to Their Pre-school Children, *J. Dent., 8,* 307, December, 1980.

Boyer, E.M. and Field, H.M.: Tissue Response to Initial Performance of Flossing and Sulcular Toothbrushing, *Dent. Hyg., 54,* 370, August, 1980.

Claus, J. and Alexander, K.: Dental Health Programs in Preschools, *Dent. Hyg., 55,* 21, February, 1981.

Frazier, P.J.: School-based Instruction for Improving Oral Health: Closing the Knowledge Gap, *Int. Dent. J., 30,* 257, September, 1980.

Gill, S. and Jorstad, M.E.: A Public School Preventive Dental Health Program, *Dent. Hyg., 54,* 281, June, 1980.

Honkala, E., Nyyssönen, V., Knuuttila, M., and Markkanen, H.: Effectiveness of Children's Habitual Toothbrushing, *J. Clin. Periodontol., 13,* 81, January, 1986.

Horowitz, A.M., Suomi, J.D., Peterson, J.K., Mathews, B.L., Voglesong, R.H., and Lyman, B.A.: Effects of Supervised Daily Dental Plaque Removal by Children After 3 Years, *Community Dent. Oral Epidemiol., 8,* 171, August, 1980.

Kleber, C.J., Putt, M.S., and Muhler, J.C.: Duration and Pattern of Toothbrushing in Children Using a Gel or Paste Dentifrice, *J. Am. Dent. Assoc., 103,* 723, November, 1981.

Korins, J.I., Sposato, A., Leske, G.S., and Ripa, L.W.: Toothbrushing Efficiency of First-grade Children, *J. Pedod., 6,* 148, Winter, 1982.

Leatherman, G.H.: Oral Hygiene for Children: A Look at What We Must Have and What We Should Do, *Int. Dent. J., 32,* 252, September, 1982.

Mescher, K.D., Brine, P., and Biller, I.: Ability of Elementary School Children to Perform Sulcular Toothbrushing as Related to Their Hand Function Ability, *Pediatr. Dent., 2,* 31, March, 1980.

Simmons, S., Smith, R., and Gelbier, S.: Effect of Oral Hygiene Instruction on Brushing Skills in Preschool Children, *Community Dent. Oral Epidemiol., 11,* 193, August, 1983.

Søgaard, A.J., Tuominen, R., Holst, D., and Gjermo, P.: The Effect of 2 Teaching Programs on the Gingival Health of 15-year-old Schoolchildren, *J. Clin. Periodontol., 14,* 165, March, 1987.

Sutcliffe, P., Rayner, J.A., and Brown, M.D.: Daily Supervised Toothbrushing in Nursery Schools, *Br. Dent. J., 157,* 201, September 22, 1984.

Torpaz, E., Noam, Y., Anaise, J.Z., and Sgan-Cohen, H.: Effectiveness of Dental Health Educational Programs on Oral Cleanliness of Schoolchildren in Israel, *Dent. Hyg., 58,* 169, April, 1984.

28 *Diet and Dietary Analysis*

Planning for a total preventive program for an individual patient involves consideration of dietary and nutritional factors. The status of oral health can be affected by nutrition, diet, and food habits. Proper nutrition improves general health, and improved general health can contribute to a higher degree of oral health.

Instruction relating to diet is coordinated with other phases of teaching. To give information about a diet conducive to oral health is a responsibility, and to help motivate a patient to adopt new eating patterns, a challenge.

Food selection by an individual is influenced by age, sex, geographic location, economic status, available foods, family traditions, religion, cultural habits, prejudices, fallacies, and advertising, as well as emotional and social factors. Instruction must be made practical and possible to apply if it is to have impact on such forceful influences.

I. Terminology

A. Nutrition

The term nutrition refers to the combination of processes by which the living organism receives and utilizes the materials (food) necessary for the maintenance of its functions and for the growth and renewal of its components.

B. Diet

The diet is the total amount of food and drink regularly consumed.

C. Nutrients

Nutrients are those chemical substances in food that are needed by the body. They are divided into six classes: proteins and amino acids, fats and fatty acids, carbohydrates, mineral elements, vitamins, and water.

D. Nutritional Deficiency

A nutritional deficiency means there is an inadequacy of nutrients in the tissues. A deficiency may be the result of inadequate dietary intake or of impairment in digestion, absorption, transport, metabolism, or excretion.

II. Periodontal Tissues[1,2,3]

A. Nutritional Deficiencies

1. Protein, vitamins, and other nutrients are essential to the health of the periodontal tissues, just as they are to the health of the tissues throughout the body.

2. A nutritional deficiency has never been shown to be the specific cause of periodontal pocket formation, gingivitis, or periodontal infections. For these conditions to develop, plaque microorganisms must be present.

3. Certain nutritional deficiencies (notably protein, ascorbic acid, and vitamin B complex) may modify gingival tissue resistance so that an inflammatory condition (initiated by plaque microorganisms) may be accelerated or increased in intensity.

4. The effects of periodontal infection can alter the capacity of the tissues to utilize available nutrients; therefore, the potential for repair is modified.

B. Consistency of Food

1. Soft sticky foods cling to the teeth and gingiva and encourage food and debris accumulation. Microorganisms are protected and nourished, thus leading to increased amounts of bacterial plaque.

2. Firm fibrous foods may stimulate the tissues and improve circulation. Fibrous foods (particularly uncooked fruits and vegetables) tend to clear away loose debris and impart a generally clean sensation. They do not remove plaque from the cervical area.[4]

C. Dietary Analysis

Patients with acute gingival disease, necrotizing ulcerative gingivitis, and most patients undergoing periodontal therapy need specific instruction in diet selection. A dietary survey with analysis is necessary if a true idea of the patient's diet is to be available for study. Procedures for the survey and analysis are described later in this chapter.

III. Mucous Membranes

A. Nutritional Deficiencies

Severe nutritional deficiencies are rare except in underdeveloped areas of the world. Deficiencies tend to produce symptoms of mixed clinical entities, but infrequently of a severe acute disease. When certain oral symptoms suggest nutritional deficiencies, most likely the patient is suffering from multiple deficiencies.

Ordinarily, the effects of a deficiency are chronic and run a slow, gradual course. The clinical manifestations are influenced by trauma, local irritation, or systemic factors, such as a chronic disease, when tissue resistance may be lowered.

B. Oral Lesions

Types of oral lesions that suggest the possibility of an underlying nutritional deficiency are stomatitis, glossitis, cheilitis, and localized ulcerations and areas of atrophic change.[5] Definitive diagnosis by the dentist is difficult or impossible, even with the patient history, a dietary analysis, and laboratory tests. Nutrients that are considered particularly associated with the health of the oral mucosa are iron, ascorbic acid, and various B vitamins.

C. Instruction

Assistance to patients through recommendations for an adequate diet for general health contribute to preserving the integrity of the oral mucosa.

IV. Dental Caries[3,6]

A. Prevention

Fluoride is the essential nutrient for dental caries prevention. A deficiency of fluoride during the years of tooth formation results in an increase in carious lesions when the teeth are exposed to a cariogenic diet.

B. Role of Cariogenic Foods

Dental caries is the result of action on the external surface of the tooth. Instead of being a deficiency disease, it can be considered the result of an excess of cariogenic foods. Dietary sugars produce acids when acted on by specific plaque microorganisms. These factors were discussed in connection with bacterial plaque, page 242.

C. Dietary Analysis and Counseling

The use of dietary analysis in the instruction of patients and, when the patients are children, also their parents relative to dental caries control has proven helpful to many people. Specific personal recommendations can be made.

Special attention must be given the patient with an eating disorder that has led to rampant dental caries.

EATING DISORDERS

Patients with eating disorders are seen frequently in dental and dental hygiene practice. As has been mentioned, the problem of the patient with rampant dental caries may be an eating disorder that has led to an excessive intake of sucrose and other cariogenic foods many times each day. Another example is the obese patient whose obesity is caused by excessive eating of highly caloric foods combined with psychologic factors of significance.

Anorexia nervosa and bulimia nervosa are other examples of serious eating disorders. When these conditions are suspected by dentists and dental hygienists, advice for referral for medical evaluation is a priority. Complex medical problems may exist and psychiatric therapy is usually indicated.

I. Anorexia Nervosa[7]

The syndrome anorexia nervosa is that of a personality disorder manifested by an extreme aversion to food that results in life-threatening weight loss. It involves self-imposed starvation resulting from an obsessive desire to be thin and an intense fear of gaining weight.

A. General Characteristics

1. Initial onset is usually in adolescence or early adult life; females are afflicted primarily; less than 5 percent of patients are males. The majority of these patients are successful, attractive people.
2. The patient's self-image is of a person wider and fatter: in reality, the person is very thin, with marked weight loss.
3. Weight loss is at least 15 percent below normal for age and height; weight loss is associated with reduction in food intake and, often, extensive exercising.
4. The patient may have bulimic episodes with self-induced vomiting. Bulimia nervosa may also be diagnosed.

B. Medical Complications[8,9]

1. Profound loss of weight followed by lowered body temperature, low blood pressure, and slowed heart rate.
2. Amenorrhea.
3. Metabolic changes related to endocrine, gastrointestinal, cardiovascular, hematologic, and renal disturbances.

II. Bulimia Nervosa[7]

The syndrome of bulimia nervosa is an eating disorder characterized by recurrent episodes of binge eating and feelings of lack of control over the eating behavior.

A. General Characteristics

1. Initial onset is usually in adolescence or early adult life. It may continue over many years, alternating with periods of normal eating or periods of fasting.
2. Binge eating is followed by self-induced vomiting, use of laxatives or diuretics, fasting, or vigorous exercise to prevent weight gain.
3. Food consumed during a binge is often cariogenic, with a high caloric content, sweet taste, and a texture that allows rapid eating.
4. The patient's weight may be within a normal range.
5. Depression is common, with the patient having feelings of guilt and self-criticism following a binge-purge session.
6. Drug and/or alcohol abuse is not uncommon.

B. Medical Complications[8,9]

1. Problems include dehydration, electrolyte imbalance, cardiac arrhythmia, and gastric dilation.
2. Self-medications include the abuse of laxatives and diuretics, which contributes to intestinal disturbances. Ipecac used to induce vomiting leads to cardiovascular and muscle tissue damage (myopathy).
3. Amenorrhea, when the patient also has a history of anorexia nervosa.
4. Aspiration pneumonia related to vomiting, particularly when the patient is in a state of decreased consciousness because of drug or alcohol abuse.

C. Oral Findings

1. Swelling of parotid glands ("puffy cheeks").
2. Trauma around the mouth from implements used to induce vomiting; when fingers are used, callouses may be present.
3. Erosion of teeth, primarily on the lingual and incisal surfaces of maxillary anterior teeth and the occlusal and palatal surfaces of maxillary molars. Restorations may appear elevated when erosion occurs around them.
4. Sensitivity of eroded teeth.
5. Xerostomia from self-medications such as diuretics.

III. Appointment Considerations

A. Guides to Recognition of the Patient's Problem

With a high level of suspicion, medical history questions concerning diet, use of laxatives and diuretics, eating habits, weight, and weight control methods and exercise may bring forth a pattern of behavior suggestive of anorexia nervosa or bulimia nervosa.

B. Dietary Analysis

Use of a dietary analysis such as described in this chapter may not bring forth honest answers from the patient, but it may suggest explanations of oral findings.

C. Recommendations for Preventive Measures

1. Immediately after vomiting, rinse with sodium bicarbonate or magnesium hydroxide solution. Do not brush after vomiting.
2. Use a multiple fluoride preventive program in an attempt to counteract dental erosion: fluoride dentifrice, neutral sodium fluoride 0.05 percent rinse preparation, and daily gel tray with neutral preparation.
3. Encourage and instruct the patient in meticulous daily personal oral care with toothbrushing and flossing.

DAILY FOOD REQUIREMENTS

Patient instruction centers around helping patients learn about the foods that make up an adequate diet and improve their food selection. Poor food habits, such as missed meals, omission of essential foods, regular use of non-nutritious snacks, or illogical, unsupervised dieting, frequently are important to recommendations related to nutritional practices for oral health. Generalities may be useful to a degree, but for daily application, specific suggestions for meal planning and food selection are needed.

The information in this chapter and the suggestions for application assume that the science of nutrition has been studied comprehensively. It is also expected that reference books and other materials are available. Knowledge of sources of informational leaflets that can be made available to provide patients with useful, practical facts about diet and meal planning is necessary. Continued review of new materials constitutes an important phase of teaching.

I. Recommended Dietary Allowances[10]

A standard of dietary adequacy was prepared by the United States National Research Council for certain nutrients. The daily allowances specified are considered adequate to meet the known nutritional needs of healthy persons.

Recommended daily dietary allowances are not the same for all, are not recommended as an ideal diet, and do not include special needs such as during illness. The figures are intended as a guide. The designations of the amounts of nutrients are impractical for patient instruction. To be meaningful, nutrients must be expressed in terms of the foods that contain them and how much of each of these foods must be consumed daily to meet the requirements.

II. The Food Groups

Fulfilling minimum requirements of nutrients for the maintenance of health and resistance to disease is not a problem when a wide variety of foods is included in the diet each day. The foods that contain the essential nutrients, called foundation or protective foods, have been divided into four groups: the milk group, the meat group, the vegetable-fruit group, and the bread-cereal group.

Table 28–1 provides a summary of the groups, examples of foods included in each, the recommended daily servings, and the major nutrients each group contributes to the diet.

III. Applications

The size of the servings of the protective foods (table 28–1, middle column) varies with age and physiologic states. Servings for children are smaller; for teen-agers, extra-large or increased in number. Nutritional requirements for teenage boys are higher than at any other time in their lives; and for girls, the only time they will be higher will be during pregnancy or lactation. Dietary requirements for pregnancy are summarized in the chapter on prenatal care, page 549.

With old age, total requirements decrease, but the

Table 28–1. Food for an Adequate Diet

Food Group	Recommended Daily Amount		Contribution to Diet
Milk Group		*Servings**	
Milk: whole, evaporated, skim, dry, buttermilk	Children under 9	2 to 3	Calcium
Cheese and other milk products	Children 9 to 12	3 or more	Protein
	Teen-age	4 or more	Riboflavin
	Adults	2 or more	Vitamin A (whole milk)
	Pregnant women	3 or more	Vitamin D (when fortified)
	Nursing mothers	4 or more	Thiamine
Meat Group			
Meats, fish, poultry	2 or more servings		Protein
Eggs			Iron
Alternates: vegetable protein	to include		Thiamine
(dry beans, dry peas, lentils,			Riboflavin
nuts)	3 to 5 eggs weekly		Niacin
			Vitamin A (egg yolk, liver)
Vegetables—Fruit Group			
All Vegetables and Fruits	4 or more servings		Vitamin A (deep yellow and green vegetables)
Divided between			
Dark green or yellow vegetables and			Ascorbic acid (citrus fruits)
Citrus fruits			
Includes potato			Other minerals and vitamins
Bread—Cereal Group			
All Breads and Cereals that are whole grain, enriched or restored	4 or more servings		Protein
			Iron
			B vitamins
			Food energy
Other Foods			
Butter, margarine	To round out meals		
Other fats	and meet energy needs		

*Servings: *Milk group:* one serving is 1 cup of fluid milk or its calcium equivalent in cheese and other milk products.
    Meat group: one serving is 2 to 3 ounces of lean meat, fish, poultry, two eggs, or 1 cup cooked dried beans or peas.
    Vegetables—Fruits group: one serving is one-half cup or portion normally used such as one apple, orange, potato.
    Bread—Cereal group: one serving is 1 slice of bread, 1 cup ready-to-eat cereal, one-half cup cooked cereal, rice, pasta.

components of the daily requirements remain the same. Tissue building and repair continue throughout life, and nutrients must be supplied accordingly. Problems of the diet of aging persons are summarized on pages 568–569.

COUNSELING FOR DENTAL CARIES CONTROL

Control of bacterial plaque and of cariogenic food intake, and strengthening of the tooth surface to resist caries activity are essentials in the control of dental caries. Figure 28–1 shows that all are necessary for dental caries to develop.

This chapter focuses on the control of cariogenic food intake. Procedures for use of a dietary analysis are described. A dental caries activity test can be used in conjunction with the dietary analysis. The caries activity test can provide information about the bacteria and their acid-forming abilities in the presence of cariogenic foods. The tests are used to monitor the progress of diet therapy, because alterations in the diet alter bacterial activity. Various caries activity tests are outlined starting on page 389.

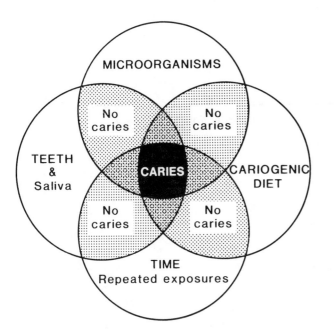

Figure 28–1. Dental Caries Process. Four overlapping circles illustrate the factors involved in the development of dental caries. All four act together and, as shown by the center, dental caries results. (Adapted from Newbrun, E.: *Cariology*, 2nd ed. Baltimore, Williams & Wilkins, 1983.)

Control of dental caries by diet accompanies procedures for the control of bacterial plaque. They are part of the total oral health program that also includes the restoration of carious teeth and the implementation of fluoride therapy.

THE DIETARY ANALYSIS

A dietary analysis is used as a guide for instruction of the patient.* Whether the analysis is made to help a patient whose major oral health problem is dental caries or a periodontal disease, the same general procedures can be followed.

I. Types of Dietary Analyses

A. Qualitative

The qualitative analysis takes into consideration the general food groups essential or detrimental to adequate oral health, but does not pretend to show precise mathematical calculations of the chemical constituents.

B. Quantitative

The nutritionist is a specialist who is skilled in making detailed quantitative analyses of diets and who works under the direction of a medical physician to provide specific therapeutic diets for physiologic and pathologic conditions.

II. Objectives of a Dietary Analysis

A. To provide an opportunity for a patient to study, objectively, personal dietary habits.

*The word "patient" is used to mean the patient and the parent when the patient is a child.

B. To obtain an overall picture of the types of food in the patient's diet, food preferences, and quantity of food eaten.

C. To study the food habits with particular reference to frequency and regularity of eating and the order in which food is taken.

D. To record for study and future comparison the types and frequency of use of potentially cariogenic food.

E. To determine the overall consistency of the diet and the fibrous foods that are regularly included.

F. To compare the frequency of cariogenic exposures with clinical and radiologic findings and the results of caries activity tests.

G. To provide a basis for making individual recommendations for changes in the diet important to the health of the oral mucosa and the periodontium and to the prevention of dental caries.

III. The Food Diary

A. Types

1. *Short.* A record of the food eaten by the patient over the previous 24 hours can be obtained by interview. Although this record is useful for discussion with the patient during instruction, a truer picture of the patient's usual diet can be obtained from a food diary kept for a week or at least 5 days.

2. *Week-long.* The week or series of consecutive days selected should be typical of ordinary daily living uncomplicated by illness, holidays, fasting, or other unusual events.

B. Characteristics of Forms to Use

1. Simple, with ample spacing.
2. Space indicated for patient's name, the day, and the date on each page.
3. Blocked off areas for each meal and between-meals.
4. Space to indicate time of eating.
5. Column to record food item and amount (figure 28–2).
6. Cover page with sample procedure for entering items (figure 28–3).

IV. Presentation to Patient

Result obtained can be expected to be directly proportional to the care taken in presentation.

A. Explain the Purpose

Avoid mention of specific foods and their relationships to oral health; the patient may not provide a true diary if what will be checked is known.

B. Explain the Form

Discuss the cover page suggestions for listing various foods and the use of household measurements for indicating quantity.

C. Complete the Current Day's Diary with the Patient

To illustrate how to itemize and how to list the foods in the order they are eaten.

NAME______________

THE DAY'S FOOD DIARY

DAY________DATE________

	AMOUNT		AMOUNT
BREAKFAST________A.M. Finished_______A.M.		BETWEEN LUNCH AND DINNER________P.M.	
BETWEEN BREAKFAST AND LUNCH_______A.M.		DINNER_______P.M. Finished_______P.M.	
LUNCH_______A.M. Finished_______P.M.		BETWEEN DINNER AND RETIRING_______P.M.	

Figure 28–2. Food Diary. Example of a form for the patient to use to record the daily diet. A booklet of 7 forms can be assembled for a week-long record. The cover for the booklet is shown in figure 28–3.

D. General Directions

1. Emphasize importance of completing each meal's record as soon after eating as possible to avoid forgetting.
2. Explain need for recording what was actually eaten in contrast to recording everything served.
3. Review details of recording the component parts of a combination dish such as a salad, sandwich, casserole.
4. Indicate need for recording vitamin concentrates, prescribed medicines, water.
5. Request that meals eaten other than at home be identified by writing "restaurant," "guest at friend's home," or "party."

V. Receiving the Completed Food Diary

The appointment for receiving the food diary should follow soon after its completion.

A. Obtain Supplemental Data

Question the patient and record additional information:

1. Whether the diary represents that of a typical week.
2. Appetite.
3. Food likes and dislikes; preferences.
4. Allergies.
5. Specially prescribed diets for the patient or other members of the family.

B. Review Patient's Food Diary

Review with the patient each day's recorded food list and supplement details that have been omitted.

1. Identify additions by using ink if the diary has been kept in pencil or vice versa.
2. Common omissions
   a. Garnishes: frosting, whipped cream, butter or margarine on vegetables, salad dressings?
   b. Size of drinking glass: 4-ounce, 8-ounce?
   c. Bread or toast: white, enriched, wheat?
   d. Chewing gum: sugarless, amount?
   e. Canned fruit: packed in water or heavy or light syrup?
   f. Fruit salad: canned, fresh?

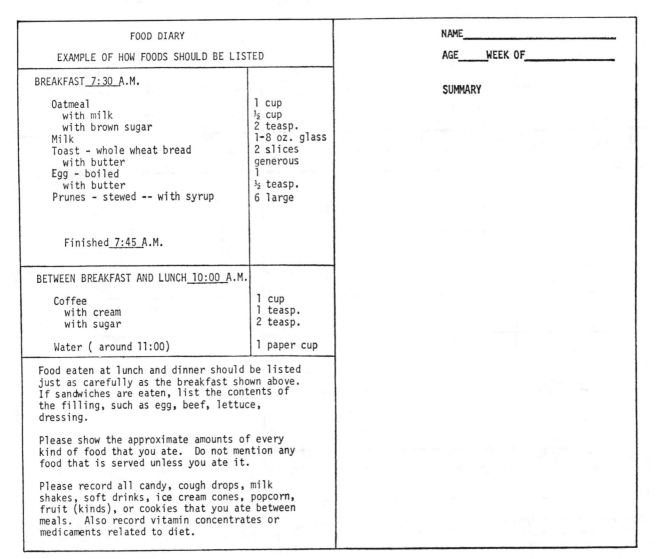

Figure 28–3. Food Diary Cover. On the cover are examples of how to list foods and indicate household measurements. The blank area on the right is for a summary prepared by the patient during the counseling appointment. Single pages for each day's diary are shown in figure 28–2.

g. Cereal: kind, milk, cream, sugar, quantity?

h. Potato: baked, buttered, fried?

i. Doughnut: sugared, glazed, plain?

VI. Summary and Analysis

Three principal parts of the food diary to analyze are the protective foods (four food groups), the cariogenic foods, and the consistency of the diet.

A. Protective Foods

1. Analysis of overall content of the diet.
   a. Comparison with four food groups (table 28–1).
   b. Approximate proportion of foods that are cariogenic compared with proportion of protective foods.
2. Suggested procedure: use check sheet to mark daily portions of each food group (figure 28–4).

a. Total for the week may be summarized for each category.

b. Gross excesses and deficiencies can be identified readily.

B. Cariogenic Foods

1. Types of sugar-containing foods included.
2. Frequency of use
   a. Daily or occasionally.
   b. Number of between-meal snacks and how many of these include sweets.
3. Time of use.
4. Consistency of sugar-containing foods relates to probable length of time food might remain on the tooth surfaces.
5. Quantity relates to frequency more than to size of individual serving (page 387).
6. Water taken at times when it could aid in rinsing sugars from the tooth surfaces.

DIETARY ANALYSIS										Name_____ Age_____ Date_____		
FOOD GROUPS	Day 1	2	3	4	5	6	7	Daily Average	Recommended Daily Amounts	Ade-quate	Inade-quate
MILK GROUP Milk									Child Adol. Adult 2-4 4+more 2+more		
Milk Products											
MEAT GROUP Meat, Fish Poultry									2 or more servings		
Eggs									(Eggs: 3-5 per week)		
VEGETABLE { Yellow & Dark Green									4 or more servings		
Other									including		
Potato									1 yellow or dark green vegetable		
& FRUIT { Raw- Citrus									1 citrus fruit		
Other											
Cooked											
BREAD & CEREALS GROUP									4 or more servings		
SWEETS								Total	NOTES AND RECOMMENDATIONS		
Liquid With Meal											
End of Meal											
Between Meal											
Soft (Sticky Retentive) With Meal											
End of Meal											
Between Meal											
Hard (Sucked- Long- Lasting) End of Meal											
Between Meal											

Figure 28–4. Dietary Analysis Recording Sheet. From the food diary kept by the patient (figures 28–2 and 28–3), each item is entered as a check in the space beside the appropriate food group. These are totaled, averaged, and compared with the recommended daily amounts on the right. The lower section provides space to categorize and count cariogenic foods.

7. Underline in red on the food diary the foods that contain sugar, or during the counseling appointment ask the patient to underline them to help learn more about the extent of the problem. The experience can be impressive to the patient, since people usually do not realize how many of the foods they are eating are cariogenic.

C. Consistency of Diet

1. Types of fibrous foods used: primarily uncooked, crisp, juicy fruits and vegetables.
2. Frequency of use: daily or occasionally.
3. Time of use
   a. During meal, end of meal, or between-meals.
   b. Relationship to providing cleansing mechanism for sugar contained in other foods.

D. Analysis

1. The patient can identify desirable and undesirable practices.

2. Compare findings with clinical findings and the patient's oral health problems.

PREPARATION FOR COUNSELING OF PATIENT

I. Define Objectives

A. To help the patient study the individual oral problems and understand the need for changing habits.
B. To explain specific changes in the diet necessary for improved general and oral health.
C. For dental caries control, to promote the elimination of sugar-containing foods, particularly those between meals, and to substitute protective foods.

II. Planning Factors

A. Patient Attitude

Consider patient's willingness and ability to cooperate in relation to other demonstrations, such as conscientiousness in keeping appointments and following personal oral care procedures.

B. Problem Areas

Identify problems that arise in presenting changes in the diet as they apply to this particular patient.

1. Difficulty in change of any habit.
2. Patient may feel dissatisfied without the usual or customary foods.
3. Lack of appreciation of need for change because of limited knowledge concerning diet and nutrition and their relationship to oral health.
4. Common misconception that concentrated sugar is an indispensable source of energy.
5. Degree of emphasis: dental disease does not kill anyone and nothing drastic is going to happen if minor deviations from the recommended diet occur.
6. Social prejudices.
7. Cultural patterns.
8. Financial considerations.
9. Emotional disturbances that have led to or contributed to specific cravings such as for sweets.
10. Parental attitude that removal of sweets from the diet would deprive the child of normal childhood pleasures.

III. Select Appropriate Teaching Aids

A. Patient's radiographs, charting, and food diary.
B. Diagrams, models, or charts applicable to material to be presented.
C. Instructive leaflets to illustrate patient's special dietary or oral health needs.
D. Printed outline of diet plan with specific suggestions for food substitutes.
E. Printed list of snack suggestions.

IV. Review

Review data and recommendations with dentist for additions and suggestions.

COUNSELING PROCEDURES

I. Setting

The conference should be held in a setting free from interruptions and distracting background sounds. Participants seated comfortably in a group will contribute to an atmosphere conducive to learning.

For a child patient, both parents should be encouraged to be present because both may supervise the child's eating and plaque control activities. For any age, it is particularly important for the person who plans and prepares the family meals to be present. To emphasize the importance of the conference

and the concern of the entire dental group for the patient's problem, the dentist should participate by opening the conference and reviewing factors related to the treatment plan.

II. Pointers for Success of a Conference

A. Be prepared—on time.
B. Plan for only a few simple visual aids.
C. Encourage parents to exclude small children (other than patient) from the conference, because they create distraction.
D. Develop a permissive atmosphere.
E. Take care not to follow a written outline of recommendations so rigidly that the conference lacks spontaneity.
F. Include all people present in the discussion.
G. Use a conversational tone of voice.
H. Make certain that all questions from patient or parent are discussed adequately.
I. Avoid note taking during the conference as much as possible.

III. Presentation

A. Review of Purposes of the Meeting

The extent of introductory detail included depends on whether parents attending the conference have already participated in previous appointments. A teen-aged patient may have been coming for appointments unattended; hence the need for clear review so the parents understand the details.

B. Clarification of "Cariogenic" Foods

The patient cannot be told simply to "cut out the sweets in your diet." The meaning of "sweets" must be made clear, and specific suggestions should be provided for "cutting them out." Many people think of sweets as candy only and do not realize the sugar content of many other foods. The meaning of cariogenic food can be illustrated by using examples from the patient's own food diary.

C. Review of Dental Caries Initiation

Discuss the principles for understanding the role of sucrose in dental caries initiation.

1. Sugar on the tooth surface is changed to acid within 5 minutes. Use figure 16–5 (page 242) as an illustration.
2. Acid left undisturbed is not cleared from the mouth for 1½ to 2 hours.

D. Frequency of Exposure

1. Each exposure of the tooth surface to sucrose in a meal or snack increases the amount of acid on the tooth. The pH drops to below the critical level for demineralization. Figure 28–5 illustrates how the frequent intake of sucrose lowers the pH for several hours in a day.
2. The actual amount of sucrose is not as important as when and how often the tooth is exposed.

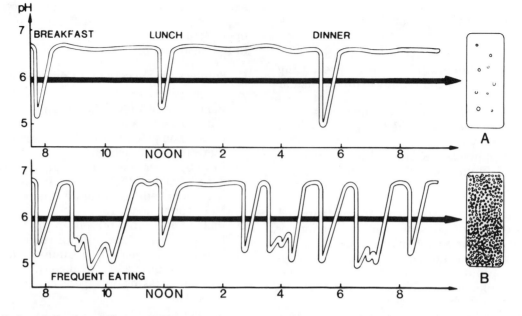

Figure 28–5. Cariogenic Foods and Plaque pH. The range of pH in the bacterial plaque from 5 to 7 pH is shown on the left. Time intervals are shown across the bottom of each graph. The double line curve represents the variations in plaque pH throughout a day. Each time sugar or a cariogenic food is taken in, the pH of the plaque drops to or below the critical pH (5.2 to 5.5). As shown in the lower graph, frequent eating keeps the pH at the critical level below which dental caries forms. On the right, **A** shows that bacterial counts are lower, whereas in **B**, aciduric microorganisms are greatly increased in numbers. (Adapted from Larmas, M.: *Int. Dent. J., 35,* 109, June, 1985.)

E. Retention

1. The texture of the food that contains the sugar influences the length of time the food stays in the mouth (whether sticky or combined with a sticky substance).
2. Vigorous rinsing after eating a concentrated sweet may help to remove part of it.
3. Sweet foods taken after brushing and flossing before retiring are not cleared readily because salivary flow decreases during sleep.

IV. Specific Dietary Recommendations

A. Examination of the Patient's Food Diary and Summary Sheet

Let the patient identify the deficiencies and excesses and suggest alternate choices. To make major changes in food habits is difficult, if not traumatic, for any individual. Application of the knowledge of the principles of learning (page 369) and the skills of a counselor are essential. One must attempt to retain as many as possible of the patient's present food habits and to make recommendations that can be adapted to the patient's pattern of living.

1. Discuss foods from each food group that are liked by the patient and can be added to the diet or substituted for more detrimental foods used.
2. Guide the patient to select those items from the present diet that need changing and to make suggestions for appropriate substitutes.

B. Basic Principles for Dietary Changes

The suggestions listed below represent basic principles to be applied. More specific recommendations should be added as they relate to an individual family. Directions must be simple and specific, because the interpretation of many new ideas is difficult for the patient.

1. Incorporate foods from the basic groups to complete the patient's diet. A diet high in protective foods frequently may imply a diet low in fermentable carbohydrate.
2. Limit the use of fermentable carbohydrates to mealtimes. Pay particular attention to the final food used in the meal which may remain on the teeth if immediate toothbrushing is not possible.
3. When a very high dental caries rate is evident, omit sweet foods even at mealtime and limit the diet to foods from the meat, milk, and vegetable–fruit groups (table 28–1). Selections from the bread-cereal group should be limited to dark bread and whole grain and enriched cereals.
4. Select between-meal snacks from protective noncariogenic foods such as plain milk, fresh fruits, and raw vegetables.
5. Use as little concentrated sweet in the preparation of foods as possible, and observe care in the purchase of prepared foods; for example, use unsweetened fruit juice, dietetically prepared canned fruits, and sugar-free ice

cream. Natural sugars are just as detrimental as refined ones (for example: honey, maple syrup).

6. Eat well at mealtime to lessen desire for between-meal snacks. Protein- and fat-containing foods are digested more slowly and should be included at each meal to prevent between-meal hunger.

7. Emphasize the need for rigid adherence to the diet features; even occasional deviations can affect the results.

EVALUATION OF PROGRESS

The success of the dental caries control diet depends on learning by the patient. Learning implies a change of behavior and progress toward goals that are clearly understood by the learner.

I. Immediate Evaluation

A. A lowered test result for caries activity at the end of the 3- to 4-week test period of restricted diet may indicate success to that date.

B. The patient's expressed interest and demonstration of cooperation in the caries control program indicate that at least temporarily the patient is motivated.

II. Overall Evaluation

A. Consistent reduction in dental caries rate in the years following the study shows sustained change in habits.

B. Patient's and parents' attitudes toward maintaining adequate oral health habits of personal care, diet containing minimum cariogenic foods, and routine professional dental care indicate application of learning.

III. 3-Months' Follow-up

A. Obtain saliva sample for caries activity test.

B. Request patient to keep a 5- to 7-day food diary for analysis and evaluation.

C. Review plaque control procedures and provide suggestions as needed.

D. Recommend return to restricted diet when indicated.

IV. 6-Months' Follow-up

A. Obtain saliva sample for caries activity test.

B. Perform examination and clinical procedures
   1. Scaling when needed.
   2. Topical application of fluoride, depending on self-applied fluoride program.
   3. Charting of carious lesions.

C. Comparing dental caries incidence with previous chartings and completed restorative dentistry.

D. Make dietary recommendations in accord with results from the test.

DENTAL CARIES ACTIVITY TESTS

A dental caries activity test may be used as an instructional and motivational aid to guide the patient toward practicing habits conducive to the prevention of dental caries. The use of test results for a visual aid can be helpful because changes in results of a series of tests can show dramatically the effects of the patient's personal efforts in carrying out dietary and oral care preventive procedures.

Caries activity tests provide information about the current oral environment. The tests are not "susceptibility" tests to predict what may occur at some future time. Various types of tests have been devised to detect dental caries activity. Evaluation may be made by counting the numbers of acid-forming bacteria or determining the acid produced or other specialized activity of the microorganisms.

Studies of the oral bacteria show that they are not distributed evenly. Microorganisms in the bacterial plaque on tooth surfaces contribute little to the pool of bacteria obtained when a saliva sample is collected. A large proportion of the organisms in the saliva is from the tongue. Such findings provide at least a partial explanation for the inconsistencies of dental caries activity tests.

I. Snyder Colorimetric Test[11]

The Snyder test agar contains the indicator brom-cresol-green and is adjusted to a pH of 5.0. Acid formation by bacteria from the saliva sample added to the medium lowers the pH. At the lowered pH, the brom-cresol-green changes from green to yellow. It is the rapidity of color change that indicates the caries activity at the time of the test.

A. Obtain Saliva Sample

The patient chews a piece of paraffin for 3 minutes and expectorates into a sterile bottle.

B. Prepare Medium and Incubate

1. Place tube of Snyder test agar in boiling water until agar melts; cool until it can be held comfortably against the cheek.

2. Shake the saliva sample well to distribute bacteria, and pipette 0.2 ml. into the agar. Mix by gentle rotation.

3. Allow to solidify and incubate at 37° C.

4. Examine daily for 3 days and record changes in color compared with uninoculated control. Hold tubes against a white background when making observations.

C. Interpret the Results

The rate of color change from green to yellow is related to the degree of caries activity. In the process of changing color, the agar will appear light green, then greenish-yellow, and finally appear a definite yellow.

No change in color indicates little or no caries activity, whereas a prompt change to yellow within 24 hours indicates significant acid formation or caries activity.

D. Color Changes in the Snyder Test

Color of Snyder Test Agar after Incubation			Suggested Degree of Caries Susceptibility
24 hours	48 hours	72 hours	
Green	Green	Green	Little or none
Green	Light green	Yellow	Slight
Green	Yellow		Moderate
Yellow			Marked or rampant

II. Modified Snyder Test[12]

A miniature version of the standard Snyder test has been used that is simpler, less expensive, and occupies less space, particularly during incubation.

A. Obtain Saliva Sample (I., A., above)

B. Prepare the Medium and Incubate

1. Shake specimen of saliva and use wire loop (flamed for sterility) to withdraw saliva (loop holds about .0113 ml.). Stab loop into the agar for inoculation.
2. Use Snyder test agar as the culture medium with the concentration of brom-cresol-green increased to facilitate the observation of the color change in the small amount of agar (0.2 ml.).
3. Incubate at 37° C for 24, 48, and 72 hours.
4. Examine daily.

C. Interpret the Results

The color changes are the same as for the original Snyder test (see I., D., above). The results are easier to read than those of the standard Snyder test, because all of the small amount of agar used changes color.

III. Swab Test[13]

The Swab test is also a modified Snyder test. Time is saved in that a saliva sample is not obtained, and the test results are evaluated after 48 hours.

A. Obtain Sample

Stroke the buccal gingival areas of the teeth in each of the four quadrants with a sterile cotton applicator.

B. Prepare the Medium and Incubate

1. Remove cap from a vial of the special medium, insert the applicator to the bottom, and rotate it about five times. Raise the applicator and break off the stick against the lip of the vial, let it drop down, and replace the cap firmly.
2. Incubate at 37° C for 48 hours.
3. Make pH reading by a color comparator or electric pH meter.

C. Interpret the Results

1. Color comparator: the brom-cresol-green changes from green to yellow as the pH declines.
2. Measurement and significance of pH (meter method):

Rampant:	pH below 4.1
Active:	pH 4.2 to 4.4
Slightly active:	pH 4.5 to 4.6
Inactive:	pH over 4.6

IV. Salivary Reductase Test[14]

This test measures the activity of the reductase enzyme present in salivary bacteria.

A. Obtain Saliva Sample (I., A., above)

B. Mix Sample with Reagent

1. Saliva sample is mixed with the dye diazoresorcinol (Resazurin reagent) and allowed to stand 15 minutes.
2. The color changes as the dye is reduced, and the caries conduciveness is interpreted after 15 minutes at room temperature.

C. Note Color Changes in the Salivary Reductase Test

Color	Caries Conduciveness
Blue in 15 minutes	Nonconducive
Orchid in 15 minutes	Slightly conducive
Red in 15 minutes	Moderately conducive
Red immediately on mixing	Highly conducive
Colorless in 15 minutes	Extremely conducive

V. Methyl Red-Plaque-Sugar Test[15]

This test is also known as the Spot Plate Colorimetric Test. A dramatic change in color of the methyl red from yellow to red occurs as the pH changes from about 6.3 to 4.2. Lowering of the pH is accomplished by the acid-producing bacteria in the plaque acting on sucrose.

A. Obtain Plaque Sample

With a curet, scrape plaque from the distofacial surfaces of maxillary molars, the lingual surfaces of mandibular molars, or other surfaces with thick plaque. Collect enough plaque to cover the working end of the curet.

B. Mix Sample with Indicator

1. Arrange the plaque sample in a small circle (about ¼ inch diameter) on a white porcelain tile.
2. Cover with 2 to 3 drops of methyl red indicator. Sprinkle a few crystals of sugar (sucrose) into the center of the circle.
3. Wait 10 to 30 minutes for the color to change.

C. Interpret the Results

1. The following criteria for scoring the color change may be used. The amount of red present determines the degree of acid production.

0 = Yellow

+1 = Yellow with a small red circle

+2 = Yellow with a red circle one half of the area

+3 = Yellow with a red circle covering all but the edges

+2 and +3 indicate the presence of a significant number of plaque bacteria that are acid producing

2. Record results in patient's record.

VI. Streptococcus Mutans Count[16]

Dental caries incidence and *Streptococcus mutans* infection have been correlated and evidence shows that an increased count may precede the development of carious lesions.

A. Obtain Saliva Sample

Insert wooden tongue depressor into the mouth and turn it several times to cover it with saliva.

B. Prepare Medium and Incubate

1. Press the wooden depressor against the selective agar plate.
2. Incubate anaerobically or in a sealed plastic bag containing expired air for 48 hours.
3. Count colony-forming units.

C. Interpret the Results

Highly infected patients may be detected readily because of the density of colonies. In a similar method using plaque samples, numbers of colonies were graded 1, 2, or 3, with group 3 being the high colony counts.[17]

FACTORS TO TEACH THE PATIENT

I. Medications, particularly those in liquid form, are often thick syrups containing sucrose. When chronically ill patients, especially children, have liquid medication that must be taken several times each day, the harm to the teeth can be severe. If the medication cannot be given in a less caries-producing form, the mouth should be cleared of sucrose immediately following each dose by toothbrushing, rinsing, and flossing.[18]

II. How dental caries forms and how the acid is produced on the tooth surface by microorganisms in the plaque. Use figure 28–1 to illustrate the interaction of the sugar and other cariogenic foods on the tooth surface and the microorganisms, and show the relation of frequency of eating to acid production, using figure 28–5.

References

1. Carranza, F.A.: *Glickman's Clinical Periodontology*, 6th ed. Philadelphia, W.B. Saunders Co., 1984, pp. 134, 154, 444–458.
2. Grant, D.A., Stern, I.B., and Listgarten, M.A., eds.: *Periodontics*, 6th ed. St. Louis, The C.V. Mosby Co., 1988, pp. 293–306.
3. *Preventive Dental Services, Practices, Guidelines and Recommendations*. Report of the Working Group on Preventive Dental Services, Health and Welfare, Canada, September, 1979, pp. 142–171.
4. Arnim, S.S.: The Use of Disclosing Agents for Measuring Tooth Cleanliness, *J. Periodontol., 34,* 227, May, 1963.
5. McCarthy, P.L. and Shklar, G.: *Diseases of the Oral Mucosa,* 2nd ed. Philadelphia, Lea & Febiger, 1980, pp. 376–388.
6. Newbrun, E.: *Cariology,* 2nd ed. Baltimore, Williams & Wilkins, 1983, pp. 86–115.
7. American Psychiatric Association: *Diagnostic and Statistical Manual of Mental Disorders,* 3rd ed. Revised (DSM-III-R). Washington, D.C., American Psychiatric Association, 1987, pp. 65–68.
8. Herzog, D.B. and Copeland, P.M.: Eating Disorders, *N. Engl. J. Med., 313,* 295, August 1, 1985.
9. Mitchell, J.E., Seim, H.C., Colon, E., and Pomeroy, C.: Medical Complications and Medical Management of Bulimia, *Ann. Intern. Med., 107,* 71, July, 1987.
10. National Research Council, Committee on Dietary Allowances, Food and Nutrition Board: *Recommended Dietary Allowances,* 9th ed. Washington, D.C., National Academy of Sciences, Office of Publications, 1980.
11. Snyder, M.L.: A Simple Colorimetric Method for the Estimation of Relative Numbers of Lactobacilli in the Saliva, *J. Dent. Res., 19,* 349, August, 1940.
12. Sims, W.: A Modified Snyder Test for Caries-activity in Humans, *Arch. Oral Biol., 13,* 853, August, 1968.
13. Grainger, R.M., Jarrett, M., and Honey, S.L.: Swab Test for Dental Caries Activity: an Epidemiological Study, *Can. Dent. Assoc. J., 31,* 515, August, 1965.
14. Rapp, G.W.: Fifteen Minute Caries Test, *Ill. Dent. J., 31,* 290, May, 1962.
15. Arnim, S.S. and Sweet, A.P.: Acid Production by Mouth Organisms. Use of Aqueous Methyl Red for Patient Education, *Dent. Radiogr. Photogr., 29,* 1, Number 1, 1956.
16. Köhler, B. and Bratthall, D.: Practical Method to Facilitate Estimation of *Streptococcus mutans* Levels in Saliva, *J. Clin. Microbiol., 9,* 584, May, 1979.
17. Woods, R.: A Dental Caries Susceptibility Test Based on the Occurrence of *Streptococcus mutans* in Plaque Material, *Aust. Dent. J., 16,* 116, April, 1971.
18. Feigal, R.J., Jensen, M.E., and Mensing, C.A.: Dental Caries Potential of Liquid Medications, *Pediatrics, 68,* 416, September, 1981.

Suggested Readings

American Dental Association, Council on Dental Therapeutics: *Accepted Dental Therapeutics,* 40th ed. Chicago, American Dental Association, 1984, pp. 151–177.

Ashpole, B.R.: Medication Caries; The Risk to Healthy Teeth of Sucrose in Medications, *Can. Dent. Hyg./Probe, 22,* 30, March, 1988.

Bibby, B.G.: Diet and Nutrition and Dental Caries, *Can. Dent. Assoc. J., 46,* 47, January, 1980.

Chandra, R.K.: Nutrition and Immunity: I. Basic Considerations. II. Practical Applications, *ASDC J. Dent. Child., 54,* 193, May-June, 1987.

de Menezes, A.C., Costa, I.M., and El-Guindy, M.M.: Clinical Manifestations of Hypervitaminosis A in Human Gingiva, A Case Report, *J. Periodontol., 55,* 474, August, 1984.

Ehrlich, A.: *Nutrition and Dental Health.* Albany, New York, Delmar Pub., 1987, pp. 158–176.

Jakush, J., ed.: Emphasis: Diet, Nutrition, and Oral Health: A Rational Approach for the Dental Practice, *J. Am. Dent. Assoc., 109,* 20, July, 1984.

Lee, M.M. and Frazier, D.M.: Biochemistry and Nutrition, in Darby, M.L. and Bushee, E.J., eds.: *Mosby's Comprehensive Review of Dental Hygiene.* St. Louis, The C.V. Mosby Co., 1986, pp. 348–387.

Newbrun, E.: Sucrose in the Dynamics of the Carious Process, *Int. Dent. J., 32,* 13, March, 1982.

Pollack, R.L., Kravitz, E., and Litwack, D.: Nutrition and Periodontal Health, *Quintessence Int., 15,* 65, January, 1984.

Shaw, J.H.: Causes and Control of Dental Caries, *N. Engl. J. Med., 317,* 996, October 15, 1987.

Shaw, J.H.: Diet and Dental Health, *Am. J. Clin. Nutr., 41*, 1117, Supplement Number 5, May, 1985.

White-Graves, M.V. and Schiller, M.R.: History of Foods in the Caries Process, *J. Am. Diet. Assoc., 86*, 241, February, 1986.

Woolfe, S.N., Hume, W.R., and Kenney, E.B.: Ascorbic Acid and Periodontal Disease: A Review of the Literature, *J. West. Soc. Periodont. Periodont. Abstr., 28*, 44, Number 2, 1980.

Diet Counseling

Bedi, R. and Brown, C.P.M.: Behavioural Principles Underlying Effective Dietary Instruction, *J. Dent., 11*, 35, March, 1983.

Hölund, U., Theilade, E., and Poulson, S.: Validity of a Dietary Interviewing Method for Use in Caries Prevention, *Community Dent. Oral Epidemiol., 13*, 219, August, 1985.

Katz, S.: A Diet Counseling Program, *J. Am. Dent. Assoc., 102*, 840, June, 1981.

Nizel, A.E. and Papas, A.S.: *Nutrition in Clinical Dentistry*, 3rd ed. Philadelphia, W.B. Saunders Co., 1989, pp. 277–308.

Pal, K.: Children's Dental Diet. The Short-term Effects of a Behavior Modification Program, *Dent. Hyg., 60*, 56, February, 1986.

Palmer, C., Cassidy, M., and Larsen, C.: *Nutrition, Diet and Dental Health: Concepts and Methods*. Chicago, American Dental Hygienists' Association, 1981, pp. 44–63.

Poplin, L.E.: Cautions in Nutritional Counseling, *Dent. Hyg., 55*, 40, February, 1981.

Scanlan, D. and Wyatt, M.: Tools for Nutrition and Preventive Dental Counselling for South East Asian Refugees, *Can. Dent. Hyg., 14*, 60, Fall, 1980.

Cariogenic Foods

Addy, M., Perriam, E., and Sterry, A.: Effects of Sugared and Sugar-free Chewing Gum on the Accumulation of Plaque and Debris on the Teeth, *J. Clin. Periodontol., 9*, 346, July, 1982.

Ayers, C.S. and Abrams, R.A.: Noncariogenic Sweeteners. Sugar Substitutes for Caries Control, *Dent. Hyg., 61*, 162, April, 1987.

Bibby, B.G., Mundorff, S.A., Zero, D.T., and Almekinder, K.J.: Oral Food Clearance and the pH of Plaque and Saliva, *J. Am. Dent. Assoc., 112*, 333, March, 1986.

Birkhed, D.: Sugar Content Acidity and Effect on Plaque pH of Fruit Juices, Fruit Drinks, Carbonated Beverages and Sport Drinks, *Caries Res., 18*, 120, Number 2, 1984.

Blinkhorn, A.S.: The Caries Experience and Dietary Habits of Edinburgh Nursery School Children, *Br. Dent. J., 152*, 227, April 6, 1982.

Bowen, W.H., Amsbaugh, S.M., Monell-Torrens, S., Brunelle, J., Kuzmiak-Jones, H., and Cole, M.F.: A Method to Assess Cariogenic Potential of Foodstuffs, *J. Am. Dent. Assoc., 100*, 677, May, 1980.

Hsu, S.C., Pollack, R.L., Hsu, A.-F.C., and Going, R.E.: Sugars Present in Tobacco Extracts, J. Am. Dent. Assoc., 101, 915, December, 1980.

Ismail, A.I., Burt, B.A., and Eklund, S.A.: The Cariogenicity of Soft Drinks in the United States, *J. Am. Dent. Assoc., 109*, 241, August, 1984.

Jalil, R.A., Cornick, D.E.R., and Waite, I.M.: Effect of Variation in Dietary Sucrose Intake on Plaque Removal by Mechanical Means, *J. Clin. Periodontol., 10*, 389, July, 1983.

Jensen, M.E.: Responses of Interproximal Plaque pH to Snack Foods and Effect of Chewing Sorbitol-containing Gum, *Dent. Hyg., 62*, 81, February, 1988.

Loesche, W.J.: The Rationale for Caries Prevention Through the Use of Sugar Substitutes, *Int. Dent. J., 35*, 1, March, 1985.

Loesche, W.J., Grossman, N.S., Earnest, R., and Corpron, R.: The Effect of Chewing Xylitol Gum on the Plaque and Saliva Levels of *Streptococcus mutans, J. Am. Dent. Assoc., 108*, 587, April, 1984.

Morrissey, R.B., Burkholder, B.D., and Tarka, S.M.: The Cariogenic Potential of Several Snack Foods, *J. Am. Dent. Assoc., 109*, 589, October, 1984.

Newbrun, E.: Criteria of Cariogenicity for Labeling Foods, *J. Am. Dent. Assoc., 105*, 627, October, 1982.

Newbrun, E., Hoover, C., Mettraux, G., and Graf, H.: Comparison

of Dietary Habits and Dental Health of Subjects with Hereditary Fructose Intolerance and Control Subjects, *J. Am. Dent. Assoc., 101*, 619, October, 1980.

Rateitschak-Plüss, E.M. and Guggenheim, B.: Effects of a Carbohydrate-free Diet and Sugar Substitutes on Dental Plaque Accumulation, *J. Clin. Periodontol., 9*, 239, May, 1982.

Sidi, A.D. and Ashley, F.P.: Influence of Frequent Sugar Intakes on Experimental Gingivitis, *J. Periodontol., 55*, 419, July, 1984.

Walker, A.R.P.: Diets for Caries Control, *J. Am. Dent. Assoc., 108*, 751, May, 1984.

Weiss, R.L. and Trithart, A.H.: Between-meal Eating Habits and Dental Caries Experience in Preschool Children, *Am. J. Public Health, 50*, 1097, August, 1960.

Caries Activity Tests

Beighton, D.: A Simplified Procedure for Estimating the Level of *Streptococcus mutans* in the Mouth, *Br. Dent. J., 160*, 329, May 10, 1986.

Birkhed, D., Edwardsson, S., and Andersson, H.: Comparison Among a Dip-slide Test (Dentocult), Plate Count, and Snyder Test for Estimating Number of Lactobacilli in Human Saliva, *J. Dent. Res., 60*, 1832, November, 1981.

Crossner, C.-G.: Salivary Lactobacillus Counts in the Prediction of Caries Activity, *Community Dent. Oral Epidemiol., 9*, 182, August, 1981.

Helminen, S.K.J., Meurman, J.H., Koskinen, K.P., and Rytömaa, I.: Use of a Chair-side Method for Salivary Lactobacillus Count, *Quintessence Int., 12*, 1321, December, 1981.

Köhler, B. and Emilson, C.-G.: Comparison Between a Micromethod and a Conventional Method for Estimation of Salivary *Streptococcus mutans, Scand. J. Dent. Res., 95*, 132, April, 1987.

Larmas, M.: Simple Tests for Caries Susceptibility, *Int. Dent. J., 35*, 109, June, 1985.

Maki, Y., Yamamoto, H., Takaesu, Y., Shibuya, M., Kinoshita, Y., and Asami, K.: A Rapid Caries Activity Test by Resazurin Disc, *Bull. Tokyo Dent. Coll., 27*, 1, February, 1986.

Newbrun, E.: *Cariology*. 2nd ed. Baltimore, Williams & Wilkins, 1983, pp. 256–273.

Newbrun, E.: Comparison of Two Screening Tests for *Streptococcus mutans* and Evaluation of Their Suitability for Mass Screenings and Private Practice, *Community Dent. Oral Epidemiol., 12*, 325, October, 1984.

Vanderas, A.P.: Bacteriologic and Nonbacteriologic Criteria for Identifying Individuals at High Risk of Developing Dental Caries: A Review, *J. Public Health Dent., 46*, 106, Spring, 1986.

Anorexia and Bulimia

Abrams, R.A. and Ruff, J.C.: Oral Signs and Symptoms in the Diagnosis of Bulimia, *J. Am. Dent. Assoc., 113*, 761, November, 1986.

Altshuler, B.D.: Anorexia Nervosa and Bulimia, A Review for the Dental Hygienist, *Dent. Hyg., 60*, 466, October, 1986.

Andrews, F.F.H.: Dental Erosion Due to Anorexia Nervosa with Bulimia, *Br. Dent. J., 152*, 89, February 2, 1982.

Barkmeier, W.W., Peterson, D.S., and Wood, L.W.: Anorexia Nervosa: Recognition and Management, *J. Oral Med., 37*, 33, April-June, 1982.

Clark, D.C.: Oral Complications of Anorexia and/or Bulimia: With a Review of the Literature, *J. Oral Med., 40*, 134, July-September, 1985.

Harrison, J.L., George, L.A., Cheatham, J.L., and Zinn, J.: Dental Effects and Management of Bulimia Nervosa, *Gen. Dent., 33*, 65, January-February, 1985.

Johnson, D.L. and Rue, V.M.: The Bulimic Dental Patient. Recognition and Recommendations, *Dent. Hyg., 59*, 372, August, 1985.

Kleier, D.J., Aragon, S.B., and Averbach, R.E.: Dental Management of the Chronic Vomiting Patient, *J. Am. Dent. Assoc., 108*, 618, April, 1984.

Negus, T.W. and Todd, J.O.: Bulimia Nervosa in a Male, *Br. Dent. J., 160*, 290, April 19, 1986.

Roberts, M.W. and Li, S.-H.: Oral Findings in Anorexia Nervosa and Bulimia Nervosa: A Study of 47 Cases, *J. Am. Dent. Assoc., 115,* 407, September, 1987.

Ruff, J.C. and Abrams, R.A.: Preventive Dental Prosthesis for the Patient with Bulimia, *Spec. Care Dentist., 7,* 218, September-October, 1987.

Sansone, R.A.: Complications of Hazardous Weight-loss Methods, *Am. Fam. Physician, 30,* 141, August, 1984.

Stege, P., Visco-Dangler, L., and Rye, L.: Anorexia Nervosa: Review Including Oral and Dental Manifestations, *J. Am. Dent. Assoc., 104,* 648, May, 1982.

Wolcott, R.B., Yager, J., and Gordon, G.: Dental Sequelae to the Binge-purge Syndrome (Bulimia): Report of Cases, *J. Am. Dent. Assoc., 109,* 723, November, 1984.

Yochim, J.R.: Anorexia and Bulimia. Where Will They End? *Can. Dent. Hyg./Probe, 21,* 173, December, 1987.

29 *Fluorides*

The use of fluorides provides the most effective method for dental caries prevention and control. Although historically associated primarily with dental caries, the action of fluoride on bacterial plaque also has important therapeutic and preventive effects on the control of periodontal infections and the maintenance of health after periodontal treatments.

Fluoride is made available at the tooth surface by two general means: *systemically,* by way of the circulation to developing teeth, and *topically,* directly to the exposed surfaces of erupted teeth. Fluoride as a systemic nutrient is available from the community drinking water, either naturally or by fluoridation, from prescribed dietary supplements, or in small amounts from certain foods.

I. Fluoride Intake[1,2]

A. Ingestion
Fluoride is taken in by way of fluoridated water, supplemental tablets, and, in small amounts, foods.

B. Absorption
1. *Stomach and Small Intestine.* Rapid absorption. Only 5 percent not absorbed is excreted in the feces.
2. *Bloodstream.* Maximum blood levels are reached within an hour of intake. The level fluctuates with intake. Normal plasma levels are very low. Fluoride in the saliva is lower than in the plasma.

C. Distribution and Retention
1. *Young Child.* About one half of the fluoride intake deposits in calcifying bones and teeth.
2. *Adult.* When the fluoride intake is continuous from daily use of fluoridated water, fluoride enters into the normal bone exchange and maintenance. Fluoride continues to accumulate in the skeleton throughout life.
3. *Storage.* Fluoride is stored in bone (95 percent of the body fluoride). The teeth store small amounts, with highest levels on the tooth surface.
4. *Fluoride in Soft Tissues.* Some tissues have fluoride levels higher than that of the plasma. Fluoride concentration in human milk is low.

D. Excretion
Most fluoride is excreted through the kidneys, with a small amount excreted by the sweat glands. Urinary fluoride concentration is reached within 2 hours of intake of a single amount of fluoride, such as a fluoride tablet.

II. Fluoride and Tooth Development
Fluoride is a nutrient essential to the formation of sound teeth and bones, as are calcium, phosphorus, and other elements obtained from food and water.

The teeth can acquire fluoride during three periods: during the *mineralization stage* of tooth development, *after mineralization* and before eruption, and *after eruption.* At this point of study, a review of the histology of tooth development and mineralization can be a helpful supplement to the information included here.[3,4]

A. Pre-eruptive: Mineralization Stage
1. Fluoride is deposited during the formation of the enamel, starting at the dentinoenamel junction, after the enamel matrix has been laid down by the ameloblasts (figure 29–1A).
2. Fluoride is incorporated as fluorapatite during mineralization.
3. Fluoride is available to the developing teeth by way of the bloodstream to the tissues surrounding the tooth buds.
4. Sources of fluoride include drinking water and other ingested fluoride, such as that from tablets, drops, and foods.
5. During mineralization, when there is excess fluoride, the normal activity of the ameloblasts may be inhibited and a defective enamel matrix can form. This mechanism can lead to dental fluorosis. Dental fluorosis is a form of hypomineralization that results from ingestion of an excess amount of fluoride during tooth development.

B. Pre-eruptive: Maturation Stage
1. After mineralization is complete and before eruption, fluoride deposition continues in the surface of the enamel (figure 29–1B).
2. Fluoride is taken up from the nutrient tissue fluids surrounding the tooth crown. Much more fluoride is acquired by the outer surface during this period than in the underlying layers of enamel during mineralization. Children who are exposed to fluoride for the first time within the 2 years prior to eruption benefit from fluoride acquired during this pre-eruptive stage.

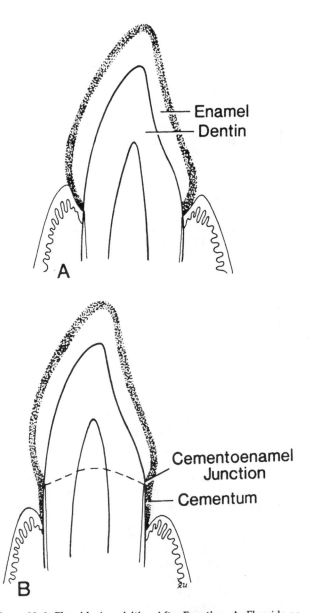

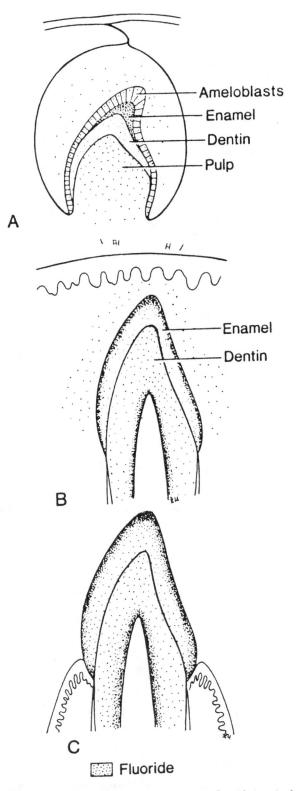

C. Posteruptive

1. After eruption and throughout the life span of the teeth, fluoride is taken up from the drinking water, dentifrice, rinse, and saliva (figure 29–2).

2. Uptake is rapid on the enamel surface during the first years after eruption. It is greater at high than at low levels of fluoride, especially from supplements used as chewable tablets or a swish-and-swallow liquid (page 400). Continuing intake of drinking water with fluoride provides a topical source as it washes over the teeth.

Figure 29–1. Systemic Fluoride. Dots represent fluoride ions in the tissues and distributed throughout the tooth. **A.** Developing tooth during mineralization shows fluoride from water and from other systemic sources deposited in the enamel and dentin. **B.** Maturation stage prior to eruption when fluoride is taken up from tissue fluids around the crown. **C.** Erupted tooth continues to take up fluoride on the surface from external sources. Note concentrated fluoride deposition on the enamel surface.

Figure 29–2. Fluoride Acquisition After Eruption. A. Fluoride on the enamel surface taken up from external sources, including dentifrice, rinse, topical application, and water from fluoridation passing over the tooth. **B.** Gingival recession exposes the cementum to external sources of fluoride for the prevention of root caries and the alleviation of sensitivity.

III. Tooth Surface Fluoride

Fluoride concentration decreases inward from the enamel surface to the dentinoenamel junction.[5]

A. Fluoride Uptake

Uptake of fluoride depends on the amount of fluoride ingested and the length of time of exposure.

B. Amount of Fluoride in the Enamel Surface

Extracted teeth from people who had used water with fluoride all their lives have been analyzed. Examples of the parts per million (ppm) fluoride in the enamel surface are shown by the following:[6]

Fluoride in Water	Fluoride in Enamel Under Age 20	Over Age 50
0.1 ppm	571 ppm	1247 ppm
1.0 ppm	889 ppm	1552 ppm
3.0 ppm	1930 ppm	2290 ppm

Fluoride is a natural constituent of enamel; even at minimal fluoride exposure (0.1 ppm), 500 to 1200 ppm fluoride are present in the enamel. The surface has the highest concentration and the amount decreases rapidly toward the interior layers of the tooth. For example, 3000 ppm may exist at the surface, but at a depth of 50 μm, only 100 ppm may be found.

FLUORIDE ACTION

Fluorides act in the following ways to provide the beneficial effects on oral health and disease control:
1. Reduction of enamel solubility.
2. Remineralization of early carious lesions.
3. Action on plaque bacteria.

Each of the three ways is reviewed in the following sections. The various modes and methods for providing fluorides to accomplish the beneficial effects then are described.

I. Reduction of Enamel Solubility

The use of fluorides is based on the knowledge that, when the fluoride content of the teeth, particularly that of the surface enamel, is increased to an optimum level, the resistance to dental caries is marked. The source of the fluoride may be systemic or topical. As described previously, fluoride becomes incorporated into the tooth structure by mineralization during tooth development.

Fluoride can be made available for uptake at the surface of the erupted tooth by professional applications of fluoride solutions or gels, as well as by self-application using mouthrinses, chewable tablets, gels, and dentifrices. Fluoride is also taken up at the tooth surface from the drinking water as it passes over the teeth.

II. Remineralization[7,8]

Remineralization of an early carious lesion is one of the principal cariostatic mechanisms of fluoride.

In early dental caries, acid formed by bacteria acting on cariogenic food, especially sucrose, causes demineralization of the hard tooth surface. Caries formation was described on page 242 and illustrated in the flow chart in figure 16–5.

Demineralization means breakdown of the tooth structure with a loss of mineral content. The acids produced in the bacterial plaque act on the enamel to form microchannels through the surface. Demineralization occurs in the subsurface layer and is visible under a microscope. Figure 29–3 shows a cross section of enamel with a subsurface demineralized area. Eventually the area can be detected on clinical examination when the spot may become chalky or discolored by food or tobacco.

When made available on the tooth surface, fluoride is readily taken into the demineralized area where it becomes concentrated. Note in figure 29–3 that the enamel over the demineralized area has the highest fluoride concentration. The presence of fluoride greatly enhances remineralization.

Low concentrations of fluorides applied frequently are the most beneficial; hence, daily use of dentifrice and mouthrinse is indicated. A constant exchange of minerals occurs at the tooth surface. Demineralization is reversed by the fluoride to remineralization and, thus, an advanced destructive carious lesion does not develop.

III. Fluoride in Bacterial Plaque

Bacterial plaque may contain from 5 to 150 ppm fluoride.[9] The content varies greatly and is influenced by the amount of fluoride in the drinking water, in dentifrices, and in all forms of fluoride taken in by the individual.[10]

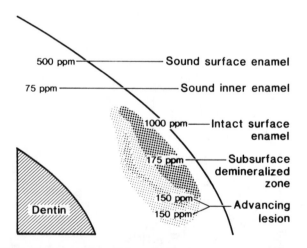

Figure 29–3. Examples of Enamel Fluoride Content. A demineralized area readily takes up available fluoride. As shown, the fluoride content (1000 ppm) of the relatively intact surface over a demineralized white spot is higher than that of the sound surface enamel (500 ppm). The body of the advancing lesion has a higher fluoride content (150 ppm) than does the sound inner enamel (75 ppm). (Drawn after Mellberg, J.R., Ripa, L.W., and Leske, G.S.: *Fluoride in Preventive Dentistry. Theory and Clinical Applications.* Chicago, Quintessence Publishing Co., 1983, p. 31.)

Fluoride has been shown to be an antibacterial and antiplaque agent.[11] The effect of fluoride on the microorganisms depends on its concentration. For example, a gel used for topical application in high concentration (12,000 ppm) is bactericidal. Lower concentrations used frequently reduce dental caries incidence possibly by inhibiting enzyme production that, in turn, can cause acid production.

Other ways that the bacteria in plaque may be affected by fluoride are interference with bacterial adherence and plaque formation on the tooth surface[12] or decrease of the acidogenic potential of bacterial plaque.[13]

FLUORIDATION

Fluoridation is the adjustment of the fluoride ion content of a domestic water supply to the optimum physiologic concentration that will provide maximum protection against dental caries and enhance the appearance of the teeth with a minimum possibility of producing objectionable enamel fluorosis.[14] Fluoridation has been established as the most efficient, effective, reliable, and inexpensive means for improving oral health.

I. Historical Aspects[15,16]

A. Mottled Enamel and Dental Caries

Early in this century Dr. Frederick S. McKay began his extensive studies to find the cause of "brown stain," which later was called mottled enamel and now is known as *dental fluorosis.* He observed that people with mottled enamel had significantly less dental caries.[17] He associated the condition with the drinking water, but tests were inconclusive until 1931 when Churchill pinpointed fluorine as the specific element related to the tooth changes.[18]

B. Background for Fluoridation

Epidemiologic studies of the 1930s sponsored by the United States Public Health Service and directed by Dr. H. Trendley Dean led to the conclusion that the level of fluoride in the water optimum for dental caries prevention averages 1 ppm. Clinically objectionable dental fluorosis is associated with levels well over 2 ppm.[19]

From this knowledge and the fact that many healthy people had lived long lives in communities where the fluoride content of the water was much greater than 1 ppm, the concept of adding fluoride to the water developed. It was still necessary, however, to show that the benefits from controlled fluoridation could parallel those of natural fluoride.

C. Fluoridation—1945

The first communities were fluoridated in 1945. Research in the communities began before fluoridation was started to obtain base-line information, and continued over the years with detailed examinations and reports in the following communities and their scientific controls:

Fluoridation	Control City
Grand Rapids, Michigan (January, 1945)	Muskegon, Michigan
Newburgh, New York (May, 1945)	Kingston, New York
Brantford, Ontario (June, 1945)	Sarnia, Ontario
Evanston, Illinois (February, 1947)	Oak Park, Illinois

Aurora, Illinois, where the natural fluoride level is optimum (1.2 ppm), was used to compare the benefits of natural fluoride in the water supply with those of fluoridation, as well as with a fluoride-free city, Rockford, Illinois.

The research conducted in these cities, as well as other research done throughout the world, has documented the influence of fluoride on oral health. The effects and benefits itemized in Section III summarize important features of fluoridation; examples of research findings are given for illustration.

II. Fluoride Level

The optimum fluoride level for water in temperate climates is 1 ppm. For warmer and colder climates, the amount can be adjusted from approximately 0.6 ppm to 1.2 ppm, adapted in accord with the amount of water consumed.[14]

In the United States, close to 9,800,000 people live in 3063 communities where natural fluoride occurs in the drinking water at 0.7 ppm or more,[20] a level that is sufficient to prevent dental caries.

III. Effects and Benefits

A. Appearance of Teeth

Teeth exposed to an optimum or slightly higher level of fluoride frequently are clear white, shining, opaque, and without blemishes. When the level is slightly more than optimum for the individual, white areas, such as bands or flecks, may be apparent. These areas can be seen professionally by drying the teeth and observing under a dental light. Without such close scrutiny, such spots may blend with the overall appearance. Dental fluorosis associated with higher than optimum fluoride levels has been classified on page 258.

B. Dental Caries: Permanent Teeth

Continuous use of fluoridated water from birth results in an average of 60 to 70 percent fewer carious lesions. The effects are similar to those found in communities with optimum levels of natural fluoride in the water. Many more individuals are completely caries-free when fluoride is in the water.

1. *Distribution.* Anterior teeth, particularly max-

illary, receive more protection from fluoride than do posterior teeth.[19] The anterior teeth are contacted by the drinking water as it passes into the mouth. Fluoride is added to the enamel after eruption.

2. *Posteruption.* Although maximum benefits are derived when fluoridated water is consumed through the entire pre-eruptive period, significant benefits also are derived by teeth that have erupted prior to exposure to fluoride.[21,22,23]

3. *Progression.* Not only are the numbers of carious lesions reduced, but the rate of decay is slowed. Caries progression is also reduced in the surfaces that receive fluoride for the first time after eruption.[24]

C. Root Caries

Root caries experience of lifelong residents of a community with fluoridated water is in direct proportion to the fluoride concentration in the water when compared with the experience of residents of a fluoride-free community.[25]

The incidence of root caries is approximately 50 percent less in lifelong residents of a fluoridated community.[26]

D. Dental Caries: Primary Teeth

With fluoridation from birth, caries incidence is reduced in the primary teeth up to 50 percent.[21] For example, children aged 6 to 9 years in Newburgh had 5 times as many caries-free primary teeth present as did the children of Kingston, where fluoride was not present in the community drinking water.[27]

E. Prenatal Fluoride

Fluoride can pass the placental barrier and become incorporated in the fetal calcifying tissues. Research on the actual effect on dental caries in the primary teeth has not been consistent.[28,29] A major portion of the calcification of primary teeth takes place after birth: the crowns of primary incisors are not fully completed until approximately 3 months, canines at 9 months, and second molars at 11 months, average. The outermost layers of the enamel are formed last, so that fluoride ingested after birth has the most influence on the primary teeth.

F. Tooth Loss

Both primary and permanent tooth loss are much greater in teeth without fluoride[27] because of increased dental caries, which progresses more rapidly.

G. Malocclusion

With fewer extractions, particularly less premature loss of primary molars, the incidence of malocclusion from local causes is less common.[30]

H. Adults

When a person resides in a fluoride area throughout life, benefits continue. In Colorado Springs, adults aged 20 to 44 years who had used water with natural fluoride showed 60 percent less caries experience than did adults in fluoride-deficient Boulder. In Boulder, adults also had had three to four times as many permanent teeth extracted.[31] In a survey of adults in Rockford, Illinois (no fluoride), there were about seven times as many edentulous persons as there were in a comparable group in Aurora (natural fluoride).[32]

I. Bone

Evidence shows that fluoride is important to the maintenance of normal bone and the improvement of calcium metabolism. Studies have shown that there are fewer bone fractures, and when they occur, they heal more quickly; less osteoporosis, especially in women; and less calcification of the aorta, especially in men, when there is increased exposure to fluoride in the water over the years.[33,34,35] Fluoride has been used to improve the bone in the treatment of osteoporosis.[36]

J. Periodontal Diseases

Favorable effects of fluoride on periodontal health have been shown. Improved bone density resulting from fluoride can affect the alveolar bone along with all bones and may have an effect on bone resorption and resistance to local factors.

Dental caries favors plaque retention and, therefore, irritation to gingival tissues, particularly lesions adjacent to the gingival margin and proximal lesions, which favor food impaction. When dental caries, tooth loss, and malocclusion are decreased, a difference can be expected in the severity of periodontal conditions.

The incidence of periodontal diseases increases with age because of the cumulative effects of etiologic factors and the disease processes. With the use of fluorides, particularly fluoridation, fewer teeth are lost because of dental caries at younger ages. Therefore, periodontal disease prevention and control must be emphasized in communities with fluoride in the drinking water.

IV. Partial Defluoridation

Several hundred communities in the United States have water supplies that contain more than twice the optimal level of fluoride. With excess fluoride, the water does not meet the requirements of the United States Public Health Service. Defluoridation can be accomplished by one of several chemical systems.

The efficacy of the methods has been shown. The water supply in Britton, South Dakota, has been reduced from almost 7 ppm to 1.5 ppm since 1948, and in Bartlett, Texas, from 8 ppm to 1.8 ppm since 1952. Examinations have shown a dramatic reduction in incidence of objectionable fluorosis in children born since defluoridation.[37,38]

V. School Fluoridation

One satisfactory method of bringing the benefits of fluoridation to children living in areas lacking a central water system has been the fluoridation of a school water supply. Because of the intermittent use of the water (only part of each day for 5 days each week during the school year), the amount of fluoride added is increased over the usual 1 ppm.

Although children are 5 or 6 years old before they go to school, definite benefits have been shown. The effect is about twice as great on late erupting teeth because they receive the benefit of systemic fluoride and topical exposure, whereas early erupting teeth have only topical benefits.[39]

After 12 years of fluoride at 5 ppm in the school drinking water of Elk Lake, Pennsylvania, children who had attended that school regularly had 39 percent fewer decayed, missing, and filled teeth than did those in the control group. The greatest benefits were found on proximal tooth surfaces.[39]

The benefits increase with increased fluoride levels. In the schools of Seagrove, North Carolina, after 12 years with fluoride level at 6.3 ppm, the children experienced a 47.5 percent decrease in decayed, missing, and filled surfaces when compared with those in the control group.[40]

VI. Discontinued Fluoridation

The control of dental caries by fluorides can be clearly shown in a community when fluoride is removed. For example, in Antigo, Wisconsin, the action of antifluoridationists in 1960 brought about the discontinuance of fluoridation, which had been installed in 1949. Examinations in the years following revealed the marked drop in the number of children who were caries-free, and the steep increases in caries rates. For example, from 1960 to 1966, the number of caries-free children in the second grade decreased by 67 percent.[41] Fluoridation was reinstated in 1966 by popular demand.

VII. Economic Benefits

A. Cost of Fluoridation

In the United States, costs after installation have been estimated to be as low as 15 cents per person per year. When the benefits are considered, and the fact that ALL children are reached, not just those whose parents make the effort to seek preventive professional care, there is little question about the need for fluoridation in all possible domestic water supplies.

No other method for the administration of fluorides has consistently shown equal benefits. All other methods require more professional time, more effort on the part of the individual, and/or more financial outlay.

B. Cost of Professional Care

1. *Influence of Fluoridation.* Individual, family, and community costs of dental care can be reduced markedly. In addition, the number of dental appointments, the extent of individual restorations, and the number of dental extractions are all reduced.

2. *Newburgh-Kingston Study.*[42] Newburgh, New York, and the control city, Kingston (without fluoridation), have been used to demonstrate a specific program of dental care. After 6 years of dental clinic operation for the 5- and 6-year-old lifelong residents of the poorest socioeconomic areas of the cities, the cost for care of the children exposed to fluoridation was shown to be less than half that required for the Kingston children.

At the initial examinations, 41 percent of the Newburgh children were caries-free, whereas only 17 percent of the Kingston children were. Of the needed restorations, about 75 percent of those for the Kingston children were compound; in Newburgh only about 55 percent involved more than 1 surface. At the annual maintenance appointment, the Kingston children consistently required more restorative services; the Newburgh children required only about one half as many appointments. These findings have marked significance for all types of dental programs for all ages.

FLUORIDES IN FOODS

I. Foods

Certain foods contain fluoride, but not enough to constitute a significant part of the day's need for caries prevention. Meat, eggs, vegetables, cereals, and fruits have very small but measurable amounts, whereas tea and fish have larger amounts.

II. Salt

Fluoridated salt has been used, particularly in Switzerland, and although reduced incidence of dental caries has been shown, effects comparable to those gained by fluoridation of water have not been attained. The use of salt as it is currently available supplies about one third to one half of the amount of fluoride ingested daily from 1 ppm fluoridated water, when average amounts of water used by individuals are compared.

DIETARY FLUORIDE SUPPLEMENTS

Approximately 23 percent of the population of the United States live in areas that do not have central water systems. Without fluoride in the drinking water, individuals and communities must resort to other means for making fluoride available. One method is the use of dietary fluoride supplements. Later in the chapter other methods will be described. Other meth-

ods are not substitutes for fluoridation but are needed as follows:
A. For people who use a private water supply that does not have natural fluoride and that is not practical to fluoridate.
B. When the fluoride in the water is less than optimum level.
C. For those whose community water supply has not yet been fluoridated.
D. At the start of fluoridation, fluoride applications and other methods are used to protect the teeth of children too old to receive the full benefits from fluoridation.
E. As a supplement to fluoridation, multiple use of fluorides has been shown to provide added benefits.

I. Administration

A. A fluoride supplement can be administered as a pill, chewable tablet, lozenge, drop, or mouthrinse for swallowing after rinsing.
B. The supplement may be prescribed on an individual patient basis for daily use at home, or it may be administered to school classroom groups as part of a total public health program.
C. Chewing and rinsing with a supplement before swallowing results in a dual action: first, locally on the tooth surface, and second, systemically in teeth that have not erupted (figures 29–1 and 29–2, page 395). After chewing, the mixture should be swished over and between the teeth for 1 minute so that optimal benefit can be obtained. The person should not eat or drink for 30 minutes after chewing the tablet. The preferred time for using the tablet is after toothbrushing before going to bed. The maximum topical effect occurs on newly erupted teeth.

II. Benefits

Studies using preschool children have shown caries incidence reduced as much as 80 percent in primary teeth. The benefit was greatest for those children who started at birth with drops and continued with tablets longer.[43] Studies in permanent teeth have been summarized to show a caries incidence reduction of 70 to 80 percent when started at birth. Results vary from approximately 15 to 70 percent when started before 6 years of age.[43]

For maximum possible effect, fluoride must be administered at least during the period of tooth development, from birth until 12 to 14 years of age or longer for the maturation of the crown of the third permanent molar.

III. Determine the Need

Prescriptions are advised only when the fluoride concentration in the drinking water used by the child is known to have a fluoride ion concentration no higher than 70 percent of the optimal level recommended for water fluoridation in that community.[44]

A. Review patient history to be certain the child is not receiving other fluoride in such preparations as vitamin-fluoride supplements.
B. Refer to list of fluoridated communities to determine patient's fluoride consumption level. Lists are available from state or local health departments.
C. Request water analysis when fluoride level in private water source has not been determined.

IV. Available Forms of Supplements

Products are classified by the American Dental Association, Council on Dental Therapeutics, and the list of approved preparations is published annually in the *Journal of the American Dental Association.*

A. Tablets and Lozenges
These may be scored or unscored. They may be chewed, rinsed, and swallowed, or dissolved slowly in the mouth as a lozenge. The resulting mix with saliva should be swished over and between the teeth for 1 minute. For infants, the tablet can be crushed to add to food.

B. Mouthrinse
A measured amount of rinse contains prescribed daily fluoride. The rinse is swished for at least 1 minute before swallowing.

C. Drops
The liquid is prepared in a concentrate with directions that specify the number of drops for the prescription equivalent. The liquid form has its primary use for the child from birth to 2 years; a drop can be placed directly into the child's mouth or in food. For other children, the tooth contact of the chewable tablet or mouthrinse is important to provide the enamel surface with protective fluoride.

V. Prescription

A. Adjust For No Fluoride in the Drinking Water[44]
1. *Over 3 Years.* 1.0 mg. (prescription: 2.2 mg. sodium fluoride. A 2.2-mg. tablet contains 1.0 mg. fluoride).
2. *Between 2 and 3 Years.* 0.5 mg. (one-half of a 2.2-mg. tablet).
3. *Birth to 2 Years.* 0.25 mg.

B. Adjust For Fluoride in The Water System Up to 0.7 ppm.
Table 29–1 shows the fluoride dosage necessary to supplement at the different levels of fluoride in the drinking water.

C. Prescription for Breast-fed Infant
The concentration of fluoride in breast milk is very low, even when the mother uses fluoridated community water. Infants who are totally breast-fed need a daily fluoride supplement of 0.25 mg. (table 29–1).

In a fluoridated community, an infant who receives other sources of liquid, such as drinking

Table 29–1. Fluoride Supplements Dosage Schedule in mg. F/day*

Age of Child (years)	Water Fluoride Concentration (ppm)		
	Less than 0.3	Between 0.3–0.7	Greater than 0.7
Birth to 2	0.25 (drops)	0**	0**
2 to 3	0.50 (drops or tablet)	0.25	0
3 to 16	1.00 (tablet)	0.50	0

*2.2 mg. sodium fluoride provide 1 mg. fluoride ions.
**Infants receiving their total diet from breast-feeding need a 0.25-mg. supplement.
(Recommendations from the American Dental Association, Chicago, Illinois.)

water or supplemental formula feedings made with fluoridated water, does not need the prescription.

D. Limitation on Total Prescription
1. Prescribe no more than 264 mg. of sodium fluoride at one time; sufficient for 4 months when 2.2 mg. are used daily.
2. The amount (264 mg.) is below the toxic or lethal doses and therefore eliminates the hazard of storing large amounts in the home.

E. Storage
Tablets should be kept out of the reach of children.

F. Vitamins with Fluoride
1. Preparations are available in liquid and tablet form.
2. The American Dental Association has not considered for acceptance vitamin fluoride combinations for several reasons:
   a. It is more difficult to adjust the prescribed fluoride to the amount already received through the water supply (table 29–1).
   b. The preparation contains a fixed amount of fluoride.
   c. There is no evidence that the vitamins enhance the effectiveness of the fluoride.
   d. The expense of buying vitamins that are not needed or prescribed is unnecessary.[44]

VI. Group Administration
Administration of fluoride supplements to groups of children as part of a school health program has been shown to be beneficial.[45,46,47] They should be started early, when the child enters kindergarten. Supervised group administration can be carried out by school personnel and adult volunteers under the supervision of a dental hygienist.

The use of tablet administration as part of a school health program has several advantages, especially when compared with prescription on an individual basis. A minimum of professional service time is needed, and no special effort is required by the individual child or the parents. The use of a daily supplement until the child is 13 to 15 years of age is difficult to supervise in the home setting.

VII. Patient Instruction

A. Individual
For those patients who receive a prescription for fluoride tablets, instruction, motivation, and supervision are needed. When prescribed on an individual basis, problems arise in the continued administration of the tablets over the years of childhood, even when parents are conscientious and highly motivated.

B. Patient Follow-up
Maintenance appointments should be planned for the time when the patient's prescription will be in need of renewal so that encouragement and supervision can be provided.

PROFESSIONAL TOPICAL FLUORIDE APPLICATIONS

Topical application of fluoride preparations frequently may be an essential part of a total preventive program, particularly when fluoridation is not available.

Research in topical applications has continued since the early 1940s, when Dr. Basil G. Bibby conducted the initial topical sodium fluoride study using Brockton, Massachusetts schoolchildren.[48] More than one-third fewer new carious lesions resulted from a 0.1% aqueous solution applied at 4-month intervals for 2 years.

That research led to extensive studies by Dr. John W. Knutson and others sponsored by the United States Public Health Service. The aim was to determine the most effective concentration of sodium fluoride, the minimum time required for application, and procedural details.[49,50] Their results still provide the basis for applications as used currently and described below.

Although several fluoride preparations have been tried and have shown caries-preventive effects, those most generally used have been *sodium fluoride* (NaF), *acidulated phosphate-fluoride* (APF), and *stannous fluoride* (SnF$_2$).

Summaries of many clinical trials show that all three are effective for dental caries prevention with a reduction in caries incidence of approximately 30 percent.[51] Table 29–2 provides a comparison of the three topical agents.

A review of research to determine retained effectiveness of the topical applications shows a gradual decrease over 2 years.[52] A retained anticaries effect

Table 29–2. Comparison of Topical Fluoride Agents for Professional Application

	NaF	APF	SnF₂
Concentration	Solution 2%	Gel or solution 1.23%	Solution 8%
Fluoride ion %	0.91%	1.23%	1.95%
ppm Fluoride	9,040 ppm	12,000 ppm	19,360 ppm
Mg. F/ml	9.04	12.0	19.36
Efficacy	29%	28%	32%
Application Frequency	4/year at ages 3, 7, 10, 13	1 or 2/year	1 or 2/year
Taste	Bland	Bitter without flavoring	Astringent
Tooth Discoloration	None	None	Brown
Gingival Reaction	None	None	Occasional

Modified from Ripa, L.W.: Professionally (Operator) Applied Topical Fluoride Therapy: A Critique. *Int. Dent. J.*, 31:105, June, 1981.

of 10 to 40 percent, however, does occur. The longest-lasting effects were shown for APF, probably because of the greater amount of fluoride deposited in the enamel.

SODIUM FLUORIDE

I. Solution

The solution is 2% aqueous sodium fluoride (basic pH 9.2).

II. Frequency of Application

A. Four Applications

As originally planned, a series of 4 applications, 2 days to 1 week apart, were given at intervals throughout childhood in accord with the tooth eruption pattern of the individual.

B. Ages

Greatest protection is afforded to newly erupted teeth. Ages 3, 7, 10, and 13 were considered average.

C. Supplemental Applications

A single application is recommended at intervals between the series of four for caries-susceptible individuals.

III. Clinical Features

A. Solution is relatively stable when kept in a polyethylene bottle.
B. Patient acceptance is favorable: solution tastes salty but is not objectionable.
C. No tooth staining or adverse gingival reactions occur.
D. Patient education is enhanced. Although the series of appointments required for four treatments has been considered a disadvantage, one distinct advantage is instruction of the patient in bacterial plaque control procedures. The fluoride appointment series gives the opportunity for continuing instruction and review. Toothbrushing and flossing practice precedes each fluoride application and thus serves to prepare the teeth by removing plaque and debris.

ACIDULATED PHOSPHATE-FLUORIDE (APF)

I. Preparations

A 1.23% sodium fluoride with 0.1 M orthophosphoric acid (pH 3.0 to 3.5).

APF has been used in three forms: an aqueous solution, a gel, and a thixotropic agent. In the gel, a carboxymethylcellulose gelling base is used. Flavoring and coloring agents are added.

A thixotropic agent is a type of gel that sets in a gel-like state, but becomes fluid-like under stress. Gels of this type can flow into interdental areas. In the gel form, they adhere to tooth surfaces.

II. Frequency of Application

At least twice annually; more frequently for caries-susceptible individuals.

III. Clinical Features

A. Stable when kept in a polyethylene bottle.
B. No staining of the tooth structure.
C. Patient acceptance favorable: taste objectionable, but commercial preparations are flavored.
D. No gingival irritation.
E. Cause surface roughening, pitting, or etching of porcelain and composite restorations. Nonacidic fluoride preparations should be used for patients with these restorations.[53]

STANNOUS FLUORIDE

I. Solution

Aqueous stannous fluoride 8% (pH 2.1 to 2.3).

II. Frequency of Application

At least twice annually; more frequently for the caries-susceptible individuals.

III. Clinical Features

A. Unstable solution. Fresh solution must be mixed for each appointment.*
B. Limited patient acceptance because of astringent quality and unpleasant taste.
C. Staining of teeth in demineralized areas, pits, fissures, and grooves.
D. Possible gingival sloughing, particularly if applied to inflamed tissue.
E. Possible discoloration of tooth-color restorations and around margins.

CLINICAL PROCEDURES FOR TOPICAL FLUORIDE APPLICATIONS

I. Appointment Planning

Appointments for topical fluoride applications should be scheduled to end more than 30 minutes before a patient's regular mealtime. The patient is instructed not to eat, drink, rinse, brush, or floss to avoid disturbing the action of the fluoride.

Planning the time is especially important to patients on a strict diet schedule, for example, a person with diabetes.

II. Explanation to Patient

A. Inform the patient (and parent of young patient) of the purposes and benefits of fluoride applications.
B. Explain the procedures and prepare the patient for any discomfort, the 4-minute timing, and the postoperative instructions (to be repeated again at the completion of the procedure).

III. Preparation of the Teeth

Research has been summarized to show that "rubber cup polishing" of the teeth is not required prior to topical fluoride application.[54] Removal of all pellicle and bacterial plaque is not necessary, because the fluoride diffuses through and is not inhibited by these deposits. Calculus and heavy stains that could prevent the fluoride from reaching the tooth should be removed.

The clinical sequence is as follows:

A. Use patient instruction time with toothbrush and dental floss to prepare the teeth by removing debris, materia alba, and bacterial plaque as the instruction is provided.
B. Perform scaling for calculus removal.
C. Apply principles of selective polishing (pages 504–506).
   1. When visible dental stains are not present, further tooth preparation is not necessary.
   2. When stains must be removed, use the rubber cup with paste selectively where the stains appear. A fluoride-containing paste may be used (page 508). Although only a small amount of fluoride may be added to the tooth surface, a fluoride paste may replace, at least in part, the fluoride removed by the polishing abrasive.[55]

IV. Procedures

A. Two Methods

One system uses cotton-roll isolation with applicators to "paint on" the gel or solution. The other system uses trays that fit over the teeth of each dental arch.

B. Benefits

Maximum benefits of reduction of dental caries incidence can be expected in proportion to the care taken to follow a well-defined, exacting application procedure.

C. Technique Objectives

1. Apply fluoride to all tooth surfaces for 4 minutes without dilution by the saliva.
2. Prevent ingestion of fluoride by swallowing of gel or solution.

PAINT-ON TECHNIQUE: SOLUTION OR GEL

I. Supplies and Preparation

A. Cotton-roll holders of appropriate size.
B. Cotton rolls of proper lengths attached to holders (see Section II., B. and C. following).
C. Cotton pellets (six to eight medium size) and cotton pliers. Cotton applicators may be used.
D. Saliva absorbers for parotid duct opening in cheeks.
E. Mouth prop for patient unable to hold the mouth open 4 minutes.
F. Fluoride solution or gel in disposable cup. (Stannous fluoride must be mixed in special container.)*
G. Saliva ejector connected and water control adjusted.
H. Air tip connected to compressed air outlet.
I. Timer set for 4 minutes (egg timer or a darkroom alarm).

---

*To mix stannous fluoride solution: Obtain capsules containing SnF_2 powder from pharmacy: 0.8 gram for 8%. Keep capsules in a tightly sealed container. When ready for use, add contents to 10 ml. distilled water and shake. Use a 25-ml. graduated cylinder to measure the water and a 25-ml. polyethylene bottle for mixing the solution. Do not add flavoring or coloring. Discard excess solution after application to dry, isolated teeth (page 404). Prompt care of equipment, including running water through the saliva ejector for at least 1 minute to prevent clogging, is important. A grayish-white deposit collects on equipment as the solution dries. Instruments prepared for sterilizing should be thoroughly rinsed to prevent contamination of sterilizing equipment and disinfecting solution. Change gloves before processing radiographs (page 147).

II. Cotton-Roll Preparation

A. Prepare in Advance

1. Cut cotton rolls into appropriate sizes; sterilize in package with cotton-roll holders and other essentials.
2. Use No. 2 cotton rolls, except in small mouths or very shallow vestibules for which a No. 1 may be fitted and maintained more effectively.
3. Bevel ends at 45 degrees to facilitate placement and retention in the mucobuccal fold and under the tongue.

B. Lengths: Continuous Cotton-roll Technique

1. *Facial* (5- to 6-inch cotton roll)
   a. Attach to facial prong of cotton-roll holder.
   b. Should extend (in the mucobuccal fold) from the mandibular labial frenum to the maxillary labial frenum (figure 29–4).
2. *Lingual Mandibular* (1¼- to 2-inch cotton roll)
   a. Attach to lingual prong of holder.
   b. Should extend from canine area to just distal to the most posterior tooth (figure 29–4).
   c. Have available an extra cotton roll (1 to 1¼ inches). For most patients a short cotton roll is needed under the side of the tongue (before the cotton-roll holder is placed) for balance. The vestibule, which is more shallow than the floor of the mouth, permits the cotton-roll holder to tip toward the lingual if not supported by an extra cotton roll.

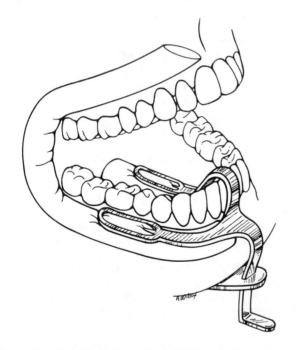

Figure 29–4. Isolation Using Cotton-Roll Holders. One half of the teeth are treated simultaneously. A continuous cotton roll extends from the mandibular anterior vestibule to the maxillary anterior. Lingual prong holds cotton roll adjacent to tongue over floor of mouth. Care is taken to maintain cotton away from tooth surfaces to assure maximum contact of fluoride solution or gel being applied. See text for details.

C. Lengths: Discontinuous Cotton-Roll Technique

1. *Indications.* The continuous method can be used only when retraction of the cotton roll from the distobuccal surfaces of the most posterior teeth can be assured during the application. Usually, when second permanent molars (and always the third) have erupted, separate facial cotton rolls are needed for the maxillary and mandibular teeth.
2. *Facial Maxillary* (3 inches)
   a. Finger-held.
   b. Should extend from labial frenum to area distal to most posterior tooth and the opening to Stensen's duct.
3. *Facial Mandibular* (3 inches)
   a. Attach to facial prong of holder.
   b. Should extend from mandibular labial frenum to the distal of the most posterior tooth.
   c. Prevent dislodgment by activity of muscles of throat or cheeks by not extending the cotton roll over the retromolar area.
4. *Lingual Mandibular.* Same as for continuous technique (B., 2 previously).

III. Isolation Procedure

A. Seat the patient upright to prevent gel or solution from passing into the throat.

B. Place single cotton roll beneath the edge of the tongue.

C. Insert holder with attached cotton rolls over the mandibular teeth. Adjust to proper position.
   1. Place lingual cotton roll beside and under the lateral margin of the tongue without pressing the tongue down.
   2. Check that the cotton rolls are positioned to protect the oral tissues from contact with the metal holder.
   3. Hold the holder with nondominant hand while adjusting the chin clamp. Fasten securely.

D. Insert saliva ejector gently in the region of the canine of the side opposite the holder.

E. Adjust maxillary. The continuous cotton roll curves up, distal to the most posterior tooth.
   1. Retract the cheek and twist the cotton roll slightly (toward the gingiva) as it is brought into position in the mucobuccal fold.
   2. Adapt the end in position beside the labial frenum (figure 29–4).

F. Hold maxillary section of the cotton roll with the fingers of the nondominant hand. When the discontinuous procedure is used, the maxillary facial cotton roll is held as described here.
   1. Hold the cotton roll away from the distal of the most posterior tooth to assure access of molar surfaces to fluoride.
   2. Maintain retraction throughout application.

G. Make a final check before application.
   1. Cotton is not on the teeth.

2. Oral tissues are protected from metal parts of the holder.
3. Cotton rolls are not extended too far distally so they can be easily displaced.

IV. Application Procedure

A. Dry Teeth

Dry teeth thoroughly with compressed air: maxillary first, then mandibular (figure 29–5). Direct the air to each surface and proximal area, because complete dryness contributes to the effectiveness of fluoride by preventing dilution.

B. Apply Fluoride Preparation

Apply quickly to moisten all teeth: mandibular teeth first, then maxillary.

C. Start the Timer

The patient may be instructed to do this so that retraction is not interrupted.

D. Keep Tooth Surfaces Wet

Maintain wet tooth surfaces by continuous application of the solution throughout the 4-minute period.

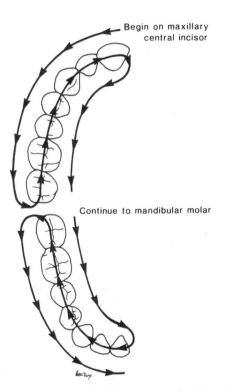

Begin on maxillary central incisor

Continue to mandibular molar

Figure 29–5. Procedure for Drying Teeth. After the teeth have been isolated using cotton in cotton-roll holder, a saliva ejector is positioned. The teeth are dried before applying the solution or gel. Because maxillary teeth can be maintained in a drier state longer, the mandibular teeth are dried with compressed air after the maxillary teeth have been dried. As shown by arrows, air is applied from maxillary facial, over occlusal, and then palatal surfaces. Proceed to mandibular lingual surfaces, over the occlusals, and finally over the facial. Apply fluoride preparation to the mandibular teeth first (see text).

E. Completion of Application

1. Remove saliva ejector.
2. Release cotton-roll holder clamp and remove holder with cotton rolls attached.
3. Remove remaining cotton rolls with cotton pliers.
4. Wipe over teeth with sponge to remove superficial gel or solution.
5. Allow the patient to expectorate.

F. Proceed to Opposite Side of Mouth

The patient does not rinse either between sides or at completion of both sides.

G. Instruct Patient

Instruct patient not to rinse, eat, drink, or brush the teeth for at least 30 minutes, preferably longer.

TRAY TECHNIQUE: GEL

I. Supplies and Preparation

A. Trays of appropriate size.
B. Saliva ejector connected and water control adjusted.
C. Air tip connected to compressed air outlet.
D. Timer set for 4 minutes (egg timer or a darkroom alarm).
E. Cotton rolls, sponges.

II. Tray Preparation

A. Characteristics of an Acceptable Tray

1. Disposable or can be sterilized.
2. Designed to aid in holding gel to prevent ingestion.
   a. Border rim to help to seal in the gel and prevent saliva from entering.
   b. Post-dam to prevent outflow.
3. Available in choice of sizes to accommodate various patients.
4. Designed to cover all the patient's dentition of both the mandible and the maxilla.
5. Deep enough to cover the cervical third. Figure 29–6 shows a mandibular tray try-in. In figure 29–6B, the tray is deep enough to cover the entire exposed enamel above the gingiva. In figure 29–6C, the patient has deep recession with areas of exposed root surface. The same tray is not deep enough to extend the fluoride gel to the important root surfaces. In such an instance, a custom-made tray is necessary.
6. Made of a material that cannot be distorted easily or altered in fit by the oral temperature or fluids, but is sufficiently flexible to receive pressure to force the gel interproximally. A custom-made tray fits closely and requires only a small serving of gel; consequently, pressing to force the gel between the teeth is not necessary.
7. Equipped with lining to aid in gel retention.
8. Cost-effective.

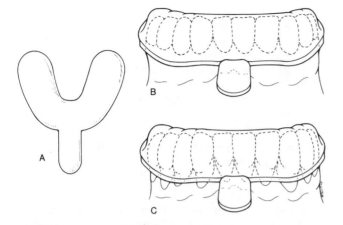

Figure 29–6. Tray Selection. A. Mandibular tray held for try-in. **B.** Tray over teeth is deep enough to cover the entire exposed enamel above the gingiva. **C.** In patient with recession and areas of root surfaces exposed, the same tray is not deep enough to cover the important root surfaces where fluoride is needed for prevention of root caries or hypersensitivity. A custom-made tray is needed.

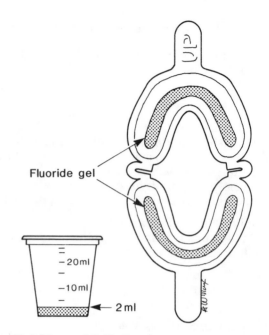

Figure 29–7. Measured Gel in Tray. No more than 2 ml. gel should be placed in each tray for small children, and no more than 2.5 ml. for larger patients with permanent teeth. A medicine cup can be used to measure the amount once, so that the correct level of gel in the tray can be determined. A minimum amount of gel is indicated to prevent ingestion by the patient.

B. Types of Trays

1. *Custom-made Thermoplastic or Vacuum-processed Vinyl.* Useful for frequent applications; patient in one of the "risk" groups may need daily fluoride application.
2. *Disposable Styrofoam.* Single arch or hinged for insertion of both arches simultaneously; pliable, comfortable, and most models are deep enough to cover most teeth.
3. *Reusable Vinyl.* Least comfortable and most are difficult to adapt.
4. *Air-cushion Fluoridator.* Has a built-in saliva ejection system; good adaptation; cannot be autoclaved; bulky.
5. *Wax.* Soft and pliable; time-consuming preparation to mold into proper fit; poor retention without border rim and may spread because of warmth of mouth and pressure from closing of teeth by patient.

C. Loading the Tray

1. May dispense directly from commercial container when the tray is prepared prior to patient contact. (Dispensing bottles can be surface disinfected when handled during the appointment.)
2. Use minimum amount
   a. No more than 2 ml. per tray or 5 ml. total are recommended by the American Academy of Pediatric Dentistry.[56]
   b. Determine correct level by measuring 2 ml. in a graduated medicine cup and then placing it in the tray. This procedure may be tried for each tray size so that measuring is not necessary on a routine basis. Figure 29–7 shows the level of a measured 2 ml. in a Styrofoam tray.

III. Application Procedure

Table 29–3 summarizes the procedures recommended to reduce fluoride ingestion by the patient during the gel tray application.

A. Seat patient in upright position to prevent gel from passing into the throat.
B. Request patient to expectorate or swallow to clear the mouth.
C. Dry maxillary teeth for single tray insertion. When both trays will be placed simultaneously, dry mandibular teeth last.
D. Insert tray or trays promptly, and place saliva ejector between trays.
E. Press tray against teeth starting over the occlusal and on the sides to force the gel between the teeth.
F. When appropriate, place a cotton roll between the trays over the premolar areas on each side to soften the pressure as the patient closes. The gentle pressure can aid in the adaptation of gel to tooth surfaces. It also prevents closure on the saliva ejector.
G. Set timer for 4 minutes.
H. On completion, remove tray(s). Patient does not rinse, but can expectorate.
I. Immediately place the second tray when a two-step operation is preferred or necessary.
J. Do not allow the patient to rinse on removal of second tray.
   1. Wipe teeth with sponge to remove excess residual gel. Apply high-power suction.
   2. Request patient to expectorate for several minutes.

Table 29–3. Procedures to Reduce Fluoride Ingestion During Topical Gel-tray Application

Patient	Seat upright
	Instruct not to swallow
	Tilt head forward with trays; tilt away from side with cotton-roll holder
Trays	Custom-made or appropriate size with absorptive liners; post-dam; border rim
	Use minimum amount of gel: 2 ml. per tray, less for small tray; no more than total of 5 ml. for large trays
Isolation	Use saliva ejector with maximum efficiency suction
	Cotton-roll holder technique: position for security, stability; place saliva absorber in cheek
Attention	Do not leave patient unattended
Timing	Use a timer; do not estimate
Completion	Tilt head forward for removal of tray or cotton-roll holder
	Request patient to expectorate for several minutes; do not allow swallowing
	Wipe excess gel from teeth with gauze sponge
	Use high-power suction to draw out saliva and gel
	Instruct patient not to rinse, eat, drink, or brush teeth for at least 30 minutes

Recommendations based on Oral Health Policies for Children: Protocol for Fluoride Therapy, American Academy of Pediatric Dentistry, 211 E. Chicago Avenue, Chicago, 60611.

K. Instruct patient not to rinse, eat, drink, brush the teeth, or perform other activity that could disturb the fluoride action for at least 30 minutes, preferably longer.[57]

SELF-APPLIED FLUORIDES

I. Methods

The three methods for self-application are by mouth tray, rinsing, and toothbrushing.

A. Mouth tray

A fluoride gel is placed in a custom-made or disposable tray and is held in the mouth for 4 minutes.

B. Rinsing

The patient swishes for 1 minute with a measured amount of a fluoride rinse. Except when used as a rinse-supplement in a nonfluoridated community, the fluoride rinse is expectorated.

C. Toothbrushing

A gel or paste is used for regular brushing 2 or 3 times daily. In addition, a brush-on gel may be used after regular brushing to provide special benefits.

II. Indications

Indications for use of mouth tray, rinsing, and/or toothbrushing depend on the individual patient problems. Patient needs are determined as a part of total treatment planning. Certain patients need multiple procedures combined with professional applications at the regular maintenance appointments. Special indications are suggested as each method is described in the following sections.

Frequent application using weak preparations of fluoride compounds is considered more beneficial than infrequent high-concentration applications. Therefore, the daily applications are recommended when performed on an individual basis. Fluoridated water, described earlier in this chapter, provides another method of self-application.

TRAY TECHNIQUE: HOME APPLICATION[58]

The original gel tray studies using custom-fitted polyvinyl mouthpieces compared the use of 1.1% acidulated NaF with plain NaF gel. The gel was applied daily over a 2-year period by schoolchildren aged 11 to 14 years during the school years. Dental caries incidence was reduced up to 80 percent.[59]

I. Indications for Use

A. Rampant enamel or root caries in persons of any age.
B. Xerostomia of any cause, particularly loss of salivary gland function.
C. Exposure to radiation therapy (pages 606–607).
D. Caries prevention under an overdenture (page 350).
E. Root surface hypersensitivity (pages 499–500).

II. Gels Used

A. Concentrations

APF 0.5%; NaF 1.1%; SnF_2 0.4%.

B. Precaution

Dispensing of large quantities is contraindicated. Prescription for 24 to 30 ml. of APF 0.5% in a dropper bottle that dispenses drops containing 0.1 ml. F is suggested.

III. Procedure

A. Use custom-made polyvinyl tray. A disposable tray can be used each day if the appropriate fit can be obtained.
B. Load tray by distributing no more than 5 drops

of the gel around each tray. Each drop is equivalent to 0.1 ml.

C. Follow patient instructions:
1. Use toothbrush and dental floss to remove thoroughly all bacterial plaque.
2. Dry the mouth by swallowing several times.
3. Prepare trays. Apply tray(s) over the teeth and close gently. When a soft tray is used, the finger can be pressed along the facial to push the gel between the teeth.
4. Time by clock for 4 minutes. *Do Not Swallow.* This instruction is particularly important for children in the tooth development years who live in a fluoridated community.
5. Expectorate several times. Do not eat or drink for 30 minutes. One application can be made immediately before retiring.

FLUORIDE MOUTHRINSES

Mouthrinsing is a practical and effective means for self-application of fluoride. The only persons excluded from the practice of this method are children under 6 years of age and those of any age who cannot rinse because of oral-facial musculature problems or other handicap. Rinsing can be part of an individual treatment plan or can be included in a group program conducted during school attendance.

Mouthrinses containing fluoride are reviewed by the American Dental Association, Council on Dental Therapeutics. Approved products are listed annually and bear the seal of the Association (figure 23–14, page 331).

I. Indications

Mouthrinsing with a fluoride preparation may have particular meaning for the following:
A. General prevention of dental caries in
1. Young persons during the high-risk preteen and adolescent years.
2. Patients with root exposure following recession and periodontal therapy.
3. Participants in a school health group program for all grades.
B. Patients with moderate to rampant dental caries who live in a fluoridated or nonfluoridated community.
C. Patients whose oral health care is complicated by plaque-retentive appliances, including orthodontics and partial dentures or space maintainers.
D. Patients with xerostomia caused by any reason, including head and neck radiation and saliva-depressing drug therapy.
E. Patients with hypersensitivity of exposed root surfaces.

II. Preparations

Rinse preparations are referred to as *low potency/high frequency rinses, high potency/low frequency rinses,* and *oral rinse supplements.*[60] Certain low po-

tency rinses may be purchased directly "over-the-counter" (OTC); all others are provided by prescription.

A. Over-the-counter: Sodium Fluoride 0.05%
1. *Fluoride Content.* 0.025% fluoride; 225 ppm.
2. *Specifications*
   a. Single container must contain no more than 264 mg. NaF (120 mg. fluoride) dispensed at one time. A 500-ml. bottle of 0.05% NaF rinse contains 100 mg. fluoride.
   b. Bottle must have child-proof cap.
   c. Label must state that the rinse is not to be used by children under 6 years of age or by children with a handicap involving oral-facial musculature. Young children do not have sufficient control to expectorate, and they tend to swallow quickly.
   d. Label must indicate that the rinse is not to be swallowed.
3. *Procedure for Use*
   a. Rinse daily with 1 teaspoonful (5 ml.) after brushing before bed.
   b. Swish between teeth with lips tightly closed for 60 seconds; expectorate.
4. *Limitations*
   a. Alcohol content of commercial preparations is not advisable for children. Alcohol-containing preparations should never be recommended for a recovering alcoholic person.
   b. Motivation of patient and/or parent to carry out faithfully the recommended procedures. Daily rinse is better than weekly rinse when practiced on an individual home basis.

B. Prescription
1. *Oral Rinse Supplement: Acidulated NaF 0.04% (low potency).* Supplements were described and the recommendation listed on pages 399–400. They are swished and swallowed to provide daily systemic supplementation to inadequate fluoride in the drinking water. For rampant caries, hypersensitive teeth, or other conditions, the preparation may be used to provide local effect only by expectorating after 1 minute of swishing.
2. *Sodium fluoride: 0.2%*
   a. Fluoride Content. .090% F; 900 ppm (high potency).
   b. Use. Weekly rinse using 5 ml. (younger children) or 10 ml. (older children) swished for 60 seconds and expectorated.
   c. School Group Program. The use of the weekly rinse is the most common school-based program in the United States. Advantages are that it requires little time (about 5 minutes once weekly for an entire class); is inexpensive; is easy to learn, and well accepted by participants; and can be

carried out by non-dental personnel. Responsibility for providing the correctly mixed 0.2% solution and for locking the fluoride in an inaccessible place can be taken by school officials and a supervising dental hygienist.[60,61]

III. Benefits

Benefits from fluoride mouthrinsing have been documented many times since the original research using various percentages of various fluoride preparations.[62,63] Frequent rinsing with low concentrations of fluoride have the following effects:

A. A 30 to 40% average reduction in dental caries incidence.
B. Greater benefit for smooth surfaces, but some benefit to pits and fissures.
C. Greatest benefit to newly erupted teeth (thus, the program should be continued through the teenage years to benefit the second and third permanent molars).
D. Added benefits have been shown in a community with fluoridation.[64]
E. Post-treatment benefits increase as the length of time of rinsing increases.[59,65]
F. Primary teeth present in school-age children benefit by as much as 42.5 percent average reduction in dental caries incidence.[66]

FLUORIDE DENTIFRICES

Historically dentifrices have been tried with various compounds, including stannous fluoride, sodium fluoride, sodium monofluorophosphate, and amine fluoride. The main research objective has been to find fluoride and abrasive systems that are compatible. Early dentifrices had problems of stability and fluoride availability for uptake by the tooth surface.

A dentifrice containing stannous fluoride 0.4% was the first fluoride-containing dentifrice to gain approval by the Council on Dental Therapeutics.[67] An excellent review by Stookey that describes the development of present formulations and the extensive research over past years is recommended for reading.[68] Guidelines for the acceptance of dentifrices by the Council are frequently updated and call for laboratory and clinical efficacy of each product.[69]

I. Indications

A. Dental Caries Prevention

A fluoride dentifrice approved by the American Dental Association should be recommended for each patient as part of the complete preventive program.

B. Caries-risk Patients

Patients with moderate to rampant dental caries should be advised to brush several times each day with a fluoride-containing dentifrice.

C. Desensitization

Certain dentifrices containing fluoride have desensitizing properties. These are included on pages 328 and 500.

II. Preparations

Fluoride dentifrices are available as gels or pastes. Sodium fluoride and sodium monofluorophosphate dentifrices are approved currently. Amine fluorides have not been developed and promoted in the United States.

A. Current Constituents

1. Sodium fluoride (NaF) 0.24% (1100 ppm).
2. Sodium monofluorophosphate (Na_2PO_3F) 0.76% (1000 ppm). An "extra strength" Na_2PO_3F contains 1500 ppm.

B. Specifications From Guidelines for Acceptance[69]

To gain approval by the American Dental Association and to use the seal of acceptance (figure 23–14, page 331), a product must meet certain criteria, including the following:

1. The active fluoride (F) agent must be chemically free and available in both fresh and aged samples to the end of the specified expiration date.
2. The ability to deliver and incorporate levels of F into both sound and demineralized enamel must be demonstrated.
3. The product must promote or enhance remineralization of enamel.
4. The product must reduce the rate of demineralization.

III. Patient Instruction: Recommended Procedures

Instruction in the selection of a dentifrice, the need for frequent use, the method for application to the tooth surfaces, and the effects of fluoride can help the patient appreciate the significant role of fluoride in oral health.

A. Select an approved fluoride-containing dentifrice.
B. Place a small amount of dentifrice on the toothbrush tips.
1. Child: Use only a small amount, the size of a pea (figure 29–8). Demonstrate this amount and explain that the child should not swallow excess amounts of dentifrice because that may cause white spots to develop in the enamel (pages 397 and 412).
2. Older children and adults: ½ inch or less.
C. Spread dentifrice over the teeth with a light touch of the brush.
D. Proceed with correct brushing for sulcular removal of bacterial plaque.
E. Keep dentifrice container out of reach of children.

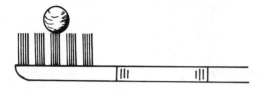

Figure 29–8. Dentifrice for a Child. To prevent ingestion of an excess amount of dentifrice, a parent must be instructed to place only a small portion of dentifrice on the brush; the size can be compared to the size of a pea.

IV. Benefits

Dentifrices are used often, at least once or twice each day as recommended. Caries-risk patients may use a dentifrice several times per day. The dentifrice is a continuing source of fluoride for the tooth surface in the control of demineralization and promotion of remineralization. Fluoride is deposited in demineralized white spots (figure 29–3).

Many research studies have shown that the incidence of dental caries can be reduced between 20 to 30 percent when NaF or Na_2PO_3F dentifrices are used regularly.

BRUSH-ON GEL

Brush-on gel has been used as an adjunct to the daily application of fluoride in a dentifrice and as a supplement to periodic professional applications. Although widely accepted, reviews of the research show limited and somewhat conflicting reports of the benefits.[70,71]

I. Preparations

A. Acidulated phosphate fluoride (APF) 0.5%.
B. Stannous fluoride (SnF_2) 0.4% in glycerin base.
C. Sodium fluoride (NaF) 1.1%.

II. Procedure

A. Use once a day, preferably at night.
B. Complete toothbrushing and flossing.
C. Place about 2 mg. of the gel over about ⅓ of the brush head and spread over all teeth.
D. Brush 1 minute, then swish before expectorating.

III. Patient Instruction

A. APF gels are not for use on porcelain or composite.[53]
B. Gels of this category are not for use as dentifrices. Teeth are cleaned first with thorough brushing and flossing.
C. Regular use has been shown to help to control demineralization about orthodontic appliances,[72] and to provide protection against post-irradiation caries in conjunction with other fluoride applications.[73]

COMBINED FLUORIDE PROGRAM

Most patients can benefit from more than one method of use of fluorides. When the preventive program is planned for an individual patient, the fluoride preparations and modes of application selected should provide the greatest possible protection against dental caries.

When self-administered methods are chosen, patient cooperation is a significant factor. Age and eruption pattern influence the method selected. Fluorides must be applied as soon after tooth eruption as possible and continued indefinitely, to control demineralization.

Maintenance appointments can be scheduled for frequent topical applications and for continuing instruction and motivation. All methods are supplemented by the use of a dentifrice with fluoride.

FLUORIDE SAFETY

Fluoride preparations and fluoridated water have wide margins of safety. Fluoride is beneficial in small amounts, but can be injurious if used without attention to correct dosage and frequency. All dental personnel should be familiar with recommended approved procedures, know potentials for toxic effects, and be prepared to administer emergency measures should accidental overdosages occur.

I. Summary of Fluoride Management

A. Use and recommend for patient use only approved fluoride preparations. Products have approval from the Food and Drug Administration and the American Dental Association in the United States.
B. Use only researched, recommended amounts and methods for delivery.
C. Know potential toxicity of the various products and be prepared for administering emergency measures for treating an accidental toxic response.
D. Instruct patients in proper care of fluoride products.
   1. Dentist will prescribe no more than 264 mg. of sodium fluoride at one time. Do not store large quantities in the home.
   2. Request parental supervision of child's brushing or other fluoride administration. Rinses, for example, are not to be used by children under 6 years of age.
   3. Fluoride products should have child-proof covers and should be kept out of reach of small children and other persons, such as the mentally or physically handicapped, who may not understand limitations.
   4. In school health programs, dispensing of the fluoride product must be supervised by responsible adults. Containers must be stored under lock and key when not in active use.

II. Acute Toxicity

Acute refers to rapid intake of an excess dose over a short time, whereas *chronic* applies to long-term ingestion of fluoride in amounts that exceed the approved therapeutic levels. An accidental ingestion of a concentrated fluoride preparation can lead to a toxic reaction. Acute fluoride poisoning is rare.[74]

A. Certainly Lethal Dose (CLD)[75]

A lethal dose is the amount of a drug likely to cause death if not intercepted by antidotal therapy.
1. *Adult Lethal Dose.* 5 to 10 grams of sodium fluoride taken at 1 time. The fluoride ion equivalent is 32 to 64 milligrams fluoride per kilogram (mg. F/kg.) body weight (table 29–4A).
2. *Child.* Approximately 0.5 to 1.0 gram variable with size and weight of the child.

B. Safely Tolerated Dose (STD): One Fourth of the CLD

1. *Adult STD.* 1.25 to 2.5 grams of sodium fluoride (8 to 16 mg. F/kg.)
2. *Child.* Table 29–4B shows STDs and CLDs for children. Weights given for each selected age are minimal, and calculations for the doses are conservative. As can be noted from the table, less than 1 gm (1000 mg.) may be fatal for children 12 years old and younger, and ½ gram (500 mg.) exceeds the STD for all ages shown. For children under 6 years of age, however, 500 mg. would be lethal.[75]

III. Signs and Symptoms of Acute Toxic Dose

Symptoms begin within 30 minutes of ingestion and may persist for as long as 24 hours.

A. Gastrointestinal Tract

Fluoride in the stomach is acted on by the hydrochloric acid to form hydrofluoric acid, an irritant to the stomach lining. Symptoms include
1. Nausea, vomiting, diarrhea.
2. Abdominal pain.
3. Increased salivation, thirst.

B. Systemic Involvement

1. *Blood.* Calcium may be bound by the circulating fluoride, thus causing symptoms of hypocalcemia.
2. *Central Nervous System.* Hyperreflexia, convulsions, paresthesias.
3. *Cardiovascular and Respiratory Depression.* If not treated may lead to death in a few hours from cardiac failure or respiratory paralysis.

IV. Emergency Treatment

A. Induce Vomiting (table 60–1, page 753)

1. *Mechanical.* Digital stimulation at back of tongue or in throat.
2. *Drug.* Ipecac syrup.

Table 29–4. Lethal and Safe Doses of Fluoride

A. *Lethal and safe dosages of fluoride for a 70 kg adult.*

Certainly Lethal Dose (CLD)
5–10 gm NaF
or
32–64 mg F/kg
Safely Tolerated Dose (STD) = 1/4 CLD
1.25–2.5 gm NaF
or
8–16 mg F/kg

B. *CLDs and STDs of fluoride for selected ages.*

Age	Weight (lbs)	CLD (mg)	STD (mg)
2	22	320	80
4	29	422	106
6	37	538	135
8	45	655	164
10	53	771	193
12	64	931	233
14	83	1,206	301
16	92	1,338	334
18	95	1,382	346

From Heifetz, S.B. and Horowitz, H.S.: The Amounts of Fluoride in Current Fluoride Therapies: Safety Considerations for Children, *ASDC J. Dent. Child.*, 51, 257, July-August, 1984.

B. Second Person.

Call emergency service; transport to hospital.

C. Administer Fluoride-binding Liquid When Patient Is Not Vomiting

1. Milk
2. Lime water ($CaOH_2$ solution 0.15%).

D. Support Respiration and Circulation (Chapter 60, pages 740–744)

E. Additional Therapy Indicated at Emergency Room

1. Calcium gluconate for muscle tremors or tetany.
2. Gastric lavage.
3. Cardiac monitoring.
4. Endotracheal intubation.
5. Blood monitoring (calcium, magnesium, potassium, pH).
6. Intravenous feeding to restore blood volume, calcium.

V. Chronic Toxicity

A. Skeletal Fluorosis[74]

Isolated instances of osteosclerosis resulting from chronic toxicity after long-term (20 or more years) use of water with 10 to 25 ppm fluoride or from industrial exposure.[74] Methods for defluoridation have been developed, as described on page 398.

B. Dental Fluorosis

Naturally occurring excess fluoride in the drinking water can produce visible fluorosis only when used during the years of development of the crowns of the teeth, namely, from birth until ages 8 or 9 or when the crowns of the second permanent molars are completed. No systemic effects result from the fluoride, and the individual will have maximum protection against dental caries. The classification of fluorosis is found on page 258.

C. Mild Fluorosis

1. *Clinical Evaluation.* In its mild and very mild forms, dental fluorosis appears as white opacities in the enamel surface. No esthetic or health problem is involved. Many such white spots are not visible except when scrutinized under a dental light and the surface is dried. Because all white spots in the enamel are not related to fluoride intake, distinction must be made by reviewing the patient's dental and fluoride-intake history, by noting the location and distribution of the white spots, and by considering the sequence of tooth development.

2. *Relation to Fluoride Sources.* Mild fluorosis or white spots may result from inadvertent ingestion of excess fluoride by young children from topical procedures both self-applied and professional. No problem exists when care is taken to follow basic rules, such as those listed in table 29–3 for professional applications and shown in figure 29–8 for daily use of dentifrice the size of a pea. Mouthrinses are not indicated for children under 6 years of age.

   Small amounts of dentifrice may be swallowed at each brushing. A child of 4 years who lives in a nonfluoridated community, uses a daily supplement (1 mg), and swallows 2 or 3 small amounts of dentifrice ingests far less than the SLD of 106 mg. shown in table 29–4B. References are provided in the *Suggested Readings* at the end of this chapter for further study of the effects of fluoride ingested from the various topical preparations.

VI. How to Calculate Amounts of Fluoride[75–77]

Figure 29–9 is a flow chart that shows the steps necessary to determine the amount of fluoride in a fluoride compound. By doing so, one then can calculate the amount ingested by the patient.

First, the percentage of fluoride ion in the compound is multiplied by the molecular weight conversion ratio, as shown in figure 29–9. The ratio was obtained by dividing the molecular weight of the compound by the atomic weight of fluoride. For example, the molecular weight of sodium fluoride is 42 (Na = 23, F = 19). When divided by 19, a 1/2.2 ratio results, as used in the example in figure 29–9.

TECHNICAL HINTS

I. Alternate Isolation Procedures for Topical Application

The procedure described on pages 404–405 is for isolation of one half of the dentition at one time. Objectives are to conserve time, but also to maintain as dry a field as possible and to prevent the fluoride solution from being absorbed by cotton rolls or the saliva from contaminating or diluting the solution. Other systems that may be applied include:

A. Rubber Dam

1. *Use.* For application of fluoride following restorative procedures or sealant placement.
2. *Preparation.* When the rubber dam has not been fitted to include the entire quadrant, additional holes may be made in the dam with an explorer.
3. *Advantages*
   a. Better control of the patient during the application, particularly a small child or handicapped patient with special problems.
   b. Saves time. Dry teeth can be maintained.
   c. Helpful when general anesthesia is used, particularly for a hospitalized patient.
   d. Stannous fluoride solution is confined and the patient does not experience the unpleasant taste.
4. *Disadvantage.* When root surface exposure needs fluoride, retraction of rubber dam may be difficult or impossible.

B. Single Quadrant

Each quadrant can be done separately by holding the cotton rolls with the fingers. In a very small mouth, a No. 1 continuous cotton roll may be held around the entire maxillary arch to make the entire application in one timing. This approach can be particularly useful for a small child.

II. Fluoride Application Following Polishing of Restorations

Because abrasive stones and polishing agents remove a layer of surface enamel and polishing procedures extend over the margins of the restoration, a topical application of fluoride can be particularly important (page 535). The removal of surface fluoride about the margin weakens the enamel, thereby rendering it more susceptible to dental caries if precautions are not taken.

III. Communities With Fluoridation

Maintain list of communities. Update annually by contacting state health department.

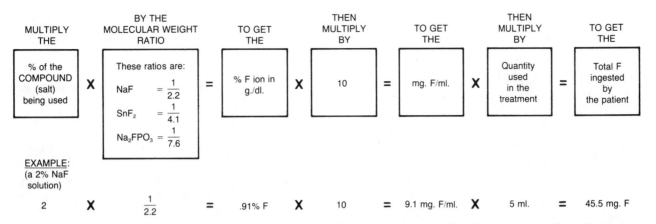

Figure 29–9. Fluoride Calculation. Flow chart shows steps in the calculation of the amount of fluoride in a compound used in treatment. The example shows that 5 ml. of a 2% solution of NaF contains 45.5 mg. F, an amount slightly greater than half of the safely tolerated dose (STD) for a 2-year-old child (Table 29–4B). (From Heifetz, S.B. and Horowitz, H.S.: The Amounts of Fluoride in Current Fluoride Therapies: Safety Considerations for Children, *ASDC J. Dent. Child., 51,* 257, July-August, 1984.)

FACTORS TO TEACH THE PATIENT

I. Personal Use of Fluorides

A. Purposes, action, and expected benefits relative to the specific forms of fluoride treatment the patient will receive.

B. Specific instruction concerning self-applied techniques that will be performed at home. Prepared printed instruction materials can be especially useful.

II. Need for Parental Supervision

A. Supervise daily care of child's teeth and mouth, including brushing of teeth using pea-sized quantity of dentifrice to prevent excess ingestion of fluoride.

B. Keep fluoride products out of reach of small children.

C. Brush teeth before using chewable dietary supplements. Avoid eating and drinking after use. Preferred time for use is just before going to bed.

III. Determining Need for Fluoride Supplements

A. Reference to list of communities with fluoride in the drinking water at optimum level.

B. Where to call to obtain information about fluoride in drinking water: health department, water department, or other community source.

C. Where to send private water source sample for fluoride analysis.

IV. Preparation for Topical Fluoride Application

When the teeth are free from plaque and the gingival tissue is firm and healthy, uptake of fluoride by the teeth is greater and the possibility of a slight tissue reaction is lessened. When the gingiva is inflamed, the patient will need instruction to understand why the topical application must be postponed until the tissue has healed.

V. Fluorides Are Part of the Total Preventive Program

Control of cariogenic foods in the diet, particularly between meals, and professional care are still necessary to supplement fluoride treatment for caries control.

VI. Fluoridation

In a nonfluoridated community, information concerning the significance of fluoridation to the entire community and its benefits and operation should be available and disseminated.

VII. Stannous Fluoride

When stannous fluoride preparations are used, the patient (or parent) should be informed about the possibility of tooth staining.

References

1. Mellberg, J.R., Ripa, L.W., and Leske, G.S.: *Fluoride in Preventive Dentistry. Theory and Clinical Applications.* Chicago, Quintessence Publishing Co., 1983, pp. 123–124.
2. Whitford, G.M.: Fluoride Metabolism, in Newbrun, E., ed.: *Fluorides and Dental Caries,* 3rd ed. Springfield, Illinois, Charles C Thomas, 1986, pp. 174–197.
3. Bhaskar, S.N., ed.: *Orban's Oral Histology and Embryology,* 10th ed. St. Louis, The C.V. Mosby Co., 1986, pp. 24–44, 71–100.
4. Melfi, R.C.: *Permar's Oral Embryology and Microscopic Anatomy,* 8th ed. Philadelphia, Lea & Febiger, 1988, pp. 41–84.
5. Brudevold, F., Gardner, D.E., and Smith, F.A.: The Distribution of Fluoride in Human Enamel, *J. Dent. Res., 35,* 420, June, 1956.
6. Brudevold, F., Steadman, L.T., and Smith, F.A.: Inorganic and Organic Components of Tooth Structure, *Ann. N.Y. Acad. Sci., 85,* 110, March 29, 1960.
7. Silverstone, L.M.: Caries and Remineralization, *Dent. Hyg., 57,* 30, May, 1983.
8. Silverstone, L.M.: Fluorides and Remineralization, in Wei, S.H.Y., ed.: *Clinical Uses of Fluorides.* Philadelphia, Lea & Febiger, 1985, pp. 153–175.
9. Jenkins, G.N. and Edgar, W.M.: Distribution and Forms of F in Saliva and Plaque, *Caries Res., 11,* 226, Supplement 1, 1977.

10. Dawes, C., Jenkins, G.N., Hardwick, J.L., and Leach, S.A.: The Relation Between the Fluoride Concentrations in the Dental Plaque and in Drinking Water, *Br. Dent. J., 119,* 164, August 17, 1965.

11. Loesche, W.J.: Topical Fluorides As An Antibacterial Agent, *J. Prev. Dent., 4,* 21, January-February, 1977.

12. Kilian, M., Larsen, M.J., Fejerskov, O., and Thylstrup, A.: Effects of Fluoride on the Initial Colonization of Teeth *in vivo, Caries Res., 13,* 319, Number 6, 1979.

13. Geddes, D.A.M. and McNee, S.G.: The Effect of 0.2 percent (48 mM) NaF Rinses Daily on Human Plaque Acidogenicity *in situ* (Stephan Curve) and Fluoride Content, *Arch. Oral Biol., 27,* 765, Number 9, 1982.

14. Richards, L.F., Westmoreland, W.W., Tashiro, M., McKay, C.H., and Morrison, J.T.: Determining Optimum Fluoride Levels for Community Water Supplies in Relation to Temperature, *J. Am. Dent. Assoc., 74,* 389, February, 1967.

15. Striffler, D.F., Young, W.O., and Burt, B.A.: *Dentistry, Dental Practice, and the Community,* 3rd ed. Philadelphia, W.B. Saunders Co., 1983, pp. 155–162.

16. Herschfeld, J.J.: Classics in Dental History. Frederick S. McKay and The "Colorado Brown Stain," *Bull. Hist. Dent., 26,* 118, October, 1978.

17. McKay, F.S.: The Relation of Mottled Enamel to Caries, *J. Am. Dent. Assoc., 15,* 1429, August, 1928.

18. Churchill, H.V.: Occurrence of Fluorides in Some Waters of United States, *J. Indust. Engin. Chem., 23,* 996, 1931.

19. Dean, H.T., Arnold, F.A., Jr., and Elvove, E.: Domestic Water and Dental Caries. V. Additional Studies of the Relation of Fluoride Domestic Waters to Dental Caries Experience in 4425 White Children, Aged 12 to 14 Years, of 13 Cities in 4 States, *Public Health Rep., 57,* 1155, August 7, 1942.

20. United States Department of Health and Human Services, Centers for Disease Control: *Fluoridation Census 1980.* Atlanta, Georgia, Centers for Disease Control, Dental Disease Prevention Activity, June, 1984, p. xi.

21. Arnold, F.A., Dean, H.T., Jay, P., and Knutson, J.W.: Effect of Fluoridated Public Water Supplies on Dental Caries Prevalence. Tenth Year of the Grand Rapids-Muskegon Study, *Public Health Rep., 71,* 652, July, 1956.

22. Hayes, R.L., Littleton, N.W., and White, C.L.: Posteruptive Effects of Fluoridation on First Permanent Molars of Children in Grand Rapids, Michigan, *Am. J. Public Health, 47,* 192, February, 1957.

23. Russell, A.L. and Hamilton, P.M.: Dental Caries in Permanent First Molars After Eight Years of Fluoridation, *Arch. Oral Biol., 6,* 50, July, 1961.

24. Backer Dirks, O., Houwink, B., and Kwant, G.W.: Some Special Features of the Caries Preventive Effect of Water Fluoridation, *Arch. Oral Biol., 4,* 187, August, 1961.

25. Burt, B.A., Ismail, A.I., and Eklund, S.A.: Root Caries in an Optimally Fluoridated and a High-fluoride Community, *J. Dent. Res., 65,* 1154, September, 1986.

26. Stamm, J.W. and Banting, D.W.: Comparison of Root Caries Prevalence in Adults With Life-long Residence in Fluoridated and Non-fluoridated Communities, *J. Dent. Res., 59,* 405, Abstract 552, Special Issue A, March, 1980.

27. Ast, D.B. and Fitzgerald, B.: Effectiveness of Water Fluoridation, *J. Am. Dent. Assoc., 65,* 581, November, 1962.

28. Mellberg, Ripa, and Leske: op. cit., pp. 133–134.

29. Kula, K. and Wei, S.H.Y.: Fluoride Supplements and Dietary Sources of Fluoride, in Wei, S.H.Y., ed.: *Clinical Uses of Fluorides.* Philadelphia, Lea & Febiger, 1985, pp. 65–71.

30. Salzmann, J.A.: The Effects of Fluoride on the Prevalence of Malocclusion, *J. Am. Coll. Dent., 35,* 82, January, 1968.

31. Russell, A.L. and Elvove, E.: Domestic Water and Dental Caries. VII. A Study of the Fluoride-Dental Caries Relationship in an Adult Population, *Public Health Rep., 66,* 1389, October 26, 1951.

32. Englander, H.R. and Wallace, D.A.: Effects of Naturally Fluoridated Water on Dental Caries in Adults, *Public Health Rep., 77,* 887, October, 1962.

33. Sognnaes, R.F.: Fluoride Protection of Bones and Teeth, *Science, 150,* 989, November 19, 1965.

34. Bernstein, D.S., Sadowsky, N., Hegsted, D.M., Guri, C.D., and Stare, F.J.: Prevalence of Osteoporosis in High- and Low-fluoride Areas in North Dakota, *J. Am. Med. Assoc., 198,* 499, October 31, 1966.

35. Fluoride, Bony Structure, and Aortic Calcification, *Nutrition Rev., 25,* 100, April, 1967.

36. Grøn, P., McCann, H.G., and Bernstein, D.: Effect of Fluoride on Human Osteoporotic Bone Mineral, *J. Bone Joint Surg., 48A,* 892, July, 1966.

37. Horowitz, H.S., Maier, F.J., and Law, F.E.: Partial Defluoridation of a Community Water Supply and Dental Fluorosis, *Public Health Rep., 82,* 965, November, 1967.

38. Horowitz, H.S. and Heifetz, S.B.: The Effect of Partial Defluoridation of a Water Supply on Dental Fluorosis—Final Results in Bartlett, Texas, After 17 Years, *Am. J. Public Health, 62,* 767, June, 1972.

39. Horowitz, H.S.: School Fluoridation for the Prevention of Dental Caries, *Int. Dent. J., 23,* 346, June, 1973.

40. Heifetz, S.B., Horowitz, H.S., and Brunelle, J.A.: Effect of School Water Fluoridation on Dental Caries: Results in Seagrove, N.C., After 12 Years, *J. Am. Dent. Assoc., 106,* 334, March, 1983.

41. Lemke, C.W., Doherty, J.M., and Arra, M.C.: Controlled Fluoridation: The Dental Effects of Discontinuation in Antigo, Wisconsin, *J. Am. Dent. Assoc., 80,* 782, April, 1970.

42. Ast, D.B., Cons, N.C., Pollard, S.T., and Garfinkel, J.: Time and Cost Factors to Provide Regular, Periodic Dental Care for Children in a Fluoridated and Nonfluoridated Area: Final Report, *J. Am. Dent. Assoc., 80,* 770, April, 1970.

43. Mellberg, Ripa, and Leske: op. cit., pp. 125–145.

44. American Dental Association, Council on Dental Therapeutics: *Accepted Dental Therapeutics,* 40th ed. Chicago, American Dental Association, 1984, pp. 399–402.

45. Aasenden, R., DePaola, P.F., and Brudevold, F.: Effects of Daily Rinsing and Ingestion of Fluoride Solutions upon Dental Caries and Enamel Fluoride, *Arch. Oral Biol., 17,* 1705, December, 1972.

46. Driscoll, W.S., Heifetz, S.B., and Brunelle, J.A.: Treatment and Posttreatment Effects of Chewable Fluoride Tablets on Dental Caries: Findings After 7½ Years, *J. Am. Dent. Assoc., 99,* 817, November, 1979.

47. Driscoll, W.S., Heifetz, S.B., and Brunelle, J.A.: Caries-preventive Effects of Fluoride Tablets in Schoolchildren Four Years After Discontinuation of Treatments, *J. Am. Dent. Assoc., 103,* 878, December, 1981.

48. Bibby, B.G.: Use of Fluorine in the Prevention of Dental Caries. II. The Effects of Sodium Fluoride Applications, *J. Am. Dent. Assoc., 31,* 317, March 1, 1944.

49. Knutson, J.W.: Sodium Fluoride Solutions: Technic for Application to the Teeth, *J. Am. Dent. Assoc., 36,* 37, January, 1948.

50. Galagan, D.J. and Knutson, J.W.: The Effect of Topically Applied Fluorides on Dental Caries Experience. VI. Experiments with Sodium Fluoride and Calcium Chloride . . . Widely Spaced Applications . . . Use of Different Solution Concentrations, *Public Health Rep., 63,* 1215, September 17, 1948.

51. Ripa, L.W.: Professionally (Operator) Applied Topical Fluoride Therapy: A Critique, *Int. Dent. J., 31,* 105, June, 1981.

52. Brudevold, F. and Naujoks, R.: Caries-preventive Fluoride Treatment of the Individual, *Caries Res., 12,* 52, Supplement 1, 1978.

53. American Dental Association, Council on Dental Materials, Instruments, and Equipment and Council on Dental Therapeutics: Status Report: Effect of Acidulated Phosphate Fluoride on Porcelain and Composite Restorations, *J. Am. Dent. Assoc., 116,* 115, January, 1988.

54. Ripa, L.W.: Need for Prior Toothcleaning When Performing a Professional Topical Fluoride Application: Review and Recommendations for Change, *J. Am. Dent. Assoc., 109,* 281, August, 1984.

55. Vrbic, V., Brudevold, F., and McCann, H.G.: Acquisition of

Fluoride by Enamel from Fluoride Pumice Pastes, *Helv. Odontol. Acta., 11,* 21, April, 1967.

56. American Academy of Pediatric Dentistry: Oral Health Policies for Children: Protocol for Fluoride Therapy, American Academy of Pediatric Dentistry, 211 E. Chicago Avenue, Chicago, 60611, May, 1985.

57. Stookey, G.K., Schemehorn, B.R., Drook, C.A., and Cheetham, B.L.: The Effect of Rinsing With Water Immediately After a Professional Fluoride Gel Application on Fluoride Uptake in Demineralized Enamel: An *in vivo* Study, *Pediatr. Dent., 8,* 153, June, 1986.

58. American Dental Association: A Guide to the Use of Fluorides for the Prevention of Dental Caries, 2nd ed., *J. Am. Dent. Assoc., 113,* 558, September, 1986.

59. Englander, H.R., Keyes, P.H., and Gestwicki, M.: Clinical Anticaries Effect of Repeated Topical Sodium Fluoride Applications by Mouthpieces, *J. Am. Dent. Assoc., 75,* 638, September, 1967.

60. Ripa, L.W.: Fluoride Rinsing: What Dentists Should Know, *J. Am. Dent. Assoc., 102,* 477, April, 1981.

61. Horowitz, H.S. and Heifetz, S.B.: Topically Applied Fluorides, in Newbrun, E., ed.: *Fluorides and Dental Caries,* 3rd ed. Springfield, Illinois, Charles C Thomas, 1986, pp. 95–99.

62. Torell, P. and Ericsson, Y.: The Potential Benefits Derived from Fluoride Mouth Rinses, in Forrester, D.J. and Schulz, E.M., eds.: *International Workshop on Fluorides and Dental Caries Reductions.* Baltimore, Maryland, 1974, pp. 114–176.

63. Birkeland, J.M. and Torell, P.: Caries-preventive Fluoride Mouthrinses, *Caries Res., 12,* 38, Supplement 1, 1978.

64. Driscoll, W.S., Swango, P.A., Horowitz, A.M., and Kingman, A.: Caries-preventive Effects of Daily and Weekly Fluoride Mouthrinsing in a Fluoridated Community: Final Results After 30 Months, *J. Am. Dent. Assoc., 105,* 1010, December, 1982.

65. Leske, G.S., Ripa, L.W., and Green, E.: Posttreatment Benefits in a School-based Fluoride Mouthrinsing Program. Final Results After 7 Years of Rinsing by All Participants, *Clin. Prevent. Dent., 8,* 19, September-October, 1986.

66. Ripa, L.W., Leske, G.S., and Varma, A.: Effect of Mouthrinsing With a 0.2 Per Cent Neutral NaF Solution on the Deciduous Dentition of First to Third Grade School Children, *Pediatr. Dent., 6,* 93, June, 1984.

67. American Dental Association, Council on Dental Therapeutics: Evaluation of Crest Toothpaste, *J. Am. Dent. Assoc., 61,* 272, August, 1960.

68. Stookey, G.K.: Are All Fluoride Dentifrices the Same? in Wei, S.H.Y., ed.: *Clinical Uses of Fluorides.* Philadelphia, Lea & Febiger, 1985, pp. 105–131.

69. American Dental Association, Council on Dental Therapeutics: Guidelines for the Acceptance of Fluoride-containing Dentifrices, *J. Am. Dent. Assoc., 110,* 545, April, 1985.

70. Tolle, S.L., Bauman, D.B., and Allen, D.S.: Effects of Fluoride Gels on Plaque and Gingival Health, *Dent. Hyg., 61,* 280, June, 1987.

71. Naleway, C.A.: Laboratory Methods of Assessing Fluoride Dentifrices and Other Topical Fluoride Agents, in Wei, S.H.Y., ed.: *Clinical Uses of Fluorides.* Philadelphia, Lea & Febiger, 1985, pp. 144–146.

72. Stratemann, M.W. and Shannon, I.L.: Control of Decalcification in Orthodontic Patients by Daily Self-administered Application of a Water-free 0.4 Per Cent Stannous Fluoride Gel, *Am. J. Orthod., 66,* 273, September, 1974.

73. Wescott, W.B., Starcke, E.N., and Shannon, I.L.: Chemical Protection Against Postirradiation Dental Caries, *Oral Surg. Oral Med. Oral Pathol., 40,* 709, December, 1975.

74. Hodge, H.C. and Smith, F.A.: Fluoride Toxicology, in Newbrun, E., ed.: *Fluorides and Dental Caries,* 3rd ed. Springfield, Illinois, Charles C Thomas, 1986, pp. 199–220.

75. Heifetz, S.B. and Horowitz, H.S.: The Amounts of Fluoride in Current Fluoride Therapies: Safety Considerations for Children, *ASDC J. Dent. Child., 51,* 257, July-August, 1984.

76. Bayless, J.M. and Tinanoff, N.: Diagnosis and Treatment of Acute Fluoride Toxicity, *J. Am. Dent. Assoc., 110,* 209, February, 1985.

77. Lyon, T.C.: Topical Fluorides: How Much Are You Using? *Dent. Hyg., 59,* 58, February, 1985.

Suggested Readings

Cawson, R.A. and Stocker, I.P.D.: The Early History of Fluorides as Anti-caries Agents, *Br. Dent J., 157,* 403, December 8, 1984.

Ericsson, Y. and Andersson, R.: Fluoride Ingestion With Fluoridated Domestic Salt Under Swedish Dietary Conditions, *Caries Res., 17,* 277, Number 3, 1983.

Frachella, J.C.: Fluoride and Bone Mineralization: An Important Issue in Dentistry, *ASDC J. Dent. Child., 51,* 417, November-December, 1984.

Hanes, C.M. and Hanes, P.J.: Effective Delivery Systems for Prolonged Fluoride Release: Review of Literature, *J. Am. Dent. Assoc., 113,* 431, September, 1986.

Haugejorden, O. and Helöe, L.A.: Fluorides for Everyone: A Review of School-based or Community Programs, *Community Dent. Oral Epidemiol., 9,* 159, August, 1981.

Heifetz, S.B.: Self-applied Fluorides for Use at Home, *Clin. Prevent. Dent., 4,* 6, March-April, 1982.

Holloway, P.J. and Levine, R.S.: The Value of Self-applied Fluorides at Home, *Int. Dent. J., 31,* 232, September, 1981.

Horowitz, H.S.: Alternative Methods of Delivering Fluorides: An Update, *Dent. Hyg., 57,* 37, May, 1983.

Hunstadbraten, K.: Fluoride in Caries Prophylaxis at the Turn of the Century, *Bull. Hist. Dent., 30,* 117, October, 1982.

König, K.G.: Fluorides in Preventive Dentistry, *Int. Dent. J., 30,* 364, December, 1980.

Love, W.D.: Fluoride Therapy in Clinical Practice, *Dent. Clin. North Am., 28,* 611, July, 1984.

National Health and Medical Research Council: Report of Working Party on Fluorides in the Control of Dental Caries, *Aust. Dent. J., 30,* 433, December, 1985.

Newbrun, E.: Systemic Fluorides. An Overview, *Can. Dent. Assoc. J., 46,* 31, January, 1980.

Shannon, I.L.: Fluoride Treatment Programs for High-caries-risk Patients, *Clin. Prevent. Dent., 4,* 11, March-April, 1982.

Whitford, G.M.: Fluorides: Metabolism, Mechanisms of Action and Safety, *Dent. Hyg., 57,* 16, May, 1983.

Fluoridation

Banoczy, J., Zimmerman, P., Pinter, A., Hadas, E., and Bruszt, V.: Effect of Fluoridated Milk on Caries: 3-year-Results, *Community Dent. Oral Epidemiol., 11,* 81, April, 1983.

Brossok, G.E., McTigue, D.J., and Kuthy, R.A.: The Use of a Colorimeter in Analyzing the Fluoride Content of Public Well Water, *Pediatr. Dent., 9,* 204, September, 1987.

Brustman, B.A.: Impact of Exposure to Fluoride-adequate Water on Root Surface Caries in Elderly, *Gerodontics, 2,* 203, December, 1986.

Burt, B.A., Eklund, S.A., and Loesche, W.J.: Dental Benefits of Limited Exposure to Fluoridated Water in Childhood, *J. Dent. Res., 65,* 1322, November, 1986.

Carmichael, C.L., Rugg-Gunn, A.J., French, A.D., and Cranage, J.D.: The Effect of Fluoridation Upon the Relationship Between Caries Experience and Social Class in 5-year-old Children in Newcastle and Northumberland, *Br. Dent. J., 149,* 163, September 16, 1980.

Carr, S.M., Dooland, M.B., and Roder, D.M.: Fluoridation II: An Interim Economic Analysis, *Aust. Dent. J., 25,* 343, December, 1980.

Doessel, D.P.: Cost-benefit Analysis of Water Fluoridation in Townsville, Australia, *Community Dent. Oral Epidemiol., 13,* 19, February, 1985.

Downer, M.C., Blinkhorn, A.S., and Attwood, D.: Effect of Fluoridation on the Cost of Dental Treatment Among Urban Scottish Schoolchildren, *Community Dent. Oral Epidemiol., 9,* 112, June, 1981.

Englander, H.R. and DePaola, P.F.: Enhanced Anticaries Action from Drinking Water Containing 5 ppm Fluoride, *J. Am. Dent. Assoc., 98,* 35, January, 1979.

Grembowski, D.: The Effect of Fluoridation on Dental Care Demand, *Compend. Cont. Educ. Dent., 5,* 689, September, 1984.

Hardwick, J.L., Teasdale, J., and Bloodworth, G.: Caries Increments Over 4 Years in Children Aged 12 at the Start of Water Fluoridation, *Br. Dent. J., 153,* 217, September 21, 1982.

Hefti, A. and Marthaler, T.M.: Bone Fluoride Concentrations After 16 Years of Drinking Water Fluoridation, *Caries Res., 15,* 85, Number 1, 1981.

Ishii, T. and Suckling, G.: The Appearance of Tooth Enamel in Children Ingesting Water With a High Fluoride Content for a Limited Period During Early Tooth Development, *J. Dent. Res., 65,* 974, July, 1986.

Johnsen, D.C., Bhat, M., Kim, M.T., Hagman, F.T., Allee, L.M., Creedon, R.L., and Easley, M.W.: Caries Levels and Patterns in Head Start Children in Fluoridated and Non-fluoridated, Urban and Non-urban Sites in Ohio, U.S.A., *Community Dent. Oral Epidemiol., 14,* 206, August, 1986.

Künzel, W.: Effect of an Interruption in Water Fluoridation on the Caries Prevalence of the Primary and Secondary Dentition, *Caries Res., 14,* 304, Number 5, 1980.

Kuthy, R.A., Naleway, C., and Durkee, J.: Factors Associated With Maintenance of Proper Water Fluoride Levels, *J. Am. Dent. Assoc., 110,* 511, April, 1985.

Löe, H.: The Fluoridation Status of U.S. Public Water Supplies, *Public Health Rep., 101,* 157, March-April, 1986.

Marthaler, T.M., Mejia, K., Toth, K., and Viñes, J.J.: Caries-preventive Salt Fluoridation, *Caries Res., 12,* 15, Supplement 1, 1978.

Roder, D.M. and Sundram, P.S.: Fluoridation. I. Effects on Children's Caries Rates and Professionally Defined Requirements for Dental Care, *Aust. Dent. J., 25,* 76, April, 1980.

Simonen, O. and Laitinen, O.: Does Fluoridation of Drinking-water Prevent Bone Fragility and Osteoporosis? *Lancet, 2,* (8452), 432, August 24, 1985.

Walvekar, S.V. and Qureshi, B.A.: Endemic Fluorosis and Partial Defluoridation of Water Supplies—A Public Health Concern in Kenya, *Community Dent. Oral Epidemiol., 10,* 156, June, 1982.

Dental Fluorosis

Driscoll, W.S., Horowitz, H.S., Meyers, R.J., Heifetz, S.B., Kingman, A., and Zimmerman, E.R.: Prevalence of Dental Caries and Dental Fluorosis in Areas With Negligible, Optimal, and Above-optimal Fluoride Concentrations in Drinking Water, *J. Am. Dent. Assoc., 113,* 29, July, 1986.

Granados, E.A.: A Synoptic Review of Fluorosis, *Dent. Hyg., 55,* 17, June, 1981.

Larsen, M.J., Richards, A., and Fejerskov, O.: Development of Dental Fluorosis According to Age at Start of Fluoride Administration, *Caries Res., 19,* 519, November-December, 1985.

Leverett, D.: Prevalence of Dental Fluorosis in Fluoridated and Nonfluoridated Communities—A Preliminary Investigation, *J. Public Health Dent., 46,* 184, Fall, 1986.

McInnes, P.M., Richardson, B.D., and Cleaton-Jones, P.E.: Comparison of Dental Fluorosis and Caries in Primary Teeth of Preschool-children Living in Arid High and Low Fluoride Villages, *Community Dent. Oral Epidemiol., 10,* 182, August, 1982.

Myers, H.M.: Dose-response Relationship Between Water Fluoride Levels and the Category of Questionable Dental Fluorosis, *Community Dent. Oral Epidemiol., 11,* 109, April, 1983.

Supplements

Allmark, C., Green, H.P., Linney, A.D., Wills, D.J., and Picton, D.C.A.: A Community Study of Fluoride Tablets for School Children in Portsmouth. Results After Six Years, *Br. Dent. J., 153,* 426, December 21, 1982.

American Academy of Pediatrics: Fluoride Supplementation. Committee on Nutrition, *Pediatrics, 77,* 758, May, 1986.

Bruun, C., Poulsen, S., Ostergaard, V., and Højbjerg, R.: Preeruptive Acquisition of Fluoride by Surface Enamel of Permanent Teeth After Daily Use of F Supplements, (Short Communication), *Caries Res., 17,* 89, Number 1, 1983.

deLiefde, B. and Herbison, G.P.: Prevalence of Developmental Defects of Enamel and Dental Caries in New Zealand Children Receiving Differing Fluoride Supplementation, *Community Dent. Oral Epidemiol., 13,* 164, June, 1985.

Dowell, T.B. and Joyston-Bechal, S.: Fluoride Supplements—Age Related Dosages, *Br. Dent. J., 150,* 273, May 19, 1981.

Driscoll, W.S.: What We Know and Don't Know About Dietary Fluoride Supplements—the Research Basis, *ASDC J. Dent. Child., 52,* 259, July-August, 1985.

Fanning, E.A., Cellier, K.M., and Somerville, C.M.: South Australian Kindergarten Children: Effects of Fluoride Tablets and Fluoridated Water on Dental Caries in Primary Teeth, *Aust. Dent. J., 25,* 259, October, 1980.

Horowitz, A.M.: Ways to Improve/Increase Appropriate Use of Dietary Fluorides, *ASDC J. Dent. Child., 52,* 269, July-August, 1985.

Hussein, N.N. and Hill, F.J.: An Assessment of Commercially Available Fluoride Supplements, *Br. Dent. J., 153,* 99, August 3, 1982.

Levy, S.M.: Expansion of the Proper Use of Systemic Fluoride Supplements, *J. Am. Dent. Assoc., 112,* 30, January, 1986.

Primosch, R.E., Weatherell, J.A., and Strong, M.: Distribution and Retention of Salivary Fluoride from a Sodium Fluoride Tablet Following Various Intra-oral Dissolution Methods, *J. Dent. Res., 65,* 1001, July, 1986.

Rigilano, J.C., Friedler, E.M., and Ehemann, L.J.: Fluoride Prescribing Patterns Among Primary Care Physicians, *J. Fam. Pract., 21,* 381, November, 1985.

Smyth, J.B.: Fluoride Tablets and Dental Health, *Aust. Dent. J., 29,* 296, October, 1984.

Widenheim, J., Birkhed, D., Granath, L., and Lindgren, G.: Preeruptive Effect of NaF Tablets on Caries in Children from 12 to 17 Years of Age, *Community Dent. Oral Epidemiol., 14,* 1, February, 1986.

Widenheim, J.: A Time-related Study of Intake Pattern of Fluoride Tablets Among Swedish Preschoolchildren and Parental Attitudes, *Community Dent. Oral Epidemiol., 10,* 296, December, 1982.

Tooth Surface Fluoride

Brewer, K.P., Retief, D.H., Wallace, M.C., and Bradley, E.L.: Cementum Fluoride Uptake from Topical Fluoride Agents, *Gerodontics, 3,* 212, October, 1987.

Grobler, S.R. and Louw, A.J.: Enamel-fluoride Levels in Deciduous and Permanent Teeth of Children in High, Medium and Low Fluoride Areas, *Arch. Oral. Biol., 31,* 423, Number 7, 1986.

Grøn, P.: Chemistry of Topical Fluorides, *Caries Res., 11,* 172, Supplement 1, 1977.

Iijima, Y. and Katayama, T.: Fluoride Concentration in Deciduous Enamel in High- and Low-fluoride Areas, (Short Communication), *Caries Res., 19,* 262, Number 3, 1985.

Keene, H.J., Mellberg, J.R., and Pederson, E.D.: Relationship Between Dental Caries Experience and Surface Enamel Fluoride Concentration in Young Men from Three Optimally Fluoridated Cities, *J. Dent. Res., 59,* 1941, November, 1980.

Margolis, H.C., Moreno, E.C., and Murphy, B.J.: Effect of Low Levels of Fluoride in Solution on Enamel Demineralization *in vitro, J. Dent. Res., 65,* 23, January, 1986.

Mellberg, J.R., Ripa, L.W., Leske, G.S., Sanchez, M., and Polanski, R.: The Relationship Between Dental Caries and Tooth Enamel Fluoride, *Caries Res., 19,* 385, September-October, 1985.

Nagagaki, H., Weatherell, J.A., Strong, M., and Robinson, C.: Distribution of Fluoride in Human Cementum, *Arch. Oral Biol., 30,* 101, Number 2, 1985.

Nasir, H.I., Retief, D.H., and Jamison, H.C.: Relationship Between Enamel Fluoride Concentration and Dental Caries in a Selected Population, *Community Dent. Oral Epidemiol., 13,* 65, April, 1985.

Pearce, E.I.F., Suckling, G.W., and Cutress, T.W.: Fluoride in the Outer Enamel of New Zealand Children. I. Its Relation to the Fluoride Concentration of the Water Supply and to the Use of Fluoride Tablets, *NZ Dent. J., 77,* 144, October, 1981.

Pearce, E.I.F., Suckling, G.W., and Cutress, T.W.: Fluoride in the Outer Enamel of New Zealand Children. II. Its Relation to Caries Experience, *NZ Dent. J., 78,* 8, January, 1982.

Weatherell, J.A., Deutsch, D., Robinson, C., and Hallsworth, A.S.: Assimilation of Fluoride by Enamel Throughout the Life of the Tooth, *Caries Res., 11,* 85, Supplement 1, 1977.

Root Caries

Burt, B.A., Ismail, A.I., and Eklund, S.A.: Root Caries in an Optimally Fluoridated and a High-fluoride Community, *J. Dent. Res., 65,* 1154, September, 1986.

Eklund, S.A., Burt, B.A., Ismail, A.I., and Calderone, J.J.: High-fluoride Drinking Water, Fluorosis and Dental Caries in Adults, *J. Am. Dent. Assoc., 114,* 324, March, 1987.

Mitchell, T.L. and Forgay, M.G.E.: Root Surface Caries: Implications for Dental Hygienists, *Can. Dent. Hyg. (Probe), 21,* 31, March, 1987.

Potter, D.E., Manwell, M.A., Dess, R., Levine, E., and Tinanoff, N.: SnF₂ As an Adjunct to Toothbrushing in an Elderly Institutionalized Population, *Spec. Care Dentist., 4,* 216, September-October 1984.

Tinanoff, N. and Zameck, R.: Alteration in Salivary and Plaque *S. mutans* in Adults Brushing With 0.4% SnF₂ Gel Once or Twice a Day, *Pediatr. Dent., 7,* 180, September, 1985.

Topical Applications

Brunn, C. and Stoltze, K.: *In vivo* Uptake of Fluoride by Surface Enamel of Cleaned and Plaque-covered Teeth, *Scand. J. Dent. Res., 84,* 268, Number 5, 1976.

Cobb, B.H., Rozier, R.G., and Bawden, J.W.: A Clinical Study of the Caries Preventive Effects of an APF Solution and APF Thixotropic Gel, *Pediatr. Dent., 2,* 263, December, 1980.

Houpt, M., Koenigsberg, S., and Shey, Z.: The Effect of Prior Toothcleaning on the Efficacy of Topical Fluoride Treatment. Two-year Results, *Clin. Prevent. Dent., 5,* 8, July-August, 1983.

Klimek, J., Prinz, H., Hellwig, E., and Ahrens, G.: Effect of a Preventive Program Based on Professional Toothcleaning and Fluoride Application on Caries and Gingivitis, *Community Dent. Oral Epidemiol., 13,* 295, December, 1985.

Markitziu, A., Gedalia, I., Stabholz, A., and Shuval, J.: Prevention of Caries Progress in Xerostomic Patients by Topical Fluoride Applications: A Study *in vivo* and *in vitro, J. Dent., 10,* 248, September, 1982.

McCall, D.R., Watkins, T.R., Stephen, K.W., and MacFarlane, G.J.: Distribution of APF Gel on Tooth Surfaces, *Br. Dent. J., 159,* 82, August 10, 1985.

Nagle, S.: Prophylaxis Prior to Topical Fluoride Application: A Questionable Procedure, *Can. Dent. Hyg., 15,* 19, Spring, 1981.

Steele, R.C., Waltner, A.W., and Bawden, J.W.: The Effect of Tooth Cleaning Procedures on Fluoride Uptake in Enamel, *Pediatr. Dent., 4,* 228, September, 1982.

Swango, P.A.: The Use of Topical Fluorides to Prevent Dental Caries in Adults: A Review of the Literature, *J. Am. Dent. Assoc., 107,* 447, September, 1983.

Mouthrinses

Ayers, C., Kolthoff, C., and Durr, D.: Fluoride Mouthrinses, *Dent. Hyg., 55,* 23, June, 1981.

Doherty, N.J., Brunelle, J.A., Miller, A.J., and Li, S.-H.: Costs of School-based Mouthrinsing in 14 Demonstration Programs in U.S.A., *Community Dent. Oral Epidemiol., 12,* 35, February, 1984.

Doherty, N.J.G. and Martie, C.W.: Analysis of the Costs of School-based Mouthrinsing Programs, *Community Dent. Oral Epidemiol., 15,* 67, April, 1987.

Leske, G.S., Ripa, L.W., Sposato, A., and Rebich, T.: Posttreatment Benefits from Participation in a School-based Fluoride Mouthrinsing Program: Results After Up to 7 Years of Rinsing, *Caries Res., 19,* 371, July-August, 1985.

Leverett, D.H. and Curzon, M.E.J.: Effect of Flossing and Brushing Immediately Prior to Weekly Fluoride Mouthrinsing, *Pediatr. Dent., 5,* 187, September, 1983.

Leverett, D.H., Sveen, O.B., and Jensen, Ø.E.: Weekly Rinsing With a Fluoride Mouthrinse in an Unfluoridated Community: Results After Seven Years, *J. Public Health Dent., 45,* 95, Spring, 1985.

Leverett, D.H., McHugh, W.D., and Jensen, Ø.E.: Effect of Daily Rinsing with Stannous Fluoride on Plaque and Gingivitis: Final Report, *J. Dent. Res., 63,* 1083, August, 1984.

Ripa, L.W., Leske, G.S., Sposato, A., and Rebich, T.: Supervised Weekly Rinsing With a 0.2 Percent Neutral NaF Solution: Final Results of a Demonstration Program After Six School Years, *J. Public Health Dent., 43,* 53, Winter, 1983.

Svanberg, M. and Rölla, G.: *Streptococcus mutans* in Plaque and Saliva After Mouthrinsing With SnF₂, *Scand. J. Dent. Res., 90,* 292, August, 1982.

van Wyk, I. and van Wyk, C.W.: The Effectiveness of a 0.2 Per Cent and 0.05 Per Cent Neutral NaF Mouthrinsing Programme, *J. Dent. Assoc. So. Africa, 41,* 35, February, 1986.

Weatherell, J.A., Strong, M., Robinson, C., and Ralph, J.P.: Fluoride Distribution in the Mouth After Fluoride Rinsing, *Caries Res., 20,* 111, March-April, 1986.

Wei, S.H. and Kanellis, M.J.: Fluoride Retention After Sodium Fluoride Mouthrinsing by Preschool Children, *J. Am. Dent. Assoc., 106,* 626, May, 1983.

Dentifrices

Barbakow, F., Cornec, S., Rozencweig, D., and Vadot, J.: Enamel Fluoride Content After Using Amine Fluoride- or Monofluorophosphate-Sodium Fluoride-Dentifrices, *ASDC J. Dent. Child., 50,* 186, May-June, 1983.

DePaola, P.F.: Clinical Studies of Monofluorophosphate Dentifrices, *Caries Res., 17,* 119, Supplement 1, 1983.

Ekstrand, J. and Ehrnebo, M.: Absorption of Fluoride from Fluoride Dentifrices, *Caries Res., 14,* 96, Number 2, 1980.

Forward, G.C.: Action and Interaction of Fluoride in Dentifrices, *Community Dent. Oral Epidemiol., 8,* 257, September-October, 1980.

Lu, K.H., Ruhlman, C.D., Chung, K.L., Sturzenberger, O.P., and Lehnhoff, R.W.: A Three-year Clinical Comparison of a Sodium Monofluorophosphate Dentifrice With Sodium Fluoride Dentifrices on Dental Caries in Children, *ASDC J. Dent. Child., 54,* 241, July-August, 1987.

Mobley, M.J.: Fluoride Uptake from *in situ* Brushing with a SnF₂ and a NaF Dentifrice, *J. Dent. Res., 60,* 1943, December, 1981.

Moran, J., Addy, M., and Newcombe, R.: The Antibacterial Effect of Toothpastes on the Salivary Flora, *J. Clin Periodontol., 15,* 193, March, 1988.

Reintsema, H., Schuthof, J., and Arends, J.: An *in vivo* Investigation of the Fluoride Uptake in Partially Demineralized Human Enamel from Several Different Dentifrices, *J. Dent. Res., 64,* 19, January, 1985.

Ripa, L.W., Leske, G.S., Forte, F., and Varma, A.: Caries Inhibition of Mixed NaF-NaPO₃F Dentifrices Containing 1,000 and 2,500 ppm: 3-year Results, *J. Am. Dent. Assoc., 116,* 69, January, 1988.

Schmid, R., Barbakow, F., Mühlemann, H., and DeVecchi, P.: Amine Fluoride and Monofluorophosphate: I. Historical Review of Fluoride Dentifrices, *ASDC J. Dent. Child., 51,* 99, March-April, 1984.

Stookey, G.K., Schemehorn, B.R., Cheetham, B.L., Wood, G.D., and Walton, G.V.: *In situ* Fluoride Uptake from Fluoride Dentifrices by Carious Enamel, *J. Dent. Res., 64,* 900, June, 1985.

Triol, C.W., Mandanas, B.Y., Juliano, G.F., Yraolo, B., Cano-Arevalo, M., and Volpe, A.R.: A Clinical Study in Children Comparing Anticaries Effect of Two Fluoride Dentifrices, A 31-Month Study, *Clin. Prevent. Dent., 9,* 22, March-April, 1987.

von der Fehr, F.R. and Møller, I.J.: Caries Preventive Fluoride Dentifrices, *Caries Res., 12,* 31, Supplement 1, 1978.

Fluoride Ingestion

Baxter, P.M.: Toothpaste Ingestion During Toothbrushing by School Children, *Br. Dent. J., 148,* 125, March 4, 1980.

Dowell, T.B.: The Use of Toothpaste in Infancy, *Br. Dent. J., 150,* 247, May 5, 1981.

Duxbury, A.J., Leach, F.N., and Duxbury, J.T.: Acute Fluoride Toxicity, *Br. Dent. J., 153,* 64, July 20, 1982.

Eisen, J.J. and LeCompte, E.J.: A Comparison of Oral Fluoride Retention Following Topical Treatments with APF Gels of Varying Viscosities, *Pediatr. Dent., 7,* 175, September, 1985.

Ekstrand, J. and Koch, G.: Systemic Fluoride Absorption Following Fluoride Gel Application, *J. Dent. Res., 59,* 1067, June, 1980.

Ekstrand, J., Koch, G., Lindgren, L.E., and Petersson, L.G.: Pharmacokinetics of Fluoride Gels in Children and Adults, *Caries Res., 15,* 213, Number 3, 1981.

Ekstrand, J., Koch, G., and Petersson, L.G.: Plasma Fluoride Concentrations in Pre-school Children After Ingestion of Fluoride Tablets and Toothpaste, *Caries Res., 17,* 379, Number 4, 1983.

Ekstrand, J., Spak, C.J., Falch, J., Afseth, J., and Ulvestad, H.: Distribution of Fluoride to Human Breast Milk Following Intake of High Doses of Fluoride, *Caries Res., 18,* 93, Number 1, 1984.

Fretwell, L.D.: Fluoride: Caution Against Abuse, *Gen. Dent., 29,* 431, September-October, 1981.

LeCompte, E.J. and Whitford, G.M.: Pharmacokinetics of Fluoride from APF Gel and Fluoride Tablets in Children, *J. Dent. Res., 61,* 469, March, 1982.

LeCompte, E.J. and Doyle, T.E.: Oral Fluoride Retention Following Various Topical Application Techniques in Children, *J. Dent. Res., 61,* 1397, December, 1982.

LeCompte, E.J. and Rubenstein, L.K.: Oral Fluoride Retention With Thixotropic and APF Gels and Foam-lined and Unlined Trays, *J. Dent. Res., 63,* 69, January, 1984.

LeCompte, E.J. and Doyle, T.E.: Effects of Suctioning Devices on Oral Fluoride Retention, *J. Am. Dent. Assoc., 110,* 357, March, 1985.

LeCompte, E.J.: Clinical Application of Topical Fluoride Products—Risks, Benefits, and Recommendations, *J. Dent. Res., 66,* 1066, May, 1987.

McCall, D.R., Watkins, T.R., Stephen, K.W., Collins, W.J.N., and Smalls, M.J.: Fluoride Ingestion Following APF Gel Application, *Br. Dent. J., 155,* 333, November 19, 1983.

McCall, D.R., Watkins, T.R., Stephen, K.W., and MacFarlane, G.J.: Distribution of APF Gel on Tooth Surfaces, *Br. Dent. J., 159,* 82, August 10, 1985.

Monsour, P.A., Kruger, B.J., Petrie, A.F., and McNee, J.L.: Acute Fluoride Poisoning After Ingestion of Sodium Fluoride Tablets, *Med. J. Aust., 141,* 503, October 13, 1984.

Newbrun, E.: Topical Fluoride Therapy: Discussion of Some Aspects of Toxicology, Safety, and Efficacy, *J. Dent. Res., 66,* 1084, May, 1987.

Ophaug, R.H., Singer, L., and Harland, B.F.: Estimated Fluoride Intake of Average Two-year-old Children in Four Dietary Regions of the United States, *J. Dent. Res., 59,* 777, May, 1980.

Ophaug, R.H. and Singer, L.: Fluoride Intake of Infants and Young Children and the Effect of Supplemental and Nondietary Sources of Fluoride, *Compend. Contin. Educ. Dent., 9,* 68, January, 1988.

Purdell-Lewis, D.J., van Dijk, H.A., Heeres, G.J., Flissebaalje, T.D., Groeneveld, A., and Booij, M.: Plasma Fluoride Levels in 9 Children With Acute Lymphatic Leukaemia Using Daily Self-applied Fluoride Gels, *Caries Res., 19,* 475, September-October, 1985.

Rubenstein, L.K. and Avent, M.A.: Frequency of Undesirable Side-effects Following Professionally Applied Topical Fluoride, *ASDC J. Dent. Child., 54,* 245, July-August, 1987.

Tinanoff, N. and Mueller, B.: Fluoride Content in Milk and Formula for Infants, *ASDC J. Dent. Child., 45,* 53, January-February, 1978.

Tyler, J.E. and Andlaw, R.J.: Oral Retention of Fluoride After Application of Acidulated Phosphate Fluoride Gel in Air-cushion Trays, *Br. Dent. J., 162,* 422, June 6, 1987.

Wei, S.H. and Kanellis, M.J.: Fluoride Retention After Sodium Fluoride Mouthrinsing by Preschool Children, *J. Am. Dent. Assoc., 106,* 626, May, 1983.

Bacterial Plaque and Periodontal Infection

Agus, H.M., Un, P.S.H., Cooper, M.H., and Schamschula, R.G.: Ionized and Bound Fluoride in Resting and Fermenting Dental Plaque and Individual Human Caries Experience, *Arch. Oral Biol., 25,* 517, Number 8–9, 1980.

Boyd, R.L., Leggott, P.J., and Robertson, P.B.: Effects on Gingivitis of Two Different 0.4% SnF_2 Gels, *J. Dent. Res., 67,* 503, February, 1988.

Camosci, D.A. and Tinanoff, N.: Anti-bacterial Determinants of Stannous Fluoride, *J. Dent. Res., 63,* 1121, September, 1984.

Harper, D.S. and Loesche, W.J.: Inhibition of Acid Production from Oral Bacteria by Fluorapatite-derived Fluoride, *J. Dent. Res., 65,* 30, January, 1986.

Loesche, W.J.: The Bacteriology of Dental Decay and Periodontal Disease, *Clin. Prevent. Dent., 2,* 18, May-June, 1980.

Newman, M.G., Perry, D.A., Carranza, F.A., and Mazza, J.E.: Fluorides in Periodontal Therapy, in Wei, S.H.Y., ed.: *Clinical Uses of Fluorides.* Philadelphia, Lea & Febiger, 1985. pp. 83–92.

Perry, D.A.: Fluorides and Periodontal Disease: A Review of the Literature, *J. Western Soc. Periodont. Periodont. Abstr., 30,* 92, Number 3, 1982.

Reddy, J., Parker, J.R., Africa, C.W., and Stephen, L.X.G.: Prevalence and Severity of Periodontitis in a High Fluoride Area in South Africa, *Community Dent. Oral Epidemiol., 13,* 108, April, 1985.

Rölla, G.: Effects of Fluoride on Initiation of Plaque Formation, *Caries Res., 11,* 243, Supplement 1, 1977.

Tinanoff, N., Hock, J., Camosci, D., and Helldén, L.: Effect of Stannous Fluoride Mouthrinse on Dental Plaque Formation, *J. Clin. Periodontol., 7,* 232, June, 1980.

Tinanoff, N., Klock, B., Camosci, D.A., and Manwell, M.A.: Microbiologic Effects of SnF_2 and NaF Mouthrinses in Subjects With High Caries Activity: Results After One Year, *J. Dent. Res., 62,* 907, August, 1983.

Yoon, N.A. and Berry, C.W.: The Antimicrobial Effect of Fluorides (Acidulated Phosphate, Sodium and Stannous) on *Actinomyces viscosus, J. Dent. Res., 58,* 1824, August, 1979.

Yoon, N.A. and Newman, M.G.: Antimicrobial Effect of Fluorides on *Bacteroides melaninogenicus subspecies* and *Bacteroides asaccharolyticus, J. Clin. Periodontol., 7,* 489, December, 1980.

Combined Fluoride Programs

Blinkhorn, A.S., Holloway, P.J., and Davies, T.G.H.: Combined Effects of a Fluoride Dentifrice and Mouthrinse on the Incidence of Dental Caries, *Community Dent. Oral Epidemiol., 11,* 7, February, 1983.

Haugejorden, O., Lervik, T., and Riordan, P.J.: Comparison of Caries Prevalence 7 Years After Discontinuation of School-based Fluoride Rinsing or Toothbrushing in Norway, *Community Dent. Oral Epidemiol., 13,* 2, February, 1985.

Heifetz, S.B., Horowitz, H.S., Meyers, R.J., and Li, S.-H.: Evaluation of the Comparative Effectiveness of Fluoride Mouthrinsing, Fluoride Tablets, and Both Procedures in Combination: Interim Findings After Two Years, *Pediatr. Dent., 9,* 121, June, 1987.

Horowitz, H.S., Meyers, R.J., Heifetz, S.B., Driscoll, W.S., and Li, S.-H.: Combined Fluoride, School-based Program in a Fluoride-deficient Area: Results of an 11-year Study, *J. Am. Dent. Assoc., 112,* 621, May, 1986.

Mallon, D.E. and Mellberg, J.R.: Inhibition of Caries Lesion Formation by an MFP Dentifrice and APF Solution, *Pediatr. Dent., 6,* 230, December, 1984.

Ripa, L.W., Leske, G.S., and Forte, F.: The Combined Use of Pit and Fissure Sealants and Fluoride Mouthrinsing in Second and Third Grade Children: Final Clinical Results After Two Years, *Pediatr. Dent., 9,* 118, June, 1987.

30 *Sealants*

As part of a complete preventive program, pit and fissure sealants are indicated for selected patients. Because topically or systemically applied fluorides protect smooth tooth surfaces more than occlusal surfaces, a method to reduce the incidence of occlusal dental caries is needed. Research studies have shown that the incidence of occlusal caries can be reduced significantly by the application of an adhesive sealant to the occlusal surfaces of caries-free molars and premolars.[1-4]

I. Definition and Action

A pit and fissure resin sealant is an organic polymer that bonds to the enamel surface mainly by mechanical retention. It acts as a physical barrier to prevent oral bacteria and their nutrients from collecting within a pit or fissure and creating the acid environment essential to the initiation of dental caries.

Before the sealant is applied, the enamel surface is treated with an acid etch process to increase the adhesion of the sealant. The acid etch creates micropores in the enamel. When the resin sealant is applied, it penetrates into the tiny pores and creates a bond or mechanical interlocking. Figure 30–1 is a diagram that shows irregularities created when an enamel surface is etched, and how the sealant resin penetrates into the tiny irregularities.

II. Types of Sealants

Currently, most sealants in clinical use are made of Bis-GMA (a reaction product of bis-phenol A and glycidyl methacrylate). The techniques of application vary slightly among available products.

The American Dental Association Council on Dental Materials, Instruments, and Equipment has a program for evaluation and acceptance of pit and fissure sealants.[5] Sealants are usually categorized by the method required for polymerization.

A. Chemical or Autopolymerization

The product is available in two bottles. When the two liquids are mixed, polymerization begins. Placement, or working time, is limited, and the setting time after placement is usually short.

B. Photopolymerization

Light-activated sealants harden when exposed to light. The lights that are used are hand held and may be ultraviolet or visible (an intense blue light source). The clinician has more working time, because polymerization does not start until the light is directed on to the sealant.

III. Selection of Teeth for Sealant Application

All caries-free pits and fissures are not necessarily indicated for sealant application. When evaluation is made and the teeth that will receive sealant are chosen selectively, several factors must be considered.

A. Location of Pits and Fissures

Sealants are indicated for permanent and primary teeth that have pits and fissures. These include occlusal pits and fissures, facial pits (such as the buccal pits of the mandibular molars), palatal pits (such as at the cusps of Carabelli), and cingulum pits (such as the palatal of maxillary anterior teeth).

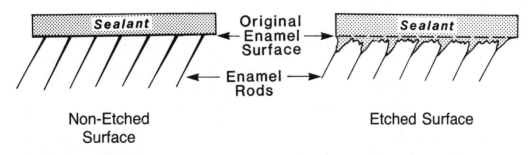

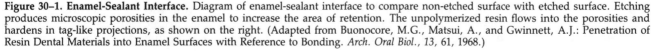

Figure 30–1. Enamel-Sealant Interface. Diagram of enamel-sealant interface to compare non-etched surface with etched surface. Etching produces microscopic porosities in the enamel to increase the area of retention. The unpolymerized resin flows into the porosities and hardens in tag-like projections, as shown on the right. (Adapted from Buonocore, M.G., Matsui, A., and Gwinnett, A.J.: Penetration of Resin Dental Materials into Enamel Surfaces with Reference to Bonding. *Arch. Oral Biol., 13*, 61, 1968.)

B. Contour of Pits and Fissures

Sealants are indicated especially for teeth with deep, narrow pits and fissures. Teeth with shallow and well coalesced pits and fissures are less likely to become carious because they are more accessible for plaque removal.

C. Relation to Eruption

Applications should be made as soon as possible following eruption. When application is delayed, caries may start, and the surface no longer can be considered for sealant. When possible, sealant can be applied before full eruption, provided there is no tissue flap over the occlusal to interfere with application procedures.

D. Relation to Dental Caries

1. Overall caries susceptibility is significant. When there are current carious lesions and previous restorations, newly erupted teeth should be treated with sealants promptly.
2. Sealant is not indicated when proximal carious lesions are present in the same tooth. When the proximal caries is restored, tooth preparation involves the occlusal surface, and the sealant would be removed.
3. Incipient pit and fissure caries is arrested by sealant placement.[6,7] Bacterial cultures under sealed lesions have been negative or insignificant because cariogenic bacteria cannot act on tooth structure without the presence of sucrose or other cariogenic substance (figure 28–1, page 383).

E. Age

The age of the patient may have particular significance. When teeth have been erupted several years and have not become carious, they are not necessarily less susceptible indefinitely. Habits may change. For example, application of a sealant to caries-free occlusal surfaces during early teenage years, when caries rates are high, may prove beneficial to the individual.

F. Prevention Program

Other preventive measures used for and by the patient are necessary. Sealant application should be part of a complete prevention program, not an isolated procedure. As an isolated procedure, patient (and parent) may misunderstand the selected area of prevention that this measure represents. Other surfaces and other teeth still need other methods of preventive protection.

IV. Detection of Pit and Fissure Caries

When selecting a tooth for which a sealant may be indicated, one can readily recognize a gross carious lesion when the tooth structure has clearly broken down and has become discolored. The more difficult lesions to discriminate are those that are small and do not have classic observable characteristics.

Criteria that have been defined for the determination of pit and fissure lesions of facial, occlusal, and lingual surfaces are as follows:[8]

A. An area is carious when the explorer "catches" or resists removal after the insertion into a pit or fissure with moderate to firm pressure and when the resistance is accompanied by one or more of the following signs of caries:
   1. A softness at the base of the area.
   2. Opacity adjacent to the pit or fissure as evidence of undermining or demineralization.
   3. Softened enamel adjacent to the pit or fissure that may be scraped away with an explorer.
B. Area is carious if the normal translucency of the enamel adjacent to a pit appears lost in contrast to the surrounding tooth structure. The condition is considered to be reliable evidence of undermining. In some of these teeth the explorer may not catch or penetrate the pit.

APPLICATION OF SEALANT[9,10,11]

Each quadrant should be treated separately. Isolation to prevent contamination and moisture can then be controlled. The precise technique is most effectively carried out when two dental team members work together.

The manufacturer's directions must be followed carefully for each specific product. Although the basic techniques are similar, characteristic steps are unique to each product.

General directions are described here in sequence, with brief explanations of the purposes of each step. The main steps are cleaning and drying the tooth surfaces, conditioning (enamel etching), applying the sealant, and polymerization. The success of treatment depends on precision in the techniques of application.

I. Clean the Tooth Surface

Although the rubber cup or bristle brush with plain pumice may have been used traditionally, research has shown successful sealant retention in pits and fissures when the surfaces had been prepared by the acid etch alone.[2,3]

A. Purposes

1. Remove deposits and debris.
2. Permit maximum contact of the sealant with enamel surface.

B. Inspect the Surfaces

Usual instrumentation for removal of calculus and heavy stain is carried out first.

C. Patient With No Stain or Calculus

1. Suction the pits and fissures with high-volume evacuator.
2. Use a sharp explorer (for example, No. 23 or other straight line at the tip) to dig out debris and bacteria from the pit or fissure.
3. Suction again to remove loosened material.
4. Additional cleaning is not necessary.

D. Cleansing Effect of Acid Etch Conditioner[12,13]

The acid etch conditioner removes a shallow layer of enamel approximately 10 μm deep. At the same time, plaque, surface pellicle, and subsurface pellicle are removed. Additional cleaning procedures are not necessary.

E. Cleansing Agent

When indicated because of heavy dental stains, fine pumice and water are used with a pointed polishing brush in a slow-speed handpiece.

1. Use only the pumice and water mix. Oil and fluoride must not be present. Commercial polishing pastes are contraindicated because frequently they contain glycerin, oils, flavoring agents, and fluorides that can interfere with bonding.
2. Apply the pumice mixture with a rotating pointed bristle brush. "Jab" the bristles into the pits and fissures to remove as much stain and debris as possible. Rinse and suction. Clean with an explorer tip.

II. Isolate the Tooth

A. Patient Position

The quadrant to be treated should be comfortably positioned for visibility and accessibility. The head is slightly tilted so saliva can flow to the opposite side of the mouth and not collect around the treatment area.

B. Purposes of Isolation

1. Keep the tooth clean and dry for optimal action and bonding of the sealant.
2. Eliminate possible contamination by saliva and moisture from the breath.
3. Keep the materials from contacting the oral tissues, being swallowed accidentally, or being unpleasant to the patient because of flavor.

C. Rubber Dam

1. Rubber dam application is the method of choice because the most complete isolation is obtained. This method is especially helpful when more than one tooth must be sealed.
2. Rubber dam is essential when profuse saliva flow and overactive tongue and oral muscles make retraction and consistent maintenance of a dry, clean field impossible.
3. Combined treatment should be planned. When a quadrant will have a rubber dam and anesthesia for restoration of other teeth, teeth indicated for sealant may be treated.
4. Rubber dam is not possible when
   a. Application of the clamp could not be tolerated by the patient without anesthesia.
   b. Tooth is not fully erupted and may not hold a rubber dam clamp.

D. Cotton-Roll Isolation

Details for cotton-roll isolation and maintenance of a dry field are described on page 404.

1. Request patient to expectorate and swallow.
2. Position cotton rolls (Garmer holder for mandibular, figure 29–4, page 404).
3. Place saliva ejector.
4. Apply triangular saliva absorber over the opening of the parotid gland in the cheek (bibulous pads: Dri-angle or Dri Aids).
5. Take great care to prevent the saliva from entering the etched area.

III. Dry the Tooth

A. Purposes

1. Prepare the tooth for the conditioner.
2. Prevent dilution and contamination of the conditioner.

B. Use Only Dry, Oil-free, Clean Air

Many syringes, particularly the multipurpose types, emit a combination of air and water spray. Some syringes may emit oil.

1. Clear the air by releasing the spray into a sink before directing it onto the tooth.
2. Test the air for water content by blowing on the back of the gloved hand or on a mirror surface.
3. Air dry for at least 10 seconds.

IV. Apply Conditioner for Enamel Etching

A. Purposes

To increase the adherence of the sealant, the conditioner (either gel or solution) is used to

1. Create surface irregularities to increase the area for retention (figure 30–1).
2. Increase the size of the microspaces between enamel rods so they are accessible to the adhesive.
3. Remove bacterial plaque and pellicle.

B. Conditioner

1. Apply the phosphoric acid (37 to 50%) with a brush, cotton pellet, or plastic sponge over the occlusal surface and the buccal and/or lingual when sealant is indicated.
2. Note the time or start timer. Total application time is as follows:
   a. 1 minute: permanent teeth.
   b. 1½ minutes: primary teeth.
   c. 1¾ minutes: fluorosed teeth (greater acid resistance).
3. Place gel over the surface and leave undisturbed.
4. For a solution use a continuous dabbing, not a rubbing, motion. Gentle dabbing does not damage the fragile enamel latticework formed during the etching process.

V. Rinse Thoroughly

A. Purposes

1. Remove all excess acid and complexes formed from the action of the minerals of the tooth and the acid.

2. Prevent saliva from reaching the etched surface. Saliva reduces the bonding strength of the sealant by depositing the salivary constituents on the surface.

B. Procedure

1. Do not permit the patient to rinse or expectorate. Contaminants must be kept from the etched area.
2. Clear the water in the tubing of the air/water syringe by releasing the water into a sink.
3. Hold wide aspirator tip between tooth and cotton. The tip should be maintained firmly against the tooth to collect the water as it flows across the occlusal surface.[11]
4. Rinse thoroughly (10 to 15 seconds for solution; 30 seconds for a gel).[10] Direct the water stream across the etched surfaces so that each portion of the surface is washed.
5. Evacuate excess water from the entire area immediately after rinsing.
6. Maintain dry area. When a rubber dam is not used, the cotton rolls are difficult to change. Two preferred procedures are suggested.
   a. Place one dry cotton roll over each wet cotton roll. Suction must be applied constantly. For some patients, with great care, the wet cotton roll can be slid out from under and then can be removed in the direction of the opposite side of the mouth.
   b. Leave the wet cotton rolls in place, and suction excess moisture from the cotton rolls.[14]
7. Should accidental contamination with saliva occur, wash, dry, and etch again for 10 seconds. Wash and dry to prepare for next step.

C. Examine the Surface

The etched surface should be a dull, chalky white. When it is not, repeat the application of the conditioner step-by-step. Primary teeth or older permanent teeth may require a repeat application.

VI. Dry the Tooth Thoroughly Again

A. Purposes

1. Prepare the tooth for the sealant application.
2. Prevent moisture from reducing the affinity of the adhesive for the enamel surface and preventing penetration of the adhesive into the microspaces created by etching.

B. Procedure

1. Dry the tooth thoroughly for 15 to 30 seconds per tooth. Use only clean, dry, oil-free air (see III above).
2. Do not blow saliva onto the etched surface.
3. Drying is continued while the assistant prepares the sealant resin.

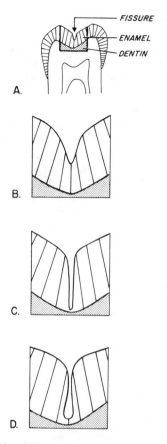

Figure 30–2. Occlusal Fissures. Drawings made from microscopic slides show variations in shape and depth of fissures. **A.** Tooth with section enlarged for B, C, and D. **B.** Wide V-shaped fissure. **C.** Long narrow groove that reaches nearly to the dentinoenamel junction. **D.** Long constricted form with a bulbous terminal portion.

VII. Apply the Sealant

A. Follow Manufacturer's Instructions

Each type of sealant has specific timing, applicator, and details for manipulation. Autopolymerized sealants are measured by drops and mixed; photopolymerized sealants are not mixed, but are initiated to polymerization when the light is placed on them.

B. Placement

1. Do the most-posterior tooth first (when more than one sealant is to be applied in a quadrant).
2. Do only two teeth per mix (when more than two sealants are to be applied in one quadrant).

C. Application

1. Use disposable applicator (brush, sponge, or other) provided.
2. Flow the sealant first into the pit or fissure that has the maximum depth. Extend and thicken. Avoid marginal ridges, cusp tips.
3. Time by the instructions. After polymerization begins, the material should not be disturbed.

D. Photopolymerization

1. Connect special light in ample time before beginning the sealant preparation.
2. Wear protective glasses to protect eyes from the light.
3. Apply sealant with special applicator.
4. Hold light tip 2 mm. from sealant surface to prevent any contact during the first few seconds.
5. Make sure all parts of the sealant are equally exposed to the light. The most posterior portion may be the most difficult to reach.

E. Observe Sealant

Before discontinuing the dry field, the sealant is examined. Voids may be filled, and portions may be added without re-etching. A fresh mix is needed.

F. Test for Retention

Run an explorer around the margin and try to pry the sealant away from the enamel. Sealants obtain optimum strength soon after polymerization, so they can be tested. Replacement can be made immediately using a 10-second re-etch.

PENETRATION OF SEALANT

The penetration of a sealant depends on the configuration of the pit or fissure, the presence of deposits and debris within the pit or fissure, and the properties of the sealant itself.[15]

I. Pit and Fissure Anatomy

A review of the anatomy of pits and fissures may be helpful in understanding the effects of sealants in the prevention of dental caries. The shape and depth of pits and fissures vary considerably even within one tooth.

There are *long narrow pits* and grooves that reach to, or nearly to, the dentinoenamel junction. Others are *wide V-shaped* or *narrow V-shaped,* whereas still others may have a *long constricted form with a bulbous terminal portion* (figure 30–2). The pit or fissure may take a wavy course; thus, it may not lead directly from the outer surface to the dentinoenamel junction.

II. Contents of a Pit or Fissure

A pit or fissure contains bacterial plaque, pellicle, debris, and sometimes relatively intact remnants of tooth development.

III. Effect of Cleaning

The narrow, long fissures are impossible to clean completely, and the conditioner cannot reach the deeper portions. Retained cleaning material can block the sealant from filling the fissure and can also become mixed with the sealant. Removal of pumice used for cleaning and thorough washing is necessary to the success of the sealant.

IV. Amount of Penetration

Wide V and shallow fissures are more apt to be filled by sealant (figure 30–3B). Although ideally the

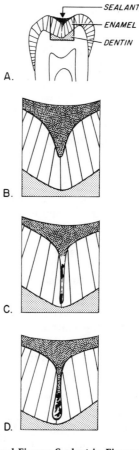

Figure 30–3. Pit and Fissure Sealant in Fissures. Drawings made from microscopic slides show extent to which sealant fills a fissure. **A.** Tooth with section enlarged for B, C, and D. **B.** Sealant fills wide V-shaped fissure and extends part way up the slopes of surrounding cusps. **C.** and **D.** Fissures partially filled as a result of narrow constriction of the groove and blockage by trapped debris.

sealant should penetrate to the bottom of a pit or fissure, such penetration is frequently impossible because of the debris. Microscopic examination of pits and fissures after sealant application has shown that the sealant does not penetrate to the bottom because residual debris, cleansing agents, and trapped air prevent passage of the material (figure 30–3C and D).

RETENTION AND REPLACEMENT

Length of time of retention depends almost entirely on the precision of technique. Although surface sealant may be lost, sealant in the pits and fissures and sealant that penetrated into the microspaces of the enamel still remain and provide protection.[16]

I. Factors That Influence Retention Time

A. Precision of Technique

Each step in the preparation of the tooth and the application of the sealant must be carefully performed. Improper technique is probably the major cause of early loss of sealant from the tooth surface.

B. Effect of Contamination

Any contact of the etched enamel surface, either by saliva, water, or any other contaminant, before application of the sealant markedly decreases the effectiveness of the sealant.

II. Reexamination

At each maintenance appointment, or at least every 6 months, the sealant should be examined for deficiencies that may have developed.

III. Replacement

Consult the manufacturer's instructions. Tooth preparation is the same as for an original application. Re-etching of the tooth surface is always essential.

FLUORIDE AND SEALANT

I. Topical Application in Conjunction with Sealant

When used, fluoride must be applied before the conditioner or after the sealant. It should not be applied between these two steps because the bond strength may be reduced between the sealant and the etched enamel surface.

II. Combined Preventive Program

Sealants are part of a total preventive program. Although sealant is applicable for occlusal surfaces, fluoride applications and other fluoride sources for self-administration are necessary for all other surfaces.

TECHNICAL HINTS

I. Eye Protection

The patient must wear safety protective glasses during the etching process. Phosphoric acid could cause loss of sight if a drop inadvertently falls into an eye.[17]

II. Occlusion

The occlusion should be checked for interferences after thick sealants have been placed. An occlusal wax or an articulating paper can be used to identify high spots, and a fine stone or finishing-type bur can be used to reshape.[9]

FACTORS TO TEACH THE PATIENT

I. Sealants are part of a total preventive program. Sealants are not substitutes for other preventive measures, including limitations of dietary sucrose, fluorides, and plaque control.

II. What a sealant is and why such a meticulous application procedure is required.

III. What can be expected from a sealant: how long it will last, how it prevents dental caries.

IV. Need for examination of the sealant at frequent, scheduled appointments and replacement when indicated.

References

1. Ripa, L.W.: The Current Status of Pit and Fissure Sealants. A Review, *Can. Dent. Assoc. J., 51,* 367, May, 1985.
2. Mertz-Fairhurst, E.J., Fairhurst, C.W., Williams, J.E., Della-Giustina, V.E., and Brooks, J.D.: A Comparative Clinical Study of Two Pit and Fissure Sealants: 7-year Results in Augusta, GA, *J. Am. Dent. Assoc., 109,* 252, August, 1984.
3. Houpt, M. and Shey, Z.: The Effectiveness of a Fissure Sealant After Six Years, *Pediatr. Dent., 5,* 104, June, 1983.
4. Vrbic, V.: Five-year Experience with Fissure Sealing, *Quintessence Int., 17,* 371, June, 1986.
5. American Dental Association, Council on Dental Health and Health Planning and Council on Dental Materials, Instruments, and Equipment: Pit and Fissure Sealants, *J. Am. Dent. Assoc., 114,* 671, May, 1987.
6. Going, R.E.: Sealant Effect on Incipient Caries, Enamel Maturation, and Future Caries Susceptibility, *J. Dent. Educ., 48,* 35, Supplement, February, 1984.
7. Mertz-Fairhurst, E.J., Schuster, G.S., and Fairhurst, C.W.: Arresting Caries by Sealants: Results of a Clinical Study, *J. Am. Dent. Assoc., 112,* 194, February, 1986.
8. Radike, A.W.: Criteria for Diagnosis of Dental Caries, in American Dental Association, Council on Dental Research and Council on Dental Therapeutics: *Clinical Testing of Cariostatic Agents.* Chicago, American Dental Association, 1968, pp. 87–88.
9. Harris, N.O. and Scheirton, L.S.: *Pit and Fissure Sealants.* Chicago, American Dental Hygienists' Association, 1985.
10. Massachusetts Department of Public Health and Massachusetts Health Research Institute: *Preventing Pit and Fissure Caries: A Guide to Sealant Use.* Boston, Massachusetts, Department of Public Health, 1986.
11. Harris, N.O. and Simonsen, R.J.: Pit and Fissure Sealants, in Harris, N.O. and Christen, A.G.: *Primary Preventive Dentistry,* 2nd ed. Norwalk, Connecticut, Appleton & Lange, 1987, pp. 235–256.
12. Main, C., Thomson, J.L., Cummings, A., Field, D., Stephen, K.W., and Gillespie, F.C.: Surface Treatment Studies Aimed at Streamlining Fissure Sealant Application, *J. Oral Rehabil., 10,* 307, July, 1983.
13. Silverstone, L.M.: Fissure Sealants: Laboratory Studies, *Caries Res., 8,* 2, Number 1, 1974.
14. Little, N.: Pit and Fissure Sealants: Pitfalls and Progress, *Horizons, 7,* 8, December, 1986.
15. Taylor, C.L. and Gwinnett, A.J.: A Study of the Penetration of Sealants into Pits and Fissures, *J. Am. Dent. Assoc., 87,* 1181, November, 1973.
16. Buonocore, M.G.: Pit and Fissure Sealing, *Dent. Clin. North Am., 19,* 367, April, 1975.
17. Colvin, J.: Eye Injuries and the Dentist, *Aust. Dent. J., 23,* 453, December, 1978.

Suggested Readings

American Society of Dentistry for Children and American Academy of Pedodontics: Rationale and Guidelines for Pit and Fissure Sealants, *Pediatr. Dent., 5,* 89, March, 1983.

British Dental Association: Fissure Sealants. Report of the Joint BDA/DHSS Working Party, *Br. Dent. J., 161,* 343, November 8, 1986.

Brooks, J.D., Azhdari, S., and Ashrafi, M.H.: A Comparative Study of Three Tinted, Unfilled Pit and Fissure Sealants. Eleven-month Results in Milwaukee, Wisconsin, *Clin. Prevent. Dent., 7,* 4, January-February, 1985.

Disney, J.A. and Bohannan, H.M.: The Role of Occlusal Sealants in Preventive Dentistry, *Dent. Clin. North Am., 28,* 21, January, 1984.

Hardison, J.R., Collier, D.R., Sprouse, L.W., Van Cleave, M.L., and

Hogan, A.D.: Retention of Pit and Fissure Sealant on the Primary Molars of 3- and 4-year-old Children After 1 Year, *J. Am. Dent. Assoc., 114,* 613, May, 1987.

Hardison, J.R.: The Clinical Effectiveness of a Transparent Visible Light-polymerized Sealant: 24-month Results, *Compend. Contin. Educ. Dent., 6,* 229, March, 1985.

Houpt, M., Shapira, J., Fuks, A., Eidelman, E., and Chosack, A.: A Clinical Comparison of Visible Light-initiated and Autopolymerized Fissure Sealant: One-year Results, *Pediatr. Dent., 8,* 22, March, 1986.

Isler, S.L. and Doline, S.: Clinical Application of Pit and Fissure Sealants, *Compend. Contin. Educ. Dent., 2,* 207, July/August, 1981.

Isler, S.L. and Doline, S.L.: Practical Application of Pit and Fissure Sealants. A Seven-year Retrospective Study, *Clin. Prevent. Dent., 3,* 18, September-October, 1981.

JADA Advances in Dental Research: Fluoride-releasing Sealants, *J. Am. Dent. Assoc., 110,* 90, January, 1985.

Jakush, J., ed.: Pit and Fissure Sealant Use: An Issue Explored, *J. Am. Dent. Assoc., 108,* 310, March, 1984.

Li, S.H., Swango, P.A., Gladsden, A.N., and Heifetz, S.B.: Evaluation of the Retention of Two Types of Pit and Fissure Sealants, *Community Dent. Oral Epidemiol., 9,* 151, August, 1981.

National Institutes of Health: Consensus Development Conference Statement on Dental Sealants in the Prevention of Tooth Decay, *J. Am. Dent. Assoc., 108,* 233, February, 1984.

Newbrun, E.: *Cariology,* 2nd ed. Baltimore, Williams & Wilkins, 1983, pp. 291–307.

Rawls, H.R. and Zimmerman, B.F.: Fluoride-exchanging Resins for Caries Protection, *Caries Res., 17,* 32, Number 1, 1983.

Richardson, A.S., Gibson, G.B., and Waldman, R.: Chemically Polymerized Sealant in Preventing Occlusal Caries, *Can. Dent. Assoc. J., 46,* 259, April, 1980.

Silverstone, L.M.: The Current Status of Adhesive Sealants, *Dent. Hyg., 57,* 44, May, 1983.

Silverstone, L.M.: Fissure Sealants: The Enamel-Resin Interface, *J. Public Health Dent., 43,* 205, Summer, 1983.

Simonsen, R.J.: Potential Uses of Pit-and-Fissure Sealants in Innovative Ways: A Review, *J. Public Health Dent., 42,* 305, Fall, 1982.

Simonsen, R.J.: Retention and Effectiveness of a Single Application of White Sealant After 10 Years, *J. Am. Dent. Assoc., 115,* 31, July, 1987.

Straffon, L.H., Dennison, J.B., and More, F.G.: Three-year Evaluation of Sealant: Effect of Isolation on Efficacy, *J. Am. Dent. Assoc., 110,* 714, May, 1985.

Sveen, O.B. and Jensen, O.E.: Two-year Clinical Evaluation of Delton and Prisma-Shield, *Clin. Prevent. Dent., 8,* 9, September-October, 1986.

Tillis, T.S.I.: Application of Pit and Fissure Sealants. Long-term Effects of a One-day Continuing Education Course, *Dent. Hyg., 60,* 300, July, 1986.

Turpin-Mair, J.S., Rawls, H.R., and Christensen, L.V.: An *in vitro* Study of Caries Prevention, Cavity Adaptation, Homogeneity and Microleakage of a New Fluoride-releasing Resin, *J. Oral Rehabil., 9,* 523, November, 1982.

Techniques

Barkmeier, W.W., Gwinett, A.J., and Shaffer, S.E.: Effects of Enamel Etching Time on Bond Strength and Morphology, *J. Clin. Orthod., 19,* 36, January, 1985.

Chosack, A., Shapira, J., Tzukert, A., and Eidelman, E.: The Parameters Influencing Time of Application of Fissure Sealants. Etching Time, Type of Polymerization, and Experience, *Clin. Prevent. Dent., 9,* 17, March-April, 1987.

Daniel, S.J., Grose, M.D., Scruggs, R.R., and Stoltz, R.F.: Examiner Reliability in Evaluating Dental Sealants, *Dent. Hyg., 61,* 410, September, 1987.

Eidelman, E., Fuks, A.B., and Chosack, A.: The Retention of Fissure Sealants: Rubber Dam or Cotton Rolls in a Private Practice, *ASDC J. Dent. Child., 50,* 259, July-August, 1983.

Eidelman, E., Shapira, J., and Houpt, M.: The Retention of Fissure Sealants Using Twenty-second Etching Time, *ASDC J. Dent. Child., 51,* 422, November-December, 1984.

Fuks, A.B., Grajower, R., and Shapira, J.: *In vitro* Assessment of Marginal Leakage of Sealants Placed in Permanent Molars with Different Etching Times, *ASDC J. Dent. Child., 51,* 425, November-December, 1984.

Garcia-Godoy, F.: Retention of a Light-cured Fissure Sealant (Helioseal®) in a Tropical Environment After 12 Months, *Clin. Prevent. Dent., 8,* 11, May-June, 1986.

Garcia-Godoy, F. and Gwinnett, A.J.: Penetration of Acid Solution and Gel in Occlusal Fissures, *J. Am. Dent. Assoc., 114,* 809, June, 1987.

Hormati, A.A., Fuller, J.L., and Denehy, G.E.: Effects of Contamination and Mechanical Disturbance on the Quality of Acid-etched Enamel, *J. Am. Dent. Assoc., 100,* 34, January, 1980.

Redford, D.A., Clarkson, B.H., and Jensen, M.: The Effect of Different Etching Times on the Sealant Bond Strength, Etch Depth, and Pattern in Primary Teeth, *Pediatr. Dent., 8,* 11, March, 1986.

Scott, L. and Greer, D.: The Effect of an Air Polishing Device on Sealant Bond Strength, *J. Prosthet. Dent., 58,* 384, September, 1987.

Silverstone, L.M., Hicks, M.J., and Featherstone, M.J.: Oral Fluid Contamination of Etched Enamel Surfaces: An SEM Study, *J. Am. Dent. Assoc., 110,* 329, March, 1985.

Speiser, A.M. and Segat, T.E.: The Influence of Technique Modifications on Sealant Leakage, *ASDC J. Dent. Child., 47,* 93, March-April, 1980.

Activating Lights

American Dental Association, Council on Dental Materials, Instruments, and Equipment: Visible Light-cured Composites and Activating Units, *J. Am. Dent. Assoc., 110,* 100, January, 1985.

American Dental Association, Council on Dental Materials, Instruments, and Equipment: The Effects of Blue Light on the Retina and the Use of Protective Filtering Glasses, *J. Am. Dent. Assoc., 112,* 533, April, 1986.

Berry, E.A., Pitts, D.G., Francisco, P.R., and von der Lehr, W.N.: An Evaluation of Lenses Designed to Block Light Emitted by Light-curing Units, *J. Am. Dent. Assoc., 112,* 70, January, 1986.

Blankenau, R.J., Kelsey, W.P., Cavel, W.T., and Blankenau, P.: Wavelength and Intensity of Seven Systems for Visible Light-curing Composite Resins: A Comparison Study, *J. Am. Dent. Assoc., 106,* 471, April, 1983.

Ellingson, O.L., Landry, R.J., and Bostrom, R.G.: An Evaluation of Optical Radiation Emissions From Dental Visible Photopolymerization Devices, *J. Am. Dent. Assoc., 112,* 67, January, 1986.

Fan, P.L., Wozniak, W.T., McGill, S., Moser, J.B., and Stanford, J.W.: Evaluation of Light Transmission Characteristics of Protective Eyeglasses for Visible Light-curing Units, *J. Am. Dent. Assoc., 113,* 770, November, 1986.

Houpt, M., Fuks, A., Shapira, J., Chosack, A., and Eidelman, E.: Autopolymerized Versus Light-polymerized Fissure Sealant, *J. Am. Dent. Assoc., 115,* 55, July, 1987.

Makinson, O.F.: Curing Lights and Eye Protection, *Aust. Dent. J., 31,* 137, April, 1986.

Moseley, H., Strang, R., and Stephen, K.W.: An Assessment of Visible-light Polymerizing Sources, *J. Oral Rehabil., 13,* 215, May, 1986.

Pollack, B.F. and Lewis, A.L.: Visible Light Resin-curing Generators: A Comparison, *Gen. Dent., 29,* 488, December, 1981.

Swartz, M.L., Phillips, R.W., and Rhodes, B.: Visible Light-activated Resins—Depth of Cure, *J. Am. Dent. Assoc., 106,* 634, May, 1983.

Sealants Over Dental Caries

Elderton, R.J.: Management of Early Dental Caries in Fissures with Fissure Sealant, *Br. Dent. J., 158,* 254, April 6, 1985.

Handelman, S.L., Leverett, D.H., Espeland, M., and Curzon, J.: Retention of Sealants Over Carious and Sound Tooth Surfaces, *Community Dent. Oral Epidemiol., 15,* 1, February, 1987.

Handelman, S.L., Leverett, D.H., Espeland, M.A., and Curzon, J.A.: Clinical Radiographic Evaluation of Sealed Carious and Sound Tooth Surfaces, *J. Am. Dent. Assoc., 113,* 751, November, 1986.

Handelman, S.L., Leverett, D.H., Solomon, E.S., and Brenner, C.M.: Use of Adhesive Sealants Over Occlusal Carious Lesions: Radiographic Evaluation, *Community Dent. Oral Epidemiol., 9,* 256, December, 1981.

Jensen, Ø.E. and Handelman, S.L.: Effect of an Autopolymerizing Sealant on Viability of Microflora in Occlusal Dental Caries, *Scand. J. Dent. Res., 88,* 382, October, 1980.

Leverett, D.H., Handelman, S.L., Brenner, C.M., and Iker, H.P.: Use of Sealants in the Prevention and Early Treatment of Carious Lesions: Cost Analysis, *J. Am. Dent. Assoc., 106,* 39, January, 1983.

Meiers, J.C. and Jensen, M.E.: Management of the Questionable Carious Fissure: Invasive vs. Noninvasive Techniques, *J. Am. Dent. Assoc., 108,* 64, January, 1984.

Swift, E.J.: The Effect of Sealants on Dental Caries: A Review, *J. Am. Dent. Assoc., 116,* 700, May, 1988.

Programs and Cost-effectiveness

American Dental Association, Council on Dental Research: Cost-effectiveness of Sealants in Private Practice and Standards for Use in Prepaid Dental Care, *J. Am. Dent. Assoc., 110,* 103, January, 1985.

Calderone, J.J. and Mueller, L.A.: The Cost of Sealant Application in a State Dental Disease Prevention Program, *J. Public Health Dent., 43,* 249, Summer, 1983.

Callanen, V.A., Weintraub, J.A., French, D.P., and Connolly, G.N.: Developing A Sealant Program: the Massachusetts Approach, *J. Public Health Dent., 46,* 141, Summer, 1986.

DiLeone, C.M.: Dental Sealants: Information and Guidelines for Insurance Carriers, *Dent. Hyg., 61,* 18, January, 1987.

Horowitz, A.M. and Frazier, P.J: Issues in the Widespread Adoption of Pit-and-Fissure Sealants, *J. Public Health Dent., 42,* 312, Fall, 1982.

Houpt, M.I. and Shey, Z.: Cost-effectiveness of Fissure Sealants, *ASDC J. Dent. Child., 50,* 210, May-June, 1983.

Jones, R.B.: The Effects for Recall Patients of a Comprehensive Sealant Program in a Clinical Dental Public Health Setting, *J. Public Health Dent., 46,* 152, Summer, 1986.

Little, N.J.: Sealant Retention Rates in a Community Children's Dental Clinic, *Dent. Hyg., 60,* 62, February, 1986.

Ripa, L.W., Leske, G.S., and Forte, F.: The Combined Use of Pit and Fissure Sealants and Fluoride Mouthrinsing in Second and Third Grade Children: One-year Clinical Results, *Pediatr. Dent., 8,* 158, June, 1986.

V

Treatment

INTRODUCTION

Instrumentation for scaling, root planing, gingival curettage, extrinsic stain removal, finishing amalgam restorations, debonding, and postoperative care is included in Part V. Postoperative procedures for placement and removal of dressings, removal of sutures, and treatment of hypersensitive teeth are outlined. Immediate evaluation of techniques and their effects, short-term follow-up, and maintenance evaluation are described. These procedures are all part of *nonsurgical periodontal therapy*.

The first objective of treatment is to create an environment in which the tissues can return to health. In the sequence of patient treatment, introduction to preventive measures is first, before professional instrumentation. After health has been attained, the patient's self-care on a daily basis is essential to keep the teeth and gingival tissues free from new or recurrent disease caused by the microorganisms of bacterial plaque. Professional instrumentation makes a limited contribution to arresting the progression of disease without daily plaque control measures performed by the patient.

I. Oral Prophylaxis: Definition Dilemma

The term *oral prophylaxis* means those specific treatment procedures aimed at removing local irritants to the gingiva, including complete calculus removal followed by root planing. A smooth tooth surface resists the retention of dental deposits. The oral prophylaxis performed with these objectives is truly a *preventive periodontal treatment procedure*.[1]

There is a definite need for clarification and new terminology for the various services performed under the title "oral prophylaxis." Through common usage, an oral prophylaxis has taken on a variety of meanings.

Because *prophylaxis* means *prevention of disease*, then *oral prophylaxis*, as the *prevention of oral disease*, would include such preventive procedures as restoring individual teeth, replacing missing teeth, adjusting the occlusion, correcting faulty proximal contacts, and many other procedures, the basic purposes of which are preventive.[2]

Unfortunately the term oral prophylaxis also is sometimes used to mean a superficial 5- to 10-minute application of a rubber polishing cup with an abrasive paste to the enamel surfaces that appear above the gingival margin. The term "oral prophylaxis" obviously must be carefully and specifically defined if it is to be applied to the comprehensive treatment services of a dental hygienist.

In the development of a meaningful concept of the oral prophylaxis upon which the techniques and anticipated outcomes described in this book could be based, the acceptable definition could only be one based on the preventive aspects of periodontal infections.

II. Objectives of Treatment

Specific objectives for each type of instrumentation are included in the chapter that describes the details of the technique. General objectives are that dental hygiene instrumentation will

A. Create an environment in which the tissues can return to health and then be maintained in health.

B. Eliminate periodontal pathogenic microorganisms and control reinfection.

C. Aid in the prevention and control of gingival and periodontal infections by removal of factors that predispose to the retention of bacterial plaque. Factors particularly implicated are dental calculus, irregular and overhanging restorations, and diseased, altered cemental tooth surfaces.

D. Comprise the total treatment needed for certain patients with uncomplicated disease, and the initial preparatory phase of treatment for others with more advanced disease.

E. Assist in the maintenance phase of care to prevent recurrence of disease.

F. Provide the patient with smooth tooth surfaces, which are easier to clean and to keep plaque-free by daily self-care procedures.

G. Assist in instructing the patient in the appearance

and feeling of a thoroughly clean mouth as a motivation toward the development of adequate habits of personal oral care.

H. Prepare the teeth and gingiva for dental procedures including those performed by the restorative dentist, prosthodontist, orthodontist, pedodontist, and oral surgeon.

I. Improve oral esthetics and sanitation.

References

1. *World Workshop in Periodontics.* Ann Arbor, University of Michigan, 1966, p. 450.
2. Bunting, R.W.: *Oral Hygiene,* 3rd ed. Philadelphia, Lea & Febiger, 1957, p. 233.

31 *Principles for Instrumentation*

Instrumentation begins with the identification of the various types of instruments for specific services to be performed and knowledge of the parts of those instruments. Then, to put the instruments into action to accomplish a particular task, requirements are stabilization by means of a correct grasp and finger rest, adaptation, angulation, lateral pressure, and stroke.

A study of oral and dental anatomy and histology necessarily accompanies techniques. Development of a thorough, efficient, and safe procedure depends on an understanding of the characteristics of the dental and periodontal tissues being influenced.

Knowledge of the specific morphology and topography of each tooth and the relationship to the other teeth in the permanent, mixed, and primary dentitions is essential to the understanding and use of the instruments. Recognition of the characteristic signs of health and disease of the periodontal tissues provides the basis for application of instruments for treatment.

A high degree of skill in the care and use of the fine instruments is required. Skill is dependent on knowledge and understanding of the goals of therapy and of how the goals can be reached through application of the fundamental principles of instrumentation.

INSTRUMENT IDENTIFICATION

I. Recognition of Instruments

The instruments needed for examination and evaluation were described in Chapter 13, page 191 and instruments for scaling, planing, and gingival curettage are described in Chapter 32, page 439. Other instruments needed for various services may be found in other chapters.

Each instrument must be recognized by sight and distinguished at a glance by the profile of the instrument on the sterile tray. The clinician must be able to designate the names and numbers, and to associate each instrument promptly with the various phases of instrumentation. Such spot identification contributes to neatness of tray arrangement and efficiency of service rendered through prompt selection of the proper instrument for the service to be performed.

A. Classification by Purpose and Use
1. *Examination Instruments.* Probe, explorer.
2. *Treatment Instruments.* Curets, scalers (sickle, hoe, chisel).

B. Description on the Instrument Handle
1. *Design Name.* The school or individual responsible for the design or development.
2. *Design Number.* The traditional number used to identify the specific instrument. The same instrument may be made by various manufacturers using the same number.

II. Instrument Parts

The three major parts are the *working end,* the *shank,* and the *handle* or shaft. The relationship of these parts is illustrated by the scaler in figure 31–1.

A. Working End
The working end refers to that part used to carry out the purpose and function of the instrument. Each working end is unique to the particular instrument.
1. *Sharp Instruments.* The working end of a sharp instrument is called a *blade.* The parts of a sharp blade are the
   a. Cutting Edge. A line where two surfaces meet. For example, the face and the lateral surfaces meet to form the sharp cutting edge of a sickle scaler (figures 32–4 and 32–6, page 441) or a curet (figure 32–1, page 439).
   b. Lateral Surfaces. The lateral surfaces meet or are continuous (as in a curet) to form the back of the instrument.
2. *Non-sharp Instruments.* The working end of a non-sharp instrument is a dull blade, or a *nib.* Although the term nib is most frequently applied to instruments for restorative dentistry, such as a condenser or burnisher, it may also apply to non-sharp ends, such as the wood point at the end of the porte polisher (page 517) and the rubber cup of the prophylaxis angle (page 509).

B. Shank
1. Connects the working end with the handle.
2. May be angled, curved, or straight; the more restricted the access to an area, the greater the number of shank angles that are usually required. Anterior teeth are more accessible; therefore, straight-shanked instruments can be used. Posterior teeth need angled-shank instruments, particularly for proximal surfaces.

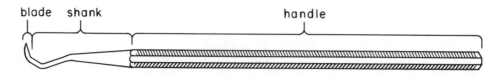

blade shank   handle

Figure 31–1. Parts of an Instrument. Scaler illustrates relationship of the blade, shank, and handle of an instrument.

C. Handle

The handle is the part of the instrument that is held (grasped) during activation of the working end. The handle is available in a wide variety of types, shapes, weights, and surface serrations (smooth, ribbed, or knurled).

1. Single-end instrument has one working end.
2. Double-ended instrument may have paired (mirror image) or complementary working ends. Paired working ends are used for access to proximal surfaces from the facial or lingual aspects.
3. Cone socket handles are separable from the shank and working end. They permit instrument exchanges and replacements.

III. Instrument Balance

A. Definition

The working end of a balanced instrument is centered in line with the long axis of the handle (figure 31–2).

B. Effect of Shank Length

The distance from the cutting edge (working end) of the blade to the junction of the shank and handle should not be greater than 35 to 40 mm. (1½ inches). Too short a distance limits action;

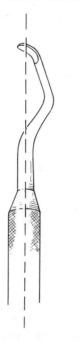

Figure 31–2. Instrument Balance. The working end of a balanced instrument is centered over the long axis of the instrument handle.

too long a distance may result in an unbalanced instrument.

INSTRUMENT GRASP

Stability is essential for effective, controlled action of an instrument. The correct use depends on maintaining *control* of the movement of the instrument through use of an effective *grasp* and the establishment and maintenance of an appropriate, firm, fulcrum *finger rest.*

I. Functions of the Instrument Grasp

A. Dominant Hand

The right hand is the dominant hand for the right-handed clinician. A few rare people are completely ambidextrous, and others are partially dexterous with the nondominant hand, a useful accomplishment when carrying out dental and dental hygiene procedures. Exercises for developing dexterity are provided on page 436.

The dominant hand is used to hold and operate the treatment instrument. The manner in which the instrument is held influences the entire procedure.

A rigid grasp, in which the instrument is gripped tightly, lessens the tactile sensitivity and, hence, the effectiveness of instrumentation. The appropriate grasp is firm, displays the confidence of the clinician in the work being done, and provides the following effects:

1. Increased fingertip tactile sensitivity.
2. Positive control of the instrument with balance and flexibility during motion.
3. Decreased hazard of trauma to the dental and periodontal tissues, which in turn results in less postoperative discomfort for the patient.
4. Prevention of fatigue to clinician's fingers, hand, and arm.

B. Nondominant Hand

The right-handed clinician uses the left hand and the left-handed clinician uses the right hand for essential supplementary functions to assist the dominant hand. Figure 31–3 shows the recommended modified pen grasp (described later) for each hand. The mouth mirror is frequently held by the nondominant hand. With the appropriate grasp and finger rest, the following effects can be provided:

1. Control of the position of the mirror for indirect vision, indirect lighting, and retraction.

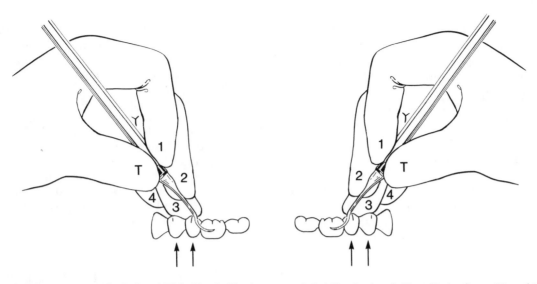

Figure 31–3. Modified Pen Grasp for Left and Right Hands. The instrument is held by the thumb (T) and index finger (1), and is supported by the middle finger (2). The ring finger (3) serves as the finger rest; the little finger (4) gives support.

2. Assistance in providing the dominant hand with an auxiliary finger rest.

II. Types
A. Modified Pen Grasp
1. *Description.* The modified pen grasp is a three-finger grasp with the tips of the thumb, index finger, and middle (second) finger all in contact with the instrument. The ring finger is the finger rest. The instrument is held by the thumb and index finger at the junction of the shank and handle. The middle (second) finger is placed on the shank to hold and guide the movement (figure 31–3).
2. *Role of Middle Finger.* The shank of the instrument is held against the pad of the middle finger. The instrument is not held across the nail or the side of the middle finger, as in a pen grasp usually used for writing. The specific position of the middle finger is extremely important to instrument control in preventing the instrument from slipping during adaptation and activation.

B. Palm Grasp
1. *Description.* The handle of the instrument is held in the palm by cupped index, middle, ring, and little fingers. The thumb is free to serve as the fulcrum (figure 31–4).
2. *Limitations of Use.* Instruments for scaling, planing, and gingival curettage are not used with a palm grasp. The possible exception is a chisel scaler when it is used to remove gross calculus by a push stroke (pages 442–443). The palm grasp limits operation in that there is less tactile sensitivity and less flexibility of movement.
3. *Examples of Uses for Palm Grasp*
   a. Air syringe.

b. Rubber dam clamp holder.
c. Handpiece grasp for instrument sharpening (figure 32–17, page 451).
d. Porte polisher for facial surfaces. A porte polisher is shown in figure 31–4.

FULCRUM: FINGER REST

A fulcrum must always be used when instruments are applied to the teeth and gingiva.

I. Definition
A. Fulcrum
The support, or point of rest, on which a lever turns in moving a body.

B. Finger Rest
The support, or point of finger rest on the tooth surface, on which the hand turns in moving an instrument.

II. Objectives
An effective, well-established finger rest is essential to the following:

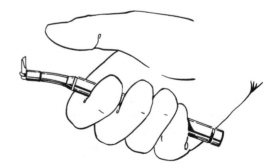

Figure 31–4. Palm Grasp. The instrument handle is held in the palm by cupped index, middle, ring, and little fingers. Thumb is free and serves as the finger rest.

A. Stability

For controlled action of the instrument.

B. Unit Control

Provides a focal point from which the whole hand can move as a unit.

C. Prevention of Injury

Injury to the patient's oral tissues can result from irregular pressure and uncontrolled movement.

D. Comfort for the Patient

Confidence in clinician's ability, which results from the feeling of securely applied instruments.

E. Control of Length of Stroke

With instrument grasp, the finger rest limits the instrumentation to where it is needed.

III. Conventional Intraoral Rests

A. Digits Used for Finger Rest

1. *Modified Pen Grasp*
   a. Ring Finger. Little finger is held close beside ring finger (fingers Nos. 3 and 4 in figure 31–3).
   b. Supplementary. Pad of middle finger rests lightly on incisal or occlusal surface of tooth to which instrument is applied; ring finger maintains regular fulcrum position and middle finger maintains its grasp on instrument.
2. *Palm Grasp.* Thumb.

B. Location of Finger Rest

1. *Purposes.* The location of a finger rest is selected for the following reasons:
   a. Convenience to area of operation.
   b. Ease in instrument adaptation.
   c. Maintenance of an effective grasp.
   d. Application of the appropriate angulation.
   e. Stability and control of instrument during the activation (strokes).
   f. Safety of the clinician. A finger rest placed in line of the stroke direction could result in a rubber glove puncture and/or a finger stab if the patient moved suddenly or the instrument slipped for any reason.
2. *Principles*
   a. The first choice for a rest is usually the tooth adjacent to the tooth being treated.
   b. Maintain the rest on firm stable tooth or teeth. The patient's chin, lips, and cheeks are mobile and flexible and therefore less reliable for stability.
   c. Where possible, the rest should be on the same arch, maxillary or mandibular, as the instrumentation; also, where possible, the rest should be in the same quadrant.

IV. Variations of Finger Rest

A basic fulcrum location cannot always be used or may require supplementation.

A. Problems

1. A patient's facial musculature, oral anatomic features, dental anatomy, or physical handicap affecting the oral cavity indirectly may interfere with customary positioning for instrumentation.
2. Tenacious calculus in difficult-access areas may not be removed and root surfaces may not be planed by the usual procedures. Greater support and pressure to the instrument are required.
3. When the problem in instrumentation seems to be related to space and accessibility, the height and position of the patient's oral cavity should be checked. Also, a change in the clinician's working position may be necessary.

B. General Categories of Variations[1,2]

When a variation in finger rest is used, apply basic rules for stability and control and avoid rests on movable tissues. Three types of variations are suggested here: *substitute, supplementary,* and *reinforced* finger rests. Any of these variations may require an external position.

1. *Substitute*
   a. Missing teeth where finger rest is usually applied. For an edentulous area, a cotton roll or gauze sponge may be packed into the area to provide a dry finger rest. Otherwise, a rest across the dental arch or in the opposite arch may be required to provide stability.
   b. Mobile teeth, or teeth with inadequate bony support. Avoid mobile teeth for finger rests or use only with minimal pressure for brief periods. Not only would the rest on a mobile tooth be unstable, but pressure, movement, and undue stress on the tooth could traumatize and tear the periodontal ligament fibers.
   c. Index finger of nondominant hand may be placed in the vestibule over a cotton roll. The usual finger rest can be placed on that to aid retraction and visibility, particularly in the mouth of a small child.
2. *Supplemental.* Place the index finger of the nondominant hand on the occlusal surfaces of teeth adjacent to the working area. The finger rest can then be applied to the index finger. Such supplements are not useful for distal surfaces where the mouth mirror is essential for vision.
3. *Reinforced*
   a. In this type, a support is placed between the instrument handle and the working end to provide additional strength and force, particularly for hard, tenacious calculus in pockets. Greater control of the instrument can result and, when applied correctly, reduce the danger of instrument breakage. A

definite rest for both hands is needed to distribute the pressure.

    b. Index finger of nondominant hand can be rested on the tooth adjacent to the one being scaled while the thumb is placed on the instrument shank (or handle) for a reinforcement.

V. Touch or Pressure Applied to Finger Rest

A. Balance

The fulcrum finger maintains a firm hold with moderate pressure to balance the action of the instrument being applied.

B. Effects of Excess Pressure

1. Decreased stability.
2. Diminished control.
3. Overtightened grasp to accommodate.
4. Fatigue caused by use of mandibular fulcrums. Heavy pressure on the movable mandible can cause fatigue in the temporomandibular joint and related muscles, and thus discomfort for the patient.
5. Fatigue in clinician's fingers and hand.

ADAPTATION

With an appropriate grasp and finger rest, the instrument is next ready for application. The working end of the instrument is adapted to the surface of the tooth or tissue where instrumentation is to take place. *Adaptation* refers to the relationship between the instrument and the surface of the tooth or soft tissue.

I. Relation to Tooth Surface

Adaptation of instruments is closely related to tooth and soft tissue contours. Adaptation depends on a knowledge of oral anatomy. The adaptation of the instrument is significant because of the need for thorough, careful instrumentation. Improperly adapted instruments can damage the tooth surface or remove excess tooth substance.

II. Characteristics of a Well-adapted Instrument

A. Working End

1. The working end of the instrument is correctly positioned for the task to be accomplished. For example, when scaling, the angle formed by the face of the instrument and the tooth surface is crucial for effective calculus removal. Angulation is described in a following section.
2. As much as possible of the working end of the instrument is used. The instrument is adapted for maximum usefulness of the working end. For example, 2 to 3 mm. of the end of a curet may be adaptable when on a "flat" surface, whereas at a line angle or convex surface of a narrow root, less than 2 mm. may be adaptable (figure 31–5).
3. The working end is applied so that it fits

closely to the surface; it is applied to conform to the contour of the surface.

4. As the instrument is activated, it can be adjusted to changes required by variations in the surface topography.

B. Soft Tissue

A properly adapted instrument will harm neither the tissue being treated nor the surrounding or adjacent tissues.

III. Problem Areas

Areas where instrument adaptation is most difficult and requires more attention, time, and careful application of skill include the following:[3]

A. Line Angles

All line angles require that the instrument be rolled between the fingers to turn the working end as the instrument is activated. At each change of direction around a line angle, the instrument must be turned to keep it adapted to the surface.

B. Convex and Rounded Surfaces

Particularly of narrow roots.

C. Cervical Area

Where the root is constricted.

D. Proximal Root Surfaces

Root surfaces may be concave, have longitudinal grooves, and have open furcations.

ANGULATION

A factor closely related to and directly influencing instrument adaptation is angulation. Angulation refers to the angle formed by a working end of an instrument with the surface to which the instrument is applied. Each instrument is applied to a surface in a specific manner for optimum operation.

I. Probe

The usual adaptation of a probe is to maintain the side of the working tip on the tooth, with the long axis of the working end nearly parallel with the tooth surface (pages 196–198).

As used for a bleeding index, the tip is placed inside the pocket wall and pressed lightly on the wall as the probe is moved horizontally around the tooth (figure 19–8, page 273).

II. Explorer

An explorer is held with the tip at a right angle to the occlusal surface when detecting occlusal pit or fissure caries. On other surfaces, the side of the tip is kept on the tooth at all times. The angle is 5 degrees or less.

III. Scalers and Curets

Angulation for a scaler or a curet means the angle formed by the face of the instrument with the surface

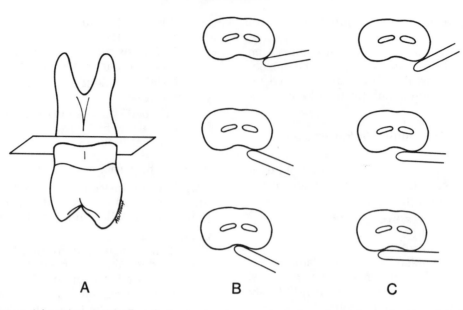

Figure 31–5. Instrument Adaptation. A. Maxillary first premolar shows cross section of root drawn for **B.** and **C. B.** Diagram of three positions of a curet shows correct adaptation at a line angle and on the concave mesial surface with 2 mm. of the instrument maintained on the tooth as the instrument is adapted. **C.** Diagram shows incorrect adaptation with toe of curet extended away from the tooth surface.

to which the instrument is applied. The relationship of the face of the instrument to the tooth surface is further described on pages 477–478 with figure 34–2.

A. Scaling and Root Planing

An angle of less than 90 degrees but of not less than 45 degrees permits effective calculus removal and root planing with removal of altered cementum. The preferred angulation is between 60 and 80 degrees. Using a markedly closed angulation under 45 degrees may result in burnishing the calculus to produce a smooth veneer.

B. Gingival Curettage

The face is turned toward the soft tissue wall of the pocket. The angle formed by the face of the curet blade and the soft tissue pocket wall being treated is less than 90 degrees but more than 45 degrees (figure 34–2, page 478).

LATERAL PRESSURE

Lateral pressure means the pressure of the instrument against the tooth surface during activation. It is described as light, moderate, or heavy pressure.

I. Detection Instruments

Explorers and probes are used with a light pressure to maximize the sense of touch in detecting irregularities.

II. Treatment Instruments

A. Exploratory Stroke

A light but secure pressure applied as a curet is passed over the tooth surface to the edge of the calculus deposit or lower border of a rough root surface.

B. Scaling Stroke

A definite controlled moderate to heavy pressure for calculus removal.

C. Root Planing Stroke

A lighter pressure applied progressively as the root surface becomes smooth (pages 463–464).

ACTIVATION: STROKE

A stroke is a single unbroken movement made by an instrument. It is the action of an instrument in the performance of the task for which it was designed.

Strokes are usually identified by the instrumentation being performed. Examples are the "probing stroke," "scaling stroke," or "root planing stroke." Technique for each type is described in the chapters covering the specific techniques.

I. Characteristics of Strokes

A. Types

1. *Pull.* Example: scaler removing calculus.
2. *Push.* Example: exploratory stroke when a curet is being positioned.
3. *Combined Push and Pull.* Example: explorer in a walking stroke, which is moving the instrument up and down with equal pressure on the surface (figure 13–15, page 205).
4. *Walking Stroke.* Example: probe is moved up and down, touching the coronal border of the periodontal attachment with each down stroke (figure 13–6, page 197).

B. Directions (figure 31–6)

1. *Vertical.* Strokes parallel with the long axis of a tooth.

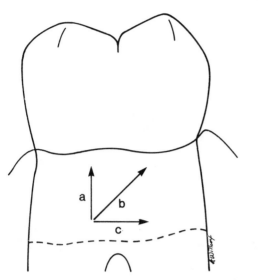

Figure 31–6. Directions of Strokes. Arrows on root surface represent **a.** vertical stroke, **b.** diagonal or oblique stroke, and **c.** horizontal stroke.

2. *Horizontal.* Strokes perpendicular to the long axis of a tooth. They are sometimes called circumferential, which should not be interpreted to mean that a stroke can be made to go around a tooth or large segment of a tooth. A horizontal stroke necessarily must be a short stroke because of the constant changes in the topography of the tooth surface.

3. *Diagonal or Oblique.* Stroke that is diagonal to the long axis of the tooth.

4. *Circular.* Stroke used with a porte polisher. A small 1- to 2-mm. diameter circular stroke is used with pressure, for example, to apply desensitizing paste (pages 500, 519).

II. Factors That Influence Selection of Stroke

A. Size, contour, and position of gingiva.
B. Surface and section of surface where the instrument is used.
C. Depth of sulcus or pocket.
D. Size and shape of instrument used.

III. Nature of Stroke

A. Grasp

The grasp of a scaler or curet is light while the working end is positioned for the stroke, and then the instrument is held more firmly during movement. An explorer and a probe should be held lightly for tactile sensitivity at all times.

B. Hand Stability

During a stroke the whole hand pivots or rotates on the fulcrum.

C. Motion

The motion for a stroke is generated by a unified action of the shoulder, arm, wrist, and hand.

D. Length

1. The length of the stroke is limited by the action of the entire arm.
2. The stroke is short, controlled, decisive, and directed to protect the tissues from trauma.
3. Instrumentation should be applied to the section of the tooth where treatment is indicated. This section is called the *instrumentation zone*. Strokes should not be long enough to pass over the whole crown when the calculus represents only a small area at the cervical third of the tooth.
4. The length of a stroke varies with each instrument and purpose. A description of strokes for each instrument is included in the respective chapters. The probe is described on page 197; the explorer, page 205; scalers and curets, pages 460 and 462–463; curettage, page 478; and handpiece, page 510.

VISIBILITY AND ACCESSIBILITY

I. Effects of Adequate Vision and Accessibility

A. Instrumentation is more thorough with minimal trauma to the oral tissues.
B. Length of time required is lessened, thereby lessening fatigue for patient and clinician.
C. Patient cooperation is increased because of shortened treatment time and less discomfort.

II. Contributing Factors

A. Patient and clinician positions (pages 64–65).
B. Efficient use of direct or reflected (by mouth mirror) illumination for each tooth surface.
C. Adequate, yet gentle, retraction of lips, cheeks, and tongue with consideration for the patient's comfort and clinician's convenience.

THOROUGHNESS OF PROCEDURE

During treatment, each particle of calculus and altered cementum must be removed from the tooth surfaces. A technique with a painstaking approach achieves both the complete removal of deposits and the comfort for the patient.

Roughness is generally associated with carelessness, and neither has any place in dental hygiene procedures. Possible effects of roughness are as follows:

1. Infliction of unnecessary pain during instrumentation.
2. Production of tissue lacerations with prolonged postoperative discomfort.
3. Gouging of tooth surfaces, which may produce a rough tooth surface subject to plaque retention and postoperative sensitivity.
4. Forcing of infected material into the deeper periodontal tissues, which can lead to in-

creased incidence of bacteremia and postoperative infection.

DEXTERITY DEVELOPMENT FOR THE USE OF INSTRUMENTS

This section is included particularly for the beginning dental hygiene student and for the graduate dental hygienist who plans to return to practice after a period of retirement. A primary objective when learning or reviewing techniques for instrumentation is to develop the ability to hold instruments correctly while employing them for use.

However generally dexterous a person may be, the use of new or unusual instruments requires different procedures for coordination. Control is essential, and guided strength contributes to control.

Proficiency during techniques comes from repeated correct use of the instruments. Exercises for the fingers, hands, and arms supplement experience. Directed exercises are needed for both hands, separately and together. Certain exercises to facilitate the development of dexterity have been selected to supplement other types of practice, such as the use of instruments on a manikin. A regular period of time each day during the training period should be set aside for exercises.

I. Squeezing a Ball
A. Purposes
    1. To develop general muscles of hand and arm.
    2. To develop strength and control for use of palm grasp.
B. Tennis Ball
    1. Hold ball in palm of hand; grip with thumb and all fingers (figure 31–7).
    2. Tighten and release grip at regular intervals.
    3. One hand rests while other is holding the ball.
    4. Use two balls, one for each hand.

II. Stretching a Rubber Band
A. Purposes
    1. To strengthen finger and hand muscles.
    2. To develop control of finger movements.

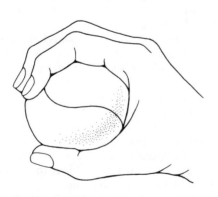

Figure 31–7. Exercise for Dexterity Development. Squeezing a ball increases strength and control.

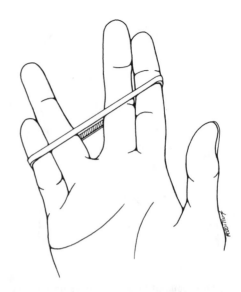

Figure 31–8. Exercise for Dexterity Development. Stretching a rubber band strengthens finger and hand muscles.

    3. To develop ability to separate ring and middle fingers, while keeping ring and little fingers together and index and middle fingers together to simulate application of a finger rest.
B. Rubber Band on Finger Joints
    1. Place rubber band at joint between first phalanx and second phalanx.
    2. Stretch band by separating middle and ring fingers (figure 31–8).
    3. Place rubber band at joint between second phalanx and third phalanx and proceed as before.
    4. Place rubber bands on both hands and do exercises together.
    5. Use rubber bands of smaller diameter as strength and control increase.
C. Rubber Band on Finger Joints with Use of Fulcrum
    1. Place rubber band on joint between first phalanx and second phalanx.
    2. Establish fulcrum finger (ring finger) on tabletop with little finger closely adjacent to it; elbow and forearm are free, as they are during instrumentation. Stretch band by separating middle and ring fingers.
    3. Touch thumb and index and middle fingers to simulate a modified pen grasp for holding an instrument. Stretch band by separating middle and ring fingers.
    4. Variations
       a. Hold instrument in modified pen grasp while doing the exercise.
       b. Do writing exercise with rubber band in place.
    5. Rest one hand while other is being exercised.

III. Writing
A. Purposes
    1. To develop correct instrument modified pen grasp.

2. To propel instrument by activation from wrist and arm, without moving fingers.
3. To practice use of instruments when mouth mirror is required.
4. To develop control and precision.

B. Circles and Vertical Lines
1. Hold long, well-sharpened, wooden lead pencil with modified pen grasp.
2. Establish fulcrum finger (ring finger) on a piece of paper on tabletop; forearm and elbow are free.
3. Inscribe counterclockwise small circles and vertical lines on paper, rapidly and lightly at first, slowly and with more pressure later.
4. Accomplish writing by activation of the hand by the upper arm, without flexing or extending the thumb and fingers holding the pencil.
5. Practice each hand separately at first; then use pencil in each hand at the same time, alternating writing action to simulate adaptation of the mirror first and then the explorer or scaler.

C. Using Mouth Mirror
1. Hold mouth mirror with modified pen grasp in nondominant hand close to pencil while practicing writing exercises (III B) through the mirror. Reverse hands.
2. Using engineer's graph paper and modified pen grasp with fulcrum as described earlier, follow the lines of the small squares while looking in mirror held with opposite hand.

D. Everyday Penmanship
1. Use modified pen grasp whenever possible for writing.
2. Practice word writing with the left hand (with the right hand for left-handed person) to increase dexterity for handling instruments.

IV. Mouth Mirror, Cotton Pliers, and Explorer

A. Purposes
1. To develop ability to turn mouth mirror at various angles.
2. To develop dexterity in holding objects with cotton pliers.
3. To establish desired grasp of explorer to assure maximum touch sensitivity.

B. Mouth Mirror
1. Hold mouth mirror with modified pen grasp, ring finger on tabletop as fulcrum finger with little finger closely adjacent to it; elbow and forearm are free. The mirror is frequently used in the non-dominant hand.
2. Practice turning mirror with fingers, adjusting as to the several surfaces of the tooth.
3. Hold a small object in the dominant hand for viewing in mirror held in non-dominant hand.
4. Practice crossing the mirror over fulcrum finger as in position for retracting lower lip while viewing lingual surfaces of mandibular anterior teeth in mouth mirror.

C. Cotton Pliers
1. Make small, tight cotton pellets with thumb and index and middle fingers of each hand; then make one in each hand simultaneously.
2. Hold cotton pliers with modified pen grasp and establish fulcrum finger on tabletop; elbow and forearm are free.
3. Practice picking up cotton pellets.
   a. Use in wiping motion on tabletop or other object.
   b. Move to different area to release pellet.

D. Explorer
1. Hold explorer with modified pen grasp and establish fulcrum finger on tabletop with upper arm and forearm free.
2. Use extracted teeth to feel with explorer tip until a light grasp permits maximum security of grasp and maximum sense of touch. Extracted teeth can be used to provide a contrast between exploring enamel, cementum, calculus, or other rough area of tooth surface (page 183).

TECHNICAL HINTS

I. Time spent on exercises should be sufficient in any one period to cause moderate (but never severe) strain and fatigue of hand muscles.
II. To relax the muscles of the hands during a practice session, wash hands in warm water.

References
1. Pattison, G.L. and Pattison, A.M.: *Periodontal Instrumentation.* Reston, Virginia, Reston Publishing Co., 1979, pp. 185–190.
2. Cooper, N.P.: *Variations in Fulcrum* (mimeographed). Albuquerque, University of New Mexico, Dental Hygiene Program, 1974.
3. Terwilliger, D. and Schwindt, S.: *Instrument Adaptation as Related to Tooth Root Morphology.* Ann Arbor, School of Dentistry, University of Michigan, 1975, 80 pp.

Suggested Readings
Byrnes, J.M.: Reaching for Excellence: A Review of the Basics, *RDH, 5,* 10, June, 1985.
Carranza, F.A.: *Glickman's Clinical Periodontology,* 6th ed. Philadelphia, W.B. Saunders Co., 1984, pp. 601–620.
Hard, D.: Oral Prophylaxis, in Bunting, R.W.: *Oral Hygiene,* 3rd ed. Philadelphia, Lea & Febiger, 1957, pp. 249–258.
Hirschfeld, L.: Subgingival Curettage in Periodontal Treatment, *J. Am. Dent. Assoc., 44,* 301, March, 1952.
Kunovich, R.S., Rosenblum, R.H., and Beck, F.M.: The Effect of Training on Indirect Vision Skills, *J. Dent. Educ., 51,* 716, December, 1987.
Lieberman, N.W.: Your Best Dental Instrument, Your Hands: Exercises to Reduce Muscle Fatigue, *Dent. Surv., 49,* 56, April, 1973.
Nield, J.S. and Houseman, G.A.: *Fundamentals of Dental Hygiene Instrumentation,* 2nd ed. Philadelphia, Lea & Febiger, 1988, pp. 165–188.
Rosenblum, R.H., Hedge, T.K., Beck, F.M., and Kunovich, R.S.:

Comparison of Three Intraoral Hand Mirror Positions, *J. Dent. Educ., 49,* 827, December, 1985.

Taylor, M.: A Comparison of Three Methods of Initial Presentation of Instrument Adaptation, *J. Dent. Educ., 39,* 163, March, 1975.

Tondrowski, V.E.: Preclinical Procedures for the Dental Hygiene Student, *J. Dent. Educ., 20,* 321, November, 1956.

Wilkins, E.M.: Instrumentation for Patient Examination and Treatment, in Darby, M.L. and Bushee, E.J., eds.: *Mosby's Comprehensive Review of Dental Hygiene.* St. Louis, The C.V. Mosby Co., 1986, pp. 497–529.

32 *Instruments and Sharpening*

Knowledge and understanding of the purpose and use of each instrument and the development of dexterity in the effective manipulation of the instruments are basic to clinical dental hygiene practice. The clinical results obtained for the patient depend in part on the proficiency and thoroughness with which the instrumentation is accomplished. *The main purpose of instrumentation is to create an environment about the teeth in which the tissues can heal and be maintained in health.*

I. Types of Instruments

Each instrument is designed for a specific type of application during treatment procedures. An instrument first can be categorized by whether it is designed primarily for supragingival treatment procedures (scalers) or for subgingival treatment (curets). Scalers and curets are then subdivided by their blade anatomy into the following types:

A. Curets
1. Universal
2. Area specific

B. Scalers
1. Sickle scaler
   a. Curved sickle scaler
   b. Straight sickle scaler
2. Hoe scaler
3. Chisel scaler
4. File scaler

II. Instrument Blade Anatomy

The parts of the blade of a scaler or a curet are the *face* (inner surface), *lateral surfaces, back, tip* (scaler) or *toe* (curet), and the *cutting edges.* The cutting edges are formed by the junction of the face and the lateral surfaces.

Figure 32–1 shows a curet with each part labeled. The parts of a scaler are the same. The differences are the pointed tip and the V-shaped back, shown in figure 32–4. Each type of instrument is described in the next sections.

CURETS

I. Characteristics

A. Blade
1. *Cutting Edges.* Two cutting edges on a curved blade (figure 32–1A); one cutting edge has a

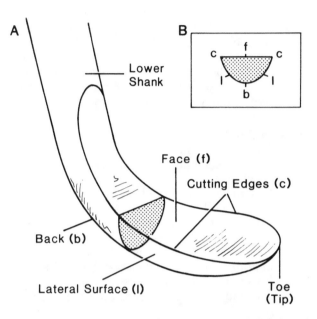

Figure 32–1. Parts of a Curet. A. Curet with parts labeled. Lower shank is also called the terminal shank. The curet has a round toe, whereas the scaler has a pointed tip. **B.** Cross section of a curet labeled f (face), c (cutting edges), l (lateral surfaces), and b (back).

wider curvature than does the other. The two cutting edges curve around to meet at the toe. In reality, a curet has one continuous cutting edge because the two sides are united without interruption by the rounded toe.

2. *Face.* Flat in cross section (figure 32–1B) and curved lengthwise.
3. *Back or Undersurface.* Rounded.
4. *Cross Section of the Blade.* Shaped like a half circle.
5. *Internal Angles.* Angles of 70 to 80 degrees are formed where the lateral surfaces meet the face. Figure 32–2 shows the cross section of a curet with the internal angles marked.

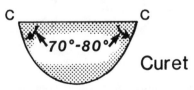

Figure 32–2. Internal Angles of a Curet. Cross section of a curet shows the 70- to 80-degree internal angles at the cutting edges.

B. Shank

1. *Anterior Teeth.* Shank, blade, and handle may be in a relatively flat plane for curets primarily adaptable to anterior teeth.
2. *Posterior Teeth.* The shank is contra-angled for access to proximal surfaces.

C. Universal Curet

A universal curet can be adapted for instrumentation on any tooth surface.

1. Designed with paired mirror-image working ends usually placed on a single handle.
2. The face of the blade is perpendicular (at a 90-degree angle) to the lower shank (figure 32–3).
3. The cutting edge (continuous around the face), used on both sides, is sharpened on both sides and around the toe. Angulation and adaptation determine the side that is correct for the surface being treated.

D. Area Specific Curet

The Gracey curets are area specific, which means that each curet is designed for adaptation to specific surfaces.

1. Designed with paired mirror-image working ends usually placed on a single handle. The seven pairs are numbered 1-2, 3-4, 5-6, 7-8, 9-10, 11-12, and 13-14.
2. The face of the blade is "off-set" (at an angle of approximately 70 degrees) in relation to the lower shank (figure 32–3).[1]
3. The cutting edge is continuous around the face.
4. Only the longer, outer cutting edge is used during instrumentation.

II. Purposes and Uses

A. Standard instrument for subgingival scaling and root planing (see also page 461).
B. After ultrasonic scaling to complete the root planing.
C. Removal of fine supragingival calculus close to the gingival margin. The rounded instrument is best adapted to the cervical area; round back does not traumatize the gingival margin.
D. Curettage of the lining of the gingival wall of the sulcus or pocket.
E. Useful for obtaining a sample of subgingival plaque to place on a glass slide for the phase microscope or for microbiologic tests.

III. Application

A. Angulation

Blade is applied to the tooth so that the face is at an angle of less than 90 degrees but more than 45 degrees with the tooth surface. The preferred angulation is between 60 and 80 degrees.

B. Adaptation

The lower third of the cutting edge (the part nearest the toe) is maintained on the tooth surface at all times to minimize soft tissue trauma from extension of the toe away from the tooth in the narrow pocket. Changes in tooth surface contour require constant attention to accomplish proper contact. On line angles, only 1 or 2 mm. near the toe may be used (figure 33–4, page 459).

C. Curet Selection

Universal curets are used for subgingival scaling for removal of as much of the calculus as possible, followed by area-specific curets for fine scaling and root planing.

D. Design

The design of the curet allows easy entrance into the sulcus, and the curved blade with rounded end permits access to the base of the sulcus or pocket. The slender shank permits entrance to the sulcus with minimal tissue distention.

E. Stroke

Pull stroke only; applied in vertical, horizontal, or oblique directions (figure 31–6, page 435).

SCALERS

I. Sickle Scaler

By usual definition a sickle is considered curved. The shapes of sickle scalers vary, however, and in some forms the blade and cutting edges are straight. When reference is made to a specific instrument with either a curved or a straight blade, the types usually are called "curved sickle" or "straight sickle."

A. Curved Sickle Scaler

1. Two cutting edges on a curved blade (figure 32–4).
2. Face is flat in cross section and curved lengthwise.
3. The face converges with the two lateral surfaces to form the *tip* of the scaler, which is a sharp point.

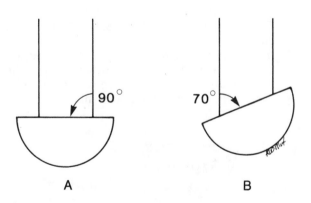

Figure 32–3. Curet Design. A. A universal curet with the blade at a 90-degree angle to the lower shank. **B.** Offset blade of an area-specific curet at a 70-degree angle to the lower shank.

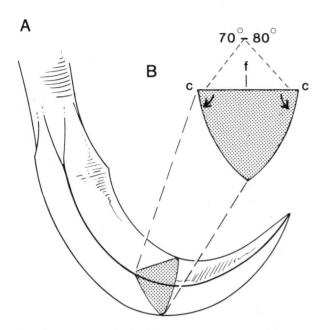

Figure 32–4. Curved Sickle Scaler. A. The curved blade terminates in a point. B. Cross section shows the face (f) and the two cutting edges (c) formed where the lateral surfaces meet the face at 70- to 80-degree angles.

4. In cross section, some blades are triangular (figure 32–4B), whereas others are trapezoidal.
5. Internal angles of 70 to 80 degrees are formed where the lateral surfaces meet the face at the cutting edges. Figure 32–5 shows the cross section of a scaler with the internal angles marked.

B. Straight Sickle Scaler
1. Two cutting edges on a straight blade (figure 32–6).
2. Face (between the cutting edges) is flat.
3. The face converges with the two lateral surfaces to form the tip of the scaler, which is a sharp point.
4. Cross section of the blade is triangular (figure 32–6B).
5. Internal angles of 70 to 80 degrees are formed where the lateral surfaces meet the face at the cutting edges (figure 32–5).

C. Angulation of the Shank
Both curved and straight sickle scalers are available with angulated or straight shanks.

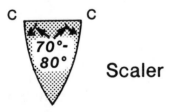

Figure 32–5. Internal Angles of a Scaler. Cross section of a scaler shows the 70- to 80-degree internal angles. These angles are restored by sharpening techniques.

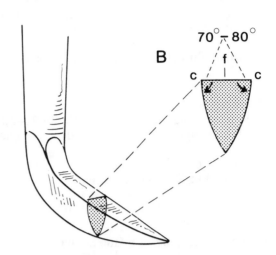

Figure 32–6. Straight Sickle Scaler. A. The straight blade converges to a point where the two cutting edges meet at the tip. B. Cross section of the scaler shows the face (f), the two cutting edges (c), and the 70- to 80-degree internal angles. This type of sickle scaler is also known as the Jacquette scaler.

1. *Straight.* Single instrument in which the relationships of the shank, blade, and handle are in a flat plane; adaptable primarily for anterior teeth, although may be used for scaling premolars when the lips and cheeks permit retraction for correct angulation.
2. *Modified or Contra-angle.* Paired instruments that are mirror images of each other to provide access to the proximal surfaces of posterior teeth; one adapts from the facial and the other from the lingual and palatal aspects.

D. Purposes and Uses of Sickle Scalers
1. Principally for the removal of supragingival calculus.
2. May be useful for removal of gross calculus that is slightly below the gingival margin when the calculus is continuous with the supragingival calculus and when the gingival tissue is spongy and flexible to permit easy insertion of the instrument.
3. Contraindications for use of sickle scalers subgingivally:
   a. Cause undue trauma to the gingival tissue because of the large size, thickness, and length of the blade.
   b. Pointed tip and straight cutting edges cannot be adapted to the curved tooth surfaces. Possibility for grooving or scratching the cemental surface is greater.
   c. Tactile sensitivity decreased with larger, heavier blades.
4. Small sickle scalers can be useful for removal of fine supragingival deposits directly under contact areas and between overlapping teeth.

E. Application
1. *Angulation.* The face of the blade is adapted to the tooth surface at an angle of approximately 70 degrees.
2. *Stroke.* Pull stroke only for this type of blade.

II. Hoe Scaler

A. Characteristics
1. Single, straight cutting edge (figure 32–7).
2. Blade turned at a 99- to 100-degree angle to the shank.
3. Cutting edge beveled at a 45-degree angle to the end of the blade (figure 32–7B).
4. Shank variously angulated for adaptation of cutting edges to accessible tooth surfaces; some are paired.

B. Purposes and Uses of a Hoe Scaler
1. Removes supragingival calculus, particularly large, accessible, tenacious pieces.
2. May be useful to remove gross calculus 2 to 3 mm. below the gingival margin provided the tissue is spongy, flexible, and easily displaced.

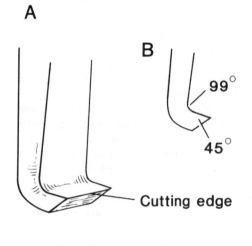

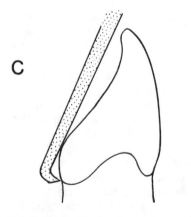

Figure 32–7. Hoe Scaler. A. The hoe has a single cutting edge. **B.** The blade is turned at an angle of 99 degrees to the shank, and the cutting edge is beveled at a 45-degree angle. **C.** Adaptation to a tooth for removal of calculus is with a two-point contact where possible.

3. Contraindications for use subgingivally
   a. Insertion of the thick-bladed instrument into the sulcus causes distention of the pocket wall.
   b. Lack of adaptability of the wide straight cutting edge to the curved root surface.
   c. Difficulty of use without gouging the cemental surface.
   d. Lack of sensitivity because of the bulk of the instrument and the marked angulation of the shanks of some hoes.
   e. Impossibility of reaching the bottom of the pocket without stretching and tearing the gingival pocket wall unnecessarily because of the size and shape of the blade.

C. Application
1. Full width of the cutting edge is in contact with the calculus, and when possible, a two-point contact is maintained with the tooth to stabilize the instrument during the positioning and activation. Two-point contact means contact of the cutting edge and the side of the shank with the tooth (figure 32–7C).
2. Hoes are not generally applied to proximal surfaces except the surface adjacent to an edentulous area.
3. Pull stroke is used toward occlusal or incisal surfaces.

III. Chisel Scaler

A. Characteristics
1. Single straight cutting edge (figure 32–8).
2. Blade is continuous with a slightly curved shank.
3. End of blade is flat and beveled at 45 degrees (figure 32–8B).

B. Purposes and Uses of a Chisel Scaler
1. Useful for removal of supragingival calculus from exposed proximal surfaces of anterior teeth where interdental gingiva is missing.
2. Well suited for quick dislodgement of heavy calculus from the proximal areas of mandib-

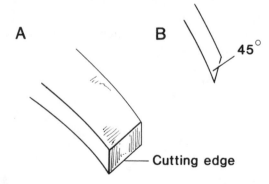

Figure 32–8. Chisel Scaler. A. A chisel scaler has a single cutting edge, and the blade is continuous with a slightly curved shank. **B.** A 45-degree bevel is at the cutting edge.

ular anterior teeth. When the calculus on the lingual forms a continuous bridge across several teeth, the chisel can be pushed horizontally from the facial to break up the large masses of calculus.

3. Useful for proximal surfaces of premolars when flexibility of the lips and cheeks permits retraction for proper positioning of the cutting edge.

C. Application

1. Full width of cutting edge should be applied, as the sharp corners can nick and groove the tooth surface.
2. Stroke is horizontal only, from facial to lingual on proximal surfaces of anterior, particularly mandibular teeth.

IV. File Scaler

A. Characteristics

1. Multiple cutting edges lined up as a series of miniature hoes on a round, oval, or rectangular base (figure 32–9A).
2. The multiple blades are at a 90- or 105-degree angle with the shank (figure 32–9B).
3. Shanks are variously angulated, similar to the hoes; some are paired instruments, others single.
4. Reduced tactile sensitivity because of the size and shape; files are wide, flat, and bulky.

B. Purposes and Uses of a File Scaler

In general, the file can be considered a supplementary instrument rather than the definitive instrument for routine use during scaling and root planing.

Although never used by some dental hygienists, the file is used by others for one or more of the following purposes:

1. Removal of calculus (accomplished by crushing or fragmentation).

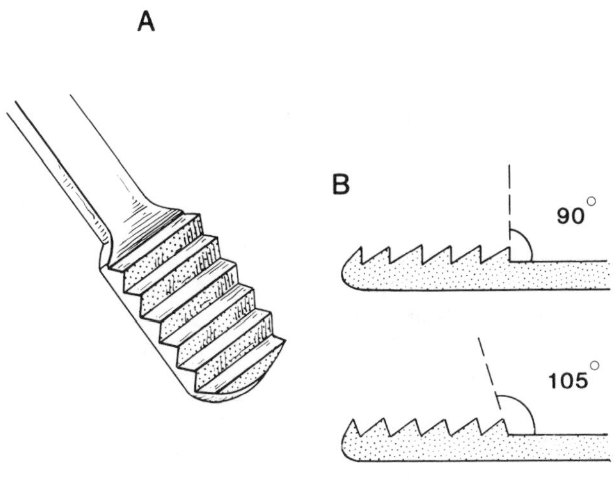

A

B

90°

105°

Figure 32–9. File Scaler. A. A file has multiple cutting edges. **B.** Each blade is at a 90- or a 105-degree angle with the shank.

2. Smoothing of the tooth at the cementoenamel junction.
3. Root planing, primarily the exposed root surface following periodontal surgery.
4. Smoothing down of overextended or rough amalgam restorations, particularly on proximal surfaces or in the cervical areas.

C. Application

1. The entire working surface is placed flat against the area to be treated.
2. Adaptation to the curved tooth surfaces is difficult. In certain relationships the file has only a tangential contact.
3. Pressure applied permits the cutting edges to grasp the surface.
4. Stroke is pull only.
5. When the file is used to assist in root planing, the file should be followed with a curet, because research has shown that a greater degree of smoothness can be attained with a curet.[2,3]

SPECIFICATIONS FOR INSTRUMENTS FOR SCALING AND ROOT PLANING

I. Basic Qualities

Each instrument is designed for a specific purpose and is intended to be used for the purpose for which it was designed. Characteristics of instruments that influence their usefulness are listed below. An instrument should

A. Be effective and efficient for calculus removal and smoothing tooth surfaces with the least possible trauma to the gingival tissue or the tooth surface.
B. Provide comfort to the clinician without causing fatigue or muscle cramp. Hollow handles have a comfortably wide diameter and are lightweight.
C. Permit maximum use of tactile sensitivity.
D. Have balance (figure 31–2, page 430).
E. Have a blade of a size in keeping with
   1. Anatomy of the tooth; root curvatures.
   2. Location and extent of calculus deposits.
   3. Anatomy of the sulcus or pocket.
F. Be easy to care for when cleaning, sterilizing, sharpening.

II. Sharp Cutting Edges

Instruments must be sharp if scaling and root planing are to be completed efficiently with minimal trauma to the tissues. When the instrument blade is maintained with its original contour and sharp cutting edges, the following may be expected:

A. Greater precision of treatment, improved quality of results, and less working time involved.
B. Increased tactile sensitivity during instrumentation. A sharp instrument does not have to be gripped as firmly as a dull one.
C. Greater control of the instrument because of the

lighter grasp needed; less pressure on the tooth being scaled or planed and decreased pressure on the finger rest are required.

D. Fewer strokes required.

E. Less possibility of burnishing rather than removing the calculus.

F. Prevention of unnecessary trauma to gingival tissues and, therefore, less discomfort experienced by the patient.

G. Decreased possibility of nicking, grooving or scratching the tooth surfaces.

H. Less fatigue for the clinician.

INSTRUMENT SHARPENING

Objectives for techniques of sharpening emphasize the *preservation of the original shape* of the instrument while restoring a sharp cutting edge. Instruments designed for a particular purpose should continue to be used in the manner for which they were designed and should not be distorted by inaccurate sharpening techniques.

Sharpening procedures are not easy to learn and require skill and patience to accomplish. More instruments undoubtedly are worn out from sharpening than from use.

This chapter includes sharpening procedures for the curet, sickle, hoe, chisel, and explorer, using various sharpening stones and devices. The principles of sharpening that are outlined and illustrated here may be applied to various types of sharpening stones and instruments.

I. Sharpening Stones

A. Materials and Their Sources

1. *Natural Abrasive Stones.* Quarried from mineral deposits, the hard Arkansas stone is used for dental instruments because of its fine abrasive particle size.

2. *Artificial Materials*
   a. Hard, nonmetallic substances impregnated with aluminum oxide, silicon carbide, or diamond particles; these are larger and coarser than particles of the Arkansas stone. Examples: ruby stone, carborundum stones, and the diamond hone.
   b. Solid aluminum oxide. Example: moonstone.[4]
   c. Steel alloys are metals that are harder than most dental instrument steel and, therefore, are capable of sharpening the instrument. Example: tungsten carbide steel used in the Neivert Whittler.

B. Categories

Sharpening stones as they are manufactured for use may be classified into two general groups: those for manual (unmounted) sharpening and those for power-driven (mandrel mounted) sharpening. Examples of procedures using both unmounted and mounted stones are supplied in this chapter.

1. *Unmounted*
   a. Stationary flat stones. Rectangular stones with square or rounded edges, or with one side grooved for the special adaptation of curved blades.
   b. Hand stones. Cylindrical (tapered or straight) or rectangular with rounded edges.
   c. Other types. Sharpening devices, such as the Neivert Whittler.

2. *Mandrel Mounted.* Cylindrical (straight or tapered) small stones of various diameters designed to fit the various sizes of instrument blades.

II. Facilities for Sharpening

The work area where instrument sharpening is accomplished should be arranged for convenience and comfort. Because sharpening is an everyday event, the procedure is planned so that available time can be utilized effectively without inconveniences.

A. Place

A definite place should be arranged where materials for sharpening can be kept together and work can be done from a seated position.

B. Lighting

A permanently fixed light that can be concentrated over the work area is needed; light must be shaded to protect the eyes.

C. Working Surface

The working surface should be firm and stationary. A bracket table or cervical tray is undesirable because of lack of stability.

D. Equipment

An adequate assortment of stones and the materials for their maintenance and cleanliness, a magnifying glass, and other incidental materials related to specific procedures should be available.

III. Dynamics of Sharpening

A. Sharpening Stone Surface

A sharpening stone acts as an abrasive to reshape a dulled blade by grinding the surface until the cutting edge is restored. The surface of the stone is made up of masses of minute crystals, which are the abrasive particles that accomplish the grinding of the instrument. A smaller particle size or a finer grain, as it is generally called, abrades or reduces more slowly and produces a finer cutting edge.

B. Cutting Edge

The cutting edge is a fine *line* formed where the face and lateral surface meet at an angle. The edge is a line and, therefore, has length but no thickness. The edge becomes dull when pressed against a hard surface (the tooth), or it may be nicked when drawn over a rough surface. A dull edge is rounded and therefore has thickness. The object in sharpening is to reshape the cutting edge to a line.

C. Sharpening

Sharpening is accomplished by grinding the surface or surfaces that form the cutting edge.

IV. Tests for Instrument Sharpness

A. Visual or Glare Test

1. Examine the cutting edge under adequate light, preferably with a magnifying glass.
2. Because the sharp cutting edge is a fine *line*, it does not reflect light.
3. The dull cutting edge presents a rounded, shiny *surface*, which reflects light.

B. Plastic Testing Stick[5]

1. Use a plastic or acrylic ¼-inch rod, 3 inches long. The hardness and texture approximate a fingernail. A plastic disposable suction tip also may be useful for this purpose.
2. Apply the instrument blade to the plastic stick at the correct angle for scaling; press lightly but firmly.
3. The sharp cutting edge engages or grips the plastic and moves with resistance if an attempt is made to draw the cutting edge over the surface.
4. The dull cutting edge does not catch without undue pressure and slides easily over the surface of the stick.
5. Test each area along an entire cutting edge because the edge is not uniformly dulled during use.

V. Some Basic Principles

A. Sharpening Before Sterilization

When sharpening before sterilization, the instruments must first be cleaned and disinfected. An ultrasonic cleaner is recommended for sanitization. As an alternate, the instruments may be scrubbed thoroughly with soap and water, provided heavy-duty household gloves are worn and other procedures are followed as described on pages 43–44. Steps for maximum precautions were outlined on page 59.

After sharpening, the instruments are prepared for sterilization. When a dry stone is used, or when plain water is used on the stone, instruments and the stone are scrubbed thoroughly before packaging for sterilization.

When oil is used during sharpening, the instruments should be placed again in the ultrasonic cleaner or scrubbed thoroughly with soap and hot water to remove all the oil. Oil on the instruments or stone can protect microorganisms and thereby prevent complete sterilization. Rather than an oil, which is penetrating and dif-

ficult to remove, petroleum jelly may be preferred because it is water soluble and therefore readily removed before sterilizing.

B. Sterilization of the Sharpening Stone

A sterile sharpening stone should be a part of the basic clinic set-up for a scaling and root planing appointment. Instruments then may be sharpened throughout the procedure as they show signs of dullness. Efficiency will increase and the patient will benefit from receiving a more thorough treatment in less time.

Sterilization of stones may be accomplished by any of the acceptable sterilization methods described in Chapter 4 (pages 46–49). A limitation of the steam autoclave is that autoclaving may dry out a stone and lead to chipping or breakage.

C. Instrument Handling

All instruments must be handled with care to preserve sharpness and prevent accidental damage to the cutting edges.

D. Preparation of Stone for Sharpening

1. *Lubricated Stone.* Spread a thin layer of lubricant over the surface of the stone. A clear, fine sterile oil or petroleum jelly may be used. An excess amount of oil or petroleum jelly can obscure the view of the cutting edge being sharpened.

   When sharpening is done during an appointment, a sterile swab is used to apply the lubricant to the sterile stone. The lubricant should be kept in a clinically clean covered jar or tube and set aside expressly for that purpose.

   The lubricant can provide the following effects:

   a. Facilitate the movement of the instrument blade over the stone and prevent scratching of the stone.
   b. Suspend the metallic particles removed during sharpening and so help to prevent clogging of the pores of the stone (glazing).

2. *Dry Stone.* Because of the problems related to maintaining a sterile stone and preventing contamination when oil, tap water, or petroleum jelly is applied, the use of a dry stone provides a particular advantage.

   A dry stone contributes to the following effects:

   a. Sharpen the cutting edge without nicks in the blade which can be created from particles of metal suspended in a lubricant.[6]
   b. Allow the stone to be completely sterilized without the problem of interference by the oil left in and on the stone.

E. Sharpening

1. *Objectives.* The objectives during sharpening are to produce a sharp cutting edge and to preserve the original shape of the blade.
2. *When to Sharpen.* Sharpen at the first sign of

dullness during an appointment. When instruments become grossly dulled, recontouring wastes the instrument. Restoration of the original contour while maintaining a strong blade is difficult to achieve.

3. *Choice of Method.* Select the sharpening method and sharpening stone or device consistent with the size and shape of the instrument being treated.

4. *Angulation.* Before starting to sharpen, analyze the cutting edge and establish the proper angle between the stone and the blade surface. Maintain the angle through the firm grasp, secure finger rest, moderate pressure, short stroke, and other features of the technique appropriate to the individual instrument.

5. *Maintain Control.* Maintain control so that the entire surface is reduced evenly. Care must be taken not to create a new bevel at the cutting edge.

6. *Prevent Grooving.* Prevent grooving of the sharpening stone by varying the areas for instrument placement. Cleaning and stain removal procedures are described on page 453.

F. After Sharpening

Gently hone or burnish the nonbeveled surface adjacent to the cutting edge.

1. By definition, a *hone* is a sharpening stone and *honing* means sharpening. In common usage, honing has been applied to the process whereby the "bur" or "wire edge" is removed from the side of the cutting edge that was not reduced.

2. During sharpening, some of the metal particles removed during grinding remain attached to the edge of the instrument and create the wire edge. If allowed to remain, the tiny particles may be removed when the instrument is applied to the tooth surface during treatment.

3. By sharpening into, toward, or against the cutting edge, the production of a wire edge will be minimized.

4. The method for removal is as follows. Using an even and light pressure, pass a flat Arkansas stone along the nonbeveled side of the cutting edge. One or two strokes is usually sufficient. If heavy pressure is applied, the bevel of the cutting edge can be altered.

SHARPENING CURETS AND SICKLES

Sharpening of both the lateral surfaces and the face preserves the original contour of the blade. For both curets and sickles, the internal angle at the cutting edge is 70 to 80 degrees (figures 32–2 and 32–5). To preserve this angle, sharpening stones must be placed and activated carefully.

Manual sharpening procedures are the methods of choice so that the blade is not reduced unnecessarily by the rapid-cutting mounted stone. Techniques in this section show the use of a flat stone for manual sharpening of lateral surfaces. When sharpening lateral surfaces, the flat stone may be used in one of two ways: the stone may be moved while the instrument is stationary, or the stone may be stationary while the instrument is moved.

MOVING FLAT STONE: STATIONARY INSTRUMENT

The side of the cutting edge formed by the lateral surface is reduced by this method. The technique described applies to both curets and sickles. Because the sickle has a pointed tip and the curet has a round toe end, a variation is necessary in the adaptation of the sharpening stone to that portion of the blade.

I. Prepare the Stone

Preparation of stones is described on page 445.

II. Examine the Cutting Edge to Be Sharpened

Test for sharpness to determine specific areas that are dull.

III. Stabilize the Instrument

A. Grasp the instrument in a palm grasp and hold the hand against the edge of an immovable workbench or table under adequate light (figure 32–10A). The instrument should be low enough to allow the clinician to see clearly the cutting edges and the angle formed by the instrument and the sharpening stone.

B. Turn the face of the instrument up and parallel with the floor.

IV. Apply Sharpening Stone

A. Apply the stone in a vertical position to the lateral surface at the heel of the cutting edge. Figure 32–10B shows the position for one side of the blade, and figure 32–10C shows the position for the other side.

B. Adjust the angle at which the stone is held to maintain the internal 70 to 80 degrees of the blade. The angle on the outside, between the instrument and the stone, is 100 to 110 degrees (figure 32–11A and B).

V. Activate the Sharpening Stone

A. Keep the stone in contact with the blade and at the proper angle throughout the procedure. The broken line in figure 32–11 represents the flat surface of the sharpening stone.

B. Move the stone up and down with short rhythmic strokes about ½ to ¼ inch high. Put more pressure on the down stroke.

C. Follow the cutting edge from heel to toe, applying several strokes to each millimeter.

D. Do not change the angle of the stone with the face

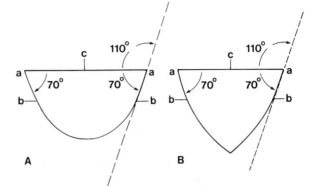

Figure 32–11. Angulation for Sharpening. Cross sections of a curet (**A.**) and a sickle scaler (**B.**) show correct angulation of the face of the blade with the flat sharpening stone (broken line) to reproduce the internal angle of the instrument at 70 degrees. Note the cutting edges (a) and the lateral surfaces (b).

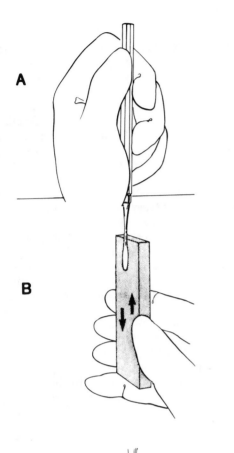

Figure 32–10. Stationary Instrument–Moving Stone Technique. A. Grasp the instrument with the nondominant hand. Stabilize the hand on the edge of a stationary table or bench and provide good light on the instrument. **B.** The stone is angled with the face of the instrument at 100 to 110 degrees (figure 32–11) to maintain the internal angle of the blade at 70 to 80 degrees. **C.** Stone reversed to sharpen the opposite cutting edge of a universal curet.

of the instrument. When the angle is varied, an irregularity is ground into the cutting edge.

E. Keep the wrist straight and use the whole arm to standardize the stroke and the adaptation of the stone to the instrument.

F. Variation at the toe-end
   1. For a sickle scaler, the stone is held straight as it nears the pointed tip.
   2. For the curet, the position of the stone is adapted so that sharpening continues around the round toe. The same angle between the stone and the face is maintained.

G. Finish with a down stroke.

VI. Test for Sharpness

Determine whether to repeat the first side before starting the second.

STATIONARY FLAT STONE: MOVING INSTRUMENT

I. Curet

A. Prepare the stone (page 445) and place it flat on a steady workbench or table.

B. Examine the cutting edges to be sharpened. Test for sharpness.

C. Hold the instrument in a modified pen grasp and establish a secure finger rest (figure 32–12B).

D. Apply the cutting edge to the stone. An angle of 110 degrees is formed by the stone and face.
   1. Because the curet is curved, only a small section of the cutting edge can be applied at one time.
   2. Sharpening is performed in a *series* of applications of the cutting edge to the stone, each overlapping the previous, as the instrument is turned and drawn steadily along the stone.
   3. The portion of the cutting edge nearest the shank is applied first (figure 32–12C, a).

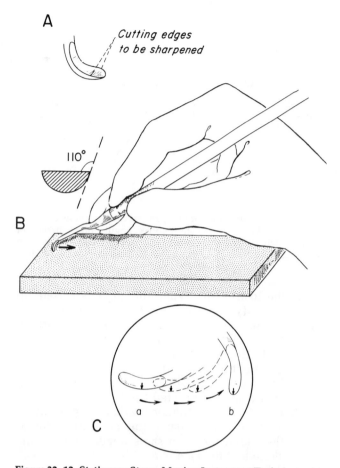

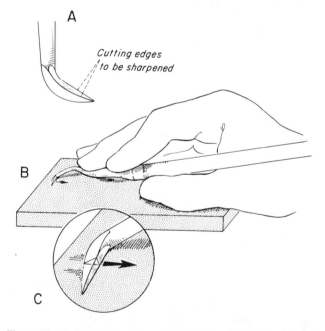

Figure 32–12. Stationary Stone–Moving Instrument Technique. A. Curet shows cutting edges to be sharpened. **B.** Stone placed flat with blade in position at the beginning of the sharpening stroke. With the finger rest stabilized on the edge of the stone, the cutting edge is maintained at the proper angulation (110 degrees) as the instrument is drawn along the stone with an even moderate pressure. **C.** The movement of the blade is shown by the arrows, which indicate each portion of the cutting edge as the blade is turned on the stone from the beginning (a) to the completion (b) of the stroke at the center of the round toe of the curet. For a universal curet, the instrument is turned over and the opposite cutting edge is sharpened.

E. Apply moderate to light but firm pressure while the instrument is activated.

F. Use a slow steady stroke to maintain control and to assure that each portion of the cutting edge receives equal treatment.

G. Move the blade forward into the cutting edge. Turn the instrument continuously until the center of the round end of the blade is reached (figure 32–12C, b).

H. Test for sharpness along the entire cutting edge; reapply to stone as necessary for ideal sharpness.

I. Turn the instrument to sharpen the second cutting edge. Overlap at the center of the round tip. Universal curets are sharpened on both sides and around the toe. Gracey curets are sharpened on one side only and around the toe.

J. Use the hand sharpening cone (described in the

next section) or the Neivert Whittler (pages 449–450) for sharpening the facial aspect.

II. Sickle Scaler

A. Prepare the stone (page 445) and place the stone flat on a firm table or bench top under adequate light. Do not tilt the stone while sharpening.

B. Examine cutting edges to be sharpened. Test for sharpness.

C. Hold the instrument with a firm pen grasp, using thumb, index, and middle (second) fingers to prevent the instrument from rotating or changing angles during sharpening (figure 32–13B).

D. Establish finger rest on side of stone using ring and little fingers.

E. Stabilize stone with fingers of opposite hand.

F. Apply cutting edge to be sharpened to the stone. Maintain 70- to 80-degree internal angle of the instrument (figure 32–11B). The portion of the cutting edge nearest the shank is applied first. Some sickles have flat lateral surfaces, and an entire side may be positioned at one time.

G. Apply moderate to light but firm pressure while instrument is in motion. Heavy pressure can reduce control of instrument, cause scratching of the stone, and produce an unfavorable bevel at the cutting edge.

H. Use a short, slow stroke to maintain the exact relation of the cutting edge to the stone.

   1. Pull blade forward, toward the cutting edge.

Figure 32–13. Stationary Stone Technique for a Scaler. A. Scaler shows cutting edges to be sharpened. **B.** With a modified pen grasp and a finger rest established on the side of the stone, the scaler is positioned for sharpening. **C.** The portion of the cutting edge nearest the lower shank is applied first with an angle of 100 to 110 degrees between the face and the stone. The instrument is turned continuously to follow the arc-like shape of the blade. The cutting edges are sharpened to the pointed tip.

2. All fingers move with the arm as a unit.
3. Use a slow, steady stroke to maintain control and to assure that each portion of the cutting edge receives equal treatment.
4. Turn the instrument continually to follow the arc-like shape of the blade to the pointed tip. A sickle with a flat lateral surface is not turned.

I. Test for sharpness after one or two strokes. Repeat as needed for ideal sharpness.

J. Turn instrument and proceed to sharpen other lateral surface. When instrument placement is awkward for a modified contra-angle sickle, use a narrow side of the stone.

K. When sharpening the face of a straight blade*
1. Position the surface over a side of the flat stone with the tip pointed down.
2. Apply entire face flat against the stone.
3. With firmly established finger rest, apply moderate to light but firm pressure for a short slow stroke while the exact relation of the flat face is maintained on the stone.

SHARPENING CONE

I. Description

A. Types
Stones are cylindrical Arkansas cones (tapered or straight) or rectangular with rounded edges, and tapered carborundum stones.

B. Uses
1. *Arkansas.* Tapered cone is recommended for curved cutting edges of sickles and curets.
2. *Carborundum.* Coarser grain is useful for preliminary shaping or sharpening of excessively dulled instruments. Use of a finer stone follows to refine the cutting edge.

II. Sharpening Procedure

A. Preparation of Stone (page 445).

B. Position
1. Hold instrument in nondominant hand across palm with fingers and thumb grasping firmly. Direct blade toward self with face of the blade up and parallel with the floor.
2. For additional support, place instrument over the edge of a firm hard block and maintain rigidly (figure 32–14).
3. Stabilize arms between the wrists and elbows on the edge of a solid table or bench top.
4. Use the following procedure for a tapered cone
   a. With a firm grasp of the sharpening cone, position the appropriate diameter of the cone to fit the curvature of the surface to be sharpened.
   b. Apply the stone straight across the face so that an even pressure can be applied to

---

*Face of a curved sickle is sharpened with a hand sharpening cone or the Neivert Whittler.

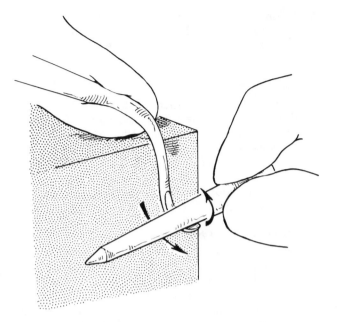

Figure 32–14. Sharpening Cone. A cylindrical Arkansas stone is applied to the face of a curet. The instrument is stabilized over a firm block, and the stone is positioned to fit the curvature of the surface to be sharpened. An even pressure is applied across the face of the instrument so that both cutting edges will be sharpened on the same plane.

both cutting edges simultaneously to produce an evenly sharpened instrument (figure 32–14).

C. Motion
1. Rotate stone counterclockwise over the instrument with even, firm pressure.
2. Continue rotation of stone upward (as in a circle) when approaching the end of the curet to prevent tapering off and reshaping (flattening) the curvature of the tip. (Figure 32–17B illustrates this for the mounted stone.)
3. Use a horizontal stroke, if preferred. The instrument is maintained stationary as previously described, and the stone is moved back and forth across the face of the blade. Care must be taken to maintain the stone straight across so that an even pressure is applied simultaneously to both cutting edges.

D. Test for Sharpness
Test for sharpness after a few applications. Repeat as necessary to obtain ideal sharpness.

THE NEIVERT WHITTLER

I. Description

A. Working End
The working end consists of five sharpening edges and a rounded burnishing edge of tungsten carbide steel.

B. Handle

The handle, which is made of stainless steel, is bulky and hexagonal for comfortable grasping (figure 32–15).

II. Uses

A. Manufacturer's instructions describe the procedure used for sharpening straight and curved blades, including those of dental instruments, scissors, and knives.
B. Particularly useful for the face of a curved scaler or curet.
C. The outer rounded edge is designed for honing (burnishing).

III. Sharpening Procedure

A. Position

Stability and control are most important.
1. Hold instrument to be sharpened firmly in the nondominant hand, across palm, grasping with all fingers and the thumb, with the surface to be sharpened turned toward self. The instrument can also be stabilized over the edge of a firm, hard surface, as shown for the cone in figure 32–14.
2. Stabilize arms between the wrists and the el-

bows on the edge of an immovable table or bench top.
3. Whittler is held in a palm grasp with thumb under handle adjacent to the working end. At the same time, the thumb rest is applied beneath the instrument blade on the nondominant hand (figure 32–16A).
4. Apply working end to the curvature of the surface to be sharpened straight across so that even pressure can be applied to both cutting edges simultaneously, thereby producing an evenly sharpened instrument (figure 32–16B).

B. Motion

1. Draw the whittler edge across the length of the face with a moderate, even pressure.
2. As the end is approached, continue in an upward motion to prevent tapering off and reshaping curvature of the tip.

C. Test for Sharpness

Test for sharpness after a few applications.

D. Hone

Hone the lateral surfaces of blade next to cutting edges.

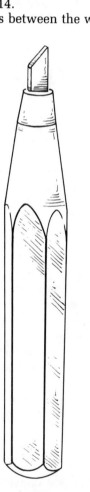

Figure 32–15. The Neivert Whittler. The working end is made of tungsten carbide steel and the handle is made of stainless steel.

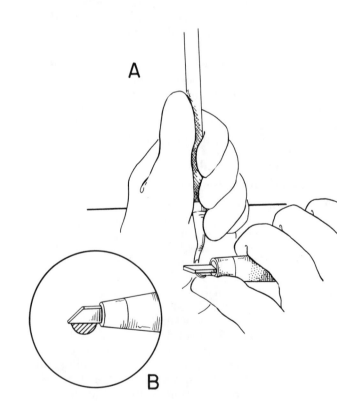

Figure 32–16. Sharpening with a Neivert Whittler. A. The instrument is stabilized in the nondominant hand, and the whittler is held in a palm grasp with the thumb rest close to the instrument to be sharpened. **B.** Close-up shows position of the blade of the sharpener across the face of the curet.

MANDREL MOUNTED STONES

I. Description

A. Types
1. *Arkansas.* Fine grain.
2. *Ruby Stone.* Coarser grain, especially useful for recontouring excessively dull instrument. When used for routine sharpening, the ruby stone should be applied conservatively.

B. Shapes
The stones are cylindrical with flat end or cone shape.

C. Use
1. Applicable to most cutting edges. Various sizes and grains of stones are selectively utilized.
2. Coarse-grained ruby stone may be useful for reshaping.
3. Stones are sterilized and may be used with water. They are useful for sharpening sterile instruments and for use during the patient's appointment.

II. Sharpening Procedure

A. Select Stone
Select a sharpening stone with a diameter appropriate to fit the blade of the instrument to be sharpened.

B. Prepare Stone
Apply sterile oil or petrolatum to Arkansas stone. Dip ruby stone in water and repeat at intervals during sharpening to aid in reducing heat production.

C. Position
1. Hold instrument to be sharpened in a palm grasp with blade face up.
2. Hold handpiece in other hand using a palm grasp with the thumb securely placed against the thumb of the hand holding the instrument (figure 32–17).
3. Stabilize arms between wrists and elbows on the edge of a solid table or bench top.
4. Apply stone to surface to be sharpened straight across so that light, even pressure can be applied to both cutting edges simultaneously, thereby producing an evenly sharpened instrument.

D. Motion
1. Use low speed to
   a. Minimize heat production (alteration of the temper of the steel can result with repeated use).
   b. Allow complete control of position of sharpening stone on blade.
2. Apply light pressure to prevent undue reduction of instrument. Pressure, however, should

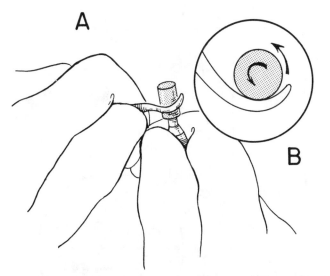

Figure 32–17. Mandrel Mounted Sharpening Stone. A. A mounted stone with a diameter appropriate for the curved blade to be sharpened is positioned across the face for even sharpening of the cutting edges. Hands and arms are stabilized for precision and control. **B.** With low speed to minimize heat production, the rotating stone is passed along the face of the instrument. Near the toe, the stone is moved upward to prevent flattening of the instrument.

be sufficiently heavy to create a smooth surface.
3. Maintain blade shape. Pass the rotating stone upward when approaching the end of the blade to prevent tapering off and reshaping the tip (figure 32–17B).

E. Test for Sharpness
Test for sharpness after one or two applications. Repeat when necessary.

F. Hone
Hone the lateral borders of the cutting edges.

III. Disadvantages of Power-Driven Sharpening

A. Inconsistent results because of variations in speed and difficulty of stabilization of instrument and sharpening stone.
B. Excess reduction of instrument during shorter period of use; less conservation of instruments than by manual methods.
C. Frictional heat may affect the temper of the steel.

SHARPENING THE HOE SCALER

Characteristics of the hoe scaler are described on page 442. The hoe has only one surface to be ground. Because placement of the small surface on the Arkansas stone is difficult to visualize, use of a magnifying glass can be particularly helpful.

I. Surface To Be Ground
Examine surface to be ground (figure 32–18A). Test for sharpness.

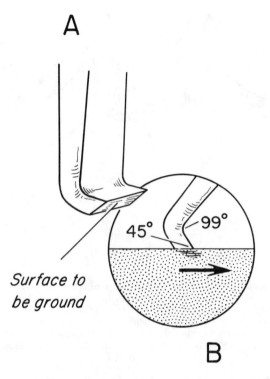

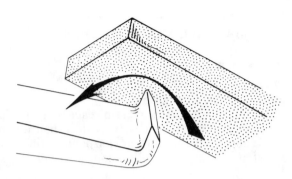

Figure 32–19. Rounding a Hoe Scaler. To round the sharp corners of the hoe scaler, a flat stone is rubbed over the instrument with a gentle rolling motion.

SHARPENING THE CHISEL SCALER

Sharpening procedures for the chisel are similar to those for the hoe. Again, the surface is small, the angulation is difficult to visualize, and the use of a magnifying glass is recommended. Review the characteristics of the chisel scaler on page 442.

I. Surface To Be Ground

Examine surface to be ground (figure 32–20A). Test for sharpness.

II. Sharpening Procedure

A. Hold instrument with a modified pen grasp, establish finger rest, and apply the surface to be ground to the stone in the correct relationship to maintain the 45-degree bevel (figure 32–20B).
B. With moderate, steady pressure, push the instru-

Figure 32–18. Sharpening a Hoe Scaler. A. Surface to be ground. B. Hoe adapted to the surface of a stationary flat stone at the proper angle to maintain the original bevel of 45 degrees. Arrow indicates direction of the sharpening stroke leading into the cutting edge.

II. Sharpening Procedure

A. Hold instrument in modified pen grasp. Establish finger rest on the stone.
B. Apply the surface to be ground to the stone in correct relationship to maintain the 45-degree bevel (figure 32–18B).
C. With moderate, steady pressure, pull the instrument toward the cutting edge a short distance. Allow the whole hand to move with the arm as a unit.
D. Release pressure and slide the instrument back. Repeat.
E. Test for sharpness and reapply as needed for ideal sharpness.
F. Hone the undersurface of the blade adjacent to the cutting edge.

III. Round Corners

Corners should be rounded at each end of the cutting edge.
A. Rounded corners help to prevent laceration of soft tissue or grooving of tooth surface.
B. Hold instrument in nondominant hand with corners of cutting edge directed inward.
C. Rub the surface of the sharpening stone across each corner with a gentle rolling motion (figure 32–19). Two or three applications are usually sufficient.

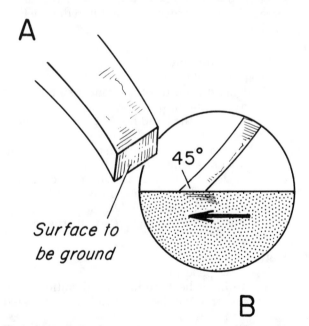

Figure 32–20. Sharpening a Chisel Scaler. A. Surface to be ground. B. Chisel is adapted to the surface of a stationary flat stone at the proper angle to maintain the original bevel of 45 degrees. Arrow indicates direction of the sharpening stroke leading into the cutting edge.

ment forward, toward the cutting edge, without changing the relationship with the stone.

C. After two or three applications, test for sharpness and reapply as necessary for an ideal cutting edge.

D. Hone the nonbeveled surface.

III. Round Corners

Round the corners at each end of the cutting edge. In a manner similar to that shown in figure 32–19 for the hoe scaler, rub the surface of the flat stone across each corner of the chisel with a gentle, even, rolling motion. Two or three applications are usually sufficient.

SHARPENING EXPLORERS

I. Tests for Sharpness
A. Visual

When examined under concentrated light, a dull explorer tip appears rounded. The tip may reflect light.

B. Plastic Testing Stick

A sharp explorer grips the plastic tester on light pressure and moves with resistance when pulled over the surface. A dull explorer does not catch. It slides.

II. Recontour

Small-nosed pliers can be used to straighten a bent tip.

III. Sharpening Procedure

A. Prepare flat stone.

B. Instrument is held with a modified pen grasp. Finger rest is established on side of stone.

C. Placement and movement of the tip over the stone resemble somewhat the procedure for the curet on the stone (figure 32–12, page 448).
1. Place side of tip on stone at approximately a 15- to 20-degree angle of stone with shank of explorer.
2. As tip is moved over the surface, the handle is rotated so that even pressure can be applied to each part of the tip.

CARE OF SHARPENING STONES

I. Flat Arkansas Stone

A. Prepare for Sterilization

Submerge in ultrasonic cleaner or scrub with soap and hot water to remove oil, petroleum jelly, and/or metal particles left from sharpening. Wrap and seal for sterilization.

B. Stain Removal

Periodically clean with ammonia, gasoline, or kerosene when stone becomes discolored. If the

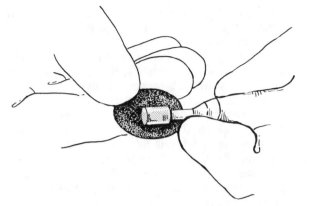

Figure 32–21. Care of a Mounted Stone. A Joe Dandy disc is used to maintain a smooth surface on the stone. Repeated sharpenings tend to make grooves in a stone.

stone becomes "glazed" by metal particles ground into the surface, rub the stone over emery paper placed on a flat, solid surface.

C. Storage

Keep in sealed, sterilized package until needed for sharpening.

II. Mounted Stones

A. Arkansas Mounted Stones

Same basic procedures as for the flat stone.

B. Ruby Stone
1. Clean by scrubbing with soap and water.
2. Maintain an ungrooved surface by frequently applying the stone to a Joe Dandy disc (figure 32–21). A sandpaper disc is too flexible for this purpose.
3. Sterilize in a sealed bag.

III. Manufacturer's Directions

Follow manufacturer's directions for all artificial stones.

TECHNICAL HINTS

I. Prevent unnecessary dulling of instruments by applying the following suggestions:

A. When handling instruments for cleaning, sterilizing, or other reasons, keep blades from hooking, bumping, or pressing against each other, as cutting edges become dull from contact with hard surfaces. Thinner instruments, such as explorers and probes, are subject to bending and breaking.

B. During instrumentation, utilize instruments at the appropriate angulation to the teeth. Avoid pressing instrument against hard surface of metallic restorations.

II. Discard instruments that have been reduced so much by frequent sharpening that even moderate to slight pressure flexes the blade. A tip could break off in a pocket or interproximally during instrumentation.

III. Sharpening of files has not been included in this chapter for several reasons. Because sharpening of files is a difficult procedure owing to the several parallel cutting edges, the amount of time consumed in sharpening with limited promise of effective results may not be justified. When sharpening of a file is required, a jeweler's tang file may be obtained for that purpose. Use of a professional sharpening service or return of the files to the manufacturer for sharpening is highly recommended.

References

1. Pattison, G.L. and Pattison, A.M.: *Periodontal Instrumentation.* Reston, Virginia, Reston Publishing Co., 1979, p. 150.
2. Barnes, J.E. and Schaffer, E.M.: Subgingival Root Planing: A Comparison Using Files, Hoes, and Curettes, *J. Periodontol., 31,* 300, September, 1960.
3. Green, E. and Ramfjord, S.P.: Tooth Roughness After Subgingival Root Planing, *J. Periodontol., 37,* 396, September-October, 1966.
4. W.R. Case & Sons Cutlery Company, Bradford, Pennsylvania 16701.
5. Hu-Friedy Manufacturing Company, 3232 N. Rockwell Street, Chicago, Illinois 60618.
6. Juranitch, J.A.: Sharpening Secrets of a Pro, *Popular Science, 210,* 118, February, 1977.

Suggested Readings

Biller, I.R. and Karlsson, U.L.: SEM of Curet Edges, *Dent. Hyg., 53,* 549, December, 1979.
Bower, R.C.: An Aid for Sharpening Periodontal Instruments, *Aust. Dent. J., 28,* 212, August, 1983.
Carranza, F.A.: *Glickman's Clinical Periodontology,* 6th ed. Philadelphia, W.B. Saunders Co., 1984, pp. 630–642.
DeNucci, D.J. and Mader, C.L.: Scanning Electron Microscopic Evaluation of Several Resharpening Techniques, *J. Periodontol., 54,* 618, October, 1983.
Green, E. and Seyer, P.C.: *Sharpening Curets and Sickle Scalers,* 2nd ed. Berkeley, California, Praxis Publishing Co., 1972, 40 pp.
Hoople, S.: Files Provide Desirable Results in Patient Treatment Procedures, *RDH, 5,* 22, November/December, 1985.
Huntley, D.E.: A Fine Edge: Instrument Sharpening, Part I, *RDH, 2,* 15, July/August, 1982.
Huntley, D.E.: Honing Your Technique. Instrument Sharpening, Part II, *RDH, 2,* 51, September/October, 1982.
Marquam, B.J.: Strategies to Improve Instrument Sharpening, *Dent. Hyg., 62,* 334, July/August, 1988.
Murray, G.H., Lubow, R.M., Mayhew, R.B., Summitt, J.B., and Usseglio, R.J.: The Effects of Two Sharpening Methods on the Strength of a Periodontal Scaling Instrument, *J. Periodontol., 55,* 410, July, 1984.
Newell, K.J., Furry, C.A., Haider, M.L., and Lange, A.L.: Evaluating Sharpness of Gracey Curets, *Educ. Directions, 5,* 25, August, 1980.
Nield, J.S. and Houseman, G.A.: *Fundamentals of Dental Hygiene Instrumentation,* 2nd ed. Philadelphia, Lea & Febiger, 1988, pp. 229–335, 471–483.
Parker, M.E.: Recontouring Instruments to Prolong Life, *RDH, 3,* 44, July/August, 1983.
Parkes, R.B. and Kolstad, R.A.: Effects of Sterilization on Periodontal Instruments, *J. Periodontol., 53,* 434, July, 1982.
Pattison, G.L. and Pattison, A.M.: *Periodontal Instrumentation.* Reston, Virginia, Reston Publishing Co., 1979, pp. 308–333.
Sasse, J.: Cutting Edges of Curets. Effect of Repeated Sterilization, *Dent. Hyg., 61,* 14, January, 1987.
Smith, B.A., Setter, M.S., Caffesse, R.G., and Bye, F.L.: The Effect of Sharpening Stones Upon Curet Surface Roughness, *Quintessence Int., 18,* 603, September, 1987.
Taylor, G.B.: Teaching Instrument Design by the Inquiry Approach: A Preliminary Report, *Educ. Directions, 6,* 25, December, 1981.
United States Department of Health, Education and Welfare, Project Acorde: *Instrument Sharpening.* Castro Valley, California, Quercus Corp., August, 1976, 107 pp.
Wehmeyer, T.E.: Chairside Instrument Sharpening, *Quintessence Int., 18,* 615, September, 1987.
Zimmer, S.E.: Instrument Sharpening—Sickle Scalers and Curettes, *Dent. Hyg., 52,* 21, January, 1978.

33 Scaling and Root Planing

Complete subgingival scaling and root planing are specific procedures in the treatment of inflammatory gingival and periodontal diseases. *Scaling* and *root planing* provide definitive or complete treatment for many patients with less advanced periodontal infections, and preparatory or initial therapy for those with more advanced disease. In addition to the patient's personal daily plaque removal program, scaling and root planing are considered the first line of treatment in nonsurgical periodontal therapy. The ultimate goals are elimination of pathogenic microorganisms and health of the tissue.

The success of treatment depends on the control of bacterial plaque by the patient. Therefore, instruction and supervision in plaque control procedures precede, continue simultaneously with, and follow instrumentation for treatment.

Scaling and planing must be thorough to be effective. When calculus is left on the teeth, surfaces are not smooth, and areas of root surface contain endotoxin and other bacterial products, gingival irritation and inflammation can persist, and the pocket microflora repopulate the pocket sooner.

Development of ability, skill, and efficiency in the successful removal of calculus through positive scaling procedures requires more than the development of dexterity for applying instruments to the tooth surfaces. In these refined and exacting techniques, the dental hygienist must apply knowledge of the anatomic, histologic, and physiologic characteristics of the teeth and gingival tissues to the fullest advantage of the patient.

I. Definitions

A. Scaling

Scaling is the basic treatment procedure by which calculus is removed from the surfaces of the teeth. Scaling is divided into supragingival and subgingival scaling, depending on the location of the calculus in relation to the gingival margin (figure 33–3, page 458).

B. Root Planing

Root planing is the meticulous treatment procedure for the removal of residual calculus and altered cementum and for smoothing the surfaces of the roots. When the root surface is exposed following gingival recession or surgery, root planing is performed supragingivally; otherwise, it is a subgingival procedure.*

II. Purposes

Complete supragingival and subgingival scaling and root planing, accompanied by the patient's therapeutic bacterial-plaque removal on a daily basis, are specific procedures for the treatment of inflammatory periodontal infections. The effects and benefits are listed here.

A. Interrupt or stop the progress of disease.

B. Induce positive changes in the count and content of the subgingival bacterial flora.
  1. Before instrumentation, the predominant microorganisms are anaerobic, gram-negative, motile forms, with many spirochetes and rods, high counts of all types of microorganisms, and many leukocytes.
  2. After instrumentation, the composition of the bacterial flora shifts to a predominance of aerobic, gram-positive, nonmotile, coccoid forms, with lowered total counts and fewer leukocytes.

C. Create an environment that encourages the tissue to heal and the inflammation to be resolved.
  1. Convert pocket (disease) to sulcus (health).
  2. Shrink previously enlarged spongy tissue.
  3. Reduce probed pocket depth.
  4. Eliminate bleeding on probing.
  5. Regenerate the gingival tissues to normal color, size, and contour (table 11–1, page 174).
  6. Change the quality of the tissues from spongy to firm.
  7. Improve the integrity of attachment.

D. Increase the effectiveness of the patient's plaque control measures.

E. Provide initial preparation (tissue conditioning) for complicated periodontal therapy required for advanced disease.
  1. Reduce or eliminate etiologic and predisposing factors.
  2. Permit reevaluation. Surgical procedures may be lessened in extent.

F. Prevent recurrence of disease through maintenance supervision and treatment.

---

*Root planing is sometimes called root curettage. In this book the term curettage is reserved for curettage of the soft tissues. Gingival curettage is the process by which the diseased tissue lining the gingival sulcus or pocket wall is removed (Chapter 34).

PREPARATION FOR INSTRUMENTATION

I. Review the Patient's Record
A. Study the data from the diagnostic work-up.
B. Note special needs and plan accordingly.

II. Check Premedication Requirements for Risk Patient

A. Bacteremia Following Instrumentation
Bacteremia means the presence of bacteria in the blood. A transient bacteremia can occur during and immediately after any type of oral surgery, periodontal therapy, scaling and root planing, or any treatment that may produce bleeding.[1,2,3]

B. Factors Affecting the Incidence of Bacteremia
1. Degree of trauma inflicted during instrumentation.[4]
2. Severity of gingival or periodontal infection present.[5,6] In one study patients with clinically healthy gingiva had a 21.6 percent incidence of bacteremia, those with gingivitis a 29.0 percent incidence, and those with periodontitis a 51.2 percent incidence following scaling and root planing.[6]

C. Premedication
1. Certain risk patients who require antibiotic premedication are listed on pages 85 and 91.
2. Ask to make sure that the patient has taken the prescribed medication 1 hour before the scheduled appointment.

III. Use of Radiographs
The radiographic survey can be a useful adjunct during scaling appointments. Radiographic findings were outlined on pages 207–209.
A. Place the radiographs on a lighted viewbox before gloving.
B. Review findings applicable during instrumentation, such as
  1. Anatomic features of roots, furcations, and bone level.
  2. Overhanging restorations that must be removed (page 529).
  3. Carious lesions that may "catch."

IV. Patient Preparation
Patient factors for the appointment were described on page 56. As the instrumentation for scaling and root planing is carried out, aseptic procedures with protection for both patient and clinician must be followed.
A. Instruct patient to rinse with a germicidal mouthrinse to reduce the numbers of oral microorganisms and, hence, the contamination of aerosols.
B. Provide protective eyewear for the patient.

V. Supragingival Examination
A. Visual
Gross and moderate deposits and surface irregularities can be seen directly. Fine, unstained, white or yellowish calculus is frequently invisible when wet with saliva. Dry calculus is seen more readily than is wet calculus. Procedures for calculus detection were described on page 248.

B. Tactile Method
Without deposits the enamel surface is smooth; an explorer passed over the surface slides freely, smoothly, and quietly. Calculus deposits are rough; the explorer does not slide freely, but meets with resistance and produces a scratchy sound.

VI. Subgingival Examination

A. Determine the Need for Instrumentation
Prior to actual scaling and root planing, a probe and subgingival explorer must be used to locate calculus and areas of root roughness, to define the extent of instrumentation that is required.

Scaling and root planing in shallow pockets (sulci) of fewer than 3 mm. can lead to loss of periodontal attachment.[7,8,9] Research has shown that repeated scaling results in detachment of periodontal ligament fibers from the root cementum and that healing does not bring them back.[9]

The use of a curet as an explorer or to clean out subgingival bacterial plaque should be discouraged.

B. Make a Direct Visual Examination
1. *Gingiva.* The following clinical appearance of the gingival tissues reveals or is highly suggestive of the presence of subgingival calculus:
   a. Gingival tissue that is soft, spongy, non-resilient, bluish-red, with enlargement of the marginal gingiva, a rolled edge that tends to be separated from the tooth surface, and a smooth shiny surface on which stippling is indistinct or missing.
   b. Dark-colored subgingival calculus that may sometimes be seen as a dark area beneath relatively translucent marginal gingiva.
2. *Subgingival calculus.* A loose and resilient pocket wall can be separated from the tooth surface. Apply compressed air gently to the gingival margin, deflect the tissue, and look into the pocket. Dark subgingival calculus can be seen.

C. Note the Position and Anatomy of Teeth
1. Close, narrow contact areas where the insertion of a curet to the bottom of a pocket may be difficult or impossible.
2. Furcation variations. Figure 33–1 shows different anatomic features that may impede access for scaling and root planing.
3. Other contributing factors are listed in Chapter 12, pages 185–186.

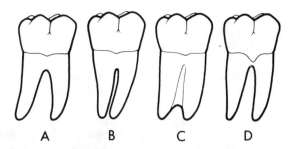

Figure 33–1. Anatomic Variations of Furcations. A. Widely separated. **B.** Separated but close together. **C.** Fused roots separated only in the apical portion. **D.** Presence of an enamel projection that may be conducive to an early furcation involvement. (From Carranza, F.A.: *Glickman's Clinical Periodontology*, 6th ed. W.B. Saunders Co., 1984, page 847.)

D. Apply Probe and Explorer Findings

1. Use pocket recordings from periodontal charting as a basic guide for scaling.
2. Perform additional probing during the immediate appointment.
   a. Anesthesia facilitates exact examination. If patient is to receive anesthesia, the clinician should probe while the anesthetic is in effect.
   b. Tissue may change between appointments. Patient's plaque control procedures often condition the tissue; bleeding is lessened, tissue may have tightened, and pockets may be more shallow.
   c. Figure 33–2 illustrates probing of irregularities of a tooth surface. A probe passing over the surface of the root may be intercepted by calculus (figure 33–2B).
   d. Tooth topography is evaluated. For example, the groove and furcation of a mandibular molar may be examined by using a horizontal stroke, as shown in figure 33–2C.
3. Use explorer before, during, and at the completion of scaling and root planing to evaluate a tooth surface.

pletion of scaling and root planing to evaluate a tooth surface.

PROCEDURE FOR SCALING

I. Clinical Approach

Criteria for the determination of treatment sequence were described on page 293 in connection with treatment planning. Application of the concept of *tissue conditioning* by the patient in preparation for scaling and root planing contributes to more efficient treatment and more predictable and rapid postoperative healing. Tissue conditioning is described on page 294.

Prerequisite to any selected procedure is the use of an efficient routine to minimize time. With respect to the use of individual instruments, one time-saver is the application of one instrument to all appropriate tooth surfaces within a quadrant or area being treated. Similar use of the next instrument follows. This procedure minimizes transfer to and from the tray. Each instrument may need supplemental sharpening during the treatment of the area.

The advantages of a systematic procedure are
A. Thoroughness in the completion of treatment.
B. Ease and smoothness of procedure.
C. Increased efficiency through repeated routine.
D. Decrease in time required to complete the treatment.
E. Increase in patient comfort.
F. Increase in patient's confidence in the clinician.

II. Overall System

A. Single Appointment

When a single appointment is expected to be sufficient to complete the scaling of the entire dentition, gross supragingival deposits throughout the dentition should be removed first by manual or ultrasonic techniques. The finer scaling for each area can then be completed.

B. Planned Multiple Appointments

When extensive scaling and root planing must be accomplished because of generalized supra- and subgingival calculus, a series of appointments can be planned, as suggested on page 295.
1. *Quadrant Scaling and Root Planing Appointments*
   a. Appointments are scheduled at 1-week intervals to permit progressive healing.
   b. Use of local anesthesia for each quadrant may be indicated.*
   c. Plaque control procedures can be reviewed and supplemented before scaling at each appointment.
2. *Complete a Selected Area*

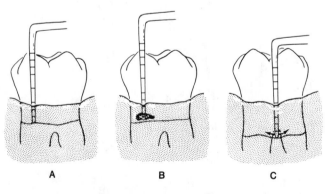

Figure 33–2. Subgingival Examination Using a Probe. A. Probe inserted to the bottom of a pocket for complete examination prior to subgingival scaling and root planing. **B.** As the probe passes over the root surface, it may be intercepted by a hard mass of calculus. **C.** Using a horizontal probe stroke to examine the topography of a furcation area.

*Local anesthesia must be provided by the dentist in states where state practice acts have not been changed to allow the dental hygienist to administer the anesthesia.

a. Scale one quadrant (or selected group of teeth) thoroughly before moving to the next. Do not move from area to area.

b. When anesthesia is used, concentrate only on the anesthetized area.

C. Incomplete Scaling

One system that has been used involves an initial "gross scaling" or "prescaling." A series of appointments then is planned for deep scaling and root planing by quadrants or sextants. Before using this system, the following should be considered:

1. *Potential for Abscess Formation.* Incomplete, superficial scaling of deep pockets can lead to abscess formation, especially when the pockets extend into furcation areas or intrabony defects.

   a. With partial healing, the tissue at the gingival margin tightens, the pocket closes, bacteria multiply within, white blood cells are attracted until pus forms, and an abscess develops (page 486).

   b. Susceptibility to abscess formation is greater in persons susceptible to infection, such as those with uncontrolled diabetes or with an immunodeficiency disease, or those being medicated with an immunosuppressive drug.

2. *Healing at the Gingival Margin.* Insertion of curets for additional deep instrumentation is difficult in chronically healed tightened tissue.

3. *Tissue Conditioning.* At the initial appointment, the patient is instructed in the care of the mouth and the need for daily plaque removal. By teaching the patient about diseased tissue and letting the patient condition the tissues, many lessons are learned.

4. *Patient Instruction.* When calculus is removed all at once, the visual lesson is taken away. With complete treatment area by area, the patient can see and feel changes and improvements that contrast with non-treated areas.

5. *Roughened Calculus.* Calculus roughened by partial removal may be a source of great irritation to the gingiva because of its increased ability to hold a covering of bacterial plaque.

6. *Patient Misunderstanding.* For the patient with limited understanding of the seriousness and extent of periodontal infection, the mouth may "feel clean and look good" at the end of the gross scaling. Thus, the patient may not return for subsequent appointments because the personal objective has been fulfilled. When severe periodontitis, with continued loss of attachment, alveolar bone loss, and the signs of mobility, later develops, the patient may claim that incomplete treatment was given at earlier appointments. By receiving repeated information at each successive treatment, the patient may be able to understand and appreciate the necessity for multiple appointments.

III. Calculus Removal

Calculus is removed by systematic scaling from tooth to tooth and section by section of the calculus deposit on each tooth surface. Each scaling stroke overlaps the previous stroke as the scaler is positioned progressively along the area of the deposit.

A. Location of Instrumentation

Figure 33–3 illustrates the location of instrumentation on the tooth surface. The type of

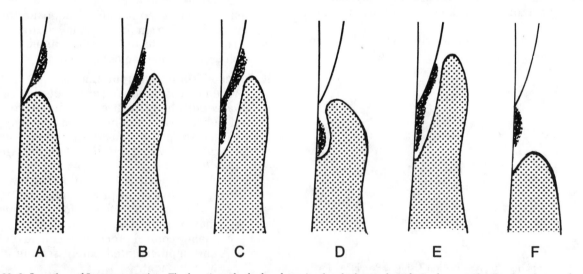

Figure 33–3. Location of Instrumentation. The location of calculus deposits, level of periodontal attachment, depth of pocket, and position of the gingival margin determine the site of instrumentation. **A.** Supragingival calculus on the enamel. **B.** Gingival pocket with both supra- and subgingival calculus on enamel. **C.** Periodontal pocket with both supra- and subgingival calculus. **D.** Periodontal pocket with subgingival calculus only on cementum. **E.** Periodontal pocket with subgingival calculus only on both enamel and cementum. **F.** Calculus on cementum exposed by gingival recession.

pocket, location of calculus, position of the margin of the free gingiva, and level of periodontal tissue attachment all determine the location of instrumentation and instrument selection for that instrumentation.

B. Effect of Mode of Calculus Attachment

Removal of calculus relates to the mode of attachment (page 250). Calculus removal from enamel is different from the calculus removal and root planing required for cementum.

C. Steps

Scaling is not a shaving process in which layers are removed. Such a procedure tends to make the surface of the calculus smooth and burnished and sometimes indistinguishable from the tooth surface. The oldest calculus, that next to the tooth surface, is the hardest calculus.

The basic principles for the five fundamental steps in the application of an instrument for calculus removal and root planing were described in Chapter 31, pages 430–435. In the sections following, the steps are described in detail for supragingival instrumentation and then are followed by additional adaptations required for subgingival instrumentation. The five steps are:

1. Grasp of instrument.
2. Establishment of finger rest.
3. Adaptation
4. Angulation
5. Activation
   a. Working Stroke. Activate the instrument.
   b. Apply lateral pressure.
   c. Completion of Stroke. Prepare for the next.

SUPRAGINGIVAL SCALING

I. Instruments

A. Scalers: Sickle, Hoe, Chisel

These instruments are designed for supragingival instrumentation. Sickles are sometimes used to remove gross calculus that may be 1 or 2 mm. below the gingival margin, provided the tissue of the gingival pocket wall is loose and the instrument can be inserted without force.

B. Curet

A curet is used primarily for subgingival instrumentation, but is recommended for supragingival scaling and planing in the following instances:

1. When a curved, rounded instrument is particularly adaptable for removing fine, hard deposits near the gingival margin.
2. When gingival recession has caused exposure of cementum, and root planing techniques are required.

II. Steps for Calculus Removal

A. Grasp the Instrument

1. Apply modified pen grasp (figure 31–3, page 431).

2. Use a light grasp while instrument is positioned and at the completion of the stroke; tighten grasp during the working stroke.

B. Establish the Finger Rest

1. Use ring and little fingers on firm tooth or teeth for the major rest; apply supplementary rests for increased stability when indicated (pages 431–433).
2. The fulcrum where the finger rest is applied must be dry for stability. Plaque and saliva make tooth surfaces slippery. Use a folded gauze sponge in the vestibular area with a corner over the fulcrum rest tooth; dry with compressed air or wipe with cotton, maintain retraction, and repeat the drying as needed for continued instrument control.
3. Finger rests are applied on the tooth adjacent to that being scaled, or as close as possible and convenient. Long stretches between the rest and the point of instrument application can decrease control.
4. Use light but firm pressure on the finger rest while the instrument is being positioned and at the end of the stroke.
5. During the working stroke, the pressure on the fulcrum increases slightly to balance the pressure of the instrument on the tooth being scaled.

C. Adaptation

The tip third of the scaler and the toe third of the curet blade are used primarily (figure 33–4). After the tip or toe is adapted, as much of the blade as can be applied to the surface being scaled is used. Adaptation is described on page 433 and illustrated in figure 31–5.

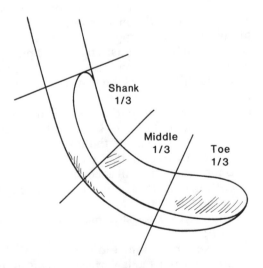

Figure 33–4. Curet Divided Into Thirds. The toe third is kept in contact with the tooth surface during instrumentation. Because of tooth contours, most strokes for scaling and root planing are accomplished using the toe third. Adaptation of the toe third is shown in figure 31–5, page 434.

D. Angulation

1. *Sickle Scaler.* Blade is applied beneath the calculus deposit so that the angle formed by the face and the tooth surface is between 60 and 80 degrees (less than 90 degrees but at least 45 degrees).
2. *Hoe Scaler.* The full width of the cutting edge is in contact with the calculus. The shank is adapted closely to the side of the tooth or is in contact with the crown of the tooth (figure 32–7, page 442).
3. *Chisel Scaler.* The full width of the cutting edge is in contact with the calculus. The shank is adapted closely to the tooth, in position for scaling from labial to lingual.
4. *Curet.* A curet is held at an angle formed by the face of the blade and the tooth surface between 60 and 80 degrees (less than 90 degrees but at least 45 degrees).

E. Activate the Instrument: Working Stroke

1. *Tighten the Grasp.* Move the instrument firmly and deliberately.
2. *Maintain the Cutting Edge.* Maintain evenly on the tooth surface during the stroke. The side of the tip or toe should always stay adapted in contact with the tooth surface.
3. *Direction of Strokes*
   a. Vertical pull strokes are used for sickle scalers and hoes; horizontal and oblique strokes may be used when away from the cervical region near the gingival margin.
   b. Vertical, horizontal, and oblique strokes may be used for the curet.
   c. Horizontal push strokes only are used for the chisel from facial to lingual at right angles with the long axis of anterior teeth.
4. *Lateral Pressure of the Instrument* (on tooth surface). When the instrument is sharp, the minimum pressure applied allows the cutting edge to grip the calculus; a balance of pressure is maintained between the pressure of the instrument, the grasp of the instrument, and the pressure on the finger rest.
5. *Control of Motion.* Without independent finger movement, the hand, wrist, and arm act as a continuum to activate the instrument.
6. *Length of Stroke.* Short.
   a. Short strokes permit accommodation of the cutting edge to changes in the topography of the tooth surface.
   b. Short strokes assist in maintaining *control* and *precision.*
   c. Strokes are confined to the area of the deposit on the tooth surface known as the *instrumentation zone.*[10] Extending the instrument up the side of the tooth in unnecessarily long strokes is time-consuming, dulls the instrument, and decreases

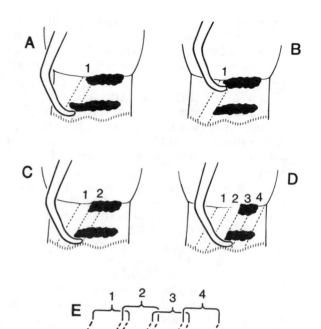

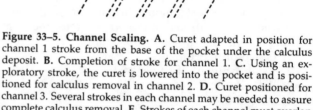

Figure 33–5. Channel Scaling. A. Curet adapted in position for channel 1 stroke from the base of the pocket under the calculus deposit. **B.** Completion of stroke for channel 1. **C.** Using an exploratory stroke, the curet is lowered into the pocket and is positioned for calculus removal in channel 2. **D.** Curet positioned for channel 3. Several strokes in each channel may be needed to assure complete calculus removal. **E.** Strokes of each channel must overlap strokes of the previous channel. (Adapted from Parr, R.W., Green, E., Madsen, L., and Miller, S.: *Subgingival Scaling and Root Planing.* Berkeley, California, Praxis Publishing Co., 1976.)

control by and concentration of the clinician.

F. Completion of Stroke

1. Hold instrument in place momentarily, maintain the finger rest, lighten the grasp on the instrument, and then return the instrument to position for a repeat stroke.
2. Repeat strokes until surface is smooth.

G. Continuation of Procedure

1. Move instrument laterally on the tooth surface to adjacent undisturbed deposit; maintain the same finger rest.
2. Overlap strokes in channels to ensure complete removal of deposit (figure 33–5). Roll the handle between the fingers of the grasp to maintain adaptation at line angles and other variations of tooth anatomy.
3. Repeat strokes until the tooth surface has been completely scaled.
4. Examine surface with explorer assisted by compressed air; repeat scaling strokes as needed to produce a smooth surface that is free of calculus.

SUBGINGIVAL INSTRUMENTATION

Dexterity, deliberateness, and diligence are key words in perfecting the techniques for subgingival areas. *The principal objectives are to remove the calculus and to plane the root surface with a minimum of trauma to the gingival tissue.* Procedures are guided by the recognized need for removal of all calculus and altered cementum to assure maximum tissue response for oral health.

Root planing follows calculus removal. It is a continuation and an integral part of subgingival scaling. Not all root planing is subgingival, because when root surfaces are exposed as a result of recession or periodontal surgery, the cemental surface is supragingival (figure 33–3F).

I. Comparison of Supragingival and Subgingival Instrumentation

Although the basic techniques and steps described previously for removal of supragingival calculus are applied in the subgingival area, subgingival techniques are complicated by several factors.

A. Accessibility
Instrumentation is necessary in areas where access is difficult.

B. Invisible Working Area
Techniques depend almost entirely on tactile sensitivity. Location and removal of minute roughnesses of the tooth surface require a keenly developed tactile sensitivity.

C. Calculus Attachment
Attachment of calculus to the cementum is more tenacious than to the enamel. On the cementum, calculus attaches to minute irregularities and in areas of cemental resorption. Direct attachment of the calculus matrix to the root surface, which makes removal difficult, may also occur. Attachment to the enamel is primarily by means of the acquired pellicle, which makes calculus removal much easier (page 250).

D. Morphology of Calculus
Subgingival calculus is irregularly deposited and occurs in nodular, ledge or ring-like, smooth veneer, and other forms (table 17–1, page 249).

E. Variations in Root Surface Topography
Although many variations can be expected as part of the normal tooth anatomy, some unusual variations complicate scaling primarily because of their invisibility. The roots and furcation areas shown in figure 33–1 are examples of differences that can be found.

F. Variations in Depth of Pockets
Pockets must be measured about each tooth because variations in depth can occur on a single surface. Instruments must be adapted to reach the bottom of the pocket around the entire periphery of each tooth.

G. Gingival Wall
The gingival wall is close to the tooth surface. Only a narrow area is available for manipulation of instruments. The width of the pocket varies; it narrows down at the base next to the attachment area.

II. Instrument Selection: Curets

As mentioned previously, gross calculus just below the gingival margin may be removed during supragingival scaling, provided the tissue is loose and resilient enough to permit easy access by the instruments without forcing them into the sulcus. The ultrasonic scaler may also be used to remove gross subgingival deposits (pages 465–468).

The curets are the instruments of choice deeper in the pocket and close to the root surface for several reasons:

A. Fine, thin instruments permit the increased tactile sensitivity that bulkier instruments cannot. Increased sensitivity is essential to thoroughness in areas with limited accessibility and visibility.

B. Root planing with curets produces smoother surfaces than does planing with other instruments.[11,12,13,14]

C. The curved, narrow, fine curets with rounded ends can be adapted to the anatomic features of the subgingival area with less trauma to the tooth surface and the gingival tissue. Supragingival sickles, hoes, and chisels have sharp points or corners and are thick, bulky, and straight.

D. The sulcus or pocket narrows in the deeper area close to the attachment. The smallest, smoothest instruments are best applied to this narrow area to prevent the need for excess stretching of the gingival wall, where a splitting of the attachment from the tooth can occur.

E. Because of the rounded toe end, a horizontal stroke can be used conservatively. The length of the horizontal stroke depends on variations in pocket depth. When used in position for a vertical stroke, the rounded back of the curet can be placed against the bottom of the pocket.

SUBGINGIVAL PROCEDURES

After root surface evaluation with probe and explorer, as described on pages 183 and 456, the same basic five steps for calculus removal are followed as for supragingival scaling. Variations are listed in the following.

A universal curet is used for convenience and efficiency to remove heavier subgingival calculus. The smaller, area-specific curets should be reserved and kept sharp for fine scaling and root planing, particularly in the narrow depth of the pocket.

I. Grasp the Instrument

A modified pen grasp is used. The grasp is lightened as increased tactile sense is needed for refinement of the root surface with continued root planing.

II. Establish the Finger Rest

1. A definite finger rest on dry, firm tooth structure as close to the tooth being treated as possible and convenient is indicated.
2. Complete control is essential.

III. Adaptation

A. Position the toe third of the blade (figure 33–4) on the tooth surface near the gingival margin where the instrument will be inserted for subgingival scaling.
B. Ascertain whether the correct curet (of the mirror-image pair) is being applied. For a scaling or root planing stroke, the face of the instrument should be against the tooth. Only the back of the blade is clearly seen. The wrong end is being used when the whole, shiny face is clearly seen. This end is impossible to angulate correctly for scaling.

IV. Angulation

A. Hold at the appropriate angulation for scaling, that is, with the face at an angle between 60 and 80 degrees with the tooth surface.
B. Note the relationship of the handle, finger rest, grasp, blade, and tooth so that after insertion the blade may be promptly reangulated for calculus removal.

V. Insertion

A. Exploratory Stroke*

1. The exploratory stroke is a preliminary stroke in which the blade is applied lightly over the calculus until the base of the deposit is located. The blade then is positioned for the working stroke.
2. Direct the tip of the curet gingivally; maintain contact with the tooth surface.
3. With light grasp, insert the curet gently under the gingival margin (figure 33–6A).
4. Keep the instrument toe third in light contact with the tooth or calculus surface. The blade is closed toward the tooth surface and held at or near an angle of 0 degrees during the exploratory stroke (figure 33–6B).
5. Pass the instrument over the surface of the deposit to the base of the pocket until tension of the soft tissue attachment is felt.
6. Adjust the blade to the correct angulation with the tooth surface (as determined before insertion) just below the calculus deposit (figure

---

*The exploratory stroke is sometimes referred to as the preliminary or preparatory stroke. When the term "exploratory" is used, it should be distinguished from the meaning of the word as it applies to the use of an explorer. The curet is not used as an explorer, and the calculus has been identified previously by using an explorer.

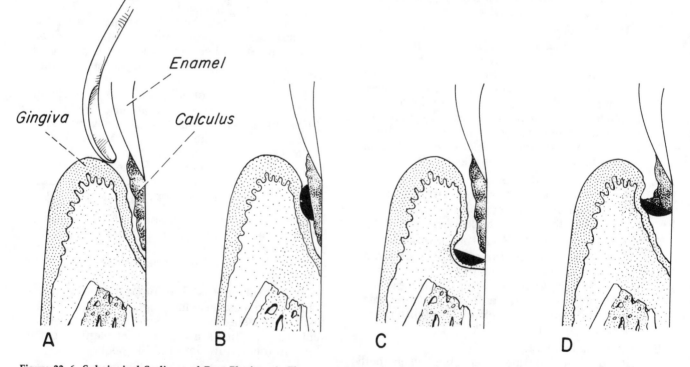

Figure 33–6. Subgingival Scaling and Root Planing. A. The curet is inserted gently under the gingival margin. **B.** With an exploratory stroke, the blade is passed over the surface of the tooth or calculus. Note 0-degree angle of the face of the curet with the calculus. **C.** The curet is lowered to the base of the pocket until the tension of the soft tissue is felt with the rounded back of the curet. The curet then is positioned at an angle of 70 to 80 degrees with the tooth surface beneath the calculus deposit. **D.** The blade is moved along the root surface in a scaling stroke to remove the calculus or in a planing stroke to smooth the surface.

33–6C). The side of the toe should be in contact with the tooth surface at all times.

VI. Activate the Instrument: Working Stroke

A. Tighten the Grasp
Move the instrument firmly and deliberately (figure 33–6D).

B. Maintain the Cutting Edge
Maintain evenly on the tooth surface during the stroke and at the completion of the stroke.

C. Direction of Strokes
1. Vertical, oblique, or horizontal strokes may be applied (figure 33–7).
2. All strokes are limited in length by the constant adjustment needed to conform with the curved tooth surfaces and the varying depths of the sulcus or pocket around the tooth.
3. Horizontal strokes cannot be applied to the bottom of the sulcus or pocket except where the probe measurements show the depth is uniform; otherwise the curet would be dragged into the attachment at the higher areas.
4. Push-pull type of stroke is not used subgingivally as it would tend to push particles and bacteria deep into the sulcus and into the soft tissue.

D. Pressure of Instrument
A balance of pressure between the pressure of the instrument, the grasp of the instrument, and the finger rest must be maintained. Undue pressure decreases control and lessens tactile sensitivity. Uncontrolled, excessive pressure causes gouges in cementum and dentin.

E. Control of Motion
Without independent finger movement, the hand, wrist, and arm act as a continuum to activate the instrument.

F. Length of Stroke
1. Use short smooth decisive strokes, the length dependent on the height of the deposit (instrumentation zone, page 460).
2. Confine the strokes within the pocket to prevent the need for repeated removal and reinsertion of the instrument.
   a. To save time.
   b. To prevent trauma to the gingival margin.

G. Completion of Stroke
Maintain finger rest, lighten grasp, and repeat exploratory stroke within the pocket. Reposition for a repeat or adjacent stroke. Several strokes are generally required for each area.

VII. Channel Strokes

A. Calculus Removal
Calculus should not be shaved off in layers. With shaving, the remaining thin veneer of calculus may be smooth and indiscernible from the tooth surface, yet contain endotoxin and other substances that can keep the gingiva from healing.

B. Overlapping Strokes (figure 33–5)
1. Repeat strokes at each channel until the area is smooth.
2. Overlap each channel with the next.
3. Roll instrument between fingers to adapt to each part of the tooth surface as scaling continues around line angles and other anatomic features.

C. Explorer
Use explorer to examine for completion of calculus removal. Some slight roughness of the cemental surface may be present. An enamel surface, however, should be completely "glassy smooth."

VIII. Plane the Root Surface

The technique for planing is basically the same as for scaling. Instrument control, adaptation and angulation at the cutting edge, directions for strokes, and other principles are not essentially different. The difference is the ultimate perfection of resulting smoothness attained because of the high degree of tactile sensitivity involved and the precise instrumentation.

Specific differences in technique are related to touch and pressure. A lighter grasp must be used to increase tactile sensitivity. Because increased pressure is not needed, a lighter shaving-like stroke can be used for smoothing or finishing the root surface.

A. Check the Sharpness of the Curets
Generally, curets dulled during scaling should be resharpened or a freshly sharpened set should be used for root planing.

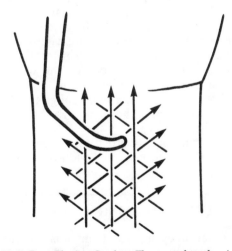

Figure 33–7. Root Planing Strokes. The use of strokes in vertical and oblique directions with light lateral pressure can eliminate grooves left after scaling. A smooth, hard surface will result. Around the cervical portion of the root, the cementum is only .02- to .05-mm thick; thus, root planing removes most of the cementum to expose the harder dentin beneath. (Adapted from Parr, R.W., Green, E., Madsen, L., and Miller, S.: *Subgingival Scaling and Root Planing.* Berkeley, California, Praxis Publishing Co., 1976, p. 42.)

B. Strokes

1. Light pressure is applied for maximum sensitivity to minute irregularities of the surface.

2. Smooth strokes with even lateral pressure that systematically overlap and cross over each other are used. As the surface becomes smoother, longer strokes with reduced pressure will help to remove small lines, scratches, or grooves without gouging the dentinal surface.

3. Vertical, then oblique, strokes are used. Then, when applicable at levels away from the attachment epithelium, horizontal strokes may be used (figure 33–7).

4. Many strokes usually are needed before a section of the root surface feels glassy smooth and hard.

5. Careful application is necessary to adapt the curet to the anatomic features of the roots. The convex rounded surfaces, the constricted cervical area, the concavities and grooves of proximal surfaces, and furcations all require precise adaptation.

6. As planing nears completion, a gradual change occurs in the sound of the instrument on the root surface. At the completion, the instrument may be nearly as quiet as when used on polished enamel.

IX. Post-treatment Procedures

A. Examine with a subgingival explorer to establish completion of instrumentation. Use strokes in vertical, oblique, and horizontal directions (figure 33–7) to check for minute grooving of the cemental or dentinal surface.

B. Irrigate all sulci or pockets. This step should be done thoroughly with warm water under mild to moderate pressure and high-velocity suction to remove particles of cementum, calculus, and all tissue debris. Research has shown that bits of calculus, debris, or microorganisms can become implanted into the underlying tissue.[15,16,17]

C. Apply pressure with a wet sponge to adapt the tissue to the tooth and minimize the blood clot for healing.

D. Give instructions for brushing, rinsing, and other pertinent care measures to be followed during the first 24 hours.

EFFECTS OF SCALING AND PLANING

An evaluation by exploring immediately after completion of instrumentation is made to ascertain that the tooth surfaces are smooth and hard and that all detectable calculus has been removed. The real evaluation, the true test of successful treatment, cannot be made until 1 to 2 weeks after the initial scaling and root planing. At that time, the response of the gingival tissue is apparent.

I. Effect on Gingiva

A. Coincidental Curettage

Without intentional curettage during scaling and root planing, some debridement (coincidental inadvertent curettage) of the lining of the sulcus or pocket occurs.[15,16,17] In the research, this effect was noted particularly in the deeper aspects, where the pocket narrows toward the attachment area. The partial curettage that occurs results from the outer or unused side of the curet blade, even though a less-than-90-degree angulation of the face of the blade to the tooth surface is maintained.

The soft tissue attachment may be partially removed, depending on the severity of the inflammation, the size of the instrument, and the amount of trauma inflicted by the clinician. The objectives of curettage are described on page 476.

B. Healing

With scaling, root planing, and plaque control, the adjacent gingival tissue heals by resolution of the inflammation. Edema recedes, necrotic cells are cleared away, and the tissue regenerates.

Healing has been shown to start with beginning epithelial regeneration within 2 days of scaling. New attachment to the tooth surface has been demonstrated as early as 5 days, and complete regeneration occurs by approximately 2 weeks.[18,19] Healing time is generally related to the severity of the periodontal inflammation at the start of treatment.

After scaling and root planing, followed by bacterial plaque control by the patient, the formation of a long junctional epithelium can be expected.[20]

C. Effect of Partial Scaling

When altered cementum or even a small amount of subgingival calculus is left on a tooth surface, an area of inflammation can persist. At examination on the subsequent appointment, tissue shrinkage may be evident, and the remaining deposit can be removed readily for complete resolution.

In contrast, partial overall scaling, sometimes referred to as "gross preliminary scaling," performed with the intent to schedule additional appointments for quadrant or sextant scalings has significant limitations (page 458).

When large or small deposits are left after incomplete scaling, particularly in a deep pocket or furcation area, an acute periodontal abscess may form as mentioned on page 486. A periodontal abscess results in pain, swelling, tooth sensitivity, and various other symptoms.[21,22] Such abscesses can be prevented by completing calculus removal and planing at the initial scaling.

Only as many teeth as can be completed in a given appointment should be undertaken. Other teeth should remain untouched except for plaque control instruction.

II. Effect on Tooth Surface

Research has shown that, following careful subgingival scaling and root planing, some calculus frequently remains. During root planing, the altered cementum and residual calculus are removed. The cementum is partly or wholly removed to obtain a smooth and hard root surface. The amount varies from surface to surface.[23,24]

Cementum must be removed because the surface, exposed after recession of the junctional epithelium during pocket formation, is rough, soft, and altered by bacterial and inflammatory substances from the contents of the pocket. Altered cementum contains endotoxin and other toxic substances that can prevent healing of the adjacent gingival tissue and can aggravate continuing inflammation.

The removal of endotoxin from diseased altered cementum has been measured.[25] When tooth surfaces were scaled but not root planed, the endotoxin content of the surface was much greater than the content of healthy, unexposed tooth surfaces. After manual root planing, however, the tooth surfaces were nearly as free of endotoxin as were the healthy, unexposed surfaces.

Teeth that had been scaled were studied by electron microscopy.[24] The tooth surfaces that were under calculus were less mineralized than were exposed root surfaces. An exchange of minerals occurs between the saliva and the tooth. Following exposure for 3 to 4 weeks after scaling, some surfaces became hypermineralized, whereas others became decalcified and carious.

Knowledge of the processes involved in the surface changes can aid in the prevention of cemental caries, hypersensitivity, and calculus. Fluoride-containing dentifrice and mouthrinse should be routinely recommended following root planing when apparent recession and exposed cementum exist.

III. Effect on Pocket Microorganisms[26,27,28,29]

The subgingival bacterial flora is changed after scaling and root planing. Prior to instrumentation for treatment of periodontitis, the subgingival microorganisms are primarily anaerobic, gram-negative, motile forms, with bacterioides and spirochetes predominating.

After scaling and root planing, the total number of subgingival organisms decreases substantially. A shift to aerobic, gram-positive, nonmotile forms occurs. Spirochetes and bacterioides are reduced, and coccoid cells become more prominent.

With the conversion of the disease-producing gram-negative pocket microorganisms to a health-producing gram-positive flora, the gingiva reflects the changes. Gingival bleeding on probing is lessened, and the color, size, shape, and other characteristics assume a normal appearance.

Without personal daily plaque control, the microorganisms can return to pretreatment levels within an average of 42 days.[28] With plaque control, the repopulation of the pocket takes much longer, even in susceptible patients. In many patients, nonsurgical periodontal therapy effects a gingival condition that can be maintained free from reinfection.

ULTRASONIC AND SONIC SCALING

Ultrasonic instrumentation and sonic instrumentation are adjuncts to, but not substitutes for, manual scaling. The powered instruments are indicated primarily for adult patients with gross calculus.

Root planing must be completed by curets. The ultrasonic method, therefore, is principally used for treatment when deposits are gross, but is not applicable for preventive scaling measures when small deposits are removed at frequent maintenance appointments.

When the energy output is low, the hand pressure light, and the tip of the instrument broad and polished where it touches the tooth, presumably no adverse effects on the tooth surfaces would be expected, at least not within a reasonable number of applications.[30]

While the instrument tip is on calculus, the tooth surface is unaffected. Consequently, tactile sensitivity of the clinician is diminished appreciably. The tooth surface, therefore, should be examined with an explorer frequently during instrumentation so that excessive application of the instrument to the tooth structure can be avoided. Also, instrument application must be minimal when small discrete calculus deposits must be removed.

In addition to the removal of heavy calculus deposits, an ultrasonic instrument may be used in various other ways, including the removal of overhanging restorations and in periodontal curettage and surgery. In orthodontics, ultrasonic instrumentation has been found effective for scaling prior to fitting and cementing appliances, and for the removal of excess cement after initial cementation and after removal of appliances.

The American Dental Association, Council on Dental Materials, Instruments, and Equipment evaluates professional scaling devices. They are classified as Acceptable or Provisionally Acceptable, and use the seal shown in figure 23–15, page 331.[30,31]

I. Mode of Action[32,33]

The two types of ultrasonic instruments are magnetostrictive and the piezoelectric. Sonic instruments are air turbine.

A. Ultrasonic: Magnetostrictive

The ultrasonic unit consists of an electric generator, a handpiece assembly, a set of interchangeable prophylaxis inserts, and a foot control. The ultrasonic principle is based on the use of high-frequency sound waves.

1. The ultrasonic machine converts high-frequency electrical energy into mechanical energy in the form of rapid vibrations.

2. The instrument tip vibrations vary for different models, but may be, for example, 25,000 cycles per second (range 25,000 to 35,000) in an elliptical motion. The vibratory action fractures the deposit and causes its removal from the tooth.

3. Ultrasonic waves are dissipated in the form of heat. The heat is reduced by keeping the handpiece cooled internally and the working end cooled by a constant flow of water, which is expelled through a metal tube or by means of an internal flow through the working end.

4. The atomized water forms minute vacuum bubbles that collapse with release of tremendous local pressure; the effect is cleansing to the area. Because the instrument must be in contact with the deposit on the tooth surface if the deposit is to be removed, the bubbling cavitational action of the water has little, if any, actual influence on deposit removal.

B. Ultrasonic: Piezoelectric

1. A quartz or metal alloy crystal transducer converts electrical energy into ultrasonic vibrations.

2. No magnetic field is present, and less heat is produced.

3. Vibrations at the tip range from 29,000 to 40,000 cycles per second in a linear action.

4. Water cooling is needed to cool the friction between the tip and the tooth surface.

C. Sonic

1. Attached to conventional handpiece operated with clean, dry air (cannot attach to an oiled air line); advantage in small size and convenience of attachment without separate unit.

2. Vibrations at the tip range from 2000 to 6500 cycles per second, a disadvantage because less power means less action for calculus removal. The tip revolves in an elliptical or an orbital path.

3. Heat is not generated, but water cooling is indicated.

4. Air turbine produces a high pitched sound.

II. Indications for Use

A. Heavy, gross calculus deposits generalized throughout the dentition.

B. Tenacious deposits of calculus and stain, provided great care is taken to avoid overheating of the tooth.

C. Initial debridement for a patient with necrotizing ulcerative gingivitis or other condition that can be relieved by removal of deposits, provided that loose debris, materia alba, and microorganisms are first removed by rinses, brushing, and flossing during patient instruction to prevent contaminated aerosol production.

D. Prescaling for oral surgery, such as tooth removal (pages 589–591).

III. Contraindications for Use

A. Patient with a known communicable disease that can be transmitted by aerosols.

B. Compromised patient with a marked susceptibility to infection. Examples of conditions are immunosuppression from disease or medication, uncontrolled diabetes, debilitation, or renal and other organ transplant.

C. Patient with a respiratory risk. Septic material and microorganisms from bacterial plaque and periodontal pockets can be aspirated into the lungs.[35]
   1. History of chronic pulmonary disease, including asthma, emphysema, or cystic fibrosis.
   2. History of cardiovascular disease with secondary pulmonary disease or breathing problem.

D. Patient with a swallowing problem or who is prone to gagging.

E. Patient with a cardiac pacemaker or other electronic life-support device.*[36] Some newer models have protective coverings. A consultation with the patient's cardiologist is necessary.

F. Children.
   1. Young, growing, developing tissues are sensitive to ultrasonic vibrations.
   2. Primary and newly erupted permanent teeth have large pulp chambers. The vibrations and heat from the ultrasonic scaler may damage the pulp tissue.

G. Characteristics of the teeth.
   1. Demineralized areas. Ultrasonic vibrations can remove the delicate remineralizing cover of a white spot.
   2. Exposed cemental surfaces. Tooth structure can be removed in excess. Mature calculus is harder than cementum.
   3. Restorative materials. Certain materials can be damaged or removed by ultrasonic instrumentation.
      a. Porcelain jacket crowns can be fractured by ultrasonic vibrations.[37]
      b. Composite resins. A laminate veneer can be removed.[38]
      c. Amalgam surface and margins can be altered.[39] Ultrasonic instruments can be used to reshape amalgam overhanging fillings, so margins can also be damaged.
   4. Patients with sensitive areas. Ultrasonic instrumentation can aggravate existing sensitivity.

H. Subgingival areas where lack of visibility and narrow pockets can interfere with proper angulation. Overinstrumentation can result.

I. Maintenance-care patients who are oriented to daily bacterial plaque removal and have minimal

---

*Attention must be paid to the proximity of any person in the dental office or clinic who may be wearing a pacemaker, whether a member of the dental team or a patient.

amounts of calculus develop between appointments.

IV. Procedure for Use[30,32,40]

The clinician and the assistant apply full barrier protection with eyeglasses, mask, and gloves. Hair covering should also be used when possible.

A. Unit Preparation
1. *Minimize Water Contamination.* Run water through the tubing of the ultrasonic unit for a full 2 minutes prior to use. Cultures of samples from water lines have shown high microbial counts, particularly in water left in the tubing overnight. The use of contaminated water provides a potential source for disease transmission. Such contaminated water forced into a pocket could produce bacteremia.[41]
2. *Unit Adjustment*
   a. Tune according to the manufacturer's specifications. Use the lowest effective power setting.
   b. Adjust water to a maximum mist about the working tip. Overheating must be prevented.
3. *Prophylaxis Tips*
   a. Sterilized tip is adapted to the handpiece after the unit water has cleared.
   b. Instrument tips must be dull; if sharp, the tooth surface could be nicked or gouged.
   c. Handle inserts with care to avoid damage to working ends or internal parts. Wrap individually for sterilization.

B. Patient Preparation
1. Review patient history and radiographs.
2. Check that risk patient has taken prescribed antibiotic medication. Prophylactic antibiotic premedication is indicated for risk patients. Bacteremia is produced in a high percentage of patients treated by ultrasonic, as well as by manual, instrumentation.[41]
3. Explain the procedure and the handpiece to the patient. Describe and demonstrate sound and spray, vibration, and the purpose for using the method. Hearing aid should be turned off.
4. Instruct the patient to use an antiseptic mouthrinse for 1 minute prior to ultrasonic scaling to lower the oral bacterial count and, hence, lower the bacterial count of the aerosols produced (page 56).
5. Use coverall and towel, and provide protective eyeglasses (patient should be requested to remove contact lenses).

C. Instrumentation
1. Place patient in supine position. In supine position, the airway is closed (figure 60–5, page 741). Use of an assistant is recommended.
2. Apply topical anesthetic or use local anesthetic as indicated and necessary.
3. Explore to review location of calculus.
4. Use high-velocity suction. When working solo, a saliva ejector must be in top running condition. Every effort must be made to prevent aspiration by the patient.
5. Plan systematic sequence. Finish one quadrant before starting another.
6. Use a modified pen grasp and apply finger rest on a tooth surface near the calculus to be removed.
7. Bring instrument to position before activating the water spray.
8. *Keep tip parallel with long axis of the tooth or at no more than a 15-degree angle with tooth surface.* Adaptation to variations in tooth topography is difficult but necessary. Maintenance of less than a 15-degree angle in all positions requires practice and concentration.
9. Stroke
   a. *Keep the tip in motion at all times.*
   b. Check to ensure that the water reaches the operating area.
   c. Brush lightly over the deposit, moving in a vertical or diagonal direction. A maximum of six strokes should be applied at one spot. Do not press. Pressure removes tooth structure.
   d. Move instrument with smooth, light, constant, and overlapping strokes.
   e. Be sure the tip is not held perpendicular to the tooth surface.
   f. Instrument may tend to bind when inserted interproximally, and the excess pressure stops the vibration. Remove and reactivate the instrument.
10. Release foot pedal switch at regular intervals to aid in water control. Stop periodically to evaluate the tooth surfaces with an explorer.
11. Complete the procedure with manual instruments directly following ultrasonic instrumentation.
    a. Check subgingival areas with a subgingival explorer.
    b. Remove remaining subgingival irregularities, and plane the surface smooth with curets.

D. Postoperative Instructions
1. Plaque control procedures should follow the usual pattern as recommended.
2. Use of fluoride dentifrice and mouthrinse is important for newly exposed tooth surfaces.
3. Counteract sensitivity to cold, hot, and condiments by avoiding extremes of temperature for a few days. If sensitivity persists, recommendations can be made at the next patient visit for use of special procedures or professional desensitization (pages 499–500).
4. When the gingiva is sensitive, rinsing with

warm weak saline solution can be recommended (page 538).

V. Advantages and Limitations

A. Advantages

1. Gross calculus removal may be accomplished with less effort than by manual instrumentation. More time can be devoted to thorough, careful root planing.
2. Requires minimum tissue manipulation for hypersensitive tissues.
3. Water flushes out pockets. Too much water pressure into the pocket can force particles into the tissue, which is a disadvantage.
4. Treatment time is reduced for removal of heavy stains and calculus.
5. Equipment requires minimal care.

B. Limitations

1. *Operational Factors*
   a. Less tactile perception.
   b. Impeded visibility during instrumentation.
   c. Use of mirror not possible for vision and reflected light because of water spray.
   d. Patient and clinician have discomfort and inconvenience of water spray and water accumulation when an assistant is not available.
   e. Accessibility for instrument adaptation and angulation in posterior oral regions is difficult.
2. *Heat Production.* Potential damage to the pulp tissue should be kept in mind during instrumentation.[42,43] One study showed that the amount of heat produced by an uncooled ultrasonic handpiece compares with that produced by an uncooled conventional high-speed handpiece.[42] Constant motion of the instrument, correct angulation, and ample water for cooling are essential to operation.
3. *Platelet Aggregation.* Human platelets are susceptible to damage by forces associated with ultrasonic cavitation at the level used clinically. If such damage were to occur in the pulp chamber of a tooth, thrombosis could result. The effect would be unlikely in large arteries, but could happen in a tooth because of the close area of enclosure. Pulpal thrombosis could lead to pulp death.[44]
4. *Aerosols.* Aerosols produced by an ultrasonic scaler may contain high bacterial counts.[45,46,47,48] The ultrasonic scaler should not be used for a patient with a communicable disease or for one susceptible to infections.[49]
5. *Hearing Shifts.* Extended exposure to noises above a certain level, such as the noise of a high-speed handpiece or an ultrasonic scaler, may be potentially damaging. Temporary hearing shifts have been demonstrated for a group of patients.[50] Noise reduction or ear protection measures are available and can be investigated by a concerned professional.[51]

EFFECTS OF ULTRASONIC INSTRUMENTATION

A review of the research literature reveals that many factors are involved when manual and ultrasonic instrumentation are compared. The instruments, their application through adaptation, angulation, lateral pressure, and strokes, and the variables related to individual clinicians can be significant. Another group of variables can be found in the teeth being treated, and in several studies, a notable difference was observed when anterior teeth were compared with posterior teeth, for which access and instrument positioning were problems.

Ultrasonic instrumentation has been compared with manual instrumentation in several published reviews of the literature.[52,53,54,55] A few of the research studies are summarized here.

In nonsurgical periodontal therapy, histologic and clinical assessments of plaque, bleeding, probed pocket depths, and probed attachment levels have shown that satisfactory healing has been obtained from treatment using either type of instrumentation.[8,56–60] Although variations occurred between studies, no real difference was apparent in the ability of the two types of instruments to remove calculus.[61–64] Roots prepared by ultrasonic instrumentation, however, had more remaining endotoxin than did those scaled manually.[65]

In one study, ultrasonic scaling was more effective than hand scaling in Class II and III furcations.[66] The reason suggested was that curets must be adapted at specific angles, whereas ultrasonic tips can work at almost any angle. When accessibility is more difficult, however, greater root damage can result, as shown in a comparison of anterior and posterior instrumentation in which posterior teeth showed the greatest damage from ultrasonic scaling.[67]

Many studies have demonstrated that manual instrumentation leaves a smoother root surface.[13,57,64,68,69,70,71] These research findings provide the basis for the need to complete subgingival instrumentation by root planing with curets after ultrasonic treatment.

Detectable roughness, gouging, and other damage to a root surface by an ultrasonic instrument clearly relate to the technique used. Scanning electron microscopy has revealed more extensive root surface damage associated with the use of the high setting of the machine.[72] The basic rules of low setting, light touch without pressure of the instrument against the tooth or deposit, smooth dull tips, and constant water cooling are important to the outcome of treatment.

USE OF A TOPICAL ANESTHETIC

A topical or surface anesthetic is a drug applied to the mucous membrane to produce a loss of sensation.

A topical anesthetic can be used with a degree of success for short-duration desensitization of the gingiva. As a soft tissue anesthetic, a topical agent does not influence sensations in the teeth and, therefore, is not a substitute for local anesthetic administered by injection.

Pain reaction varies from person to person and even in the same person, depending on emotional state and degree of fatigue. A person with a low reaction to pain, who is hypo-reactive, is said to have a *high pain threshold*. The person with a high reaction is hyper-reactive and has a *low pain threshold*.

In addition to emotional state and fatigue, other factors that influence pain threshold are age, sex, fear, and apprehension. Older individuals tend to have a higher pain threshold than that of younger individuals, and men tend to have a higher threshold than that of women. In fear or apprehension, however, the pain threshold for either sex at any age is lowered.

I. Indications for Use

A *local anesthetic* should be used when indicated by the extent of the procedure, by the patient's pain threshold, or by evidence of fear and apprehension. Although a local anesthetic would be indicated primarily for deep subgingival scaling, root planing, and curettage, it may be indicated for any degree of scaling requirement.

Pain threshold can usually be detected during initial examination. A patient who hyper-reacts to gentle, careful probing may indeed have a low pain threshold. A note should be made on the record to indicate possible need for anesthesia during clinical treatments.

A *topical anesthetic* can be used conservatively for many dental hygiene and dental services, including the following:
A. Prior to injection for local anesthesia.
B. Prevention of gagging in radiographic techniques and impression making.
C. Relief of pain from localized diseased areas, such as oral ulcers, wounds, or injuries.
D. During instrumentation for probing, exploring, scaling, and, sometimes, root planing and gingival curettage. When root planing and curettage are deep and generalized, a local anesthetic is usually indicated.
E. Suture removal.
F. Replacement of a dressing after removal. When light pressure is needed for adaptation of the dressing, a topical application can provide relief.

II. Action of a Topical Anesthetic

The purpose of a topical anesthetic is to desensitize the mucous membrane by anesthetizing the terminal nerve endings. A superficial anesthesia is produced that is related to the amount of absorption of the drug by the tissue.

The absorption varies with the thickness of the stratified squamous epithelial covering and the degree of keratinization. The skin and lips are highly resistant; the attached gingiva and cheek and palatal mucosa absorb drugs slowly; and the tissues without keratinization absorb promptly.

III. Requirements for an Adequate Topical Anesthetic

A. Produces effective lasting anesthesia.
B. Is miscible and stable in vehicle used.
C. Anesthetizing agent readily released from the preparation when applied.
D. Is nonirritating to the tissues.
E. Does not induce hypersensitivity reaction or other toxic effect at the concentration required for anesthesia.
F. Does not delay healing.
G. Can be readily washed off with water.

IV. Preparations Used: Characteristics

Several preparations have been used in the form of gels, ointments, solutions, troches, or sprays. The American Dental Association, Council on Dental Therapeutics evaluates and classifies topical anesthetics.[73]

General properties and characteristics of anesthetics for surface use follow.
A. Oils, alcohols, or glycols are used as the vehicle because most of the anesthetizing substances are only slightly soluble in water.
B. Most topical anesthetics are prepared in fairly concentrated form to allow for the resistance of the thick epithelial covering and viscid coating of saliva on the tissues. They are generally more concentrated than their counterparts used for local anesthesia. An example is lidocaine. For injection, a 2% solution is used, whereas for a topical preparation, the concentration is 5 or 10%.
C. The rate of absorption of a drug depends on solubility and the resistance of the mucous membrane.
D. Alcohols or glycols in concentrated solutions may be irritating to the sensitive mucous membranes and, therefore, are inferior vehicles (percent of alcohol or glycol should not be greater than 10 percent).
E. Carbowaxes used as vehicles for topical anesthetics are somewhat hygroscopic; thus, the jar in which the ointment is kept should be closed tightly.
F. Pressurized spray preparations must be used with caution because the amount of material expelled is difficult to control and the area of application is difficult to limit. Inhalation of the fine spray into the lungs can produce a toxic reaction. When the liquid flows into the throat (as may be possible with application of any type of preparation), coughing may be initiated.

V. Agents Used in Surface Anesthetic Preparations

The six drugs most commonly contained in surface anesthetics for dental use are listed here with brief notes about their characteristics.[73,74,75,76]

A. **Benzocaine** (ester type)
   1. Slow absorption; may be applied to abrasions or open lesions.
   2. May produce localized allergic reactions after prolonged or repeated use.

B. **Tetracaine** (ester type)
   1. Rapid absorption and high toxicity; not for use on open abraded tissue.
   2. Use in small quantities; avoid spray media where quantity used cannot be controlled. Not recommended.

C. **Butacaine** (ester type)
   1. Good action through mucous membrane.
   2. Toxic; should be used cautiously.

D. **Lidocaine** (amide type)
   1. Allergy is rare; aqueous form is more toxic than nonaqueous lidocaine base.
   2. May be applied to lacerated or incompletely healed tissue.

E. **Chlorbutanol** (aliphatic compound)
   1. Has both antiseptic and anesthetic properties.
   2. Has been used in preparations for alleviation of pain from pulpitis in a near pulp exposure and in dressings for relief from postsurgical discomfort.

F. **Dyclonine** (ketone)
   1. May be applied to lacerated or incompletely healed tissue because it is absorbed slowly.
   2. Has low systemic toxicity; useful when other agents cannot be used.

VI. Technique for Application of a Topical Anesthetic

A. Consult history and other records for pertinent information concerning a patient's previous experiences with anesthetics. A patient with an allergy to a local anesthetic may also be allergic to a surface anesthetic.

B. Explain purpose and anticipated effect to the patient.

C. Dry area with gauze sponge or cotton roll. Compressed air may be used, with consideration for sensitive tissues.

D. Apply anesthetic.
   1. Ointment
      a. A syringe with a bent needle may be used to introduce an ointment into a sulcus or pocket.
      b. Apply a small amount to a limited area with a cotton pellet and rub into the proximal area.
   2. Liquid
      a. Use a cotton swab or pellet for application.
      b. Apply a small amount directly over the dry tissues.

E. Wait briefly for anesthetic to take effect before proceeding.

VII. Adverse Reactions[77]

A. **Causes and Symptoms**
   1. *Allergic Response*
      a. Cause. Ingredients of the preparation have high allergenicity (the ability to produce an allergic reaction). The ester-type drugs have a greater tendency to produce allergic reactions than do other anesthetics.
      b. Symptoms. Erythema or angioedema of mucous membranes and lips.
   2. *Overdose*
      a. Cause. When a large quantity of the agent is spread over a large area and rapid absorption through the mucous membranes occurs, an immediate elevation of the anesthetic blood level results.
      b. Symptoms. Patient agitation, apprehension, excitement, speech irregularity, and tremors that progress to a mild convulsion. Pulse rate, blood pressure, and respiratory rate are elevated (table 60–1, pages 751–752).

B. **Precautions and Prevention**[77]
   1. Use amide-type topical anesthetic.
   2. Apply small amount to a limited area. For example, the anesthetic should not be spread over a whole quadrant for probing or scaling.
   3. Use metered or measured dose forms, especially if a liquid spray is to be used. The metered-dose container has a dispenser that limits the amount that can be expelled.
   4. Avoid areas of sepsis and open traumatized tissue unless the particular agent is specifically recommended for safe application on an open wound.
   5. Prevent inspiration (inhalation) by avoiding spray preparations. A spray must never be directed toward the throat.

C. **Adverse Reactions**[77]
   1. Allergic-type reactions may occur. Such reactions are related to a topical anesthetic preparation that contains an ester-type agent.
   2. Agents that are rapidly absorbed may cause an overdose reaction.

TECHNICAL HINTS

I. Maintain Sharp Instruments

Examine curets and scalers for sharpness at frequent intervals during instrumentation. Keep a sterile stone with each instrument set so that instruments can be sharpened during an appointment. Curets that are used most frequently may be packaged individually so a new package can be opened, or two curets of each type can be sterilized with the regular adult package.

II. Replace Curets Frequently

While sharpening, examine for wear. Discard a curet with a thin weak blade to prevent breakage during a treatment.

III. Broken Instrument

The procedure to follow when an instrument blade tip breaks in a patient's mouth during treatment should be in accord with the dentist's own policy. Therefore, the procedure should be discussed and clarified before an accident happens.

The principal objective in the location of a broken instrument tip is to *know positively that the tip has been removed.* With this in mind, rinsing, use of suction or compressed air, or initiation of other procedures that could cause the removal of the tip unknowingly would be out of order. A general procedure is suggested here.

A. Cease procedure, retain retraction without moving the patient's head unnecessarily, and isolate with gauze or cotton roll.

B. Do not alarm patient by describing the accident.

C. Examine the immediate field of operation, the floor of the mouth, and the mucobuccal fold. Blot the gingival tissue dry with a cotton roll and examine around the tooth.

D. Apply transilluminator or mouth light when available.

E. The gingival sulcus can be gently examined using a curet in a spooning-like stroke, but take care not to push the tip into the base of the sulcus (should the tip be there).

F. Consult the dentist for assistance in accord with previously discussed policy.

G. When the tip is not removed by any means mentioned thus far, make a periapical radiograph of the area.

IV. Summary: Methods to Minimize Patient Discomfort

A. Tissue Sensitivity

1. For gingival tissue, use topical anesthetic and/or local anesthetic as needed.
2. For exposed cementum or dentin, apply desensitizing agent (Chapter 37).
3. Protect lips and corners of mouth from irritation during instrumentation by application of petrolatum, cocoa butter, or other appropriate lubricant.
4. Use only *warm* water for rinsing.

B. Preventive Instrumentation

1. Use appropriate instrument, applied at the correct angulation, for each tooth surface.
2. Curets applied to base of sulcus or pocket must be small to prevent undue stretching of gingival wall and, hence, unnecessary detachment of the soft tissue attachment.

3. Instruments must be sharp, but the cementum can be scratched if sharp curets are not applied correctly and discriminately.
4. Maintain control of instrument at all times through effective grasp, appropriate finger rest, and correctly applied strokes to prevent accidental trauma to gingival tissue.
5. Apply minimum effective pressure on finger rest and of instrument on tooth to prevent patient from developing tired muscles and a stressed temporomandibular joint.
6. Finger rests on soft tissue give the patient a feeling of more pressure than do finger rests on the teeth and, consequently, may give the impression that the clinician is heavy-handed.

C. Postoperative Care (page 538)

1. Massage of gingival tissue at completion of instrumentation can be soothing and restful for the patient.
2. An antiseptic may be applied or the patient may be requested to use a fluoride mouthrinse.
3. Provide instruction for personal care, such as rinsing with warm saline solution and other appropriate measures for post-appointment follow-up.

V. Maintenance of a Clear Field

A. Use of saliva ejector and evacuator as needed.

B. Use of rolled gauze sponge or cotton rolls.
1. A gauze sponge rolled in the long dimension and placed in the mucobuccal fold beneath the teeth being treated can assist by
   a. Retracting the cheek or lip.
   b. Keeping teeth dry for secure finger rest.
   c. Drying the individual area for better vision.
2. Aid in retraction of tongue and keeping field free from saliva by placing cotton roll under tongue.

C. Maintenance of clear field and/or control of bleeding.
1. Application of pressure with cotton roll or pellet.
2. Application of 3% hydrogen peroxide with cotton pellet, followed by patient rinsing and/or dry pellet applied with pressure.
3. Use of compressed air to deflect tissue and remove debris.

FACTORS TO TEACH THE PATIENT

I. The nature, occurrence, and etiology of calculus.

II. The importance of the complete removal of calculus to the health of the oral tissues in the prevention of periodontal infections.

III. Relationship of the accumulation of plaque to the patient's personal oral hygiene procedures.

IV. Basic reasons for need and advantages of more than one appointment to complete the scaling and root planing.

V. Needed frequency of maintenance appointments in relation to oral health.

References

1. De Leo, A.A., Schoenknecht, M.D., Anderson, M.W., and Peterson, J.C.: The Incidence of Bacteremia Following Oral Prophylaxis on Pediatric Patients, *Oral Surg., 37,* 36, January, 1974.

2. Korn, N.A. and Schaffer, E.M.: Comparison of the Postoperative Bacteremias Induced Following Different Periodontal Procedures, *J. Periodontol., 33,* 226, July, 1962.

3. Royer, R., Gaines, R., and Kruger, G.: Bacteremia Following Exodontia, Prophylaxis, and Gingivectomy, *J. Dent. Res., 43,* 877, September-October, 1964, (Supplement).

4. Bender, I.B., Seltzer, S., Tashman, S., and Meloff, G.: Dental Procedures in Patients With Rheumatic Heart Disease, *Oral Surg., 16,* 466, April, 1963.

5. Winslow, M.B. and Kobernick, S.D.: Bacteremia After Prophylaxis, *J. Am. Dent. Assoc., 61,* 69, July, 1960.

6. Connor, H.D., Haberman, S., Collings, C.K., and Winford, T.E.: Bacteremias Following Periodontal Scaling in Patients with Healthy Appearing Gingiva, *J. Periodontol., 38,* 466, November-December, 1967.

7. Knowles, J.W., Burgett, F.G., Nissle, R.R., Shick, R.A., Morrison, E.C., and Ramfjord, S.P.: Results of Periodontal Treatment Related to Pocket Depth and Attachment Level. Eight Years, *J. Periodontol., 50,* 225, May, 1979.

8. Badersten, A., Nilvéus, R., and Egelberg, J.: Effect of Nonsurgical Periodontal Therapy. I. Moderately Advanced Periodontitis, *J. Clin. Periodontol., 8,* 57, February, 1981.

9. Lindhe, J., Nyman, S., and Karring, T.: Scaling and Root Planing in Shallow Pockets, *J. Clin. Periodontol., 9,* 415, September, 1982.

10. Carranza, F.A.: *Glickman's Clinical Periodontology,* 6th ed. Philadelphia, W.B Saunders Co., 1984, p. 613.

11. Barnes, J.E. and Schaffer, E.M.: Subgingival Root Planing: A Comparison Using Files, Hoes and Curettes, *J. Periodontol., 31,* 300, September, 1960.

12. Green, E. and Ramfjord, S.P.: Tooth Roughness After Subgingival Root Planing, *J. Periodontol., 37,* 396, September-October, 1966.

13. Kerry, G.J.: Roughness of Root Surfaces After Use of Ultrasonic Instruments and Hand Curettes, *J. Periodontol., 38,* 340, July-August, 1967.

14. Walker, S.L. and Ash, M.M.: A Study of Root Planing by Scanning Electron Microscopy, *Dent. Hyg., 50,* 109, March, 1976.

15. Ramfjord, S. and Kiester, G.: The Gingival Sulcus and the Periodontal Pocket Immediately Following Scaling of Teeth, *J. Periodontol., 25,* 167, July, 1954.

16. Moskow, B.S.: Response of the Gingival Sulcus to Instrumentation: A Histological Investigation. I. The Scaling Procedure, *J. Periodontol., 33,* 282, July, 1962.

17. Schaffer, E.M., Stende, G., and King, D.: Healing of Periodontal Pocket Tissues Following Ultrasonic Scaling and Hand Planing, *J. Periodontol., 35,* 140, March-April, 1964.

18. Stahl, S.S., Weiner, J.M., Benjamin, S., and Yamada, L.: Soft Tissue Healing Following Curettage and Root Planing, *J. Periodontol., 42,* 678, November, 1971.

19. Tagge, D.L., O'Leary, T.J., and El-Kafrawy, A.H.: The Clinical and Histologic Response of Periodontal Pockets to Root Planing and Oral Hygiene, *J. Periodontol., 46,* 527, September, 1975.

20. Caton, J.G. and Zander, H.A.: The Attachment Between Tooth and Gingival Tissues After Periodic Root Planing and Soft Tissue Curettage, *J. Periodontol., 50,* 462, September, 1979.

21. Carranza, F.A.: op. cit., p. 259.

22. Armitage, G.C.: *Biologic Basis of Periodontal Maintenance Therapy.* Berkeley, California, Praxis Publishing Co., 1980, pp. 154–156.

23. Schaffer, E.M.: Histological Results of Root Curettage of Human Teeth, *J. Periodontol., 27,* 296, October, 1956.

24. Selvig, K.A.: Biological Changes at the Tooth-saliva Interface in Periodontal Disease, *J. Dent. Res., 48,* 846, September-October, 1969, (Supplement).

25. Jones, W.A. and O'Leary, T.J.: The Effectiveness of *in vivo* Root Planing in Removing Bacterial Endotoxin from the Roots of Periodontally Involved Teeth, *J. Periodontol., 49,* 337, July, 1978.

26. Listgarten, M.A. and Hellden, L.: Relative Distribution of Bacteria at Clinically Healthy and Periodontally Diseased Sites in Humans, *J. Clin. Periodontol., 5,* 115, May, 1978.

27. Listgarten, M.A., Lindhe, J., and Hellden, L.: Effect of Tetracycline and/or Scaling on Human Periodontal Disease. Clinical, Microbiological, and Histological Observations, *J. Clin. Periodontol., 5,* 246, November, 1978.

28. Mousquès, T., Listgarten, M.A., and Phillips, R.W.: Effect of Scaling and Root Planing on the Composition of the Human Subgingival Microbial Flora, *J. Periodont. Res., 15,* 144, March, 1980.

29. Slots, J., Mashimo, P., Levine, M.J., and Genco, R.J.: Periodontal Therapy in Humans. I. Microbiologic and Clinical Effects of a Single Course of Periodontal Scaling and Root Planing, and of Adjunctive Tetracycline Therapy, *J. Periodontol., 50,* 495, October, 1979.

30. American Dental Association, Council on Dental Materials, Instruments, and Equipment: Status Report on Professional Scaling and Stain-removal Devices, *J. Am. Dent. Assoc., 111,* 801, November, 1985.

31. American Dental Association, Council on Dental Materials, Instruments, and Equipment, and Council on Dental Therapeutics: Accepted Dental Products, *J. Am. Dent. Assoc., 116,* 249, February, 1988.

32. Clark, S.M.: The Ultrasonic Dental Unit: A Guide for the Clinical Application of Ultrasonics in Dentistry and in Dental Hygiene, *J. Periodontol., 40,* 621, November, 1969.

33. Ewen, S. and Glickstein, C.: *Ultrasonic Therapy in Periodontics.* Springfield, Illinois, Charles C Thomas, 1968, pp. 12–45.

34. Odlum, O.: Dentistry and Immunosuppression, (Letter to the Editor), *J. Am. Dent. Assoc., 114,* 12, January, 1987.

35. Suzuki, J.B. and Delisle, A.L.: Pulmonary Actinomycosis of Periodontal Origin, *J. Periodontol., 55,* 581, October, 1984.

36. Adams, D., Fulford, N., Beechy, J., MacCarthy, J., and Stephens, M.: The Cardiac Pacemaker and Ultrasonic Scalers, *Br. Dent. J., 152,* 171, March 2, 1982.

37. American Dental Association, Council on Dental Materials, Instruments, and Equipment: *Dentist's Desk Reference: Materials, Instruments, and Equipment,* 2nd ed. Chicago, American Dental Association, 1983, pp. 361–362.

38. Carr, E.H.: Laminate Veneers. Restoration Alternative Means Special Care, *RDH,* 2, 11, July-August, 1982.

39. Rajstein, J. and Tal, M.: The Effect of Ultrasonic Scaling on the Surface of Class V Amalgam Restorations—A Scanning Electron Microscopy Study, *J. Oral Rehabil., 11,* 299, May, 1984.

40. Nield, J.S. and Houseman, G.A.: *Fundamentals of Dental Hygiene Instrumentation,* 2nd ed. Philadelphia, Lea & Febiger, 1988, pp. 341–356.

41. Bandt, C.L., Korn, N.A., and Schaffer, E.M.: Bacteremias from Ultrasonic and Hand Instrumentation, *J. Periodontol., 35,* 214, May-June, 1964.

42. Frost, H.M.: *Heating Under Ultrasonic Dental Scaling Conditions,* HEW Publication (FDA) 78-8048, Rockville, Maryland, Public Health Service, Bureau of Radiological Health, pp. 64–76, December, 1977.

43. Abrams, H., Barkmeier, W.W., and Cooley, R.L.: Temperature Changes in the Pulp Chamber Produced by Ultrasonic Instrumentation, *Gen. Dent., 27,* 62, September-October, 1979.

44. Williams, A.R. and Chater, B.V.: Mammalian Platelet Damage *in vitro* by an Ultrasonic Therapeutic Device, *Arch. Oral Biol., 25,* 175, Number 3, 1980.

45. Larato, D.C., Ruskin, P.F., and Martin, A.: Effect of an Ultrasonic Scaler on Bacterial Counts in Air, *J. Periodontol., 38,* 550, November-December, 1967.

46. Holbrook, W.P., Muir, K.F., MacPhee, I.T., and Ross, P.W.:

Bacteriological Investigation of the Aerosol from Ultrasonic Scalers, *Br. Dent. J., 144,* 245, April 18, 1978.

47. Muir, K.F., Ross, P.W., MacPhee, I.T., Holbrook, W.P., and Kowolik, M.J.: Reduction of Microbial Contamination from Ultrasonic Scalers, *Br. Dent. J., 145,* 76, August 1, 1978.

48. Williams, G.H., Pollok, N.L., Shay, D.E., and Barr, C.E.: Laminar Air Purge of Microorganisms in Dental Aerosols: Prophylactic Procedures With an Ultrasonic Scaler, *J. Dent. Res., 49,* 1498, November-December, 1970.

49. Gross, A., Devine, M.J., and Cutright, D.E.: Microbial Contamination of Dental Units and Ultrasonic Scalers, *J. Periodontol., 47,* 670, November, 1976.

50. Moller, P., Grevstad, A.O., and Kristoffersen, T.: Ultrasonic Scaling of Maxillary Teeth Causing Tinnitus and Temporary Hearing Shifts, *J. Clin. Periodontol., 3,* 123, May, 1976.

51. Coles, R.R.A. and Hoare, N.W.: Noise-induced Hearing Loss and the Dentist, *Br. Dent. J., 159,* 209, October 5, 1985.

52. Green, G.H. and Sanderson, A.D.: Ultrasonics and Periodontal Therapy—A Review of Clinical and Biologic Effects, *J. Periodontol., 36,* 232, May-June, 1965.

53. Suppipat, N.: Ultrasonics in Periodontics, *J. Clin. Periodontol., 1,* 206, Number 4, 1974.

54. Brown, F.H., Lubow, R.M., and Cooley, R.L.: A Review of Applied Ultrasonics in Periodontal Therapy, *J. West. Soc. Periodont. Periodont. Abstr., 35,* 53, Number 2, 1987.

55. Zitterbart, P.A.: Effectiveness of Ultrasonic Scalers: A Literature Review, *Gen. Dent., 35,* 295, July-August, 1987.

56. Bhaskar, S.N., Grower, M.F., and Cutright, D.E.: Gingival Healing After Hand and Ultrasonic Scaling—Biochemical and Histologic Analysis, *J. Periodontol., 43,* 31, January, 1972.

57. Rosenberg, R.M. and Ash, M.M.: The Effect of Root Roughness on Plaque Accumulation and Gingival Inflammation, *J. Periodontol., 45,* 146, March, 1974.

58. Walsh, T.F. and Waite, I.M.: A Comparison of Postsurgical Healing Following Debridement by Ultrasonic or Hand Instruments, *J. Periodontol., 49,* 201, April, 1978.

59. Badersten, A., Nilvéus, R., and Egelberg, J.: Effect of Nonsurgical Periodontal Therapy. II. Severely Advanced Periodontitis, *J. Clin. Periodontol., 11,* 63, January, 1984.

60. Schwarcz, J., Caffesse, R.G., Kerry, G.J., Smith, B.A., and Morrison, F.C.: Clinical Evaluation of Hand and Ultrasonic Instrumentation in Root Preparation, *J. Dent. Res., 67,* 158, Abstract 361, March, 1988.

61. Stende, G.W. and Schaffer, E.M.: A Comparison of Ultrasonic and Hand Scaling, *J. Periodontol., 32,* 312, October, 1961.

62. Moskow, B.S. and Bressman, E.: Cemental Response to Ultrasonic and Hand Instrumentation, *J. Am. Dent. Assoc., 68,* 698, May, 1964.

63. Jones, S.J., Lozdan, J., and Boyde, A.: Tooth Surfaces Treated *in situ* with Periodontal Instruments, *Br. Dent. J., 132,* 57, January 18, 1972.

64. Hunter, R.K., O'Leary, T.J., and Kafrawy, A.H.: The Effectiveness of Hand Versus Ultrasonic Instrumentation in Open Flap Root Planing, *J. Periodontol., 55,* 697, December, 1984.

65. Nishimine, D. and O'Leary, T.J.: Hand Instrumentation Versus Ultrasonics in the Removal of Endotoxins from Root Surfaces, *J. Periodontol., 50,* 345, July, 1979.

66. Leon, L.E. and Vogel, R.I.: A Comparison of the Effectiveness of Hand Scaling and Ultrasonic Debridement in Furcations as Evaluated by Differential Dark-field Microscopy, *J. Periodontol., 58,* 86, February, 1987.

67. D'Silva, I.V., Nayak, R.P., Cherian, K.M., and Mulky, M.J.: An Evaluation of the Root Topography Following Periodontal Instrumentation—A Scanning Electron Microscopic Study, *J. Periodontol., 50,* 283, June, 1979.

68. Wilkinson, R.F. and Maybury, J.E.: Scanning Electron Microscopy of the Root Surface Following Instrumentation, *J. Periodontol., 44,* 559, September, 1973.

69. Meyer, K. and Lie, T.: Root Surface Roughness in Response to Periodontal Instrumentation Studied by Combined Use of Microroughness Measurements and Scanning Electron Microscopy, *J. Clin. Periodontol., 4,* 77, May, 1977.

70. Bye, F.L., Ghilzon, R.S., and Caffesse, R.G.: Root Surface Roughness After the Use of Different Modes of Instrumentation, *Int. J. Periodontics Restorative Dent., 6,* 986, Number 5, 1986.

71. Barnes, C., Russell, C.M., and McDaniel, S.: An *in vitro* Comparison of Piezoelectric Ultrasonic Scaling and Hand Instrumentation, *J. Dent. Res., 67,* 158, Abstract 365, March, 1988.

72. Breininger, D.R., O'Leary, T.J., and Blumenshine, R.V.H.: Comparative Effectiveness of Ultrasonic and Hand Scaling for the Removal of Subgingival Plaque and Calculus, *J. Periodontol., 58,* 9, January, 1987.

73. American Dental Association, Council on Dental Therapeutics: *Accepted Dental Therapeutics,* 40th ed. Chicago, American Dental Association, 1984, pp. 194–196.

74. Holroyd, S.V., ed.: *Clinical Pharmacology in Dental Practice,* 3rd ed. St. Louis, The C.V. Mosby Co., 1983, p. 186.

75. Snyder, N.C.: *Dental Hygiene Clinical Applications in Pharmacology.* Philadelphia, Lea & Febiger, 1987, p. 73.

76. Requa, B.S. and Holroyd, S.V.: *Applied Pharmacology for the Dental Hygienist,* St. Louis, The C.V. Mosby Co., 1982, pp. 163–164.

77. Malamed, S.F.: *Handbook of Medical Emergencies in the Dental Office,* 3rd ed. St. Louis, The C.V. Mosby Co., 1987, pp. 259, 274–275.

Suggested Readings

Armitage, G.C.: *Biologic Basis of Periodontal Maintenance Therapy.* Berkeley, California, Praxis Publishing Co., 1980, pp. 79–115.

Badersten, A., Nilvéus, R., and Egelberg, J.: Effect of Nonsurgical Periodontal Therapy. III. Single Versus Repeated Instrumentation, *J. Clin. Periodontol., 11,* 114, February, 1984.

Badersten, A., Nilvéus, R., and Egelberg, J.: Effect of Nonsurgical Periodontal Therapy. IV. Operator Variability, *J. Clin. Periodontol., 12,* 190, March, 1985.

Carranza, F.A.: *Glickman's Clinical Periodontology,* 6th ed. Philadelphia, W.B. Saunders Co., 1984, pp. 545–553, 601–620, 660–670.

Daly, C.G., Seymour, G.J., Kieser, J.B., and Corbet, E.F.: Histological Assessment of Periodontally Involved Cementum, *J. Clin. Periodontol., 9,* 266, May, 1982.

Daly, C.G., Seymour, G.J., and Kieser, J.B.: Bacterial Endotoxin: A Role in Chronic Inflammatory Periodontal Disease? *J. Oral Pathol., 9,* 1, January, 1980.

Garrett, J.S.: Root Planing: A Perspective, *J. Periodontol., 48,* 553, September, 1977.

Grant, D.A., Stern, I.B., and Listgarten, M.A., eds.: *Periodontics,* 6th ed. St. Louis, The C.V. Mosby Co., 1988, pp. 650–715.

Hirschfeld, L.: Subgingival Curettage in Periodontal Treatment, *J. Am. Dent. Assoc., 44,* 301, March, 1952.

Magnusson, I., Runstad, L., Nyman, S., and Lindhe, J.: A Long Junctional Epithelium—A Locus Minoris Resistentiae in Plaque Infection? *J. Clin. Periodontol., 10,* 333, May, 1983.

Nakib, N.M., Bissada, N.F., Simmelink, J.W., and Goldstine, S.N.: Endotoxin Penetration into Root Cementum of Periodontally Healthy and Diseased Human Teeth, *J. Periodontol., 53,* 368, June, 1982.

O'Leary, T.J. and Kafrawy, A.H.: Total Cementum Removal: A Realistic Objective? *J. Periodontol., 54,* 221, April, 1983.

Parr, R.W., Green, E., Madsen, L., and Miller, S.: *Subgingival Scaling and Root Planing.* Berkeley, California, Praxis Publishing Co., 1976, 90 pp.

Parr, R.W., John, R., and Ratcliff, P.A.: *Tooth Preparation.* Berkeley, California, Praxis Publishing Co., 1974, 52 pp.

Pattison, G.L. and Pattison, A.M.: *Periodontal Instrumentation.* Reston, Virginia, Reston Publishing Co., 1979, pp. 143–306.

Rabbani, G.M., Ash, M.M., and Caffesse, R.G.: The Effectiveness of Subgingival Scaling and Root Planing in Calculus Removal, *J. Periodontol., 52,* 119, March, 1981.

Rawlinson, A.: Periodontally Involved Cementum: Some Aspects of Its Management Old and New, *Br. Dent. J., 159,* 153, September 7, 1985.

Reinhardt, R.A., Johnson, G.K., and Tussing, G.J.: Root Planing

With Interdental Papilla Reflection and Fiber Optic Illumination, *J. Periodontol., 56,* 721, December, 1985.

Stahl, S.S.: Repair Potential of the Soft Tissue-Root Interface, *J. Periodontol., 48,* 545, September, 1977.

Tal, H., Panno, J.M., and Vaidyanathan, T.K: Scanning Electron Microscope Evaluation of Wear of Dental Curettes During Standardized Root Planing, *J. Periodontol., 56,* 532, September, 1985.

Waerhaug, J.: Healing of the Dento-epithelial Junction Following Subgingival Plaque Control. I. As Observed in Human Biopsy Material, *J. Periodontol., 49,* 1, January, 1978.

Waerhaug, J.: Healing of the Dento-epithelial Junction Following Subgingival Plaque Control. II. As Observed on Extracted Teeth, *J. Periodontol., 49,* 119, March, 1978.

Wirthlin, M.R.: The Current Status of New Attachment Therapy, *J. Periodontol., 52,* 529, September, 1981.

Instrumentation in Shallow Pockets

Knowles, J., Burgett, F., Morrison, E., Nissle, R., and Ramfjord, S.: Comparison of Results Following Three Modalities of Periodontal Therapy Related to Tooth Type and Initial Pocket Depth, *J. Clin. Periodontol., 7,* 32, February, 1980.

Lindhe, J., Westfelt, E., Nyman, S., Socransky, S.S., Heijl, L., and Bratthall, G.: Healing Following Surgical/Non-surgical Treatment of Periodontal Disease. A Clinical Study, *J. Clin. Periodontol., 9,* 115, March, 1982.

Linde, J., Socransky, S.S., Nyman, S., Haffajee, A., and Westfelt, E.: "Critical Probing Depths" in Periodontal Therapy, *J. Clin. Periodontol., 9,* 323, July, 1982.

Pihlstrom, B.L., Ortiz-Campos, C., and McHugh, R.B.: A Randomized Four-Year Study of Periodontal Therapy, *J. Periodontol., 52,* 227, May, 1981.

Pihlstrom, B.L., McHugh, R.B., Oliphant, T.H., and Ortiz-Campos, C.: Comparison of Surgical and Nonsurgical Treatment of Periodontal Disease. A Review of Current Studies and Additional Results After 6½ Years, *J. Clin. Periodontol., 10,* 524, September, 1983.

Anatomic Features

Bower, R.C.: Furcation Morphology Relative to Periodontal Treatment. Furcation Entrance Architecture, *J. Periodontol., 50,* 23, January, 1979.

Bower, R.C.: Furcation Morphology Relative to Periodontal Treatment. Furcation Root Surface Anatomy, *J. Periodontol., 50,* 366, July, 1979.

Gher, M.E. and Vernino, A.R.: Root Morphology—Clinical Significance in Pathogenesis and Treatment of Periodontal Disease, *J. Am. Dent. Assoc., 101,* 627, October, 1980.

Harris, J.H. and Overton, E.E.: Cementoenamel Defects in an Unusual Location, *J. Am. Dent. Assoc., 97,* 221, August, 1978.

Holton, W.L., Hancock, E.B., and Pelleu, G.B.: Prevalence and Distribution of Attached Cementicles on Human Root Surfaces, *J. Periodontol., 57,* 321, May, 1986.

Ultrasonic Scaling

Catherman, J.L.: Power-Driven Scaling and Polishing Instruments, in Clark, J.W., ed.: *Clinical Dentistry,* Volume 3, Chapter 5A. Philadelphia, J.B. Lippincott Co., Revised 1984, pp. 1–17.

Clinical Research Associates: Sonic and Ultrasonic Scalers, *Newsletter, 6,* 1, July, 1982.

Glick, D.H. and Freeman, E.: Postsurgical Bone Loss Following Root Planing by Ultrasonic and Hand Instruments, *J. Periodontol., 51,* 510, September, 1980.

Lie, T. and Meyer, K.: Calculus Removal and Loss of Tooth Substance in Response to Different Periodontal Instruments, *J. Clin. Periodontol., 4,* 250, November, 1977.

Pearlman, B.A.: Ultrasonic Root Planing, *Aust. Dent. J., 27,* 109, April, 1982.

Reinhardt, R.A., Bolton, R.W., and Hlava, G.: Effect of Nonsterile Versus Sterile Water Irrigation With Ultrasonic Scaling on Postoperative Bacteremias, *J. Periodontol., 53,* 96, February, 1982.

Thilo, B.E. and Baehni, P.C.: Effect of Ultrasonic Instrumentation on Dental Plaque Microflora *in vitro, J. Periodont. Res., 22,* 518, November, 1987.

Thornton, S. and Garnick, J.: Comparison of Ultrasonic to Hand Instruments in the Removal of Subgingival Plaque, *J. Periodontol., 53,* 35, January, 1982.

Torfason, T., Kiger, R., Selvig, K.A., and Egelberg, J.: Clinical Improvement of Gingival Conditions Following Ultrasonic Versus Hand Instrumentation of Periodontal Pockets, *J. Clin. Periodontol., 6,* 165, June, 1979.

Walmsley, A.D., Williams, A.R., and Laird, W.R.E.: Acoustic Absorption Within Human Teeth During Ultrasonic Descaling, *J. Dent., 14,* 2, February, 1986.

Walmsley, A.D., Laird, W.R.E., and Williams, A.R.: Inherent Variability of the Performance of the Ultrasonic Descaler, *J. Dent., 14,* 121, June, 1986.

Walmsley, A.D., Laird, W.R.E., and Williams, A.R.: Investigation Into Patient's Hearing Following Ultrasonic Scaling, *Br. Dent. J., 162,* 221, March 21, 1987.

Sonic Scaling

Gankerseer, E.J. and Walmsley, A.D.: Preliminary Investigation Into the Performance of a Sonic Scaler, *J. Periodontol., 58,* 780, November, 1987.

Gellin, R.G., Miller, M.C., Javed, T., Engler, W.O., and Mishkin, D.J.: The Effectiveness of the Titan-S Sonic Scaler Versus Curettes in the Removal of Subgingival Calculus. A Human Surgical Evaluation, *J. Periodontol., 57,* 672, November, 1986.

Lie, T. and Leknes, K.N.: Evaluation of the Effect on Root Surfaces of Air Turbine Scalers and Ultrasonic Instrumentation, *J. Periodontol., 56,* 522, September, 1985.

Loos, B., Kiger, R., and Egelberg, J.: An Evaluation of Basic Periodontal Therapy Using Sonic and Ultrasonic Scalers, *J. Clin. Periodontol., 14,* 29, January, 1987.

Smith, S.J., Eberhart, A., Killoy, W., and Cobb, C.: Comparing Ultrasonic and Sonic Instrumentation, *Dent. Hyg., 55,* 32, July, 1981.

Woodruff, H.C., Levin, M.P., and Brady, J.M.: The Effects of Two Ultrasonic Instruments on Root Surfaces, *J. Periodontol., 46,* 119, February, 1975.

34 *Gingival Curettage*

Gingival curettage is a selective procedure. When indicated it is used to supplement the patient's disease control program (daily therapeutic plaque removal) and to enhance thorough professional scaling and root planing.

Soft tissue curettage contributes to the control of disease and may be the definitive treatment by which a pocket can be reduced in depth or eliminated. It also may be part of the preparatory or initial phase of treatment. Reevaluation can then be made to determine whether more complex periodontal therapy will be required.

To contribute to healing and the return of the tissues to health, gingival curettage must be preceded by subgingival scaling and root planing. The root surface must be smooth and free from diseased, altered cementum with endotoxin and other irritants to the gingiva. Gingival curettage promotes healing by aiding the body in the removal of tissue debris and microorganisms from the pocket.

I. Types of Curettage

In periodontics an attempt has been made to identify types of gingival curettage by the anatomic extent (gingival, subgingival), by the objective to be attained (definitive, nondefinitive), and by the clinical procedure used (open, closed).

A. Closed Gingival Curettage (gingival curettage, soft tissue curettage, free gingival curettage)

Closed gingival curettage is a planned, systematic procedure used to remove the diseased lining of the soft tissue wall, including pocket and junctional epithelium and the underlying inflamed connective tissue.

B. Closed Subgingival Curettage

Closed subgingival curettage is a planned, systematic procedure used to remove the diseased lining of the soft tissue wall, including pocket and junctional epithelium as well as the deep connective tissue attachment down to the crest of the bone. The objective is reattachment.

C. Open Subgingival Curettage (surgical curettage, open-flap curettage, modified Widman flap,[1] excisional new attachment procedure [ENAP][2])

Open subgingival curettage is a surgical flap procedure in which the diseased pocket epithelium, the junctional epithelium, and the underlying inflamed connective tissue below the base of the pocket are removed down to the crest of the bone.

D. Definitive Curettage

In general, a definitive treatment corrects the defect and eliminates the disease. Definitive curettage, therefore, is curettage that is expected to have a direct role in elimination of inflammation and reduction of the pocket to maintainable levels.

E. Nondefinitive Curettage

1. For reduction of inflammation and conditioning of gingival tissue as a preparation for subsequent surgery.
2. For maintenance therapy when extensive surgery cannot be performed for various reasons, such as systemic health problems, personal reasons, or emotional disturbances.

F. Coincidental Curettage (inadvertent, incidental, unpremeditated curettage)

Curettage is considered coincidental when debridement of the soft tissue pocket wall is caused by the back and lateral surface of the offset cutting edge of a curet during the strokes for scaling and root planing. *Coincidental* contrasts with *deliberate,* which means a planned open, closed, definitive, or nondefinitive procedure.

II. The Pocket Wall

A. In Health

The lining of the sulcus is nonkeratinized stratified squamous epithelium. The average depth of a healthy sulcus is 1.8 mm., and it is sealed at the base by the junctional epithelium attached to the tooth (page 168).

B. In Disease

1. *Epithelium*
   a. Ulceration of the sulcular epithelium with areas of exposed inflamed connective tissue.
   b. Proliferation of epithelium into the connective tissue.
   c. Apical migration of the junctional epithelium.
2. *Connective Tissue*
   a. Destruction of connective tissue fibers of the gingiva and the periodontal ligament.
   b. Vascular changes with disintegration of vessel walls, increased permeability, and resulting edema into the tissue.

PLAQUE/BACTERIA

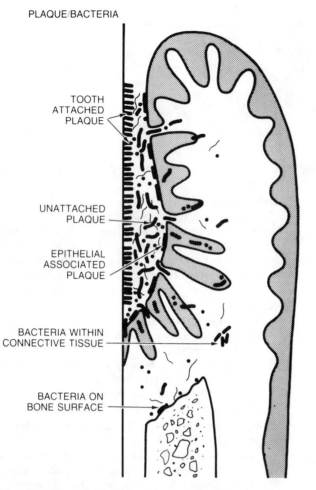

TOOTH
ATTACHED
PLAQUE

UNATTACHED
PLAQUE

EPITHELIAL
ASSOCIATED
PLAQUE

BACTERIA WITHIN
CONNECTIVE TISSUE

BACTERIA ON
BONE SURFACE

Figure 34-1. Bacterial Invasion. Diagram of a periodontal pocket shows bacteria of attached and unattached plaque bacteria within the pocket epithelium, in the connective tissue, and on the surface of the bone. (From Carranza, F.A.: *Glickman's Clinical Periodontology*, 6th ed. Philadelphia, W.B. Saunders Co., 1984, p. 368.)

C. Bacterial Invasion[3,4]

Microorganisms from the pocket plaque can invade the periodontal tissues by way of the epithelial breaks or ulcerations. Figure 34-1 shows the microorganisms of a periodontal pocket and in tissue invasion.

III. Purposes of Gingival Curettage

A. Overall Objectives

As a part of the treatment for the restoration of gingival health, with complete scaling and root planing and effective plaque control, curettage can contribute to

1. Reduction or elimination of inflammation.
2. Reduction or eradication of gingival or periodontal pockets.

B. Specific Objectives

Removal of the inflamed, ulcerated soft tissue of the pocket wall can

1. Allow inflammation to subside by establishing drainage for edema.

2. Cause shrinkage of the free gingiva and, hence, reduce pocket depth.
3. Remove area of soft tissue invaded by bacteria to discourage recolonization and disease redevelopment.
4. Promote fibrosis and healing.
5. Permit replacement of the diseased pocket lining with newly formed connective tissue and sulcular epithelium that can be maintained in health.
6. Contribute to a return of the gingiva to a normal contour.

IV. Treatment Plan

The overall periodontal treatment plan may include gingival curettage during the following:[5]
A. Initial therapy or Phase I to assist in the elimination of etiologic factors causing inflammation.
B. Presurgical preparation of the tissues. Gingival curettage may increase fibrosis, thereby allowing easier management of the tissue during surgical intervention.
C. Treatment of patients compromised by health problems that may limit total periodontal therapy.
D. Maintenance for the treated patient.

TREATMENT

I. Appointment Plan

At an appointment, treatment is confined to one or possibly two quadrants. The plan for treatment, however, depends on the severity of the condition, depth of pockets, and whether treatment is localized or generalized. The extent of treatment is also influenced by the use of anesthesia and by whether topical or local anesthetic is to be administered.

The treatment plan outlined on page 295 is illustrative of the steps needed. With local anesthetic and the use of periodontal dressings, several appointments are needed in a series over several weeks for continuing evaluation.

II. Selection of Treatment Areas

A. Indications for Definitive Curettage

1. Gingival tissue with a soft, spongy consistency and other signs of inflammation (table 11-1, page 174).
2. Pockets that are relatively shallow (4 to 5 mm.) and are suprabony.
3. Persistence of hyperemia, edema, and pocket depth after complete scaling and root planing.

B. Contraindications for Definitive Curettage

1. Gingival tissue with a firm, fibrous consistency contains fibrotic, collagenous elements that do not permit shrinkage of a pocket wall.
2. Thin, fragile pocket walls that could be punctured easily during instrumentation.

3. Acute periodontal inflammatory lesions, particularly necrotizing ulcerative gingivitis.
4. Periodontal conditions that require specific surgical treatment, such as
   a. Pockets that are deep and/or intrabony.
   b. Areas of narrow attached gingiva or mucogingival involvement.
   c. Furcation involvement.

C. Indications for Nondefinitive Curettage
1. As preparation for pocket elimination by surgical methods. Reduces inflammation and increases fibrosis.
2. As maintenance therapy. Aids in the control of recurrent infection.

III. Preparation for Instrumentation

A. Prerequisites
1. Adequate bacterial plaque removal must be performed daily. Otherwise, benefits from non-surgical periodontal therapy will be short-lived.
2. Complete scaling and root planing.
3. Removal of overhanging fillings.

B. Patient Preparation
1. *Explanation to Patient*
   a. Procedures.
   b. Possible postoperative discomforts.
   c. Expected results.
   d. Personal care responsibilities.
2. *Review of Patient's Medical History*
   a. Need for administration of antibiotic for prevention of bacteremia, or of other premedication, for certain risk patients.
   b. Limitations and special concerns.
3. *Anesthesia*
   a. Topical Anesthesia. A topical application may be sufficient when the curettage is confined to an isolated area or when shallow pockets are present.
   b. Local Anesthesia. Infiltration may be sufficient for certain patients and for limited areas. Block anesthesia is indicated for quadrant treatment of deep pockets.
4. *Root Planing*
   a. Same Appointment. When part or all of the scaling and root planing are performed on the same day as curettage, the pockets must be carefully irrigated followed by high-powered suction to remove particles of calculus, cementum, and other debris so that they cannot be driven into the tissue during curettage.
   b. Previous Appointment. When curettage is not performed at the same appointment as scaling and root planing, the tooth surfaces should be carefully checked and replaned in preparation for tissue adaptation and healing.

C. Instruments
1. Curets for curettage should be kept separate from scaling and root planing curets. Marking tapes may prove helpful.
2. Curets must be very sharp for efficient instrumentation to prevent excess pressure and numbers of strokes.
3. When the same instruments are used for scaling and planing, they must be resharpened. A sterile stone for sharpening is part of every instrument set-up.

IV. Steps for Clinical Instrumentation

A. Technique Objectives
The instrumentation is planned to remove
1. The diseased pocket lining epithelium and underlying inflamed connective tissue.
2. Tissue debris and chronic granulation tissue.
3. Particles of calcified debris not removed by irrigation and suction after scaling and planing.
4. Microorganisms embedded within the tissue.

B. Arrange Instruments and Equipment
Maintain aseptic field.

C. Isolate the Area
Use sterile sponges and adjust the saliva ejector.

D. Re-examine and Review
Use a probe to note pocket depths and pocket contour.

E. Select and Apply the Appropriate Curet
1. Use a modified pen grasp.
2. Establish a finger rest on a tooth near the area to be curetted. Fulcrum finger (ring finger supported by little finger) is applied and maintained.

F. Sequence
Begin with the most posterior tooth of the quadrant. For convenience of retraction and efficient continuity, work from posterior to anterior, facial surfaces, then lingual or palatal.

G. Angulation and Adaptation
1. Position the blade over the pocket to be treated. Blade is open and held at an angle of greater than 90 degrees. For scaling and root planing, the blade is closed toward the tooth (figure 34–2).
2. Note the relation of the handle, grasp, rest, and blade angle. By maintaining this relationship, one can promptly reposition the curet after insertion.
3. Insertion
   a. Direct the toe toward the opening of the pocket. Open the blade and slide under the margin.
   b. Move the curet to the base of the pocket. Use the round back to determine the base, where tension of the soft tissue can be felt.

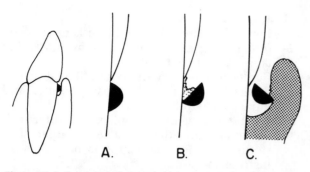

Figure 34–2. Curet Angulation. A. Enlargement of pocket area from the tooth on the left shows a cross section of the blade of a curet in black. The curet is angulated at 0 degrees with the tooth surface when used with an exploratory or insertion stroke. **B.** Blade angulated for scaling and root planing at approximately 70 degrees with the tooth surface. **C.** Blade angulated with the gingival wall of a pocket in position for closed gingival curettage. The face of the blade forms approximately a 70-degree angle with the soft tissue pocket wall.

4. Reposition the blade to correct angulation at approximately 70 degrees between the face of the blade and the soft tissue pocket wall (figure 34–3).

H. Strokes

1. *Maintain the Finger Rest.* Tighten the grasp slightly to permit definitive moderate pressure for removal of the pocket lining.
2. *Support the Pocket Wall*
   a. Facial and Lingual or Palatal. Apply a finger of the nonworking hand to the outer surface of the pocket wall to offset pressure

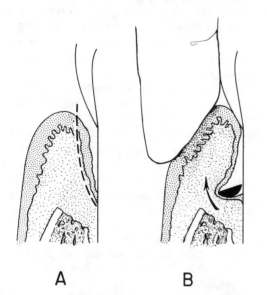

Figure 34–3. Gingival Curettage. A. Broken line shows pocket tissue to be removed during gingival curettage, namely the pocket epithelium and the underlying inflamed connective tissue. **B.** Curet positioned at the bottom of the pocket with the cutting edge toward the gingival tissue wall. Pressure applied with a finger on the outside of the pocket provides support for the pressure of the curet as it is activated. The curet is angled for a vertical stroke as shown by the cross section of the blade and the arrow.

of the curet and to produce effective cutting action (figure 34–3B).
   b. Interdental Papilla. Press the curet toward the proximal surface of the adjacent tooth.
3. *Strokes.* Use even smooth strokes to minimize excess instrumentation.
   a. Vertical and Oblique. Work toward the gingival margin to treat the walls of the pocket. Overlap deep strokes with those nearer the margin.
   b. Horizontal. Direct strokes circumferentially. Use a horizontal stroke to curet an entire facial or lingual surface.
      i. At the base of a pocket, keep the curet above the probing depth to prevent unnecessary detachment of attached connective tissue fibers under the epithelium.
      ii. A horizontal stroke is used near the gingival margin to finish off the ends of the vertical and oblique strokes.
   c. Removal of Junctional Epithelium. Research has shown that the attachment area is usually removed, or at least changed, during scaling and root planing when no deliberate strokes are applied to the attachment;[6] therefore, only conservative strokes need to be applied.
   d. Length of Strokes
      i. Longer, continuous strokes produce clean areas of debrided pocket wall.
      ii. Length of strokes is governed by the tooth contour.
   e. Precaution. Evaluate the tissue. Do not pierce or tear the pocket wall.
4. *Proceed Systematically Around Each Tooth.* Overlap strokes at line angles.

I. Completion

1. *Determination.* An experienced sense of touch can distinguish the soft mushy granulation tissue from the underlying firm connective tissue. When the curet is sharp, only a few strokes are needed.
2. *Removal of Debris from Pocket.* Use suction.
3. *Test for Residual "Tags."* Use suction to pull "tags" of tissue out of the pocket. Remove with a sharp curet.

J. Irrigation

Irrigate with sterile water to limit the possibility of bacteremia.

K. Tissue Adaptation and Hemostasis

1. Press the area with a damp sponge to adapt the tissue closely and stop the bleeding.
2. Press to reduce the size of the blood clot. A thin clot is beneficial during healing.

L. Place a Dressing When Needed (pages 489–491)

1. To hold detached papillary tissue over the interdental area (dentist may choose to place a suture).

2. To protect the healing tissue from trauma that might cause excess bleeding and thereby extend the healing period.
3. To minimize the size of the clot.

POSTOPERATIVE CARE

I. Postoperative Instructions

A. Dressing Placed

Printed instructions are advisable. Suggestions for care following dressing placement are found on page 492 (table 36–1).

B. Without Dressing

1. Plaque removal is important. Use soft toothbrush with end-rounded filaments. Definite plaque removal with care taken not to traumatize the healing tissue is necessary.
2. Rinse with warm weak saline solution (page 538).

II. Follow-up

A. Dressing Removal

Dressing should be removed in approximately 1 week. Specific plaque removal instructions are given.

B. Tooth Sensitivity

Advise the patient that most sensitivity is transient. Toothbrushing with a fluoride dentifrice and daily use of a fluoride mouthrinse can be most effective. Desensitizing agents can be applied to persistent spots (pages 499–500).

C. Stain Removal

Stain removal is not advised immediately following dressing removal because curettage leaves a wide healing area. An abrasive would be an irritant. Instruction for daily complete plaque removal by the patient is necessary to prevent reinfection.

HEALING

I. Effects of Instrumentation

Removal of the chronically inflamed ulcerated pocket lining and underlying inflamed connective tissue creates a surgical wound. Healing follows a pattern of epithelialization and collagenation and resolution of inflammation in the connective tissue. The effects are as follows:

A. Shrinkage of the gingival walls with fluid drainage.
B. Re-epithelialization with coverage of the exposed connective tissue.
C. Formation of a long junctional epithelium.
D. Formation of new connective tissue beneath the new epithelial lining of the sulcus and attachment.
E. Return to normal circulation.

II. Steps in Healing[7]

A. Formation of a blood clot immediately after curettage. The clot fills the pocket area, which is adapted against the tooth by pressure and a dressing.
B. Initial tissue reaction of inflammation as with any wound.
C. Proliferation of fibroblasts and new vessels to form granulation tissue.
D. Epithelial cells arise from the epithelium at the margin of the gingiva. The epithelium migrates in and over the granulation tissue by approximately 4 hours following the curettage.
E. New epithelium covers the sulcus lining within 5 to 6 days, and the new junctional epithelium begins to develop by 5 days.
F. Connective tissue healing proceeds and is well organized by 2 weeks.
G. Keratinization of oral (outer) epithelium may be observed by 2 weeks and reaches normal thickness by 28 to 40 days.

III. Factors Affecting Healing

A. Residual and newly formed calculus. Repeated root planing is frequently necessary.
B. Plaque and other local irritants. Meticulous self-care must be supervised over several weeks following curettage.
C. Systemic factors may be involved when healing delay cannot be otherwise accounted for, but local factors must be rechecked first.

IV. Clinical Appearance of the Healed Tissue

When healing is complete, the usual signs of healthy gingiva as outlined in table 11–1 on page 174 should be evident. Probe measurement in the sulcus should be minimal, the sulcus should be free from bleeding on probing, and the color, size, shape, and other characteristics should be normal.

FACTORS TO TEACH THE PATIENT

I. Why pockets need to be treated; how curettage contributes to pocket reduction or elimination.
II. Reasons for periodontal dressing placement.
III. Postoperative care with and without a dressing. Care of teeth and gingiva not involved in the curettage.
IV. Relationship of bacterial plaque and plaque control to healing.
V. Desensitization, using proper toothbrushing technique applied to cervical areas, and a fluoride dentifrice and mouthrinse.

References

1. Ramfjord, S.P. and Ash, M.M.: *Periodontology and Periodontics.* Philadelphia, W.B. Saunders Co., 1979, pp. 602–610.

2. Fedi, P.F., ed.: *The Periodontic Syllabus.* Philadelphia, Lea & Febiger, 1985, pp. 105–108.

3. Frank, R.M.: Bacterial Penetration in the Apical Pocket Wall of Advanced Human Periodontitis, *J. Periodont. Res., 15,* 563, Number 6, 1980.

4. Saglie, F.R., Carranza, F.A., and Newman, M.G.: The Presence of Bacteria Within the Oral Epithelium in Periodontal Disease. I. A Scanning and Transmission Electron Microscopic Study, *J. Periodontol., 56,* 618, October, 1985.

5. Barrington, E.P.: An Overview of Periodontal Surgical Procedures, *J. Periodontol., 52,* 518, September, 1981.

6. Ramfjord, S. and Kiester, G.: The Gingival Sulcus and the Periodontal Pocket Immediately Following Scaling of Teeth, *J. Periodontol., 25,* 167, July, 1954.

7. Goldman, H.M. and Cohen, D.W.: *Periodontal Therapy,* 6th ed. St. Louis, The C.V. Mosby Co., 1980, pp. 677–682.

Suggested Readings

Bradley, R.E.: The Rationale and Technique of Subgingival Curettage in the Treatment of Periodontal Disease, *Tex. Dent. J., 101,* 14, November, 1984.

Buethe, C.G., Kalkwarf, S.R., Kalkwarf, K.L., and Tussing, G.J.: Gingival Curettage. Is It a Viable Therapy Alternative? *Dent. Hyg., 60,* 24, January, 1986.

Carranza, F.A. and Perry, D.A.: *Clinical Periodontology for the Dental Hygienist.* Philadelphia, W.B. Saunders Co., 1986, pp. 221–224.

Echeverria, J.J. and Caffesse, R.G.: Effects of Gingival Curettage When Performed 1 Month After Root Instrumentation, A Biometric Evaluation, *J. Clin. Periodontol., 10,* 227, May, 1983.

Grant, D.A., Stern, I.B., and Listgarten, M.A., eds.: *Periodontics,* 6th ed. St. Louis, The C.V. Mosby Co., 1988, pp. 740–760, 823–837.

Green, M.L. and Green, B.L.: Aggressive Curettage, *Dent. Hyg., 53,* 409, September, 1979.

Knowles, J., Burgett, F., Morrison, E., Nissle, R., and Ramfjord, S.: Comparison of Results Following Three Modalities of Periodontal Therapy Related to Tooth Type and Initial Pocket Depth, *J. Clin. Periodontol., 7,* 32, February, 1980.

Kuren, S., Bissada, N., Maybury, J., and Bhat, M.: Comparative Effectiveness of Gingival Curettage With and Without Root Planing on Periodontal Health, *J. Dent. Res., 65,* 270, Abstract 912, Special Issue, 1986.

Meador, H.L., Lane, J.J., and Suddick, R.P.: The Long-term Effectiveness of Periodontal Therapy in a Clinical Practice, *J. Periodontol., 56,* 253, May, 1985.

Pattison, G.L. and Pattison, A.M.: *Periodontal Instrumentation.* Reston, Virginia, Reston Publishing Co., 1979, pp. 351–363.

Pawlak, E.A. and Hoag, P.M.: *Essentials of Periodontics,* 3rd ed. St. Louis, The C.V. Mosby Co., 1984, pp. 180–185.

Pollack, R.P.: Curettage: A New Look at an Old Technique, *Int. J. Periodontics Restorative Dent., 4,* 24, Number 5, 1984.

Smith, B.A. and Echeverri, M.: The Removal of Pocket Epithelium.

A Review, *J. West. Soc. Periodont. Periodont. Abstr., 32,* 45, Number 2, 1984.

Sterry, K.A., Langeroudi, M., and Dolby, A.E.: Metronidazole as an Adjunct to Periodontal Therapy with Sub-gingival Curettage, *Br. Dent. J., 158,* 176, March 9, 1985.

Bacterial Invasion

Allenspach-Petrzilka, G.E. and Guggenheim, B.: Bacterial Invasion of the Periodontium; An Important Factor in the Pathogenesis of Periodontitis? *J. Clin. Periodontol., 10,* 609, November, 1983.

Carranza, F.A., Saglie, R., Newman, M.G., and Valentin, P.L.: Scanning and Transmission Electron Microscopic Study of Tissue-invading Microorganisms in Localized Juvenile Periodontitis, *J. Periodontol., 54,* 598, October, 1983.

Gillett, R. and Johnson, N.W.: Bacterial Invasion of the Periodontium in a Case of Juvenile Periodontitis, *J. Clin. Periodontol., 9,* 93, January, 1982.

Manor, A., Lebendiger, M., Shiffer, A., and Tovel, H.: Bacterial Invasion of Periodontal Tissues in Advanced Periodontitis in Humans, *J. Periodontol., 55,* 567, October, 1984.

Nisengard, R. and Bascones, A.: Bacterial Invasion in Periodontal Disease (Workshop Abstracts), *J. Periodontol., 58,* 331, May, 1987.

Saglie, F.R., Carranza, F.A. Jr., Newman, M.G., Cheng, L., and Lewin, K.J.: Identification of Tissue-invading Bacteria in Human Periodontal Disease, *J. Periodont. Res., 17,* 452, Number 5, 1982.

Saglie, R. and Elbaz, J.J.: Bacterial Penetration Into the Gingival Tissue in Periodontal Disease, *J. West. Soc. Periodont. Periodont. Abstr., 31,* 85, Number 3, 1983.

Saglie, R., Newman, M.G., Carranza, F.A., and Pattison, G.L.: Bacterial Invasion of Gingiva in Advanced Periodontitis in Humans, *J. Periodontol., 53,* 217, April, 1982.

Chemical Curettage

Adcock, J.E., Berry, W.C., and Kalkwarf, K.L.: Effect of Sodium Hypochlorite Solution on the Subgingival Microflora of Juvenile Periodontitis Lesions, *Pediatr. Dent., 5,* 190, September, 1983.

Forgas, L.: Soft Tissue Curettage. Literature Review, *Dent. Hyg., 60,* 402, September, 1986.

Forgas, L.B. and Gound, S.: The Effects of Antiformin-Citric Acid Chemical Curettage on the Microbial Flora of the Periodontal Pocket, *J. Periodontol., 58,* 153, March, 1987.

Kalkwarf, K.L., Tussing, G.J., and Davis, M.J.: Histologic Evaluation of Gingival Curettage Facilitated by Sodium Hypochlorite Solution, *J. Periodontol., 53,* 63, February, 1982.

Melnyk, R. and Himrichs, J.: Clinical and Microbiological Evaluation of Sodium Hypochlorite Periodontal Curettage, *J. Dent. Res., 65,* 308, Abstract 1255, Special Issue, March, 1986.

Vieira, E.M., O'Leary, T.J., and Kafrawy, A.H.: The Effect of Sodium Hypochlorite and Citric Acid Solutions on Healing of Periodontal Pockets, *J. Periodontol., 53,* 71, February, 1982.

35 *Acute Gingival Conditions*

The dental hygienist frequently participates in clinical treatment procedures for acute gingival lesions. The dentist determines the diagnosis and treatment plan and supervises and directs the instruction and clinical techniques to be carried out.

NECROTIZING ULCERATIVE GINGIVITIS

Necrotizing ulcerative gingivitis (NUG) or necrotizing gingivitis (NG) is an acute, inflammatory, destructive disease of the periodontium. Other names that have been used include acute necrotizing ulcerative gingivitis (ANUG), trench mouth, Vincent's infection, Vincent's disease, and ulceromembranous gingivitis.

The condition may be superimposed over existing periodontitis, or with recurrent attacks of the disease, bone loss and other symptoms of periodontitis may develop.

Although NUG may occur at any age, it is usually seen among young people between ages 15 and 30. It is rare in children under 10 years of age in the United States, but is not uncommon in young children from low socioeconomic groups studied in South America and in some developing countries.[1,2] Malnutrition and lowered resistance to infection are significant predisposing factors. Individuals with Down's syndrome have been shown to have an increased incidence of NUG, as described on page 651.

I. Clinical Recognition

A. Initial Signs and Symptoms
The patient reports
1. Sudden onset.
2. Pain and soreness caused by slight pressure such as during chewing and toothbrushing; may be intensified by hot or highly seasoned foods. Gentle probing may produce an exaggerated pain response.
3. Bleeding: spontaneous or on slight pressure.
4. Poor appetite.
5. Metallic or other unpleasant taste.

B. Characteristic Clinical Findings
1. Interdental necrosis with ulceration of the papillae produces crater-like defects in the col area. In early disease, only the tips of papillae are involved, followed by progressive destruction of the entire papillae and extension to the marginal gingiva facially and lingually (figure 35–1).

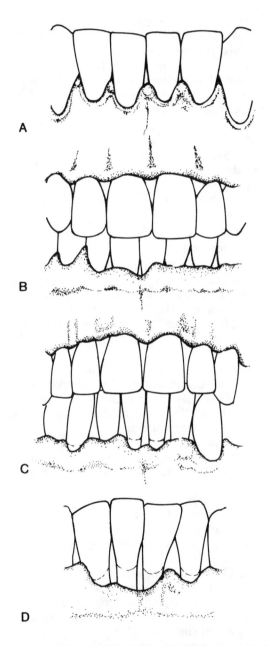

Figure 35–1. Necrotizing Ulcerative Gingivitis. A. Early lesion with blunted papillae and interdental necrosis. **B.** Increased destruction with loss of interdental tissue; rolled margins of the gingiva. **C.** More advanced destruction with recession and interdental cratering. **D.** Very advanced lesions, with loss of attached gingiva, recession, and tooth mobility.

2. A pseudomembrane may form over the necrotic area. It is a gray, loose, necrotic slough that, when wiped off, exposes a red and shiny hemorrhagic gingiva.

3. The membranous ulceration may be seen locally, that is, between two or three teeth, or it may be generalized throughout both maxillary and mandibular arches.

C. Other Clinical Findings

The following usually accompany the characteristic signs and symptoms:

1. Debris, materia alba, and plaque collect profusely because the patient avoids brushing the sensitive teeth and gingiva.

2. Fetor oris (bad breath) is often severe. It is caused by necrotic tissue, stagnant saliva, and breakdown products of blood and debris.

3. Increased salivation.

D. Systemic Signs

A few patients have signs of systemic involvement. Examination should always be made to detect the presence of the following:

1. Malaise.

2. Lymphadenopathy of submaxillary and cervical nodes.

3. Possible slight elevation of body temperature.

II. Predisposing Factors

NUG is an infectious disease caused by a fuso-spirochetal complex of microbes that develops and increases in association with predisposing factors that have lowered the body's defenses. Major predisposing factors are stress, very poor oral hygiene, and smoking. Other related factors are listed here.

A. Local Factors

NUG is rarely, if ever, seen in a clean, healthy, cared-for, and professionally supervised mouth. Many of the factors that can be considered predisposing are the same as those that predispose to chronic marginal gingivitis.

Predisposing factors include

1. Preexisting gingivitis and/or periodontitis.

2. Inadequate personal oral care with general neglect.

3. Tobacco use.

4. Factors related to retention of microorganisms and deposits

   a. Calculus as a retainer for plaque and debris.

   b. Open contacts, which encourage food impaction and stagnation.

   c. Oral habits, for example, mouth breathing.

   d. Periodontal pockets, which retain microorganisms and debris.

   e. Malposition of teeth; overcrowding.

   f. Iatrogenic causes, such as overhanging fillings.

   g. Tissue flap; for example, over a partially erupted third mandibular molar.

   h. Open carious lesions.

B. Stress Factors

1. Acute anxiety related to life situations is a common characteristic of patients with NUG. In susceptible people, the condition has been found to occur or recur during periods of stress. Examples include students during examination periods, military men in combat, and people at times of important decision-making.

2. Emotional stress is frequently accompanied by poor oral care, improper diet, excessive smoking, overexertion, interrupted sleep, and other deviations in health habits.

C. Systemic: Disease-resistance Factors

1. Dietary and nutritional inadequacies; vitamin deficiencies.

2. Recent illnesses; frequent upper respiratory infections; debilitating diseases such as infectious mononucleosis, pernicious anemia, hepatitis or human immunodeficiency virus (HIV) infection.

3. Fatigue; insufficient sleep.

III. Etiology

Bacteriologic and immunologic factors are implicated. For many years, bacteriologic smears were made from the NUG lesion and examined by microscope for the presence of fusiform bacilli and spirochetes. The smear test is no longer considered significant for making a diagnosis.

NUG has not been identified as a communicable disease. Research has shown that a transfer of organisms from an infected patient does not produce the typical disease.

A. Microbiologic Factors[3,4,5]

Of the many types of organisms found in NUG lesions, fusiform bacilli and medium-sized spirochetes predominate. The constant flora has been shown to include *Treponema* and *Selenomonas* species, *Bacteroides intermedius, Bacteroides gingivalis,* and *Fusobacterium* species.

B. Immune Factors[5,6]

Patients with NUG may have depressed polymorphonuclear leukocyte (PMN) responsiveness in chemotaxis and phagocytosis as well as other signs of altered host response. A high incidence of NUG has been shown in patients with acquired immune deficiency syndrome (AIDS).[6] Such an altered immune response permits opportunistic microorganisms to flourish and destructive periodontal infections to develop (page 23).

IV. Course of Development

A. Description of the Lesion

1. NUG is superimposed on gingivitis or periodontitis.

2. Ulceration and necrosis begin in the col area.

3. Both epithelial tissue and connective tissue are involved.

4. The disease process progresses to involve the entire papilla, and eventually, to the marginal gingiva on the facial and lingual surfaces.

5. The pseudomembrane covering the lesion is a necrotic slough of the surface epithelium. It contains leukocytes, bacteria, epithelial cells, and fibrin.

6. Connective tissue shows the signs of acute inflammation. It is hyperemic and filled with leukocytes, and its capillaries are engorged. When the pseudomembrane is lifted, the red inflamed connective tissue can be seen.

B. Microscopic Examination

The four layers in the lesion have been described from observations made by electron microscopy.[7] All layers contain spirochetes.

1. *Bacterial Zone.* The most superficial zone consists primarily of a mass of varied bacteria, including a few spirochetes.

2. *Neutrophil-rich Zone.* Under the bacterial zone is a layer of leukocytes, predominantly neutrophils. Microorganisms, including many spirochetes, are found among the leukocytes.

3. *Necrotic Zone.* This zone contains disintegrating tissue cells, many spirochetes, and other bacteria.

4. *Spirochetal Infiltration Zone.* In this non-necrotized layer where tissue components are still preserved, spirochetes have invaded, but other microorganisms have not. The action of toxins and other bacterial products was described with pocket formation on pages 181–182.

TREATMENT

Patient instruction and motivation for self-care are needed along with skillful subgingival instrumentation. After the initial symptoms have subsided, complete therapy must be carried out. The tissue destruction usually has left the gingiva deformed, with interdental flattening or cratering. Surgical treatment may be needed to restore a physiologic form that can be maintained by the patient in the plan to prevent recurrence of the disease.

I. Preparation for Diagnosis

Initially, certain data must be collected for use by the dentist in making the diagnosis and treatment plan. Preparation of a complete diagnostic work-up may be impractical, considering the emergency nature of the patient's condition. Basic information needed is suggested by the steps described here.

A. History

1. *Record the Chief Complaint.* The history of the current disease is described by date of onset, duration, symptoms as reported, and what self-treatment the patient had already performed.

2. *Record Whether This is a Recurrence.* If so, note details of previous episodes, and the treatment given.

3. *Obtain Information Needed for Preliminary Treatment*
   a. Conditions needing medical consultation.
   b. Need for premedication for prevention of bacteremia (see the list on pages 85 and 91).
   c. Allergies.

4. *Use Knowledge of Predisposing Factors for NUG to Gather Pertinent Information*
   a. Tobacco habits.
   b. Recent illnesses or types of therapy may explain a lowered resistance.
   c. Record of immediately previous 24-hour food intake. When the mouth has been sore and eating has been painful, a diet recording may not be typical of the patient's usual intake. Later, a 5-day or week-long food diary will be requested as part of the continuing preventive program.
   d. Variations of normal sleeping hours and routine.

B. Examination

1. *Record the Patient's Temperature* (pages 95–96).

2. *Extraoral Examination*
   a. Palpate submaxillary and cervical nodes (figure 8–4, page 105).
   b. Observe face and skin: flushed, damp.
   c. Observe signs of malaise.

3. *Oral Examination.* Without instrumentation, a preliminary examination can be made and the overall appearance of the gingival tissue recorded. The dentist may prefer to see the gingiva as it appeared initially, before instrumentation or rinsing, to make the diagnosis and prepare the treatment plan. Instrumentation may be temporarily delayed for patients requiring premedication.

II. Treatment Plan

The dental hygiene treatment plan is formulated within the total treatment plan. Only a partial treatment plan is made until after the acute phase of the disease has passed. After the initial treatment, the diagnostic work-up can be completed and full evaluation made.

A. Systemic Treatment

1. Directions concerning diet, rest, and other systemic influences.

2. Multivitamin supplements are sometimes prescribed.

3. Antibiotics. After the diagnosis is made, the dentist determines whether systemic therapy is indicated. Except for a patient who requires antibiotic coverage to prevent bacteremia, antibiotics are prescribed conservatively.

B. Relief of Acute Symptoms

1. Personal care instructions for rinsing, brushing, and limiting use of tobacco.

2. Debridement of teeth and gingiva.
3. Begin subgingival scaling and root planing.

C. Basic Therapy
1. Complete diagnostic work-up.
2. Reevaluation and preparation of total treatment plan.
3. Preventive program.
   a. Instruction for prevention of recurrence of NUG.
   b. Dietary analysis and counseling.
   c. Self-care fluoride, professional application when indicated.
4. Complete scaling and root planing.
5. Reduction or elimination of predisposing factors to NUG
   a. Removal of overhanging margins and other retention factors.
   b. Restoration of teeth and contact areas.
6. Evaluation for periodontal surgery; need for restoration of tissue contour and elimination of craters.
7. Restoration of occlusion; prosthetic replacements and all other dental needs.

DENTAL HYGIENE CARE

A series of appointments for a typical NUG patient is outlined here. The number of appointments and the exact procedure at each appointment depend on the severity of the disease and the response of the gingiva as treatment progresses.

Usually 4 or 5 appointments are needed during the acute stage, and at least the first 3 should be at 24-hour intervals. After that, when the acute stage has subsided, a regular appointment is established for continued supervision and for proceeding with basic therapy.

I. Acute Phase: First Appointment

The first part of this appointment has been described under the discussion of history in preparation for diagnosis on page 483. After the dentist has examined the patient and made the diagnosis, the dental hygienist will be directed to follow a procedure such as described here.

A. History Review
Check the history for a patient requiring prophylactic premedication for prevention of bacteremia and arrange accordingly. Parenteral administration may be indicated, which should be discussed with the patient's physician.

B. Patient Instruction
1. Explain local causes and control measures.
2. Demonstrate plaque with a disclosing agent.
3. Show plaque removal procedures, using a soft brush moistened with warm water.

C. General Debridement
1. Apply hydrogen peroxide (3% solution with equal parts of water) with cotton pellets at proximal areas; request patient to rinse. Avoid use of compressed air or water spray to prevent dispersion of contaminated aerosols.
2. Apply topical anesthetic and, when painful, treat by quadrants, using block anesthesia.
3. Use ultrasonic or manual instruments or a combination for supragingival scaling. Use warm water for frequent irrigation while scaling.

D. Subgingival Instrumentation
The gingiva will respond sooner if subgingival scaling can be started at the first visit.
1. Perform instrumentation carefully to prevent tissue damage.
2. Have assistant evacuate continuously when an ultrasonic instrument is used to prevent contaminated aerosols and to protect the patient from inhaling microorganisms.
3. Irrigate and evacuate frequently to clear all debris and calculus removed during instrumentation.

E. Patient Instruction
1. *Instructions for Home Use.* Instructions for home procedures must be carefully explained. Written directions are needed.
2. *Instructions for Continuing Care.* Inform the patient that treatment will not be complete when the pain is eliminated. Explain the underlying gingival or periodontal infection and how NUG recurs if the periodontal condition is not treated.
3. *Rinsing Directions.* Vigorous rinsing with hot water or weak saline solution (page 329) is necessary every hour during the period of acute symptoms.

   Rinsing with hydrogen peroxide 3% with equal parts of water is preferred by some dentists. This should be recommended for only the first 2 or 3 days and then discontinued.
4. *Toothbrushing.* Use a soft nylon brush gently, but thoroughly. Clean the teeth as much as possible after each meal and before going to bed. When a brush is not given the patient at the clinic or office, write down the names of specific brushes for the patient to purchase.
5. *Avoiding Tobacco Products.* The heavy smoker can be asked to limit the amount.
6. *Diet*[8]
   a. Recommend frequent small nutritious meals that incorporate daily requirements from the Basic 4 (table 28–1, page 382).
   b. A liquid or soft bland diet is advised for the first day, particularly for the patient with systemic symptoms or pronounced sensitivity when chewing. A diet of soft solids can be used on the second day. Examples of foods to include in a liquid and a soft solid diet are listed on page 598.
   c. The choice of foods should include in-

creased amounts of meat and milk products and of fruits and juices.

d. Avoid highly seasoned foods and alcoholic beverages.

II. Acute Phase: Second Appointment

A. Patient Examination

A remarkable improvement can usually be seen within 24 hours, with pain and discomfort lessened, the pseudomembrane gone, and tissue enlargement reduced.

B. Scaling and Root Planing

Continue these procedures from the previous appointment after checking areas previously treated. The objective is to be as thorough as possible, because plaque retained over residual calculus and altered cementum can keep the tissues from healing completely.

C. Instruction: Second Day

1. *Rinsing.* When healing is progressing favorably, change rinsing schedule to every 2 hours.
2. *Toothbrushing.* Emphasize thorough coverage of the entire dentition, using sulcular brushing.
3. *Proximal Surfaces.* The use of floss is advised and should be demonstrated at this or the third appointment, depending on the readiness of the patient and the tissue. Other proximal cleaning devices may be useful. When the interdental embrasures are open as a result of papillary necrosis (figure 35–1C and D), an interdental brush or other device is usually indicated. The importance of complete plaque removal must be explained.
4. *Diet.* A liquid diet is not usually indicated after the first day and the patient can use the soft solids diet or a regular diet adapted with bland foods that will not irritate the healing tissues.
5. *Instructions.* Provide specific written instructions.

III. Acute Phase: Third Appointment

A. Observe and Evaluate the Gingival Tissues

Continued improvement should be expected each day. Areas where healing has not progressed need additional attention to personal plaque control and further professional scaling and root planing.

B. Instruction in Self-care Procedures

Instructions are continued. Follow Lesson I or Lesson II (pages 372–373), depending on the extent of previous instruction.

C. Scaling and Root Planing

Treatment is continued, with particular attention paid to areas where healing has not been complete.

D. Home Care Instruction

1. *Rinsing.* Discontinue peroxide if that was the selected rinse. Request the patient to use warm mild saline solution vigorously after brushing and flossing.
2. *Review Instructions.* Review and emphasize previous instruction.

IV. Successive Appointments

After daily supervision during the acute stage, regular appointments for basic treatment are planned. The gingiva is evaluated, and repeated scaling and root planing are performed as needed to complete that part of the treatment.

A. Preparation of a Diagnostic Work-up

The complete diagnostic work-up is prepared as directed by the dentist, and the patient is instructed for continued treatment.

B. Recurrence of NUG

When the gingival and bony craters that remain after the initial healing phase are not treated, they are vulnerable to continuing disease and recurrence of NUG. Plaque and debris can collect readily in the misshapen proximal areas, and these areas are difficult to clean with plaque control techniques. Gingival craters invite further tissue breakdown, leading to periodontal pocket formation.

Surgical treatment may involve gingivoplasty when the bone is not involved. When bony craters exist, treatment may involve flap surgery with osseous reshaping.

PERIODONTAL ABSCESS

An abscess is a collection of pus in a circumscribed or walled-off area. Gingival and periodontal abscesses occur within the periodontal tissues. An abscess is called *gingival* when it is located in the marginal area, and *periodontal* when it is in the deeper periodontal tissues. They may also be known as *lateral abscesses* because they occur along the lateral surfaces of a tooth, in contrast to a periapical abscess which is usually associated with the apex.

I. Development of a Periodontal Abscess

Pus collects in the tissue as a result of bacterial infection. The infection may be a complication of an existing periodontal disease or it may be an immediate result of purulent microorganisms forced into the tissue by some form of trauma. The body's reaction is to send large numbers of defense cells to the area, particularly polymorphonuclear leukocytes (PMNs), which are major constituents of the purulent exudate (pus) that collects.

Pus is a thick fluid product of inflammation. It contains many living and dead PMNs mixed with debris from cells and tissues that have been destroyed by the enzymes released by the PMNs. Unless there is a means for drainage, the pus collects and forms an abscess.

A sinus or fistula may form. A *fistula* is a pathologic sinus or abnormal passage that leads from an abscess to the surface of the gingiva or mucosa. Drainage may occur through this sinus and release the pressure within the abscess, which in turn, can relieve the pain the patient may experience.

II. Etiologic Factors

A. Periodontal Pockets

Deep pockets of chronic inflammatory periodontal disease provide an environment for abscess formation. Special anatomic variations predispose to abscess formation. Instrumentation applied within the pocket and the effects of the instrumentation may be the precipitating factors that initiate abscess formation.

1. *Anatomic Features.* Intrabony pockets, pockets that extend into bi- or trifurcation areas and complex pockets that develop in winding or irregular shapes are particularly susceptible to becoming closed and therefore susceptible to abscess formation.
2. *Instrumentation.*[9] Incomplete scaling and root planing in the depth of a pocket may allow the tissue at the opening of the pocket to heal, tighten, and prevent drainage from the infectious material deep in the pocket. Plaque and calculus remaining in the sealed off part of the pocket attract the collection of more PMNs, and an abscess develops.

B. Trauma

Foreign objects may enter by way of the sulcus or pocket and become embedded along with microorganisms. The infection leads to abscess formation.

1. *Implanted or Impacted Material*[10]
   a. Popcorn husk, small fish bone or shellfish fragment, seeds, seed coverings, or other material from food.
   b. Oral hygiene devices include toothbrush bristle or filament or a sliver from a toothpick.
2. *Instrumentation.* Trauma during subgingival instrumentation may force infectious material into the pocket wall.

C. Patient Susceptibility to Infection

The possibility for abscess formation within the gingival tissue is increased from any of the etiologic factors that have been mentioned when the patient's resistance to infection is lowered. Patients with uncontrolled diabetes or those who are receiving immunosuppressive medication are examples.

III. Clinical Signs and Symptoms

Even though clinical manifestations may vary, the classic signs and symptoms are listed here.

A. Clinical Appearance

The area of the abscess is enlarged, with a red, shiny, smooth surface. It may appear dome-like or pointed, and on slight digital pressure, pus may appear.

B. The Tooth

1. *Sensitivity.* The tooth may be sensitive to percussion. When extruded, it may be sensitive to touching the tooth in the opposing jaw. It may be slightly mobile.
2. *Pulp Vitality Test.* Pulp testing usually reveals a vital tooth, responding within the normal range.
3. *Radiographs.* A radiolucency may be noted along the lateral wall beside the tooth but such a finding is variable. No bone loss shows in early lesions. The amount of bone destruction and the location of the abscess influence the possible radiographic findings.

C. General Physical Condition

Occasionally, a patient shows evidence of systemic involvement, such as a slight elevation in body temperature, malaise, and lymphadenopathy.

D. Chronic Abscess

In the chronic state, a sinus tract usually opens on the gingival surface and drains periodically. Before drainage, the patient may have a dull pain from the pressure of the fluid within the abscess area. Acute symptoms may be expected from time to time unless definitive periodontal therapy is completed.

IV. Comparison of Periapical and Periodontal Abscesses

The dentist must often differentiate between a periapical and a periodontal abscess. Certain signs and symptoms are nearly the same for both. A few of the potentially distinguishing findings are noted here.

A. Pulp Test

The tooth with a periapical lesion does not respond normally to a pulp tester.

B. Sinus Tract Formation

The opening of a sinus tract from a periapical abscess usually is positioned more apically; whereas the opening from a periodontal abscess is more coronal.

C. Pain

Sharp steady pain is typical of a periapical lesion; whereas the pain from a periodontal abscess varies.

D. Periodontal Examination

A tooth with a periapical lesion is not necessarily periodontally involved. Probing may reveal no pocket depth of note, and no bone loss may be apparent in the radiograph.

Occasionally, a combined periodontic and endodontic lesion occurs. Communication between a deep periodontal pocket and an apical lesion is not unusual. Communication may also exist from a periodontal pocket into the pulp by way of a lateral or accessory canal through the dentin.

E. Dental Caries

A diseased pulp leading to a periapical abscess is caused by either trauma to the tooth or dental caries extending inward until the pulp becomes infected. A carious lesion may also be present with a periodontal abscess, which may complicate the differential diagnosis.

F. Radiographic Examination

Early stages of either a periapical or a periodontal abscess will not be evident in a radiograph. A widening of the periodontal ligament space may appear.

V. Treatment

Two phases of treatment are used for the patient with a periodontal abscess. The first is for immediate relief of acute symptoms, and the second is the definitive treatment followed by preventive maintenance. The entire plan should be explained to the patient at the outset.

A. Objectives of Emergency Treatment
1. Relieve pain.
2. Establish drainage.
3. Determine need for systemic antibiotic therapy.

B. Review Medical History

Determine necessary preappointment precautions such as the need for antibiotic premedication (pages 85 and 91).

C. Examination for Systemic Involvement

Antibiotic medication is frequently prescribed by the dentist when systemic involvement is definite.
1. Determine and record the patient's body temperature (pages 95–96).
2. Examine submaxillary and neck lymph nodes for adenopathy.

D. Provide Anesthesia

When the abscess is confined to the gingival area, and the drainage may be expected to cause little if any discomfort, a topical anesthetic may suffice. Usually, block anesthesia is indicated.

E. Methods for Drainage[11,12,13]
1. *Via Pocket or Sulcus Opening.* Isolate the area, swab with a topical antiseptic, and use a probe to gain admission into the sulcus or pocket. Gently probe circumferentially until an opening into the abscess is found. Drainage usually begins promptly.

   Use a curet to open the area and locate and remove a foreign body irritant when it is known to be present from the history obtained from the patient. Scaling and root planing are performed as needed.
2. *Direct Incision.* The type of incision varies. A horizontal or semilunar incision may be made

directly over the abscess. A drain may be needed to keep the incision open long enough to drain completely. A piece of rubber dam or iodophor gauze may be used.

All incisions should be avoided, if possible, to prevent gingival recession from a vertical incision, unsightly scars from any type of incision, or complications during healing.

F. Postoperative Instructions

Rinsing with hot saline solution every 2 hours is advised. The patient should return for observation in 24 to 48 hours. Relief from pain and discomfort can be expected and appointments for definitive treatment planned. Plaque control instruction is initiated or continued, and scaling and root planing are completed.

G. Anticipated Results
1. Acute symptoms are resolved.
2. Pain relief occurs within a short time following the initiation of drainage, because the pressure is released from within the abscessed area.
3. Extruded tooth returns to its normal position.
4. Swelling is reduced.
5. Temporary comfort is obtained for the patient; the lesion is reduced to a standard chronic lesion that requires additional treatment.
6. If drainage is not complete, an acute lesion may develop into a lesion with a chronic sinus.

VI. Definitive Therapy

Whatever pocket elimination procedures are indicated should be completed within a reasonable time to prevent further complications. Careful and regular plaque control with scaling and root planing are usually needed.

TECHNICAL HINTS

I. Provide explicit directions concerning rinsing with hydrogen peroxide. Extended use of oxygenating drugs can cause tissue changes.
II. Instructions for patients can be printed or written. Because instructions change each day during the acute phase, individual slips should be prepared, using paper of different colors. Printed instructions can be personalized with added written notations.

FACTORS TO TEACH THE PATIENT

I. Premature discontinuation of treatment for NUG because acute signs have subsided can lead to recurrence of the infection.
II. The role of diet, rest, and plaque control in the prevention of NUG.
III. The avoidance of an oral irrigating device in the presence of acute inflammatory conditions.[14] Mi-

croorganisms may be forced into the tissues beneath a pocket, and bacteremia can be produced.

References

1. Jiménez L., M. and Baer, P.N.: Necrotizing Ulcerative Gingivitis in Children: A 9 Year Clinical Study, *J. Periodontol., 46,* 715, December, 1975.
2. Enwonwu, C.O.: Infectious Oral Necrosis (cancrum oris) in Nigerian Children: A Review, *Community Dent. Oral Epidemiol., 13,* 190, June, 1985.
3. Loesche, W.J., Syed, S.A., Laughon, B.E., and Stoll, J.: The Bacteriology of Acute Necrotizing Ulcerative Gingivitis, *J. Periodontol., 53,* 223, April, 1982.
4. Cogen, R.B., Stevens, A.W., Jr., Cohen-Cole, S., Kirk, K., and Freeman, A.: Leukocyte Function in the Etiology of Acute Necrotizing Ulcerative Gingivitis, *J. Periodontol., 54,* 402, July, 1983.
5. Falker, W.A., Martin, S.A., Vincent, J.W., Tall, B.D., Nauman, R.K., and Suzuki, J.B.: A Clinical Demographic and Microbiologic Study of ANUG Patients in an Urban Dental School, *J. Clin. Periodontol., 14,* 307, July, 1987.
6. Dennison, D.K., Smith, B., and Newland, J.R.: Immune Responsiveness and ANUG, *J. Dent. Res., 64,* 197, Abstract 204, March, 1985.
7. Listgarten, M.A.: Electron Microscopic Observations on the Bacterial Flora of Acute Necrotizing Ulcerative Gingivitis, *J. Periodontol., 36,* 328, July-August, 1965.
8. Nizel, A.E.: *Nutrition in Preventive Dentistry: Science and Practice,* 2nd ed. Philadelphia, W.B. Saunders Co., 1981, pp. 485–488.
9. Armitage, G.C.: *Biologic Basis of Periodontal Maintenance Therapy.* Berkeley, California, Praxis Publishing Co., 1980, pp. 154–159.
10. Gillette, W.B. and Van House, R.L.: Ill Effects of Improper Oral Hygiene Procedures, *J. Am. Dent. Assoc., 101,* 476, September, 1980.
11. Fedi, P.F., ed.: *The Periodontic Syllabus.* Philadelphia, Lea & Febiger, 1985, pp. 151–153.
12. Carranza, F.A.: *Glickman's Clinical Periodontology,* 6th ed. Philadelphia, W.B. Saunders Co., 1984, p. 900.
13. Grant, D.A., Stern, I.B., and Listgarten, M.A., eds.: *Periodontics,* 6th ed. St. Louis, The C.V. Mosby Co., 1988, pp. 429–431.
14. American Dental Association, Council on Dental Materials, Instruments, and Equipment: *Dentist's Desk Reference: Materials, Instruments and Equipment,* 2nd ed. Chicago, American Dental Association, 1983, pp. 421–422.

Suggested Readings

Necrotizing Ulcerative Gingivitis

Armitage, G.C.: *Biologic Basis of Periodontal Maintenance Therapy.* Berkeley, California, Praxis Publishing Co., 1980, pp. 146–154.

Becker, S.L.: Treating ANUG Patients, *Quintessence Int., 11,* 75, February, 1980.

Carranza, F.A.: *Glickman's Clinical Periodontology,* 6th ed. Philadelphia, W.B. Saunders Co., 1984, pp. 146–157, 643–650.

Chung, C.P., Nisengard, R.J., Slots, J., and Genco, R.J.: Bacterial IgG and IgM Antibody Titers in Acute Necrotizing Ulcerative Gingivitis, *J. Periodontol., 64,* 557, September, 1983.

Courtois, G.J., Cobb, C.M., and Killoy, W.J.: Acute Necrotizing Ulcerative Gingivitis. A Transmission Electron Microscope Study, *J. Periodontol., 54,* 671, November, 1983.

Fedi, P.F., ed: *The Periodontic Syllabus.* Philadelphia, Lea & Febiger, 1985, pp. 153–160.

Grant, D.A., Stern, I.B., and Listgarten, M.A., eds.: *Periodontics,* 6th ed. St. Louis, The C.V. Mosby Co., 1988, pp. 398–412.

Harding, J., Berry, W.C., Marsh, C., and Jolliff, C.R.: Salivary Antibodies in Acute Gingivitis, *J. Periodontol., 51,* 63, February, 1980.

Jaworski, C.P., Koudelka, B.M., Roth, N.A., and Marshall, K.J.: Acute Necrotizing Ulcerative Gingivitis in a Case of Systemic Lupus Erythematosus, *J. Oral Maxillofac. Surg., 43,* 43, January, 1985.

Johnson, B.D. and Engel, D.: Acute Necrotizing Ulcerative Gingivitis. A Review of Diagnosis, Etiology and Treatment, *J. Periodontol., 57,* 141, March, 1986.

Kowolik, M.J. and Nisbet, T.: Smoking and Acute Ulcerative Gingivitis. A Study of 100 Patients, *Br. Dent. J., 154,* 241, April 23, 1983.

Lander, P.E. and Seymour, G.J.: Differential Dark Field Microscopy of Acute Ulcerative Gingivitis. Case Report, *Aust. Dent. J., 30,* 33, February, 1985.

Maltha, J.C.: Necrotizing Ulcerative Gingivitis in Beagle Dogs. III. Distribution of Spirochetes in Interdental Gingival Tissue, *J. Periodont. Res., 20,* 522, September, 1985.

Meister, F., Rank, D.F.P., and Davies, E.E.: Importance of Patient Motivation in the Treatment of Acute Necrotizing Ulcerative Gingivitis, *Quintessence Int., 12,* 199, February, 1981.

Page, L.R., Bosman, C.W., Drummond, J.F., and Ciancio, S.G.: Acute Recurrent Gingivitis, *Oral Surg. Oral Med. Oral Pathol., 49,* 337, April, 1980.

Reinhardt, R.A., Cohen, D.M., and Lewis, J.E.S.: Unusual Sequelae to Necrotizing Ulcerative Gingivitis (NUG)-Like Lesions, *J. Oral Med., 37,* 109, October-December, 1982.

Ryan, M.E., Hopkins, K., and Wilbur, R.B.: Acute Necrotizing Ulcerative Gingivitis in Children with Cancer, *Am. J. Dis. Child., 137,* 592, June, 1983.

Sabiston, C.B.: A Review and Proposal for the Etiology of Acute Necrotizing Gingivitis, *J. Clin. Periodontol., 13,* 727, September, 1986.

Stevens, A.W., Jr., Cogen, R.B., Cohen-Cole, S., and Freeman, A.: Demographic and Clinical Data Associated with Acute Necrotizing Ulcerative Gingivitis in a Dental School Population, *J. Clin. Periodontol., 11,* 487, September, 1984.

Periodontal Abscess

Abrams, H. and Kopczyk, R.A.: Gingival Sequela from a Retained Piece of Dental Floss, *J. Am. Dent. Assoc., 106,* 57, January, 1983.

Ahl, D.R., Hilgeman, J.L., and Snyder, J.D.: Periodontal Emergencies, *Dent. Clin. North Am., 30,* 459, July, 1986.

Collins, J.F.: Surgical Treatment of Acute Periodontal Abscess, *Gen. Dent., 29,* 297, July-August, 1981.

Dello Russo, N.M.: The Post-prophylaxis Periodontal Abscess: Etiology and Treatment, *Int. J. Periodontics Restorative Dent., 5,* 28, Number 1, 1985.

Fuss, Z., Bender, I.B., and Rickoff, B.D.: An Unusual Periodontal Abscess, *J. Endod., 12,* 116, March, 1986.

Goldman, H.M. and Cohen, D.W.: *Periodontal Therapy,* 6th ed. St. Louis, The C.V. Mosby Co., 1980, pp. 307–308, 744–745, 1018–1019.

Harrison, G.A., Schultz, T.A., and Schaberg, S.J.: Deep Neck Infection Complicated by Diabetes Mellitus, *Oral Surg. Oral Med. Oral Pathol., 55,* 133, February, 1983.

Kon, S., Garcia, V.G., Valente, L., and Pustiglioni, F.E.: Acute Periodontal Lesions—Simplified Treatment, *Quintessence Int., 14,* 641, June, 1983.

Kryshtalskyj, E.: Management of the Periodontal Abscess, *Can. Dent. Assoc. J., 53,* 519, July, 1987.

Palmer, R.M.: Acute Lateral Periodontal Abscess, *Br. Dent. J., 157,* 311, November 10, 1984.

Smith, R.G. and Davies, R.M.: Acute Lateral Periodontal Abscesses, *Br. Dent. J., 161,* 176, September 6, 1986.

Vence, M.-G. and Benfenati, S.P.: Treatment of Periodontal Abscess: A Rationalized Approach, *Quintessence Int., 15,* 219, February, 1984.

36 *Dressings and Sutures*

A dressing may be placed over the surgical wound following periodontal surgery. A dressing is frequently indicated after gingival curettage.

I. Purposes and Uses
A. Provide mechanical protection for the surgical wound and therefore facilitate healing.
B. Prevent postoperative bleeding by maintaining the initial clot in place.
C. Support mobile teeth during healing.
D. Aid in shaping or molding the newly formed tissues; aid in holding a flap in place or immobilizing a graft.
E. Provide patient comfort during the healing period by isolating the wound from external irritations and injuries.

II. Characteristics of Acceptable Dressing Material
An acceptable periodontal dressing should have the following characteristics:
A. Pose no risk for dental team member or patient.
B. Be nontoxic and nonirritating to oral tissues.
C. Contain no asbestos or other ingredient that may be injurious to the health of the person who prepares the dressing.
D. Be conveniently prepared, placed, and removed with minimal discomfort for the patient.
E. Be able to maintain adhesion to itself and to the teeth and tissue where it is placed.
F. Should not damage or stain restorative materials.

TYPES OF DRESSINGS

Dressings are usually classified into two groups: those that contain eugenol and those that do not contain eugenol. Healing has been shown to progress at about the same rate under either type of dressing, so selection by the dentist can be based on such factors as firmness of the material, durability, consistency, ease of manipulation, or personal preference.

Commercial preparations are available as a ready-mix or as two pastes to mix or as a liquid and a powder to mix. Products are reviewed by the American Dental Association Council on Dental Therapeutics (page 331), and the list of accepted products is published annually.

I. Eugenol-containing Dressing
A. Basic Ingredients
1. *Powder.* Zinc oxide, powdered rosin, and tannic acid. Formerly, asbestos fiber was used as a binder in some formulas. Because airborne asbestos is a recognized pulmonary health hazard, dental team members responsible for mixing periodontal dressings frequently and in quantity may become over-exposed. Asbestos fiber is no longer an acceptable ingredient of dressings.[1]
2. *Liquid.* Eugenol, with an oil such as peanut or cottonseed, and thymol.

B. Examples
Well-known dressings are Ward's (Wonderpack), Periodontal Dressing Powder and Liquid ("PPC"), and Kirkland. Formulas for the last two are given below as examples of the ingredients and their proportions.

1. *Kirkland Periodontal Pack*
   Powder: each 100 grams contains

Zinc oxide	40.00 g.
Rosin	40.00 g.
Tannic acid	20.00 g.

   Liquid: each 100 milliliters contains

Eugenol	46.50 ml.
Peanut oil	46.50 ml.
Rosin	7.70 g.

2. *Periodontal Dressing Powder and Liquid (PPC)*
   Powder: each 100 grams contains

Zinc oxide	42.90 g.
Powdered rosin	38.10 g.
Tannic acid	9.50 g.
Kaolin	2.40 g.
Mica	7.10 g.

   Liquid: each 100 milliliters contains

Eugenol	98.00 ml.
Thymol	2.00 g.
Color	

C. Advantages
1. *Consistency.* Firm and heavy; provides good support and protection for tissues and flaps.
2. *Slow setting.* Good working time.
3. *Preparation and Storage.* Can be prepared in quantity and stored (frozen) in work-size pieces.

D. Disadvantages
1. *Taste.* Sharp, unpleasant taste.
2. *Tissue Reaction.* Irritating to membranes; sensitivity reactions can occur.[2]
3. *Consistency.* Dressing is hard, brittle, and breaks easily.

II. Non-Eugenol-containing Dressing

Because of the negative qualities of eugenol, researchers have long worked at finding a substitute. Other formulas have been developed, containing such ingredients as antibiotics, that would provide bacteriostatic effects.

A. Coe-Pak

Coe-Pak is prepared by mixing pastes from two tubes: one containing metallic oxides with a fungicide and the other nonionizing carboxylic acids with a germicide-fungicide.

When a firmer dressing is desirable, some powder from a eugenol-containing dressing can be added to the Coe-Pak during mixing.

B. Advantages

1. *Taste.* Acceptable taste.
2. *Consistency.* Pliable and easy to place with light pressure.
3. *Smooth Surface.* Comfortable to patient, and plaque and debris do not stick readily.
4. *Ease of Removal.* Often comes off in one piece.

C. Disadvantages

1. *Prompt Setting.* Affected by higher room temperatures.
2. *Preparation and Storage.* Cannot be prepared in advance and stored.

CLINICAL APPLICATION

I. Eugenol-containing Dressing

A. Mixing

1. Mix powder and liquid on a paper mixing pad, incorporating the powder gradually to form a thick paste. Use a metal spatula or wooden tongue depressor.
2. Knead additional powder into the paste until the consistency is firm and thick, but not sticky.
3. Divide the mass into quantities appropriate for application to a quadrant or other specific area. Wrap pieces in foil or waxed paper for storage in freezer.

B. Application

1. Roll the mixed dressing into a round strip.
2. Examine area to be sure bleeding has stopped.
3. Use small sections of dressing to mold into wedge shapes to press interproximally from facial and lingual aspects when the patient has open interproximal embrasures with missing papillae and recession. It is important that the proximal gingiva be completely and firmly covered. A strip of dressing can then be added facially and lingually for complete coverage.
4. Apply continuously (one strip) from the lingual to the facial surface; or two strips may be used to cover a quadrant, the first to extend from the distal of the most posterior tooth over the facial surfaces, and the second to overlap the first on the distal and extend along the lingual surfaces.
5. Press at the interproximal areas to gain retention and provide complete coverage for the treatment area. Adapt with a plastic instrument.
6. Edentulous areas can usually be filled to make the dressing continuous between the teeth unless too great a gap exists.
7. Muscle trim (border mold) the cheeks, lips, and tongue to prevent movement or dislodgment of the dressing.
8. Check frena for freedom of movement.
   a. Lingual: request patient to touch palate with tip of tongue.
   b. Buccal: retract cheek up and out over maxillary premolars and out from mandibular premolars.
   c. Anterior: retract upper lip up and out over maxillary central incisors and retract lower lip out and up for mandibular midline frenum.
   d. Adjust dressing by rolling and folding back the border; remove gross excess.
9. Check the occlusion by having the patient close gently. The dressing should extend only to the height of the contour of the teeth and should not be in occlusal contact during closure.

II. Non-Eugenol-containing Dressing (Coe-Pak)

A. Mixing

1. Place equal lengths of material from each tube beside each other (but not touching) on the mixing pad. Prepare only the amount needed, which can be estimated readily after a few experiences.
2. Because working time is relatively brief, prepare the patient by stabilizing the head and placing a gauze sponge over the area that will receive the dressing. Request the patient to close.
3. Mix the two pastes together quickly until the colors are blended and neither color is perceptible. Mix over a small area, not across width of pad.
4. When mixing is complete, gather the material together with the spatula and place on the edge of a tongue depressor. If using a metal spatula, wipe it clean promptly, before dressing hardens.

B. Application

1. After 1 minute, touch the mixture with a gloved finger coated with petroleum jelly. As soon as the mixture feels warm, it usually can be managed and should be placed promptly.
2. Roll the dressing into a strip the approximate length and thickness needed for the specific area. Application of excess material should be

avoided because removal of the excess is unnecessarily time-consuming and awkward.

3. Apply in a continuous piece. For a quadrant, place center of the roll at the posterior surface of the most posterior tooth and bring around to the facial and lingual surfaces. Press the dressing at the interproximal areas (lingual and facial surfaces can be done simultaneously).

4. Mold the dressing into place to the height of contour, and border mold to prevent displacement by the tongue, cheeks, lips, or frena.

5. Smooth the dressing by gently rubbing over the surfaces with a little petroleum jelly.

6. Check the occlusion. Patient may feel the excess, or teeth prints will show the location. When excess dressing is removed, use a cutting motion with a plastic instrument or scaler. Do not pull on a section of the dressing because the whole dressing is cohesive and can be dislodged in one piece.

III. Characteristics of a Well-Placed Dressing (figure 36–1)

Dressings must be placed in keeping with biologic principles, which will contribute to healing and yet be tolerated by the patient. A satisfactory dressing has the following characteristics:

A. Is secure and rigid. A movable dressing is an irritant and can promote bleeding.

B. Has as little bulk as possible, yet is bulky enough to give strength.

C. Is locked mechanically interdentally and cannot be displaced by action of tongue, cheek, or lips.

D. Covers all of the surgical wound without unnecessary overextension.

E. Fills interdental area to cover the treated area and discourage retention of debris and bacterial plaque.

F. Has a smooth surface to prevent irritation to cheeks and lips and to discourage debris and plaque retention.

IV. Patient Dismissal and Instructions

A. Patient must not be dismissed until bleeding or oozing from under the dressing has ceased.

B. Written instructions are more effective than ver-

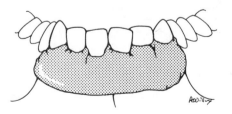

Figure 36–1. Periodontal Dressing. A dressing must cover the surgical wound without unnecessary overextension, and fill interdental areas to lock the dressing between the teeth. It should be molded in the vestibule and around frena to allow movement of the lips, cheeks, and tongue with no displacement of the dressing.

bal. Table 36–1 lists items for which instructions should be given to a patient who has a periodontal dressing. Printed instructions can be prepared from these items. Other instructions for the patient after general oral surgery or tooth removal may be found on page 592.

DRESSING REMOVAL AND REPLACEMENT

During healing, epithelium will cover a wound in 6 days, and complete restoration of epithelium and connective tissue can be expected by 21 days. The dressing may be left in place from 7 to 10 days as predetermined by the dentist.

If the dressing breaks or falls off before the appointed time for removal, the healing tissue should be evaluated. After 4 or 5 days, dressing replacement may not be needed, and the patient should proceed with daily frequent plaque removal. When replacement is indicated, the dressing should be wholly replaced rather than patched because the remaining segment usually is loose.

I. Patient Examination

A. Question patient about and record postoperative effects or discomfort. Record length of time the dressing stayed in place.

B. Examine the mucosa around the dressing and record its appearance.

II. Procedure for Removal

A. Insert a large scaler, hoe, or plastic instrument under the border of the dressing (coronal or apical border or both); apply lateral pressure.

B. Watch for sutures that may be caught in the dressing. They may need to be cut for release. Use principles for suture removal as described on pages 494–496.

C. Remove pieces of dressing gently with cotton pliers to avoid scratching the thin epithelial covering of the healing tissue with the rough edges of the dressing.

D. Observe tissue and record its appearance. Note any deviations from the normal healing expected in the length of time since the treatment.

E. Use a scaler for removal of pieces attached to tooth surfaces; use curet for particles near the gingival margin. Some root planing may be indicated, and all calculus and roughness should be eliminated to prevent plaque retention.

F. Syringe with a gentle stream of *warm* water, and provide *warm* diluted mouthrinse for the patient's comfort.

III. Indications for Dressing Replacement

A. Dressing broken or displaced before time for removal.

B. A second dressing for an extended period of time may be indicated and depends on the following:

Table 36–1.   Instructions for Postoperative Care

Factor	Instructions to Patient	Purpose of Instruction
Information about the Dressing	Dressing to protect the surgical wound and to help it heal Do not disturb it; keep it on until the next appointment	Understanding and cooperation by the patient
Care During the First Few Hours	Dressing will not be hard for a few hours. Do not eat anything that requires chewing Use only cool liquids Keep quiet; get rest	Dressing must harden and be undisturbed
Anesthesia	Be careful not to bite the lip or cheek Avoid foods that require chewing until the anesthesia has worn off	Prevent trauma to lip or cheek
Discomfort After the Anesthesia Wears Off	When a prescription is given, have the prescription filled and follow the directions for taking the medication; do not take more than directed Do not take aspirin	Pain control Aspirin can interfere with blood clotting
Ice Pack or Cold Compress	Use as directed only Apply every 30 minutes for 15 minutes; or 30 minutes on and 30 minutes off	Prevent swelling from edema
Bleeding	Slight temporary bleeding within the first few hours is not unusual Do not suck on the area or use straws. The blood clot should be left undisturbed Persistent or excessive bleeding should be reported to the dentist for treatment as indicated	Alleviate patient alarm over small amount of bleeding, but assure patient of help as needed
Dressing Care and Retention	Avoid pressing the dressing with the tongue or trying to clean under it. Small particles may chip off during the week: no problem, unless the sharp edge bothers the tongue or the dressing seems to have loosened. Call the dentist if the whole dressing or a large portion of it falls off before the fifth day: it should be replaced. If after the fifth day, call for an early replacement appointment when area is unusually sensitive: otherwise rinse with saline solution and cover the area with white petrolatum	Dressing needed for wound protection Epithelium covers wound by fifth day in normal healing
Use of Tobacco and Tobacco Products	Do not smoke. Avoid all tobacco products A heavy smoker should make every effort to decrease quantity of tobacco used	Heat and smoke irritate the gingiva and delay healing

Table 36–1. *continued*

Factor	Instructions to Patient	Purpose of Instruction
Rinsing	Do not rinse on the day of the treatment Second day: use saline solution made with one-half teaspoon (measured) in one-half cup of warm water every 2 to 3 hours Third and subsequent days: use the saline solution or a pleasant tasting mouthrinse diluted one-third mouthrinse to two-thirds water	Might disturb clot Saline may aid healing Pleasant flavored mouthrinse may reduce mouth odors from debris on the dressing
Toothbrushing and Flossing	Use better-than-usual brushing and flossing procedures on untreated areas Brush occlusal surface over dressing Use soft brush with water carefully on surface of dressing to clean off debris and film Brush the tongue	Bacterial plaque control Oral sanitation Odor and taste control Reduce number of oral microorganisms
Eating	Highly nutritious food is needed during healing. Check the Basic 4 Use soft-textured diet Omit foods that are highly seasoned, spicy, hot Avoid sticky, crunchy or coarse foods that could break the dressing	Healing Protect the dressing from breakage or displacement
Mastication	Avoid foods that require excessive chewing. Use ground meat, or cut meat into small pieces Chew only on untreated side Take small bite-sized pieces at a time	Dressing protection

1. Extent of the surgery and degree of periodontal disease involvement.
2. Need for additional healing period for certain types of surgery.

IV. Procedural Suggestions for Dressing Replacement

A. Use a topical anesthetic to prevent patient discomfort.
B. Use a soft dressing with minimal pressure during application over a partly healed area.

V. Bacterial Plaque Control Follow-up

Plaque control follow-up is essential after the final dressing removal.
A. Use a soft brush on the treated area, paying careful attention to plaque removal at the gingival margin. Use usual methods for all other areas of the mouth.
B. Increase intensity of care on the treated area each day, with a return to complete procedures by 3 or 4 days.
C. Rinse with warm mild saline solution, forcing the liquid between the teeth, to encourage healing.
D. When teeth are sensitive, a dentifrice containing a desensitizing agent may be advisable. Other suggestions for coping with sensitivity may be found on pages 499–500.

VI. Follow-up

Return for observation of complete healing in 1 week to 1 month, depending on the individual patient's progress and total treatment plan.

SUTURE REMOVAL

A suture is a strand or fiber used to unite parts of the body. Sutures are necessary in many oral operations wherever a surgical wound must be closed, a flap positioned, or tissue grafted.

I. Purposes of Sutures

A. Sutures maintain the healing tissues in position.
B. By holding and stabilizing the replaced and readapted tissue, sutures contribute to the following:
1. Maintaining the clot during the initial healing period.
2. Reducing the size of the wound, therefore lessening the time required for healing.

3. Protecting the area from foreign debris and trauma.

II. Types of Sutures and Needles

Sutures are classified as *absorbable* and *nonabsorbable.* Absorbable sutures are digested by body tissue fluids and enzymes, carried away by phagocytic action, and with the normal healing process, are replaced by scar tissue. In medical surgery, absorbable sutures can be used internally. Nonabsorbable sutures are made of inert materials and, when used on the surface, must be removed after 5 to 10 days as indicated by the type of surgery.

A. Absorbable Sutures
1. *Surgical Gut.* Prepared from the submucosa of sheep intestines, for use as plain or chrome.
   a. Plain are processed, sterilized, and tested.
   b. Chrome indicates special treatment of the suture material with chromic acid to control and lengthen the absorption time.
2. *Polyglycolic Acid (PGA).* Synthetic material that tends to produce a milder tissue reaction than surgical gut or nonabsorbable materials; it inhibits bacterial growth.

B. Nonabsorbable Sutures
1. *Surgical Silk.* Black, twisted or braided. Most widely used, particularly in oral surgery.
2. *Surgical Cotton and Linen.*
3. *Wire.* Tantalum, silver, stainless steel, vitallium.
4. *Synthetic Fibers.* Polyester, nylon, or orlon.

C. Characteristics
1. *Braided, Twisted, Plain.* Braiding provides more retention, but the suture is more permeable to bacteria.
2. *Monofilament or Multifilament.* Monofilament gives less tissue reaction, but multifilament gives better retention.
3. *Sizes.* Described from 0 to 8–0; for example, 4–0 silk is frequently used in periodontal surgery.

D. Needles
Many types of suturing needles are available, and their use and selection are based on the patient's needs and the dentist's preference. The three basic characteristics of suture needles are as follows:
1. *Shape of Needle.* Straight, half circle, 3/8 circle, half curved.
2. *Cross-sectional Shape.* Round or triangular (has cutting edge). The tip may be a tapered point or a trocar (triangular) point.
3. *Eye*
   a. Regular eye: eye may be round or square, or a French spring eye which grips suture material.
   b. Atraumatic: No eye. The needle and an end of the suture material are swaged. The suture and needle are a continuous unit.

III. Suturing Techniques

Many different patterns of suturing are used. A dental hygienist who will be removing sutures as part of postoperative patient care must become familiar with the methods preferred by the dentist-surgeon. Assisting and observing at the time of the operation can be especially educational. When the patient is one for whom the hygienist participated in the initial preparation, knowledge of the surgical procedures used adds to the continuity of treatment.

At the time of the treatment, the number and type or description of the sutures placed should be recorded in the patient's record. At the time of removal, the information is necessary, because during healing, sutures may become loosened, misplaced, or sometimes covered with tissue. All sutures should be accounted for at the time of removal.

General types of sutures frequently used in the oral cavity are described here briefly.

A. Blanket
Each stitch is brought over a loop of the preceding one, thus forming a series of loops on one side of the incision and a series of stitches over the incision (figure 36–2A). It is also called a continuous lock. It is used, for example, to approximate the gingival margins after alveolectomy.

B. Interrupted
Each stitch is taken and tied separately (figure 36–2B).

C. Continuous Uninterrupted
A series of stitches tied at one or both ends. Examples of sutures that may be applied in a series are the sling or suspension and the blanket.

D. Circumferential
A term applied to a suture that encircles a tooth for suspension and retention of a flap.

E. Interdental
Where the flaps are on both the lingual and facial sides, interdental ligation joins the two by passing the suture through each interdental area (figure 36–2C). Coverage for the interdental area can be accomplished by coapting the edges of the papillae.

F. Sling or Suspension
When a flap is only on one side, facial or lingual, the sutures are passed through the interdental papilla, through the interdental area, and around the tooth, and then into the adjacent papilla (figure 36–2D). The suture is adjusted so that the flap can be positioned for correct healing.

IV. Procedure for Removal

When a dressing has been placed over sutures, the steps will overlap with II., B., Dressing Removal, page 491. A suture can become caught in dressing material, and may need to be cut and removed while the dressing is being removed. The same principles for removal are to be observed.

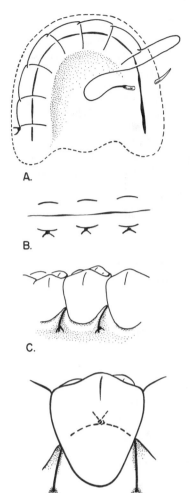

Figure 36–2. Types of Sutures. A. Blanket stitch. **B.** Interrupted, individual sutures. **C.** Interdental individual sutures. **D.** Sling or suspension suture tied on the lingual (dotted line).

A. Supplies for Suture Removal

Mouth mirror
Cotton pliers
Curved sharp scissors with pointed tip (suture scissors)
Gauze sponge
Topical anesthetic: Use type that can be applied safely on an abraded or incompletely healed area (pages 469–470).
Topical antiseptic
Cotton pellets
Saliva ejector tip

B. Patient History Check

Suture removal can cause bacteremia.[3] High-risk patients need antibiotic premedication for suture removal (pages 85 and 91).

C. Patient Examination

1. Observe healing tissue around the suture(s).
2. Record any deviations of color, size, shape of the tissue, adaptation of a flap, or coaptation of an incision healing by first intention.

D. Preparation of the Patient

1. Debride area: rinse the area and remove debris particles, using a cotton-tipped applicator or a cotton pellet dipped in 3% peroxide. Follow with another rinse, or wipe gently with a gauze sponge.
2. Place and adjust saliva ejector.
3. Retract and pat area with gauze sponge to remove surface moisture.
4. Swab area with topical antiseptic. Maintain retraction to prevent dilution.
5. Apply topical anesthetic.

E. Retraction

Three hands are really needed: one for retraction, one for cotton pliers to hold and remove the suture, and one for cutting the suture. When an assistant is not available, a cotton roll placed in the vestibule may provide enough retraction along with the finger rest and little finger of the nondominant hand holding the cotton pliers.

F. Steps for Removal

The suture removal procedure described here and illustrated in figure 36–3, is for a single interrupted suture. The same principles apply for the ends and each segment of a continuous suture, wherever septic suture material could pass through the soft tissue.

1. Grasp the suture knot with the cotton plier held in the nondominant hand. Gently draw the suture up about 2 mm. and hold with slight tension. A finger rest is needed for control.
2. Insert tip of sharp scissors under the suture, slightly depress the tissue with the back of the scissor blade, and cut the suture in the part that was previously buried in the tissue.
3. Hold knot end up with the cotton plier and pull gently to allow suture to come out through the side opposite where it was cut (figure 36–3C). This prevents any part of the external segment of the suture from passing through the tissue and introducing infectious material.
4. Withdraw gently and steadily (figure 36–3D).
5. Place each suture on a sponge for final counting and proceed to remove the next suture.
6. Count total sutures and confirm with the patient's record of the surgical procedures of the previous appointment.
7. Apply gauze sponge with slight pressure on bleeding spots.
8. Request dentist to observe the area.
9. Request patient to close on the sponge while dressing is readied (when a dressing replacement is indicated).

G. Precautions

In summary of the points brought out in the preceding description, precautions are as follows:

1. Count sutures; record number placed and number removed.

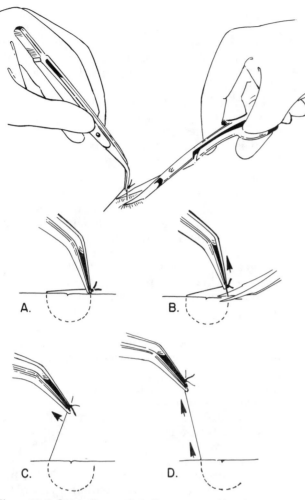

Figure 36–3. Suture Removal. A. Suture grasped by pliers near the entrance into tissue. **B.** Suture pulled gently up while scissor is inserted close to the tissue. Suture is cut in the part previously buried in the tissue. **C.** Suture is held up for vertical removal. **D.** Suture is pulled gently to bring it out on the side opposite from where it was cut. The object is to prevent the external part of the suture from passing through the tissue and introducing infectious material.

2. Record all observations of the tissues by dentist and hygienist and note any adverse reactions or bleeding problems. Record comments made by the patient.

3. Sutures should not be left longer than 5 to 10 days. Make special arrangements for removal for the patient who cannot return for a scheduled appointment.

4. Take care when removing a periodontal dressing to prevent ripping out a suture that may have become embedded in the dressing.

5. Provide proper postappointment instructions for the patient.

TECHNICAL HINTS

I. Sutures placed without a dressing may have a crust over them at the time of removal. Apply

mineral oil with a cotton swab or pellet, and in a short time, the crust will soften and can be wiped away. Removing the suture with the crust can cause unnecessary discomfort for the patient.

II. Adaptation and retention of a dressing can be improved by covering the dressing with a well-adapted adhesive periodontal foil when this is in accord with the dentist's philosophy. Place the foil over the lingual, occlusal, and facial surfaces, but do not cover the margins of the dressing to prevent irritating the mucosa.

III. When prolonged or excessive bleeding occurs (or may be anticipated because of occurrences during previous appointments) an extra-stiff dressing should be placed.[4]

FACTORS TO TEACH THE PATIENT

I. Care of the mouth during the period of treatment while wearing dressings. See table 36–1.

II. Maintenance and follow-up care after treatment is formally over.

References

1. American Dental Association, Council on Dental Therapeutics: *Accepted Dental Therapeutics,* 40th ed. Chicago, American Dental Association, 1984, p. 330.
2. Barkin, M.E., Boyd, J.P., and Cohen, S.: Acute Allergic Reaction to Eugenol, *Oral Surg. Oral Med. Oral Pathol., 57,* 441, April, 1984.
3. King, R.C., Crawford, J.J., and Small, E.W.: Bacteremia Following Intraoral Suture Removal, *Oral Surg. Oral Med. Oral Pathol., 65,* 23, January, 1988.
4. Baumhammers, A.: Control of Excessive Bleeding Following Periodontal Surgery, *Gen. Dent., 31,* 384, September-October, 1983.

Suggested Readings

Carranza, F.A.: *Glickman's Clinical Periodontology,* 6th ed. Philadelphia, W.B. Saunders Co., 1984, pp. 763–768, 807–817.
Castano, F.A. and Alden, B.A., eds: *Handbook of Expanded Dental Auxiliary Practice,* 2nd ed. Philadelphia, J.B. Lippincott Co., 1980, pp. 186–189.
Grant, D.A., Stern, I.B., and Listgarten, M.A., eds: *Periodontics,* 6th ed. St. Louis, The C.V. Mosby Co., 1988, pp. 731–733, 806–819.
Levin, M.P.: Periodontal Suture Materials and Surgical Dressings, *Dent. Clin. North Am., 24,* 767, October, 1980.
Pattison, G. and Pattison, A.M.: *Periodontal Instrumentation.* Reston, Virginia, Reston Publishing Co., 1979, pp. 369–392.
Ramfjord, S.P. and Ash, M.M.: *Periodontology and Periodontics.* Philadelphia, W.B. Saunders Co., 1979, pp. 504–519, 699–703.

Dressings

Allen, D.R. and Caffesse, R.G.: Comparison of Results Following Modified Widman Flap Surgery with or without Surgical Dressing, *J. Periodontol., 54,* 470, August, 1983.
American Dental Association, Council on Dental Therapeutics and Council on Dental Materials and Devices: Hazards of Asbestos in Dentistry, *J. Am. Dent. Assoc., 92,* 777, April, 1976.
Geiger, B., Goral, V., and Meister, F.: Periodontal Dressings: Rationale and Procedures, *Dent. Hyg., 55,* 21, September, 1981.
Hume, W.R.: The Pharmacologic and Toxicological Properties of Zinc Oxide-eugenol, *J. Am. Dent. Assoc., 113,* 789, November, 1986.

Jones, T.M. and Cassingham, R.J.: Comparison of Healing Following Periodontal Surgery with and without Dressings in Humans, *J. Periodontol., 50,* 387, August, 1979.

McGraw, V.A. and Caffesse, R.G.: Cyanoacrylates in Periodontics, *J. West. Soc. Periodont. Periodont. Abstr., 26,* 4, Number 1, 1978.

Nezwek, R.A., Caffesse, R.G., Bergenholtz, A., and Nasjleti, C.E.: Connective Tissue Response to Periodontal Dressings, *J. Periodontol., 51,* 521, September, 1980.

Rubinoff, C.H., Greener, E.H., and Robinson, P.J.: Physical Properties of Periodontal Dressing Materials, *J. Oral Rehabil., 13,* 575, November, 1986.

Sachs, H.A.: Current Status of Periodontal Dressings, *J. Periodontol., 55,* 689, December, 1984.

Sutures

American Dental Association, Council on Dental Materials, Instruments, and Equipment: *Dentist's Desk Reference: Materials, Instruments and Equipment,* 2nd ed. Chicago, American Dental Association, 1983, pp. 334–335.

Castelli, W.A., Nasjleti, C.E., Caffesse, R.E., and Diaz-Perez, R.: Gingival Response to Silk, Cotton, and Nylon Suture Materials, *Oral Surg. Oral Med. Oral Pathol., 45,* 179, February, 1978.

Manor, A. and Kaffe, I.: Unusual Foreign Body Reaction to A Braided Silk Suture: A Case Report, *J. Periodontol., 53,* 86, February, 1982.

Prato, G.P.P., Cortellini, P., Agudio, G., and Clauser, C.: Human Fibrin Glue versus Sutures in Periodontal Surgery, *J. Periodontol., 58,* 426, June, 1987.

Project Acorde, United States Department of Health, Education, and Welfare: *Assisting with Suture Placement and Sutures: Placing and Removing Medication for Dry Sockets.* Castro Valley, California, Quercus Corp., 1979, pp. 7–61.

37 *Hypersensitive Teeth*

Sensitivity in the cervical area of a tooth can produce considerable discomfort. Care must be taken during instrumentation and application of air to prevent a hypersensitive reaction. Because tooth sensitivity frequently is related to the accumulation of bacterial plaque in the exposed cervical area, instruction in exacting plaque removal techniques is indicated.

Patients are appreciative of clinical procedures directed at desensitizing the area involved. Several chemical and mechanical means have been used successfully to reduce or eliminate pain. Methods available are not consistently effective for all patients.

I. Factors Contributing to Hypersensitivity

A. Exposure of Cementum and Dentin

1. *Gingival Recession*[1,2]
   a. Pathologic (localized or generalized): inflammation that may initiate proliferation of the junctional epithelium along the root surface.
   b. Traumatic: toothbrush with abrasive dentifrice.
2. *Periodontal Procedure.* For pocket elimination.

B. Anatomy of the Cementoenamel Junction

A zone of dentin occurs between the enamel and the cementum in approximately 10 percent of teeth[3] (figure 12–2, page 183).

C. Loss of Cementum

Cementum is lost through abrasion, erosion, dental caries, scaling, root planing, or polishing with an abrasive agent or airbrasive instrument. The dentin is uncovered and the dentinal tubules are exposed.

D. Loss of Enamel

Sensitivity can be associated with areas where enamel is lost because of dietary erosion, fractures, toothbrush abrasion, occlusal wear, and parafunctional habits. When enamel erosion results from the repeated induced vomiting of bulimia, the teeth may be extremely sensitive (pages 380–381).

II. Types of Pain Stimuli[4]

A. Mechanical

Toothbrush filaments or bristles, eating utensils, periodontal and dental hygiene instruments, friction from denture clasps or other appliances.

B. Chemical

Acids formed from fermentable carbohydrates by bacteria in plaque, citrus fruit acids, or condiments.

C. Thermal

Hot or cold foods or beverages; air entering the oral cavity.

III. Pain Impulse Conduction

A. Theories[5]

The exact mechanism of pain transmission from the tooth surface to the pulp has not been completely defined. Several theories have been the subjects of extensive research.

1. *Nerve Endings in the Dentin.* Nerve endings extend from the pulp near the cells of the odontoblasts (figure 37–1). No nerves have been demonstrated in the periphery of the dentin near the dentinoenamel junction.
2. *Odontoblast as a Special Sensory Cell.* Other research has suggested that the odontoblast might be a special sensory cell that could pass the sensations on to the pulpal nerves. Odontoblasts do not have the characteristics of spe-

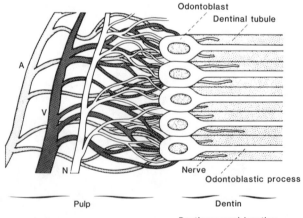

Figure 37–1. Relationship of Odontoblasts and Nerve Endings. Nerve endings from the pulp lie side by side with odontoblasts lined up at the edge of the pulp. A few nerve endings extend short distances into dentinal tubules. According to the hydrodynamic theory of dentinal sensitivity, pain is created by stimulation of the free nerve endings by rapid fluid flow in the tubules after a stimulation from the surface. (Adapted from Bennett, C.R.: *Monheim's Local Anesthesia and Pain Control in Dental Practice*, 7th ed. St. Louis, The C.V. Mosby Co., 1984.)

cial neurons such as those for the senses of vision or smell.

3. *Hydrodynamic Mechanism.*[6,7] This theory has been the most widely accepted. Stimuli such as hot, cold, or air blast on the surface of the exposed dentin set up rapid movement of the fluid in the dentinal tubule. That fluid then stimulates nerve endings in the pulp. The fluid may expand with heat and contract with cold.

B. Dentin Structure[8]
1. *Composition.* Dentin is composed of calcified tissue surrounding dentinal tubules.
2. *Tubules*
   a. Number: Millions of tubules penetrate the dentin. They follow the paths taken by the odontoblasts during dentin formation.
   b. Route: In the crown and cervical areas, the tubules follow an "S" line from the pulp to the dentinoenamel and dentinocemental junctions (figure 37–2 A). In the root, the tubules are in straight lines.
   c. Branching: The tubules branch near the dentinoenamel and the dentinocemental junctions (figure 37–2 B). Cross connections (anastomoses) also exist between the tubules.
3. *Odontoblastic Process.* Each dentinal tubule contains a cytoplasmic cell process that extends from the odontoblast cell body at the edge of the pulp. In young teeth, the process extends to the dentinoenamel or dentinocemental junction. In older teeth, the processes may have withdrawn.
4. *Exposed Surface at the Dentinocemental Junction.* After exposure to the oral environment for a few weeks or months, the dentin usually becomes sclerotic. This can explain why tooth

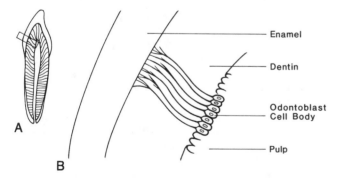

Figure 37–2. Odontoblasts. Cell body of an odontoblast is on the edge of the pulp. Each cell has an odontoblastic process that extends from the cell to the dentinoenamel junction. **A.** In the crown, the processes run in an "S" line, whereas in the root they are straight across. **B.** The processes may branch near the dentino-enamel and cementoenamel junctions to give more exposure when enamel or cementum is lost. (Redrawn from Brand, R.W. and Isselhard, D.E.: *Anatomy of Orofacial Structures.* 3rd ed. St. Louis, The C.V. Mosby Co., 1986.)

sensitivity following root planing disappears when it is kept plaque-free on a daily basis.

ACTION OF DESENSITIZING AGENTS

I. Modes of Action
Reviews that have been written about the various desensitizing agents are recommended for a complete study.[7,9,10,11]

A. Closure of Dentinal Tubules
Sensation cannot pass into the dentinal tubule and set the hydrodynamic mechanism into action. Mechanical blockage of the tubules may result from
1. Coagulation; protein precipitation.
2. Mineralization; building a calcific barrier.
3. Surface coating.

B. Formation of Secondary Dentin
Irritation and stimulation from external agents over time result in build up of secondary dentin.

II. Characteristics of a Desensitizing Agent[12]
When selecting a method for desensitization, practical aspects are important. When possible, the patient's daily personal care can be used to incorporate treatment on a self-care basis. When an agent is applied professionally, the following considerations are suggested. An agent needs
A. Rapidity of action.
B. Ease of application.
C. Biologic acceptance by the body tissues.
D. Long-lasting or permanent effects.
E. No side effects such as tooth discoloration, gingival irritation, or pulpal changes.
F. No pain to patient during application.
G. Consistent effectiveness.

METHODS FOR DESENSITIZATION

Few patients respond to a single form of treatment. For all, keeping the teeth as free of bacterial plaque as possible, particularly at the gingival third where sensitivity areas occur, and the use of a form of self-applied topical fluoride are basic procedures. Specific agents can be selected on an individual basis for professional application to persistent areas of sensitivity.

I. Self-care by the Patient

A. Plaque Control
Root surfaces subjected to vigorous plaque control measures by brushing, flossing, and the use of other selected aids develop a smooth hard surface with increased luster and less hypersensitivity. The dentinal tubules are blocked off by increased mineralization.

When bacterial plaque is retained at the cervical third of the tooth, the root surfaces may develop root caries and usually are hypersensitive because of acid formed from cariogenic substances. A concentrated program of instruction and supervision is indicated.

B. Dentifrice

The Council on Dental Therapeutics of the American Dental Association has established guidelines for the evaluation of the efficacy of agents to reduce dentinal hypersensitivity.[13]

Dentifrices containing strontium chloride, potassium nitrate, and sodium citrate have been evaluated and use the stamp of approval (figure 23–14, page 331).

C. Self-applied Fluoride

In addition to the desensitizing dentifrice, the patient's treatment plan should include daily applications of fluoride by mouth rinsing, custom tray with gel, brushing with a gel, or other mode for regular use. The various procedures were described on pages 407–410. With an increase in surface fluoride, hypersensitivity usually decreases.

D. Diet

A food diary kept for 5 to 7 days, from which a dietary analysis is made with the patient, can be valuable. Foods that aggravate the hypersensitivity can be identified, and substitutes can be selected with the patient. Excessive fermentable carbohydrates, citrus fruits, or condiments with pronounced flavors may initiate a reaction.

II. Professional Applications

Without effective personal plaque removal measures, professional applications have limited, and frequently temporary, effects. Dentists have used albumin precipitants such as 40% formalin, 40% zinc chloride, or 40% silver nitrate to seal the dentinal tubules and hence reduce sensitivity.

Cavity varnishes, thin mixes of crown and bridge cement, zinc oxide and eugenol packs, or Gottlieb's solution have been used to protect the tooth surface against thermal shock. Impregnation using composite resin preceded with acid etch has been successful to a degree.[14]

A. Preparation for Desensitization

1. *Complete Scaling and Planing.* Removal of deposits and altered cementum may be needed to provide access of the agent for desensitization directly onto the tooth surface.
2. *Anesthesia.* When teeth are too sensitive for application of the agent, a local anesthetic is indicated. Note areas where a desensitizing agent is to be applied before the anesthetic is given.

B. Sodium Fluoride Desensitizing Paste[15]

1. *Composition.* 33% sodium fluoride, 33% kaolin, and 33% glycerin.

2. *Preparation*
   a. Clean and isolate the sensitive tooth, using cotton rolls, cotton roll holder for the mandibular arch, and saliva ejector.
   b. Wipe exposed area with cotton pellet moistened in 2% sodium fluoride solution.
   c. Dry area thoroughly, using cotton pellets or cotton roll.
3. *Application*
   a. Place a small amount of desensitizing paste on the area with the tip of a wood point in a porte polisher. A narrow wood point may fit the cervical area more effectively than a wide one.
   b. Massage paste on the area gently but firmly with a wood point, using small circular strokes. If patient suffers acute pain response at beginning of application, wipe off paste, have patient rinse with warm water, and begin again immediately.
   c. Continue massage for 3 minutes: use timer.
   d. Wipe off excess paste with cotton pellet.
   e. Remove cotton rolls and saliva ejector and request patient to rinse with warm water.
   f. Repeat at future appointment if desensitization has not been accomplished.

C. Iontophoresis[16,17]

Iontophoresis is the impregnation of tissue with ions from dissolved salts with the aid of an electric current. Iontophoresis utilizes a direct current to promote ionic transport of fluoride, a negatively charged ion, onto a tooth surface.

The actual mechanism of action may be deposition of fluoride ions deeper into the dentin to obtain more extensive protoplasmic precipitation or formation of secondary dentin. A short-lived paresthesia of the odontoblastic processes may be produced. Manufacturer's instructions should be followed for use of the equipment.

1. Isolate with rubber dam or cotton rolls.
2. Low-voltage batteries (1½ to 9 volts) supply positive current to patient's tooth. A special direct-current source has been developed.[16]
3. Circuit completed by contact of brush applicator for negatively charged aqueous fluoride solution (2% sodium fluoride).
4. Check patient's medical history before use of a current. A patient wearing a pacemaker should not receive treatment by such means as a pulp tester, ultrasonic, or other current-producing instrument (page 693).

TECHNICAL HINTS

I. Do not use compressed air on sensitive teeth. Dry only with cotton pellets or cotton roll.
II. Sodium fluoride desensitizing paste contains enough fluoride to cause nausea if swallowed in excess. Prevent this by using only small

amounts, wiping off excess with cotton pellets before removing cotton rolls, requesting the patient to rinse thoroughly, and using the saliva ejector to prevent the need for swallowing before the mouth can be rinsed.

III. Keep jar containing sodium fluoride desensitizing paste tightly closed. Its shelf-life can be indefinite because of its glycerin base.

FACTORS TO TEACH THE PATIENT

I. General causes of gingival recession.

II. Causes of hypersensitivity of teeth.

III. Importance of correct toothbrushing using a soft brush for plaque removal in the cervical area as a method of desensitization.

IV. Probability that the hypersensitivity will subside in time with daily bacterial plaque removal whether a desensitizer is applied or not.

V. Specific foods that should and should not be used in the diet if relief from sensitivity is to be obtained.

References

1. Grant, D.A., Stern, I.B., and Listgarten, M.A., eds.: *Periodontics,* 6th ed. St. Louis, The C.V. Mosby Co., 1988, pp. 460–467.
2. Carranza, F.A.: *Glickman's Clinical Periodontology,* 6th ed. Philadelphia, W.B. Saunders Co., 1984, pp. 114–117.
3. Bhaskar, S.N., ed.: *Orban's Oral Histology and Embryology,* 10th ed. St. Louis, The C.V. Mosby Co., 1986, p. 188.
4. Grant, Stern, and Listgarten: op. cit., pp. 638–641.
5. Bennett, C.R.: Understanding Dental Pain: Part I, *Compend. Contin. Educ. Dent., 6,* 121, February, 1985.
6. Brännström, M., Lindén, Å., and Aström, A.: The Hydrodynamics of the Dental Tubule and of Pulp Fluid. A Discussion of Its Significance in Relation to Dentinal Sensitivity, *Caries Res., 1,* 310, Number 4, 1967.
7. Greenhill, J.D. and Pashley, D.H.: The Effects of Desensitizing Agents on the Hydraulic Conductance of Human Dentin *in vitro, J. Dent. Res., 60,* 686, March, 1981.
8. Melfi, R.C.: *Permar's Oral Embryology and Microscopic Anatomy,* 8th ed. Philadelphia, Lea & Febiger, 1988, pp. 111–130.
9. Addy, M. and Dowell, P.: Dentine Hypersensitivity—A Review. Clinical and *in vitro* Evaluation of Treatment Agents, *J. Clin. Periodontol., 10,* 351, July, 1983.
10. Berman, L.H.: Dentinal Sensation and Hypersensitivity. A Review of Mechanisms and Treatment Alternatives, *J. Periodontol., 56,* 216, April, 1985.
11. Ong, G.: Desensitizing Agents. A Review, *Clin. Prevent. Dent., 8,* 14, May-June, 1986.
12. Grossman, L.I.: A Systematic Method For the Treatment of Hypersensitive Dentin, *J. Am. Dent. Assoc., 22,* 592, April, 1935.
13. American Dental Association, Ad Hoc Advisory Committee on Dentinal Hypersensitivity: Council on Dental Therapeutics: Recommendations for Evaluating Agents for the Reduction of Dentinal Hypersensitivity, *J. Am. Dent. Assoc., 112,* 709, May, 1986.
14. Brännström, M., Johnson, G., and Nordenvall, K.-J.: Transmission and Control of Dentinal Pain: Resin Impregnation for the Desensitization of Dentin, *J. Am. Dent. Assoc., 99,* 612, October, 1979.
15. Hoyt, W.H. and Bibby, B.G.: Use of Sodium Fluoride for Desensitizing Dentin, *J. Am. Dent. Assoc., 30,* 1372, September 1, 1943.
16. Gangarosa, L.P. and Park, N.H.: Practical Considerations in Iontophoresis of Fluoride for Desensitizing Dentin, *J. Prosthet. Dent., 39,* 173, February, 1978.
17. Holman, D.J.: Desensitizing of Dentin by Iontophoresis: A Review, *Gen. Dent., 30,* 481, November-December, 1982.

Suggested Readings

Absi, E.G., Addy, M., and Adams, D.: Dentine Hypersensitivity. A Study of the Patency of Dentinal Tubules in Sensitive and Non-sensitive Cervical Dentine, *J. Clin. Periodontol., 14,* 280, May, 1987.

Addy, M., Mostafa, P., and Newcombe, R.G.: Dentine Hypersensitivity: the Distribution of Recession, Sensitivity, and Plaque, *J. Dent., 15,* 242, December, 1987.

Collins, J.F., Gingold, J., Stanley, H., and Simring, M.: Reducing Dentinal Hypersensitivity with Strontium Chloride and Potassium Nitrate, *Gen. Dent., 32,* 40, January-February, 1984.

Dowell, P. and Addy, M.: Dentine Hypersensitivity—A Review. I. Aetiology, Symptoms and Theories of Pain Production, *J. Clin. Periodontol., 10,* 341, July, 1983.

Dowell, P. and Addy, M.: Dentine Hypersensitivity. A Quantitative Comparison of the Uptake of Metal Salts and Fluoride by Dentine and Hydroxyapatite, *J. Periodont. Res., 19,* 530, September, 1984.

Dowell, P., Addy, M., and Dummer, P.: Dentine Hypersensitivity: Aetiology, Differential Diagnosis and Management, *Br. Dent. J., 158,* 92, February 9, 1985.

Hodosh, M., Hodosh, S., Hodosh, A., and Shklar, G.: Potassium Nitrate Gel-sleeve: An Effective Procedure for Dentinal Hypersensitivity, *Quintessence Int., 13,* 1251, November, 1982.

Javid, B., Barkhordar, R.A., and Bhinda, S.V.: Cyanoacrylate—A New Treatment for Hypersensitive Dentin and Cementum, *J. Am. Dent. Assoc., 114,* 486, April, 1987.

Jensen, M.E. and Doering, J.V.: A Comparative Study of Two Clinical Techniques for Treatment of Root Surface Hypersensitivity, *Gen. Dent., 35,* 128, March-April, 1987.

Krauser, J.T.: Hypersensitive Teeth. Part I: Etiology, *J. Prosthet. Dent., 56,* 153, August, 1986.

Krauser, J.T.: Hypersensitive Teeth. Part II: Treatment, *J. Prosthet. Dent., 56,* 307, September, 1986.

McFall, W.T.: A Review of the Active Agents Available for Treatment of Dentinal Hypersensitivity, *Endod. Dent. Traumatol., 2,* 141, Number 4, 1986.

Newman, G.V.: Sealant Impregnation for Treatment of Hypersensitive Dentin, *J. Clin. Orthod., 16,* 457, July, 1982.

Orchardson, R. and Collins, W.J.N.: Thresholds of Hypersensitive Teeth to 2 Forms of Controlled Stimulation, *J. Clin. Periodontol., 14,* 68, February, 1987.

Orchardson, R. and Collins, W.J.N.: Clinical Features of Hypersensitive Teeth, *Br. Dent. J., 162,* 253, April 11, 1987.

Overman, P.R.: Calcium Hypophosphate As a Root Desensitizing Agent, *Dent. Hyg., 57,* 30, August, 1983.

Pashley, D.H.: Dentin Permeability, Dentin Sensitivity, and Treatment through Tubule Occlusion, *J. Endod., 12,* 465, October, 1986.

Pashley, D.H., Leibach, J.G., and Horner, J.A.: The Effects of Burnishing NaF/Kaolin/Glycerin Paste on Dentin Permeability, *J. Periodontol., 58,* 19, January, 1987.

Touyz, L.Z.G.: The Mechanism and Management of Dental Cervical Sensitivity, *Dent. Health (London), 22,* 5, Number 4, 1983.

Wycoff, S.J.: Current Treatment for Dentinal Hypersensitivity. In-office Treatment, *Compend. Contin. Educ. Dent.,* S 113, Supplement 3, 1982.

Dentifrices

Blong, M.A., Volding, B., Thrash, W.J., and Jones, D.L.: Effects of a Gel Containing 0.4 Percent Stannous Fluoride on Dentinal Hypersensitivity, *Dent. Hyg., 59,* 489, November, 1985.

Clark, D.C., Hanley, J.A., Geoghegan, S., and Vinet, D.: The Effectiveness of a Fluoride Varnish and a Desensitizing Toothpaste in Treating Dentinal Hypersensitivity, *J. Periodont. Res., 20,* 212, March, 1985.

Clark, D.C., Al-Joburi, W., and Chan, E.C.S.: The Efficacy of a New Dentifrice in Treating Dentin Sensitivity: Effects of Sodium

Citrate and Sodium Fluoride as Active Ingredients, *J. Periodont. Res., 22,* 89, March, 1987.

McFall, W.T. and Hamrick, S.W.: Clinical Effectiveness of a Dentifrice Containing Fluoride and a Citrate Buffer System for Treatment of Dentinal Sensitivity, *J. Periodontol., 58,* 701, October, 1987.

McFall, W.T. and Morgan, W.C.: Effectiveness of a Dentifrice Containing Formalin and Sodium Monofluorophosphate on Dental Hypersensitivity, *J. Periodontol., 56,* 288, May, 1985.

Minkoff, S. and Axelrod, S.: Efficacy of Strontium Chloride in Dental Hypersensitivity, *J. Periodontol., 58,* 470, July, 1987.

Pashley, D.H., O'Meara, J.A., Kepler, E.E., Galloway, S.E., Thompson, S.M., and Stewart, F.P.: Dentin Permeability. Effects of Densensitizing Dentifrices *in vitro, J. Periodontol., 55,* 522, September, 1984.

Silverman, G.: The Sensitivity-reducing Effect of Brushing with a Potassium Nitrate—Sodium Monofluorophosphate Dentifrice, *Compend. Contin. Educ. Dent., 6,* 131, February, 1985.

Tarbet, W.J., Silverman, G., Fratarcangelo, P.A., and Kanapka, J.A.: Home Treatment for Dentinal Hypersensitivity: A Comparative Study, *J. Am. Dent. Assoc., 105,* 227, August, 1982.

Uchida, A., Wakano, Y., Fukuyama, O., Miki, T., Iwayama, Y., and Okada, H.: Controlled Clinical Evaluation of a 10% Strontium Chloride Dentifrice in Treatment of Dentin Hypersensitivity Following Periodontal Surgery, *J. Periodontol., 51,* 578, October, 1980.

Wei, S.H.Y., Lainson, P.A., Henderson, W., and Wolfson, S.H.: Evaluation of Dentifrices for the Relief of Hypersensitive Tooth Surfaces, *Quintessence Int., 11,* 67, January, 1980.

Iontophoresis

Brough, K.M., Anderson, D.M., Love, J., and Overman, P.R.: The Effectiveness of Iontophoresis in Reducing Dentin Hypersensitivity, *J. Am. Dent. Assoc., 111,* 761, November, 1985.

Carlo, G.T., Ciancio, S.G., and Seyrek, S.K.: An Evaluation of Iontophoretic Application of Fluoride for Tooth Desensitization, *J. Am. Dent. Assoc., 105,* 452, September, 1982.

Gangarosa, L.P.: Iontophoretic Application of Fluoride by Tray Techniques for Desensitization of Multiple Teeth, *J. Am. Dent. Assoc., 102,* 50, January, 1981.

Johnson, R.H., Zulgar-Nain, B.J., and Koval, J.J.: The Effectiveness of an Electro-ionizing Toothbrush in the Control of Dentinal Hypersensitivity, *J. Periodontol., 53,* 353, June, 1982.

Lutins, N.D., Greco, G.W., and McFall, W.T.: Effectiveness of Sodium Fluoride on Tooth Hypersensitivity with and without Iontophoresis, *J. Periodontol., 55,* 285, May, 1984.

Wilson, J.M., Fry, B.W., Walton, R.E., and Gangarosa, L.P.: Fluoride Levels in Dentin After Iontophoresis of 2% NaF, *J. Dent. Res., 63,* 897, June, 1984.

38 *Extrinsic Stain Removal*

After treatment by scaling, root planing, and other periodontal therapy, the teeth are evaluated for the presence of stains. The use of polishing agents for stain removal is a selective procedure, one that not every patient needs, especially on a routine basis.

Stains on the teeth are not etiologic factors for any disease or destructive process. Therefore, the removal of stains is for esthetic, not for health reasons. The need to remove stains by polishing should be evaluated after the plaque is under control, because some stains are incorporated in plaque and can be removed during brushing and flossing by the patient.

The objectives for stain removal may need to be clarified, because polishing has been a routine procedure in many offices and clinics. Information should be provided for each patient concerning individual needs.

When the evaluation is made, several factors must be taken into consideration. These factors will be described in this chapter.

EFFECTS OF POLISHING

Because of the potentially detrimental effects, the needs of an individual patient must be reviewed before stain removal. Professional judgment based on patient need decides when a service is to be included in a treatment plan.

I. Bacteremia

Because bacteremia can be created during the use of power-driven stain removal instruments, the *medical history* must be recorded initially and then reviewed and updated at succeeding appointments.

Bacteremias result from manipulation of the gingival tissues. In one research study, 11 of 39 children (mean age, 9 years) developed bacteremia following application of a rubber cup with a prophylaxis paste.[1] It is recommended that use of a rubber cup be withheld until the plaque is under control and the gingiva do not bleed when the patient brushes.

For patients at risk, particularly those with damaged or abnormal heart valves, prosthetic valves, joint replacements, rheumatic heart disease, and other conditions listed on pages 85 and 91, antibiotic prophylaxis as outlined by the American Heart Association is needed.

II. Environmental Factors

A. Aerosol Production

Aerosols are created during use of all rotary instruments, including a prophylaxis handpiece with a polishing paste and the air and water sprays used during rinsing.[2] The biologic contaminants of aerosols stay suspended for long periods and provide a means for disease transmission to dental personnel as well as to succeeding patients (pages 10–11).

Rotary instruments should be avoided when a patient is known to have a communicable disease. Precautions for hepatitis B and other diseases were described on pages 58–59.

B. Splatter

Protective eyeglasses are needed for all dental team members and for the patient. Serious eye damage has occurred as a result of splatter in the eye from a polishing paste or from instruments. Constituents of commercial prophylaxis pastes may include various chemicals such as oils that can aggravate a severe inflammatory response.[3]

III. Effect on Teeth

A. Removal of Tooth Structure

Polishing for 30 seconds with a pumice paste may remove as much as 4 μm of the outer enamel.[4] Performed repeatedly over the years, the tooth loss could be substantial. The effect has particular significance for children because the surfaces of young, newly erupted teeth are incompletely mineralized.

Cementum and dentin are softer and more porous, so greater amounts of these can be removed during polishing than of the enamel.[5,6] When cementum is exposed because of gingival recession, polishing of the exposed surfaces should be avoided. Also to be avoided are areas of demineralization. Nearly three times more surface enamel is lost from abrasive polishing over white spots than over intact enamel.[7]

B. Increased Roughness

A coarse abrasive may create a rougher tooth surface than existed before polishing. Grooves and scratches created by an abrasive applied with a rubber cup have been studied microscopically.[8,9]

C. Areas of Thin Enamel

Certain patients have teeth with thin enamel, such as those with amelogenesis imperfecta (page 257) or overdemineralized areas (figure 29–3, page 396).

Removal of tooth structure in the cervical portion of the tooth, where enamel is thin and cementum is exposed, can create unnecessary sensitivity. Special treatment problems may follow. These areas should not be polished.

D. Removal of Fluoride-rich Surface

More important than the amount of enamel lost during polishing is that the outermost layer of tooth structure contains the greatest amounts of fluoride.[10] The surface fluoride protects against dental caries. The concentration of fluoride drops quickly inward toward the dentin, so that, if the surface layer is polished away, the protection is greatly diminished.

The *fluoride-rich surface* is important and should not be removed. Certain conditions increase caries susceptibility and therefore preclude the removal of this surface through polishing. Patients with *xerostomia* from any cause, for example drug or radiation therapy, cannot afford to have the enamel surface weakened by polishing. In contrast, their therapy must include daily addition of concentrated fluoride, usually through self-applied methods such as rinsing or gel tray.

When upon evaluation it appears that polishing is required and therefore loss of the fluoride-rich surface is unavoidable, topical fluoride (gel or solution) must be applied in an attempt to replace the lost protection.[11] Fluoride uptake is minimal from prophylaxis pastes as compared with that from topical solutions or gels; therefore, a paste is not a substitute. In addition to topical application, daily self-applied fluoride should be recommended and prescribed. All patients need a fluoride-containing dentifrice, and in addition, a rinse, chewable tablet, or gel tray can be used, depending on the patient's age and caries susceptibility.

E. Heat Production

Steady pressure with a rapidly revolving rubber cup or bristle brush and a minimum of wet abrasive agent can create sufficient heat to cause pain and discomfort for the patient. Damage to the pulp by the heat has not been documented, but the pulps of young people are large and may be more susceptible to heat.

IV. Effect on Gingiva

Trauma to the gingival tissue can result, especially when the prophylaxis angle is run at a high speed and the rubber cup is applied for an extended period. In one study, a rubber cup with pumice rotated for 2 minutes caused a total removal of the epithelium inside the crest of the free gingiva.[12] Complete healing from such a wound would take from 8 to 14 days. The patient's sore and sensitive tissues could prevent adequate plaque removal during that time and a severe inflammation could result, along with calculus reformation.

With the fast rotation of a rubber cup, particles of a polishing agent can be forced into the subepithelial tissues and create a source of irritation. Polishing after gingival and periodontal treatments, including scaling, root planing, and curettage, is not recommended on the same day. The diseased lining of the pocket usually has been removed, and the pocket wall is wide open and can receive particles that may become embedded, out of reach of the most careful irrigation and rinsing.

By rotation of the rubber cup, microorganisms can be forced into the tissues. An inflammatory response can be expected, and bacteria may gain access to the blood stream to create a bacteremia.

Foreign-body reactions to abrasives have been tested. Several agents have been shown to have potential for creating reactions. Some explanation for delayed healing following tissue trauma may be found in this concept.[13]

V. Effect on Restorations

A. Existing Restorations

Abrasive pastes can leave rough surfaces on various types of restorative materials, including gold, amalgam, and composites.[14,15]

B. Newly Placed Restorations

Procedures for finishing and polishing newly placed amalgam restorations are described in Chapter 41, pages 531–535. In the polishing process, a coarse abrasive is used first, followed by abrasives of finer grits. It is important that the tooth surface around the restoration be left as intact as possible. Remineralization of the surface with fluoride is necessary after polishing the restoration.

INDICATIONS FOR STAIN REMOVAL

I. To Remove Extrinsic Stains not Otherwise Removed During Toothbrushing and Scaling

A. Scaling and Root Planing

When the stain is to be removed by the professional person, as much stain as possible must first be removed with the calculus during scaling. Certain stains can be scaled away readily even without being incorporated within calculus.

Black line stain, for example, has been identified as a type of calculus. It resembles calculus in that it is composed of microorganisms, has a similar mode of attachment to enamel, and similar signs of mineralization under a microscope.[16] Another reason why black line stain should be scaled rather than polished is that it is most commonly found on the teeth of children. Newly erupted teeth are more porous and less mineralized and should not be damaged by polishing. The effect of heat created by power-driven instruments is not completely known, except that excess heat can produce pulp damage.

For stains on adult teeth that are not removed with calculus, the least abrasive paste should be selected. The toothpaste manufactured for daily home use may be amply abrasive for professional use when very little stain removal is needed.

B. Patient Instruction

The source of an extrinsic stain should be discussed with the patient and a preventive plan initiated. When the recurrence of a stain is preventable, or when the etiologic factor is controllable, the patient should be encouraged to make the necessary habit changes to prevent the stain from collecting again. Improved techniques of personal plaque removal and more frequent attention to oral hygiene can result in significant improvement.

II. To Prepare the Teeth for Caries Preventive Agents

A. Pit and Fissure Sealant

Although the manufacturer's directions should be followed relative to preparation of the teeth for sealant application, research has shown that sealants have been successfully placed without the initial cleaning of the teeth (page 420). Because commercial prophylaxis pastes contain oils, fluoride, flavoring substances, or other agents that may interfere with the integrity of the sealant, a plain, fine pumice with water is indicated when precleaning is needed (pages 420–421).

B. Professional Application of Fluoride Solutions or Gels

Traditionally, tooth polishing after scaling has preceded topical application of fluoride because of the original history-making research of Knutson.[17] Current research shows that plaque and debris removal can be accomplished adequately by the patient using a toothbrush and dental floss, rather than requiring the more drastic means of professional polishing with a rubber cup and abrasive cleaning agent. New evidence has shown that the pellicle on the tooth surface does not act as a barrier to fluoride, and that fluoride uptake in the enamel from a fluoride application is similar whether the teeth are brushed by the patient or polished with pumice.[18,19]

Having a patient brush and floss prior to a topical application provides an excellent opportunity to combine patient instruction with treatment and utilize the educational principle of participation of the learner. Such an objective has unquestionable value.

Excellent benefits, many similar or better for caries prevention than those accomplished by professional topical applications, have been obtained from home and school fluoride-rinsing programs.[20,21] When considering whether the use of a rubber cup with prophylaxis paste is necessary before topical application, the effects of rinsing on a weekly or daily basis without prior polishing should be recognized.

A stain removal procedure may be deemed necessary prior to professional fluoride application when stains are not removed during scaling. In that case, it is advised that a fluoride-containing prophylaxis paste with minimal abrasiveness be used. The fluoride from the paste may replace in part that removed by the abrasive action.[4]

III. To Contribute to Patient Motivation

Removal of plaque must be a *daily* procedure carried out *by the patient.* It must be accomplished thoroughly at least once or twice daily, and for some patients, three times daily if disease is to be controlled and the sanitation of the mouth maintained.

A one-time removal of soft deposits from the teeth at a dental hygiene appointment does not accomplish any purpose because deposits return promptly. It is known that pellicle returns to cover the teeth within minutes after complete polishing, and that plaque bacteria begin to collect on the pellicle within 1 or 2 hours, increasing in thickness, until by 12 to 24 hours, plaque is thick enough to show clearly when a disclosing agent is applied. Undisturbed, plaque may begin to calcify within a few days in a calculus-susceptible patient (page 248).

Except for a minority of patients who practice superior plaque control, the deposits return promptly. Effects of stain removal as a preventive measure for gingival disease or dental caries have not been proven.

Smooth polished tooth surfaces may contribute in part to the following effects:
A. Help the instructed patient to obtain more satisfactory results from self-care procedures. A smooth surface should be easier to clean.
B. Show the patient the appearance and feeling of a clean mouth for motivational purposes. The greatest change in behavior, however, the true learning, can usually be obtained through patient participation in the use of a disclosing agent and personal removal of plaque with floss and toothbrush.

CLINICAL APPLICATION OF SELECTIVE POLISHING

Polishing should never be a substitute for complete calculus removal and root planing as a means for making the tooth surfaces smooth. Smoothing of tooth surfaces is a part of the basic instrumentation and is performed during the final series of strokes for scaling and planing.

Because of the numbers of health and safety factors involved, as have been described, the decision to polish should be based on consideration for the individual patient. Instruction for stain prevention is important, as is minimizing for all patients, or omitting for selected ones, the use of the abrasive paste with the rubber cup.

I. Summary of Contraindications for Polishing

The following list suggests some of the specific instances in which polishing either should be postponed or is contraindicated indefinitely.

A. No Unsightly Stain

The principle of selective polishing is not to polish unless necessary. Appearance is important to patients, but maintaining the integrity of the tooth surface for disease prevention is also important. When stain is noted on specific tooth surfaces, polishing can be applied to selected areas without having to cover all the teeth in a generalized procedure.[22]

B. Patients at Risk for Dental Caries

1. Rampant caries: nursing bottle caries; root caries; all ages.
2. Thin enamel: amelogenesis imperfecta.
3. Demineralized areas.
4. Radiation to head, particularly involving the salivary glands.
5. Xerostomia for any reason.

C. Patients with Respiratory Problems

Power-driven instruments are contraindicated.

D. Tooth Sensitivity

Abrasive agent will uncover ends of dentinal tubules on area of thin cementum or dentin.

E. Restorations

Restorations may be scratched by polishing abrasive.

F. Newly Erupted Teeth.

Incomplete mineralization of surface.

G. Conditions Requiring Postponement for Later Evaluation

1. When instruction for personal plaque removal (daily care) has not yet been given or when the patient has not demonstrated adequate plaque control.
2. Soft spongy tissue that bleeds on brushing or gentle instrumentation.
3. Immediately following deep subgingival scaling, root planing, and gingival curettage, because abrasive particles can become embedded in the pocket wall and interfere with healing.

II. Suggestions for Clinic Procedure

A. Remove Stain by Scaling

Whenever possible, stains can be removed during scaling. Unsightly stains should be removed for the new patient initially. At that time, an explanation of the selective polishing principle can be presented and assistance given for a preventive plan for stain control.

B. Remove Stain during Root Planing

The end product of root planing is a smooth, hard surface that does not need further polishing. Abrasive action of polishing paste can scratch the finely planed surface.

C. Minimize Instrumentation

Use a light intermittent stroke with the rubber cup. Factors affecting the rate of abrasion are described in the next section.

D. Substitute Nonabrasive Agent

Use over-the-counter toothpaste with very light pressure when stain is missing or minimal but the patient requests the treatment in spite of education.

CLEANING AND POLISHING AGENTS

Abrasive agents are applied with polishing instruments to remove extrinsic dental stains. Abrasives selected should produce smooth tooth surfaces but not remove tooth structure unnecessarily, abrade gingival epithelium, or produce excessive frictional heat.

I. Definitions

A. Abrasive

A material composed of particles of sufficient hardness and sharpness to cut or scratch a softer material when drawn across its surface.

B. Abrasion

The wearing away of surface material by friction. Marked or severe abrasion would be destructive to a tooth surface.[23]

C. Polishing

The production, especially by friction, of a smooth, glossy, mirror-like surface that reflects light.[23] A very fine agent is used for polishing after a coarser agent is used for cleaning.

II. Factors Affecting Abrasive Action

During polishing, sharp edges of abrasive particles are moved along the surface of a material, abrading it by producing microscopic scratches or grooves. The rate of abrasion, or speed with which structural material is removed from the surface being polished, is governed by characteristics of the abrasive particles as well as by the manner in which they are applied.

A. Characteristics of Abrasive Particles[23]

1. *Shape.* Irregularly shaped particles with sharp edges produce deeper grooves and thus abrade faster than rounded particles with dull edges.
2. *Hardness.* Particles must be harder than the

surface to be abraded; harder particles abrade faster.

3. *Body Strength.* Particles that fracture into smaller sharp-edged particles during use are more abrasive than those that wear down with use and become dull and rounded.

4. *Attrition Resistance.* Effective abrasive particles do not dull or become embedded in the surface being abraded; particles with greater attrition resistance abrade faster.

5. *Particle Size (Grit)*
   a. The larger the particles, the more abrasive they are and the less polishing ability they have. Finer abrasive particles achieve a glossier finish.
   b. Abrasive and polishing agents are graded from coarse to fine based on the size of the holes in a standard sieve through which they will pass. The finer abrasives are called powders or flours and are graded in order of increasing fineness as F, FF, FFF, etc. Particles embedded in papers are graded 0, 00, 000, etc.

B. Method of Application of Abrasives

1. *Quantity Applied.* The more particles applied per unit time, the faster the rate of abrasion.
   a. Particles suspended in water or other vehicles are present in quantities proportional to the thickness of the paste. These vehicles act as lubricants to reduce the amount of frictional heat produced.
   b. Dry powders or flours represent the greatest quantity that can be applied per unit of time. Frictional heat produced is proportional to the rate of abrasion; therefore, the use of *dry agents* is *contraindicated* for polishing natural teeth because of the potential danger of thermal injury to the dental pulp.

2. *Speed of Application.* The greater the speed of application, the faster the rate of abrasion.
   a. With increased speed of application, pressure must be reduced.
   b. *Rapid abrasion* is *contraindicated* because it increases frictional heat.

3. *Pressure of Application.* The heavier the pressure applied, the faster the rate of abrasion.
   a. Particles to which pressure is applied produce deep grooves at first, but fracture according to their impact strength. With sufficient pressure, the particles may disintegrate.
   b. *Heavy pressure* is *contraindicated* because it increases frictional heat.

4. *Summary.* When cleaning and polishing are indicated after patient evaluation, the following should be observed:
   a. Use wet agents.
   b. Apply a rubber polishing cup, using low speed.
   c. Use a light, intermittent touch.

III. Abrasive Agents[23]

The abrasives listed here are examples of commonly used agents. Some are available in several grades, and the specific use varies with the grade. For example, while a superfine grade might be used for polishing enamel surfaces and metallic restorations, a coarser grade would be used for laboratory purposes only.

Abrasives for use daily in a dentifrice must necessarily be of a finer grade than those used for professional polishing accomplished a few times each year. Dentifrice abrasives are described on pages 326–328.

A. Silex (Silicon Dioxide)
1. *XXX Silex.* Fairly abrasive.
2. *Super-fine Silex.* Can be used for stain removal from enamel.

B. Pumice
Powdered pumice is of volcanic origin and consists chiefly of complex silicates of aluminum, potassium, and sodium. The specifications for particle size are listed in the *National Formulary*[24] as follows:
1. *Pumice Flour or Superfine Pumice.* Least abrasive, and may be used to remove stains from enamel.
2. *Fine Pumice.* Mildly abrasive.
3. *Coarse Pumice.* Not for use on natural teeth.

C. Calcium Carbonate (Whiting, Calcite, Chalk)
Various grades are used for different polishing techniques.

D. Tin Oxide (Putty Powder, Stannic Oxide)
Polishing agent for teeth and metallic restorations.

E. Emery (Corundum)
Not used directly on the enamel.
1. *Aluminum Oxide (Alumina).* The pure form of emery.
2. *Levigated Alumina.* Consists of extremely fine particles of aluminum oxide, which may be used for polishing metals but are destructive to tooth surfaces.

F. Rouge (Jeweler's Rouge)
Iron oxide, a fine red powder sometimes impregnated on paper discs. It is useful for polishing gold and precious metal alloys in the laboratory.

IV. Preparation of Abrasives

Agents used for polishing the natural teeth and restorations are mixed with water or other lubricant to facilitate particle movement across the tooth surface and to reduce frictional heat. A quantity of polishing paste can be prepared in advance and kept in a closed jar. Glycerin is added to help as a spreading factor and to prevent splashing during application of the polishing cup.

A. Preparation of Single Quantity
1. Place water or flavored mouthrinse in a dappen dish. Some agents require a specific amount of water.
2. Add the dry agent to saturation and stir.

B. Consistency
The paste should be as moist as possible, but transportable between dappen dish and the teeth.

C. Containers
Two separate containers and rubber cups are used when a cleaning abrasive is used first and followed by a polishing agent.

V. Commercial Preparations

Numerous dental prophylactic cleaning and polishing preparations are available. Some of these have been studied for their relative abrasive effect on enamel and dentin, and their cleaning properties.[15,25]

A. Constituents
Most commercially prepared polishing pastes contain an abrasive, water, a humectant, a binder, and agents for sweetening, flavoring, and color. Approximate proportions and purposes of each constituent with examples are as follows:
1. *Abrasive* 50 to 60 percent, main ingredient. Examples: pumice, silicon dioxide.
2. *Water* 10 to 20 percent, solvent, and to provide desired consistency.
3. *Humectant* 20 to 25 percent, moisture-retainer, stabilize the ingredients. Examples: glycerin, sorbitol.
4. *Binder* 1.5 to 2.0 percent, prevent separation, non-splatter. Examples: agar-agar, sodium silicate powder.
5. *Sweetener,* artificial, noncariogenic.
6. *Flavoring,* coloring agents.

B. Packaging
Commercial preparations are in the forms of pastes, powders, or tablets. Some are available in measured amounts, contained in small plastic or other individual packets that contribute to the cleanliness and sterility of the procedure.

Selection of a preparation has been based on its qualities of abrasiveness, consistency for convenient use, or flavor for patient pleasure.

C. Fluoride Prophylaxis Pastes[26,27]
Application of fluoride by pastes cannot be considered a substitute for conventional topical application on the basis of present-day research. Reviews of the research show that, while moderate caries-preventive effects have been demonstrated, other studies have had minimal or no statistically significant results.

Incompatibility of the fluoride agent with the abrasive or other paste ingredients has been a problem with certain combinations. It is not merely a question of adding a fluoride solution to a cleaning paste. When mixed, agents may react, and the effect of the fluoride can be neutralized or the shelf-life may be limited.

Another limitation of the paste preparations is that certain abrasives can remove a thin layer of enamel during polishing. With the removal of the enamel, the outer layer of fluoride is also removed, possibly as fast as it is added from the paste, but this concept has not been researched.

To be able to evaluate fluoride preparations that become available on the market, a continuing review of the new research is needed as additional studies are reported. Because the caries prevention that can be expected from the use of prophylaxis pastes is minimal, other means for applying fluoride must be used if the patient is to receive optimum protection by fluorides.

PROCEDURES FOR STAIN REMOVAL (CORONAL POLISHING)

I. Patient Preparation for Stain Removal

Preparation of the patient includes instruction in plaque control procedures, complete scaling and root planing, and overhang removal. The patient should be informed of the limited value of polishing and why it is a selective procedure performed as needed.

A. Plaque Control
Stain removal should be withheld until the patient's plaque removal on a daily basis is adequate, so that the deposition of stains can be controlled. When a patient is informed of the relationship between self-care and the recurrence of stains, cooperation may be obtained. When a stain such as tobacco stain returns, polishing frequency should be limited and, with each polishing, topical fluoride should be applied.

B. Scaling
As much stain as possible should be removed during scaling for calculus removal from the enamel. All stain should be removed during root planing, because the stain is located within the diseased, altered cementum.

C. Evaluation
After scaling and other periodontal treatment, an evaluation is made to determine the need to polish teeth, restorations, and dental prostheses.

II. Environmental Preparation

Environmental factors were described in Chapters 3 and 4. A topical summary is provided here.

A. Procedures to Lessen the Extent of Contaminated Aerosols
1. Avoid use of power-driven instruments for a patient with a communicable disease that could be disseminated by way of aerosols.

2. Clear the water that will be used for rinsing. Flush water through the tubing for 5 to 6 minutes at the beginning of each work period, and for 30 seconds after each appointment.
3. Request patient to rinse with an antimicrobial mouthrinse to reduce the numbers of oral microorganisms before starting instrumentation.
4. Use high-velocity evacuation.

B. Protective Barriers

The patient must wear protective eyeglasses and coverall. The clinician wears the usual barrier protection, namely, eyeglasses, mask, and gloves.

III. Instruments

Both power-driven and manual instruments may be useful when polishing. All polishing instruments should be used with discretion and in a manner requiring minimal abrasion of the tooth surface. Because tooth structure is removed when an abrasive is used on the enamel and still more when it is used on dentin or cementum, only a mild abrasive agent is appropriate.

Power-driven implements, floss, and finishing strips will be outlined first, followed by procedures for cleaning a removable prosthesis. In Chapter 40, the removal of bonding agents will be outlined, and in Chapter 41, the finishing of amalgam restorations will be described.

THE INSTRUMENTS

I. Handpiece

A handpiece is used to hold rotary instruments in the dental unit. It is connected by an arm, cable, belt, or tube to the source of power. Rotary instruments have been classified according to their rotational speeds, designated by revolutions per minute (r.p.m.) as high speed, mid speed, and low speed.[28]

A. Ultra or High Speed (Type I)
Class A: Greater than 160,000 r.p.m.
Class B: 100,000 to 160,000 r.p.m.

B. Mid Speed (Type II)
Between 20,000 and 100,000 r.p.m. Some high-speed handpieces can be adjusted to speeds from zero to their capacity, which makes it possible to use them with the proper attachments for tooth polishing.

C. Low Speed (Type III)
Typical range under 20,000 r.p.m. Lowest speeds are used for polishing and finishing procedures.

II. Prophylaxis Angle

Contra or right-angle attachment for the handpiece to which polishing devices (rubber cup, bristle brush) are attached.

A. Characteristics

Many types of prophylaxis angles are available. Some are disposable and others are made of stainless steel and may have hard chrome, carbon steel, or brass bearings. Unless they are disposable, only instruments that can be sterilized should be selected.

B. Service Life

The length of time a prophylaxis angle is serviceable is related in part to the quality of materials used and the manner of construction. Primarily, however, *the length of life is directly proportional to the care provided.*

III. Prophylaxis Angle Attachments

A. Rubber Polishing Cups
1. *Types* (figure 38–1)
   a. Slip-on: with ribbed cup to aid in holding polishing agent.
   b. Slip-on: with bristles inside cup.
   c. Threaded (screw type): with plain ribbed cup or flange (webbed) type.
2. *Materials*
   a. Natural rubber: more resilient and will not stain the teeth.
   b. Synthetic: stiffer than natural rubber; white cups must be used because synthetic black may stain the teeth.

B. Bristle Brushes

1. *Types*
   a. For prophylaxis angle: slip-on or screw type.

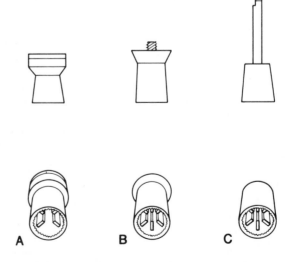

Figure 38–1. Rubber Cup Attachments. A. Slip-on or Snap-on for button-end prophylaxis angle. **B.** Threaded for direct insertion in right angle. **C.** Mandrel stem for latch-type angle.

b. For handpiece: mandrel mounted.

2. *Materials.* Nylon or natural bristles.

IV. Uses for Attachments

A. Handpiece with Straight Mandrel

1. Dixon bristle brush (Type C, soft) for polishing removable dentures (page 514).
2. Mounted stone for sharpening instruments (page 451).
3. Rubber cup on mandrel for polishing facial surfaces of anterior teeth.

B. Prophylaxis Angle with Rubber Cup or Brush

1. *Rubber Cup.* For removal of stains from the tooth surfaces and polishing restorations.
2. *Brush*
   a. For removing stains from deep pits and fissures and enamel surfaces away from gingival margin. A brush is not recommended for use on exposed cementum or dentin, because they are easily grooved by such an instrument.
   b. For preliminary polishing of amalgam restorations.

USE OF THE PROPHYLAXIS ANGLE

I. Effects on Tissues: Precautions

The use of power-driven instruments can cause discomfort for the patient if care and consideration for the oral tissues are not exercised to prevent unnecessary trauma.

Awareness of the potential tissue damage is important. Tactile sensitivity of the clinician while using a thick, bulky handpiece is diminished and unnecessary pressure may be applied inadvertently. Frictional heat may cause pain or discomfort.

Some loss of tooth structure occurs during polishing when an abrasive agent is used. Research on the effects on tooth structure was reviewed on pages 503–504.

The greater the speed of application of a polishing agent, the faster the rate of abrasion (page 507). Therefore, the speed at which the handpiece is operated should be a low r.p.m.

Trauma to the gingival tissue can result from too high a speed, extended application of the rubber cup, or use of an abrasive polishing agent. Tissue damage and the need for antibiotic premedication for risk patients was described on page 503.

II. Prophylaxis Angle Technique

The first technique principle is to apply the polishing agent only where it is needed, that is, where there is unsightly stain. Contraindications were listed on page 506.

As with all oral procedures, a systematic order of polishing should be followed. A variety of skills must be learned in using and caring for the equipment.

A. Instrument Grasp

Modified pen (page 431)

B. Finger Rest (pages 431–432)

1. Establish firmly on tooth structure.
2. Use a wide fulcrum area when practical to aid in the balance of the large instrument. Example: place cushion of fulcrum finger across occlusal surfaces of premolars while polishing the molars.
3. Avoid use of mobile teeth as finger rests.

C. Speed of Handpiece

1. Use lowest available speed to minimize frictional heat.
2. Adjust r.p.m. by changing the position of the rheostat foot pedal.

D. Use of Rheostat Pedal

1. Apply steady pressure with foot to produce an even, low speed.
2. Keep sole of the foot that activates rheostat pedal flat on the floor. Use toe to activate rheostat pedal.

E. Preparation of Polishing Agent

1. Agent is mixed as wet as possible, but not so wet that it cannot be carried conveniently in the rubber cup from the dappen dish to the teeth.
2. Wetness aids in alleviating the frictional heat produced.

F. Rubber Cup: Stroke and Procedure

1. Observe where polishing is needed to prevent unnecessary rubber cup application.
2. Fill rubber cup with polishing agent, and distribute agent over tooth surfaces to be polished.
3. Establish finger rest and bring rubber cup almost in contact with tooth surface before activating power source.
4. Using slowest r.p.m., apply revolving cup lightly to tooth surface for 1 or 2 seconds. Use a light pressure so that the edges of the rubber cup flare slightly.
5. Move cup to adjacent area on tooth surface, using a patting or brushing motion.
6. Replenish supply of polishing agent frequently.
7. Turn handpiece to adapt rubber cup to fit each surface of the tooth, including proximal surfaces and gingival surfaces of fixed partial dentures.
8. Start with the distal surface of the most posterior tooth of a quadrant and move forward toward the anterior. For each tooth, work from the gingival third toward the incisal third of the tooth.
9. When two polishing agents of different abrasiveness are to be applied, use a separate rubber cup for each.
10. Cups that cannot be sterilized are used only once. Disposable one-use cups are preferred.

G. Bristle Brush

Bristle brushes should be used selectively and limited to occlusal surfaces. Lacerations of the gingiva and grooves and scratches in the tooth surface, particularly the roots, may result.

1. Soak stiff brush in hot water to soften bristles.
2. Distribute mild abrasive polishing agent over occlusal surfaces of teeth to be polished.
3. Place fingers of nondominant hand in a position that will both retract and protect cheek and tongue from the revolving brush.
4. Establish a firm finger rest and bring brush almost in contact with the tooth before activating power source.
5. Using slowest r.p.m., apply revolving brush lightly to the occlusal surface only, avoiding contact of bristles with soft tissues.
6. Use a short stroke in a brushing motion, following the inclined planes of the cusps.
7. Move from tooth to tooth to prevent generation of excessive frictional heat. Replenish supply of polishing agent frequently.

H. Irrigation

Teeth and interdental areas should be irrigated thoroughly several times with water from the syringe to remove abrasive particles. The rotary movement of the rubber cup or bristle brush tends to force the abrasive into the gingival sulci, which may be a source of irritation to the soft tissues.

POLISHING PROXIMAL SURFACES

Considerable care must be exercised in the use of floss, tape, and finishing strips. Understanding the anatomy of the interdental papillae and their relationship to the contact areas and proximal surfaces of the teeth is prerequisite to the prevention of tissue damage. Inadequate contacts between teeth provide potential areas of food impaction and plaque retention. These contacts should be charted for consideration by the dentist during treatment planning.

As much polishing as possible of accessible proximal surfaces is accomplished during the use of the rubber cup in the prophylaxis angle. This is followed by the use of dental tape with polishing agent when necessary. Finishing strips are used only in selected instances when all other techniques fail to remove a stain.

The use of dental floss or tape for bacterial plaque control on proximal tooth surfaces is an essential part of self-care by the patient.

I. Dental Tape and Floss

A. Description

Floss and tape are made of spun silk or nylon thread and are available unwaxed or coated with wax. The wax covering affords some protection for the tissues, facilitates the movement of the floss or tape, prevents excessive absorption of moisture, and helps to prevent shredding.

Tape is flat and has relatively sharp edges, whereas floss is round. Either floss or tape may injure the tissue when used incorrectly or carelessly.

B. Uses

1. *Tape for Polishing*
   a. Proximal tooth surfaces.
   b. Gingival surface of fixed partial denture.
2. *Floss for Removing*
   a. Debris and food particles. Patient instruction and review at beginning of appointment prepares the teeth for scaling.
   b. Particles of polishing agents at completion of polishing procedures.
      i. From interproximal areas and gingival sulci.
      ii. From gingival surface of fixed partial dentures.
   c. Retained abrasive particles after use of finishing strips.

C. Technique for Dental Floss and Tape

Techniques for tape and floss application are described on pages 318–319 and illustrated in figures 23–1, 23–2, and 23–3. The same principles apply whether the patient or the clinician is using the floss. Finger rests must be used to prevent snapping through contact areas.

1. *Polishing with Dental Tape.* Polishing agent is applied to the tooth, and the tape is moved gently back and forth over the area where stain was observed.
2. *Polishing Gingival Surface of a Fixed Partial Denture.* A floss threader is used to position the floss or tape over the gingival surface. Floss threaders are described and illustrated on page 342. Polishing agent is applied under the pontic, and the floss or tape is moved back and forth.
3. *Flossing after Polishing.* Particles of abrasive agent should be removed by irrigation and by using a clean length of floss applied in the usual manner.
4. *Rinsing and Irrigation.* Irrigate with water-spray syringe to clean out all abrasive agent.

II. Finishing Strips

A. Description

Finishing strips are also known as linen abrasive strips. They are thin, flexible, tape-shaped, and are available in four widths—extra narrow, narrow, medium, and wide.

Finishing strips are made of linen or plastic with one smooth side and the other that serves as a carrier for abrasive agents bonded to the side. "Gapped" strips are available with an abrasive-free portion to permit sliding the strip through the contact area without abrading the enamel.

They are available in extra fine, fine, medium, or coarse grit. *Only extra narrow or narrow strips with fine grit are suggested for stain removal and then only with discretion.*

B. Use

1. *For Stain Removal on Proximal Surfaces of Anterior Teeth.* When other polishing techniques are unsuccessful.
2. *Precautions for Use*
   a. Edge of strip is sharp and may cut gingival tissue or lip.
   b. Rough working side of strip is capable of removing tooth structure and may make nicks or grooves, particularly in the cementum.
   c. Use of a finishing strip should be limited to enamel surfaces.

C. Technique for Finishing Strip

1. *Grasp and Finger Rest.* A strip no longer than 6 inches is most conveniently applied. The grasp and fulcrum must be well controlled. Protection of the lip by retraction with the thumb and index finger holding the strip is mandatory.
2. *Positioning*
   a. Direct the abrasive side of strip toward the proximal surface to be treated, as the strip is worked slowly and gently between the teeth with a slight sawing motion. Bring strip just through the contact area. If the strip breaks, immediately use floss to remove particles of abrasive.
   b. When a space is clearly visible through an interproximal area and the interdental papilla is missing, a narrow finishing strip may be threaded through. Prepare strip by cutting the end on a diagonal to facilitate threading.
3. *Stain Removal*
   a. Press abrasive side of strip against tooth. Draw back and forth in a ⅛-inch arc 2 or 3 times, rocking on the established fulcrum.
   b. Remove strip. Do not attempt to turn the strip while it is in the interdental area.
4. *Dental Floss.* Follow each application of a finishing strip with dental floss to remove abrasive particles.

AIRBRASIVE FOR POLISHING

The airbrasive machines are known by several names, including air-polishing, air-powder abrasive, air-powered slurry, or airabrasive system or device. As applied in principles of selective polishing, after patient instruction in plaque control, scaling and root planing are completed to be followed by an evaluation of a need for stain removal.

I. Description

A. Definition

The airbrasive is an air-powered device using air and water pressure to deliver a controlled stream of a specially processed sodium bicarbonate in a slurry through the handpiece nozzle.[29]

B. Operation

Only a 3- to 5-second application of the spray is advisable at any specific spot on a tooth surface. The stream must be kept in constant circular motion with the nozzle tip about 4 to 5 mm. away from the enamel surface.

The spray is angled away from the gingival margin (figure 38–2). The periphery of the spray may be near the gingival margin, but the center should be directed at an angle less than 90 degrees away from the margin.

Complete directions for care of equipment and preparation for use of the device are provided by the various manufacturers.[29]

C. Mode of Action

The fine particles of sodium bicarbonate are propelled by compressed air in a warm spray. They debride the tooth surface by mechanical abrasion. The air pressure is 50 to 60 pounds per square inch (psi).

II. Recommendations and Precautions

A. Aerosol Production[30,31]

A copious spray containing oral debris and microorganisms is produced. As with all contaminated aerosols, a health hazard can exist. Sug-

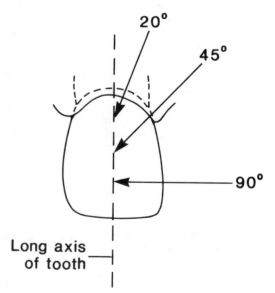

Figure 38–2. Airbrasive Spray. The spray should focus on areas of extrinsic stain, using principles of selective polishing. To protect the gingival tissue from the impact, to avoid exposed cementum, and to prevent direct application of the spray into a pocket, the spray should be directed away from the gingiva.

gestions for minimizing contamination as well as the effects of the aerosols include the following:

1. Patient should use a preoperative antibacterial mouthrinse.
2. High-volume suction should be applied, using a wide tip held near the tooth where the spray is applied from the nozzle. A saliva ejector has been shown to be insufficient to reduce bacterial counts in the aerosol.[31]
3. Protective patient procedures
   a. Remove contact lens; wear eye protection.
   b. Lubricate lips to prevent drying effect of the sodium bicarbonate.
   c. Wear complete coverall and cover for hair.
4. Clinician should wear usual mask, gloves, and eye-safety glasses. Uniform cover is also recommended.

B. Risk Patients: Airbrasive Contraindicated

The information from the patient's medical history must be reviewed and appropriate applications made. Antibiotic premedication is indicated for all the same patients who are at risk for any dental hygiene procedure (pages 85 and 91). The airbrasive is not used for a patient with a

1. Restricted sodium diet.[32]
2. Respiratory disease or other condition that limits swallowing or breathing.
3. Communicable infection that can contaminate the aerosols produced.

C. Other Contraindications

1. *Root Surfaces.* Cementum and dentin should be avoided. They can be readily removed by an airbrasive.[33,34,35]
2. *Soft, Spongy Gingiva.* The airbrasive irritates and traumatizes the free gingival tissue.[36] When heavy stain calls for use of an airbrasive, the patient should be instructed in daily bacterial plaque removal, scaling and root planing should be completed, and the stain removal should be postponed until the soft tissue has healed.
3. *Restorative Materials.* The use of airbrasive on composite resins, cements, and other non-metallic materials causes removal or pitting.[37,38] Less damage occurs to the harder restorative materials.

CLEANING THE REMOVABLE DENTURE

A complete patient service includes the scaling and polishing of all natural teeth and their replacements. Complete and partial dentures may accumulate calculus, soft deposits, and stains, which may affect the adaptation of the dentures in the mouth as well as afford a source of irritation to adjacent mucous membranes. The parts of a complete denture are illustrated in figure 24–14, page 345, and the parts of a partial in figure 24–12, page 343.

A learning experience in the proper care of the dentures can be provided for the patient while the dentures are cleaned professionally. Specific instruction for the patient is described on pages 344 and 347.

I. Objectives

With professional cleaning of a removable denture, the following benefits can be expected:

A. Aid in preserving the natural teeth associated with a removable partial denture.
B. Removal of calculus and stains, thereby smoothing the surfaces of the denture to lessen plaque and debris retention.
C. Improvement of the appearance and sanitation of the denture.
D. Provide the patient with a feeling of complete oral cleanliness.
E. Understanding by the patient of the importance of routine personal and professional care of the denture.

II. Removal of Denture

Usually, the patient removes the denture. The dental hygienist will have occasion to remove dentures for certain patients, particularly those who may be handicapped or helpless, or as an emergency measure.

Although denture removal may be complicated by anatomic features of an individual mouth, a general procedure is outlined here. The procedure should be reviewed with the dentist in order to follow a preferred technique.

A. Complete Maxillary Denture

1. Grasp the denture firmly with the thumb on the facial surface at the height of the border of the denture under the lip, and the index finger on the palatal surface.
2. With the other hand, elevate the lip to expose the border of the denture to break the seal.
3. Remove the denture gently in a downward and forward direction.
4. If the retention of the denture cannot be overcome by elevation of the lip, request the able patient to blow into the mouth with the lips closed. This usually breaks the seal.

B. Complete Mandibular Denture

1. Grasp the denture firmly on the facial surface with the thumb and on the lingual surface with the index finger.
2. With the other hand, retract the lower lip forward and remove the denture gently.

C. Partial Denture with Clasps

Exert an even pressure on both sides of the denture simultaneously as the clasps are lifted over their abutment teeth. Usually, the line of insertion and removal of a partial denture is designed and constructed for an even, vertical movement.

III. Care of Dentures During Intra-oral Procedures

A. Provide a cleansing tissue for the patient's use when requesting the patient to remove or insert the denture.

B. Receive removable denture in a paper cup or container with a fitted cover.

C. Immerse in antimicrobial solution.

D. Place container in a safe place away from working area to minimize hazard of breakage.

IV. Procedure for Cleaning

Ultrasonic cleaning is the procedure of choice for the safety of the denture, for the preservation of the surface finish, to eliminate the possibility of scratching the denture surface through the use of scalers, polishing agents, or other devices, and for the time saved. When ultrasonic equipment is not available, manual and power-driven instruments must be used.

A. Ultrasonic

1. Principles and procedures were described on pages 44–45.
2. Use the solution designated for stain and calculus removal and follow the manufacturer's directions specifically.
3. Rinse thoroughly and scrub free of solution and loosened debris with a moderately stiff brush before returning the denture to the patient. Brushes reserved for this purpose should be sterilized.

B. Manual and Power-driven

1. *Removal of Calculus.* Remove calculus by careful scaling. Care must be taken not to scratch the denture.
2. *Method for Holding Denture.* Grasp firmly and securely in the palm of the nondominant hand (figure 24–15, page 348); avoid excessive pressure on a partial denture bar or clasps to prevent bending.
3. *Polishing the Denture.* Polish only the external polished surface of a denture; abrasive applied to the internal impression surface could alter the fit of the denture.
4. *Polishing at the Dental Chair*
   a. With a conventional dental chair, polishing over the cuspidor (lined with a towel) is sometimes convenient. Focus the dental light over the work area.
   b. Polish nonmetal parts with a mounted brush (Dixon C softened in warm water), using very wet superfine pumice or other appropriate abrasive. The finger rest is maintained on the denture.
   c. Polish metal parts lightly with a rubber polishing cup. A fine polishing agent should be used to prevent scratching the metal.
5. *Polishing on the Dental Lathe in the Laboratory*
   a. Prevention of cross contamination in the laboratory.

      i. Wear a mask and safety glasses while working over a lathe.

      ii. Use sterile rag wheel and pumice.

      iii. Soak the prosthesis in an antiseptic solution for 2 to 3 minutes before returning it to the patient. The solution should be fresh for each patient.

    b. Use a wet rag wheel with fine wet abrasive for nonmetal parts, and whiting or tin oxide on a separate rag wheel for the metal parts other than clasps. Keep denture and polishing agent wet at all times.

    c. Hold the denture in a two-handed grip. Cover the clasps and denture teeth with fingers to prevent abrasive from scratching the teeth and the clasps from hooking into the rag wheel. The clasps are cleaned later with a wood point in the porte polisher.

    d. Run the lathe at low speed and apply denture carefully. Constantly change the surface applied to the rag wheel to prevent excess frictional heat.

6. *Rinsing the Denture.* Rinse the denture thoroughly under warm (never hot) running water.
   a. Line the sink with a towel, or fill half-full with water to avoid breakage in case the denture is dropped.
   b. Brush the internal impression surface of the denture using a mild soap or a detergent; rinse thoroughly.
7. *Evaluation.* Evaluate the cleanliness of the denture: examine under bright light and apply compressed air stream to detect calculus or denture plaque.
8. *Disinfection.* Disinfect, rinse and return the denture to the patient on a paper towel. The denture should be wet for comfortable insertion.

TECHNICAL HINTS

I. Maintain several prophylaxis angles in practice to facilitate use during successive appointments.

II. Prevent rheostat from sliding on highly polished floor by placing one or two drops of carbon tetrachloride under the rheostat.

III. Protect patient's lips and intraoral soft tissues during the use of floss, tape, finishing strips, and discs.

FACTORS TO TEACH THE PATIENT

I. How plaques and stains form on the natural teeth and their replacements and why too frequent polishing in the dental office is not advisable.

II. The meaning of selective polishing and why it is not necessary to polish all teeth at every appointment.

III. Stains and bacterial plaque removed by polishing can return promptly if plaque is not removed faithfully on a schedule of two or three times each day.

IV. Polishing agents utilized in the dental office or clinic are too abrasive for daily home use.

V. The need for adapting toothbrushing and flossing techniques to clean abutment teeth.

VI. The importance of regular cleaning of dentures with special attention to clasps.

VII. How to handle and clean a denture.

References

1. DeLeo, A.A.: The Incidence of Bacteremia Following Oral Prophylaxis on Pediatric Patients, *Oral Surg., 37,* 36, January, 1974.

2. Micik, R.E., Miller, R.L., Mazzarella, M.A., and Ryge, G.: Studies on Dental Aerobiology: I. Bacterial Aerosols Generated During Dental Procedures, *J. Dent. Res., 48,* 49, January-February, 1969.

3. Hartley, J.L.: Eye and Facial Injuries Resulting from Dental Procedures, *Dent. Clin. North Am., 22,* 505, July, 1978.

4. Vrbic, V., Brudevold, F., and McCann, H.G.: Acquisition of Fluoride by Enamel from Fluoride Pumice Pastes, *Helv. Odontol. Acta, 11,* 21, April, 1967.

5. Whitehurst, V.E., Stookey, G.K., and Muhler, J.C.: Studies Concerning the Cleaning, Polishing, and Therapeutic Properties of Commercial Prophylactic Pastes, *J. Oral Ther. Pharm., 4,* 181, November, 1967.

6. Stookey, G.K.: *In vitro* Estimates of Enamel and Dentin Abrasion Associated with a Prophylaxis, *J. Dent. Res., 57,* 36, January, 1978.

7. Zuniga, M.A. and Caldwell, R.C.: The Effect of Fluoride-containing Prophylaxis Pastes on Normal and "White-spot" Enamel, *J. Dent. Child., 36,* 345, September-October, 1969.

8. Brasch, S.V., Lazarou, J., Van Abbé, N.J., and Forrest, J.O.: The Assessment of Dentifrice Abrasivity *in vivo, Br. Dent. J., 127,* 119, August 5, 1969.

9. Jefferies, R.W.: Polishing Dental Enamel, *N.Z. Dent. J., 69,* 167, July, 1973.

10. Brudevold, F., Gardner, D.E., and Smith, F.A.: The Distribution of Fluoride in Human Enamel, *J. Dent. Res., 35,* 420, June, 1956.

11. Vrbic, V. and Brudevold, F.: Fluoride Uptake From Treatment with Different Fluoride Prophylaxis Pastes and from the Use of Pastes Containing a Soluble Aluminum Salt Followed by Topical Application, *Caries Res., 4,* 158, Number 2, 1970.

12. Löe, H.: Reactions of Marginal Periodontal Tissues to Restorative Procedures, *Int. Dent. J., 18,* 759, December, 1968.

13. Miller, W.A.: Experimental Foreign Body Reactions to Toothpaste Abrasives, *J. Periodontol., 47,* 101, February, 1976.

14. Roulet, J.F. and Roulet-Mehrens, T.K.: The Surface Roughness of Restorative Materials and Dental Tissues After Polishing with Prophylaxis and Polishing Pastes, *J. Periodontol., 53,* 257, April, 1982.

15. Heath, J.R., Davenport, J.C., and Jones, P.A.: The Abrasion of Acrylic Resin by Cleaning Pastes, *J. Oral Rehabil., 10,* 159, March, 1983.

16. Theilade, J., Slots, J., and Fejerskov, O.: The Ultrastructure of Black Stain on Human Primary Teeth, *Scand. J. Dent. Res., 81,* 528, Number 7, 1973.

17. Knutson, J.W.: Sodium Fluoride Solutions: Technique for Application to the Teeth, *J. Am. Dent. Assoc., 36,* 37, January, 1948.

18. Tinanoff, N.: The Significance of the Acquired Pellicle in the Practice of Dentistry, *J. Dent. Child., 43,* 20, January-February, 1976.

19. Tinanoff, N., Wei, S.H.Y., and Parkins, F.M.: Effect of a Pumice Prophylaxis on Fluoride Uptake in Tooth Enamel, *J. Am. Dent. Assoc., 88,* 384, February, 1974.

20. Birkeland, J.M. and Torell, P.: Caries-preventive Fluoride Mouthrinses, *Caries Res., 12,* 38, Supplement 1, 1978.

21. Jones, J.C., Murphy, R.F., and Edd, P.A.: Using Health Education in a Fluoride Mouthrinse Program: The Public Health Hygienist's Role, *Dent. Hyg., 53,* 469, October, 1979.

22. Sheiham, A.: Prevention and Control of Periodontal Disease, in *International Conference on Research in the Biology of Periodontal Disease.* Chicago, University of Illinois, June, 1977, p. 332.

23. Phillips, R.W.: *Skinner's Science of Dental Materials,* 8th ed. Philadelphia, W.B. Saunders Co., 1982, pp. 578–589.

24. American Pharmaceutical Association: *National Formulary XIII.* Washington, D.C., American Pharmaceutical Association, 1970, p. 611.

25. Krouse, M. and Gladwin, S.C.: Identification and Management of Restorative Dental Materials During Patient Prophylaxis, *Dent. Hyg., 58,* 456, October, 1984.

26. Wei, S.H.Y., Ngan, P.W.K., Wefel, J.S., and Kerber, P.: Evaluation of Fluoride Prophylaxis Pastes, *J. Dent. Res., 60,* 1297, July, 1981.

27. Ripa, L.W.: The Roles of Prophylaxis and Dental Prophylaxis Pastes in Caries Prevention, in Wei, S.H.Y., ed.: *Clinical Uses of Fluorides.* Philadelphia, Lea & Febiger, 1985, pp. 45–49.

28. American Dental Association, Council on Dental Materials, Instruments, and Equipment: *Dentist's Desk Reference: Materials, Instruments, and Equipment,* 2nd ed. Chicago, American Dental Association, 1983, pp. 279–282.

29. Dentsply/Cavitron: *Instruction Manual, Dentsply/Cavitron Prophy-Jet C-300, Dental Prophylaxis Unit,* York, Pennsylvania, Dentsply International, 1983.

30. Glenwright, H.D., Knibbs, P.J., and Burdon, D.W.: Atmospheric Contamination During Use of an Air Polisher, *Br. Dent. J., 159,* 294, November 9, 1985.

31. Worrall, S.F., Knibbs, P.J., and Glenwright, H.D.: Methods of Reducing Bacterial Contamination of the Atmosphere Arising from Use of an Airpolisher, *Br. Dent. J., 163,* 118, August 22, 1987.

32. Rawson, R.D., Nelson, B.N., Jewell, B.D., and Jewell, C.C.: Alkalosis as a Potential Complication of Air Polishing Systems. A Pilot Study, *Dent. Hyg., 59,* 500, November, 1985.

33. Willmann, D.E., Norling, B.K., and Johnson, W.N.: A New Prophylaxis Instrument: Effect on Enamel Alterations, *J. Am. Dent. Assoc., 101,* 923, December, 1980.

34. Atkinson, D.R., Cobb, C.M., and Killoy, W.J.: The Effect of an Air-Powder Abrasive System on *in vitro* Root Surfaces, *J. Periodontol., 55,* 13, January, 1984.

35. Galloway, S.E. and Pashley, D.H.: Rate of Removal of Root Structure by the Use of the Prophy-Jet Device, *J. Periodontol., 58,* 464, July, 1987.

36. Mishkin, D.J., Engler, W.O., Javed, T., Darby, T.D., Cobb, R.L., and Coffman, M.A.: A Clinical Comparison of the Effect on the Gingiva of the Prophy-Jet and the Rubber Cup and Paste Techniques, *J. Periodontol., 57,* 151, March, 1986.

37. Patterson, C.J.W. and McLundie, A.C.: A Comparison of the Effects of Two Different Prophylaxis Regimes *in vitro* on Some Restorative Dental Materials, *Br. Dent. J., 157,* 166, September 8, 1984.

38. Cooley, R.L., Lubow, R.M, and Patrissi, G.A.: The Effect of An Air-Powder Abrasive Instrument on Composite Resin, *J. Am. Dent. Assoc., 112,* 362, March, 1986.

Suggested Readings

Christensen, R.P.: Brand Names and Characteristics of Polishing Products Used by Dental Hygienists in the U.S., Results of a Survey, *Dent. Hyg., 58,* 222, May, 1984.

Christensen, R.P. and Bangerter, V.W.: Determination of rpm, Time, and Load Used in Oral Prophylaxis Polishing *in vivo, J. Dent. Res., 63,* 1376, December, 1984.

Christensen, R.P. and Bangerter, V.W.: Immediate and Long-term *in vivo* Effects of Polishing on Enamel and Dentin, *J. Prosthet. Dent., 57,* 150, February, 1987.

Eames, W.B., Reder, B.S., Smith, G.A., Satrom, K.D., and Dwyer,

B.M.: Ten High-speed Handpieces: Evaluation of Performance, *Gen. Dent., 28,* 22, March-April, 1980.

Eaton, K.A., Kieser, J.B., and Davies, R.M.: The Removal of Root Surface Deposits, *J. Clin. Periodontol., 12,* 141, February, 1985.

Hunter, E.L., Biller-Karlsson, I.R., Featherstone, M.J., and Silverstone, L.M.: The Prophylaxis Polish—A Review of the Literature, *Dent. Hyg., 55,* 36, September, 1981.

Mellberg, J.R.: The Relative Abrasivity of Dental Prophylactic Pastes and Abrasives on Enamel and Dentin, *Clin. Prevent. Dent., 1,* 13, January-February, 1979.

Nagle, S.: Prophylaxis Prior to Topical Fluoride Application: A Questionable Procedure? *Can. Dent. Hyg., 15,* 19, Spring, 1981.

Nield, J.S. and Houseman, G.A.: *Fundamentals of Dental Hygiene Instrumentation,* 2nd ed. Philadelphia, Lea & Febiger, 1988, pp. 361–374.

Putt, M.S., Kleber, C.J., and Muhler, J.C.: Enamel Polish and Abrasion by Prophylaxis Pastes, *Dent. Hyg., 56,* 38, September, 1982.

Smith, B.A., Shanbour, G.S., Caffesse, R.G., Morrison, E.C., and Dennison, J.D.: *In vitro* Polishing Effectiveness of Interdental Aids on Root Surfaces, *J. Clin. Periodontol., 13,* 597, July, 1986.

Stephens, R.R.: The Dental Handpiece—A History of Its Development, *Aust. Dent. J., 31,* 165, June, 1986.

Thompson, R.E. and Way, D.C.: Enamel Loss Due to Prophylaxis and Multiple Bonding/Debonding of Orthodontic Attachments, *Am. J. Orthod., 79,* 282, March, 1981.

Tillis, T.S.I. and Hicks, M.J.: Enamel Surface Morphology Comparison. Polishing with a Toothpaste and a Prophylaxis Paste, *Dent. Hyg., 61,* 112, March, 1987.

Torres, H.O. and Ehrlich, A.: *Modern Dental Assisting,* 3rd ed. Philadelphia, W.B. Saunders Co., 1985, pp. 491–500.

Waring, M.B., Horn, M.L., Ames, L.L., Williams, N.J., and Lyne, S.M.: Plaque Reaccumulation Following Engine Polishing or Toothbrushing. A 90-day Clinical Trial, *Dent. Hyg., 62,* 282, June, 1988.

Waring, M.B., Newman, S.M., and Lefcoe, D.L.: A Comparison of Engine Polishing and Toothbrushing in Minimizing Dental Plaque Reaccumulation, *Dent. Hyg., 56,* 25, December, 1982.

Winston, A.E. and Lehne, R.K.: The Effect of Concentration on the Abrasivity of Baking Soda, A Brief Overview, *Clin. Prevent. Dent., 5,* 21, November-December, 1983.

Selective Polishing

Cross, G.N. and Carr, E.H.: Patients' Acceptance of Selective Polishing, *Dent. Hyg., 57,* 20, December, 1983.

Haeseler, G.A.: Is Scaling and Polishing Children's Teeth Justified? *N.Y. State Dent. J., 45,* 71, February, 1979.

Hassell, B.L. and Kohut, R.D.: Survey on Selective Polishing, *Dent. Hyg., 55,* 27, September, 1981.

Primosch, R.E.: Rubber Cup Prophylaxis: A Reevaluation of Its Use in Pediatric Dental Patients, *Dent. Hyg., 54,* 525, November, 1980.

Rohleder, P.V. and Slim, L.H.: Alternatives to Rubber Cup Polishing, *Dent. Hyg., 55,* 16, September, 1981.

Schifter, C.C., Hangorsky, C.A., and Emling, R.C.: A Philosophy of Selective Polishing, *RDH, 1,* 34, March, 1981.

Walsh, M.M., Heckman, B.H., and Moreau-Diettinger, R.: Polished and Unpolished Teeth. Patient Responses After an Oral Prophylaxis, *Dent. Hyg., 59,* 306, July, 1985.

Walsh, M.M., Heckman, B., Moreau-Diettinger, R., and Buchanan, S.A.: Effect of a Rubber Cup Polish After Scaling, *Dent. Hyg., 59,* 494, November, 1985.

Wilkins, E.M.: Removal of Extrinsic Dental Stains. "Selective Polishing," *Can. Dent. Hyg., 20,* 59, Summer, 1986.

Airbrasive Polishing

Barnes, C.M., Hayes, E.F., and Leinfelder, K.F.: Effects of an Airbrasive Polishing System on Restored Surfaces, *Gen. Dent., 35,* 186, May-June, 1987.

Berkstein, S., Reiff, R.L., McKinney, J.F., and Killoy, W.J.: Supragingival Root Surface Removal During Maintenance Procedures Utilizing an Air-Powder Abrasive System or Hand Scaling, An *in vitro* Study, *J. Periodontol., 58,* 327, May, 1987.

Boyde, A.: Airpolishing Effects on Enamel, Dentine, Cement and Bone, *Br. Dent. J., 156,* 287, April 21, 1984.

Boyle, M.A., Ferguson, M.M., MacFadyen, E.E., McGady, J., and Scothorne, R.J.: Airpolishing Effects on Soft Tissue, *Br. Dent. J., 157,* 4, July 7, 1984.

deWet, F.A., Holtzhausen, T., and Nel, J.J.: Evaluation of a New Prophylaxis Device, *J. Dent. Assoc. S. Afr., 39,* 207, March, 1984.

Finlayson, R.S. and Stevens, F.D.: Subcutaneous Facial Emphysema Secondary to Use of the Cavi-Jet, *J. Periodontol., 59,* 315, May, 1988.

Horning, G.M., Cobb, C.M., and Killoy, W.J.: Effect of an Air-Powder Abrasive System on Root Surfaces in Periodontal Surgery, *J. Clin. Periodontol., 14,* 213, April, 1987.

Lubow, R.M. and Cooley, R.L.: Effect of Air-Powder Abrasive Instrument on Restorative Materials, *J. Prosthet. Dent., 55,* 462, April, 1986.

Newman, P.S., Silverwood, R.A., and Dolby, A.E.: The Effects of an Airbrasive Instrument on Dental Hard Tissues, Skin and Oral Mucosa, *Br. Dent. J., 159,* 9, July 6, 1985.

Orton, G.S.: Clinical Use of an Air-Powder Abrasive System, *Dent. Hyg., 61,* 513, November, 1987.

Petersson, L.G., Hellden, L., Jongebloed, W., and Arends, J.: The Effect of a Jet Abrasive Instrument (Prophy-Jet®) on Root Surfaces, *Swed. Dent. J., 9,* 193, Number 5, 1985.

Toevs, S.E.: Root Topography Following Instrumentation, A SEM Study, *Dent. Hyg., 59,* 350, August, 1985.

Walmsley, A.D., Williams, A.R., and Laird, W.R.E.: The Air-Powder Dental Abrasive Unit—An Evaluation Using a Model System, *J. Oral Rehabil., 14,* 43, January, 1987.

Weaks, L.M., Lescher, N.B., Barnes, C.M., and Holroyd, S.V.: Clinical Evaluation of the Prophy-Jet as an Instrument for Routine Removal of Tooth Stain and Plaque, *J. Periodontol., 55,* 486, August, 1984.

39 *The Porte Polisher*

The porte polisher is a prophylactic hand instrument constructed to hold a wood polishing point at a contra-angle. Figure 39–1A shows an assembled porte polisher.

Manual polishing is accomplished by applying pressure with the wood point on the tooth surfaces as a moist abrasive is applied. The firm, carefully directed, rhythmic strokes impart a vigorous massage to the periodontal tissues. This is considered beneficial to the periodontal ligament because the periodontal fibers serve as a cushion for the slight movement of the tooth that occurs with the pressure of the instrument. Fones described the beneficial effects to the gingival margin.[1] He suggested that the gentle bumping of the wood point on the tissue causes a light pressure and release that has a massaging effect in producing a stimulation of the peripheral circulation.

I. Purposes and Uses

The entire polishing procedure may be accomplished with the porte polisher, although this is unusual in routine practice because of the time factor. The porte polisher and the prophylaxis angle are compared in table 39–1.

Patients can be highly appreciative of smooth, quiet, manual instrumentation. For certain patients, under particular circumstances and for selected procedures, porte polishing is specifically indicated. Functions, purposes, and uses of the porte polisher are suggested as follows:

A. Removes stains from the natural and restored surfaces of the teeth.
B. Provides a high, smooth polish, which may help the tooth surfaces to resist deposit accumulation.
C. Effective for cervical areas and exposed cementum or dentin of teeth that are hypersensitive to the heat produced by even a slowly revolving rubber polishing cup. A superfine, unflavored abrasive mixed with water only is appreciated by the patient and causes less abrasion of tooth structure.
D. Adapts to tooth surfaces that are inaccessible to a prophylaxis angle, such as the following:
   1. Exposed proximal surfaces of the teeth of patients who have undergone periodontal surgery.
   2. Lingual surfaces of lingually inclined mandibular molars, or distal surfaces of maxillary third permanent molars.

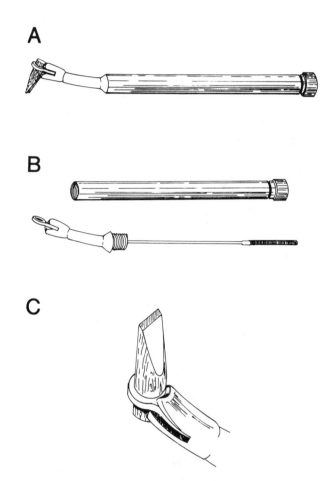

Figure 39–1. Porte Polisher. A. Assembled instrument, shows position of wood point ready for instrumentation. **B.** Disassembled, ready for autoclave. **C.** Working end showing wedge-shaped wood point inserted.

E. Indicated for a patient with an infectious disease to prevent aerosol production and hence disease dissemination.
F. Method of choice for application of certain desensitizing agents for exposed cementum and dentin (page 500).
G. Useful for the homebound or bedridden patient when portable power-driven equipment is not available.
H. Helpful for orientation of small children, disabled patients, or other patients apprehensive of power-driven equipment.

Table 39–1.   Comparison of the Porte Polisher and the Prophylaxis Angle

Characteristic	Porte Polisher	Prophylaxis Angle
Aerosol Production	None; useful for special cases, especially infectious disease	Aerosols produced, as with all powered instruments
Protection of Gingiva from Trauma	Easy by use of slow, even strokes	Difficult because of speed at which rubber cup is moving
Danger of Abrading Enamel and Cementum	Minimized	Greater because of faster speed and decreased sense of touch
Stain Removal	Removes all stains	Time saved in the removal of gross stains, but steady application of rubber cup could produce heat and remove excess tooth surface fluoride
Heat	None	Much heat produced
Accessibility to Tooth Surface	Readily adapted to all surfaces	Limited because of size and weight of handpiece
Operator's Sense of Touch	Greater control of instrument is possible because sense of touch is present	Sense of touch is decreased because of weight and size of handpiece
Comfort to Patient	Increased because of quietness and lack of discomfort from heat	Decreased because of noise, vibration, and heat produced
Comfort to Operator	Light instrument, less tiring to trained hands	Heavy instrument is tiring to hold
Polishing Agent	Less damage because of fewer strokes; agent must be applied wet	Only very fine grain powder should be used; must be applied very wet
Portability	Is portable, therefore useful at any time (for example, for bedridden patient)	Useful only in dental office or with portable motor with power source
Care of Instrument	Simple to sterilize	More time required for sterilization and maintenance

II. Characteristics of a Porte Polisher

Several types of porte polishers are available for use. Practical features that influence selection are suggested below.

A. Can be taken apart conveniently for cleaning and sterilization (figure 39–1B).
B. Will not rust or discolor when given ordinary care.
C. Has convenient adjustment for attachment of wood points of various widths.
D. Is light weight for comfort of the clinician during use.
E. Has handle of diameter convenient to type of instrument grasp required.
F. Has handle with a finish that resists slipping in the hand during operation.

III. Selection and Preparation of Wood Points

Although several kinds of wood, including cedar, maple, and hard pine, have been used for polishing points, orangewood is preferred because it is hard enough to withstand pressure without fraying readily, yet porous enough to hold polishing agents.

Ready-made wood points are available commercially in standard sizes and shapes.

A supply of wood points of routinely used sizes and shapes should be cut, sterilized, and stored in small sealed packages. Wood points should be included in a package or tray for sterilization.

A. **Length**
   1. *Short*
      a. To maintain rigidity of wood.
      b. To prevent unnecessary retraction of cheek and tongue.
   2. *Long.* Enough to gain access to tooth surfaces without interference of shank of the porte polisher.

B. **Width**
   1. *Narrow*
      a. To adapt to the variety of tooth surfaces and contours.
      b. To prevent damage to the gingival margins as the point is adapted to the curved tooth surfaces.
   2. *Wide.* Enough for efficiency in stain removal.
   3. *Recommended Average Width.* Equal to the

diameter of the circular wood point holder of the porte polisher.

C. Shape
1. *Wedge.* For facial, lingual, and proximal surfaces, and inclined planes of cusps. Figure 39–1C shows a wedge-shaped wood point.
2. *Cone (Pointed).* For occlusal pits and grooves.

D. Position in Handle
Place wood point flush with porte polisher attachment to prevent possible irritation to cheek, lip, or tongue.

IV. Techniques for Use of Porte Polisher

The principles of technique described in Chapter 31 are applied during manual instrumentation. A systematic order of procedure from one tooth surface to the next surface is prerequisite to thoroughness. Applications of the general principles are included here.

A. Instrument Grasps (pages 430–431)
1. *Modified Pen*
   a. Recommended for all surfaces except maxillary anterior facial.
   b. Hold middle finger as near working end of instrument as possible as a guide and support.
2. *Palm* (figure 31–4, page 431)
   a. Recommended for maxillary anterior facial surfaces.
   b. Adapt to posterior maxillary facial surfaces when indicated by existing stains.

B. Finger Rest
Securely maintained on firm tooth.

C. Strokes
1. *Circular.* Diameter $\frac{1}{16}$ to $\frac{1}{8}$ inch. Apply at cervical third and when adjacent to gingival margin.
2. *Linear*
   a. Horizontal: back and forth on facial and lingual surfaces of posterior teeth and to proximal surfaces as applicable.
   b. Vertical: up and down over facial and lingual surfaces of anterior teeth.
3. *Selection of Type and Size*
   a. Provide greatest protection for gingiva.
   b. Provide greatest efficiency in technique in accord with the anatomy of the tooth and the nature and location of the stains.

D. Manner of Operation
1. Apply appropriate grasp and finger rest, then position wood point on the tooth surface.
2. Hand, wrist, and arm rotate to propel the porte polisher.
   a. Fulcrum remains positioned as hand pivots around it.
   b. Fingers remain immobile, except to turn the instrument for adaptation.

E. Pressure Applied
1. Apply a directed, firm, moderate pressure with slow deliberate strokes.
2. Apply increased pressure when circular stroke is directed away from the free gingiva; decrease pressure when the stroke is directed toward the free gingiva.
3. Vary pressure with the tenacity of the deposit or stain to be removed.
4. Balance pressure applied to wood point with finger rest pressure.
5. Effect of excess pressure.
   a. Increases hazard of injury to the margin of the free gingiva.
   b. Decreases stability and control during stroke.

TECHNICAL HINTS
I. Edges of wood points should be trimmed and the wood grain smoothed to minimize splinters that may harm the gingival tissues.
II. Change wood point frequently during polishing procedure as it becomes saturated with moisture and splintered.
   A. To prevent wood slivers from damaging free gingiva.
   B. To increase efficiency by having well-shaped wedge for polishing.
III. When more than one polishing agent is to be applied, use fresh wood points for each to prevent mixing the abrasives.
IV. Avoid undue pressure on pontics and mobile teeth.
V. Thorough flossing and irrigation of sulci following instrumentation is important because retained particles of polishing agent can be a source of irritation to the gingiva and increase postoperative discomfort.
VI. An iodine disclosing solution applied to green stain prior to polishing tends to facilitate its removal.

FACTORS TO TEACH THE PATIENT

I. The nature, occurrence, and causes of stains.
II. Reasons for dental stain removal.
III. Benefits of manual instrumentation.
IV. Relationship of plaque and stain accumulation to the frequency and thoroughness of patient's personal oral care habits.

Reference
1. Fones, A.C.: *Mouth Hygiene,* 4th ed. Philadelphia, Lea & Febiger, 1934, p. 277.

Suggested Readings
Alper, M.N.: An Evaluation of Tooth Polishing Techniques, *J. Am. Dent. Hyg. Assoc., 43,* 137, 3rd Quarter, 1969.
Carranza, F.A.: *Glickman's Clinical Periodontology,* 6th ed. Philadelphia, W.B. Saunders Co., 1984, pp. 592–593.

Fones, A.C.: *Mouth Hygiene,* 4th ed. Philadelphia, Lea & Febiger, 1934, pp. 277–289.

Hard, D.: Oral Prophylaxis, in Bunting, R.W.: *Oral Hygiene,* 3rd ed. Philadelphia, Lea & Febiger, 1957, pp. 255–258.

Miller, S.C.: *Textbook of Periodontia,* 3rd ed. Philadelphia, Blakiston, 1950, pp. 278–280.

Nield, J.S. and Houseman, G.A.: *Fundamentals of Dental Hygiene Instrumentation,* 2nd ed. Philadelphia, Lea & Febiger, 1988, pp. 363–366.

Sorrin, S., ed.: *The Practice of Periodontia.* New York, Blakiston Division, McGraw-Hill, 1960, pp. 182–183.

40 *Debonding*

Brackets bonded to the teeth are used widely in orthodontic treatment. The brackets serve to retain arch wires and to aid in the application and control of the applied forces needed to accomplish the necessary tooth movement and bone remodeling for orthodontic therapy.

I. Comparison of Cemented Bands and Bonded Brackets

Formerly, fixed appliances mainly were circumferential stainless steel bands cemented to the teeth. Bands are illustrated in figure 24–2, page 338. Currently, cemented bands commonly are placed on molars and premolars and bonded brackets are placed on anterior teeth. Banding may be recommended for maxillary and mandibular first permanent molars because of the need for their strength to hold orthodontic auxiliaries for palatal bars, elastics, or other special devices.

A. Advantages of Bonded Appliances[1,2]
1. Improved esthetics.
2. Improved gingival condition because they provide access for control of bacterial plaque at the cervical third of the teeth.
3. Proximal surface dental caries can be detected and treated without band removal.
4. Patient can be aware immediately when a bracket loosens, whereas undermining of a band can go undetected.
5. Placement factors
   a. No need for tooth separation (as required for band placement) and no band spaces to close at the end of treatment.
   b. Bonded appliances can be placed on partially erupted teeth, so no wait for tooth eruption is necessary before treatment can be started.
   c. Lingual brackets ("invisible braces") may be used for specially selected cases.

B. Disadvantages of Bonded Brackets
1. Attachment may be weaker because less surface area is in contact with tooth. Bracket may detach more readily than a band.
2. Rebonding a loose bracket is more time consuming and requires more tooth preparation than recementing a loose band.
3. Debonding at the end of treatment is more time consuming than debanding, with more danger of damage to the tooth surface.

II. Bonding and Debonding: Definitions*
A. Bonding
Bonding is the process by which orthodontic attachments are affixed to the tooth surface. An acrylic resin is used to provide a mechanical or a physiochemical union.
1. *Direct Bonding.* A single-step intraoral procedure in which orthodontic attachments are oriented and bonded individually.
2. *Indirect Bonding.* A two-step process by which orthodontic attachments are affixed temporarily to the teeth of a study cast. They are then transferred to the mouth all at one time by means of a molded matrix or template that preserves the predetermined orientation and permits them to be bonded simultaneously.

B. Debonding
Debonding is the removal of bonded orthodontic attachments, followed by removal of residual surface adhesive resins to restore the surface as closely as possible to its pretreatment condition with minimal iatrogenic damage.

III. Fixed Appliance System
Figure 40–1 shows the bonded brackets with arch wire held in place by elastomeres.

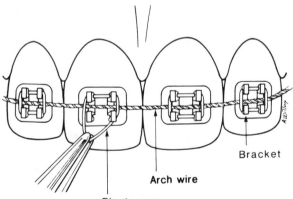

Figure 40–1. Fixed Appliance System. Bonded brackets with arch wire held in place by elastomeres.

*Definitions in this chapter are taken or adapted from and in accord with the *Glossary of Dentofacial Orthopedic Terms, Orthodontic Glossary,* 1987 edition, American Association of Orthodontists, 460 N. Lindbergh Boulevard, St. Louis, Missouri 63141-7883.

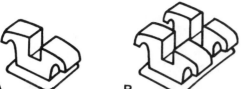

Figure 40–2. Orthodontic Brackets. A. Single bracket with an incisal and a cervical wing. **B.** Twin, or Siamese, with two wings on each side of the central groove where the arch wire is held. The shape and style of each bracket vary with the tooth where the bracket will be located.

A. Brackets

A bracket is an orthodontic attachment that is bonded to the enamel for the purpose of holding an arch wire.

1. *Materials*
   a. Metal (stainless steel).
   b. Plastic (polycarbonate).
   c. Plastic with metal reinforcements.
   d. Ceramic.
2. *Forms.* Brackets are made in many styles, shapes, and sizes for different teeth, each designed to accomplish a specific objective of treatment. The basic forms are *single* or *twin* (figure 40–2).
3. *Base.* The base of the bracket is prepared with a mesh backing to assist in retaining the acrylic bonding agent. The mesh backing, or bonding pad as it is also called, is made to the exact size of the bracket so that no area of tooth is left uncovered where demineralization can occur.

   Mesh backing retains less bacterial plaque than other types of backing.[3,4]

B. Arch Wire

An arch wire is a curved wire held in place in a bracket by elastomeres or ligatures (figure 40–1). The arch wire is used to generate or distribute forces that cause or guide orthodontic tooth movement. Arch wires are made of stainless steel or an alloy of chromium or titanium, and may be round, rectangular, or multistranded.

C. Elastomere

An elastomere is an elasto-plastic ring or latex elastic used
1. To hold wires in the brackets (figure 40–1).
2. To apply force to close spaces between teeth.

IV. Clinical Procedures for Bonding

The principles described in Chapter 30 (pages 420–423) for pit and fissure sealants apply for bonding orthodontic brackets. Details will not be included here.

The basic procedural steps are *cleaning the tooth surface, conditioning the enamel surface,* and *applying the bonding agent.* After the bonding, the area around the bracket must be cleaned of excess resin.

A. Tooth-Surface Cleaning

Plain pumice and water are used with a rubber cup to remove all surface plaque and pellicle. Commercial preparations of polishing agents should not be used because they are contaminated with additives. Thorough rinsing is important after the cleaning.

B. Enamel Conditioning (Etching)

1. Isolate.
2. Dry with clean, dry air.
3. Apply 37 to 65% phosphoric acid solution or gel for 60 timed seconds.
4. Rinse, keeping the teeth free from contamination by saliva.
5. Dry, using clean, dry air.

   The etched surface must not be treated roughly, such as by wiping vigorously with a cotton pellet or gauze sponge with pressure. The etched irregularities in the enamel surface may have many delicate projections that can fracture and fall off.

C. Bonding Procedure

1. *Use of Sealant.* Depending on the resin system used, a low-viscous, unfilled sealant may be placed before the bonding resin. The results of research vary regarding the need for the intermediate layer,[5] but the manufacturer's instructions should be followed. The purposes are to protect the enamel against demineralization, to enhance bond strength, and to minimize permeability between the enamel and the bonding resin.[5]
2. *Types of Bonding Resins.*[5,6] The adhesives used in orthodontics are acrylic or diacrylic resins. They may be filled or unfilled. The filler particles are silicate glass or quartz of various sizes: microsize, minisize, or macrosize. Filler resins are categorized as follows:
   a. Unfilled: contain no filler particles.
   b. Lightly filled: contain up to 30% fillers.
   c. Heavily filled: contain more than 30% fillers. These are known as composites.

D. Characteristics of Bonding Relating to Debonding

1. *Nature of the Bond*
   a. Metal brackets: mechanical locking of the resin to irregularities in the enamel surface that result from the etching. The acid etch exposes the prism structure and creates microclefts (figure 30–1, page 419). The average depth of the microclefts ranges from 50 to 80 μm.[7,8,9] Some fine tag extensions have been observed to depths of 100 to 170 μm.[9] On the bracket side, the resin becomes locked into the mesh base.
   b. Plastic bracket: a chemical bond is created.
2. *Effect of Filling Particles*
   a. Physical property values increase from unfilled to heavily filled resins. Fillers in-

crease bond strength, hardness, and wear resistance.

b. Heavily filled resins (composites) perform better for the posterior teeth because posterior attachments are subject to high forces of mastication.

c. Ease of debonding can be related to the type of resin. Heavily filled composites are thicker and less viscous; they may be the more difficult to remove.

d. The bond is stronger when a smaller (thinner) layer of resin is placed between the tooth surface and the bracket.

e. In summary, anterior brackets may be bonded with a lightly filled resin, whereas posterior teeth need a heavily filled resin to prevent detachment.

CLINICAL PROCEDURES FOR DEBONDING

Debonding can be divided into three basic steps, namely, bracket removal, reduction of the resin bulk, and restoration of the pretreatment characteristics of the tooth surface.[10] In addition, postoperative anticaries preventive care and patient instruction are essential.

I. Research

The aim in debonding is to remove the bracket and the residual resin with minimal damage to the enamel surface. Scratches and gouges of the enamel surface, as well as fractures of the enamel, have resulted from improperly applied techniques. To minimize enamel damage, an efficient and effective procedure is needed.

Researchers have used manual, power-driven, and ultrasonic methods in an attempt to determine which instruments can cause the least damage.[10–19] To evaluate instrument effects, studies have been made to measure the amount of enamel lost during each step of debonding. The appearance of the enamel surface after debonding with various bond-removing pliers, scalers, disks, rubber wheels, diamond and carbide burs, and pumice has been observed by scanning electron microscope, stereoscopic microscope, and other methods. Everett provided an excellent review of the literature.[10]

The clinical procedures for debonding outlined in the following were derived from the research. Each clinician must keep in mind that all of the instruments and materials can lead to scratches, grooves, or other irregularities of the tooth surface and that rotary instruments create heat that affects the pulp. Careful application of the instruments as well as frequent visual and tactile examination of the surface are necessary.

II. Bracket Removal[10,19]

A. Technique Objectives

1. Create a fracture within the resin bonding material or between the bracket and the resin.

2. Leave the enamel surface intact.

3. Leave the arch wire in position with ligatures or elastomeres.
   a. When all brackets have been released, the entire assemblage can be removed together.
   b. Threat of the patient swallowing or aspirating a loosened bracket is eliminated by having the brackets remain connected to the arch wire.

B. The "Squeeze-Release" Technique[10,19]

1. Use a small plier with blunt beaks.

2. Apply the beaks to outside edges of the mesial and distal bracket wings (arrow A, figure 40–3).

3. Squeeze the beaks together; do not twist
   a. The wings bend together and cause the mesial and distal of the bracket base to pull away.
   b. The break is at the adhesive-bracket interface, leaving the enamel undisturbed.
   c. Varying amounts of adhesive are left on the tooth surface; some may be attached to the mesh bracket base.

C. Precautions

1. *For Mechanical Removal.* Do not twist in a shearing stroke for the following reasons:
   a. Potential fracture of enamel. The fragile projections of the etched enamel are susceptible to breaking.
   b. Traumatic for patient. Teeth following orthodontic treatment are often mobile. Twisting can be painful.
   c. Potential damage to periodontal ligament. Twisting stretches the fibers.

2. *For Selection and Positioning of Pliers*
   a. Dull pliers are preferred to prevent scratching or gouging.
   b. Pliers should be positioned for the A and B sites in figure 40–3, at the adhesive-

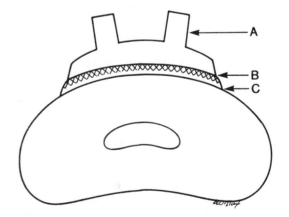

Figure 40–3. Cross-Section of a Bracket. Viewed from the incisal aspect of a tooth: **A.** Bracket wing. **B.** Junction of bracket and mesh backing with resin at the adhesive-bracket interface. **C.** Junction of resin and enamel. (Adapted from Bennett, Shen, and Waldron, J. Clin. Orthodont., *18*: 330, 1984.)

bracket interface. When cutting pliers are placed between the resin adhesive and the tooth (arrow C, in figure 40–3) and used in a cutting stroke, the damage to the enamel can be severe.

III. Removal of Residual Adhesive

A. Technique Objectives
1. Remove resin bulk.
2. Avoid damage to enamel surface.

B. Examination
Varying amounts of resin remain after the bracket is removed, particularly in normal anatomic grooves. During debonding, frequent examination is necessary, using visual and tactile methods.
1. *Identification of Residual Resin*
   a. Visual. When dry, the resin appears dull and opaque, as compared with clean, shiny, enamel.
   b. Tactile. Application of an explorer reveals a rough surface, sometimes with catches along the margin of a resin tag.
2. *Use of Loupes for Magnification of the Tooth Surface.* A more accurate evaluation of enamel surface can be made.
3. *Prevention of Over-instrumentation.* Examine surface frequently during instrumentation to prevent over-instrumentation.

C. Pretest for Possible Removal of Large Bulk
1. *Scaler.* Occasionally, a whole section of residual resin can be removed safely by catching a scaler at the edge of the deposit and applying gentle force. Do not continue to use the scaler if the resin deposit is resistant. Scalers can gouge and scratch the tooth surface and are not recommended.[11,15,18]
2. *Debonding or Debanding Pliers*
   a. Dull, debanding pliers are preferred. Place the nylon cover tab on the incisal or occlusal edge and apply the plier tip to the outer margin of the resin. Do not continue when resistance of the resin suggests the possibility of tearing away enamel.
   b. Proceed to next step. When no edge exists to "catch" the scaler or pliers, proceed directly to the next step. Wedging or forcing can fracture the enamel.[20]

D. Use of Tungsten Carbide Bur[1,10]
1. *Bur Selection*
   a. Use a rounded, tapering, plain-cut or 12-bladed tungsten carbide finishing bur.
   b. Select a new bur for each patient.
2. *Speed.* Use only low to medium speed to control heat.
3. *Technique*
   a. Use a smooth, evenly applied stroke to prevent faceting.
   b. Adapt the side of the bur to the tooth surface.
   c. Move the bur over the resin with short, light continuous movements. The resin is removed in fine white shavings.

IV. Final Finish

A. Objective
Restore pretreatment surface finish.

B. Examination
1. Visual and tactile examination for areas of normal enamel and irregularities.
2. Request patient to examine by rubbing the tongue over the surface.

C. Application of Rubber Cup
1. Use fine pumice slurry.
2. Polish in a wet field to prevent overheating.
3. Adapt interrupted application of rubber cup, and move from area to area.
4. Check progress by rinsing and drying. Avoid overinstrumentation.

D. Expected Effects
1. Reduce roughness.
2. Reduce small areas of residual resin left after other instrumentation.
3. Round off defects. Deep grooves and scratches, or fractured areas of enamel detachment are too deep for complete reshaping.[13,18] The etching may leave microclefts as deep as 80 μm on the average, but some may be as deep as 100 to 170 μm. An enamel fracture from careless debonding may be 100 μm or deeper. Unless an excess of enamel is removed during the finishing procedures, such a defect could not be reduced completely; it must be rounded off.[9]

E. Finishing
Apply tin oxide for fine finish. Use a clean rubber cup.

POST-DEBONDING EVALUATION

I. The Tooth Surface After Debonding
Each step in bonding and debonding has an effect on the enamel surface. Realization that the enamel surface can be damaged can help the clinician avoid unnecessary trauma during the various procedures.

A. Enamel Loss
Total enamel loss from etching, bracket removal, residual resin removal, surface finishing, and application of pumice averages approximately 55 to 80 μm.[9,12,14,17] Enamel loss is greater when filled resins (composites) are used for bonding than when unfilled resins are used. The loss is also greater when a rotating bristle brush is used with the abrasive for finishing rather than a rubber cup.

The outer layer of enamel is the most significant. The fluoride-rich surface enamel is approximately 50 μm deep. Therefore, the entire protective layer can be removed. When multiple bonding and debonding procedures are done, such as when a bracket becomes detached, the enamel loss is compounded. As much as 72 μm of enamel may be lost during a complete multiple procedure.[21]

The need for careful selection of instruments and abrasives, along with minimal instrumentation, to prevent unnecessary enamel loss, is apparent.

B. White Spots (Demineralization)

White spots or dental caries have been relatively common findings after orthodontic treatment. Patients with teeth that have been banded or bonded tend to develop the spots significantly more often than do patients who have not had orthodontic therapy. Maxillary anterior teeth, particularly the lateral incisors, were found to be involved most frequently.[22,23]

Bacterial plaque retention by the appliances and the resin, along with the difficulty of plaque removal by the patient, contribute to demineralization and dental caries.

C. Etched Enamel Not Covered by Adhesive

Surface areas etched but not covered with adhesive resin may be incompletely repaired.[9] The etched area may be affected by the following:
1. Covered by pellicle.
2. Filled or partially filled with organic or inorganic precipitates.
3. Graded or smoothed by toothbrush and dentifrice.
4. Remineralized when the fluoride contact is high through personal and professional applications. Etched enamel has a high fluoride uptake.[24]

D. Stains
1. *Yellowish Discoloration of the Bonding Resin.* Stains of the residual resin can be related to the patient's habits such as the use of tobacco and certain foods or beverages.
2. *Greenish Black Stain.* Enamel staining can result after corrosion of metal brackets. Most of the staining has been found in patients who practiced inadequate oral hygiene and bacterial plaque control.[25,26,27] Because of the indelible quality of the stain, care must be taken during any attempts to remove the spots. An undue amount of enamel could be removed.

POST-DEBONDING PREVENTIVE CARE

I. Periodontal Evaluation

A complete examination with careful probing and charting is necessary, because many changes take place during treatment. Calculus removal should be completed as needed.

II. Dental Caries

Examination for demineralization (white spots) and dental caries is essential. Bacterial plaque retention by orthodontic appliances can be extensive. The configurations of the appliances make plaque control efforts by the patient extremely difficult. Plaque collects on brackets and some resins even when the patient's oral hygiene is generally good.[4]

Composite resin may be left on the tooth surface around the bracket. The surface of resins is difficult to make smooth, so that plaque collects. It is the bacteria of the plaque, not the rough surface, that causes the gingival inflammatory response and the white spots, or demineralization.

After debonding, the use of a retainer provides another source for retention of bacterial plaque. Special instruction for cleaning the retainer is needed (page 339).

III. Fluoride Therapy

A complete program of fluoride treatments professionally at frequent maintenance appointments and by the patient on a daily basis is prerequisite. With the loss of the fluoride-rich enamel surface during bonding and debonding procedures, the need for remineralization and replenishment of fluoride is clear.

TECHNICAL HINTS

I. Document any irregularities of the patient's teeth, such as white spots or cracks, before orthodontic treatment begins and appliances are affixed, to prevent misunderstanding by the patient after debonding.[28]
II. Make periodic photographs to compare gingival tissue changes and teeth before and after disclosing agent application for documentation and patient instruction.

FACTORS TO TEACH THE PATIENT

I. The significance of plaque around orthodontic appliances and the teeth.
II. How to apply the toothbrush and auxiliary devices to remove plaque from the bracket, the arch wire, and the teeth (Chapters 23 and 24).
III. How, when, and why to use fluoride rinse, toothpaste, and brush-on gel.
IV. The frequency of follow-up after debonding.

References
1. Zachrisson, B.U.: Bonding in Orthodontics, in Graber, T.M. and Swain, B.F.: *Orthodontics, Current Principles and Techniques.* St. Louis, The C.V. Mosby Co., 1985, pp. 485–487.
2. Maijer, R.: Bonding Systems in Orthodontics, in Smith, D.C. and Williams, D.F., eds.: *Biocompatibility of Dental Materials,* Volume II. Boca Raton, Florida, CRC Press, Inc., 1982, pp. 51–76.

3. Zachrisson, B.U. and Brobakken, B.O.: Clinical Comparison of Direct versus Indirect Bonding with Different Bracket Types and Adhesives, *Am. J. Orthod., 74,* 62, July, 1978.

4. Gwinnett, A.J. and Ceen, R.F.: Plaque Distribution on Bonded Brackets: A Scanning Microscopic Study, *Am. J. Orthod., 75,* 667, June, 1979.

5. Gwinnett, A.J. for the American Dental Association, Council on Dental Materials, Instruments, and Equipment: State of the Art and Science of Bonding in Orthodontic Treatment, *J. Am. Dent. Assoc., 105,* 844, November, 1982.

6. Craig, R.G., O'Brien, W.J., and Powers, J.M.: *Dental Materials, Properties and Manipulation,* 4th ed. St. Louis, The C.V. Mosby Co., 1987, pp. 60–65.

7. Buonocore, M.G., Matsui, A., and Gwinnett, A.J.: Penetration of Resin Dental Materials into Enamel Surfaces with Reference to Bonding, *Arch. Oral Biol., 13,* 61, January, 1968.

8. Retief, D.H.: Effect of Conditioning the Enamel Surface with Phosphoric Acid, *J. Dent. Res., 52,* 333, March-April, 1973.

9. Diedrich, P.: Enamel Alterations from Bracket Bonding and Debonding: A Study with the Scanning Electron Microscope, *Am. J. Orthod., 79,* 500, May, 1981.

10. Everett, M.S.: Debonding Orthodontic Adhesives, *Dent. Hyg., 59,* 364, August, 1985.

11. Gwinnett, A.J. and Gorelik, L.: Microscopic Evaluation of Enamel After Debonding: Clinical Application, *Am. J. Orthod., 71,* 651, June, 1977.

12. Fitzpatrick, D.A. and Way, D.C.: The Effects of Wear, Acid Etching, and Bond Removal on Human Enamel, *Am. J. Orthod., 72,* 671, December, 1977.

13. Burapavong, V., Marshall, G.W., Apfel, D.A., and Perry, H.T.: Enamel Surface Characteristics on Removal of Bonded Orthodontic Brackets, *Am. J. Orthod., 74,* 176, August, 1978.

14. Brown, C.R.L. and Way, D.C.: Enamel Loss During Orthodontic Bonding and Subsequent Loss During Removal of Filled and Unfilled Adhesives, *Am. J. Orthod., 74,* 663, December, 1978.

15. Retief, D.H. and Denys, F.R.: Finishing of Enamel Surfaces After Debonding of Orthodontic Attachments, *Angle Orthod., 49,* 1, January, 1979.

16. Zachrisson, B.U. and Arthun, J.: Enamel Surface Appearance After Various Debonding Techniques, *Am. J. Orthod., 75,* 121, February, 1979.

17. Pus, M.D. and Way, D.C.: Enamel Loss Due to Orthodontic Bonding with Filled and Unfilled Resins Using Various Cleanup Techniques, *Am. J. Orthod., 77,* 269, March, 1980.

18. Rouleau, B.D., Marshall, G.W., and Cooley, R.O.: Enamel Surface Evaluations After Clinical Treatment and Removal of Orthodontic Brackets, *Am. J. Orthod., 81,* 423, May, 1982.

19. Bennett, C.G., Shen, C., and Waldron, J.M.: The Effects of Debonding on the Enamel Surface, *J. Clin. Orthodont., 18,* 330, May, 1984.

20. Andreasen, G.F. and Chan, K.C.: A Hazard in Direct Bonding Bracket—A Case Report, *Quintessence Int., 12,* 569, June, 1981.

21. Thompson, R.E. and Way, D.C.: Enamel Loss Due to Prophylaxis and Multiple Bonding/Debonding of Orthodontic Attachments, *Am. J. Orthod., 79,* 282, March, 1981.

22. Gorelick, L., Geiger, A.M., and Gwinnett, A.J.: Incidence of White Spot Formation After Bonding and Banding, *Am. J. Orthod., 81,* 93, February, 1982.

23. Mizrahi, E.: Enamel Demineralization Following Orthodontic Treatment, *Am. J. Orthod., 82,* 62, July, 1982.

24. Kochavi, D., Gedalia, I., and Anaise, J.: Effect of Conditioning with Fluoride and Phosphoric Acid on Enamel Surfaces as Evaluated by Scanning Electron Microscopy and Fluoride Incorporation, *J. Dent. Res., 54,* 304, March-April, 1975.

25. Ceen, R.F.: Indelible Iatrogenic Staining of Enamel Following Debonding. A Case Report, *J. Clin. Orthod., 14,* 713, October, 1980.

26. Maijer, R. and Smith, D.C.: Corrosion of Orthodontic Bracket Bases, *Am. J. Orthod., 81,* 43, January, 1982.

27. Gwinnett, A.J.: Corrosion of Resin-bonded Orthodontic Brackets, *Am. J. Orthod., 82,* 441, June, 1982.

28. Zachrisson, B.U., Skogan, Ö., and Höymyhr, S.: Enamel Cracks in Debonded, Debanded, and Orthodontically Untreated Teeth, *Am. J. Orthod., 77,* 307, March, 1980.

Suggested Readings

American Dental Association, Council on Dental Materials, Instruments, and Equipment: *Dentists' Desk Reference: Materials, Instruments and Equipment,* 2nd ed. Chicago, American Dental Association, 1983, pp. 182–192.

Artun, J. and Thylstrup, A.: Clinical and Scanning Electron Microscopic Study of Surface Changes of Incipient Caries Lesions after Debonding, *Scand. J. Dent. Res., 94,* 193, June, 1986.

Brobakken, B.O. and Zachrisson, B.U.: Abrasive Wear of Bonding Adhesives: Studies During Treatment and After Bracket Removal, *Am. J. Orthod., 79,* 134, February, 1981.

Bryant, S., Retief, D.H., Bradley, E.L., and Denys, F.R.: The Effect of Topical Fluoride Treatment on Enamel Fluoride Uptake and the Tensile Bond Strength of an Orthodontic Bonding Resin, *Am. J. Orthod., 87,* 294, April, 1985.

Casperson, I.: Residual Acrylic Adhesive After Removal of Plastic Orthodontic Brackets: A Scanning Electron Microscopic Study, *Am. J. Orthod., 71,* 637, June, 1977.

Ceen, R.F.: Orthodontic Bonding—An Overview, *J. Pedod., 5,* 62, Fall, 1980.

Ceen, R.F. and Gwinnett, A.J.: Plaque Patterns and Crevicular Fluid Flow Related to Orthodontic Bracket Bonding, *J. Prev. Dent., 6,* 229, June, 1980.

Ceen, R.F. and Gwinnett, A.J.: White Spot Formation Associated with Sealants Used in Orthodontics, *Pediatr. Dent., 3,* 174, June, 1981.

Dragiff, D.A.: A New Debonding Procedure, *J. Clin. Orthod., 13,* 107, February, 1979.

Everett, M.S. and Krouse, M.A.: Teaching Debonding in Dental Hygiene Programs, *J. Dent. Educ., 50,* 540, September, 1986.

Fields, H.W.: Bonded Resins in Orthodontics, *Pediatr. Dent., 4,* 51, March, 1982.

Gorelick, L.: Bonding. The State of the Art. A National Survey, *J. Clin. Orthod., 13,* 39, January, 1979.

Graber, T.M.: Orthodontics in the Mid-1980's, *Quintessence Int., 16,* 73, January, 1985.

Kajander, K.C., Uhland, R., Ophaug, R.H., and Sather, A.H.: Topical Fluoride in Orthodontic Bonding, *Angle Orthod., 57,* 70, January, 1987.

Lehman, R. and Davidson, C.L.: Loss of Surface Enamel after Acid Etching Procedures and Its Relation to Fluoride Content, *Am. J. Orthod., 80,* 73, July, 1981.

Lehman, R., Davidson, C.L., and Duijsters, P.P.E.: *In vitro* Studies on Susceptibiity of Enamel to Caries Attack After Orthodontic Bonding Procedures, *Am. J. Orthod., 80,* 61, July, 1981.

Mizrahi, E.: Surface Distribution of Enamel Opacities Following Orthodontic Treatment, *Am. J. Orthod., 84,* 323, October, 1983.

O'Reilly, M.M. and Featherstone, J.D.B.: Demineralization and Remineralization Around Orthodontic Appliances: An *in vivo* Study, *Am. J. Orthod. Dentofac. Orthop., 92,* 33, July, 1987.

Saloum, F.S. and Sondhi, A.: Preventing Enamel Decalcification After Orthodontic Treatment, *J. Am. Dent. Assoc., 115,* 257, August, 1987.

Viazis, A.D.: Direct Bonding of Orthodontic Brackets, *J. Pedod., 11,* 1, Fall, 1986.

41 *Amalgam Restorations*

Finishing an amalgam restoration includes the procedures that collectively produce a restoration with normal tooth contours, refined margins, smooth, corrosion-resistant surfaces, functional effectiveness, and an acceptable appearance. With such characteristics, the restoration can be expected to contribute to the patient's oral health for a long time. The economic benefit is especially notable when preventive measures are emphasized.

The two applications for finishing procedures are for the newly placed restoration and for the previously placed restoration that, for various reasons, has irregular margins and surfaces. Basic procedures to follow when treating both old and new restorations are similar.

The extent of finishing necessary for a new restoration depends on the carving and burnishing performed at the time the restoration was placed. The neatly and carefully carved restoration that fulfills ideal, normal anatomic and functional requirements needs little smoothing of margins and surfaces before polishing. On the other hand, an "old" filling may have many irregularities of the margins and surfaces that have resulted either from inadequate finishing when the restoration was placed originally or from changes over the years.

Principles and procedures are presented in this chapter. A study of amalgam and its properties should precede learning to finish and polish.[1,2,3]

RATIONALE FOR FINISHING AND POLISHING

Finishing and polishing amalgam restorations contribute to the following effects:
A. Increased length of service of the restoration by eliminating factors that lead to surface changes and recurrent dental caries.
B. Decreased amalgam tarnish and corrosion.
C. Increased integrity of the junction of tooth surface and amalgam.
D. Improved gingival health because of less plaque retention by amalgam irregularities.
E. Improved maintenance by the patient: plaque is more easily removed by brush and floss from smooth surfaces.
F. Improved compatibility of the restorative material with the oral soft tissues.

G. Increased comfort for the patient because the restorations are smooth to the tongue.
H. Improved appearance of the restorations.

THE AMALGAM RESTORATION

A large majority of restorations for both primary and permanent teeth are made of dental amalgam. Amalgam is an important restorative material, and when scientific principles are used while a restoration is placed and the restored tooth is cared for daily by the patient, the restoration can be expected to last many years, some, even a lifetime.

A review of selected amalgam properties and changes with age that are pertinent to finishing and polishing will be considered. That will be followed by descriptive definitions of types of marginal irregularities of an amalgam restoration encountered during examination.

I. Longevity of Amalgam Restorations[1]

The initial factors that influence the length of time an amalgam restoration maintains its form and function include the following:
A. Design of the cavity preparation.
B. Mix and manipulation of the dental material.
C. Condensation during placement of the restoration.
D. Prevention of contamination and moisture.
E. Finishing and polishing.
F. Care of the completed restoration by a daily preventive program of bacterial plaque control, low cariogenic diet, and fluoride application daily, combined with maintenance supervision at professional appointments.

II. Amalgam Properties and Age Changes

A. Surface Changes
1. *Tarnish.* Tarnish is a surface discoloration, principally a sulfide. It is usually caused by lack of oral cleanliness, with resultant plaque collection, and certain foods, especially foods containing sulfur. Tarnish is less frequently found on properly finished and polished restorations.
2. *Corrosion.* Corrosion is an actual chemical deterioration of the metal, which usually begins as a tarnish and is caused by environmental factors such as air, moisture, acid or alkaline

solutions, and other chemicals.[4] Smoothly polished amalgam resists corrosion.

Corrosion at the margin of a restoration can cause deterioration and fracture of the margin. An open gap where plaque can collect is the usual result. The products of corrosion may be carried into the dentinal tubules, and the entire area around the restoration may appear bluish-black.

B. Dimensional Changes[1,2]

Expansion can occur as a result of incomplete trituration and condensation or contamination from moisture entering the amalgam during the mixing and placing of the restoration. When expansion occurs in excess, the filling appears extruded above the cavosurface margin. Expansion can also produce postoperative pain or tooth sensitivity because of pressure on the pulp.

When contraction occurs, the amalgam may pull away from the cavosurface margin. Contraction is one of the causes of "ditching," a term used to describe a space between the filling material and the tooth structure, as defined on page 529.

C. Amalgam Strength

Fractures are a result of insufficient strength. A fracture may be seen as a gross irregularity, a crack-line across an entire restoration, or a marginal chip. Several factors can be involved in amalgam fractures, including the following:

1. *Manipulation of the Filling Material.* Undertrituration of amalgam results in low strength.
2. *Overload of Pressure on a Restoration Before Setting is Complete.* Strength of the amalgam is low during the first few hours after placement. After carving, the occlusal relationship should be checked for high contact spots, which if subjected to masticatory stress, can lead to fracture.
3. *Inadequate Strength of Surrounding Tooth Structure.* Strength and support for an amalgam restoration depend in part on the strength of the surrounding tooth structure. When dental caries requires wide extension of the cavity preparation, the tooth walls may be subject to fracture. Both the amalgam and the tooth may fracture together.

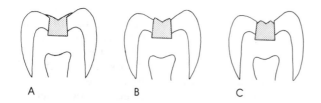

Figure 41–1. Amalgam Irregularities. A. Flash on the occlusal surface related to a Class 1 restoration. Flash refers to a thin layer of amalgam that extends over the margin of the cavity preparation. **B.** Irregular margin results when the flash breaks off. **C.** Ditching that results from broken off flash.

4. *Improper Carving of the Restoration.* Marginal strength can be compromised when a thin excess of amalgam is left extending over the cavosurface margin. If the small overhang (flash) breaks off, a part of the margin of the restoration may also break off with the flash (figure 41–1). The fracture may be caused by occlusal pressures or finishing procedures.

III. Types of Marginal Irregularities: Definitions

When an amalgam restoration is to be finished and polished, it is first examined by moving an explorer over the surfaces and margins. A variety of irregularities or defects may be found. The defects represent excesses or deficiencies of amalgam.

The finished functional restoration follows the normal contours of the tooth. All cavosurface junctions should feel smooth to an explorer.

Excesses and deficiencies must be recognized and differentiated, so that finishing and polishing procedures can be carried out effectively. When deficiencies of amalgam occur, correction by finishing techniques may require removal of excess tooth structure. Usually, deficiencies must be corrected by replacement of the restoration.

The common irregularities and defects of amalgam restorations are defined and described in the following section.

A. Overhanging Margin

An amalgam overhang is an area of excess amalgam that extends beyond the cavosurface margin of a cavity preparation (figure 41–2A). Proximal overhangs result primarily from improper placement of the matrix band and wedge. Overhangs may occur on any tooth surface, supra- or subgingivally, in any class of cavity. They may be caused by errors of manipulation, carving, and/or finishing.

B. Flash

A flash is a type of overhang in which a thin layer of amalgam extends beyond the cavosurface margin. It is sometimes referred to as a feather ledge.

1. *Occlusal.* Figure 41–1A illustrates a feather ledge or flash that was left during carving. Carving, correctly performed, brings the cavosurface margin into view and makes the filling material flush with the enamel.
2. *Proximal-Gingival.* A flash-type overhang can result when an amalgam is packed between a matrix band and the tooth surface below the cavity preparation (figure 41–2B). The irregularity can occur when a proximal wedge is not used or not positioned to adapt the matrix tightly against the tooth surface. A tooth with a concave proximal surface is most vulnerable to flash.

C. Open Margin

An open margin is found when there is a distinct space between the amalgam and the wall of

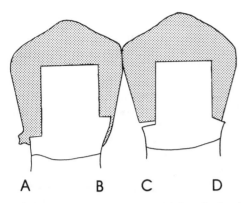

Figure 41–2. Irregularities of Amalgam Margins. A. Overhang. **B.** Flash on a proximal surface. **C.** Open or deficient margin. **D.** Undercontoured margin that can result from an improperly placed matrix band or misdirected carving.

the cavity preparation (figure 41–2C). The causes include the following:

1. Too much time elapses after trituration before condensation. The amalgam material begins to set and becomes difficult to condense properly.
2. Too large an amount of the amalgam mix is inserted into the cavity preparation at one time.

D. Undercontoured

The opposite of an overhang is a deficiency of amalgam between the margin of the amalgam and the cavity wall as shown in figure 41–2D. On the proximal surface causes may be related to improper placement of the matrix or wedge or both or to misdirected carving with poorly selected instruments.

Undercontouring is exemplified also by missing contact areas, flattened cervical ridges, incomplete marginal ridges, and incomplete filling of the cavity preparation.

E. Overcontoured

An overcontoured restoration has an excess of amalgam in such a position as to change the normal anatomic form of the restoration. Interproximally overcontoured surfaces may widen the contact area or narrow the embrasure. When the crown is overcontoured, the effect can be plaque retention and pressure on the gingival margin.

In figure 25–1C, on page 355, overcontoured crowns of a double abutment have narrowed the embrasure. Problems of plaque control for the overcontoured crowns are illustrated in figure 25–4 on page 356.

F. Ditch or Groove

The formation of a gap between the cavity preparation margin and the amalgam, as shown in figure 41–1C, is usually referred to as ditching. Plaque retention can lead to recurrent caries in such an area.

OVERHANGING RESTORATIONS

Recontouring overhanging restorations is an essential part of the dental and periodontal treatment of patients. Treatment planning for initial therapy, or Phase I periodontal therapy, must include the correction of overhangs if inflammation is to be controlled.[5]

I. Description

An overhang is identified by its relation to the gingival margin, location on a specific tooth surface, and size or extent. From these data, the required finishing procedures can be selected for a specific treatment plan.

A. Relation to Gingival Margin
1. Supragingival.
2. Subgingival.

B. Location on Tooth Surface
1. Occlusal, mesial, distal, facial, lingual, palatal, or combination.
2. Tooth surface margin
   a. Enamel only.
   b. Enamel and cementum.
   c. Cementum only.

C. Size Determined by Visual and Tactile Examination[6]

Overhangs are found by running a sharp explorer back and forth over the junction between the tooth and the amalgam.
1. *Type I.* Small overhang; slight catch with explorer in at least one section.
2. *Type II.* Moderately large overhang with definite catch with explorer, usually involving more than one side of the restoration.
3. *Type III.* Large, gross overhang clearly apparent by exploration and often visually apparent on direct observation.

II. Radiographic Examination

Overhangs on surfaces other than proximal are rarely visible on radiographic examination. Visibility of proximal surface overhangs depends on angulation of the x-ray. In other words, radiographic examination for overhangs should be a supplementary procedure to examination using an explorer. The entire outline of each restoration can be explored.

A magnifying glass is recommended for examining radiographs for small type I overhangs. Adjacent and undermining carious lesions are more definitively seen when magnification is used.

III. Effects of Overhangs

A. Relation to Periodontal Disease

Because overhanging restorations harbor plaque and hinder plaque removal by the patient, they are considered significant iatrogenic contributing factors in periodontal disease development. In the presence of overhangs, plaque collects in greater amounts and inflammation is more severe than in teeth that do not have overhangs.[7,8,9] Increased bone loss adjacent to overhangs has been demonstrated.[7,10]

Removal of overhangs is beneficial to the periodontal tissues. Combined with scaling and plaque control, a marked improvement in the periodontal condition has been shown after overhang removal.[8,11]

B. Problems of Plaque Control

1. Irregular margins of overhangs catch and tear dental floss.
2. Inaccessible areas
   a. Area under the ledge of the overhang, particularly a proximal overhang, is inaccessible for the direct application of a toothbrush and other plaque removal aids.
   b. Gingival enlargement can result from inflammation caused by bacterial plaque held by the overhang and may cover a portion of the overhang. After shrinkage of the soft-tissue pocket wall and overhang removal, the restoration may be wholly supragingival and, therefore, accessible for maintenance.
3. Debris retention contributes to a general lack of oral sanitation and to halitosis from breakdown products in bacterial plaque and food debris held by the overhang.

C. Dental Caries

Marginal irregularities harbor microorganisms and sucrose in an environment conducive to the formation of secondary caries. The caries process is described on pages 242–243.

IV. Indications and Contraindications for Removal of Overhangs

All overhanging restorations should be corrected or removed and replaced for the health of the periodontium. Large overhangs cannot usually be treated by finishing procedures and are, therefore, an indication for total removal of the restoration. If replacement will be delayed, the gross overhang should be reshaped and smoothed to make plaque control possible. The periodontal tissues can recover, inflammation can be reduced, and continuing treatment can be more satisfactory.

Whether a certain overhang can be removed by finishing techniques or whether it must be removed and replaced with a new properly prepared, contoured, and finished restoration, is the professional decision that must be made. Guidelines for selection of the correct procedure are suggested here. Contraindications for finishing procedures apply to restorations of any size or location.

A. Indications for Finishing

1. Tooth anatomy can be maintained or improved to conform with normal contour.

2. The overhang is small or moderate in size.
3. Proximal contact is intact.
4. No adjacent secondary dental caries can be detected.
5. There are no fractures of the cavity margin either of the tooth or the filling, and no large fractures of the bulk of the restoration.
6. The overhang is accessible for the instrumentation necessary for finishing and polishing without damaging the adjacent tooth structure or unduly traumatizing the gingival tissues.

B. Indications for Removal and Restoration

1. The overhang is extensive and would require an excessively long time to completely recontour.
2. Secondary marginal or undermining dental caries is present.
3. The contact area must be restored.
4. Fractures, chips, cracks, or broken margins are apparent that could not be corrected by finishing and polishing procedures.

CLINICAL MANAGEMENT: MERCURY HYGIENE

The mercury vapor level in a dental treatment room can be higher than in the normal atmosphere when many amalgam restorations are completed during each day. Although members of the dental team rarely exhibit symptoms of toxicity, the potential danger exists, and certain precautions are necessary.

I. Mercury Pollution of Environment

The American Dental Association lists sources of mercury that include the following:[12]
A. Direct contact or handling of mercury.
B. Inhalation of vapors from mercury.
C. Exposure to accidental spills and leaky or contaminated amalgamator capsules and amalgamators.
D. Wringing excess mercury from amalgam.
E. Vaporization of mercury from contaminated instruments in sterilizers.
F. Amalgam condensation, especially with ultrasonic compactors.
G. Scrap amalgam improperly stored.
H. Milling old amalgam restorations.

II. Mercury Hygiene Practices

Recommendations from the American Dental Association include the following:[12]
A. Work in well ventilated areas.
B. Wear mask, eyeglasses, gloves for protection from mercury vapor and amalgam dust.
C. Avoid carpeting or porous materials for treatment room floors.
D. Monitor the office or clinic periodically for atmospheric mercury.

E. Require yearly urinalysis for mercury for all personnel.
F. Store mercury in unbreakable, tightly sealed containers away from heat sources.
G. Keep amalgam scrap in a tightly sealed container.
H. Handle amalgam with caution and without direct contact; clean up spilled mercury immediately.
I. Use water stream and high-volume evacuation when removing or finishing amalgam restorations.
J. Avoid heating mercury, amalgam, or mercury-containing solutions.
K. Do not eat, drink, or smoke in dental and dental hygiene treatment rooms.

FINISHING PROCEDURES

I. Definitions

A. Carving
Carving is the removal of excess filling material, using specially designed instruments, immediately after condensation of the amalgam into the cavity preparation. The goal of carving is to produce accurate anatomic contours that approximate normal for the particular tooth.

B. Contouring
Contouring includes procedures to reproduce the size, shape, grooves, and other details of tooth form in the restoration. The term *contouring* is usually used when a new restoration is being prepared, whereas the term *recontouring* is used when an old or previously placed restoration is being corrected and reshaped.

C. Burnishing
Burnishing is the production of a smooth, lustrous surface of a restoration by rubbing lightly (to prevent heat production) with a metal, specially designed instrument for amalgam burnishing or rubbing with a cotton pellet. The effects are improved marginal adaptation, increased hardness, and increased resistance to corrosion.

D. Margination
Margination procedures are carried out to remove excess restorative material and apply finishing techniques to establish a smooth, well-adapted junction between the enamel surface (or cementum in a restoration of root surface) and the restoration. The resultant enamel–amalgam junction should conform in shape to the normal anatomic characteristics of the particular tooth.

E. Polishing
Polishing procedures are applied after other finishing techniques to produce a visually smooth, unscratched, lustrous, homogeneous amalgam surface. Abrasive agents are used during polishing to remove final surface roughness, make the surface resistant to corrosion, and eliminate grooves or pits left after carving.

II. Technique Objectives
At the completion of finishing procedures, the restoration and the tooth have the following characteristics:
A. Normal anatomic tooth form has been restored or preserved and no signs of gouges or other damage are evident.
B. Margins between tooth structure and restoration are smooth, so that no irregularity is detectable when a fine explorer is passed back and forth over the entire outline of the restoration. Neither an area of deficient margin nor an overhanging margin exists.
C. Contact is maintained with the adjacent tooth.
D. Embrasures provide normal spacing and appear functional.
E. The surface of the restoration is smooth, lustrous, glossy, free from visible and tactile irregularities, and functionally adequate.

APPOINTMENT PLANNING

I. Patient Preparation

A. Patient History Review
A review of the patient's medical and dental history and the entire current appointment record reveals essential appointment features that will be required. For a risk patient, prophylactic antibiotic premedication may be indicated.

B. Protective Glasses and Mask
Both patient and clinician must wear protective eyeglasses. The use of rotary instruments and polishing agents creates a potential hazard of splatter and aerosols (pages 10–11).

II. Sterile Procedures
Procedures to prevent disease transmission are followed as described in Chapters 3 and 4. A specific tray arrangement is planned. The specific instruments, burs, and stones can be kept in sealed sterilized packages, or a preset tray system can be used.

III. Patient Instruction
A. Explain the purposes and need for finishing restorations.
B. Explain possible detrimental effects of rough restorations, particularly in relation to plaque retention, gingival disease, and dental caries.
C. For new restorations, describe why finishing procedures are to be performed 24 to 48 hours after the restoration is placed.

IV. Examination
A. Review charting and treatment plan for restoration to be treated.
B. Make certain that a new restoration has been placed for a minimum of 24 hours and preferably for 48 hours.[1,2]

C. Study the radiographs for available information to supplement the clinical visual examination.

D. Visually evaluate an unpolished restoration by noting small shiny spots that may indicate specific occlusal contacts. Call the spots to the attention of the dentist to check the occlusal relationship before the spots are obliterated during finishing procedures.

E. Examine with an explorer to determine the nature of any irregularities such as the following:
1. Margins with excess amalgam.
2. Roughness of amalgam surfaces.
3. Entire outline of the restoration.

V. Technique Selection

A. Assessment

During careful examination by direct observation, radiographs, and exploration, the need for finishing is determined and the technique treatment plan is outlined. As mentioned previously, a newly placed, neatly carved restoration may require only polishing, whereas much more instrumentation is required to recontour overhanging margins.

The extent of instrumentation is limited to that required. Overinstrumentation must be avoided.

B. Procedural Plan

Many technique routines are used in practice.[6,13,14,15,16] Procedures may be carried out using manual instruments primarily, power-driven instruments primarily, or a combination of manual and power-driven. It is important to work out a practical routine for efficiency and time conservation.

General suggestions are provided below, describing procedures for finishing in which the excess amalgam and overhanging margins are removed, margins and surfaces are smoothed, and a careful check with an explorer is made before the polishing procedures are carried out.

VI. Rubber Dam Placement

A. Purposes

A rubber dam should be placed whenever possible, particularly when several restorations must be polished in a given quadrant. The rubber dam serves to
1. Protect the patient's soft tissues.
2. Aid in control of debris, moisture, and aerosols created during the finishing procedures to prevent inhalation of particles of amalgam and polishing agents.
3. Improve vision and accessibility.
4. Decrease treatment time by eliminating difficulties in maintaining a clear field.

B. Problems of Isolation

1. *Anesthesia.* Although the use of anesthesia can be helpful while finishing restorations, patients are not routinely anesthetized. Placing a rubber dam clamp without anesthesia may cause discomfort for the patient.

2. *Tooth Temperature.* Keeping the tooth cool during finishing may be more difficult with the rubber dam in place. The use of air spray for cooling may lead to scattering of amalgam particles; central suction evacuation is required.

3. *Use of Cotton Rolls*
   a. Rotating instruments catch the cotton rolls.
   b. Repeated need for cooling and rinsing away debris from finishing and polishing procedures requires considerable time in changing cotton rolls.

VII. Selection of Instruments

Development of a workable set of instruments is accomplished with experience. As knowledge of normal dental anatomy is applied during finishing and polishing, instruments will be used with increased skill and efficiency. Not all of the instruments listed in the following are needed for each restoration.

A. Factors Affecting Selection of Instruments

1. *Location of the Restoration.* Accessibility and visibility.
2. *Instrument Size, Shape, and Form.* To fit the tooth surface and area without traumatizing adjacent tooth structure and gingival tissues.
3. *Abrasiveness of Discs and Polishing Agents.* The character of the surface of the restoration defines the degree of abrasiveness. As mild an abrasive as possible should be used to prevent unnecessary removal of amalgam and tooth structure adjacent to the cavosurface margin. Replenishment of tooth surface fluoride will be described later in this chapter.

B. Manual Instruments

Amalgam or gold knives
Files (heavy, medium, fine)
Cleoid-discoid carver
Scaler, curet
Finishing strips (fine grit, single surface, narrow)
Waxed dental tape

C. Power-driven Instruments

1. *Bladed Instruments*
   Finishing burs (12-bladed)
2. *Abrasive*
   Stones: green or white
   Discs: waterproof, fine grit, in garnet or cuttle
3. *Polishing*
   Rubber cup
   Mandrel-mounted brushes

VIII. Principles and Precautions

A. Anatomic Considerations

1. *Cementum.* When a restoration extends near or into the cementum, care must be taken to prevent ditching or grooving the cementum. Cementum is softer than enamel and therefore is damaged more easily.

2. *Tooth Form and Position.* Concave surfaces such as the mesial of the maxillary first premolars and the mesials of the mandibular first molars require special adaptations of instruments. Other problem areas are created by tooth rotations, inclinations, and other malpositions.

3. *Gingival Tissues.* Restorations may be partially or wholly covered by enlarged gingival tissue related to plaque accumulation as described previously.

When the papillae are bulbous, enlarged, and bleed easily on manipulation, plaque control instruction and supervision should be provided first to improve the health of the tissue before undertaking margination procedures. Waxed floss can be used by the patient so less tearing and shredding will occur when the floss is passed under the overhang.

B. Instrumentation

1. *Finger Rests.* Use secure finger rests to allow precision techniques. Prevention of damage to surrounding tooth structure as well as preservation of tooth anatomy is essential.

2. *Contact Area.* Avoid the contact area. It was created for a new restoration by a smooth, polished matrix band and usually requires no additional smoothing. Polishing agents can remove amalgam and alter the contour and contact.

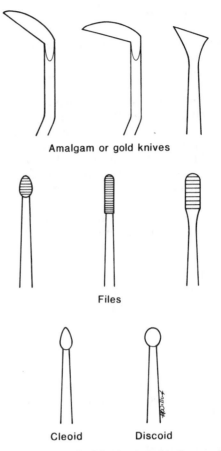

Amalgam or gold knives

Files

Cleoid   Discoid

Figure 41–3. Instruments for Margination. Amalgam and gold foil knives, various shapes of files, and the amalgam carvers, cleoid and discoid, are especially useful for margination.

MARGINATION

I. Margination Procedures Summarized

A. Remove excess amalgam and overhangs.

B. Finish all cavosurface margins to assure continuous, uninterrupted smooth relationships.

C. Smooth all surfaces of the restoration.

II. Manual Instruments

A. General Suggestions for Use of Manual Instruments

1. Maintain sharp instruments. The object is to cut, not burnish, excess amalgam in small increments and prevent amalgam fracture.

2. Work deliberately and carefully to prevent damage to gingival tissue and uninvolved tooth surfaces, especially cementum.

3. Use the tooth surface as a guide to the contour of the restoration. The instrument is moved parallel with or diagonal to the margin.

B. Amalgam Knife (figure 41–3)

1. Hold the knife blade across the tooth structure and amalgam, and activate the knife diagonally across the junction.

2. Use short, overlapping, shaving strokes to remove amalgam in small increments. Prevent risk of fracture of the margins.

3. For proximal adaptation, move the knife away from the gingiva to prevent amalgam bits from being pushed into the pocket. Continuous evacuation is recommended.

C. File (figure 41–3)

1. Determine from the design of each file whether it is intended for a pull or a push stroke, and position the file accordingly.

2. The bulk of the amalgam is removed by coarser files; margin smoothness can be refined with finer files.

3. Overlap tooth and amalgam together during a stroke to prevent ditching, gouging, or leaving a deficiency (undercontour).

D. Cleoid–Discoid Carver (figure 41–3)

1. Refine fossae and fissures with a small sharp cleoid (the pointed tip). The discoid is not used in occlusal fossae because the effect would be one of scooping out and making a round channel.

2. Use discoid as aid for refining cavosurface margins.

E. Finishing Strips

1. Use narrow, fine or medium strips after gross amalgam has been removed by amalgam knife or file.
2. Avoid contact area with abrasive finishing strip
   a. Cut end of strip on diagonal to thread the strip through the embrasure. The slanted tip may be dipped in cavity varnish to facilitate sliding the strip through.[17]
   b. Strips with a gap or middle area without abrasive are available to make it possible to position the strip from the occlusal or incisal aspect.
3. Position strip over the amalgam at the cavosurface margin. Avoid pressure of the abrasive strip on the adjacent tooth structure, especially cementum, because grooves can be made.
4. Curve the strip and move gently and carefully to prevent damage to the interdental gingival tissue.

F. Scaler

Only a strong scaler should be used. A scaler tip can be broken easily if applied with much force. It should also be remembered that using a metal cutting edge on metal (the amalgam) will dull the instrument rapidly.

III. Power-driven Instruments

A. General Suggestions for Power-driven Instruments

Power-driven instruments can create heat, which is detrimental. Pressure and heat can produce mercury vapor and amalgam dust. With careful techniques, ill effects can be minimized.
1. Effects of overheating
   a. Irreversible pulp damage.
   b. Alteration of the chemical structure of the amalgam. Properties of the amalgam can be changed and the longevity of the restoration can be decreased.
   c. Patient discomfort from tooth sensitivity.
2. Use only low speed handpiece, with intermittent, light strokes.
3. Use water and/or air for cooling.
4. Use high-velocity evacuation.

B. Finishing Burs and Stones

1. Select the shape appropriate for accessibility and visibility.
2. Position the bur or stone to permit the remaining enamel to guide the contour produced. The instrument is held across the cavosurface margin and then moved diagonally to prevent fracture or ditching.
3. Keep the bur or stone in constant motion, with a light, sweeping movement to reduce the possibility of leaving marks and grooves.

C. Discs[14]

1. Select abrasivity of disc in accord with objective. Coarse discs will remove bulk more readily, but also may be more damaging to surrounding tissues and tooth structure.
2. Do not reduce tooth structure.
3. Activate the disc for contouring and smoothing the proximal surface in a position that prevents flattening of the restoration and removing amalgam near the contact area.
4. Use short, overlapping strokes with a sweeping motion diagonally across the cavosurface margin. Rotate the disc from the tooth structure to the amalgam to reduce chance of ditching.

D. Ultrasonic

Certain models of ultrasonic machines have special tips designed for removal of overhanging amalgam. The device can be helpful for removal of gross amalgam prior to the use of finer instruments. The precautions for use of ultrasonics are listed on page 468.

POLISHING

After margination and surface smoothing, the amalgam is polished.

I. General Suggestions for Polishing Amalgam

A. Use Very Wet Polishing Agents

1. Heat factors described previously for power-driven instruments apply alike to polishing instruments.
2. Avoid dry polishing powders and discs.
3. Avoid rubber devices such as rubber polishing or finishing points because of heat production. Rubber polishing cups should always be separated from the tooth and restoration by a wet abrasive agent.

B. Do Not Overpolish

Overpolishing, even with a fine abrasive agent, can alter the contour of the restoration, destroy the contact area, and remove excess surrounding tooth structure, especially when cementum is involved.

C. Use Low Speed

Use light, intermittent strokes.

D. Do Not Extend Polishing Brushes or Cups Over the Cementum

The abrasive polishing agent can groove and scratch the cementum.

II. Instruments

A. Bristle brushes: pointed, cup-shaped, disc-shaped.

B. Rubber cups
C. Waxed dental tape.

III. Procedures

A. Initial Polish

1. *Agent.* Fine silex or fine pumice in a very wet slurry with water.
2. *Bristle Brushes*
   a. Prepare by soaking in warm water.
   b. Apply with copious amounts of the slurry.
3. *Application*
   a. Apply the agent over the tooth and restoration before starting the power-driven instrument.
   b. Use the pointed brush in the pits and fissures and cup-shaped brush or rubber cup for convex surfaces.
   c. Keep the brush or cup in constant motion with light, intermittent strokes to prevent heat generation. Replenish slurry often.
   d. Apply polishing agent to proximal surfaces with waxed dental tape. Avoid the contact area. Curve the tape around the tooth to prevent damage to the interdental gingival tissue.
4. *Examination.* Rinse and inspect frequently to prevent overpolishing.

B. Fine Finish

1. *Agent.* Apply tin oxide in a thin, wet slurry with water.
2. *Selection of Polisher.* Use a new rubber cup or brush to prevent mixing the agents.
3. *Application.* Apply with light, intermittent strokes.
4. *Examination.* Rinse and inspect to prevent overpolishing.

IV. Final Evaluation

The finished and polished restoration has the characteristics described in Technique Objectives, page 531.

FLUORIDE APPLICATION

The use of abrasive stones and polishing agents at the margin of a restoration removes a layer of the surface enamel and, with it, the concentration of fluoride that is protective against dental caries. Commercially prepared paste containing fluoride may restore in part the lost fluoride (page 508), and can be used during the polishing procedure.

After polishing, a topical application of fluoride should be made, followed by periodic applications at succeeding maintenance appointments, depending on individual needs. Self-application on a daily basis, using a mouthrinse, custom tray, or brush-on gel, may also be recommended to supplement fluoride derived from the use of a dentifrice.

FACTORS TO TEACH THE PATIENT

I. Advantages of having restorations smooth and well finished.
II. Reasons for having to wait 24 to 48 hours to have finishing procedures completed for the newly placed restoration.
III. The importance of having inadequate contact areas restored rather than using floss repeatedly to alleviate the discomforts of food impaction.
IV. The need for daily and professional applications of fluoride to preserve the tooth structure around each restoration. Daily mouthrinse, brush-on gel, gel in a tray, or other form of fluoride is advised.
V. Advantages of maintaining all restorations by daily plaque control measures, limiting cariogenic foods, and all possible preventive procedures.

References

1. Phillips, R.W.: *Skinner's Science of Dental Materials*, 8th ed. Philadelphia, W.B. Saunders Co., 1982, pp. 302–354.
2. Craig, R.G., O'Brien, W.J., and Powers, J.M.: *Dental Materials. Properties and Manipulation*, 4th ed. St. Louis, The C.V. Mosby Co., 1987, pp. 94–113.
3. American Dental Association, Council on Dental Materials, Instruments and Equipment: *Dentist's Desk Reference: Materials, Instruments and Equipment*, 2nd ed. Chicago, American Dental Association, 1983, pp. 53–68.
4. Phillips: op. cit., pp. 290–301.
5. Carranza, F.A.: *Glickman's Clinical Periodontology*, 6th ed. Philadelphia, W.B. Saunders Co., 1984, pp. 664–666.
6. Langslet, J.: *Margination—Rationale and Technique.* Seattle, Washington, Department of Dental Hygiene, University of Washington, 1976, 28 pp.
7. Gilmore, N. and Sheiham, A.: Overhanging Dental Restorations and Periodontal Disease, *J. Periodontol., 42,* 8, January, 1971.
8. Highfield, J.E. and Powell, R.N.: Effects of Removal of Posterior Overhanging Metallic Margins of Restorations Upon the Periodontal Tissues, *J. Clin. Periodontol., 5,* 169, August, 1978.
9. Gorzo, I., Newman, H.N., and Strahan, J.D.: Amalgam Restorations, Plaque Removal and Periodontal Health, *J. Clin. Periodontol., 6,* 98, April, 1979.
10. Jeffcoat, M.K. and Howell, T.H.: Alveolar Bone Destruction Due to Overhanging Amalgam in Periodontal Disease, *J. Periodontol., 51,* 599, October, 1980.
11. Rodriguez-Ferrer, H.J., Strahan, J.D., and Newman, H.N.: Effect on Gingival Health of Removing Overhanging Margins of Interproximal Subgingival Amalgam Restorations, *J. Clin. Periodontol., 7,* 457, December, 1980.
12. American Dental Association, Council on Dental Materials, Instruments and Equipment: op. cit., pp. 41–43.
13. Goldfogel, M.H., Smith, G.E., and Bomberg, T.J.: Amalgam Polishing, *Operative Dent., 1,* 146, Autumn, 1976.
14. Project Acorde, United States Department of Health, Education, and Welfare: *Recontouring, Finishing, and Polishing.* Castro Valley, California, Quercus, 1976, 85 pp.
15. Murphy, M.P.: *Finishing and Polishing Dental Amalgam.* Halifax, Nova Scotia, School of Dental Hygiene, Dalhousie University, 1978, 16 pp.
16. Muhler, S.A.: *Amalgam Polish.* Pennsylvania EFDA Faculty Institute, Philadelphia, University of Pennsylvania, 1979.
17. Chapman, M.K.: Role of the Auxiliary in Restorative Dentistry, in Castano, F.A. and Alden, B.A., eds.: *Handbook of Clinical Dental Auxiliary Practice*, 2nd ed. Philadelphia, J.B. Lippincott Co., 1980, pp. 96–102.

Suggested Readings

Bader, J.D., Mullins, R., and Lange, K.: Technical Performance on Amalgam Restorations by Dentists and Auxiliaries in Private Practice, *J. Am. Dent. Assoc., 106,* 338, March, 1983.

Biller-Karlsson, I. and Sheaffer, J.K.: Class II Amalgam Overhangs—Prevalence, Significance, and Removal Techniques, *Dent. Hyg., 62,* 180, April, 1988.

Blanchard, J.S.: The Periodontal Curet and the Ultrasonic Scaler. Their Effectiveness in Removing Overhangs from Amalgam Restorations, *Dent. Hyg., 58,* 450, October, 1984.

Bower, C.F., Reinhardt, R.A., and DuBois, L.M.: Evaluation of Interproximal Finishing Techniques for Silver Amalgam Restorations, *J. Prosthet. Dent., 56,* 274, September, 1986.

Bryant, R.W.: Marginal Fracture of Amalgam Restorations. A Review, *Aust. Dent. J., 26,* 222, August, 1981.

Creaven, P.J., Dennison, J.B., and Charbeneau, G.T.: Surface Roughness of Two Dental Amalgams After Various Polishing Techniques, *J. Prosthet. Dent., 43,* 289, March, 1980.

Eide, R. and Tveit, A.B.: A Comparison of Different Techniques for Finishing and Polishing Amalgam, *Acta Odontol. Scand., 45,* 147, Number 3, 1987.

Givens, E.G., Gwinnett, A.J., and Boucher, L.J.: Removal of Overhanging Amalgam: A Comparative Study of Three Instruments, *J. Prosthet. Dent., 52,* 815, December, 1984.

Goldberg, J., Tanzer, J., Munster, E., Amara, J., Thal, F., and Birkhed, D.: Cross-sectional Clinical Evaluation of Recurrent Enamel Caries, Restoration of Marginal Integrity, and Oral Hygiene Status, *J. Am. Dent. Assoc., 102,* 635, May, 1981.

Lang, N.P., Kiel, R.A., and Anderhalden, K.: Clinical and Microbiological Effects of Subgingival Restorations with Overhanging or Clinically Perfect Margins, *J. Clin. Periodontol., 10,* 563, November, 1983.

Leidal, T.I. and Dahl, J.E.: Marginal Integrity of Amalgam Restorations, *Acta Odontol. Scand., 38,* 81, Number 2, 1980.

Letzel, H. and Vrijhoef, M.M.A.: The Influence of Polishing on the Marginal Integrity of Amalgam Restorations, *J. Oral Rehabil., 11,* 89, March, 1984.

Miranda, F.J.: Why Don't We Polish Our Amalgam Restorations? *Can. Dent. Assoc. J., 49,* 131, February, 1983.

Neumeyer, S.: Work Simplification in Carving, Burnishing, and Finishing of Amalgam Restorations, *Quintessence Int., 17,* 209, April, 1986.

Nuckles, D.B., Miller, R.A., and Olson, J.C.: Early and Delayed Finishing of Amalgam with Different Polishing Procedures, *J. Prosthet. Dent., 47,* 612, June, 1982.

Paarmann, C.S. and Christie, C.R.: A Clinical Comparison of Amalgam Polishing Agents, *Dent. Hyg., 60,* 316, July, 1986.

Reavis-Scruggs, R. and Wilder, A.D.: An Alternative Method for Polishing Amalgam Restorations, *Dent. Hyg., 59,* 458, October, 1985.

Richeson, J.S. and Sarrett, D.C.: Profilometric and Scanning Electron Microscopic Analyses of Amalgam Polishing Techniques, *Gen. Dent., 34,* 481, November-December, 1986.

Spinks, G.C., Carson, R.E., Hancock, E.B., and Pelleu, G.B.: An SEM Study of Overhang Removal Methods, *J. Periodontol., 57,* 632, October, 1986.

Straffon, L.H., Corpron, R.E., Dennison, J.B., Carron, S.H., and Asgar, K.: A Clinical Evaluation of Polished and Unpolished Amalgams: 18-month Results, *Pediatr. Dent., 5,* 177, September, 1983.

Tate, P.S. and Schierling-Wilkes, J.: Margination is an Uncommon

Hygiene Practice with Common Applications, *RDH, 7,* 37, November/December, 1987.

van Dijken, J.W.V. and Ruyter, I.E.: Surface Characteristics of Posterior Composites After Polishing and Toothbrushing, *Acta Odontol. Scand., 45,* 337, Number 5, 1987.

Restorations and Gingival Health

Blank, L.W., Caffesse, R.G., and Charbeneau, G.T.: The Gingival Response to Well-finished Composite Resin Restorations, *J. Prosthet. Dent., 42,* 626, December, 1979.

Chen, J.J., Burch, J.G., Beck, F.M., and Horton, J.E.: Periodontal Attachment Loss Associated with Proximal Tooth Restorations, *J. Prosthet. Dent., 57,* 416, April, 1987.

Dunkin, R.T. and Chambers, D.W.: Gingival Response to Class V Composite Resin Restorations, *J. Am. Dent. Assoc., 106,* 482, April, 1983.

Eid, M.: Relationship Between Overhanging Amalgam Restorations and Periodontal Disease, *Quintessence Int., 18,* 775, November, 1987.

Fayyad, M.A. and Ball, P.C.: Bacterial Penetration Around Amalgam Restorations, *J. Prosthet. Dent., 57,* 571, May, 1987.

Grasso, J.E., Nalbandian, J., Sanford, C., and Bailit, H.: Effect of Restoration Quality on Periodontal Health, *J. Prosthet. Dent., 53,* 14, January, 1985.

Hadavi, F., Caffesse, R.G., and Charbeneau, G.T.: A Study of the Gingival Response to Polished and Unpolished Amalgam Restorations, *Can. Dent. Assoc. J., 52,* 211, March, 1986.

Hodges, K.O. and Bowen, D.M.: Effectiveness of Margination Procedures in Relation to Periodontal Status, *Dent. Hyg., 59,* 320, July, 1985.

Laurell, L., Rylander, H., and Pettersson, B.: The Effect of Different Levels of Polishing of Amalgam Restorations on the Plaque Retention and Gingival Inflammation, *Swed. Dent. J., 7,* 45, Number 2, 1983.

Lervik, T., Riordan, P.J., and Haugejorden, O.: Periodontal Disease and Approximal Overhangs on Amalgam Restorations in Norwegian 21-year-olds, *Community Dent. Oral Epidemiol., 12,* 264, August, 1984.

Waerhaug, J.: Effect of Rough Surfaces Upon Gingival Tissue, *J. Dent. Res., 35,* 323, April, 1956.

Waerhaug, J.: Presence or Absence of Plaque on Subgingival Restorations, *Scand. J. Dent. Res., 83,* 193, July, 1975.

Mercury Hygiene

Abraham, J.E., Svare, C.W., and Frank, C.W.: The Effect of Dental Amalgam Restorations on Blood Mercury Levels, *J. Dent. Res., 63,* 71, January, 1984.

Brodsky, J.B., Cohen, E.N., Whitcher, C., Brown, B.W., and Wu, M.L.: Occupational Exposure to Mercury in Dentistry and Pregnancy Outcome, *J. Am. Dent. Assoc., 111,* 779, November, 1985.

Cooley, R.L. and Lubow, R.M.: Mercury Vapor Emitted from Disposable Capsules Placed in Trash Containers, *Gen. Dent., 33,* 498, November-December, 1985.

Gough, J.E.: Amalgam Material as an Occupational Hazard, *Dent. Assist., 50,* 28, March/April, 1981.

Hatch, R., Berry, T., Stach, D., and Newman, S.: Mercury Safety and Media Mania, *RDH, 6,* 16, January/February, 1986.

Richards, J.M. and Warren, P.J.: Mercury Vapour Released During the Removal of Old Amalgam Restorations, *Br. Dent. J., 159,* 231, October 5, 1985.

Ship, I.I. and Shapiro, I.M.: Preventing Mercury Poisoning in Dental Practice, *Anesth. Prog., 30,* 76, May/June, 1983.

Vimy, M.J. and Lorscheider, F.L.: Intra-oral Air Mercury Released from Dental Amalgam, *J. Dent. Res., 64,* 1069, August, 1985.

42 *Evaluation and Maintenance*

The objective of treatment is oral health for the patient; individually performed services are steps toward total health. To evaluate the health of the gingival tissues, a period of time must be allowed for healing to take place and for the benefits of the professional treatment and the patient's self-care on a daily basis to become apparent. After health has been attained, it must be maintained. Dental hygiene care is an integral part of total care and cannot be considered as isolated appointment procedures.

Evaluation consists of three basic phases. The *first* is the immediate observation at the completion of each appointment; the *second* is short-term follow-up 1 week to 10 days after completion of a treatment or series of treatments; and the *third* is long-term to evaluate maintenance.

IMMEDIATE EVALUATION

I. Objectives

A. Teeth

Observation and exploration reveal the immediate effects of instrumentation on the teeth. An objective has been to produce a smooth hard tooth surface, free from deposits and stains. The effect of specific instrumentation is to facilitate the patient's self-care by removing signs of disease and local factors, particularly calculus and overhanging fillings, which encourage plaque retention.

B. Gingiva

The gingival changes are not apparent immediately after instrumentation. Tissue regeneration and healing takes approximately 1 week to 10 days for initial healing and even longer for maturation of connective tissue and keratinization of epithelium.

The objective at the treatment appointment is to *create an environment in which the gingival tissue can heal and be maintained in health by the patient.*

II. Examination

When scaling is accomplished over a series of appointments, each previously scaled quadrant or area is examined and rescaled as needed at each appointment. For the final evaluation, visual and tactile methods are applied carefully to each tooth surface. Instruments, methods, and procedures were described on pages 456–457.

A. Visual

1. Compressed air should be used with a mouth mirror and adequate lighting to examine the supragingival areas and just below the gingival margins.
2. Transillumination methods are applied.
3. A disclosing agent can reveal small areas of remaining deposits.

B. Tactile

A subgingival explorer is used to assure smoothness of tooth surfaces to the bottom of each pocket (page 203).

III. Appearance of the Teeth after Instrumentation

The experienced eye recognizes the bright luster of thoroughly clean teeth. All deposits have been removed and the surfaces are smooth to tactile examination.

To evaluate completion of instrumentation, the following observations are made:

A. Supragingival Nondemineralized Tooth Surfaces

1. Surfaces are visually clean and lustrous.
2. No calculus or extrinsic stains are evident after drying the surfaces with compressed air.
3. Metallic restorations are free from tarnish.
4. Enamel surfaces are smooth to tactile examination; root surfaces in areas of gingival recession feel smooth and hard.
5. Gingival surfaces of pontics are free of deposits.

B. Subgingival Nondemineralized Tooth Surfaces

1. Surfaces feel free of calculus and diseased altered cementum.
2. Surfaces are smooth and hard to tactile examination with a subgingival explorer.

C. Overhanging Fillings

1. Excess amalgam has been removed.
2. Junctions between restorations and tooth surfaces are smooth and uninterrupted when an explorer tip is passed over.
3. Normal tooth contour has been restored.

D. Removable Appliance

1. Outer polished surfaces have no visible calculus, soft deposits, or stains, and are smooth and unscratched.

2. Impression surfaces are free of deposits and unmarred.
3. Attachments or metal parts are smooth and shiny.

POSTOPERATIVE PROCEDURES

Postoperative care immediately following instrumentation includes flossing, careful irrigation, and postoperative instructions for the patient to carry out after leaving the office or clinic. Depending on the service performed, postoperative care may also include the placing of a periodontal dressing or application of a topical antiseptic. An extension of professional postoperative care may be a postappointment telephone contact later that day or the next concerning patient comfort and adherence to instructions.

Long-range postoperative care may include suture and dressing removal and dressing replacement. These have been described on page 491.

Postoperative care and instruction can have a direct bearing on the progress of healing and, hence, the follow-up evaluation that is planned for 1 week to 10 days after treatment is completed. Healing may be influenced by rinsing, brushing, and other self-care measures by the patient.

I. Application of an Antiseptic

When an antiseptic is applied by irrigation or topical swab, the limitations should be realized. Although some temporary reduction in bacterial count may be expected, sterilization would be impossible. The antiseptic may contribute to reducing postoperative discomfort.

A. Surface Application

1. *Agents Used.* The antiseptics usually used for postoperative applications are iodine or mercury preparations in the proper dilutions for application to the oral mucous membrane. Thimerosal (Merthiolate) (1:1000), nitromersal (Metaphen) (1:200), or merbromin (Mercurochrome) (2%) are examples of those used for this purpose.
2. *Technique for Application*
   a. Hold small cotton pellet with cotton pliers and saturate it in the antiseptic to be used. Express excess solution.
   b. Provide adequate retraction of lip, cheek, and tongue, and apply solution to the crest of each interdental papilla on both facial and lingual surfaces. Solution will flow into sulcus/pocket.
   c. Do not allow the patient to rinse.

B. Irrigation[1]

Several chemicals have been researched for use as irrigating antiseptics. These include chlorhexidine, stannous fluoride, tetracycline, metronidazole, and hydrogen peroxide. When root plan-

ing without irrigation was compared with root planing followed by irrigation, root planing was shown to be the main factor in obtaining healing of the gingiva.[2,3]

II. Postoperative Instruction

Instruction pertaining to periodontal dressings is outlined in table 36–1 on page 492. Many of the same principles can be applied for postoperative instruction when a dressing has not been applied.

Postoperative instruction is essential following scaling, particularly when the patient's gingiva has been hypersensitive or has hemorrhaged excessively or when extensive subgingival instrumentation has been completed. Directions for postoperative care include suggestions for rinsing and toothbrushing. An explanation of what discomfort may be expected should also be given.

Dietary and nutritional factors may be discussed. The temporary use of bland foods lacking in strong, spicy seasonings, as well as continuing use of nutritional foods to promote healing can be helpful.

It is best to prepare directions for postoperative care in printed form. This can prevent incomplete or inaccurate interpretation of orally delivered directions.

A. Rinsing

A warm solution is soothing to the tissues and improves the circulation, which helps healing. A suggested solution would be one that provides the appropriate concentration for osmotic balance of the salts of the solution with the salts of the oral tissue fluids.

1. *Solutions Suggested for Use*
   a. Hypertonic salt solution: level ½ teaspoonful of table salt in ½ cup (4 ounces) of warm water.
   b. Sodium bicarbonate solution: level ½ teaspoonful of baking soda in 1 cup (8 ounces) of warm water.
2. *Directions for Rinsing*
   a. Every 2 hours; after eating; after toothbrushing; before retiring.
   b. Use the rinse mouthful by mouthful, forcing the solution between the teeth.

B. Toothbrushing

The use of a soft brush is recommended after scaling and root planing. The patient must clearly understand the need for complete bacterial plaque removal.

FOLLOW-UP EVALUATION

To observe the response of the gingival tissues to treatment and the patient's personal daily care, an appointment is planned for approximately 10 days to 1 month after instrumentation has been completed. Such reevaluation after an interval in which the tissues can heal provides the opportunity to locate areas where additional treatment and instruction may be indicated.

One should not assume that, because the teeth were apparently free from deposits and were smooth and hard at the immediate evaluation following instrumentation, gingival healing, pocket wall shrinkage, resolution of inflammation, and other favorable treatment effects will inevitably result. Follow-up examination may reveal a variety of complications that may point to a need for additional root planing, curettage, self-care instruction, or referral for periodontal therapy.

A six-step evaluation plan is described here.

I. Evaluate the Gingival Tissue

A. Examine with the patient to observe
  1. Color, size, shape, consistency, and surface texture. By 10 days, the tissues should assume normal characteristics. Use table 11–1 on pages 174–175 for guidelines.
  2. Areas of damage to the gingiva, resulting from incorrect brushing or flossing.
B. Compare findings and indices with those from previous examination.

II. Evaluate Pocket Depths

A. Use probe to measure around each tooth.
B. Record and compare with initial measurements. Shrinkage of pockets when tissue is spongy and soft can be expected as healing progresses.

III. Evaluate Gingival Bleeding

A. Run the probe along the inside of the pocket wall. The technique is illustrated in figure 19–8 on page 273. If bleeding was apparent during probing for pocket depth in Step II (preceding), evaluation can be made without additional probing for bleeding.
B. Ask the patient whether bleeding occurred during toothbrushing. Healthy tissue does not bleed. As healing progresses, bleeding should be eliminated.

IV. Evaluate Plaque

A. Apply disclosing agent and examine with the patient for areas where plaque has not been removed by the patient's personal care.
B. Relate areas of plaque on the teeth to the areas of gingival redness, enlargement, and other signs of infection.

V. Evaluate Plaque Control Methods and Techniques

A. Request patient to demonstrate techniques, with emphasis on areas where the disclosing agent revealed plaque and where the gingiva has not responded.
B. Help the patient to evaluate and make corrections.
C. Introduce or substitute new methods when applicable. Learning is a slow process; repeated review and encouragement are usually needed.

VI. Examine for Residual Calculus

A. A subgingival explorer is used to examine tooth surfaces adjacent to gingiva where gingival redness and enlargement have persisted.
B. Remaining particles of calculus or areas of root surface roughness, however small, may be sufficient to encourage plaque collection and prevent complete healing.
C. Because the detection and removal of calculus in a pocket requires intricate and exacting instrumentation, even the most skilled operator must expect to recheck and complete the scaling and planing as indicated. The most frequent areas for residual calculus are proximal surfaces of molars, premolars, and crowded anteriors.

VII. Continue Evaluation

In practice, a patient should not be placed in the maintenance category until complete healing has occurred and the dentist and dental hygienist are satisfied that optimum tissue health has been obtained. Sometimes, a series of short appointments can be arranged in conjunction with dental appointments for restorative procedures. At each appointment, the patient may meet with the dental hygienist for continuing supervision of self-care procedures and observation of tissue response.

Notes concerning the status of gingival health and the instruction for the patient should be made in the patient's permanent record at each appointment. The observations are important to long-range planning for continuing patient care.

THE MAINTENANCE PHASE

Through common usage, the term "recall" has been applied to the system of appointments for the long-term maintenance phase of patient care, which has as its primary objectives the *prevention of new disease* as well as *of the recurrence of disease* through supervised control. This program requires the cooperative efforts of the patient and all members of the dental team.

Initially, the success of the program depends on the understanding by the patient of the maintenance procedure. The patient must realize that oral diseases do recur, but *control* is possible by combined personal and professional care.

I. Appointment Interval

No fixed schedule by which all patients can be maintained in oral health is possible because the frequency depends on the needs of each patient. Appointments may vary from 2 to 6 months. The time interval must be reevaluated periodically and changed in accord with changing needs.

Factors that determine the appointment frequency include the following:

A. The patient's ability to control bacterial plaque.
B. The rate of calculus formation.
C. The nature and extent of the previous infection.
D. The type and extent of previous treatment and the response to and outcome of it.
E. Restorative complications and considerations, including prosthetic replacements.
F. Systemic factors that may alter the patient's susceptibility to infection.

II. The First Maintenance Appointment

The gingival or periodontal treatment may be completed or nearly completed by the time appointments for restorative phases of treatment are under way. The first maintenance appointment should be dated from the completion of the gingival and periodontal treatment. When extensive restorative, prosthetic, or other treatment is to follow, tissue maintenance during long-term therapy is essential.

III. Frequent Appointment Requirements

Intervals of 2 and 3 months are required by many patients. Examples of patients in this category are described throughout this book. Only a few will be mentioned here.

A. Rampant Dental Caries

Appointment for continuation of a caries control effort, which includes topical fluoride applications, dietary supervision, and personal care factors for bacterial plaque control.

B. Orthodontic Therapy

Appliances make cleaning and plaque control difficult; frequent topical fluoride applications may be indicated; response of gingival tissue to irritants can be marked.

C. Mentally or Physically Handicapped

Managing the toothbrush may be difficult; when the handicap involves the mouth area, opening the mouth may be a problem.

D. Diabetes

Diabetes or other disease that predisposes to lowered resistance to infection; tissues must not be allowed to develop advanced disease.

E. Cardiovascular Disease or Other Condition

Brushing is a difficult procedure to carry out and only short appointments at the dental office can be tolerated because of the fatigue factor.

F. Periodontal Maintenance Therapy (PMT)[4]

Any of the types of patients who have been mentioned and any of the "special" patients to be described in Section VI following this chapter may have a potentially recurrent periodontal infection or may have had periodontal corrective surgical therapy. Four categories of PMT have been defined:

1. *Preventive PMT.* To prevent the initiation of disease in individuals without periodontal infection.

2. *Trial PMT.* For borderline patients with conditions that must be observed and further evaluated before a decision can be made as to whether corrective surgery may be necessary or whether maintenance is possible without further advanced disease development.

3. *Compromise PMT.* To slow the progress of disease in patients for whom corrective surgery and other advanced treatment is indicated but cannot be implemented for reasons of health, economics, or other personal factors.

4. *Post-treatment PMT.* To prevent the recurrence of disease and maintain the state of periodontal health attained during periodontal therapy. Such therapy may have been nonsurgical or surgical.

IV. Maintenance Appointment Procedures

Preparation of data follows the same plan as for a new patient. A diagnostic work-up is prepared. At least annually, every patient needs a medical history review, an intraoral and extraoral examination for soft tissue lesions, particularly for cancer, and a blood pressure determination.

At every appointment, whether at 3, 6, or other number of months, a patient of any age needs a complete pocket probing and special evaluations for the particular problems of previous treatments.

Basic to all examinations are the periodontal examination (pages 201 and 286) and the dental examination (page 289) with charting.

Steps in preparation of a maintenance appointment diagnostic workup include the following:

A. Review Patient History

Supplementary questions are asked to determine the present state of health, recent illnesses, present medications, and other pertinent data (page 83).

B. Blood Pressure Determination (pages 98–101)

C. Extraoral and Intraoral Examination

A thorough extraoral and intraoral examination for oral disease, particularly cancer (page 105 and table 8–1, pages 106–107), must be made and recorded.

D. Radiographs

The frequency of radiographic surveys is in accord with the dentist's determination of an individual patient's need.[5]

E. Periodontal Examination

Details are outlined on pages 286–289. Minimum examination includes clinical tissue examination of color, size, shape, consistency, and surface texture, pocket charting, determination of tooth mobility, examination of the mucogingival junction, furcations, occlusion, and dental deposits. Bleeding on probing should be correlated with a bleeding index.

F. Examination of the Teeth (page 289)

A new charting with notations of restorations and caries, examination for pulp vitality when indicated, and a record of tooth sensitivity, if reported by the patient or detected during examination, should be made.

G. Evaluation of Oral Cleanliness and Adequacy of Self-care Measures

Relate plaque on teeth as observed after applying a disclosing agent to areas of gingival redness, enlargement, and other signs of infection.

H. Examination of Specific Areas by the Dentist

Areas of special problems include endodontically treated teeth, postsurgical areas, occlusal factors, and prosthetic appliances.

I. Treatment Plan

The dentist reviews the data collected and a treatment plan is outlined, based on the new diagnosis and evaluation of the patient's oral condition. For the dental hygienist's treatment plan, scaling, planing, topical fluoride or other preventive application, and patient instruction provide the basis for the continuing preventive program.

TECHNICAL HINTS

Methods for administration of a maintenance plan vary. For any plan, individual file information includes name, address, telephone numbers, and instructions concerning appointment frequency and available or preferred day and time. The data may be kept on 3 × 5 or 4 × 6 inch file cards or in a computer.

I. Pre-book Method

Make each patient's appointment before the patient leaves the current appointment. An appointment card is given the patient, who is asked to enter it on the calendar ahead of time. An envelope is prepared for mailing a duplicate card 10 days to 1 week before the scheduled appointment. The card should request the patient to call to confirm. For unconfirmed appointments, a call to the patient the day before must be made.

II. Monthly Reminders

By this system, individual data are filed alphabetically by the last name of the patient under the month when the patient is due. Each month the cards are pulled and appointment reminders are mailed or telephoned well in advance.

III. Computer Assisted

Computers can be helpful in maintaining appointment systems. Either the pre-book or the monthly reminders can be used in combination with a computer.

Information stored in a computer can be accessible readily. Computers are capable of printing address labels so that postal cards can be mailed monthly or envelopes containing the pre-book appointment card can be sent at the appropriate time.

FACTORS TO TEACH THE PATIENT

I. Appearance and feeling of a clean mouth.
II. Relationship of personal oral care habits to the maintenance of cleanliness provided through professional scaling and planing.
III. Purposes of postoperative care by the dental hygienist and the patient.
IV. How to prepare solutions for postoperative rinsing.
V. Directions for postoperative care by the patient.
VI. Purposes of follow-up and maintenance appointments.

References

1. Greenstein, G.: Effects of Subgingival Irrigation on Periodontal Status, *J. Periodontol., 58,* 827, December, 1987.
2. MacAlpine, R., Magnusson, I., Kiger, R., Crigger, M., Garrett, S., and Egelberg, J.: Antimicrobial Irrigation of Deep Pockets to Supplement Oral Hygiene Instruction and Root Debridement. I. Bi-weekly Irrigation, *J. Clin. Periodontol., 12,* 568, August, 1985.
3. Braatz, L., Garrett, S., Claffey, N., and Egelberg, J.: Antimicrobial Irrigation of Deep Pockets to Supplement Non-surgical Periodontal Therapy. II. Daily Irrigation, *J. Clin. Periodontol., 12,* 630, September, 1985.
4. Schallhorn, R.G. and Snider, L.E.: Periodontal Maintenance Therapy, *J. Am. Dent. Assoc., 103,* 227, August, 1981.
5. American Dental Association, Council on Dental Materials, Instruments, and Equipment: Recommendations in Radiographic Practices: An Update, 1988, *J. Am. Dent. Assoc., 118,* 115, January, 1989.

Suggested Readings

Axelsson, P. and Lindhe, J.: The Significance of Maintenance Care in the Treatment of Periodontal Disease, *J. Clin. Periodontol., 8,* 281, August, 1981.
Badersten, A., Nilvéus, R., and Egelberg, J.: 4-Year Observations of Basic Periodontal Therapy, *J. Clin. Periodontol., 14,* 438, September, 1987.
Becker, W., Becker, B.E., and Berg, L.E.: Periodontal Treatment without Maintenance. A Retrospective Study in 44 Patients, *J. Periodontol., 55,* 505, September, 1984.
Blunt, L.L.: Evaluate the Success of Periodontal Therapy in Your Practice, *Dent. Hyg., 58,* 26, January, 1984.
Buckley, L.A. and Crowley, M.J.: A Longitudinal Study of Untreated Periodontal Disease, *J. Clin. Periodontol., 11,* 523, September, 1984.
Carranza, F.A.: *Glickman's Clinical Periodontology,* 6th ed. Philadelphia, W.B. Saunders Co., 1984, pp. 620, 946–952.
DeVore, C.H., Duckworth, J.E., Beck, F.M., Hicks, M.J., Brumfield, F.W., and Horton, J.E.: Bone Loss Following Periodontal Therapy in Subjects without Frequent Periodontal Maintenance, *J. Periodontol., 57,* 354, June, 1986.
Goldman, H.M. and Cohen, D.W.: *Periodontal Therapy,* 6th ed., St. Louis, The C.V. Mosby Co., 1980, pp. 1155–1178.
Goldman, M.J., Ross, I.F., and Goteiner, D.: Effect of Periodontal Therapy on Patients Maintained for 15 Years or Longer. A Retrospective Study, *J. Periodontol., 57,* 347, June, 1986.
Grant, D.A., Stern, I.B., and Listgarten, M.A., eds.: *Periodontics,* 6th ed. St. Louis, The C.V. Mosby Co., 1988, pp. 1095–1124.
Johansson, L.-Å., Öster, B., and Hamp, S.-E.: Evaluation of Cause-related Periodontal Therapy and Compliance with Mainte-

nance Care Recommendations, *J. Clin. Periodontol., 11,* 689, November, 1984.

Kristoffersen, T. and Meyer, K.: The Maintenance Phase of Periodontal Therapy, in Lindhe, J.: *Textbook of Clinical Periodontology.* Copenhagen, Munksgaard, 1983, pp. 520–540.

Lang, N.P., Joss, A., Orsanic, T., Gusberti, F.A., and Siegrist, B.E.: Bleeding on Probing. A Predictor for the Progression of Periodontal Disease? *J. Clin. Periodontol., 13,* 590, July, 1986.

Lindhe, J. and Nyman, S.: Long-term Maintenance of Patients Treated for Advanced Periodontal Disease, *J. Clin. Periodontol., 11,* 504, September, 1984.

Listgarten, M.A., Levin, S., Schifter, C.C., Sullivan, P., Evian, C.I., Rosenberg, E.S., and Laster, L.: Comparative Longitudinal Study of 2 Methods of Scheduling Maintenance Visits; 2-year Data, *J. Clin. Periodontol., 13,* 692, August, 1986.

Listgarten, M.A., Schifter, C.C., Sullivan, P., George, C., and Rosenberg, E.S.: Failure of a Microbial Assay to Reliably Predict Disease Recurrence in a Treated Periodontitis Population Receiving Regularly Scheduled Prophylaxes, *J. Clin. Periodontol., 13,* 768, September, 1986.

Morrison, E.C., Ramfjord, S.P., Burgett, F.G., Nissle, R.R., and Shick, R.A.: The Significance of Gingivitis During the Maintenance Phase of Periodontal Treatment, *J. Periodontol., 53,* 31, January, 1982.

Morsey, S.L.: Effective Utilization of the Dental Hygienist in Continuing Care, *Quintessence Int., 15,* 551, May, 1984.

Ogilvie, A.L.: Maintenance of the Periodontal Patient, in Schluger, S., Yuodelis, R.A., and Page, R.C.: *Periodontal Disease.* Philadelphia, Lea & Febiger, 1977, pp. 704–721.

Parr, R.W.: *Periodontal Maintenance Therapy.* Berkeley, California, Praxis Publishing Co., 1974, 86 pp.

Parr, R.W., Green, E., and Miller, S.R.: *Hygienists in Periodontal Maintenance Therapy.* Berkeley, California, Praxis Publishing Co., 1978, 67 pp.

Pertuiset, J.H., Saglie, F.R., Rezende, M., and Sanz, M.: Recurrent Periodontal Disease and Bacterial Presence in the Gingiva, *J. Periodontol., 58,* 553, August, 1987.

Pruthi, V.K.: Reevaluation Following Initial (Non-surgical) Periodontal Therapy. Its Significance, *Can. Dent. Assoc. J., 52,* 773, September, 1986.

Ramfjord, S.P.: Maintenance Care for Treated Periodontitis Patients, *J. Clin. Periodontol., 14,* 433, September, 1987.

Ramfjord, S.P., Caffesse, R.G., Morrison, E.C., Hill, R.W., Kerry, G.J., Appleberry, E.A., Nissle, R.R., and Stults, D.L.: 4 Modalities of Periodontal Treatment Compared Over 5 Years, *J. Clin. Periodontol., 14,* 445, September, 1987.

Ramfjord, S.P., Morrison, E.C., Burgett, F.G., Nissle, R.R., Shick, R.A., Zann, G.J., and Knowles, J.W.: Oral Hygiene and Maintenance of Periodontal Support, *J. Periodontol., 53,* 26, January, 1982.

Renner, R.P., Gomes, B.C., Shakun, M.L., Baer, P.N., Davis, R.K., and Camp, P.: Four-year Longitudinal Study of the Periodontal Health Status of Overdenture Patients, *J. Prosthet. Dent., 51,* 593, May, 1984.

Roberts, B.W.: The Recall System. A Necessary Part of a Partial Denture Service, *Br. Dent. J., 149,* 46, July 15, 1980.

Rosling, B.: Periodontally Treated Dentitions: Their Maintenance and Prognosis, *Int. Dent. J., 33,* 147, June, 1983.

Saxén, L. and Aula, S.: Periodontal Bone Loss in Patients with Down's Syndrome: A Follow-up Study, *J. Periodontol., 53,* 158, March, 1982.

Schmid, M.O.: The Maintenance Phase of Dental Therapy, *Dent. Clin. North Am., 24,* 379, April, 1980.

Shick, R.A.: Maintenance Phase of Periodontal Therapy, *J. Periodontol., 52,* 576, September, 1981.

Westfelt, E., Nyman, S., Socransky, S., and Lindhe, J.: Significance of Frequency of Professional Tooth Cleaning for Healing Following Periodontal Surgery, *J. Clin. Periodontol., 10,* 148, March, 1983.

Wilson, T.G., Glover, M.E., Schoen, J., Baus, C., and Jacobs, T.: Compliance with Maintenance Therapy in a Private Periodontal Practice, *J. Periodontol., 55,* 468, August, 1984.

Wilson, T.G., Glover, M.E., Malik, A.K., Schoen, J.A., and Dorsett, D.: Tooth Loss in Maintenance Patients in a Private Periodontal Practice, *J. Periodontol., 58,* 231, April, 1987.

VI

Applied Techniques for Patients with Special Needs

INTRODUCTION

An understanding of each patient's general and/or oral health problems requires particular study. Actually, each patient is a "special" patient and must be considered according to individual needs. Certain patients, however, have problems peculiar to their age group and/or unusual health factors that may complicate the routine of care generally provided. These special patients require more skillful application of dental hygiene knowledge and ability to accomplish a comparably favorable result than do what might be called "normal" patients.

Optimum oral health is frequently an important contributing factor in maintaining or restoring the patient's physical, emotional, vocational, economic, and social usefulness to the extent of individual capabilities. *The dental hygienist's obligation is to see that no patient needs special rehabilitative dental services because of any condition that could have been prevented by dental hygiene care.*

Consideration of the patient as a whole requires attention to general physical and emotional problems as well as oral problems. Basic psychologic needs for affection, belonging, independence, achievement, recognition, and self-esteem frequently influence the outcome of treatment, as does the patient's whole attitude toward dental and dental hygiene care.

With certain disabilities, oral health has assumed less importance in the mind of the patient because other health problems have demanded so much attention. For some of these patients, neglect has intensified the need for oral care.

The patients with special needs who will be considered in the chapters following include patients with oral and general systemic conditions. Variations with respect to age and degree of disability are considered.

SPECIAL ORAL PROBLEMS

In each specialty of dentistry, patients present problems that can be helped by the services performed by the dental hygienist. For example, patients with fixed or removable dentures require particular attention. Patients with dentofacial handicaps who have missing teeth or congenital malformations, patients requiring surgery, and patients afflicted with habits conducive to the initiation of dental caries need special adaptations of the preventive care and instruction the dental hygienist can provide.

SYSTEMIC DISEASES

Oral manifestations may be evident in association with certain acute and chronic systemic diseases, particularly nutritional deficiencies, endocrine disturbances, blood diseases, and many chronic degenerative diseases. The presence of oral diseases may complicate and delay the rehabilitation of a patient with systemic illness. When an oral manifestation suggests the possibility of an undiagnosed systemic disease, dental personnel have a responsibility to refer the patient for medical examination.

Patients with chronic conditions may or may not be able to go to a dental office or clinic for appointments. Certain conditions, particularly during the advanced stages of a disease, require the patient to remain confined and, in some instances, bedridden. Dental hygienists must understand the special procedures for care in these instances.

The basic approach to oral problems of the patient with a chronic disease or a physical or mental disability is through prevention. Individual initiative is vital if the impact of preventive measures is to be understood and necessary action taken. The public, including dental personnel, must incorporate into daily living fundamental health practices that contribute to optimum health and, hence, to the prevention of chronic disease. Dental hygiene care can improve the general health and influence the resistance to infection of the oral cavity.

INTEGRATION OF APPLICATIONS TO SPECIAL NEEDS

A patient may have more than one special need. For example, the patient who requires dental hygiene care prior to oral surgery may have a blood disorder. The pregnant patient may be diabetic. The use of the patient's medical history plays an important role when the total needs of the patient are outlined.

Part VI attempts to integrate learning from other areas of medical and social sciences into the dental and dental hygiene aspects. The dental hygienist is encouraged to supplement knowledge and appreciation of the special needs of patients through the use of additional readings such as those suggested at the end of each chapter. By application of understanding of the patient's needs, clinical techniques and patient instruction may be directed more skillfully to provide *complete dental hygiene care.*

43 The Pregnant Patient and the Newborn Infant

During pregnancy, attention is focused on good health practices for the mother. She is concerned for the health of her baby and for herself. This alertness to total health, of which oral health is an important part, provides an unusual opportunity to help the patient learn principles that may be applied to the future care of the child.

The term *prenatal care* refers to the supervised preparation for childbirth that helps the mother enjoy optimum health during and after her pregnancy and provides the maximum chance for the baby to be born healthy. Such a program involves the combined efforts of the obstetrician and/or midwife, nurse, dentist, dental hygienist, and the expectant parents.

Certain women who do not receive routine dental care may appear for emergency dental service and may be receptive to a program of care and instruction to prevent further emergencies. The dental hygienist in public health participates in community educational programs with public health nurses, whereby some less informed or less motivated women may learn of the need for professional dental care and advice during pregnancy.

Obstetricians should recommend dental examination early in pregnancy. This brings to the dental office or clinic many women who previously would not have had a regular plan for obtaining professional service. Many of these women have not known the advantages of personal habits of daily care and diet related to the health of the oral tissues. Numerous misconceptions must be counteracted when providing up-to-date information about the relationship of pregnancy and oral health.

I. Fetal Development

Pregnancy is arbitrarily divided into 3 periods of 3 months each, called the first, second, and third trimesters. Normal pregnancy, or period of *gestation,* is approximately 40 weeks. *Premature birth* refers to a birth before 37 weeks' gestation.

Physiologic changes in the mother are related to the endocrine, urinary, cardiovascular, hematologic, gastrointestinal, and respiratory systems.[1] Early development of the embryo is greatly influenced by heredity, infections, and drug intake.

The developing organism is called an *embryo* from conception through approximately the end of the second month. From the beginning of the third month until birth, it is referred to as the *fetus.*

A. First Trimester

During the first trimester, the embryo is highly susceptible to injuries and malformations. Teratogenic effects can be produced by many sources, including tobacco, radiation, infections, and particularly drugs.

All organ systems are formed (organogenesis) during the first trimester. By 12 weeks, the fetus moves and swallows. In the oral cavity, the following occurs:
1. *Teeth*
   a. Tooth buds develop between the fourth and fifth weeks.
   b. Initial mineralization occurs from the ninth to the twelfth weeks.
2. *Lips and Palate*
   a. Lips form during the fourth to the seventh weeks.
   b. Palate forms between the eighth and twelfth weeks.
   c. Cleft lip is apparent by the eighth week; cleft palate by the twelfth week (page 582).

B. Second and Third Trimesters

The organs are completed, and growth and maturation continues. Fetal weight changes from 1 ounce at 3 months to 7.5 pounds average normal birthweight.

II. Factors That Can Damage the Fetus

A. Infections

Protection from infectious diseases is necessary because damage to and infection of the fetus can result. Women of child-bearing age should avail themselves of all available vaccines prior to becoming pregnant.

Defects, deformities, and life-threatening infections can result from infection acquired during pregnancy or during delivery and after birth. Rubella (German measles), rubeola, varicella, herpes viruses, hepatitis B (page 18), acquired immunodeficiency syndrome (page 22), syphilis (congenital syphilis), and gonorrhea all can have serious effects on the baby.

B. Drugs

Nearly all drugs pass through the placenta to a degree. Many drugs can cause teratogenic effects.[1,2] Table 43–1 lists drugs with proven and suspected teratogenicity.[2]

Tetracycline is well known for intrinsic stain-

Table 43–1. Drugs During Pregnancy

Proved Teratogenicity

Antineoplastic agents: various anomalies
    Aminopterin
    Busulfan (Myleran)
    Chlorambucil (Leukeran)
    Colchicine
    Cyclophosphamide (Cytoxan)
    Methotrexate

Radioiodine: anomalies (early), congenital hypothyroidism (later)
Diethylstilbestrol: subsequent to puberty, daughters may develop vaginal adenosis or clear cell carcinoma of the vagina or cervix
Alkyl (methyl) mercury: cerebral palsy, microcephaly
Progestins: masculinization of female fetus
Oral contraceptives: anomalous genitalia, limb reduction defects
Phenytoin (diphenylhydantoin): cleft lip and palate, microcephaly, congenital heart disease
Tetracyclines: enamel pigmentation of hypoplasia, congenital cataract
Warfarin: chondrodysplasia punctata (nasal hypoplasia and stippled epiphysealis)
Suspected Teratogenicity
Coumarins: various anomalies
Alcohol: small for gestational age; rarely, microcephaly or maxillary hypoplasia
Lithium: various anomalies
Quinine: limb reduction defects, congenital deafness
Reserpine: congenital lung cysts
Streptomycin: congenital deafness
Tobacco smoking: small for gestational age
Trimethadione: various anomalies
Vitamin D (massive doses): supravalvular aortic stenosis, elfin facies, mental retardation
X-ray (diagnostic): maximum total safe dose to the embryo has been stated to be 10 rads by the National Committee on Radiation Protection; this group suggests an increased risk of leukemia by age 10 years if the exposure is >15 rads
Still Under Investigation (Less Evidence Than Above)
Chlordiazepoxide (Librium) and diazepam (Valium): various anomalies from exposure during first 6 weeks only
Isoniazid: isolated case reports of anomalies
Meprobamate (Equanil, Miltown): various anomalies from exposure during first 6 weeks only

From Gier, R.E. and Janes, D.R.: Dental Management of the Pregnant Patient, *Dent. Clin. North Am.*, 27, 419, April, 1983.

ing of the tooth structure. The effect occurs during mineralization of the primary teeth, beginning at about 4 months of gestation, and of the permanent teeth near and after birth (page 257). If an antibiotic is required during pregnancy, tetracycline should be avoided.

III. Oral Findings During Pregnancy

The condition of the gingiva is the result of an exaggerated response of the tissues to bacterial plaque. When the mouth is in good health and the patient uses adequate personal oral care measures for plaque control, no adverse gingival changes may be expected.

The hormones of pregnancy tend to aggravate existing gingival conditions, and therefore, act as secondary or conditioning factors. Because the principal gingival reaction in pregnancy is an inflammatory one, the pregnancy itself cannot be the cause.

Exaggerated symptoms abate after the birth of the child, but a completely healthy condition does not necessarily result. A patient with a gingival disturbance during pregnancy continues to have the disturbance, even if to a somewhat lessened degree, after the birth.

A. Generalized Gingival Enlargement[3,4,5]

1. *Clinical Appearance.* The appearance varies and shows characteristics of inflamed tissues, including enlargement, shiny surface, bleeding readily on probing, and color changes.
2. *Predisposing Factors*
   a. Local irritation because of an unhygienic oral condition and bacterial plaque on the teeth and gingiva.
   b. Hormonal changes during pregnancy that may alter the tissue reaction.

B. Isolated Gingival Enlargement

An isolated or discrete gingival enlargement may occur, which has been called a "pregnancy tumor." The use of the word tumor is misleading because the lesion is not a tumor but a hyperplasia, and may correctly be called an epulis gravidarum, pregnancy granuloma,[6] or pyogenic granuloma.[7]

1. *Clinical Appearance*

   The enlargement is located superficially on the free gingiva, usually associated with an interdental papilla. It forms in a mushroom-like flattened mass, with a smooth, glistening surface.

   The color depends on the vascularity and may be purplish-red, magenta, or deep blue, sometimes dotted with red.
2. *Symptoms*
   a. Bleeds readily with slight trauma.
   b. Painless unless it becomes large enough to interfere with occlusion and mastication.

C. Enamel Erosion

Morning sickness with vomiting over an extended period can lead to demineralization and acid erosion primarily of the lingual surfaces of the teeth. Nausea associated with early pregnancy can be relieved by frequent eating of small amounts of food. Careful selection of nutritious yet noncariogenic foods is necessary to avoid dental caries.

ASPECTS OF PATIENT CARE

The first few months are often the most difficult for the mother-to-be, because pregnancy provides an emotional experience with many adjustments that must be made.

I. Oral Examination and Treatment Planning

The patient should be seen as early in her pregnancy as possible. Consultation with the patient's physician is particularly important to integrate total prenatal care.

II. Radiography

Radiographs are not made unless absolutely necessary. When they are required, the patient is covered with a lead apron, a thyroid collar, and a second apron for the back to prevent secondary radiation from reaching the abdomen. All current methods for radiation safety and protection are applied, including optimum filtration, collimation, use of E film, and extended target film distance.

Determine the minimum number of film exposures that will produce the required diagnostic information. The use of a paralleling technique should not require angulation directed toward the patient's abdomen, as compared with steep angulation needed for a bisection technique. Careful and skillful film placement, angulation, processing, and all phases of technique will prevent the need for remaking radiographs that are not acceptable for diagnosis.

III. Periodontal Treatment

Areas of food impaction should be corrected and all overhanging restorations reshaped or replaced. All scaling and root planing procedures should be carefully and thoroughly completed. Elective complicated periodontal treatment should be deferred until after the baby is born.

IV. Restorative Dentistry

Restorations should be completed with permanent restorative materials. One important contraindication for the use of temporary restorations is that, after the baby is born, the mother may be too busy to attend to appointments, because of added family responsibilities and/or a return to career employment.

DENTAL HYGIENE CARE

The dental hygienist should be well informed about dental care in order to motivate the patient and alleviate fears related to certain services. The patient may consult with the dental hygienist for reassurance and interpretation of the dentist's recommendations and procedures.

Gingival disease need not be expected when the patient is motivated to practice conscientious self-care procedures for oral cleanliness and plaque control. This calls for a specific appointment plan for scaling and instruction.

A concentrated plan for dental caries control is indicated. A multiple fluoride program and limitation of cariogenic foods are basic to the preventive efforts.

I. Appointment Planning

A. Frequency

Monthly appointments or appointments 3 times during the 9-month period may be required, depending on the patient's motivation to maintain a healthy oral environment.

B. Length of Individual Appointments

An appointment should be short, for patient comfort. A series of appointments is indicated when calculus is heavy.

C. Maintenance Appointments Postpartum

For the patient who has not been on a regular maintenance plan prior to pregnancy, emphasis must be placed on motivating the patient to continue regular appointments for dental hygiene and dental care after the baby is born.

II. Appointment Procedures

A. Patient History

The medical history must be reviewed carefully at each appointment to identify changes and adapt procedures accordingly. The prenatal patient may require applied techniques for conditions other than pregnancy. For example, diabetes or cardiovascular diseases can involve serious complications.

When the expectant mother is an adolescent, consideration for her own health takes on a different perspective than for the mature woman. Aspects of adolescent development and psychology will be described on pages 553–554.

B. Consultation with Physician

The dentist and the physician benefit mutually through discussion of the patient's treatment plan with the agreement of the patient. The need for particular precautions before, during, or after treatment becomes evident.

When a patient seeks dental and dental hygiene care and is not under the care of a physician, she should be urged to obtain medical supervision, have examinations, and thereby improve her health as well as that of the baby.

III. Clinical Aspects

It is not within the scope of this book to review all of the physiologic changes that occur during pregnancy. Common physical changes should be identified because they can affect appointment procedures. Nearly every woman is bothered by one or more minor complaints at some time during her pregnancy.

Attention to details provides the patient with comfort and motivates her to continue oral care. Table 43–2 lists the more common physical changes of pregnancy and suggests a few appointment considerations.

A. Instrumentation

When a patient has gingival enlargement and inflammation, it is usually advisable to spend the first appointment on instruction in plaque control and other preventive measures. At the second

appointment, evaluation is made and instruction continued.

Careful instrumentation for scaling and planing is indicated. Bleeding may be excessive. If stain removal is needed, the use of the abrasive cleaning paste should be postponed until the tissue has responded to the plaque control measures.

B. Fluoride Program

1. *Professional Topical Application.* All patients can benefit from a topical application of fluoride solution or gel after scaling and root planing. Applications can be indicated especially for patients with a tendency toward ram-

Table 43–2.   Appointment Adaptations for the Prenatal Patient

Characteristic	*Dental Hygiene Implication*
Fatigues easily, may even fall asleep	Short appointments; several in series, as needed Work with an assistant to accomplish more at each appointment
Discomfort of remaining in one position too long	Interrupt in middle of appointment to change chair position Assistance with evacuation during intraoral instrumentation can shorten appointment time
Backache	Adjust chair appropriately for comfort
Frequent urination	Allow long enough appointment time for interruptions Suggest at beginning of appointment that patient mention need for interruption
General awkwardness because of new shape and weight gain	Attend to details such as gently lowering chair and straightening it for patient to get out Make sure rinsing facilities are convenient; or preferably, an assistant attends to evacuation
Dyspnea (aggravated by supine chair position)	Adapt chair for patient comfort
Faintness and dizziness	Be prepared for emergency (table 60–1, pages 747–748). Place the patient on her *side* and not in supine or Trendelenburg position because pressure from the enlarged uterus and the abdominal organs on the inferior vena cava can interfere with venous return; placental separation could result

Nausea and vomiting (first trimester)
  a. Unpleasant taste in mouth
  b. Gagging
 	
  c. Exaggerated reactions to odors and flavors of medicaments and other office materials
 	
  d. Physician's recommendations for alleviation of symptoms: frequent eating of small amounts of foods
	
	Suggest toothbrushing or rinsing at frequent intervals
	Turn head down over sink while brushing helps to relax throat and allow saliva to flow out
	Take care in instrument and radiographic film placement
	Determine particularly obnoxious odors for an individual patient and remove them
	Pay attention to cleanliness of cuspidor
	Encourage use of noncariogenic foods

Unusual food cravings	If cravings are for sweets, clearly define relationship of frequent nibbling of cariogenic foods to dental caries Provide list of nutritious noncariogenic snacks

pant caries, who have numerous restorations. The fluoride agents and techniques are described in Chapter 29, pages 401–406.

2. *Self-application.* A fluoride dentifrice is recommended for all patients. A daily mouthrinse, gel tray, or other mode of application is essential, depending on the individual evaluation. A concentrated fluoride effort can be particularly important to the teeth of the adolescent mother-to-be.

PATIENT INSTRUCTION

The emphasis on general health during pregnancy provides the ideal situation for the dental hygienist to give instruction relative to many aspects of oral health for the mother and her expected child, as well as for other members of the family. New developments in disease prevention and control should be explained.

Printed materials concerning the prevention of periodontal diseases and dental caries and the development and care of children's teeth are available from the American Dental Association.* Reading material to supplement personal discussions can contribute to patient understanding and cooperation.

I. Bacterial Plaque Control

A rigid schedule for self-care must be demonstrated and supervised. A series of instructional periods is usually needed.

Emphasis should not be placed on the hormonal changes of pregnancy as influential in producing gingival changes. The patient may be all too willing to use the systemic factor as an excuse for her lack of attention to adequate self-care.

II. Diet

Instruction must be provided in prevention of dental caries and maintenance of the health of the supporting structures of the teeth. The use of a varied diet containing the essential protective basic four food groups, with a minimum of cariogenic foods, is necessary.

A. Purposes of Adequate Diet During Pregnancy

1. To maintain daily strength and feeling of well-being.
2. To provide the essential building materials for the developing fetus.
3. To protect and promote the health of the oral tissues of the mother.
4. To minimize any problems postpartum.

B. Dietary Needs During Pregnancy

The *Recommended Dietary Allowances* of the Food and Nutrition Board of the National Research Council specifies the increased allow-

ances during pregnancy and lactation. Because the embryo or fetus is a parasite and thrives at the mother's expense, the mother's diet must be adequate to maintain her own nutritional status and to meet the needs of the fetus.

The particular needs of the fetus are
1. Proteins, for general tissue construction.
2. Minerals, especially calcium and phosphorus, for bone and tooth mineralization; and iron for blood corpuscles.
3. Vitamins.

C. Dietary Adjustments[9,10]

Foods from the four food groups (table 28–1, page 382) are selected. To meet the needs for calcium, phosphorus, and riboflavin, a quart of milk or its equivalent in milk products is sufficient, except for the teen-age mother who needs a quart and one-half, if her own maturing body requirements are to be met.

An added citrus fruit or other good source of vitamin C, a dark green or deep yellow vegetable daily for vitamin A, and sources for iron, thiamine, and vitamin D are indicated. Proteins of high physiologic value are important; that is, proteins from meat, eggs, fish, and fowl rather than of vegetable origin only.

Calories may be increased in accord with exercise and tendency for weight gain. A decreased use of cariogenic foods is important for general nutrition and weight problems, as well as for the prevention of dental caries.

III. Dental Caries Control

A. Incidence During Pregnancy

Some patients believe that they have more dental caries during and because of pregnancy. Research has shown that this is not true, and that any relationship is an indirect one. Factors that result in dental caries formation are the same during pregnancy as at other times (pages 242–243).

B. Factors That May Contribute to Apparent Increase in Dental Caries Rate

1. *Previous Neglect.* A patient may not have kept a regular appointment plan, so that the existing dental caries during pregnancy represents an accumulation, possibly even of years.
2. *Diet During Pregnancy.* Possible increase in intake of fermentable carbohydrates
   a. Unusual cravings may be for sweet foods.
   b. Frequency of eating: patient may be eating every few hours for prevention of nausea and these foods may be cariogenic.
3. *Neglect of Personal Oral Care Procedures.* Lack of interest or laxity in toothbrushing or rinsing immediately following intake of a cariogenic food.

C. Calcium and the Mother's Teeth

The misconception concerning the withdrawal of calcium from the mother's teeth and its rela-

---

*An American Dental Association catalog for the current year may be obtained by writing the Order Section, 211 East Chicago Avenue, Chicago, Ill. 60611.

tionship to dental caries is widespread. It is important to review the known facts, because the patient's beliefs may need clarification. In discussing the problem with the patient, a summary of the process of dental caries initiation can be helpful (pages 242–243).

1. Minerals contained in the erupted tooth enamel and dentin are not available, and no removal of minerals can occur by way of the pulp.
2. Minerals contained within the alveolar bone are available as they are from other bones of the body. When the mother's diet does not contain sufficient calcium and phosphorus, her own reserve is utilized.
3. The majority of calcium and phosphorus of bones and teeth is added to the fetus during the third trimester. The incidence of dental caries in the mother is not different during that period, although the carious lesions may be larger if the teeth have been neglected throughout the pregnancy.
4. The teeth of the fetus tend to develop and mineralize normally in spite of the diet of the mother, because the reserve in her bones is used.

D. Relationship of Fluoride

No direct evidence shows that prenatal fluoride intake influences the rate of dental caries in the child.[11,12] When the community water supply is not fluoridated, dietary fluoride by prescription brings the fluoride intake to the optimum level and provides some benefit for the mother.

PARENT INSTRUCTION FOR THE NEWBORN

The goal is a dental caries-free child, with optimum gingival health. Parents can be helped to understand the importance of the oral health of the newborn and how habits practiced during the first year can influence future years.

Counseling for parents starts before and continues after the birth of the baby. Before birth, the parents are looking ahead and planning for the very best care for their baby. They are most receptive to meaningful recommendations.

Four areas for parental attention are described here. These are fluoride, the first dental appointment, diet and feeding practices, and daily bacterial plaque removal. Each child and family need individual adaptations.

I. Fluoride

Fluoride must be present in the infant's daily diet soon after birth while mineralization of the teeth is taking place.
A. Determine the fluoride content of the water supply used by the family (page 400).
B. Determine whether the baby is given water from the water supply. Children sometimes are given commercially bottled water.
C. Analyze the need for prescription
1. Totally breastfed infant needs .25 mg. sodium fluoride daily supplement (drops). When breast feeding is terminated, fluoride supplement continues if no fluoride is present in the drinking water (pages 400–401).
2. Bottle-fed baby receives formula made with fluoridated water; a supplement is prescribed when the water is nonfluoridated.

II. Infant's First Dental Visit

A. Age
The first appointment should be planned between ages 6 and 12 months, but no later than the first birthday.[13]

B. Purposes[14,15]
1. Discover, intercept, and change any practices applied by the parents that may be detrimental to the infant's oral health.
2. Initiate positive preventive measures: fluoride, feeding practices, and bacterial plaque removal.
3. Develop rapport with the baby and the family.

C. Record Medical and Dental History[14]
The forms for the histories are best filled out before the appointment. They can be mailed to the parents.

D. Appointment Procedures
1. *Oral Examination*
   a. Patient position: clinician and parent sit knee-to-knee with infant positioned on their laps. The clinician cradles the baby's head; the parent gently holds the baby's hands, and may stabilize the baby's legs with the elbows if necessary (figure 50–9D, page 627).
   b. Extra- and intraoral examination.
2. *Instruction for Bacterial Plaque Removal*
   a. Clinician demonstrates cleaning the teeth with a soft toothbrush; patient is held as described for the oral examination. Flossing will be needed when teeth are in close contact.
   b. Parent demonstrates the cleaning procedure: the baby is turned around so that the clinician holds the hands.
3. *Counseling*
   All aspects of significance for the particular child are discussed with the parents: fluoride, diet and feeding, daily oral care. Reading materials are provided.

E. Maintenance.
Plan for periodic preventive appointments.

III. Daily Bacterial Plaque Removal

A. Home Routine
Parents must plan a specific routine for cleaning the infant's teeth each day; usually at bath

time, when total body cleaning is accomplished, is most satisfactory.

B. Position of the Infant

Two family members can work together to make this a pleasant and easy experience. A system as has been described for the dental appointment can be used (figure 50–9, page 627).

IV. Diet and Feeding

A. Prevention of Nursing Bottle Caries

1. Describe nursing bottle caries and how it is caused.[16] Many parents do not realize that small babies can develop severe dental caries.
2. Advise no sweet juices or milk in naptime or bedtime bottles; only plain water should be used.
3. Recommend discontinuance of bottle feeding at least by the age of 12 months. The child can be taught to use a cup.[17]
4. Avoid "on demand" breast nursing practices. When the infant falls asleep, milk collects around the teeth. Dental caries can result (page 218).

B. Snacks

Non-sucrose-containing snacks must be used. Frequency and consistency of snack foods are most significant.

References

1. Fiese, R. and Herzog, S.: Issues in Dental and Surgical Management of the Pregnant Patient, *Oral Surg. Oral Med. Oral Pathol., 65,* 292, March, 1988.
2. Gier, R.E. and Janes, D.R.: Dental Management of the Pregnant Patient, *Dent. Clin. North Am., 27,* 419, April, 1983.
3. Ramfjord, S.P. and Ash, M.M.: *Periodontology and Periodontics.* Philadelphia, W.B. Saunders Co., 1979, pp. 196, 438, 441.
4. Carranza, F.A.: *Glickman's Clinical Periodontology,* 6th ed. Philadelphia, W.B. Saunders Co., 1984, pp. 132–133, 469–470, 904.
5. Goldman, H.M. and Cohen, D.W.: *Periodontal Therapy,* 6th ed. St. Louis, The C.V. Mosby Co., 1980, pp. 161–164.
6. Pindborg, J.J.: *Atlas of Diseases of the Oral Mucosa,* 4th ed. Philadelphia, W.B. Saunders Co., 1986, pp. 226–229.
7. Shafer, W.G., Hine, M.K., and Levy, B.M.: *A Textbook of Oral Pathology,* 4th ed. Philadelphia, W.B. Saunders Co., 1983, p. 359.
8. National Research Council, Committee on Dietary Allowances, Food and Nutrition Board: *Recommended Dietary Allowances,* 9th ed. Washington, D.C., National Academy of Sciences, Office of Publications, 1980.
9. Nizel, A.E.: *Nutrition in Preventive Dentistry,* 2nd ed. Philadelphia, W.B. Saunders Co., 1981, pp. 364–368.
10. Whitehead, R.G.: Pregnancy and Lactation, in Shils, M.E. and Young, V.R., eds.: *Modern Nutrition in Health and Disease,* 7th ed. Philadelphia, Lea & Febiger, 1988, pp. 931–943.
11. Driscoll, W.S.: A Review of Clinical Research on the Use of Prenatal Fluoride Administration for Prevention of Dental Caries, *ASDC J. Dent. Child., 48,* 109, March-April, 1981.
12. Thylstrup, A.: Is There a Biological Rationale for Prenatal Fluoride Administration? *ASDC J. Dent. Child., 48,* 103, March-April, 1981.
13. American Academy of Pediatric Dentistry: Oral Health Policies for Children: Policy Statement on Infant Dental Care, American Academy of Pediatric Dentistry, 211 E. Chicago Avenue, Chicago, Illinois 60611, May, 1986.
14. Goepferd, S.J.: Infant Oral Health: A Rationale, *ASDC J. Dent. Child., 53,* 257, July-August, 1986.
15. Goepferd, S.J.: Infant Oral Health: A Protocol, *ASDC J. Dent. Child., 53,* 261, July-August, 1986.
16. Yasin-Harnekar, S.: Nursing Caries. A Review, *Clin. Prevent. Dent., 10,* 3, March-April, 1988.
17. American Academy of Pediatric Dentistry and American Academy of Pediatrics: VI. Nursing Bottle Caries, American Academy of Pediatric Dentistry, 211 E. Chicago Avenue, Chicago, Illinois 60611, January, 1978.

Suggested Readings

American Dental Association, Council on Dental Therapeutics: *Accepted Dental Therapeutics,* 40th ed. Chicago, American Dental Association, 1984, pp. 54–55, 169–170, 288, 397, 400.

Beck-Coon, R.J. and Beck-Coon, K.A.: Dental Treatment in the Pregnant or Nursing Patient, *Gen. Dent., 30,* 237, May-June, 1982.

Blinkhorn, A.S.: Dental Preventive Advice for Pregnant and Nursing Mothers—Sociological Implications, *Int. Dent. J., 31,* 14, March, 1981.

Chiodo, G.T. and Rosenstein, D.I.: Dental Treatment During Pregnancy: A Preventive Approach, *J. Am. Dent. Assoc., 110,* 365, March, 1985.

Chiodo, G.T. and Rosenstein, D.I.: Pregnancy and Risks in the Dental Office, *Dent. Assist., 55,* 9, March-April, 1986.

Donegan, W.L.: Cancer and Pregnancy, *CA, 33,* 194, July/August, 1983.

Jankowski, C.B.: Radiation and Pregnancy. Putting the Risks in Proportion, *Am. J. Nurs., 86,* 260, March, 1986.

Jensen, J., Liljemark, W., and Bloomquist, C.: The Effect of Female Sex Hormones on Subgingival Plaque, *J. Periodontol., 52,* 599, October, 1981.

Karolus, J.A.: A Dental Hygienist's Approach to Pregnancy and Nutrition, *Dent. Hyg., 54,* 267, June, 1980.

Kornman, K.S. and Loesche, W.J.: The Subgingival Microbial Flora During Pregnancy, *J. Periodont. Res., 15,* 111, March, 1980.

Little, J.W. and Falace, D.A.: *Dental Management of the Medically Compromised Patient,* 2nd ed. St. Louis, The C.V. Mosby Co., 1984, pp. 226–232.

Littner, M.M., Kaffe, I., Tamse, A., and Moskona, D.: Management of the Pregnant Patient, *Quintessence Int., 15,* 253, February, 1984.

Löe, H.: Periodontal Changes in Pregnancy, *J. Periodontol., 36,* 209, May-June, 1965.

Martin, B.J., Stewart, J.S., and Stone, M.N.: Pregnancy Gingivitis and the Dental Hygienist's Intervention, *Can. Dent. Hyg., 19,* 121, Winter, 1985.

National Health and Medical Research Council: Guidelines for Dental Treatment: Dentistry and Pregnancy, *Aust. Dent. J., 29,* 265, August, 1984.

Rothwell, B.R., Gregory, C.E.B., and Sheller, B.: The Pregnant Patient: Considerations in Dental Care, *Spec. Care Dentist., 7,* 124, May-June, 1987.

Sahu, S.: Risks of Drugs to the Fetus and the Neonate, *Am. Fam. Physician, 24,* 147, October, 1981.

Schwartz, M., Holmes, H.I., and Schwartz, S.S.: Care of the Pregnant Patient, *Can. Dent. Assoc. J., 53,* 299, April, 1987.

Sexton, M. and Hebel, J.R.: A Clinical Trial of Change in Maternal Smoking and Its Effect on Birth Weight, *JAMA, 251,* 911, February 17, 1984.

Smith, N.J.D.: Dental Radiography During Pregnancy, *Br. Dent. J., 152,* 346, May 18, 1982.

Sonis, S.T., Fazio, R.C., and Fang, L.: *Principles and Practice of Oral Medicine.* Philadelphia, W.B. Saunders Co., 1984, pp. 199–205.

Adolescent Pregnancy

Alton, I.R.: Nutrition Services for Pregnant Adolescents within a Public High School, *J. Am. Dietet. Assoc., 74,* 667, June, 1979.

Bekenstein, S., Carter, M.H., LaRoche, M., Smith, K.E., and Francis, B.J.: Pregnant Adolescent Group for Education and Support—Illinois, *MMWR, 36,* 549, August 28, 1987.

Berg, M., Taylor, B., Edwards, L.E., and Hakanson, E.Y.: Prenatal Care for Pregnant Adolescents in a Public High School, *J. School Health, 49,* 32, January, 1979.

Steinman, M.E.: Reaching and Helping the Adolescent Who Becomes Pregnant, *Am. J. Maternal Child Nurs., 4,* 35, January/February, 1979.

Thwaites, M.S. and Cox, G.M.: The Psychosocial Aspects of Adolescent Pregnancy: A Dental Perspective, *ASDC J. Dent. Child., 53,* 371, September-October, 1986.

Infant Care

Berkowitz, R.J. and Jones, P.: Mouth-to-Mouth Transmission of the Bacterium *Streptococcus mutans* Between Mother and Child, *Archs. Oral Biol., 30,* 377, Number 4, 1985.

Brams, M. and Maloney, J.: "Nursing Bottle Caries" in Breast-fed Children, *J. Pediatr., 103,* 415, September, 1983.

Coll, J.A. and Conlan, J.G.: The Pediatric Dental Office, *Pediatr. Clin. North Am., 29,* 743, June, 1982.

Doshi, S.B.: A Study of Dental Habits, Knowledge and Opinions of Nursing Mothers, *Can. Dent. Assoc. J., 51,* 429, June, 1985.

Finocchi, L.L.: Breast Feeding, Bottle Feeding and Their Impact on Oral Habits. A Review of the Literature, *Dent. Hyg., 56,* 21, November, 1982.

George, D.I. and O'Toole, T.J.: A Review of Drug Transfer to the Infant by Breast-feeding: Concerns for the Dentist, *J. Am. Dent. Assoc., 106,* 204, February, 1983.

Goepferd, S.J.: An Infant Oral Health Program: The First 18 Months, *Pediatr. Dent., 9,* 8, March, 1987.

Gordon, Y. and Reddy, J.: Prevalence of Dental Caries, Patterns of Sugar Consumption and Oral Hygiene Practices in Infancy in S. Africa, *Community Dent. Oral Epidemiol., 13,* 310, December, 1985.

Johnson, J. and Bawden, J.W.: The Fluoride Content of Infant Formulas Available in 1985, *Pediatr. Dent., 9,* 33, March, 1987.

Kuster, C.G.: The Modern Pediatric Dental Office Experience, *Pediatr. Ann., 14,* 148, February, 1985.

Loesche, W.J.: Nutrition and Dental Decay in Infants, *Am. J. Clin. Nutr., 41,* 423, February, 1985.

Roberts, G.J.: Is Breast Feeding a Possible Cause of Dental Caries? *J. Dent., 10,* 346, December, 1982.

Sanger, R.G. and Bystrom, E.B.: Breast Feeding: Does It Affect Oral Facial Growth? *Dent. Hyg., 56,* 44, June, 1982.

Seow, W.K.: Oral Complications of Premature Birth, *Aust. Dent. J., 31,* 23, February, 1986.

Seow, W.K., Brown, J.P., Tudehope, D.A., and O'Callaghan, M.: Dental Defects in the Deciduous Dentition of Premature Infants with Low Birth Weight and Neonatal Rickets, *Pediatr. Dent., 6,* 88, June, 1984.

Wood, N. and Turner, J.W.: Fetal Alcohol Syndrome: A Review, *ASDC J. Dent. Child., 48,* 198, May-June, 1981.

44 *Preadolescent to Postmenopausal Patients*

The endocrine glands are glands of internal secretion. They secrete highly specialized substances—the hormones—which, with the nervous system, maintain body homeostasis.

A hormone is a chemical product of an organ or of certain cells within an organ, which has a specific regulatory effect upon cells remote from its origin. Hormones are transported by the blood or lymph. They may act directly on body cells or may act to control the hormones of other glands. Their complex and unified action augments and regulates many vital functions, including growth and development, energy production, food metabolism, reproductive processes, and the responses of the body to stress.

The major endocrine glands are the pituitary, thyroid, parathyroids, pancreas, adrenals, and gonads. The anterior pituitary is called the master gland, because it is the regulator of the output of hormones by other glands. In turn, the pituitary itself is regulated by the hormones of the other glands.

Both hyposecretion and hypersecretion of a hormone can cause physical and mental disturbances. Regulation of hormonal secretion is complex, and the mechanisms are not fully known. Normally, hormones are secreted when needed. The external temperature, for example, can influence the production of thyroxin of the thyroid gland. The calcium level of the blood affects parathyroid activity.

Hormones of the reproductive system have a controlling influence on the development and function of the individual. Some of the relationships to oral health and patient care are discussed in this chapter.

PUBERTY AND ADOLESCENCE[1,2]

Puberty is the period during which the gonads mature and begin to function. *Adolescence* is the period extending from time of puberty to the attainment of maturity.

I. Pubertal Changes

Chronologic age is an unreliable indicator, because puberty may begin normally in either sex between 9 and 17 years of age, depending on other factors such as race, heredity, and nutritional status. Generally, the secondary sex characteristics begin to appear between 10 and 13 years of age in girls; changes appear later in boys, starting at about 13 or 14 years. The major changes are usually complete in 3 to 4 years.

A. Hormonal Influences

Pituitary hormones control the hormones produced by the ovaries and the testes. The several hormones produced by the ovaries are known collectively as *estrogens,* and those produced by the testes are called *androgens.* They are responsible for the development of the sex organs, the accessory sex organs, and the secondary sex characteristics, and have strong physical, mental, and emotional influences throughout the body.

B. Female Development
1. Beginning of menstruation and ovulation. Menstruation may precede the first ovulation.
2. Development of the sex organs: fallopian tubes, uterus, vagina, and breasts.
3. Appearance of secondary sex characteristics
   a. Growth of pubic and axillary hair.
   b. Skeletal development: especially enlargement of the pelvis.
   c. Fat deposition on the hips.
   d. Voice drops one or two tones.

C. Male Development
1. Increase in size of testes and scrotum and beginning of spermatogenesis.
2. Development of the sex organs: vas deferens, seminal vesicles, prostate, and penis.
3. Appearance of secondary sex characteristics
   a. Growth of beard and pubic and axillary hair.
   b. Voice deepens.

II. Characteristics of Adolescence

A. Growth Spurt
1. Varies in age of occurrence, extent, and duration; usually occurs in boys between 12 and 16, girls 11 to 14.
2. Marked by rapid, extensive growth in height, weight, and muscle mass.
3. Overeating with underexercise along with psychologic problems make obesity a difficult and serious problem.
4. Poor coordination and awkwardness in young adolescents may result from irregular, uneven stages of growth.

B. Nutritional Requirements
1. Highest of any time in life for boys; will be exceeded only during pregnancy for girls.
2. Undernutrition is common; in boys, because

of overactivity and poor food selection; in girls, because of voluntary diet restrictions with poor food selection and fad diets in the attempt to keep slim.

3. Iron-deficiency anemia is not uncommon among teen-age girls, particularly after the onset of menstruation.

C. Skin Disorders

Acne vulgaris is common. Sebaceous and sweat glands are more active.

III. Personal Factors

Adolescents are no longer children, and yet they have not reached adulthood. They may respond and wish to be treated as adults or as children at different times. They are learning to adapt to body changes, sexual impulses, and secondary sex characteristics. The most likely causes of anxiety in adolescents are sex, performance in school, family relationships, peer pressures, substance abuse, confusion over their beliefs, and concern about their futures.

No fixed picture can be described, but characteristics listed here are exhibited to one degree or another by many adolescents.

A. Increased Self-interest

1. Adolescents have a great deal of concern for themselves and respond best to those who show concern for them.
2. They want attention and tend to reject those who do not listen.

B. Growing Independence

1. Adolescence is a period of rapidly growing independence of thought and action with conflicts between feelings of dependence and independence.
2. Childhood dependence on parents is gradually given up; the idea of infallibility of parents is lost; teachers and others in authority are questioned.
3. Personal identity is sought; adolescents are uncertain about their place and role in society.
4. Independence from parents frequently means increased confidence in and respect for other adults outside the family.

C. Concern over Physical Characteristics

1. Girls mature earlier than boys, and young female adolescents are usually taller than males, which presents social problems.
2. Increased interest in personal appearance; adolescents want to dress and be like their peers.
3. Problems such as delayed growth and sexual development and obesity can be extremely important.

IV. Oral Conditions

A. Dental Caries

The incidence of dental caries is often higher during adolescence than in other age groups in communities without fluoridation. This can be related to the dietary and eating habits of most adolescents. Appetite becomes intensified by the demands of rapid growth as well as by the emotional problems confronted, which leads to frequent eating. Many cariogenic foods are eaten, particularly between meals and in social settings.

B. Periodontal Infections

Young people under 20 years of age are subject to all categories of periodontal infections (table 12–1, page 180).

1. *Gingivitis.* A large majority of adolescents has gingivitis. An exaggerated response to local irritants sometimes occurs during puberty and is believed to be related to hormonal influences that may be conditioning factors.[3,4]

   The gingiva enlarge, particularly the papillae; pockets form; and the tissue appears bulbous and bluish-red. Local contributing factors include mouth breathing, erupting teeth, and orthodontic appliances.

2. *Chronic Periodontitis.* Loss of periodontal attachment and supporting bone is evident in 5 to 47 percent of adolescents examined around the world.[5–10] Careful probing and study of radiographs are indicated for each patient so that precautions may be taken, preventive measures introduced, and early treatment initiated.

3. *Juvenile Periodontitis.* Localized juvenile periodontitis, a rare condition formerly called periodontosis, is characterized by early bone destruction during circumpubertal and mid-teen years.[11] Symmetrical bone loss associated with the incisors and first permanent molars occurs more severely than can usually be explained by bacterial plaque and local predisposing factors. As the disease progresses and when plaque and calculus accumulate, chronic inflammatory periodontitis becomes clearly apparent, with tooth mobility and migration, deep pockets, and other typical signs of severe periodontal disease.

4. *Necrotizing Ulcerative Gingivitis.* Although found infrequently in children, necrotizing ulcerative gingivitis has its highest frequency in older adolescents and young adults. Stress, undernutrition, lack of plaque control, neglect of oral health, as well as psychosomatic factors are implicated as predisposing influences in its development (page 482).

DENTAL HYGIENE CARE

Dental and dental hygiene care during adolescence can influence oral health throughout the patient's lifetime. As future parents and community participants, the knowledge, attitudes, and practices acquired and developed during adolescence can have wide-reaching significance.

I. Patient Approach

Adolescence is a period of transition. Working with adolescents offers a real challenge, and each situation requires its own approach. Some of the physical and psychologic characteristics have been listed in this chapter to provide a framework for what may be expected. A few basic suggestions for approach include the following:

A. Treat adolescents as adults. Physically many of them are mature, although their emotional development may be at various levels.

B. Set the stage to let them know of your interest in them and their problems. Encourage them to talk, and then listen.

C. Suggest and advise, but do not become impatient or take offense when they try to make their own decisions.

D. They are usually interested in health matters and details about their physical condition, although they may act indifferent. Cleanliness and attractiveness are important to the teen-age patient.

E. Health, including oral health, may be a real concern. Adolescents need to be well informed about their oral conditions, and explanations on a scientific basis are generally appreciated.

II. Patient History

Adolescents should provide their own information for the medical and dental histories. It may also be necessary to consult the parents for information, but not in the same interview with the patient and not without the patient's knowledge.

Adolescents need to begin to take increasing responsibility for their own health. Although the initial dental visit may be at the insistence of the parents, every effort of the dentist and dental hygienist should be to focus the evaluation and treatment on the patient, not the parents.

The adolescent patient may also have other health problems. The patient with diabetes, heart disease, a mental, physical, or sensory handicap, or other systemic involvement requires special methods for approach as described in the various chapters of this book. Medical clearance by parent or legal guardian is necessary for conditions requiring antibiotic coverage or other medication for a patient under legal adult age.

III. Oral Health Problems in Adolescence[12]

Dental caries and periodontal infections of the adolescent years have been described. Some examples of other oral problems related to adolescent development and behavior characteristics are listed here.

A. Oral manifestations of sexually transmitted diseases (STD).

B. Effects of tobacco: leukoplakia, periodontal damage from smokeless tobacco products.

C. Effects of oral contraceptives on periodontal tissues (pages 556–557).

D. Oral findings of anorexia nervosa or bulimia (page 381).

E. Traumatic injury to teeth and oral structures from athletic activities, as well as from driving accidents.

IV. Bacterial Plaque Control

A clear explanation of the causes of dental caries and periodontal conditions, with the methods for their prevention, is basic. Adolescents need to understand the effects of the accumulation of bacterial plaque, the purposes of professional calculus removal, and the relation of the daily self-care plaque-control program to the health status of the gingiva.

For dental caries prevention, adolescents must appreciate the effects of fluoride and the need to restrict cariogenic foods that cling to the teeth. The program is outlined and conducted on the basis of these clear-cut preventive measures.

A. Instruction in self-care procedures.

B. Continuing review over a series of appointments is necessary to develop daily practices that can be carried on into adult life.

V. Instrumentation

A series of appointments frequently is required, depending on pocket depth and extent of calculus deposits. Careful and complete scaling and root planing and removal of all local irregularities and predisposing factors are the basic treatment procedures.

VI. Fluoride Treatment Program

A combined fluoride program is indicated for most adolescent patients, particularly for those who have not lived in a community with a fluoridated water supply. In addition to the topical applications made in conjunction with dental hygiene professional appointments, self-administered methods should include a fluoride dentifrice along with a mouthrinse following toothbrushing. A daily application of a fluoride gel in a custom-made tray may even be necessary for remineralization (page 407). The methods are described in Chapter 29.

VII. Diet Control

A. Dietary Analysis (pages 383–389)

A study of the patient's diet and counseling relative to general nutrition and dental caries control can provide important learning experiences for many adolescents. The parent or other person who is in charge of shopping and food preparation must be included, in order that appropriate foods will be available for selection. As much responsibility as possible should be placed on the patient.

B. Instruction Suggestions

1. *Advise Foods from the Four Food Groups* (page 382). For growth, energy, clear complexion, and prevention of illness.

2. *Emphasize a Good Breakfast.* Teen-agers tend to slight or omit breakfast, particularly if they have to prepare it for themselves.

3. *Snack Selection.* From the nutritious foods, with recognition of cariogenic foods. Snacks suggested can include raw fruits and vegetables, nuts, milk, use of sugar-free foods when possible, and sugarless chewing gum if used.

MENSTRUATION

The menstrual cycle refers to the cyclic structural changes in the uterus, instigated by hormones, which represent periodic preparation of the lining of the uterus for fertilization of the ovum and pregnancy. When fertilization does not take place, changes in the mucous membrane lining the uterus (the endometrium) lead to the menstrual discharge. The fluid discharged is composed primarily of blood with fragments of the disintegrated endometrium.

I. Characteristics

A. Occurrence

The cyclic changes occur from puberty to menopause except during pregnancy and part of breast feeding. Although the average cycle is complete in about 28 days, the normal range is from 22 to 34 days.

B. Menarche

Menstruation may begin at any time from ages 9 to 17. The mean age in the United States is between 12 and 13 years.

Menarche, the beginning of menstruation, frequently occurs before ovulation, that is, before the pituitary and ovarian hormones are synchronized and ovulation becomes a part of the menstrual cycle. Timing and extent of flow may be irregular for several months or even a few years after the onset of menstruation.

II. Irregularities

Variations in the menstrual cycle are common. The pattern of the cycle may be upset by such factors as changes in climate, changes in work schedule, emotional trauma, acute or chronic illnesses, weight loss, and excessive exercise.

Menstruation may have strong emotional impact, and associated disturbances may have psychologic bases. Intense emotional conflicts may be related to the inability to accept the feminine role and assume the responsibilities of womanhood. Some or all of the symptoms of premenstrual tension and dysmenorrhea described in the following may continue beyond adolescence and even to menopause.

A. Premenstrual Tension

This disorder is associated with fluid retention in the body and psychologic depression occurring within 10 days prior to menstruation. Symptoms may include headache, fatigue, weight gain, heaviness in the lower abdomen, and fullness and tenderness of the breasts. Feelings of depression and irritability with mood variations are common. The symptoms disappear when menstrual flow begins.

B. Dysmenorrhea

Difficult or painful menstruation may be caused by conditions such as tumors or inflammatory diseases in women past adolescence. In adolescents, causes are generally related to physiologic and/or psychologic factors. Dysmenorrhea is frequently an indication of the adolescent's emotional status, which may result from poor preparation for the arrival of puberty and menstruation, or from parental example.

Although a high percentage of women have some discomfort, a smaller percentage suffer severe pain with "cramps," sometimes accompanied by nausea and vomiting.

III. Dental Hygiene Care

A. Patient History

Menstruation is a normal process and should not be referred to as a "sick period" or a "monthly illness." When presenting questions for the patient history, use of terms such as the "period" or "monthly period" is preferable. A question about the regularity of menstruation should be included in each review medical history. When the menstrual period of a woman of child-bearing age, especially one who has indicated that she is trying to get pregnant, is delayed, treatment should be limited until it is known whether she is pregnant.

The menstrual history may provide indications of a woman's general health. Regularly excessive menstrual flow may be related to an anemic state, and medical examination and treatment are indicated.

B. Oral Findings[4]

No specific gingival changes are related to the menstrual cycle. An exaggerated response to local irritants or unusual gingival bleeding during or following scaling may be noted in an occasional patient. With control of local irritants by plaque control, self-care measures, and removal of calculus at regular maintenance appointments, bleeding can be controlled.

Recurrent aphthous ulcers have been associated with the menstrual cycle in susceptible patients. A recurrence of more severe symptoms of necrotizing ulcerative gingivitis when treatment has not been completed has been observed.

ORAL CONTRACEPTIVES

Birth control pills are recognized as the most effective method of contraception when they are taken as prescribed. Because of their convenience, they are used by millions of women worldwide.

I. Types

A. Combination Preparations

1. *Estrogen and Progesterone.* The combination of synthetically produced hormones estrogen and progesterone is nearly 100 percent effective in preventing ovulation. Estrogen inhibits the secretion of follicle-stimulating hormone (FSH) and progesterone inhibits the release of luteinizing hormone (LH) by the anterior pituitary gland. Without the hormones FSH and LH, the ovum cannot be released from the ovary.

2. *Schedule of Administration.* One pill is taken each day for 20 or 21 days starting 5 days after the onset of the menstrual flow. Then, for a period of 7 days, no pill is taken. The routine is followed regardless of when menstruation starts or stops.

B. Single Preparations

1. *Minipill.* Progesterone alone is effective 97 to 98 percent of the time. When this type of pill is used, menstrual cycles tend to be more irregular and side effects more frequent.

2. *Postcoital ("Morning After Pill").* The drug in this preparation, diethylstilbestrol, is not used except in emergency situations such as rape or incest.

II. Contraindications[13]

Contraceptives containing hormones should not be taken when the woman has a history of the following:

A. Thromboembolic disorders.
B. Impaired liver function.
C. Known or suspected cancer of the breast or other estrogen-dependent neoplasia.
D. Undiagnosed genital bleeding.
E. Smoking.

III. Side Effects

Many side effects have been reported, and not all have been researched. Visual problems, mental depression, rashes, and bleeding irregularities occur in some women. The most significant effects are the following:

A. Cardiovascular (including increased blood pressure).
B. Induction of tumors.
C. Decreased effectiveness of the contraceptive when certain drugs are used, including the following:[14,15]
1. Antibiotics.
2. Anticonvulsants.
3. Rifampin (used in treatment of tuberculosis).

IV. Effect on the Gingiva

An exaggerated response to bacterial plaque and other local irritants has been noted, especially when the personal oral hygiene is less than adequate. The gingivitis is similar to that described for pregnancy (page 546). There appears to be an increase in the extent of gingival reaction associated with extended use of the contraceptive over several years.[16]

V. Appointment Considerations

A. Medical History

A record of the use of oral contraceptives should be made and reviewed with each history review.

B. Patient Information

1. Explain the need for exceptional personal oral care and regular professional maintenance appointments to prevent complications from gingivitis.
2. Explain the need for additional contraception when antibiotic premedication or other use of antibiotics is indicated.
3. Alert patient to side effects and advise medical evaluation if side effects become troublesome.

MENOPAUSE AND CLIMACTERIC

Menopause is the cessation of menstruation. It occurs normally between the ages of 42 and 55, with the average between 47 and 49. It may be induced by surgical removal of the ovaries or by radiation therapy.

The female *climacteric* is that period of change during the gradual decline of ovarian efficiency when ovulation is less regular and finally ends, through the menopause, and including the period after menopause when the body is adjusting to endocrine and other changes. While adolescence is considered the transitional period from childhood into maturity, the climacteric has been described as the transitional period from maturity into senescence.

I. Characteristics

Prior to menopause, menstruation decreases in frequency, duration, and amount of flow over a period of about 12 to 24 months. Although many women may experience minor symptoms, only about 10 percent have any pronounced effects from menopause.

A. General Symptoms

With diminishing estrogen, as ovarian function declines, physiologic changes in body function take place. Vasomotor reactions in the form of hot flashes, in which sudden, periodic surges of heat involving the whole body and accompanied by drenching sweats may occur during the day or night. Although a strict distinction is not always made between flush and flash, the term hot flush may be used to mean a reaction of lesser degree in which a wave of warmth is felt over the face, neck, and upper thorax. Headaches, heart palpitations, and sleeplessness may occur.

Emotional disturbances are not caused specifically by estrogen deficiencies but are frequently related to personal and family circumstances and concern over growing old. Anxiety, tension, irritability, with depression and feelings of uselessness may appear.

B. Postmenopausal Effects

1. Reproductive organs atrophy.
2. Changes in bones may lead to osteoporosis. This condition is less frequent among people who have used drinking water containing fluoride over the years.
3. Skin and mucous membranes decrease in thickness and keratinization.
4. Predisposition to other conditions includes atherosclerosis, diabetes, and hypothyroidism.

II. Oral Findings

Oral disturbances that can be related to the menopause are relatively uncommon. Findings are nonspecific.

A. Gingiva

Gingival changes associated with menopause usually represent an exaggerated response to local irritation, which reflects the conditioning influence of the hormonal changes taking place. When local factors are controlled through preventive dental hygiene appointments for maintenance to supplement daily personal oral care, unusual gingival changes are uncommon.

Rarely, a condition that has been called menopausal gingivostomatitis may develop.[17] It may also occur after removal of, or radiation therapy to, the ovaries.

B. Mucous Membranes and Tongue

1. Dryness with burning or unusual taste sensations may be present.
2. Epithelium may become thin and atrophic with decreased keratinization; tolerance for removable prostheses may lessen.
3. Inadequate diet and eating habits may contribute to the adverse changes of the mucosal tissues. The appearance and symptoms frequently resemble those associated with vitamin deficiencies, particularly B vitamins.

III. Dental Hygiene Care

In the approach to the patient, a specific relationship of oral conditions to menopause should not be made, because the patient may tend to overemphasize such a relationship and de-emphasize the need for self-care measures. Because of the importance of local factors, attention should be directed to the need for regular and frequent professional care as well as to increased efforts for daily plaque control.

A. Appointment Suggestions

The symptoms of physical and emotional changes should be kept in mind when planning and conducting the appointment. The patient's possible tenseness and irritability can be antici-

pated, and attention to details, such as not keeping the patient waiting unduly, handling materials and instruments with calm assurance, and maintaining conservativeness in conversation to prevent annoyances, may be significant.

B. Instruction of Patient

Preservation of oral health is particularly important to the woman who has her natural teeth. Because of the possible difficulties and discomforts of wearing prostheses, every effort should be made to prevent the need for tooth removal. A saliva substitute may provide a degree of relief from xerostomia (pages 187–188).

Measures for the prevention of periodontal infections should be carefully explained, and emphasis placed on reasons for frequent calculus removal supplemented by meticulous daily care. Because good general health practices are very important to this age group, the relationship of general and oral health can be brought out.

C. Diet

A dietary survey may prove to be a helpful teaching-learning experience (page 383), by helping the patient to identify and correct inadequately balanced food selection. When a patient tends to indulge in between-meal eating, caries prevention through selection of nutritious and noncariogenic foods is emphasized.

References

1. Adams, W.: Adolescence, in Gabel, S. and Erickson, M.T., eds.: *Child Development and Developmental Disabilities.* Boston, Little, Brown & Co., 1980, pp. 59–81.
2. DeAngelis, C.: Special Aspects of Care for Adolescents, in Harvey, A.M., Johns, R.J., McKusick, V.A., Owens, A.H., and Ross, R.S., eds.: *The Principles and Practice of Medicine*, 21st ed. Norwalk, Connecticut, Appleton-Century-Crofts, 1984, pp. 1473–1483.
3. Pawlak, E.A. and Hoag, P.M.: *Essentials of Periodontics*, 3rd ed. St. Louis, The C.V. Mosby Co., 1984, pp. 44–45.
4. Carranza, F.A.: *Glickman's Clinical Periodontology*, 6th ed. Philadelphia, W.B. Saunders Co., 1984, pp. 133–134, 467–468, 904.
5. MacGregor, I.D.M.: Radiographic Survey of Periodontal Disease in 264 Adolescent Schoolboys in Lagos, Nigeria, *Community Dent. Oral Epidemiol., 8,* 56, February, 1980.
6. Mann, J., Cormier, P.P., Green, P., Ram, C.A., Miller, M.F., and Ship, I.I.: Loss of Periodontal Attachment in Adolescents, *Community Dent. Oral Epidemiol., 9,* 135, June, 1981.
7. Latcham, N.L., Powell, R.N., Jago, J.D., and Seymour, G.J.: A Radiographic Study of Chronic Periodontitis in 15 Year Old Queensland Children, *J. Clin. Periodontol., 10,* 37, January, 1983.
8. Hansen, B.F., Gjermo, P., and Bergwitz-Larsen, K.R.: Periodontal Bone Loss in 15-year-old Norwegians, *J. Clin. Periodontol., 11,* 125, March, 1984.
9. Gjermo, P., Bellini, H.T., Santos, V.P., Martins, J.G., and Ferracyoli, J.R.: Prevalence of Bone Loss in a Group of Brazilian Teenagers Assessed on Bite-wing Radiographs, *J. Clin. Periodontol., 11,* 104, February, 1984.
10. Wolfe, M.D. and Carlos, J.P.: Periodontal Disease in Adolescents: Epidemiologic Findings in Navajo Indians, *Community Dent. Oral Epidemiol., 15,* 33, February, 1987.
11. Newman, M.G.: Localized Juvenile Periodontitis (Periodontosis), *Pediatr. Dent., 3,* 121, May, 1981.
12. Machen, J.B.: Guidelines for Dental Health of the Adoles-

cent—May, 1986, 1985–86 AAPD Clinical Affairs Committee, *Pediatr. Dent., 9,* 247, September, 1987.

13. Murad, F. and Haynes, R.C.: Estrogens and Progestins, in Gilman, A.G., Goodman, L.S., Rall, T.W., and Murad, F., eds.: *Goodman and Gilman's The Pharmacological Basis of Therapeutics,* 7th ed. New York, MacMillan Publishing Co., 1985, pp. 1430–1439.
14. Orme, M.L.E. and Back, D.J.: Drug Interactions Between Oral Contraceptive Steroids and Antibiotics, *Br. Dent. J., 160,* 169, March 8, 1986.
15. Bainton, R.: Interaction Between Antibiotic Therapy and Contraceptive Medication, *Oral Surg. Oral Med. Oral Pathol., 61,* 453, May, 1986.
16. Pankhurst, C.L., Waite, I.M., Hicks, K.A., Allen, Y., and Harkness, R.D.: The Influence of Oral Contraceptive Therapy on the Periodontium—Duration of Drug Therapy, *J. Periodontol., 52,* 617, October, 1981.
17. Carranza: op. cit., p. 470.

Suggested Readings

Cureton, S.L.: Premenstrual Syndrome and Dentistry, *Gen. Dent., 34,* 364, September-October, 1986.
Neimi, M.-L., Ainamo, J., and Sandholm, L.: The Occurrence of Gingival Brushing Lesions During 3 Phases of the Menstrual Cycle, *J. Clin. Periodontol., 13,* 27, January, 1986.

Puberty and Adolescence

Albino, J.E., Tedesco, L.A., and Phipps, G.T.: Social and Psychological Problems of Adolescence and Their Relevance to Dental Care, *Int. Dent. J., 32,* 184, June, 1982.
Bergendal, B. and Hamp, S.-E.: Dietary Pattern and Dental Caries in 19-year-old Adolescents Subjected to Preventive Measures Focused on Oral Hygiene and/or Fluorides, *Swed. Dent. J., 9,* 1, Number 1, 1985.
Chertkow, S.: Tooth Mineralization as an Indicator of the Pubertal Growth Spurt, *Am. J. Orthod., 77,* 79, January, 1980.
Cipes, M.H., Kegeles, S.S., Lund, A.K., and Otradovec, C.L.: Differences in Dental Experiences, Practices and Beliefs of Inner-city and Suburban Adolescents, *Am. J. Public Health, 73,* 1305, November, 1983.
Crossner, C.-G. and Unell, L.: A Longitudinal Study of Dental Health and Treatment Need in Swedish Teenagers, *Community Dent. Oral Epidemiol., 14,* 10, February, 1986.
de Wet, F.A.: The Prevention of Orofacial Sports Injuries in the Adolescent, *Int. Dent. J., 31,* 313, December, 1981.
Garon, M.W., Merkle, A., and Wright, J.T.: Mouth Protectors and Oral Trauma: A Study of Adolescent Football Players, *J. Am. Dent. Assoc., 112,* 663, May, 1986.
Gröndahl, H.-G., Andersson, B., and Tortensson, T.: Caries Increment and Progression in Teenagers When Using a Prevention-Rather than Restoration-Oriented Treatment Strategy, *Swed. Dent. J., 8,* 237, Number 5, 1984.
Hamp, S.-E. and Johansson, L.-Å.: Dental Prophylaxis for Youths in Their Late Teens. I. Clinical Effect of Different Preventive Regimes on Oral Hygiene, Gingivitis and Dental Caries, *J. Clin. Periodontol., 9,* 22, January, 1982.
Hodge, H.C., Holloway, P.J., and Bell, C.R.: Factors Associated with Toothbrushing Behaviour in Adolescents, *Br. Dent. J., 152,* 49, January 19, 1982.
Howe, S.M. and Vaden, A.G.: Factors Differentiating Participants and Nonparticipants of the National School Lunch Program. I. Nutrient Intake of High School Students, *J. Am. Dietetic Assoc., 76,* 451, May, 1980.
Kampe, T., Edman, G., and Molin, C.: Personality Traits of Adolescents with Intact and Restored Dentitions, *Acta Odontol. Scand., 44,* 23, Number 1, 1986.
Lauer, R.M., Akers, R.L., Massey, J., and Clarke, W.R.: Evaluation of Cigarette Smoking Among Adolescents: The Muscatine Study, *Prev. Med., 11,* 417, July, 1982.
MacGregor, I.D.M. and Balding, J.W.: Toothbrushing Frequency, Cleanliness, and Smoking Habits in Young Adolescents, *Clin. Prevent. Dent., 9,* 18, January-February, 1987.

Marino, D.D. and King, J.C.: Nutritional Concerns During Adolescence, *Pediatr. Clin. North Am., 27,* 125, February, 1980.
Roberts, M.W., Li, S.H., Comite, F., Hench, K.D., Pescovitz, O.H., Cutler, G.B., and Loriaux, D.L.: Dental Development in Precocious Puberty, *J. Dent. Res., 64,* 1084, August, 1985.
Spencer, A.J.: Past Association of Fluoride Vehicles with Caries Severity in Australian Adolescents, *Community Dent. Oral Epidemiol., 14,* 233, October, 1986.

Periodontal Disease During Adolescence

Asikainen, S., Alaluusua, S., Kari, K., and Kleemola-Kujala, E.: Subgingival Microflora and Periodontal Conditions in Healthy Teenagers, *J. Periodontol., 57,* 505, August, 1986.
Cutress, T.W.: Periodontal Health and Periodontal Disease in Young People: Global Epidemiology, *Int. Dent. J., 36,* 146, September, 1986.
Ngan, P.W.H., Tsai, C.-C., and Sweeney, E.: Advanced Periodontitis in the Primary Dentition: Case Report, *Pediatr. Dent., 7,* 255, December, 1985.
Nordblad, A., Kallio, P., Ainamo, J., and Dusadeepan, A.: Periodontal Treatment Needs in Populations Under 20 Years of Age in Espoo, Finland and Chiangmai, Thailand, *Community Dent. Oral Epidemiol., 14,* 129, June, 1986.
Teiwik, A., Johansson, L.-Å., and Hamp, S.-E.: Marginal Bone Height in Adolescents Participating in Different Preventive Dental Care Programs, *J. Clin. Periodontol., 11,* 590, October, 1984.
Yanover, L. and Ellen, R.P.: A Clinical and Microbiologic Examination of Gingival Disease in Parapubescent Females, *J. Periodontol., 57,* 562, September, 1986.

Juvenile Periodontitis

Hangorsky, C.: Juvenile Periodontitis/Periodontosis: Historical Overview and Update, *Dent. Hyg., 56,* 29, June, 1982.
Liljenberg, B. and Lindhe, J.: Juvenile Periodontitis. Some Microbiological, Histopathological and Clinical Characteristics, *J. Clin. Periodontol., 7,* 48, February, 1980.
Mandell, R.L., Siegal, M.D., and Umland, E.: Localized Juvenile Periodontitis of the Primary Dentition, *ASDC J. Dent. Child., 53,* 193, May-June, 1986.
Rowat, J.S. and Rowe, D.J.: The Role of Impaired Host Defense Mechanisms in the Pathogenesis of Juvenile Periodontitis, *Dent. Hyg., 54,* 529, November, 1980.
Saxén, L.: Juvenile Periodontitis. A Review, *J. Clin. Periodontol., 7,* 1, February, 1980.
Saxén, L.: Heredity of Juvenile Periodontitis, *J. Clin. Periodontol., 7,* 276, August, 1980.
Sonis, A.L.: Periodontosis of the Primary Dentition: A Case Report, *Pediatr. Dent., 2,* 53, March, 1980.
Spektor, M.D., Vandesteen, G.E., and Page, R.C.: Clinical Studies of One Family Manifesting Rapidly Progressive, Juvenile and Prepubertal Periodontitis, *J. Periodontol., 56,* 93, February, 1985.
Zambon, J.J., Christersson, L.A., and Genco, R.J.: Diagnosis and Treatment of Localized Juvenile Periodontitis, *J. Am. Dent. Assoc., 113,* 295, August, 1986.

Oral Contraceptives

Barnett, M.L.: Inhibition of Oral Contraceptive Effectiveness by Concurrent Antibiotic Administration, A Review, *J. Periodontol., 56,* 18, January, 1985.
Catellani, J.E., Harvey, S., Erickson, S.H., and Cherkin, D.: Effect of Oral Contraceptive Cycle on Dry Socket (Localized Alveolar Osteitis), *J. Am. Dent. Assoc., 101,* 777, November, 1980.
Hertz, R.S., Beckstead, P.C., and Brown, W.J.: Epithelial Melanosis of the Gingiva Possibly Resulting from the Use of Oral Contraceptives, *J. Am. Dent. Assoc., 100,* 713, May, 1980.
Lorio, G.P.: Effects of Oral Contraceptives on the Oral Structures: A Review, *Gen. Dent., 30,* 140, March-April, 1982.
Murray, T.L.: Paying for the Pill: Side Effects Associated with Oral Contraceptives, *Dent. Assist., 51,* 20, May-June, 1982.
Vennetti, C.M. and Miller, S.S.: Oral Contraceptive Therapy. Effects on the Oral Tissues, *Dent. Hyg., 61,* 168, April, 1987.

Menopause

Kerr, D.A., Ash, M.M., and Millard, H.D.: *Oral Diagnosis,* 6th ed. St. Louis, The C.V. Mosby Co., 1983, pp. 63–64.

Snyder, M.B.: Endocrine Disease and Dysfunction, in Lynch, M.A., Brightman, V.J., and Greenberg, M.S., eds.: *Burkett's Oral Medicine,* 8th ed. Philadelphia, J.B. Lippincott Co., 1984, p. 840.

Wingrove, F.A., Rubright, W.C., and Kerber, P.E.: Influence of Ovarian Hormone Situation on Atrophy, Hypertrophy, and/or Desquamation of Human Gingiva in Premenopausal and Postmenopausal Women, *J. Periodontol., 50,* 445, September, 1979.

45 *The Gerodontic Patient*

Preventive measures for the aging population through care and instruction require greater emphasis as the number of people involved in this group increases steadily. By the year 2000, the population over age 65 is expected to represent nearly 13 percent of the total population of the United States, and by the year 2030, it will have increased to nearly 21 percent.[1]

Only 5 percent of persons 65 or over are in institutions such as mental hospitals, chronic disease hospitals, nursing homes, and other long-term care institutions for the aged.[1]

Members of the dental team are challenged by the need to help the aging population learn about personal care and seek professional care that will provide continuing oral comfort and function. As the percentage of people in the older group has increased, the total number of patients in a general or adult practice has grown. An increasing number of dental hygienists specialize in the care of the elderly and are employed in long-term care and resident facilities for the aged.

Tooth loss increases with age, but not because of age. Dental caries and periodontal diseases are the major causes of tooth loss. Periodontal diseases in the older population represent the cumulative effects of long-standing, undiagnosed, untreated, or neglected chronic infection, which may have had its origin in childhood. With application of current knowledge of preventive measures for all oral diseases in younger age groups, it is anticipated that future generations of older people will not be subjected to the severe effects of uncontrolled and untreated oral diseases.

AGING

When aging is defined from a chronologic viewpoint, the aging population may be recognized as the "older population" (age 55 and over), the "elderly" (age 65 and over), the "aged" (75 years and older), and the "very old" (85 years and over).[2] The elderly population has also been subgrouped as the young-old, the old-old, the active and well, the frail and homebound, and the handicapped, institutionalized, and noninstitutionalized.[3]

Biologic age is not synonymous with chronologic age, and hence, signs of aging appear at different chronologic ages in different individuals. In other words, some people are old at 45 years, while others are not old at 75 years.

Senescence, the process or condition of growing old, has sociocultural, as well as physiologic and chronologic implications. Normal aging should not be confused with the effects of pathologic influences that accelerate the aging process. Each age period brings changes in body metabolism, activity of the cells, endocrine balance, and mental processes.

An older person's health status is influenced by many factors. Both biologic and environmental factors influence longevity. Genetically, a person may belong to a family of healthy people who have exhibited great resistance to disease factors. Another person may have inherited a specific disease state. Even inherited diseases, for example diabetes or sickle cell anemia, may be controllable through treatment or genetic counseling.

CHARACTERISTICS OF AGING

Changes with aging vary among individuals and among organs and tissues of the same individual. It may be difficult to separate physiologic manifestations of aging from those of disease or the after effects of disease.

I. General Physiologic Changes

During aging, an overall reduction in functional capacities occurs in most organs, with a decrease in cell metabolism and numbers of active cells. The tissues may show signs of dehydration, atrophy, fibrosis, reduced elasticity, and diminished reparative ability, although many of these characteristics cannot be separated from pathologic changes.

A. Skeletal System
1. Skeletal integrity is significantly influenced by an insufficient intake of calcium, phosphorus, and fluoride (page 398).
2. Bone volume (mass) decreases gradually after the age of 40, depending on diet, nutrition, and exercise.
3. Osteoporosis is common in individuals over age 60, and the incidence increases with age. It is described on page 562.

B. Basal Metabolism
Basal metabolism is lowered.

C. Skin

The skin becomes thin, wrinkled, and dry, with pigmented spots, loss of tone, and atrophy of the sweat glands.

D. Locomotor System

Older patients may experience loss of muscle mass, development of unsteadiness and tremor, diminishing of muscular strength, decreased speed of response. Posture may become stooped; joints may stiffen as a result of loss of elasticity in the ligaments.

E. Gastrointestinal System

1. Production of hydrochloric acid and other secretions gradually decreases.
2. Peristalsis is slowed; absorptive functions decrease.

F. Cardiovascular System (Chapter 56)

Effects of aging on the cardiovascular system include the following:

1. Tendency toward increased blood pressure usually secondary to disease.
2. Arteriosclerosis, with decreased circulation to the tissues.
3. Reduced cardiac output; increased heart size.
4. Postural hypotension; with dizziness or weakness when sitting up from recumbent position.

G. Respiratory System

1. Vital capacity is progressively diminished.
2. Pulmonary efficiency is decreased.

H. Special Senses (Chapter 55)

1. *Vision.* Decline in accommodation, color and depth perception, and difficulty in adapting from light to dark.
2. *Hearing.* Reduced hearing ability, with a loss of sensitivity to high tones.

II. Diseases in the Elderly

With increasing age, the incidence of chronic mental and physical diseases increases. A patient may have more than one condition. Examples of diseases that are common among the elderly are cardiovascular (pages 682–694), osteoarthritis (page 670), diabetes (page 715), and vision and hearing impairment (pages 674–680). Osteoporosis is also a frequently occurring condition.

A. Response to Disease

1. *Course and Severity.* Although the diseases that affect the elderly also occur in younger persons, the course and effects of the diseases may differ. In the elderly, disease may occur with greater severity and have a longer course, with slower recovery.
2. *Pain Sensitivity.* May be lessened.
3. *Temperature Response.* May be altered so that a patient may be very ill without an expected body temperature increase.
4. *Healing*
   a. Decreased healing capacity.
   b. More prone to secondary infection.

B. Causes of Disability

According to the World Health Organization,[2] the most prevalent long-term diseases that cause the greatest incapacity or disability in persons over 65 years of age include the cardiovascular and cerebrovascular diseases, cancer, diseases of the locomotor system, mental illness, accidents, alcoholism, and pathologic conditions affecting hearing and vision. Handicapping conditions, such as hemiplegia, Parkinsonism, osteoarthritis, fracture, or amputation, are not uncommon.

C. Osteoporosis

Osteoporosis is a bone disease involving loss of mineral content and bone mass. Osteopenia means a deficiency of bone. Although most prominent in postmenopausal women, the condition may also occur at other ages and in males.

1. *Causes*
   a. Endocrine: hormonal disturbances; depletion of estrogen after menopause.
   b. Calcium deficiency; defective absorption of calcium.
   c. Steroid therapy or hypercortisonism.
2. *Risk Factors.*[4] A number of risk factors have been identified, several of which usually work together. From this list of risk factors, a list of methods for long-term prevention can be derived.
   a. Female sex.
   b. Caucasian or Asian ethnicity (worldwide, blacks are least affected).
   c. Positive family history.
   d. Low calcium intake (life-long).
   e. Early menopause or early surgical removal of ovaries.
   f. Sedentary lifestyle; lack of exercise.
   g. Alcohol abuse.
   h. High sodium intake.
   i. Cigarette smoking.
   j. High caffeine intake.
3. *Symptoms.*[5] Osteoporosis develops over many years; therefore a long asymptomatic period of bone change occurs with no clinical symptoms.
   a. Back ache; stooping of the posture.
   b. Fractures; may have spinal crush fractures with periodic acute pain.
   c. Evidence of bone changes in the mandible; residual ridge resorption.[6]
4. *Treatment.* A patient with osteoporosis may be treated with medications such as calcium, sodium fluoride, vitamin D, or possibly, estrogens. Activity and exercise require caution and preventive measures to avoid accidental falls.

Severe involvement of the spine may require orthopedic support and medication for pain.

Questions regarding the patient's medical history can elicit factors of importance to dental and dental hygiene appointments.

D. Alzheimer's Disease[7,8]

Alzheimer's disease is one of the nonreversible types of dementia. Dementia is severe impairment of the intellectual abilities, notably thinking, memory, and personality. At least one half of the patients with dementia have Alzheimer's disease. Other causes include cerebrovascular disease and alcoholism (page 727).

1. *Symptoms.* The common impairments of Alzheimer's disease may be divided into three or four overlapping stages that may extend over many years. In table 45–1, characteristics

Table 45–1. Common Impairments Associated with Alzheimer's Disease

Early Stage
Forgetfulness
Personality changes
Employment performance difficulty
Social withdrawal
Apathy
Errors in judgement
Inattentiveness
Personal hygiene neglect
Middle Stage
Disorientation
Loss of coordination
Restlessness/Anxiety
Language difficulty
Sleep pattern disturbance
Progressive memory loss
Catastrophic reactions
Pacing
Advanced Stage
Profound comprehension difficulty
Gait disturbances
Bladder and bowel incontinence
Hyperoralia
Inability to recognize family members
Seizures
Aggression
Lack of insight into deficits
Terminal Stage
Physical immobility
Contractures
Dysphagia
Emaciation
Mutism
Pathological reflexes
Unawareness of environment
Total helplessness

(From Fabiszewski, K.J.: Caring for the Alzheimer's Patient, *Gerodontology* 6, 53, Summer, 1987, © Beech Hill Enterprises, Inc. Used by Permission.)

are divided into early, middle, advanced, and terminal stages.[7]

2. *Appointment Considerations.* During the early stages, perhaps even before a diagnosis of Alzheimer's disease has been made, the patient will be attending routine dental and dental hygiene appointments.

   a. An early sign of the disease may be a slow decline of interest in oral hygiene and personal care. Review of the patient's medical and dental history at each maintenance appointment may reveal lapses in memory and other items listed under the "Early Stage" in table 45–1. An opportunity may be found to help a patient seek professional evaluation and care.

   b. Later stages may require that the patient reside in a long-term care facility. Dental hygienists in specialized facilities develop particular techniques for the variety of patients to be served.

ORAL FINDINGS

As mentioned earlier in this chapter, it is important to separate changes related to aging from the long-term effects of chronic diseases.

I. Soft Tissues

A. Lips

1. *Tissue Changes.* Dry, purse-string opening results from dehydration and loss of elasticity within the tissues.

2. *Angular Cheilitis.*[9,10] Angular cheilitis is not specifically an age-related lesion, but is frequently seen among the elderly. It appears as skin folds with fissuring at the angles of the mouth, and is related to reduced vertical dimension or inadequate support of the lips. Contributing factors are summarized on page 577.

B. Oral Mucosa

Degenerative changes take several forms. The surface texture is affected by changes in lubrication of the tissue with decreased secretion of the salivary and mucous glands. Xerostomia is not a result of aging, but is associated with certain diseases and medications.

1. *Atrophic Changes.* The tissue may become thinner and less vascular, with a loss of elasticity. Clinically, the smooth shiny appearance is related to thinning of the epithelium.

2. *Hyperkeratosis.* White, patchy areas develop as a result of irritation from sharp edges of broken teeth, restorations, or dentures, and from use of tobacco.

3. *Capillary Fragility.* Facial bruises and petechiae of the mucosa are common.

C. Tongue

1. *Atrophic Glossitis (Burning Tongue).* The tongue appears smooth, shiny, and bald, with atrophied papillae. The condition is related to anemia that results from a deficiency of iron or combinations of deficiencies. Elderly people have deficiency anemias more frequently than other age groups, because of nutritional factors but not because of aging specifically.
2. *Taste Sensations.* Taste may be reduced or abnormal taste reactions may occur, primarily in people with a disease condition, but changes are not routinely observed in the healthy elderly.[11]
3. *Sublingual Varicosities*
   a. Clinical appearance: deep red or bluish nodular dilated vessels on either side of the midline on the ventral surface of the tongue.
   b. Significance: although frequently occurring, these varicosities do not necessarily have a direct relation to systemic conditions.

D. Xerostomia

Dryness of the mouth is found frequently in older people in conjunction with pathologic states, drug-induced changes, or radiation-induced degeneration of the salivary glands. Healthy people continue to have normal salivary flow.[12] Xerostomia is described in detail on page 187.

II. Teeth

A. Color

The teeth may show color changes from long use of tobacco or foods with coloring agents such as tea or coffee. Dark intrinsic stains from dental restorations may be evident.

B. Attrition

The teeth of elderly people frequently show signs of wear, which may be the long-term effects of diet, occupational factors, or bruxism. Figure 14–3, page 213, illustrates incisal wear. Attrition may be accompanied by chipping; teeth may seem more brittle, particularly when compared with teeth of young people.

C. Abrasion

Abrasion at the neck of a tooth may be the result of extended use of a hard toothbrush in a horizontal direction with an abrasive dentifrice. With current preventive measures, use of soft-textured brushes, and attention to abrasiveness of dentifrices, future generations will be less likely to exhibit such tooth alterations.

D. Dental Caries

1. *Root Caries.* With roots exposed by periodontal infections, an increase in caries of the cementum can result. Root caries is described on page 217. Studies have shown an increase in cemental caries with age because of root exposure, not the age. In one report, the prevalence was 27 to 36 percent in those from 30 to 39 years of age, compared with 58 to 64 percent in the 50- to 59-year-old age group.[13]

   Periodontal therapy with continuing maintenance may influence the extent of cemental caries after age 60. In one group of patients with untreated moderate to severe periodontitis, root caries steadily increased with age, until in the over-60 age group, 86 percent were affected. In another group, comparable by age and disease severity but who had received periodontal treatment and regular maintenance, the dental caries incidence tapered off after 60 years, from 51 percent in the 50- to 59-year-old age group to 42 percent in those over 60.[14]
2. *Rampant Caries.* Sometimes called "retirement caries."[15] A noticeable increase in dental caries may occur after age 65. Factors influencing the development of dental caries include the following:
   a. Xerostomia. Tooth-protection factors of the saliva are missing (pages 187–188).
   b. Masticatory abilities. Oral conditions and, possibly, tooth loss make mastication difficult. This leads to changes in food selections.
   c. Life style. After retirement, without a daily work schedule, snacking and irregular mealtimes may lead to poor food selections and an excessively cariogenic diet.

E. Dental Pulp[16]

Whether pulpal changes can be considered results of aging is questionable. The pulpal changes develop as reactions to dental caries, restorations, bruxism, and other assaults during the elderly person's long life. The changes noted here may be observed at younger ages, but are seen more frequently in older people.

1. Narrowing of pulp chambers and root canals; increased deposition of secondary dentin.
2. Progressive deposition of calcified masses (pulp stones or denticles).[17]

III. Periodontium

A. Clinical Findings

The periodontal tissues reflect the health and disease of the patient over the years. One of the following may apply to any patient.

1. *The Healthy Periodontium.* Healthy tissues that have been maintained over the years may have had a minimum of disease. The radiographs show little if any bone recession, the gingiva are firm, and the appearance is normal in every way. Probing reveals minimal sulcus depth with no bleeding. The teeth are not mobile.
2. *The Treated Patient.* Although the patient was

subject to periodontal infection, treatment was completed, and the tissues were maintained in health through personal care and professional supervision. The tissues may show the effects of the treated disease, such as scar tissue. Areas of recession with exposed cementum may also be evident. The teeth are not mobile.

3. *The Patient with Periodontal Infection.* Neglect or omission of preventive measures and therapy over the years may have resulted in a chronic periodontal infection with extension of tissue destruction into the bone, periodontal ligament, and cementum. Loss of attachment, deep periodontal pockets, tooth mobility, and radiographic signs of periodontitis may be present.

B. **Tissue Changes Related to Aging**
  1. *Bone.*
    a. Osteoporosis may be present; related to nutritional and hormonal factors.
    b. Depressed vascularity, a reduction in metabolism, and reduced healing power affect bone.
  2. *Cementum.* Increased thickness has been demonstrated. In one series of measurements, the average overall thickness of the cementum at 20 years of age was 0.095 mm., while cementum from 60-year-olds measured 0.215 mm.[18]
  3. *Gingiva.* Most gingival changes can be traced to the effects of disease or to anatomic factors. For example, gingival recession is common in older individuals. Predisposing factors may be a lack of sufficient attached gingiva or malposition of the teeth.

    Precipitating factors may be vigorous, inappropriate toothbrushing, laceration, inflammation, or dental treatment such as the placement of a rubber dam on an area with minimum attached gingiva.[19]

PERSONAL FACTORS

The following list should not be considered typical of all elderly patients, because many are well adjusted. These characteristics are suggested to help the dental hygienist understand an older person's attitudes and actions.

I. **Insecurity**

A. Related to reduced economic status, self-respect, and feeling of being needed.
B. Inability to work.
C. Reduced activity
  a. Physical limitations.
  b. Overprotection by family.

D. Rejection by family.
E. Anxiety over health.

II. **Depression**

A. Limited physical power; sensitivity about shortcomings of impaired vision, hearing, and lack of motor control.
B. Changes in physical appearance.
C. Loneliness.
  1. Loss of spouse and friends.
  2. Need for attention and concern from others; companionship.

III. **Inability to Adjust to Changes in Mode of Life**

Tendency to develop fixed habits and ideas.

IV. **Slowing of Voluntary Responses**

Voluntary responses, association of thoughts, and speed of vocalization may all be slowed.

V. **Tendency to Introspection**

Narrowing of interests; living in the past.

DENTAL HYGIENE CARE

When planning and conducting appointments for an older patient, many of the procedures included in Chapter 50 (page 610) can be applied. Certain aging patients have physical and sensory limitations, and for those, adaptations are needed. It should be appreciated, however, that many members of the elderly population are independent, agile, and healthy people without systemic disease, who are not dependent on medications.

Care for the older patient should be planned in terms of comprehensive, not palliative treatment. Long-term maintenance for the prevention of oral disease must be the basic objective.

Many elderly people do not seek dental and dental hygiene care except when an emergency arises. A primary reason for the limited attention to professional care is a lack of perceived need. Other reasons relate to physical and mental disabilities, chronic disease, and physical barriers, such as transportation or accessibility of the dental office. Financial resources have not been a major reason.[20]

I. **Appointment Factors**

A. **Office or Clinic Facilities**

Attention to dental office arrangement that eliminates physical barriers is important. An aged person's impaired vision, feebleness, or lack of motor control must be considered.

Hazards can be eliminated such as small rugs, which can slide on polished floors, corners of rugs, which can be tripped over, and irregularities in floor levels. Other considerations related to architectural barriers and how to assist an elderly person who may be disabled are described on pages 612–617.

B. Patient History

Preparation of a careful and detailed medical and dental history takes on particular significance. Basic procedures for preparation of the history are described in Chapter 6.

1. *Suggestions for Good Communication*
   a. Eliminate distracting background music or sounds.
   b. Sit facing the patient, because hearing may be a problem. Other suggestions for the hearing-impaired patient are described on page 680.
   c. Do not shout, just increase volume and speak slowly and clearly.
   d. Be courteous at all times; show respect for age. Do not call the patient by his/her first name unless the patient suggests it.
   e. Present one idea at a time; be a good listener; older people do not like to be hurried.
   f. Develop trust; reduce anxiety.
2. *Medications.* Asking the patient to bring in either the bottles containing the various medications (over-the-counter as well as prescription items) or a written copy of the labels can aid in obtaining a more accurate listing when the patient is not sure. The patient's physician is the best source for an accurate list of prescribed medications.

   Neuroleptic medications are prescribed frequently for psychotherapy.[21] In addition to their calming influence, which aids in management of the patient during a dental or dental hygiene appointment, side effects after long-term administration include development of perioral dyskinesia. The condition is marked by repetitive involuntary movements of the lips, tongue, and jaws, which make providing clinical services difficult.
3. *Need for Antibiotic Premedication.* Many conditions that require prophylactic coverage are found fairly frequently in the elderly. Those with diabetes or those who receive chemotherapeutic or steroid treatments may have an increased susceptibility to infection. When the patient has a prosthetic joint replacement, heart valve or aortic prosthesis, or a history of other conditions listed on pages 85 and 91, premedication is indicated.

C. Vital Signs

Blood pressure determination is recommended for each visit (pages 98–101).

D. Intraoral and Extraoral Examination

The need for careful, periodic examination of the oral mucosa from lips to throat cannot be overstressed at any age, but especially for the elderly, because oral cancer occurs with increasing frequency with advancing years. Many, in fact most, oral lesions exist without the patient being aware of them.

For some early surface lesions, biopsy is definitely indicated. For others, the dental hygienist may prepare the cytologic smear as directed by the dentist (pages 111–113).

II. Preventive Treatment Program

Older patients need to have frequent appointments to maintain their oral health at a high level through supervision on a regular basis. The contents of a treatment plan resemble that for other age groups, and emphasis on plaque control dominates. Appointment suggestions are summarized in table 45–2. The dental hygiene appointments may include the following:

A. Plaque Control

Plaque control is described in detail in III later in this section.

B. Periodontal Care

Treatment with complete scaling, root planing, and follow-up to assess need for additional therapy.[22]

C. Dental Caries Control

1. Diet survey covering several days (page 383).
2. Diet adjustment to eliminate cariogenic foods and make appropriate substitutions.
3. Emphasis on prevention of rampant root caries.[15]
4. Fluoride therapy by use of daily self-applied preparations by dentifrice, rinse, or brush-on gel as needed (pages 407–410).

D. Xerostomia

Use of a saliva substitute (page 188).

III. Bacterial Plaque Control

A. Objectives

Basic objectives do not differ from those for younger people: infection must be eliminated and controlled.

Older individuals need to be as interested in their health and appearance as do people of any age. Esthetic deterioration may create emotional unhappiness, and when the aged feel insecure or unwanted, they may lose their interest in personal oral care and diet. Motivation through expression of sincere interest on the part of dental personnel can be an influencing factor in helping the patient to better health.

In the younger age groups, many still believe it inevitable and normal to lose the teeth eventually. Older people who still have their teeth tend to resist the loss of them.

Certain people fear dentures because they associate them with "old" people. Patients with partial dentures may already have been impressed with the need for preserving the remaining teeth. Here, in the desire to save the teeth,

Table 45–2. Adaptations in Treatment Procedures for the Gerodontic Patient

Appointment Factors	Characteristic of the Gerodontic Patient	Suggested Procedure Effect During an Appointment
Medical History Review	Many forms of chronic diseases Variety of medications used	Poor medical prognosis may limit extent of total treatment Need for antibiotic premedication for decreased immune response
Appointment Planning	Low stress tolerance Tires more easily than younger patient	Morning appointments Shorter appointments Need for frequent maintenance appointments to provide high-level preventive care Appreciation of the real effort patient has made to get there
	Slower voluntary responses Sensitivity about shortcomings of lack of motor control	Do not rush Do not make the patient feel old by obvious physical assistance
	Lowered tolerance to extremes of heat and cold; less body cooling through perspiration Impaired hearing; difficulty in hearing when there are distractions	Adjust room temperature Speak clearly and slowly; provide written memorandum of date and time of each appointment Eliminate background noises and music
Instrumentation	Loss of elasticity of lips and oral mucosa	Difficulty in retraction may provide patient discomfort
	Slowing of voluntary responses Cannot adjust to sudden muscular demands	Do not demand quick response to request for change of position of head, rinsing
	Pulp recession: variable pain threshold	Ask patient before administering anesthesia; the patient may not need it
	Reduction in growth and repair processes Decreases resistance to infection Healing slowed	Provide as little trauma to gingiva as possible during instrumentation Suggest postoperative care procedures to promote healing
	Inability to recover readily from stresses and strains Unsteadiness; tendency to postural hypotension	At completion of appointment, straighten chair back slowly and let patient sit up for short time before dismissing; assist out of chair

lies the appeal for preventive measures for both the teeth and their supporting structures, and good use should be made of this very real motivating force.

B. Approach to Instruction

In patient instruction, it is important not to try to change all life-long habits because this may create frustration and unhappiness. Self-confidence, which has diminished because of lowering of physical capabilities and emotional satisfaction, must be built up. Major changes required because previous habits were detrimental must be brought about gradually if cooperation is to be expected. A more optimistic attitude is needed about the degree of oral health the elderly patient can be expected to achieve.

C. Dental Plaque Formation

The incidence and severity of periodontal diseases increase with age as an effect of disease accumulation. The amount of periodontal destruction reflects the length of time the tissues have been exposed to disease-producing factors, primarily plaque microorganisms.

Experimental gingivitis studies have compared plaque accumulation and gingivitis development over a 21-day period (pages 243–244). In another study, young and aged individuals were compared. The older people developed plaque more rapidly and with more severe inflammation than did the younger people.[23] After 21 days, when oral hygiene procedures were reinstated, the rate of healing and the reduction of inflammation clinically was not different between the age groups. It was also shown that the microbial population of plaque was different in young and elderly persons.[24] The 4- and 9-day-old plaque of the elderly persons had a reduced number of viable organisms.

Several factors can contribute to a more rapid accumulation of plaque in the older patient. Some of these are listed here.

1. *Anatomic*
   a. Gingival recession with wide embrasures that result from periodontal destruction provides a larger surface area for plaque retention.
   b. Exposed cementum with areas of abrasion or dental caries at the neck of a tooth can create undercut areas where special adaptation of plaque removal devices are needed.
2. *Plaque Retention and Removal*
   a. Exposed untreated cementum may hold plaque more readily than does enamel. Cementum planed to a glassy smoothness is less likely to hold plaque, and plaque removal efforts are more successful.
   b. Decreased saliva production reduces or eliminates the cleansing and lubricating effects of saliva.
   c. Restorations and prostheses provide a more complex dentition for personal care. Plaque removal requires more time, patience, and motivation.
   d. Deficient restorations may have overhanging margins that provide areas of plaque retention.
   e. Lack of dexterity related to handicapping conditions resulting from chronic diseases such as arthritis and Parkinsonism makes plaque removal more difficult.

D. Specific Recommendations

Toothbrushing and other plaque control procedures as well as methods for the care of fixed and removable prostheses are selected as for other adult patients. A powered brush may help certain patients, particularly those with impaired motor function. Adaptations to alter the handle of a manual brush are described on pages 622–624.

Because of increased exposure of root surfaces, attention must be paid to dentifrice selection to prevent effects of abrasion and to prevent root caries. Certain patients may need instruction in desensitizing procedures (pages 499–500). The use of a fluoride dentifrice and a daily fluoride mouthrinse can contribute to both dental caries prevention and desensitization.

When a saliva substitute is recommended for patients with dry mouth, specific instructions must be given. Information about where to obtain available preparations is needed.

Instruction and motivation techniques are best applied gradually and regularly, at frequent intervals. Suggestions for adaptations of instruction to the physical and personal characteristics of the patient are listed in table 45–3.

IV. Diet and Nutrition

A. Dietary Habits

1. *Nutritional Deficiencies.* Dietary and resulting nutritional deficiencies are common in older people. For example, characteristic changes such as burning tongue, angular cheilitis, and atrophic glossitis may be related to vitamin B deficiencies. Unfortunately, many people believe that a diet rich in nutritive elements is important only for children.
2. *Factors Contributing to Dietary and Nutritional Deficiencies*
   a. Limited budget.
   b. Lives alone or eats alone.
   c. Does not eat regular meals; frequently uses non-nutritious snacks and foods for entertaining.
   d. Lacks interest in shopping for food or preparing it.
   e. Acuteness of senses lowered; may seek highly seasoned or sweetened foods.
   f. Childish likes and dislikes; unusual cravings.
   g. Tendency to follow food habits of lifetime; ignores newer knowledge of food preparation methods and dietary needs.
   h. Inadequate masticatory efficiency because of tooth loss or dentures that no longer fit properly.
   i. Adverse food selection may result from social embarrassment over inability to chew.
   j. Adaptations in eating habits, made to compensate for deficiency, may interfere with adequate digestion and absorption of nutrients.
   k. May follow dietary fads that provide only a limited and unbalanced diet.
   l. Loss of appetite; which may have physiologic, social, or economic causes.
   m. Lack of self-discipline; feeling that aging brings privilege to eat only preferred foods.

B. Dietary Needs of the Aged

The total nutritional needs of older persons are not different from those of younger persons, but

Table 45–3. Characteristics Affecting Instruction for the Gerodontic Patient

Characteristic of the Gerodontic Patient	Suggested Relation to Appointment Procedure
Tendency for introspection; desire for attention	Patience needed in taking time to listen to complaints and accounts of past experiences
Feelings of insecurity Deprivation of physical capabilities Touchy sensitiveness, exaggerated imaginary or real pains, or attitudes of suspicion	Sympathetic understanding needed Build up self-confidence
Resistance to change; tendency to maintain fixed habits	Should not attempt to change all life-long habits, only detrimental ones
Vision impaired	For the patient who wears prescription eyeglasses, make sure the glasses are worn while instruction is being given Recommend that eyeglasses be worn at home while performing plaque control procedures
Hearing impaired; loss of sensitivity to higher tones	Speak distinctly in normal voice. Look directly at patient while speaking; many are lip readers (page 680)
Slowing of voluntary responses Slowing of speed of thought associations Difficulty in timing sequential events; skills become separate movements, as by a child Least comfortable when must respond quickly to demanding sequential stimuli Rate of learning changed, ability to learn not changed Changes in speed of vocalization	Make suggestions gradually, over a series of appointments Do not demand learning a completely new procedure; adapt procedure already used Guide patient's demonstration of toothbrushing to prevent embarrassment Do not expect perfection; go slowly, anticipate difficulties, give cues, clues Distinguish between slowness of learning and inability to learn
Memory shortened, due mainly to lack of attention, lack of interest, or more selection of what patient wants to remember	Use motivating factors carefully. Provide written instructions; spoken instructions may be forgotten or misunderstood
Need for personal achievement	Help patient gain sense of accomplishment; commend for any success, however minor Never compare the patient's condition with other patients

they should cut down the quantity, particularly of calories. Caloric intake must be decreased to control weight. Protein, vitamins, and minerals are particularly important for body function, repair, and resistance to disease.

A necessary objective in geriatric nutrition is to retard the progression of diet-induced chronic diseases. Examples of these are arteriosclerosis related to disorders of glucose and lipid metabolism, anemias related to iron and folic acid deficiencies, and osteoporosis resulting from calcium and fluoride deficiency.

In addition to a better intake of calcium in the diet, recent research has shown that fluoride intake over the years is beneficial in the prevention of osteoporosis and fractures of the bones.[25] The relationship between fluoride in the drinking water and the decreased prevalence of osteoporosis was described on page 398.

C. Instruction in Diet and Oral Health

1. *Dietary Analysis.* A 4- or 5-day record of the patient's diet can provide information to guide recommendations to be made. Difficulties in showing the procedure to the patient and obtaining accurate results may seem insurmountable. Inaccuracy of recent memory is a problem with some elderly people, so that even the 24-hour dietary record prepared during the appointment may not be complete.

   The first consideration in making recommendations for aging patients is that a well-balanced diet be used with limited amounts of cariogenic foods for dental caries prevention. Food for an adequate diet is listed in table 28–1 on page 382.

2. *Motivation.* Appeal to the patient is made through personal concerns for the relationships of dietary deficiencies to appearance,

lowered resistance to disease, and premature aging, which may inspire the patient to improve daily habits. Educational materials are available to study with, and to give to, the patient.

TECHNICAL HINTS

Sources of Materials

American Dental Association
Order Department
211 E. Chicago Avenue
Chicago, Illinois 60611

W142 *Keeping Your Smile in the Later Years*

Barbara L. Wilson
Department of Dental Hygiene
University of Rhode Island
Kingston, Rhode Island 02881

The Why, When, and How, Preventive Oral Hygiene Care for the Elderly, Homebound or Nursing Home Residents

References

1. American Association of Retired Persons and the Administration on Aging, United States Department of Health and Human Services: *A Profile of Older Americans, 1985.* American Association of Retired Persons, 1909 K Street, N.W., Washington, D.C. 20049.
2. World Health Organization: Planning and Organization of Geriatric Services. Geneva, World Health Organization, Technical Report Series, Number 548, 1974, p. 11.
3. United States National Institute on Aging, National Institute of Dental Research, and the Veterans Administration: *A Research Agenda on Oral Health in the Elderly.* Washington, D.C., Veterans Administration, March, 1986, 38 pp.
4. Silverberg, S.J. and Lindsay, R.: Postmenopausal Osteoporosis, *Med. Clin. North Am., 71,* 41, January, 1987.
5. Berkow, R. and Fletcher, A.J., eds.: *The Merck Manual of Diagnosis and Therapy,* 15th ed. Rahway, N.J., Merck & Co., 1987, pp. 1000–1001.
6. Kribbs, P.J., Smith, D.E., and Chesnut, C.H.: Oral Findings in Osteoporosis. Part II: Relationship Between Residual Ridge and Alveolar Bone Resorption and Generalized Skeletal Osteopenia, *J. Prosthet. Dent., 50,* 719, November, 1983.
7. Fabiszewski, K.J.: Caring for the Alzheimer's Patient, *Gerodontology, 6,* 53, Summer, 1987.
8. Niessen, L.C. and Jones, J.A.: Alzheimer's Disease: A Guide for Dental Professionals, *Spec. Care Dentist., 6,* 6, January-February, 1986.
9. Shafer, W.G., Hine, M.K., and Levy, B.M.: *A Textbook of Oral Pathology,* 4th ed. Philadelphia, W.B. Saunders Co., 1983, pp. 556–557.
10. Pindborg, J.J.: *Atlas of Diseases of the Oral Mucosa,* 4th ed. Copenhagen, Munksgaard, 1985, pp. 58, 66.
11. Baum, B.J.: Current Research on Aging and Oral Health, *Spec. Care Dentist., 1,* 105, May-June, 1981.
12. Baum, B.J.: Age Changes in Salivary Glands and Salivary Secretion, in Holm-Pedersen, P. and Löe, H., eds: *Geriatric Dentistry.* St. Louis, The C.V. Mosby Co., 1986, pp. 114–122.
13. Sumney, D.L., Jordan, H.V., and Englander, H.R.: The Prevalence of Root Surface Caries in Selected Populations, *J. Periodontol., 44,* 500, August, 1973.
14. Hix, J.O. and O'Leary, T.J.: The Relationship Between Cemental Caries, Oral Hygiene Status and Fermentable Carbohydrate Intake, *J. Periodontol., 47,* 398, July, 1976.
15. Chase, R.H.: The Management of "Retirement Caries," *J. Mich. Dent. Assoc., 57,* 178, April, 1975.
16. Seltzer, S. and Bender, I.B.: *The Dental Pulp. Biologic Con-*
siderations in Dental Procedures, 3rd ed. Philadelphia, J.B. Lippincott Co., 1984, pp. 324–348.
17. Shafer, Hine, and Levy: op. cit., pp. 325–328.
18. Zander, H.A. and Hurzeler, B.: Continuous Cementum Apposition, *J. Dent. Res., 37,* 1035, November-December, 1958.
19. Hall, W.B.: Present Status of Soft Tissue Grafting, *J. Periodontol., 48,* 587, September, 1977.
20. Kiyak, H.A.: Barriers to the Utilization of Dental Services by the Elderly, in Chauncey, H.H., Epstein, S., Rose, C.L., and Hefferren, J.J., eds.: *Clinical Geriatric Dentistry. Biomedical and Psychosocial Aspects.* Chicago, American Dental Association, 1985, pp. 157–168.
21. Snyder, N.C.: *Dental Hygiene Clinical Applications in Pharmacology.* Philadelphia, Lea & Febiger, 1987, pp. 190–191.
22. Robinson, P.J.: Periodontal Therapy for the Ageing Mouth, *Int. Dent. J., 29,* 220, September, 1979.
23. Holm-Pedersen, P., Agerbaek, N., and Theilade, E.: Experimental Gingivitis in Young and Elderly Individuals, *J. Clin. Periodontol., 2,* 14, February, 1975.
24. Holm-Pedersen, P., Folke, L.E.A., and Gawronski, T.H.: Composition and Metabolic Activity of Dental Plaque from Healthy Young and Elderly Individuals, *J. Dent. Res., 59,* 771, May, 1980.
25. Simonen, O. and Laitinen, O.: Does Fluoridation of Drinking-water Prevent Bone Fragility and Osteoporosis? *Lancet, 2,* (8452), 432, August 24, 1985.

Suggested Readings

Baum, B.J.: Current Research on Aging and Oral Health, *Spec. Care Dentist., 1,* 105, May-June, 1981.
Baum, B.J.: Characteristics of Participants in the Oral Physiology Component of the Baltimore Longitudinal Study of Aging, *Community Dent. Oral Epidemiol., 9,* 128, June, 1981.
Baum, B.J.: Research on Aging and Oral Health: An Assessment of Current Status and Future Needs, *Spec. Care Dentist., 1,* 156, July-August, 1981.
Baum, B.J.: Salivary Gland Function During Aging, *Gerodontics, 2,* 61, April, 1986.
Bomberg, T.J. and Ernst, N.S.: Physical Assessment of the Elderly Patient, *Gen. Dent., 32,* 198, May-June, 1984.
Bomberg, T.J., Shapiro, S., and Benson, B.W.: Developing the Health History of the Elderly Dental Patient, *Gerodontics, 1,* 165, August, 1985.
Dolinsky, E.H. and Dolinsky, H.B.: Infantilization of Elderly Patients By Health Care Providers, *Spec. Care Dentist., 4,* 150, July-August, 1984.
Gambert, S.R.: Aging–An Overview, *Spec. Care Dentist., 3,* 147, July-August, 1983.
Gunn, W.G.: Radiation Therapy for the Aging Patient, *CA, 30,* 337, November/December, 1980.
Lang, W.P., Kerschbaum, W.E., and Kerns, K.M.: A Community-based Dental Program for Older Adults, *J. Public Health Dent., 44,* 141, Fall, 1984.
Mandel, I.D.: Preventive Dentistry for the Elderly, *Spec. Care Dentist., 3,* 157, July-August, 1983.
Marinelli, R.D.: Oral Health Care for the Elderly Patient. The Role of Dental Hygienists, *Dent. Hyg., 57,* 14, October, 1983.
Norman, B.J., Robinson, E., and Razzoog, M.E.: Societal Determinants of Cultural Factors Related to the Dental Health of a Selected Older Black Population, *Spec. Care Dentist., 6,* 120, May-June, 1986.
Odrich, J. and Levine, J.: Dental Health Knowledge in a Group of Inner-city Older Adults, *Spec. Care Dentist., 7,* 275, November-December, 1987.
Rowe, J.W.: Health Care of the Elderly, *N. Engl. J. Med., 312,* 827, March 28, 1985.
Rowland, K.K. and Mayberry, W.E.: Assessment of the Dental Attitudes of the Non-institutionalized Older Adult, *Dent. Hyg., 57,* 32, October, 1983.
Shannon, S.A.: Needs of Geriatric Females in Private Practice Settings, *Dent. Hyg., 57,* 18, October, 1983.
Shipman, B. and Teitelman, J.L.: Learned Helplessness and the

Older Dental Patient, *Spec. Care Dentist.*, *5,* 261, November-December, 1985.

Taintor, J.F., Karp, G., Taintor, M.J., and Rosenthal, A.B.: Geriatric Patient Care: Medical Aspects for Dentists, *Compend. Contin. Educ. Dent.*, *5,* 339, April, 1984.

Wycoff, S.J. and Epstein, S.: Geriatric Dentistry, in Lynch, M.A., Brightman, V.J., and Greenberg, M.S., eds.: *Burket's Oral Medicine,* 8th ed. Philadelphia, J.B. Lippincott Co., 1984, pp. 560–575.

Medications

Edwards, G.B. and Piepho, R.W.: Pharmacokinetic and Pharmacodynamic Aspects of Geriatric Drug Therapy, *Gerodontics,* *1,* 160, August, 1985.

Gambert, S.R.: Drugs and the Elderly, *Spec. Care Dentist.*, *4,* 102, May-June, 1984.

Handelman, S.L., Baric, J.M., Espeland, M.A., and Berglund, K.L.: Prevalence of Drugs Causing Hyposalivation in an Institutionalized Geriatric Population, *Oral Surg. Oral Med. Oral Pathol.*, *62,* 26, July, 1986.

Patton, L.L.: Special Considerations in Drug Therapy for Elderly Dental Patients, *Spec. Care Dentist.*, *5,* 24, January-February, 1985.

Shapiro, S., Avery, K.T., and Carpenter, R.D.: Drug Utilization by a Non-institutionalized Ambulatory Elderly Population, *Gerodontics,* *2,* 99, June, 1986.

Pathology

Alder, S.S.: Anemia in the Aged: Causes and Considerations, *Geriatrics,* *35,* 49, April, 1980.

Desmeules, H., Fournier, L., and Tremblay, P.-R.: Systemic Changes in the Elderly Patient and Their Anaesthetic Implications, *Can. Anaesth. Soc. J.*, *32,* 184, March, 1985.

Hand, J.S. and Whitehill, J.M.: The Prevalence of Oral Mucosal Lesions in an Elderly Population, *J. Am. Dent. Assoc.*, *112,* 73, January, 1986.

McGowan, J.M.: Age and Changes in Oral Tissues, *RDH,* *3,* 22, July-August, 1983.

Thomas, J.E. and Lloyd, P.M.: Oral Candidiasis in the Elderly, *Spec. Care Dentist.*, *5,* 222, September-October, 1985.

van der Waal, I.: Diseases of the Oral Mucosa in the Aged Patient, *Int. Dent. J.*, *33,* 319, December, 1983.

Osteoporosis

Altshuler, B.D. and Altshuler, S.L.: Boning Up on Osteoporosis, *RDH,* 5, 38, June, 1985.

Baxter, J.C.: Osteoporosis: Oral Manifestations of a Systemic Disease, *Quintessence Int.*, *18,* 427, June, 1987.

Hall, F.M., Davis, M.A., and Baran, D.T.: Bone Mineral Screening for Osteoporosis, *N. Engl. J. Med.*, *316,* 212, January 22, 1987.

McKenna, M.J. and Frame, B.: Hormonal Influences on Osteoporosis, *Am. J. Med.*, *82,* 81, Supplement 1 B, January 26, 1987.

Radica, B.: The Enigma of Osteoporosis, *Dent. Assist.*, *56,* 12, January/February, 1987.

Shapiro, S., Bomberg, T.J., Benson, B.W., and Hamby, C.L.: Postmenopausal Osteoporosis: Dental Patients at Risk, *Gerodontics,* *1,* 220, October, 1985.

Alzheimer's Disease

Charatan, F.B.: The Geropsychiatric Patient, *Spec. Care Dentist.*, *5,* 213, September-October, 1985.

Katzman, R.: Alzheimer's Disease, *N. Engl. J. Med.*, *314,* 964, April 10, 1986.

Kiyak, H.A.: The Dentist's Role, *Spec. Care Dentist.*, *3,* 8, January-February, 1983.

McClain, D.L.: Dental Hygiene Care for the Alzheimer's Patient, *Dent. Hyg.*, *61,* 500, November, 1987.

Montelaro, S.: Alzheimer's Disease: A Growing Concern in Geriatric Dentistry, *Gen. Dent.*, *33,* 494, November-December, 1985.

Niessen, L.C. and Jones, J.A.: Oral Health and the Patient with Dementia, *Spec. Care Dentist.*, *7,* 36, January-February, 1987.

Niessen, L.C., Jones, J.A., Zocchi, M., and Gurian, B.: Dental Care for the Patient with Alzheimer's Disease, *J. Am. Dent. Assoc.*, *110,* 207, February, 1985.

Rousseau, P.C.: Alzheimer's Disease. What Is Known, What Can Be Done, *Postgrad. Med.*, *80,* 99, July, 1986.

Schmahl, S.R.: Depression in the Geriatric Population—Implications for the Dental Practitioner, *Spec. Care Dentist.*, *4,* 16, January-February, 1984.

Shapiro, S., Hamby, C.L., and Shapiro, D.A.: Alzheimer's Disease: An Emerging Affliction of the Aging Population, *J. Am. Dent. Assoc.*, *111,* 287, August, 1985.

Periodontics

Ambjørnsen, E.: Remaining Teeth, Periodontal Condition, Oral Hygiene and Tooth Cleaning Habits in Dentate Old-age Subjects, *J. Clin. Periodontol.*, *13,* 583, July, 1986.

Anderson, D.L.: Periodontal Disease and Aging, *Gerodontology,* *1,* 19, January, 1982.

Brecx, M., Holm-Pedersen, P., and Theilade, J.: Early Plaque Formation in Young and Elderly Individuals, *Gerodontics,* *1,* 8, February, 1985.

Carranza, F.A.: *Glickman's Clinical Periodontology,* 6th ed. Philadelphia, W.B. Saunders Co., 1984, pp. 82–86.

Douglass, C., Gillings, D., Sollecito, W., and Gammon, M.: The Potential for Increase in the Periodontal Diseases of the Aged Population, *J. Periodontol.*, *54,* 721, December, 1983.

Feldman, R.S., Alman, J.E., and Chauncey, H.H.: Periodontal Disease Indexes and Tobacco Smoking in Healthy Aging Men, *Gerodontics,* *3,* 43, February, 1987.

Grant, D.A., Stern, I.B., and Listgarten, M.A., eds.: *Periodontics,* 6th ed. St. Louis, The C.V. Mosby Co., 1988, pp. 119–134.

Lindhe, J., Socransky, S., Nyman, S., Westfelt, E., and Haffajee, A.: Effect of Age on Healing Following Periodontal Therapy, *J. Clin. Periodontol.*, *12,* 774, October, 1985.

Potter, D.E., Manwell, M.A., Dess, R., Levine, E., and Tinanoff, N.: SnF_2 As An Adjunct to Toothbrushing in an Elderly Institutionalized Population, *Spec. Care Dentist.*, *4,* 216, September-October, 1984.

Rowe, D.J.: Bone Loss in the Elderly, *J. Prosthet. Dent.*, *50,* 607, November, 1983.

Socransky, S.S. and Manganiello, S.D.: The Oral Microbiota of Man from Birth to Senility, *J. Periodontol.*, *42,* 485, August, 1971.

van der Velden, U.: Effect of Age on the Periodontium, *J. Clin. Periodontol.*, *11,* 281, May, 1984.

van der Velden, U., Abbas, F., and Hart, A.A.M.: Experimental Gingivitis in Relation to Susceptibility to Periodontal Disease. I. Clinical Observations, *J. Clin. Periodontol.*, *12,* 61, January, 1985.

Ketterl, W.: Age-induced Changes in the Teeth and Their Attachment Apparatus, *Int. Dent. J.*, *33,* 262, September, 1983.

Dental Caries and Dental Care

Aragon, S.B., Buckley, S.B., and Tilson, H.B.: Oral Surgery Management of the Geriatric Patient, *Spec. Care Dentist.*, *4,* 124, May-June, 1984.

Banting, D.W.: Special Restorative Needs of Older Adults: Fractured Teeth, Root Caries, and Recurrent Caries, *Spec. Care Dentist.*, *7,* 15, January-February, 1987.

Banting, D.W., Ellen, R.P., and Fillery, E.D.: Prevalence of Root Surface Caries Among Institutionalized Older Persons, *Community Dent. Oral Epidemiol.*, *8,* 84, April, 1980.

Bomberg, T.J. and Averbach, R.E.: Local Anesthesia and the Elderly Dental Patient, *Gerodontics,* *2,* 157, October, 1986.

Epstein, S. and Corvin, S.S.: Special Considerations for Restorative Dentistry in Geriatric Patients, *Dent. Clin. North Am.*, *29,* 413, April, 1985.

Giangrego, E. and Marshall, J.Y.: Dentistry and the Older Adult, *J. Am. Dent. Assoc.*, *114,* 298, March, 1987.

Johnson, D.L. and Stratton, R.J.: Special Considerations in the Elderly Prosthodontic Patient, *Quintessence Int.*, *11,* 47, February, 1980.

Kitamura, M., Kiyak, H.A., and Mulligan, K.: Predictors of Root Caries in the Elderly, *Community Dent. Oral Epidemiol.*, *14,* 34, February, 1986.

Laskin, D.M.: Age: A Barrier to Oral Surgery? *Int. Dent. J., 33,* 313, December, 1983.

Massler, M.: Geriatric Dentistry: Root Caries in the Elderly, *J. Prosthet. Dent., 44,* 147, August, 1980.

Mulligan, R.: Pretreatment for the Cardiovascularly Compromised Geriatric Patient, *Spec. Care Dentist., 5,* 116, May-June, 1985.

Poswillo, D.: Conservative Management of Degenerative Temporomandibular Joint Disease in the Elderly, *Int. Dent. J., 33,* 325, December, 1983.

Diet and Nutrition

Baxter, J.C.: The Nutritional Intake of Geriatric Patients with Varied Dentitions, *J. Prosthet. Dent., 51,* 164, February, 1984.

Chauncey, H.H. and Wayler, A.H.: The Modifying Influence of Age on Taste Perception, *Spec. Care Dentist., 1,* 68, March-April, 1981.

Chernoff, R. and Lipschitz, D.A.: Nutrition and Aging, in Shils, M.E. and Young, V.R., eds.: *Modern Nutrition in Health and Disease,* 7th ed. Philadelphia, Lea & Febiger, 1988, pp. 982–1000.

Dodd, C.S. and Vernino, D.: Geriatric Nutrition for Edentulous and Dentulous Patients, *Gen. Dent., 32,* 103, March-April, 1984.

Duthie, E.H., Lloyd, P.M., and Gambert, S.R.: Nutrition and the Elderly: Implications for Oral Health Care, *Spec. Care Dentist., 3,* 201, September-October, 1983.

Kalu, D.N. and Masorò, E.J.: Metabolic and Nutritional Aspects of Aging, *Gerodontics, 2,* 121, August, 1986.

Nizel, A.E. and Papas, A.S.: *Nutrition in Clinical Dentistry,* 3rd ed. Philadelphia, W.B. Saunders Co., 1989, pp. 339–365.

Papas, A.S., Palmer, C.A., McGandy, R., Hartz, S.C., and Russell, R.M.: Dietary and Nutritional Factors in Relation to Dental Caries in Elderly Subjects, *Gerodontics, 3,* 30, February, 1987.

Ramsey, W.O.: Nutritional Problems of the Aged, *J. Prosthet. Dent., 49,* 16, January, 1983.

Sandstead, H.H.: Nutrition in the Elderly, *Gerodontics, 3,* 3, February, 1987.

Schachtele, C.F., Rosamond, W.D., and Harlander, S.K.: Diet and Aging: Current Concerns Related to Oral Health, *Gerodontics, 1,* 117, June, 1985.

Schafer, S.: Malnutrition in the Aged, *Dent. Hyg., 54,* 233, May, 1980.

Schneider, E.L., Vining, E.M., Hadley, E.C., and Farnham, S.A.: Recommended Dietary Allowances and the Health of the Elderly, *N. Engl. J. Med., 314,* 157, January 16, 1986.

Truesdale, K.: Nutrition to Meet the Needs of the Elderly, *Can. Dent. Hyg., 18,* 40, Summer, 1984.

Wical, K.: Commonsense Dietary Recommendations for Geriatric Dental Patients, *J. Prosthet. Dent., 49,* 162, February, 1983.

Young, V.R.: Nutrition, in Steinberg, F.U., ed.: *Cowdry's The Care of the Geriatric Patient,* 6th ed. St. Louis, The C.V. Mosby Co., 1983, pp. 216–230.

Communication; Psychologic Factors

Giddon, D.B. and Hittelman, E.: Psychologic Aspects of Prosthodontic Treatment for Geriatric Patients, *J. Prosthet. Dent., 43,* 374, April, 1980.

Hamby, C.L. and Shapiro, S.: Communicating with Elderly Patients, *RDH, 4,* 52, September/October, 1984.

Handleman, S.L., Stege, P.M., Baric, J.M., Espeland, M.A., and Saunders, R.H.: Dentists' Verbal Communication Leads During an Interview with Geriatric Patients, *Spec. Care Dentist., 6,* 253, November-December, 1986.

Kiyak, H.A.: Psychological and Social Factors in the Dental Care of the Elderly, *Int. Dent. J., 33,* 281, September, 1983.

Kiyak, H.A.: Psychosocial Factors in Dental Needs of the Elderly, *Spec. Care Dentist., 1,* 22, January-February, 1981.

Levenson, A.J.: Psychiatric Implications in the Treatment of the Geriatric Dental Patient, *Spec. Care Dentist., 3,* 4, January-February, 1983.

Portnoy, E.J.: Successful Communication with Older Patients, *Spec. Care Dentist., 5,* 180, July-August, 1985.

Zier, B.: Factors Influencing Dental Health Education for the Aged, *Can. Dent. Hyg., 16,* 110, Winter, 1982.

46 *The Edentulous Patient*

The completely edentulous patient needs an appointment at least annually for careful observation of the oral tissues, as well as for supervision of bacterial plaque control for the dentures and care of the mucosa. Instruction for the patient who receives new dentures is also a concern, because preventive procedures are necessary for the patient's general and oral health.

Of the completely edentulous population, particularly in the older age groups, some individuals have dentures they do not wear, others have full dentures but wear only one of them, whereas others have no dentures. When there is a single denture, more frequently it is the maxillary denture that is worn. It is not unusual to find that the same dentures have been worn for many years without having the dentures or the supporting oral tissues examined.

Dentures occasionally must be constructed to replace primary teeth. The teeth may be congenitally missing (anodontia) or may have required extraction because of rampant caries or trauma. Nursing bottle caries which can result in severe breakdown of the teeth soon after eruption, was described on page 218.

To provide esthetics and function, dentures can be constructed for the accepting child who is able to cooperate. As the permanent teeth begin to erupt, parts of the denture will be cut away (figure 46–1). A supervised caries prevention program is initiated for protection of the permanent dentition.

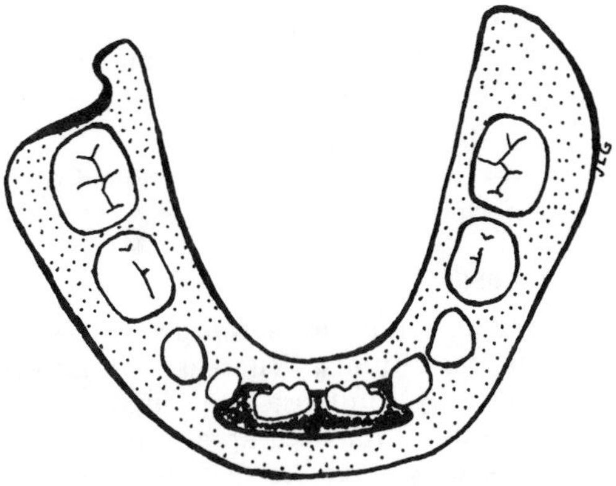

Figure 46–1. Denture for a Young Child. As permanent teeth erupt, parts of the denture are cut away. Shown are denture alterations for the mandibular right first permanent molar and the mandibular incisors.

I. Types of Complete Dentures[1]

A. Complete Denture

A complete denture is a dental prosthesis that replaces the entire dentition and associated structures of the maxilla or mandible. The components of a complete denture are described on page 345.

B. Immediate Denture

When a denture is constructed for insertion immediately following the removal of natural teeth, it is called an immediate denture.

C. Overdenture

An overdenture is supported by both retained natural teeth and the mucosa. The overdenture is described on pages 349–350.

D. Implant Denture

An implant denture receives its stability and retention from a substructure that is partially or wholly implanted under the soft tissues of the denture basal seat. Implants are described on pages 359–361.

E. Obturator

A prosthesis used to close a congenital or acquired opening in the palate is known as an obturator. When the teeth are missing, the obturator is connected to the complete denture.

II. The Edentulous Mouth

A. Bone

1. *Residual Ridges.* After the teeth are removed, the residual ridges enter into a continuing process of remodelling. The alveolar bone, which had supported the teeth, undergoes resorption. The rate and amount of bony resorption varies with each individual. The major bony changes occur during the first year after the teeth are removed, but changes continue throughout life. Mandibular bone loss is generally as much as four times greater than maxillary.[2] Because of the oral changes, it is usually necessary to have dentures rebased or remade at intervals.

2. *Tori.* Tori are benign bony outgrowths of varying shapes. A *torus palatinus* may be present in the midline of the palate. A *torus mandibularis* is generally seen on the lingual side of the mandibular arch in the premolar area. Because of size, shape, or location, it may be necessary to remove a torus surgically before a denture is constructed.

573

B. Mucous Membrane

As described on pages 166–167, the oral mucosa is composed of masticatory, lining, and specialized mucosa. The edentulous ridges and the hard palate are covered with masticatory mucosa, which is continuous with the lining mucosa that covers the floor of the mouth, vestibules, and cheeks.

The mucous membrane covering the bony ridges is made up of two layers, the lamina propria and the surface stratified squamous epithelium, which is keratinized in the healthy mouth. Underneath the mucous membrane is the submucosa, which is attached to the underlying bone.

The submucosa is composed of connective tissue with vessels, nerves, adipose tissue, and glands. The support or cushioning effect for the denture depends on the makeup of the submucosa, which varies in different parts of a mouth.

When an edentulous mouth is examined clinically, and the lips and cheeks are retracted using a tension test technique (page 199), a line of demarcation similar to the mucogingival junction is apparent, separating the attached tissue over the bony ridge and the loose lining mucosa of the vestibule. Frenal attachments can be observed readily.

III. The Patient with New Dentures

A. Patient Counseling

The preparation for denture insertion has to begin well in advance of the day the dentures are delivered. The patient needs a clear idea of what to expect and what procedures will be followed. Successful after-care and denture satisfaction depend to a large extent on conditioning the patient to the adjustments to be made and the period of practice and learning with the new dentures that can be expected.[3]

Many dentists prepare their own printed educational materials, whereas others use those available from outside sources.

The preliminary counseling is followed through the initial postinsertion appointments, particularly to teach denture hygiene and to arrange for continuing maintenance appointments during the following years.

B. Postinsertion Care

1. *Immediate Denture.* The patient receiving an immediate denture will be instructed to leave the denture in place for 24 to 48 hours to aid in the control of bleeding and swelling. When the patient returns and the denture is removed, the mouth is rinsed and appropriate instructions are given. After initial healing, the denture care and other instructions are similar to those presented in table 46–1.
2. *New Dentures over Healed Ridges*
   a. Appointments. Following insertion, adjustment appointments are scheduled routinely because adjustments can be expected. The first appointment is made within 48 hours of the time of insertion, and additional appointments are made in accord with individual needs.
   b. Instructions.[4] Too many instructions given on the day of insertion may only confuse the patient. Basic denture care and other procedures of immediate concern can be reviewed. Slow repetition over several periods will help the patient to develop adequate denture management and hygiene habits.

Basic information for the new denture wearer is provided in table 46–1. Denture cleaning methods are described with other plaque control procedures for the care of dental appliances on pages 346–349.

DENTURE-RELATED ORAL CHANGES

The condition of the mucous membranes, salivary glands, and alveolar bone is influenced by dietary and nutritional deficiencies, age, and various chronic diseases. Tissue alterations for an older patient were described on pages 561–562. Some of the denture-related changes are listed here.

I. Bone Changes

A. Alveolar Ridge Remodeling[5]

The continuing reduction in the size of the residual ridge may lead to loss of denture support, loss of facial height and lip support, increased prominence of the chin, possible temporomandibular joint manifestations, and occlusal disharmony.

B. Compensations by the Patient

1. Patients may adapt to the bone changes by making compensating adjustments in the way they wear and manage the dentures.
2. Other patients may resort to drugstore remedies such as pads, adhesives, or self-reline materials, which may be detrimental and cause further oral damage.[6]

C. Treatment by the Dentist

Dentures will need relining, rebasing, or remaking periodically.

II. Oral Mucosa

The tissue reaction under a denture varies considerably among individuals. Whereas one mouth may have thinning of the mucosa, submucosa, and particularly the epithelium with an absence of keratinization, others may have normal keratinization or hyperkeratinization.

Factors that influence the mucosa include systemic conditions that alter host response, aging, denture and tissue hygiene, wearing the denture constantly,

Table 46–1. Patient Instruction for Complete Dentures

Item	Factors to Teach

Food Selection	Use foods from the Basic 4 food groups (page 382)
	Check each day's diet to fulfill needs for a balanced diet
	Older patients: use foods to prevent diet-induced chronic diseases (pages 568–570)
	
	New denture wearer:
	  Avoid foods that need incising
	  Avoid raw vegetables, fibrous meats, and sticky foods until experience has been gained
	  Cut food into small pieces
	
	Practiced denture wearer:
	  Select a variety of foods, but do not expect the same efficiency as with the natural teeth

Incision or Biting	Use the canine and premolar area. Insert for biting at the angle of the mouth. Push back as the food is incised; do not pull or tear the food in a forward direction
Chewing	Take small portions Try to chew with some food on each side at the same time to stabilize the denture Be patient and practice
Salivary Flow	Anticipate an increased flow of saliva when a new denture is worn
Speaking	Speak slowly and quietly Practice by reading aloud at home, preferably in front of a mirror Repeat and practice words that seem the most difficult
Sneezing, Coughing, Yawning	Anticipate loss of denture retention Cover mouth with hand and handkerchief
Denture Hygiene	Thoroughly clean dentures twice each day Immerse dentures in chemical solution and brush for plaque removal. Rinse thoroughly Complete denture care is described on pages 346–349 Devices to aid a handicapped person are shown on pages 622–625
Mucosa	Tissues need to rest each day. Preferable to leave the dentures out while sleeping Brush and massage the mucosa to clean away plaque and debris and stimulate circulation
Storage of Dentures	After careful cleaning to remove all bacterial plaque, store the dentures in water (or cleaning solution) in a covered container Place in a safe place inaccessible to children or house pets Change water or cleaning solution daily and wash the container
Over-the-Counter Products	Never attempt to alter the denture for relief of discomfort Do not buy and use self-reline materials, adhesives, or other additives without consulting the dentist. They may be harmful to the dentures and/or the oral tissues. Consult the dentist for advice about all denture problems
Maintenance	Understand the importance of the dentist's examination of the denture fit, occlusion, and wear, and the condition of the oral mucosa First year: expect reline, rebase, or remake of dentures because bone remodeling is greatest during the first year. Subsequent appointment: an examination each year for most patients, provided the denture hygiene is ideal. Other patients in the cancer-susceptible category need a three months' examination.

xerostomia, and fit and occlusion of the denture itself.

III. Xerostomia

The causes of xerostomia were described on page 188. Diminished salivary flow can influence denture retention and tissue lubrication as well as reduce the resistance of the oral mucosa to trauma and infection.

A. Lubrication
The oral mucosa needs saliva for protection against frictional irritation by the denture.

B. Retention
The film of saliva between the denture and the mucosa contributes to retention of the denture.

IV. Sensory Changes

A. Tactile Sense
With the dentures in place, sensitivity may be diminished to small objects in the mouth such as small bones or bits of nut shells.

B. Taste
Occasionally, patients indicate that, since they have been wearing dentures, food has a different taste for them. Although the taste buds that are located in the tongue papillae are not affected by the dentures, the taste buds of the palate are covered by the maxillary denture and therefore are ineffective for taste perception. Denture hygiene must be meticulous to assure that the denture does not develop thick odoriferous plaque, which may alter food flavors.

DENTURE-INDUCED ORAL LESIONS

When the mouth is examined extraorally and intraorally, the dentures are removed and the mucosa is carefully and thoroughly examined. The patient may tell of an area that has been sensitive and thus helpfully call attention to a specific visible lesion. On the other hand, a patient may be unaware of chronic mucosal lesions, which are often asymptomatic. Because tissue changes may be important indicators of serious disease such as oral cancer, the intraoral examination must be conducted thoroughly with good illumination.

I. Principal Causes of Lesions Under Dentures

The factors that singly or in combination cause most oral lesions under dentures are infection, trauma, ill-fit of the dentures, inadequate oral hygiene, and wearing the dentures all the time, without relief for the tissues.

A. Ill-fitting Dentures
Because tissue changes under dentures occur gradually over a long period, the patient may not be aware of developing disease. The patient may not realize or may not have been informed of the importance of having regular professional examinations of the dentures and the oral mucosa.

B. Lack of Oral Hygiene
The dentures and the oral mucosa need daily care. Neglected dentures can accumulate heavy plaque and calculus that may irritate the mucosa.

C. Continuous Wearing of Dentures
Dentures need to be removed for a part of every 24 hours so that the mucosa can have a rest from the pressure of the hard acrylic during occlusion, bruxism, and clenching. The rest period also allows the tissue to recover in its natural environment, where the tongue and saliva provide a cleansing effect.

II. Inflammatory Lesions

A. Localized Inflammation (Sore Spots)
1. *Appearance.* Isolated red inflamed area, sometimes ulcerated.
2. *Contributing Factors.* Trauma from an ill-fitting denture, rough spot on a denture surface, tongue bite.

B. Generalized Inflammation
1. *Other Names.* "Denture sore mouth," "denture stomatitis."
2. *Appearance.* Generalized redness over the tissues that support the denture. The patient may have pain and a burning sensation. This occurs more frequently in the maxilla.
3. *Contributing Factors*
   The following may occur singly or in combinations.
   a. Denture trauma from the fit, occlusion, or parafunctional habits.
   b. Inadequate denture hygiene and care of the mucosa.
   c. Chemotoxic effect from residual cleansing paste or solution not thoroughly rinsed from the denture.
   d. Allergy to the denture base (rare).
   e. Continuous denture wearing without relief for the tissues.
   f. Patient self-treatment with over-the-counter products for relining.
   g. Systemic influence on the tolerance of the tissues to trauma and lowered resistance to infection; for examples, vitamin and other nutritional deficiencies and immunosuppressant therapy, such as chemotherapy.
   h. *Candida albicans* infection.[7] *C. albicans* is a customary member of the oral flora of people with or without teeth. In denture stomatitis, or in recognizable candidiasis or moniliasis, the numbers of the yeast-like fungus increase. Conditions that promote *C. albicans* overgrowth are depression of defense mechanisms by immunosuppressants, radiation therapy, or prolonged antibiotic therapy.

III. Ulcerative Lesions

Localized ulcer-shaped lesions usually are related to an overextended denture border. The ulcer may resemble a cancerous lesion and should be biopsied if it persists longer than expected of a healing traumatic ulcer.

IV. Papillary Hyperplasia

A. Appearance

Papillary hyperplasia is located on the palatal vault, rarely outside the confines of the bony ridges (figure 46–2). The overall lesion appears as a group of closely arranged pebble-shaped, red, edematous projections.

B. Contributing Factors

The cause is unknown but it is associated with poor denture hygiene, ill-fitting dentures, and possible *Candida albicans* infection.

V. Denture Irritation Hyperplasia (Epulis fissuratum)

Long-standing, chronic inflammatory tissue appears in single or multiple elongated folds related to the border of an ill-fitting denture.

VI. Angular Cheilitis[8]

A. Appearance

Angular cheilitis appears as fissuring at the angles of the mouth, with cracks, ulcerations, and erythema. Sometimes it is dry with a crust; other times, it is moist from saliva.

B. Contributing Factors

It is usually initiated by lack of support of the commissure because of overclosure, and moistness from drooling. Secondarily, a riboflavin deficiency or an infection by *Candida albicans* or other organisms may be involved.

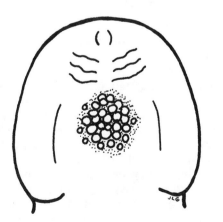

Figure 46–2. Papillary Hyperplasia. Outline of an edentulous palate to show the characteristic location of papillary hyperplasia within the bony ridges.

PREVENTION AND MAINTENANCE

I. Development of Attitude and Understanding by the Patient

For continuing oral health and appropriate denture service, the patient needs to understand the following:

A. Purposes of regular maintenance appointments for finding early signs of disease, particularly chronic irritations and oral cancer.

B. Reasons why the dentist must supervise the function and fit of the dentures.

C. Damage that can result from wearing ill-fitting dentures for long periods of time (years) without tissue and denture examination.

D. Harmful effects to the oral tissue and damage to the dentures that can result from the unsupervised use of commercial products for denture retention or relief, or of home repair kits.

II. Daily Preventive Measures

A. Denture Hygiene

Dentures must be cleaned after each meal. Details were explained on pages 346–349. Cleansing solutions must be changed daily.

B. Oral Mucosa

1. Brush to clean and massage.
2. Digital massage (page 349).

C. Rest for the Tissues

For most patients, having the dentures out while sleeping is the best procedure to provide rest for the oral tissues. When this is impossible, the patient should remove the denture for as long a daytime period as possible, such as while bathing. While the dentures are out of the mouth, they can be placed in a container with cleaning solution, and the mucosa can be cleaned and massaged.

D. Diet and Nutrition

The teaching of food selection cannot be overemphasized. For denture wearers, an emphasis on using foods from the Basic Four food groups is necessary. Control of weight and avoidance of foods that are related to specific chronic conditions are important. A dietary analysis can provide a foundation for making specific recommendations.

The diet problems of the elderly patient have been described on pages 568–569. Factors that contribute to dietary deficiencies in patients of any age are magnified when dentures are ill-fitting and masticatory efficiency is decreased. The patient tends to overlook food value and select foods that are within the limits of chewing ability or that can be swallowed without chewing.

E. Relief from Xerostomia

The use of saliva substitute may be recommended (page 188).

III. Professional Supervision

A. Appointment Frequency

1. *First Year.* After the initial adjustments, the patient can expect the dentures to need reline, rebase, or remake in 6 months to 1 year.
2. *Subsequent Maintenance Period*
   a. For most patients, one appointment each year is adequate.
   b. For patients who are careless with denture and tissue care, at least two appointments each year are recommended.
   c. For patients who are at high cancer risk because of age, tobacco use, and alcohol-drinking habits or have a previous history of cancer, examination three to four times per year should be scheduled.

B. Maintenance Appointment

Maintenance procedures as described on pages 540–541 are followed with necessary adaptations for the edentulous patient.

1. *Procedures for the Dental Hygienist*
   a. Review patient history; make necessary additions to the record.
   b. Determine blood pressure.
   c. Perform an extraoral and intraoral examination and record suspicious lesions for the dentist's review.
   d. Examine dentures for cleanliness and evidences of patient care
      i. Ask patient to describe the personal hygiene care procedures used routinely.
      ii. Supplement with additional demonstration and instruction when the care is less than adequate.
   e. Clean the dentures to remove calculus and stain. Procedures are described on pages 513–514.
2. *Procedures for the Dentist*
   a. Review all findings recorded by the dental hygienist.
   b. Examine the oral tissues and the fit and occlusion of the dentures.
   c. Treatment as needed.
3. *Subsequent Appointment*
   Make necessary appointments for continuing current treatment or for maintenance.

DENTURE MARKING FOR IDENTIFICATION[9]

The need for denture marking is apparent in a variety of situations. A universal system for marking would be ideal. Marking is required by law in some countries and in certain states of the United States. In forensic dentistry, or for identification of victims of war, disasters such as flood or fire, or transportation catastrophe, the dentition has been used increasingly as a means of identification.

Dentures provide a method for immediate identification. Prompt identification can be urgent when an individual is found unconscious from illness or injury or suffering from amnesia as a result of psychiatric or traumatic causes as well as from senility.

The dentures of people in long-term residence or care facilities should be marked. Mislaid dentures can be returned and mix-ups by the direct care staff can be prevented. Dental hygienists are able to make an important contribution to an oral health program by introducing a plan for denture marking.

I. Criteria for an Adequate Marking System

Information on the denture must be specific so that rapid identification is possible.

A. Relative to the Denture

1. Must have no adverse effects on denture material.
2. Must not change the strength, surface texture, or fit of the denture.
3. Must be cosmetically acceptable: the label placed in an inobtrusive position.

B. Relative to the Procedure

1. Readily learned and simple to carry out.
2. Inexpensive.
3. Durable result. When the information is incorporated during denture processing, indefinite durability can be expected. A surface marker for a denture already in use should be able to withstand denture cleaning methods for a reasonable period of time.

C. Characteristics of the Material Used

1. *Fire and Humidity Resistant.* When the label is placed inside the posterior section of a denture, the surrounding tongue and maxillofacial parts offer protection except in the most severe conflagration.
2. *Radiopaque.* A metal marker can be of use as a means of identification by radiographic examination in the event the radiolucent acrylic denture is accidentally swallowed.[10]

II. Methods for Marking

The types used fall into two general categories, inclusion and surface markers.

A. Inclusion

1. *New Dentures.* A typewritten or printed enclosure is inserted as a denture is being processed. Labels are positioned on the impression surfaces of the maxillary and mandibular dentures (figure 46–3). They are covered, just before the final closure of the flask, with a clear acrylic material.

   A label may be typewritten on onionskin paper or the tissue paper that separates sheets of packaged baseplate wax.[9,11,12] Another system uses a thin metal strip for the insert. Stainless steel matrix bands, orthodontic bands, and thin metal strips (shim stock) have been used.[10,13]

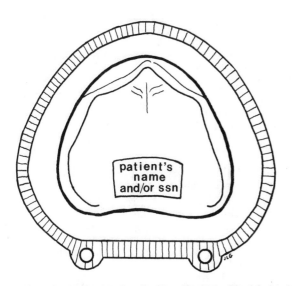

Figure 46–3. Inclusion Marker for New Denture. The label is inserted on the impression surface as the denture is being processed. On the flasked maxillary denture shown, the marker is positioned near the posterior border.

2. *Existing Dentures*[14]
   a. Clean the dentures thoroughly.
   b. Use a Number 6 or 8 round bur and an inverted cone to cut small, shallow, box-like preparations in the posterior buccal flange of the maxillary denture and the lingual posterior flange of the mandibular denture (figure 46–4). Do not go through to the impression surface.
   c. Typewrite two copies of the patient's initials (or other choice of identification) on onionskin paper, and trim the papers to fit the box-like preparations.
   d. Cover the paper with cold-cure clear acrylic and fill to a slight excess; after the acrylic has cured, polish to a smooth finish.

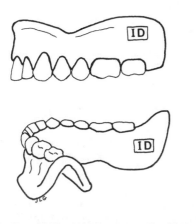

Figure 46–4. Surface Markers for Dentures. The labels are placed on the external denture surfaces for existing dentures. As shown, the markers are on the maxillary buccal flange and the mandibular lingual flange.

B. Surface Markers

Surface markers are not as durable, but instruction can be provided for persons not trained in dental laboratory methods. In a skilled nursing facility or other long-term institution that has no resident dentist or dental hygienist, it may be important to teach a nurse or other staff member to mark dentures of residents as they are admitted. The two methods described below have been used for this purpose.

1. *Indelible Pen.* After cleaning and drying the denture, a small area near the posterior of the outer or polished denture surface is rubbed with an emery board until it is rough (figure 46–4). The name, initials, or other identification is printed on the roughened area with an indelible pen and dried. Two or three coats of a finger nail acrylic (heavy nail protector) are painted over the area; each layer is dried before applying the next. Surface markings have been found to last at least 6 months.[15]

2. *Engraving Tool.* An engraving tool is used to enter the name on the denture, and the grooves created are darkened with a special pencil before a sealing liquid is applied. Materials are available in a commercial kit.[16]

III. Information to Include on a Marker

For residents of a home or institution, using only the person's name and initials should suffice for temporary surface marking.

In a community, country, or international situation, the name alone would not provide enough identification, and the social security number, armed services serial number, or the equivalent in other countries, should be included.

Other identification such as blood type and vital drug or disease condition has been suggested. In certain countries, the dentist's registration or hospital number has been used. In Sweden, the patient's date of birth and national registration number have been marked on the dentures. The markings that can provide *immediate* identification are the most significant.

FACTORS TO TEACH THE PATIENT

I. Dentures are not permanent appliances.
II. Dentures and tissues must be examined at least once a year. Teach frequency of maintenance appointments for the individual, depending in part on that individual's ability to clean the dentures and maintain them free from plaque, stain, and calculus.
III. Dentures may need replacement periodically. Tissues under the denture change.
IV. Avoid use of drugstore remedies, reliners, and other home-applied materials unless the dentist has provided specific instruction.

V. Specific methods of care for dentures.
VI. Leaving the dentures out of the mouth overnight in accord with dentist's directions.
VII. Where to obtain and how to use a saliva substitute.

References

1. American Academy of Denture Prosthetics, Nomenclature Committee: *Glossary of Prosthodontic Terms*, 5th ed. *J. Prosthet. Dent., 58,* 717, December, 1987.
2. Tallgren, A.: The Continuing Reduction of the Residual Alveolar Ridges in Complete Denture Wearers: A Mixed-Longitudinal Study Covering 25 Years, *J. Prosthet. Dent., 27,* 120, February, 1972.
3. American Dental Association, Council on Dental Health: Guidelines on After Care for Denture Patients, *J. Am. Dent. Assoc., 94,* 1187, June, 1977.
4. Gallagher, J.B.: Insertion and Postinsertion Care, in Clark, J.W., ed.: *Clinical Dentistry, Volume 5,* Chapter 14. Philadelphia, J.B. Lippincott, 1984, pp. 1–27.
5. Atwood, D.A.: Bone Loss of Edentulous Alveolar Ridges, *J. Periodontol., 50,* 11, Special Issue, 1979.
6. Welker, W.A.: Prosthodontic Treatment of Abused Oral Tissues, *J. Prosthet. Dent., 37,* 259, March, 1977.
7. Renner, R.P., Lee, M., Andors, L., and McNamara, T.F.: The Role of *C. albicans* in Denture Stomatitis, *Oral Surg., 47,* 323, April, 1979.
8. Shafer, W.G., Hine, M.K., and Levy, B.M.: *A Textbook of Oral Pathology,* 4th ed. Philadelphia, W.B. Saunders Co., 1983, pp. 556–557.
9. American Dental Association, Council on Prosthetic Services and Dental Laboratory Relations: *Operation Ident.* Chicago, American Dental Association, March, 1982.
10. Jerman, A.C.: Denture Identification, *J. Am. Dent. Assoc., 80,* 1358, June, 1970.
11. Dentsply International, Inc.: *Method for Placing Permanent Record Data in Denture Base, without Affecting Tissue Adaptation,* Technical Bulletin. Dentsply International, Inc., York, Pennsylvania, 17404.
12. Woodward, J.D.: Denture Marking for Identification, *J. Am. Dent. Assoc., 99,* 59, July, 1979.
13. Turner, C.H., Fletcher, A.M., and Ritchie, G.M.: Denture Marking and Human Identification, *Br. Dent. J., 141,* 114, August 17, 1976.
14. Bauer, T.L.: Technique for Denture Identification, *J. Indiana Dent. Assoc., 58,* 28, Number 6, 1979.
15. Deb, A.K. and Heath, M.R.: Marking Dentures in Geriatric Institutions. The Relevance and Appropriate Methods, *Br. Dent. J., 146,* 282, May 1, 1979.
16. Identure, Geri, Inc., P.O. Box 9086, North St. Paul, Minnesota, 55109.

Suggested Readings

Berthold, P. and Segal, H.: Some Aspects of Emergency Treatment of Complete Denture Patients, *Compend. Contin. Educ. Dent., 6,* 322, May, 1985.
Catelli, W.F., Engstrom, H.I.M., Hollender, L.G., and Feller, R.P.: Panoramic Radiographic Examination of Patients Who Are Edentulous, *Spec. Care Dentist., 7,* 114, May-June, 1987.
DePaola, L.G., Meiller, T.F., Leupold, R.J., Balciunas, B.A., and Williams, G.C.: The Relationship of Medical Problems and Medications to Treatment of the Denture Patient, *Gerodontics, 2,* 53, April, 1986.
Hoffman, W., Bomberg, T.J., and Hatch, R.A.: Considerations for the Elderly Denture Patient, *Gen. Dent., 33,* 489, November-December, 1985.
Hurst, T.L., Tye, E.A., and Byrd, C.: Snorkel or Scuba Diver's Denture, *J. Prosthet. Dent., 55,* 597, May, 1986.
Keur, J.J.: Radiographic Screening of Edentulous Patients: Sense or Nonsense? A Risk-Benefit Analysis, *Oral Surg. Oral Med. Oral Pathol., 62,* 463, October, 1986.

Kreher, J.M., Graser, G.N., and Handelman, S.L.: The Relationship of Drug Use to Denture Function and Saliva Flow Rate in a Geriatric Population, *J. Prosthet. Dent., 57,* 631, May, 1987.
Mersel, A. and Lowenthal, U.: Anxious Anticipation of Complete Dentures, *Spec. Care Dentist., 6,* 129, May-June, 1986.
Osterberg, T. and Mellström, D.: Tobacco Smoking: A Major Risk Factor for Loss of Teeth in Three 70-year-old Cohorts, *Community Dent. Oral Epidemiol., 14,* 367, December, 1986.
Payne, S.D.W. and Henry, M.: Radiolucent Dentures Impacted in the Oesophagus, *Br. J. Surg., 71,* 318, April, 1984.
Razzoog, M.E., Bloem, T., and Lang, B.: The Edentulous Patient: Attitudes Toward Oral Health Status, *Spec. Care Dentist., 3,* 214, September-October, 1983.
Toljanic, J.A. and Schweiger, J.W.: Fabrication of an Artificial Saliva Reservoir Denture System for Xerostomia Management, *Quintessence Dent. Technol., 9,* 355, June, 1985.
Zarb, G.A.: The Edentulous Milieu, *J. Prosthet. Dent., 49,* 825, June, 1983.

Denture Pathology

Arendorf, T.M. and Walker, D.M.: Denture Stomatitis: A Review, *J. Oral Rehabil., 14,* 217, May, 1987.
Arendorf, T.M., Walker, D.M., Kingdom, R.J., Roll, J.R.S., and Newcombe, R.G.: Tobacco Smoking and Denture Wearing in Oral Candidal Leukoplakia, *Br. Dent. J., 155,* 340, November 19, 1983.
Bergendal, T. and Isacsson, G.: A Combined Clinical, Mycological and Histological Study of Denture Stomatitis, *Acta Odontol. Scand., 41,* 33, Number 1, 1983.
Budtz-Jørgensen, E.: Oral Mucosal Lesions Associated with the Wearing of Removable Dentures, *J. Oral Pathol., 10,* 65, April, 1981.
Dorey, J.L., Blasberg, B., MacEntee, M.I., and Conklin, R.J.: Oral Mucosal Disorders in Denture Wearers, *J. Prosthet. Dent., 53,* 210, February, 1985.
Fouché, M.H., Slabbert, J.C.G., and Coogan, M.M.: Bacterial Antibodies in Patients Undergoing Treatment for Denture Stomatitis, *J. Prosthet. Dent., 58,* 63, July, 1987.
Fouché, M.H., Slabbert, J.C.G., and Coogan, M.M.: Candidal Antibodies in Patients Undergoing Treatment for Denture Stomatitis, *J. Prosthet. Dent., 57,* 587, May, 1987.
Gorsky, M. and Silverman, S.: Denture Wearing and Oral Cancer, *J. Prosthet. Dent., 52,* 164, August, 1984.
Katz, J., Benoliel, R., and Leviner, E.: Burning Mouth Sensation Associated with Fusospirochetal Infection in Edentulous Patients, *Oral Surg. Oral Med. Oral Pathol., 62,* 152, August, 1986.
Mikkonen, M., Nyyssönen, V., Paunio, I., and Rajala, M.: Oral Hygiene, Dental Visits and Age of Denture for Prevalence of Denture Stomatitis, *Community Dent. Oral Epidemiol., 12,* 402, December, 1984.
Phelan, J.A. and Levin, S.M.: A Prevalence Study of Denture Stomatitis in Subjects with Diabetes Mellitus or Elevated Plasma Glucose Levels, *Oral Surg. Oral Med. Oral Pathol., 62,* 303, September, 1986.
Russotto, S.B.: The Role of *Candida albicans* in the Pathogenesis of Angular Cheilosis, *J. Prosthet. Dent., 44,* 243, September, 1980.
Watkinson, A.C., McCreight, M.C., and Warnock, D.W.: Prevalence and Persistence of Different Strains of *Candida albicans* in Treatment of Denture Stomatitis, *J. Prosthet. Dent., 53,* 365, March, 1985.

Denture Plaque; Patient Instruction

Ambjørnsen, E., Valderhaug, J., Norheim, P.W., and Fløystrand, F.: Assessment of An Additive Index for Plaque Accumulation on Complete Maxillary Dentures, *Acta Odontol. Scand., 40,* 203, Number 4, 1982.
Bauman, R.: Survey of Dentists' Attitudes Regarding Instructions for Home Care for Patients Who Wear Dentures, *J. Am. Dent. Assoc., 100,* 206, February, 1980.
Bergman, B. and Carlsson, G.E.: Clinical Long-term Study of Complete Denture Wearers, *J. Prosthet. Dent., 53,* 56, January, 1985.
Bloem, T.J.: An Index for Assessment of Oral Health in the Eden-

tulous Population, *Spec. Care Dentist., 2,* 121, May-June, 1982.

Budtz-Jörgensen, E., Theilade, E., Theilade, J., and Zander, H.A.: Method for Studying the Development, Structure, and Microflora of Denture Plaque, *Scand. J. Dent. Res., 89,* 149, April, 1981.

Cabot, L.B. and Roberts, B.J.: Aftercare for the Complete Denture Patient, *Br. Dent. J., 157,* 72, July 21, 1984.

Chamberlain, B.B., Bernier, S.H., Bloem, T.J., and Razzoog, M.E.: Denture Plaque Control and Inflammation in the Edentulous Patient, *J. Prosthet. Dent., 54,* 78, July, 1985.

DePaola, L.G., Minah, G.E., Leupold, R.J., Faraone, K.L., and Elias, S.A.: The Effect of Antiseptic Mouthrinses on Oral Microbial Flora and Denture Stomatitis, *Clin. Prevent. Dent., 8,* 3, September-October, 1986.

Dukes, B.S.: An Evaluation of Soft Tissue Responses Following Removal of Ill-fitting Dentures, *J. Prosthet. Dent., 43,* 251, March, 1980.

Polyzois, G.L.: The Wearing of Complete Dentures: Guidance to Patients, *J. Oral Rehabil., 10,* 229, May, 1983.

Poulsen, S., Budtz-Jørgensen, E., Knudsen, A.M., Nielsen, L., and Kelstrup, J.: Evaluation of Two Methods of Scoring Denture Plaque, *Acta Odontol. Scand., 41,* 283, October, 1983.

Tarbet, W.J.: Denture Plaque: Quiet Destroyer, *J. Prosthet. Dent., 48,* 647, December, 1982.

Tautin, F.S.: The Beneficial Effects of Tissue Massage for the Edentulous Patient, *J. Prosthet. Dent., 48,* 653, December, 1982.

Wendt, D.C.: How to Promote and Maintain Good Oral Health in Spite of Wearing Dentures, *J. Prosthet. Dent., 53,* 805, June, 1985.

Denture Sanitation

DePaola, L.G. and Minah, G.E.: Isolation of Pathogenic Microorganisms from Dentures and Denture-soaking Containers of Myelosuppressed Cancer Patients, *J. Prosthet. Dent., 49,* 20, January, 1983.

Kahn, R.C., Lancaster, M.V., and Kate, W.: The Microbiologic Cross-contamination of Dental Prostheses, *J. Prosthet. Dent., 47,* 556, May, 1982.

Moore, T.C., Smith, D.E., and Kenny, G.E.: Sanitization of Dentures by Several Denture Hygiene Methods, *J. Prosthet. Dent., 52,* 158, August, 1984.

Radue, J.T., Unger, J.W., and Molinari, J.A.: Avoiding Cross-contamination in Immediate Denture Treatment, *J. Prosthet. Dent., 49,* 576, April, 1983.

Stafford, G.D., Arendorf, T., and Huggett, R.: The Effect of Overnight Drying and Water Immersion on Candidal Colonization and Properties of Complete Dentures, *J. Dent., 14,* 52, April, 1986.

Nutrition

Baxter, J.C.: Nutrition and the Geriatric Edentulous Patient, *Spec. Care Dentist., 1,* 259, November-December, 1981.

Chauncey, H.H., Muench, M.E., Kapur, K.K., and Wayler, A.H.: The Effect of the Loss of Teeth on Diet and Nutrition, *Int. Dent. J., 34,* 98, June, 1984.

Nizel, A.E. and Papas, A.S.: *Nutrition in Clinical Dentistry*, 3rd ed. Philadelphia, W.B. Saunders Co., 1989, pp. 359–365.

Denture Identification

Chalian, V.A., Sayoc, A.M., Ghalichebaf, M., and Schaeffer, L.: Identification of Removable Dental Prosthesis, *J. Prosthet. Dent., 56,* 254, August, 1986.

Davis, D.J.: "Invisible" Denture Identification: A Forensic Aid, *J. Prosthet. Dent., 48,* 221, August, 1982.

Dippenaar, A.P.: Denture Marking: An Aesthetic Inclusion, *J. Dent. Assoc. S. Afr., 41,* 13, January, 1986.

Fiske, J., Graham, T., and Gelbier, S.: Denture Identification for Elderly People, *Br. Dent. J., 161,* 448, December 20, 1986.

Harrison, A.: A Simple Denture Marking System, *Br. Dent. J., 160,* 89, February 8, 1986.

Heath, J.R.: Denture Identification—A Simple Approach, *J. Oral Rehabil., 14,* 147, March, 1987.

Johanson, G. and Ekman, B.: Denture Marking, *J. Am. Dent. Assoc., 108,* 347, March, 1984.

Kenney, J.P.: Forensic Dentistry: From Denture Identification to Murder Investigations, *Dent. Assist., 51,* 17, November-December, 1982.

Key, M.C. and Forcucci, C.: A Simplified Identification Technique for Removable Prostheses, *Gen. Dent., 28,* 59, November-December, 1980.

Seals, R.R. and Seals, D.J.: The Importance of Denture Identification, *Spec. Care Dentist., 5,* 164, July-August, 1985.

Stevenson, R.B.: Marking Dentures for Identification, *J. Prosthet. Dent., 58,* 255, August, 1987.

Yamagata, P.A.B., Haley, C.A.C., and Tomasseti, S.L.: Can Your Patients Recognize Their Dental Prostheses? A Step-by-step Identification System, *RDH, 2,* 30, January, 1982.

Denture Adhesives and Self Repair

American Dental Association, Council on Dental Materials, Instruments, and Equipment: *Dentist's Desk Reference: Materials, Instruments, and Equipment,* 2nd ed. Chicago, American Dental Association, 1983, pp. 422–426.

Getz, I.I.: The Dangers of Do-it-yourself Dentistry, *Gen. Dent., 35,* 361, September-October, 1987.

Koudelka, B.M., Nelson, J.F., and Webb, J.G.: Denture Self-repair: Experimental Soft Tissue Response to Selected Commercial Adhesives, *J. Prosthet. Dent., 43,* 143, February, 1980.

Lamb, D.J.: Denture Adhesives: A Side Effect, *J. Dent., 8,* 35, March, 1980.

Tarbet, W.J. and Grossman, E.: Observations of Denture-supporting Tissue During Six Months of Denture Adhesive Wearing, *J. Am. Dent. Assoc., 101,* 789, November, 1980.

47 The Patient with a Cleft Lip or Palate

The patient with a cleft lip and/or cleft palate may be a dental cripple unless extensive rehabilitative supervision is available. Treatment and care require the united efforts of nearly all of the dental specialists as well as the family physician, plastic surgeon, speech therapist, psychologist, otolaryngologist, audiologist, social worker, and vocational counselor. The dental hygienist is an important member of the team responsible for oral care.

Speaking ability and appearance are among the first factors considered when the long-range treatment program is planned, because the objective is to help the patient lead a normal life. Dental personnel need to maintain a current list of the health agencies, clinics, and other community resources where the patient and family may obtain assistance for the various phases of treatment and habilitation.

DESCRIPTION

I. Definitions[1]

A. Cleft Lip

A cleft lip is a unilateral or bilateral congenital fissure in the upper lip, usually lateral to the midline. The defect can extend into the nares and may involve the alveolar process. A cleft lip is caused by a defect in the fusion of the maxillary and nasal processes. It may be accompanied by a cleft palate.

B. Cleft Palate

A cleft palate is a unilateral or bilateral congenital fissure in the palate caused by a failure of the palatal shelves to fuse. It may be accompanied by a cleft lip.

II. Classification

The classification is based on disturbances in the embryologic formation of the palate as it develops from the premaxillary region toward the uvula in a definite pattern. Interference with normal development of the palate may occur at one age level of the embryo, and the normal pattern may be reestablished at a later age. Such interferences would modify the classification suggested in this chapter.

All degrees are found, from an insignificant notch in the mucous membrane of the lip or uvula, which produces no functional disability, to the complete cleft defined by Class 6 of this classification. The first six classes are illustrated in figure 47–1.

Class 1. Cleft of the tip of the uvula.
Class 2. Cleft of the uvula (bifid uvula).
Class 3. Cleft of the soft palate.
Class 4. Cleft of the soft and hard palates.
Class 5. Cleft of the soft and hard palates that continues through the alveolar ridge on one side of the premaxilla; usually associated with cleft lip of the same side.
Class 6. Cleft of the soft and hard palates that continues through the alveolar ridge on both sides, leaving a free premaxilla; usually associated with bilateral cleft lip.
Class 7. Submucous cleft in which the muscle union is imperfect across the soft palate. The palate is short; the uvula is often bifid; a groove is situated at the midline of the soft palate; and the closure to the pharynx is incompetent.

III. Etiology

A. Embryology[2]

Cleft lip and palate represent a failure of normal fusion of embryonic processes during development in the first trimester of pregnancy. Figure 47–2 shows the locations of the globular process and the right and left maxillary processes. These fuse normally and no cleft of the lip results.

Formation of the lip occurs between the fourth and seventh weeks in utero. The development of the palate takes place during the eighth to twelfth weeks. Fusion begins in the premaxillary region and continues backward toward the uvula.

A cleft lip becomes apparent by the end of the second month. A cleft palate is evident by the end of the third month in utero.

B. Predisposing Factors

Heredity (genetic predisposition) is believed to exert a major influence. Several other factors have been considered, and some of these have been shown effective in animal experimentation. Examples are infectious diseases in the mother, nutritional deficiencies, or mechanical interferences in the fetus. It is generally believed that both genetic and environmental forces are involved.

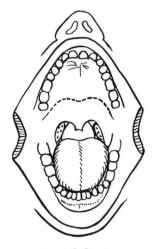

CLASS 1

Cleft of the tip of the uvula.

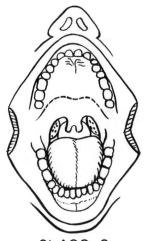

CLASS 2

Cleft of the uvula (bifid uvula).

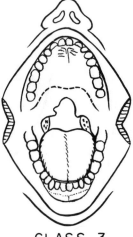

CLASS 3

Cleft of the soft palate.

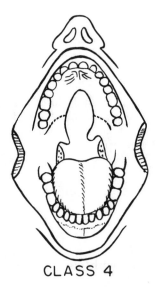

CLASS 4

Cleft of the soft and hard palates.

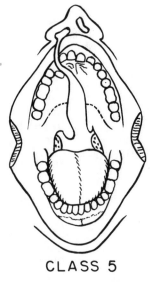

CLASS 5

Cleft of the soft and hard palates that continues through the alveolar ridge on one side of the premaxilla. Usually associated with cleft lip of the same side.

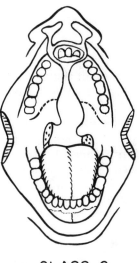

CLASS 6

Cleft of the soft and hard palates that continues through the alveolar ridge on both sides, leaving a free premaxilla. Usually associated with bilateral cleft lip.

Figure 47–1. Classification of Cleft Lip and Cleft Palate. (Courtesy of O.E. Beder.)

ORAL CHARACTERISTICS

I. Tooth Development

Disturbances in the normal development of the tooth buds occur more frequently in patients with clefts than in the general population. There is a higher incidence of missing and supernumerary teeth, as well as abnormalities of tooth form.

II. Malocclusion

A high percentage of patients with cleft lip and palate require orthodontic care.

III. Open Palate

Before surgical correction, an open palate provides direct communication with the nasal cavity.

IV. Muscle Coordination

A lack of coordinate movements of lips, tongue, cheeks, floor of mouth, and throat may exist and lead

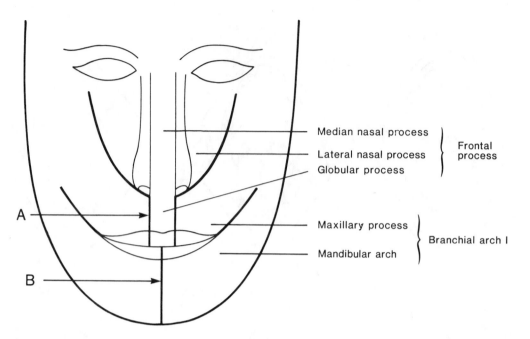

Figure 47–2. Developmental Processes of the Face. The derivations of parts of the face from the frontal process and the branchial arch. **A.** Location of cleft lip when fusion of the globular process and a maxillary process fails. **B.** Cleft of the mandible can occur at the midline. (Redrawn from Melfi, R.C.: *Permar's Oral Embryology and Microscopic Anatomy*, 8th ed. Lea & Febiger, 1988.)

to compensatory habits formed in the attempt to produce normal sounds while speaking.

V. Gingival Disturbances

These are created by effects of bacterial plaque accumulation influenced by irregularly positioned teeth, displaced teeth, inability to keep lips closed, and difficulties in accomplishing adequate personal oral care. Early periodontal disease with loss of bone and attachment is common in adolescents.[3]

VI. Dental Caries

The incidence of dental caries should be no different from noncleft patients, except that predisposing factors such as irregularly positioned teeth, problems of mastication, and dietary selection factors may be intensified.

VII. Treated Patient

A. Suture lines from surgical correction may be evident.
B. Patient may have a removable prosthodontic appliance. Types of appliances are defined on page 585.

GENERAL PHYSICAL CHARACTERISTICS

I. Other Congenital Anomalies

Incidence is higher than in noncleft people. In more than 150 disorders, cleft lip, cleft palate, or both, represent one feature of a syndrome.[4]

II. Facial Deformity

Facial deformities may include depression of the nostril on the side with the cleft lip; deficiency of upper lip in which it may be short or retroposed; overprominent lower lip.

III. Infections

Predisposition to upper respiratory and middle ear infections is common.

IV. Hearing Loss

The incidence of hearing loss is significantly higher in individuals with cleft palate than in the non-cleft population.

V. Speech

Patients with cleft lip and/or cleft palate have difficulty in making certain sounds and may produce nasal tones. Anatomic structure is not considered the only contributing factor to the speech problem. It may be related to the hearing loss or to psychologic factors related to inferior feelings or parental attitude.

VI. Undernourishment

Undernourishment may result when feeding problems continue for a long period.

PERSONAL FACTORS

Most cleft lip and palate patients do not have personality problems, but realization of the social effects of speech and appearance makes it easy to understand why some of them exhibit evidences of maladjustment. The ridicule of contemporaries soon leads even small children to think they are "different." Parental acceptance or rejection no doubt can be a strong influence in adjustment. A few possible characteristics are suggested here.

I. Self-consciousness

Hypersensitivity to taunts or obvious pity.

II. Feelings of Inferiority

The result may be a person who is quiet, unresponsive, and withdrawn or one who is openly brash or rebellious until rapport is established.

TREATMENT

Treatment is coordinated by a team of specialists and based on the patient's progress at each age period. Several reviews provide overviews of the types of treatment and the objectives of each.[5,6,7]

I. Cleft Lip

Surgical union of the cleft lip is made early, for example when the child weighs 10 pounds and is 10 weeks old. The infant's general health is a determining factor, and some surgeons wait until the birth weight is regained or the weight has reached 12 pounds. Another timetable is to repair the cleft lip within 48 hours after birth and the cleft palate by 16 weeks.[8]

The closure aids in feeding, development of the premaxilla, and growth of the lip, and may also help to partially close the palatal cleft. The operation has a favorable effect on parents and family members in that it helps to lessen their apprehension and concern.

At the time of lip surgery, an obturator may be made for the palate to make feeding easier and provide support for the lip and premaxilla. It is remade periodically to accommodate for the growth and development of the child. For each step in treatment, the parents, or other person responsible, need instruction for the daily care of the patient's oral cavity and frequent, meticulous cleaning and care of the appliance.

II. Cleft Palate

It is generally agreed that repair of the palate should be undertaken between ages 1 and 2 years. Occlusion has a strong influence on the development of palatal dimensions and growth is rapid during this period. Surgical intervention too early could interfere with normal growth. The combined efforts of many specialists are required.

A. Purposes for Early Treatment
1. Improve child's appearance.
2. Aid child's mental development.
3. Prevent malnourishment by improving the feeding apparatus.
4. Aid in development of the speech pattern.
5. Reduce possibilities of repeated infections of the nasopharyngeal region.

B. Maxillofacial Surgery
Closure of the palate is accomplished by surgery or prosthodontics or both. Surgery provides direct union of the existing tissue that has been moved to a more desirable position for function.

III. Prosthodontics

A removable appliance is designed to provide closure of the palatal opening and/or to complete the palatopharyngeal valving required for speech.

A. Types of Appliances
1. *Prosthesis.* Artificial replacement for a missing part.
2. *Obturator.* Removable appliance designed to close an opening such as a cleft of the hard palate.
3. *Speech Aid.* A removable appliance related to the soft palate that provides a means for palatopharyngeal valving for speech.

B. Purposes of the Appliance
It may be designed to accomplish one or all of the following factors:
1. Closure of the palate.
2. Replacement of missing teeth.
3. Scaffolding to fill out the upper lip.
4. Masticatory function.
5. Restoration of vertical dimension.
6. Postorthodontic retainer.

IV. Orthodontics

Treatment may be initiated as early as 3 years of age, depending on the problems of dentofacial development.

V. Speech Therapy

Training may be started with very young children, and is particularly emphasized after the surgical or prosthodontic treatment has been accomplished.

VI. Operative Dentistry (Pedodontist or General Dental Practitioner)

A major problem can be dental caries, leading to tooth loss. With missing teeth, major difficulties arise related to all phases of treatment, particularly the retention of a prosthesis. Preservation of the primary teeth is very important.

DENTAL HYGIENE CARE

Preventive measures for preservation of the teeth and their supporting structures are essential to the success of the special care needed for the habilitation of the cleft palate patient. Each phase of dental hygiene care and instruction, important for all patients, takes on even greater significance in the light of the magnified problems of the patient with a cleft lip and/or cleft palate.

Every attempt should be made to avoid the need for removal of teeth because the patient has enough oral problems without also being edentulous. Primary and permanent teeth are needed for the stabilization of a speech aid or obturator and for the success of all treatment procedures. Understanding by the patient and the parents of the value of preventive procedures is accomplished through explanation and instruction.

When the patient has not had specialized care, the dental hygienist has a responsibility in working with the dentist to arrange referral to an available agency, clinic, or private practice specialist.

I. Objectives for Appointment Planning

Frequent appointments, scheduled every 3 or 4 months, are usually needed during the maintenance phase of the patient's care.
A. To review plaque control measures and provide encouragement for the patient in maintaining the health of the supporting structures and the cleanliness of the obturator or speech aid.
B. To remove all calculus and smooth the tooth surfaces as a supplement to the patient's personal daily care procedures.
C. To make topical fluoride applications at proper intervals for both primary and permanent dentitions, and to supervise self-application of daily fluoride.

II. Appointment Considerations

A. A patient who has often been in a hospital for oral surgery may be very apprehensive about dental and dental hygiene care.
B. Speech may be almost unintelligible, although with repeated contact, understanding can be developed.
   1. Avoid embarrassment produced by constantly asking the patient to repeat what has been said.
   2. Provide pencil and paper for the older child to write requests or comments.
   3. Let parent or other person accompanying small child interpret.
C. Depending on the severity of hearing loss, the approach is similar to that for speech difficulties. Suggestions for care of patients with hearing problems are described on page 680.
D. Avoid solicitousness or obvious pity. Approach as a normal patient.
E. Provide motivations for quiet unresponsive or bold rebellious types that will help them gain an objective approach to the care of their mouths.

III. Sterile Techniques

Although procedures for asepsis should be the same for all patients, it should be remembered that the open fissure lines make the cleft palate patient particularly susceptible to infections.

IV. Instrumentation

Techniques are adapted to the oral characteristics. All objectives of scaling and other instrumentation have particular implications for the patient with a cleft palate.

A. Malaligned Teeth
Adjust scaling and root planing procedures.

B. Free Premaxilla (Unoperated Older Patient)
Related to bilateral cleft of alveolar ridge; avoid undue pressure with finger rests or instrument to prevent movement of the part.

C. Area of Recent Surgery
Avoid pressure.

D. Sensitive, Enlarged Gingival Tissue That Bleeds Readily
1. Begin plaque control instruction first before any instrumentation.
2. Continue plaque control instruction as small sections of scaling are done over several appointments.
3. Arrange follow-up appointments to check response of tissue.

E. Open Fissures
Prevent debris or pieces of calculus from passing into or being retained in the clefts. Whenever possible, use rubber dam for indicated procedures.

F. Lack of Coordinated Movements
Small children especially may need instruction in how to rinse when this is a new procedure for them.

G. Prosthesis or Speech Aid
Use same procedures and precautions as for cleaning a removable denture (pages 513–514).

V. Topical Application of Fluoride

Free premaxilla or short upper lip may complicate cotton roll or tray placement.

VI. Patient Instruction

A. Personal Oral Care Procedures
The self-conscious patient may actually fear or exhibit rejection toward the oral cavity. With a small child, the parents may be afraid of damaging the deformed areas or hurting the child if cleaning methods are employed. The dental hygienist must have an empathetic and sympathetic approach and plan for continued instruction over a long period of time.
1. *Teeth and Gingiva*
   a. Select toothbrush, brushing method, and auxiliary aids according to the individual needs.
   b. Adapt techniques for patient with free premaxilla to prevent its movement. A soft nylon brush with end-rounded filaments is indicated.

c. Instigate daily self-application of fluoride: mouth rinse, fluoride dentifrice, and diet supplements for a young child in a non-fluoridated community (pages 400 and 407).

2. *Prosthesis or Speech Aid.* Halitosis may be a real problem when the prosthesis forms the soft palate and the floor of the nasal cavity because of the accumulation of mucus secreted by the nasal cavity surfaces.

a. Instruct patient in the need for frequent removal of appliance for cleaning, particularly following eating.

b. Method for cleaning the prosthesis is the same as for a removable partial denture (pages 346–349).

B. Diet

1. *Need for a Varied Diet.* Should include adequate proportions of all essential food groups (table 28–1, page 382).

2. *Need for Prevention of Dental Caries.* Limitation of cariogenic foods, particularly for between-meal snacks.

VII. Dental Hygiene Care Related to Oral Surgery

A. Presurgery (pages 589–592, 599)

Objectives have particular significance because the cleft palate patient is unusually susceptible to infections of the upper respiratory area and middle ear. Every precaution should be taken to prevent complications.

B. Postsurgery Personal Oral Care

In certain of the palate operations, arm restraints are applied to prevent accidental damage to the repaired region. After each feeding (liquid diet for several days, soft diet for the next week), the mouth must be rinsed carefully. Brushing must be accomplished with great care, usually by the parent or hospital attendant, to avoid damage to the healing suture lines. In some cases, a toothbrush with suction attachment may be useful (page 638).

References

1. American Association of Orthodontists: *Glossary of Dentofacial Orthopedic Terms. Orthodontic Glossary.* St. Louis, American Association of Orthodontists, 1987.
2. Melfi, R.C.: *Permar's Oral Embryology and Microscopic Anatomy,* 8th ed. Philadelphia, Lea & Febiger, 1988, pp. 25–39.
3. Brägger, U., Schürch, E., Gusberti, F.A., and Lang, N.P.: Periodontal Conditions in Adolescents with Cleft Lip, Alveolus and Palate Following Treatment in a Co-ordinated Team Approach, *J. Clin. Periodontol., 12,* 494, July, 1985.
4. Cohen, M.M.: Syndromes with Cleft Lip and Cleft Palate, *Cleft Palate J., 15,* 306, October, 1978.
5. Berkowitz, S.: State of the Art in Cleft Palate Orofacial Growth and Dentistry. A Historical Perspective, *Am. J. Orthod., 74,* 564, November, 1978.
6. Krogman, W.M.: The Cleft Palate Team in Action, in Cooper, H.K., Harding, R.L., Krogman, W.M., Mazaheri, M., and Millard, R.T., eds.: *Cleft Palate and Cleft Lip: A Team Approach to Clinical Management and Rehabilitation of the Patient.* Philadelphia, W.B. Saunders Co., 1979, pp. 145–161.
7. Harris, R.: Summary of a Conference on Cleft Lip and Cleft Palate, *J. Am. Dent. Assoc., 100,* 396, March, 1980.
8. Desai, S.N.: Early Cleft Palate Repair Completed Before the Age of 16 Weeks: Observations on a Personal Series of 100 Children, *Br. J. Plast. Surg., 36,* 300, July, 1983.

Suggested Readings

Burman, N.T.: Epidemiological Aspects of Teratogenesis—A Review, *Aust. Dent. J., 29,* 159, June, 1984.

Christ, J.E. and Meininger, M.G.: Ultrasound Diagnosis of Cleft Lip and Cleft Palate Before Birth, *Plast. Reconstr. Surg., 68,* 854, December, 1981.

Goyal, B.K.: Impression Procedures for the Cleft Palate Patient, *Compend. Contin. Educ. Dent., 4,* 423, September–October, 1983.

Hairfield, W.M., Warren, D.W., and Seaton, D.L.: Prevalence of Mouthbreathing in Cleft Lip and Palate, *Cleft Palate J., 25,* 135, April, 1988.

Johnsen, D.C. and Dixon, M.: Dental Caries of Primary Incisors in Children with Cleft Lip and Palate, *Cleft Palate J., 21,* 104, April, 1984.

Jones, M.C.: Etiology of Facial Clefts: Prospective Evaluation of 428 Patients, *Cleft Palate J., 25,* 16, January, 1988.

Khoury, M.J., Weinstein, A., Panny, S., Holtzman, N.A., Lindsay, P.K., Farrel, K., and Eisenberg, M.: Maternal Cigarette Smoking and Oral Clefts: A Population-based Study, *Am. J. Public Health, 77,* 623, May, 1987.

Lynch, H.T. and Kimberling, W.J.: Genetic Counseling in Cleft Lip and Cleft Palate, *Plast. Reconstr. Surg., 68,* 800, November, 1981.

McIntee, R.A., Moore, I.J., and Yonkers, A.J.: A General Review of Maxillofacial Cleft Deformities with Emphasis on Dental Anomalies, *Ear Nose Throat J., 65,* 286, July, 1986.

McKinstry, R.E.: Cleft Palate Patients and Local Anesthesia, *Gen. Dent., 30,* 420, September–October, 1982.

Moore, I.J., Moore, G.F., and Yonkers, A.J.: Otitis Media in the Cleft Palate Patient, *Ear Nose Throat J., 65,* 291, July, 1986.

Mosher, G.: Genetic Counseling in Cleft Lip and Palate, *Ear Nose Throat J., 65,* 9, August, 1986.

Nizel, A.E.: *Nutrition in Preventive Dentistry: Science and Practice,* 2nd ed. Philadelphia, W.B. Saunders Co., 1981, pp. 521–523.

Ranta, R.: A Review of Tooth Formation in Children with Cleft Lip/Palate, *Am. J. Orthod. Dentofacial Orthop., 90,* 11, July, 1986.

Robertson, N.R.E.: Facial Form of Patients with Cleft Lip and Palate. The Long-term Influence of Presurgical Oral Orthopaedics, *Br. Dent. J., 155,* 59, July 23, 1983.

Schjelderup, H. and Johnson, G.E.: A Six-year Follow-up Study of 155 Children with Cleft Lip and Palate, *Br. J. Plast. Surg., 36,* 154, April, 1983.

Shaw, W.C. and Humphreys, S.: Influence of Children's Dentofacial Appearance on Teacher Expectations, *Community Dent. Oral Epidemiol., 10,* 313, December, 1982.

Starr, P.: Facial Attractiveness and Behavior of Patients with Cleft Lip and/or Palate, *Psychol. Rep., 46,* 579, April, 1980.

Strauss, R.P.: Culture, Rehabilitation, and Facial Birth Defects: International Case Studies, *Cleft Palate J., 22,* 56, January, 1985.

Whitaker, L.A., Pashayan, H., and Reichman, J.: A Proposed New Classification of Craniofacial Anomalies, *Cleft Palate J., 18,* 161, July, 1981.

Infant Care

Asher, C.: Neonatal Care of Infants with Clefts of the Lip and Palate. Report of a WHO Study Tour to West Germany and Scandinavia, *Br. Dent. J., 160,* 438, June 21, 1986.

Balluff, M.A.: Nutritional Needs of an Infant or Child with a Cleft Lip or Palate, *Ear Nose Throat J., 65,* 311, July, 1986.

Balluff, M.A. and Udin, R.D.: Using a Feeding Appliance to Aid the Infant with a Cleft Palate, *Ear Nose Throat J., 65,* 316, July, 1986.

Clarren, S.K., Anderson, B., and Wolf, L.S.: Feeding Infants with Cleft Lip, Cleft Palate, or Cleft Lip and Palate, *Cleft Palate J., 24,* 244, July, 1987.

Goldberg, W.B., Ferguson, F.S., and Miles, R.J.: Successful Use of a Feeding Obturator for an Infant with a Cleft Palate, *Spec. Care Dentist., 8,* 86, March-April, 1988.

Jacobson, B.N. and Rosenstein, S.W.: Early Maxillary Orthopedics for the Newborn Cleft Lip and Palate Patient. An Impression and An Appliance, *Angle Orthod., 54,* 247, July, 1984.

Jones, J.E.: Early Management of Severe Bilateral Cleft Lip and Palate in an Infant, *ASDC J. Dent. Child., 48,* 50, January-February, 1981.

Jones, J.E., Henderson, L., and Avery, D.R.: Use of a Feeding Obturator for Infants with Severe Cleft Lip and Palate, *Spec. Care Dentist., 2,* 116, May-June, 1982.

Razek, M.K.A.: Prosthetic Feeding Aids for Infants with Cleft Lip and Palate, *J. Prosthet. Dent., 44,* 556, November, 1980.

Weatherly-White, R.C.A., Kuehn, D.P., Mirrett, P., Gilman, J.I., and Weatherly-White, C.C.: Early Repair and Breast-feeding for Infants with Cleft Lip, *Plast. Reconstr. Surg., 79,* 879, June, 1987.

Adolescents

Beder, O.E. and Weinstein, P.: Explorations of the Coping of Adolescents with Orofacial Anomalies Using the Cornell Medical Index, *J. Prosthet. Dent., 43,* 565, May, 1980.

Hall, R.K.: Care of Adolescents with Cleft Lip and Palate: the Role of the General Practitioner, *Int. Dent. J., 36,* 120, September, 1986.

Henry, P.J. and Tan, A.E.S.: Prosthodontic Implications of the Adolescent Cleft Palate Patient, *Aust. Dent. J., 30,* 104, April, 1985.

Richman, L.C.: Self-reported Social, Speech, and Facial Concerns and Personality Adjustment of Adolescents with Cleft Lip and Palate, *Cleft Palate J., 20,* 108, April, 1983.

Starr, P.: Cleft Type, Age, and Sex Differences in Teen-agers' Ratings of Their Own Behavior, Self-esteem, and Attitude Toward Clefting, *Rehabil. Lit., 4,* 177, July-August, 1980.

Tan, A.E.S. and Henry, P.J.: Periodontal Implications of the Adolescent Cleft Palate Patient, *Aust. Dent. J., 30,* 8, February, 1985.

Psychological and Behavioral

Clifford, E. and Clifford, M.: Social and Psychological Problems Associated with Clefts: Motivations for Cleft Palate Treatment, *Int. Dent. J., 36,* 115, September, 1986.

Heller, A., Rafman, S., Zvagulis, I., and Pless, I.B.: Birth Defects and Psychosocial Adjustment, *Am. J. Dis. Child., 139,* 257, March, 1985.

Jones, J.E.: Self-concept and Parental Evaluation of Peer Relationships in Cleft Lip and Palate Children, *Pediatr. Dent., 6,* 132, September, 1984.

Kapp-Simon, K.: Self-concept of Primary-school-age Children with Cleft Lip, Cleft Palate, or Both, *Cleft Palate J., 23,* 24, January, 1986.

Madison, L.S.: Psychologic Aspects of Cleft Lip and Palate, *Ear Nose Throat J., 65,* 16, August, 1986.

Renalli, D.N.: Psychosocial Considerations in the Dental Treatment of Individuals with Congenital Orofacial Clefting: A Summary for Clinicians, *Spec. Care Dentist., 1,* 65, March-April, 1981.

Richman, L.C. and Eliason, M.: Psychological Characteristics of Children with Cleft Lip and Palate: Intellectual, Achievement, Behavioral and Personality Variables, *Cleft Palate J., 19,* 249, October, 1982.

Richman, L.C. and Harper, D.C.: Personality Profiles of Physically Impaired Young Adults, *J. Clin. Psychol., 36,* 668, July, 1980.

Schneiderman, C.R. and Harding, J.B.: Social Ratings of Children with Cleft Lip by School Peers, *Cleft Palate J., 21,* 219, July, 1984.

Tobiasen, J.M. and Hiebert, J.M.: Parents' Tolerance for the Conduct Problems of the Child with Cleft Lip and Palate, *Cleft Palate J., 21,* 82, April, 1984.

Treatment

Carl, W.: Anterior Fixed Prosthetics for Cleft Palate Patients, *Quintessence Int., 15,* 721, July, 1984.

Dorf, D.S. and Curtin, J.W.: Early Cleft Palate Repair and Speech Outcome, *Plast. Reconstr. Surg., 70,* 74, July, 1982.

Dorf, D.S., Reisberg, D.J., and Gold, H.O.: Early Prosthetic Management of Cleft Palate. Articulation Development Prosthesis: A Preliminary Report, *J. Prosthet. Dent., 53,* 222, February, 1985.

Drago, C.J. and Parel, S.: Overdenture Treatment of an Adult Cleft Palate Patient, *Gen. Dent., 32,* 438, September-October, 1984.

Droschl, H.: Orthodontic Therapy of Clefts of the Lips, Jaw, and Palate, *Quintessence Int., 12,* 27, January, 1981.

Groetsema, W.R.: An Overview of the Maxillofacial Prosthesis as a Speech Rehabilitation Aid, *J. Prosthet. Dent., 57,* 204, February, 1987.

Kwon, H.J., Waite, D.E., Stickel, F.R., Chisholm, T., and McParland, F.: The Management of Alveolar Cleft Defects, *J. Am. Dent. Assoc., 102,* 848, June, 1981.

McKinstry, R.E. and Aramany, M.A.: Prosthetic Considerations in the Management of Surgically Compromised Cleft Palate Patients, *J. Prosthet. Dent., 53,* 827, June, 1985.

Shah, C.P. and Wong, D.: Management of Children with Cleft Lip and Palate, *Can. Med. Assoc. J., 122,* 19, January 12, 1980.

Strohaver, R.A.: Button Obturator for a Soft Palate Defect, *J. Prosthet. Dent., 43,* 229, February, 1980.

48 The Oral Surgery Patient and the Patient with a Fractured Jaw

A mouth is not considered a good surgical risk when the teeth are covered with debris and calculus and the gingiva show signs of inflammation and possible nutritional deficiency. Unless emergency surgery is required, the appointment should be postponed until the mouth is in a better state of cleanliness and health.

I. Overview of Oral and Maxillofacial Surgery

The term *oral and maxillofacial surgery* has been defined professionally as the diagnosis and treatment, surgical and adjunctive, of the diseases, injuries, and defects of the human jaws and associated structures.

Included among the many types of operations performed are (1) the removal of hopelessly diseased or impacted teeth; (2) the removal of cysts, tumors, and obstructions of the salivary glands; (3) correction of congenital or developmental defects such as cleft lip and palate; (4) reduction and fixation of fractured jaws and other facial bones; and (5) procedures to prepare the mouth for orthodontic or prosthodontic treatments.

Surgery for treatment of diseases and correction of defects of the periodontal tissues is categorized specifically as *periodontal surgery*. Within the scope of periodontal surgery are procedures for pocket elimination, gingivoplasty, treatment of furcation involvements, correction of mucogingival defects, and treatment for bony defects about the teeth. Preparation for periodontal surgery is not specifically described in this chapter.

II. Objectives

Dental hygiene care and instruction prior to oral and maxillofacial surgery may contribute to the patient's health and well-being by one or more of the following:

A. Remove Debris and Reduce Oral Bacterial Count[1]
1. Aid in the preparation of an aseptic field of operation.
2. Make postoperative infection less likely or less severe.

B. Reduce Inflammation of the Gingiva and Improve Tissue Tone
1. Lessen local bleeding at the time of the operation.
2. Promote postoperative healing.

C. Remove Calculus Deposits
1. Remove a source of plaque retention and thus improve gingival tissue tone.
2. Prevent interference with placement of surgical instruments.
3. Prevent pieces of calculus from breaking away during tooth removal.
   a. Danger of inhalation, particularly when a general anesthetic is used.
   b. Possibility of calculus falling into socket or other surgical area and acting as a foreign body to inhibit healing.

D. Instruct in Preoperative Personal Oral Care Procedures
This will contribute to reducing inflammation and thus improve tissue tone and help prepare the patient for postoperative care.

E. Instruct in the Use of Foods
The patient should be instructed about those foods that provide the elements essential to tissue building and repair during pre- and postoperative periods.

For the patient who will have teeth removed and complete or partial dentures inserted, the importance of a diet containing all essential food groups should be emphasized.

F. Interpret the Dentist's Directions
This should be done for the immediate preoperative preparation with respect to rest and dietary limitations, particularly when a general anesthetic is to be administered.

G. Motivate the Patient Who Will Have Teeth Remaining
The patient who will have teeth remaining after surgery should be motivated to prevent further tooth loss through routine dental and dental hygiene professional care and personal oral care procedures.

III. Personal Factors
The extent of the operation to be performed and previous experiences will affect the patient's atti-

tude. Many patients who are in the greatest need of preoperative dental hygiene care and instruction may be people who have neglected their mouths for many years. They have been indifferent to or unaware of the importance of obtaining adequate care. Their only visits to a dentist may have been to have a toothache relieved by extraction. Their knowledge of preventive measures may be limited. A few of the characteristics are suggested here.

A. Apprehensive and Fearful
1. Apprehensive and indifferent toward need for personal care of teeth that are to be removed.
2. Fearful of all dental procedures, particularly oral surgery and anesthesia.
3. Fearful of cancer or other disease.
4. Fearful of personal appearance after surgery.

B. Impatient
When teeth have caused discomfort and pain, the patient may have difficulty understanding the need for delay while oral hygiene procedures are accomplished.

C. Ashamed
Of appearance or of having neglected the teeth.

D. Resigned
Feeling of inevitableness of the situation; lack of appreciation for natural teeth.

E. Discouraged
Over tooth loss or development of soft tissue lesions.

F. Resentful
1. Toward time lost from work.
2. Toward the financial aspects of dental care.
3. Toward inconvenience and discomfort.

DENTAL HYGIENE CARE

A review of the patient's record will show preliminary procedures that need to be completed. For example, a thorough intraoral and extraoral examination, a recording of vital signs, photographs, and additional radiographs may be required. The patient's medical and dental history will reveal essential information relative to the need for prophylactic antibiotics or other precautions.

I. Presurgery Treatment Planning

The pending date for the operation and the patient's attitude may limit the time to be spent.

A. First Appointment
Develop rapport with the patient; explain and demonstrate initial plaque control principles; present a dietary record form for completion before the next appointment; and remove calculus deposits. Scaling may be limited to one quadrant or one side, depending on the severity of the periodontal condition, and especially the need for tissue conditioning by the patient.

B. Second Appointment
1. Observe gingival tissue response; apply disclosing agent; and review disease control procedures. Introduce the use of dental floss or other interdental aids when applicable.
2. Receive the dietary record and review it with the patient (pages 383–386). Present diet recommendations.
3. Complete or continue the scaling. More than two appointments may be needed for patients who will have surgery for oral cancer, cardiovascular or other condition in which it is necessary to complete all periodontal and dental treatment. When radiation or chemotherapy will be used following surgery for oral cancer, or when a prosthetic heart valve or total joint replacement will be involved, complete oral care is necessary as described on pages 601–603.

II. Patient Instruction

A. Bacterial Plaque Control
1. *Brush.* Soft.
2. *Technique.* For a patient who may not have practiced careful brushing on a regular plan, a simple brushing technique is preferred. Time for establishing habits may be limited until postoperative healing is complete. Use of disclosing agent for the patient's own evaluation is important.

B. Auxiliary Procedures
Interdental plaque removal and care of fixed and removable appliances are included in instruction (Chapters 23 and 24). The patient who will have multiple extractions for the placement of an immediate denture or other appliance, such as an obturator or other prosthesis following cleft palate, tumor, or other surgery, will need postoperative instruction for the specific care of the appliance.

III. Instrumentation

Scaling techniques are of primary importance. Stain removal procedures may be contraindicated because of the condition of the gingival tissues.

A. Scaling
1. *Problems*
   a. Teeth with large carious lesions.
   b. Mobile teeth.
   c. Edentulous areas.
   d. Sensitive, enlarged gingival tissue that bleeds readily.
2. *Suggestions for Technique*
   a. Use topical or local anesthetic.
   b. Maintain a clear field, using evacuation techniques.
   c. Use alternate finger rests to adapt to mobile teeth or edentulous areas; stabilize mobile teeth during scaling strokes.
   d. Ultrasonic scaling techniques may be con-

traindicated because of the potential for contaminated aerosols. When used, an antimicrobial mouthrinse is used first to lessen the bacterial count of the aerosols produced.

B. Stain Removal

1. *Contraindications*
   a. Enlarged, inflamed, sensitive gingiva.
   b. Deep pockets.
   c. Profuse hemorrhage.
2. *Effects*
   a. Irritation to tissue by polishing abrasive and action of rubber polishing cup.
   b. Movement of rubber cup forces abrasive particles into the gingival tissues.

C. Rinsing Instruction

1. *Objectives.* To promote tissue healing following scaling and to remove debris; to initiate the habit of rinsing for postoperative care later.
2. *Rinsing Solution.* Warm, mild, hypertonic salt solution (page 538).
3. *Frequency.* Recommended for several times each day; after the surgical procedure as instructed by oral surgeon.

D. Follow-up Evaluation

Scaling and planing should be planned for a few weeks after oral surgery. Such an appointment should not be scheduled until healing has progressed favorably.

IV. Patient Instruction: Diet Selection[2]

The nutritional state can influence the resistance to infection and wound healing, as well as general recovery powers. Nutritional deficiencies can occur because of the inability to ingest adequate nutrients orally.

Specific recommendations of what to include and not to include in the diet should be given to the patient. Postoperative suggestions may differ from preoperative; for example, when difficulty in chewing is a postoperative problem, a liquid or soft diet may be required. When major oral surgery requires hospitalization, tube feeding may be necessary during the initial healing period. Tube feeding is described on page 598.

A. Nutritional and Dietary Needs

Diets outlined are designed to include the essential foods from the Basic Four Food Groups (table 28–1, page 382).

1. *Essential for Promotion of Healing.* Protein and vitamins, particularly vitamin A, vitamin C, and riboflavin.
2. *Essential for Building Gingival Tissue Resistance.* A varied diet that includes adequate portions of all essential food groups.
3. *Essential for Providing Gingival Stimulation.* Firm, fibrous foods that require mastication, especially fresh fruits and vegetables. Possi-

bilities for making recommendations in this area are limited by the patient's masticatory deficiencies.

4. *Essential for Dental Caries Prevention.* Foods without fermentable carbohydrate. When a patient has not been able to masticate properly, the diet employed frequently may have included many soft and cariogenic foods.

B. Suggestions for Instruction

1. Provide instruction sheets that show specific meal plans for pre- and postsurgery. Foods for liquid and soft diets are listed on page 598.
2. Express nutritional needs in terms of quantity or servings of foods so that the patient clearly understands.
3. For the patient who will receive dentures, careful instruction must be provided over a period of time. At the preoperative appointment, only an introduction can be given, particularly because the patient is probably more concerned about the operation than about the after effects.

   When the patient will lose the teeth because of dental caries, the diet has likely been high in fermentable carbohydrates. Emphasis should be placed on helping the patient include nutritious foods for the general health of the body and more specifically the health of the alveolar processes that will support the dentures.

V. Preoperative Instructions[3]

At the appointment just prior to the oral surgery appointment, instructions relative to the surgical procedure should be discussed with the patient. The objective is to let the patient know what to expect so that full cooperation is possible. The patient may have concerns about the anesthesia, the surgical procedure, and the outcome.

A. Explain the general procedures for anesthesia and surgery.

B. Provide printed preoperative instructions. Information in the printed instructions should include the following:

1. *Food and Liquid Intake.* Specify the number of hours before the time of the operation when the patient should stop further intake of food or fluids.
2. *Alcohol and Medications Restrictions.* Certain proprietary self-medications are not compatible with the anesthetic and drugs to be used during and following the surgical procedure. The patient should be instructed to discontinue use.
3. *Transport To and From the Appointment.* When a general anesthetic is used, the patient should not drive. Plans for someone to accompany and assist the patient should be made.
4. *The Night Before the Appointment.* In addi-

tion to food and alcohol restrictions, a good night's rest is advocated.

    5. *Personal Items*
        a. Clothing: the clothing worn should be loose and comfortable. The sleeves should be easily drawn up over the elbows.
        b. Care of contact lens and prostheses: the patient will be asked to remove contact lens and prostheses, and should bring containers for their safe keeping.

VI. Postoperative Care

A. Immediate Instructions

Printed postoperative instructions are provided following all oral operations. The prepared material is reviewed with the patient after surgery. Specific details vary, but basic information for postoperative instruction sheets includes the following:

    1. *Control Bleeding.* Keep the sponge in the mouth over the surgical area for one-half hour, then discard it. When bleeding persists at home, place a gauze pad or cold wet teabag over the area and bite firmly for 30 minutes.

    2. *Rinsing.* Do not rinse for 24 hours after the surgical appointment. Then use warm salt water (½ teaspoonful salt in ½ cup (4 oz) of warm water), after toothbrushing and every 2 hours.

    3. *Plaque Control.* Brush the teeth even more thoroughly than usual. Avoid the surgery site.

    4. *Rest.* Get plenty of rest: at least 8 to 10 hours sleep each night. Avoid strenuous exercise during the first 24 hours, and keep the mouth from excessive movement.

    5. *Diet.* Use a liquid or soft solid diet high in protein. Drink water and fruit juices freely. Avoid foods that require excessive chewing.

    6. *Pain.* If needed, use a pain-relieving preparation prescribed by the dentist. Adhere to directions.

    7. *Icepack.* Following a flap operation or when swelling is likely to occur, apply icepack (ice cubes in a plastic bag) for 30 minutes followed by 30 minutes off, or apply for 15 minutes after 30 minutes off, as directed by the dentist. Heat is not used for swelling.

    8. *Complications.* Instructions should include the telephone number to call after office hours, should complications arise; complications may include uncontrollable pain, marked bleeding, temperature rise, difficulty in opening the mouth, or unusual swelling a few days after the surgery.

B. Follow-up Care

The dental hygienist may participate in suture removal, irrigation of sockets, and other postoperative procedures when the patient returns. Appropriately, instruction concerning plaque control, rinsing, oral irrigation, and other personal care as well as diet supervision can be continued.

PATIENT WITH A FRACTURED JAW

The limited access for personal oral care procedures and the effect of the liquid diet required for most cases define the need for special dental hygiene care for the patient with a fractured jaw. Attention to rehabilitation of the oral tissues during the period following the removal of appliances takes on particular significance lest permanent tissue damage result or inadequate oral care habits be continued indefinitely.

The patient with a fractured jaw may be hospitalized. A dental hygienist employed in a hospital would be called upon to assume a part of the responsibility for patient care or to give oral hygiene instruction to direct-care personnel. After dismissal from the hospital, the patient may require special attention in the private dental office for a long period of time.

Treatment of a fractured jaw may be complex, and the patient may suffer considerably, both physically and mentally. Some basic knowledge of the nature of fractures and their treatment is helpful in understanding the patient's needs.

I. Causes

A. Traumatic

From automobile, bicycle, and sports injuries, industrial accidents, and physical violence (blows, fistfights).

B. Predisposing

Pathologic conditions such as tumors, cysts, osteoporosis, or osteomyelitis weaken the bone; thus, slight trauma or even tooth removal can cause fracture.

II. Emergency Care

Immediate attention must be paid to measures for care of the patient's general condition. Emergency care is given for airway, breathing, and circulation ("A-B-C," figure 60–4, page 740). Hemorrhage, shock, and skull or internal head injuries are next in the sequence of concern.

Almost any category of emergency care may be required (table 60–1, pages 747–754). Although treatment for the fractured jaw must not be postponed for any great length of time, its immediate care takes second place to the vital aspects of patient care.

Tetanus prophylaxis may be indicated as soon as medical treatment is available.

III. Recognition

A. History

Except for a pathologic fracture, a history of trauma should be available.

B. Clinical Signs

The patient has pain, especially on movement, and tenderness on slight pressure over the area of the fracture. Teeth may be displaced, fractured, or mobile. Because of muscle pull or contraction, segments of the bones may be displaced, and the occlusion of the teeth may be irregular.

Muscle spasm is a common finding, particularly when the fracture is at the angle or ramus of the mandible. Crepitation can be heard if the parts of bone are moved.

The soft tissue in the area of the fracture may show laceration and bleeding, discoloration (ecchymosis), and enlargement.

IV. Types

A fracture is classified by using a combination of descriptive words for its *location, direction, nature,* and *severity.* Fractures may be single or multiple, bilateral or unilateral, complete or incomplete.

A. Classification by Nature of the Fracture (figure 48–1)
1. *Simple.* Has no communication with outside.
2. *Compound.* Has communication with outside.
3. *Comminuted.* Shattered.
4. *Incomplete.* "Greenstick" fracture has one side of a bone broken and the other side bent. It occurs in incompletely calcified bones (young children, usually). The fibers tend to bend rather than break.

B. Mandibular (described by location)
1. Alveolar process.
2. Condyle.
3. Angle.
4. Body.
5. Symphysis.

C. Maxillary
1. *Alveolar Process.* The alveolar process fracture does not extend to the midline of the palate.
2. *Le Fort I.*[4] The Le Fort classification is used widely to identify the three general levels of maxillary fractures, as shown in figure 48–2.

   Le Fort I is a horizontal fracture line above the roots of the teeth, above the palate, across the maxillary sinus, below the zygomatic process, and across the pterygoid plates.
3. *Le Fort II.* The midface fracture extends over the middle of the nose, down the medial wall of the orbits, across the infraorbital rims, and posteriorly, across the pterygoid plates.
4. *Le Fort III.* The high level craniofacial fracture extends transversely across the bridge of the nose, across the orbits and the zygomatic arches, and across the pterygoid plates.

TREATMENT OF FRACTURES[5,6]

Each fracture differs from the next, and the methods used in treatment vary with the individual case. Many factors are involved when the oral surgeon selects the methods to be used, particularly the location of the fracture or fractures, the presence or absence of teeth, existing injuries to the teeth, other head injuries, and the general health and condition of the patient.

Treatment of a fracture consists of *reduction* of the fracture, *fixation* of the fragments, and *immobilization* of the jaw. A temporary, removable splint may be necessary when a patient must be transported to another location for specialized treatment. An accident or war casualty may occur many miles from a professional treatment facility.

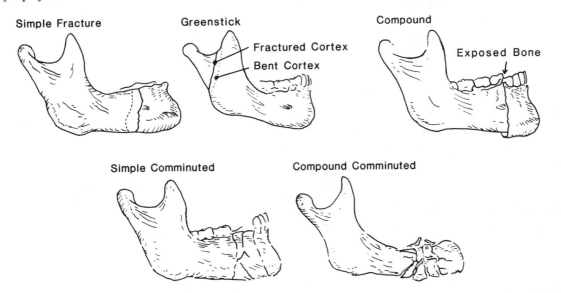

Figure 48–1. Types of Fractures. (From Kruger, G.O.: *Textbook of Oral and Maxillofacial Surgery,* 6th ed. St. Louis, The C.V. Mosby Co., 1984.)

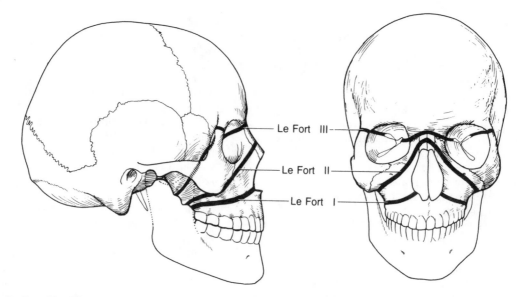

Figure 48–2. Le Fort Classification of Facial Fractures. Le Fort I, horizontal fracture above the roots of the teeth, below the zygomatic process, and across the pterygoid plates. Le Fort II, midface fracture over the middle of the nose and across the infraorbital rims. Le Fort III, transversely across the bridge of the nose, across the orbits and the zygomatic bone. (From Archer, W.H.: *Oral and Maxillofacial Surgery,* 5th ed. Philadelphia, W.B. Saunders Co., 1975; from Committee on Trauma, American College of Surgeons: Early Care of the Injured Patient. Philadelphia, W.B. Saunders Co., 1972.)

I. Reduction

Reduction means the positioning of the parts on either side of the fracture so they are in apposition for healing and restoration of function. The closure of the teeth is the guide for position in the dentulous patient.

A. Closed Reduction
1. Manual manipulation of the parts.
2. Elastic traction. The most common traction is applied with elastic bands hooked to arch bars, which are also part of the method for fixation. The method is described under the topic intermaxillary fixation.

B. Open Reduction
The bone fracture ends are exposed surgically by a flap procedure, and the two ends are brought together. They are then fixed as described under transosseous wires or bone plate.

II. Fixation

The fracture is first reduced or positioned, and then fixed or stabilized in that position. Fractures take several weeks to heal, and fixation apparatus is left in place long enough to assure union of the bony parts.

A. Transosseous Wires or Metal Plate
When the bony parts are reduced by open reduction, they are fastened together by either a wire suture threaded through holes drilled on either side of the fracture line (figure 48–3) or by a metal plate. The metal plate is designed to cross over the fracture line and is held in place by screws on either side.

B. Intermaxillary Fixation

Intermaxillary fixation is fixation obtained by applying wires or elastic bands between the maxillary and mandibular arches. This is sufficient treatment for many fractures. More complicated types of fractures may require additional or supplemental types of therapy.

Ready-made, contoured, metal arch bars are available, or wires may be custom made with loops on which to hook wires or elastics to connect the mandible and maxilla in occlusion. The arch bars are adapted carefully to fit accurately to each tooth, and then wired into place so that the hooks project up in the maxilla and down in the mandible.

Elastics are positioned to provide a steady, gradual pull to aid in reducing the fracture (figure 48–4). A

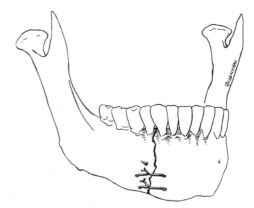

Figure 48–3. Open Reduction for Mandibular Fracture. Transosseous wiring is shown to hold bony parts in position for healing at the fracture line. (From Waite, D.E.: *Practical Oral Surgery.* 2nd ed. Philadelphia, Lea & Febiger, 1978.)

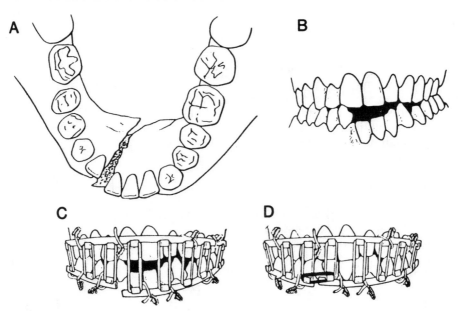

Figure 48–4. Intermaxillary Fixation. A. Location of fracture of the mandible. **B.** Segments of bone on either side of the fracture are displaced by muscle pull or contraction. **C.** Metal arch bars are held in place with rubber bands positioned to provide a steady pull for fracture reduction. **D.** Note small horizontal rubber band extending from the hook at the mandibular right central incisor to the mandibular right canine to reduce the lateral displacement. (From Archer, W.H.: *Oral and Maxillofacial Surgery,* 5th ed. Philadelphia, W.B. Saunders Co., 1975.)

small horizontal elastic may be positioned across the fracture to reduce the lateral displacement (figure 48–4D).

C. External Skeletal Fixation (figure 48–5)

1. *Indications.* Management of a fracture cannot always be accomplished satisfactorily by intermaxillary wiring alone. The following are indications for external skeletal fixation:
   a. Insufficient number of teeth in good condition for intermaxillary fixation.

   b. As a supplement to intermaxillary fixation when no teeth are present in the fractured portion of the mandible.
   c. Loss of bone substance. When bone substance is lost because of an accident, a gunshot wound, or a pathologic condition, a bone graft may be indicated. The extraoral fixation is used first to hold the fractured parts in a normal relationship, and then to immobilize the area during healing following the bone graft surgery.

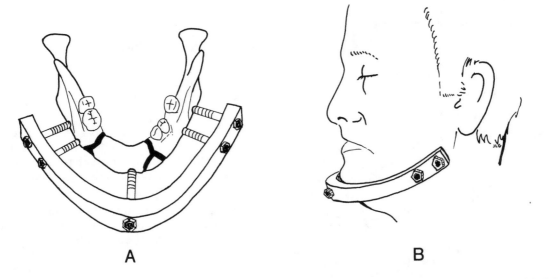

Figure 48–5. External Skeletal Fixation. A. Precision bone screws placed on either side of the fractures, shown in heavy black lines. **B.** Acrylic bar molded, positioned over the bone screws, and locked into position with nuts.

d. Patients may be unable to have the jaws closed for a long period. Examples of these are

   i. Patient with a vomiting problem, such as during pregnancy.

   ii. Patient with a mental or physical disability such as cerebral palsy, epilepsy, or mental retardation.

e. Edentulous mandible when the fracture fragments are greatly displaced, when the fracture is at the angle of the mandible, or when the mandible is atrophic or thinned.

2. *Description.* Two special bone screws are placed via skin incisions on either side of the fracture. An acrylic bar is molded, and while still pliable, is pressed over the threads of the bone screws and locked into position with the screw nuts (figure 48–5).

III. Edentulous Patient

The use of external skeletal fixation for an edentulous mandible was described earlier. Other procedures are included here.

A. Open Reduction Using Transosseous Wiring

Transosseous wiring for an edentulous mandible is similar to that described for the dentulous mandible in II., A. page 594. The bony parts are brought together and held in place by wire sutures (figure 48–6).

B. Circumferential Wiring

The patient's denture is used for a splint. If the denture was broken when the mandible was fractured, it may be repaired immediately or a temporary edentulous splint may be fabricated. Wires are placed around the denture and the arch together by threading the wire, using surgical procedures (figure 48–7). The line of fracture must be under the denture-covered area, or additional procedures are needed for the uncovered portion.

Because considerable trauma may be associated with the fracture, swelling may occur that

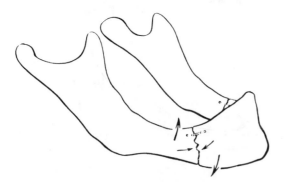

Figure 48–6. Edentulous Mandible to Show the Use of Open Reduction. Transosseous wiring placed. (From Archer, W.H.: *Oral and Maxillofacial Surgery,* 5th ed. Philadelphia, W.B. Saunders Co., 1975; From Dingman, R.A. and Natvig, P.: *Surgery of Facial Fractures,* Philadelphia, W.B. Saunders Co., 1964.)

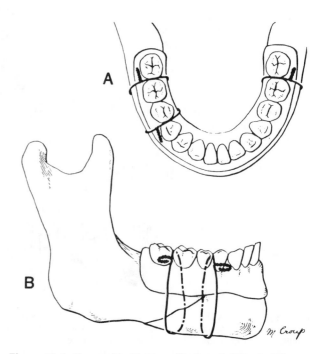

Figure 48–7. Removable Denture Used as Splint. A. Wires are placed around the denture and the edentulous arch and twisted together to stabilize the reduction. **B.** Note the line of fracture with the denture positioned to cover it. (From Archer, W.H.: *Oral and Maxillofacial Surgery,* 5th ed. Philadelphia, W.B. Saunders Co., 1975.)

prevents denture placement. In addition, the insertion of circumferential wires may cause more trauma to the soft tissues. An external skeletal fixation may be a preferred treatment.

C. Intermaxillary Fixation

The mandibular denture may be wired to the maxillary complete denture for additional mobilization. Mandibular anterior teeth may be cut away to allow the patient to feed by straw or glass feeding tube.

IV. Maxillary Fracture

Maxillary fractures are more difficult to handle because of the number of bones, the associated anatomy, and the complications of basal skull fractures.

A. Intermaxillary Fixation

Whether the fracture is Le Fort I, II, or III (figure 48–2), intermaxillary fixation is completed first to establish the occlusal relationship (figure 48–4). The next step is to accomplish craniomaxillary immobilization.

B. Craniomaxillary Immobilization

A rigid craniomaxillary fixation is necessary. A variety of methods has been used, some internal and others external.

1. *Cranial Suspension to the Nearest Superior Unfractured Bone.* Pins are used to provide a connection for the attachment of wires from a

stable bone, such as the supraorbital area, to the mandibular arch bar.

2. *Head Cap.* A plaster headcap can provide a means for extraoral traction. This method is used infrequently.

3. *Internal Suspension Wires.* A maxilla with a Le Fort I fracture may be suspended by internal wires over the zygoma. In the oral cavity, the wires are connected to the mandibular arch bar. When the zygoma is also fractured, another method must be selected.

V. Alveolar Process Fracture

The most common fracture of all is of the alveolar process, maxillary or mandibular.

A. Clinical Appearance

Lacerations of lips and gingiva, mobility, fracture or displacement of teeth, swelling, bruising, and hemorrhage are usual signs.

B. Treatment[7]

1. Replantation of displaced teeth.
2. Immobilization with interdental wiring. A temporary fixed splint of acrylic may be placed over the wires. The teeth must be tested periodically for vitality.
3. Endodontic therapy may be required later.

VI. Healing

Union is affected by the location and character of the fracture. Much depends on the patient's general health and resistance and cooperation. Six weeks is considered the average for the uncomplicated mandibular fracture and 4 to 6 weeks for the maxillary. The major cause of complication is infection.

DENTAL HYGIENE CARE

I. Problems

Fixation apparatus, however carefully placed to prevent tissue irritation, interferes with normal function. The length of time the appliances must be in place is sufficient for considerable disturbance of tissue metabolism. Identification of possible effects of treatment provides the basis for planning dental hygiene care.

A. Development of Gingivitis or Periodontal Complications

1. Thick plaque formation and food debris accumulation provide sources of irritation to the gingiva.
2. Gingivitis develops in 9 to 19 days.[8]
3. Lack of normal stimulation to the circulation of the periodontium and cleansing effects usually provided by the action of the tongue, lips, and facial muscles, contribute to stagnation of saliva and to bacterial plaque accumulation.
4. Tender, sensitive gingiva make plaque control more difficult even on available surfaces.

B. Dental Caries Initiation

It is difficult to plan an appetizing soft or liquid diet using limited cariogenic foods for dental caries prevention.

C. Loss of Appetite

Loss of appetite related to monotonous liquid or soft diet may lead to weight loss and lowered physical resistance. Secondary infections, including those of the oral tissues, may result.

D. Difficulty in Opening the Mouth

1. When the temporomandibular joint has been injured, the patient wearing fixation appliances that involve only the mandible has difficulty in applying a toothbrush to the lingual surfaces of teeth.
2. After removal of appliances, all patients have a degree of muscular trismus that hinders toothbrushing and mastication.

II. Instrumentation

A. Preoperative

Gross calculus is removed, insofar as possible, before wiring or the placement of metal or acrylic splints. Trauma to surrounding soft tissues of lip, tongue, and cheeks limits accessibility.

B. During Treatment

Periodic scaling in conjunction with plaque control contributes to oral health. Although access is only from the facial aspect for a patient with intermaxillary wiring, some benefit can be obtained. It is essential to have an assistant to provide continual suction during treatment.

C. After Removal of Appliances

A few weeks after removal of appliances, when the patient can open the mouth normally and plaque control procedures have been initiated, complete scaling and planing can be performed.

III. Diet

Many patients with fractured jaws tend to lose weight, which is generally related to an inadequate nutrient and caloric intake. Objectives in planning the diet are to help the patient maintain an adequate nutritional state, to promote healing, and to increase resistance to infection.

Attention must be given to the patient's willingness and ability to follow the recommendations made. The patient may be in the hospital for a few days to a few weeks depending on the severity of other injuries. A greater length of time is spent as an outpatient, when the diet is much more difficult to supervise. The patient's understanding of dietary instructions and what is expected appears to be much more significant than the specific components of diet recommended.

A. Nutritional Needs

After a surgical fixation procedure, the diet must be planned to promote tissue building and repair.[2]

1. All essential food elements.
2. Emphasis on protein, vitamins, particularly A and C, and minerals, particularly calcium and phosphorus.
3. Usual caloric requirements for patient's age, taking into consideration lack of physical exercise and loss of appetite while ill.

B. Methods of Feeding
1. *Plastic Straw.* Liquid is sucked through the teeth or through an edentulous area. Straw can be bent to accommodate a patient who cannot sit up.
2. *Spoon Feeding.* When a patient's arms are not functional, direct assistance is needed. The mouth may have injuries that prevent sucking food through a straw.
3. *Tube Feeding.* Tube feeding may be indicated following various types of extensive oral surgery, facial trauma, burns, immobilized fractured jaw, and other conditions that prevent ingesting sufficient calories and nutritional foods by way of the mouth.

    A nasogastric tube is used (figure 48–8). Blenderized food can be prepared or special tube formulas are available commercially. When commercial preparations are used, contents can be selected to meet the specific nutritional and caloric requirements of an individual patient.

C. Liquid Diet
1. *Indications*
   a. All patients with jaws wired together.
   b. All patients with no appliance or single-jaw appliance who have difficulty in opening the mouth because of a condition such as temporomandibular joint involvement or tongue or lip injury that hinders insertion of food or manipulation of food in the mouth.
2. *Examples of Foods.* Fruit juices; milk; eggnog;

meat juices and soups; cooked thin cereals; canned baby foods. Strained vegetables and meats (baby foods) may be added to meat juices and soups.

3. *Use of a Blender.* Regular table foods can be mixed in a food blender. With liquid such as clear soup or milk added, a fluid consistency can be obtained that will pass through a straw (figure 48–9).

D. Soft Solids Diet
1. *Indications*
   a. Patient with no appliance or with single-jaw appliance without complications in opening the mouth or in movement of the lips and tongue.
   b. Patient who has been maintained on liquid diet throughout treatment period: after appliances are removed, the soft diet is recommended for several days to 1 week to provide the stomach with foods that are readily digestible rather than making a drastic change to a regular diet. A soft solids diet can also aid by protecting tender oral tissues from the rough textures of a regular diet until the tissues have had a chance to respond to softer foods and a regular plaque control routine.
2. *Examples of Foods.* Soft-poached, scrambled, or boiled eggs; cooked cereals; mashed soft-cooked vegetables, including potato; mashed fresh or canned fruits; soft, finely divided meats; custards; plain ice cream.

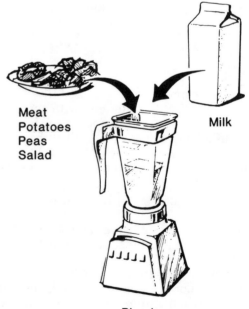

Meat
Potatoes
Peas
Salad

Milk

Blender

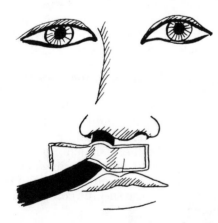

Figure 48–8. Nasogastric Feeding Tube. To prevent injury to the nasopharyngeal passages, the tube is taped securely between the upper lip and the nares. (From Lewis, C.M.: *Nursing Considerations in Tube-fed Patients.* Philadelphia, F.A. Davis Co., 1976.)

Figure 48–9. Preparation of a Liquid or Semi-solid Diet. Regular table foods can be blenderized with milk or other nutritious liquid. (From Schultz, R.C.: *Facial Injuries,* 2nd ed. Copyright © 1977 by Yearbook Medical Publishers, Inc., Chicago.)

E. Hints for Diet Planning with the Nonhospitalized Patient

1. Provide instruction sheets that show specific meal plans.
2. Express nutritional needs in quantities or servings of foods.
3. Show methods of varying the diet. A liquid or soft diet is at best monotonous because of the sameness of texture.
4. Suggest limitation of cariogenic foods as an aid to prevention of dental caries.

IV. Personal Oral Care Procedures

Every attempt to keep the patient's mouth as clean as possible for comfort and sanitation, and as plaque-free as possible for disease prevention should be made. The extent of possible care depends on the appliances, the condition of the lips, tongue, and other oral tissues, and the cooperation of the patient.

Encouragement must be given to the patient to begin toothbrushing as soon as possible after the surgical procedure but until the patient is able, a plan for care is outlined for an attendant.

A. Irrigation

1. *Indications.* During the first few days after the surgical procedure while the mouth may be too tender for brushing, frequent irrigations are required; irrigation also serves as an adjunct to toothbrushing.
2. *Method.* In a hospital, irrigations with suction are possible. At home, the patient irrigates with the head lowered over a sink (pages 324–326).
3. *Mouthrinse Selection.* The oral surgeon should be consulted for specific instructions.
   a. Physiologic saline.
   b. Chlorhexidine gluconate (pages 330–331).
   c. Fluoride rinse after toothbrushing after each meal and before going to sleep.

B. Early Mouth Cleansing

Before a toothbrush can be used effectively, a premoistened swab or toothette to clean and lubricate the lips, mucosa, and gingiva may be necessary. Because plaque removal should be attempted as soon as possible, a very soft toothbrush with suction can be applied. The toothbrush with suction is described on page 638.

C. Personal Care by the Patient

As soon as possible, the patient is instructed in personal care. A toothbrushing method and other aids such as are used for orthodontic appliances are recommended and demonstrated (pages 338–339). Because interdental and proximal tooth-surface care is limited to access only from the facial approach, the choice of devices is limited.[9] Some spaces permit insertion of an interdental brush. With instruction, most patients can use a toothpick in a holder (pages 321–322). The patient must be shown why care must be taken not to entangle the toothbrush filaments in the wires. When the tongue is not injured, the patient can be instructed to use the tongue as an aid in cleaning the lingual surfaces of the teeth and massaging the gingiva.

The ambulatory patient can use a water irrigator. Specific instructions must be provided, showing the patient how to lower the head over a sink. A low pressure setting is used and the spray is directed carefully to prevent tissue injury (pages 324–326).

D. After Appliances Are Removed

A step-by-step series of lessons is usually necessary before the patient can carry out adequate plaque control.

A method for daily self-applied fluoride, such as a mouthrinse or brush-on gel, should be introduced along with the use of a fluoride dentifrice. Demineralization and dental caries can result from plaque retention about the appliances.

DENTAL HYGIENE CARE PRIOR TO GENERAL SURGERY

Completing dental and dental hygiene treatment and bringing the oral cavity to a state of health has special significance for certain patients who will have surgical procedures other than oral. When emergency surgery is performed, preparation of the mouth is not possible, and postoperative examination and care may be complicated by various limitations.

When surgery is elective, or planned well in advance, the patient can be encouraged to have complete dental and periodontal treatment. Protection against complications related to broken appliances or restorations can be very meaningful to the hospitalized patient. Types of patients will be discussed briefly here. Other examples are to be found in the various special patient chapters throughout this book section.

I. Patients in Whom Surgical Procedures Affect Their Risk Status

Susceptibility to infection is greatly increased in certain patients, for example, those with prosthetic heart valves, prostheses for joint replacement, and transplanted organs. Patients who receive chemotherapeutic agents as partial treatment after surgery for various types of cancer, and others who use immunosuppressant drugs, require special management to prevent complications during dental and dental hygiene appointments. Antibiotic premedication to prevent infective endocarditis and other infections is mandatory for certain patients (pages 85 and 91).

Prior to general surgery for prostheses, transplants, cancer, and other serious conditions, patients can be informed of the need for completing oral care treatments and practicing preventive daily personal care.

II. Preparation of the Mouth Prior to General Inhalation Anesthesia

Plaque control and professional instrumentation aid in reducing the oral bacterial count.[1] Because the mouth is the entrance to the respiratory chamber, the possibility always exists that debris and fluids may be inhaled from the mouth. This could occur during the administration of an anesthetic or when the patient coughs.

III. Patient with a Long Convalescence

Patients whose surgery will require a long convalescence will be unable to keep a regular maintenance appointment. When the patient has a healthy mouth before the hospitalization and convalescence, the problems of postoperative oral care are lessened, but not eliminated.

Instruction for the person who will provide direct care may be needed. A home visit by the dentist and dental hygienist may be required.

TECHNICAL HINTS

I. Written Consent

Surgical treatment is not provided to minors without consent of parent or guardian. Written consent is mandatory.

II. Accident Prevention

Encourage patients to use the seat belts in their cars. Professional people should set the example by using their own seat belts.

References

1. Whitacre, R.J., Robins, S.K., Williams, B.L., and Crawford, J.J.: *Dental Asepsis.* Seattle, Stoma Press, 1979, p. 50.
2. Nizel, A.E.: *Nutrition in Preventive Dentistry: Science and Practice, 2nd ed.* Philadelphia, W.B. Saunders Co., 1980, pp. 507–521.
3. Atterbury, R.A.: Preoperative Guidelines for Oral Surgery Patients, *Dent. Surv., 52,* 35, October, 1976.
4. Haskell, R.: Applied Surgical Anatomy, in Rowe, N.L. and Williams, J.L.: *Maxillofacial Injuries.* London, Churchill Livingstone, 1985, pp. 21–24.
5. Cawson, R.A. and Rowe, N.L.: Fracture of the Jaws and Facial Skeleton, in Cawson, R.A.: *Essentials of Dental Surgery and Pathology,* 3rd ed. Edinburgh, Churchill Livingstone, 1978, pp. 252–273.
6. Kruger, G.O., ed.: *Textbook of Oral and Maxillofacial Surgery,* 6th ed. St. Louis, The C.V. Mosby Co., 1984, pp. 364–435.
7. Quinn, T.: Department of Oral Surgery, Tufts University School of Dental Medicine, Boston, Massachusetts, personal communication, July, 1980.
8. Löe, H., Theilade, E., and Jensen, S.B.: Experimental Gingivitis in Man, *J. Periodontol., 36,* 177, May-June, 1965.
9. Phelps-Sandall, B.A. and Oxford, S.J.: Effectiveness of Oral Hygiene Techniques on Plaque and Gingivitis in Patients Placed in Intermaxillary Fixation, *Oral Surg., 56,* 487, November, 1983.

Suggested Readings

Bell, C.N.A.: Prevention of Tooth Decalcification Under Acrylic Splints Used in Orthognathic Surgery, *J. Oral Maxillofac. Surg., 43,* 650, August, 1985.
Boyne, P.J.: Early Treatment of Facial Trauma, *Postgrad. Med., 77,* 99, April, 1985.
Falender, L.G., Leban, S.G., and Williams, F.A.: Postoperative Nutritional Support in Oral and Maxillofacial Surgery, *J. Oral Maxillofac. Surg., 45,* 324, April, 1987.
Huelke, D.F. and Compton, C.P.: Facial Injuries in Automobile Crashes, *J. Oral Maxillofac. Surg., 41,* 241, April, 1983.
Karlson, T.A.: The Incidence of Hospital-treated Facial Injuries from Vehicles, *J. Trauma, 22,* 303, April, 1982.
Mardirossian, G.: Intermaxillary Fixation—Torture or Therapy? *Clin. Prevent. Dent., 4,* 22, May-June, 1982.
Nash, E.S. and Addy, M.: The Use of Chlorhexidine Gluconate Mouthrinses in Patients with Inter-maxillary Fixation, *Br. J. Oral Surg., 17,* 251, March, 1980.
Sandor, G.K.B. and Collins, F.J.V.: The Potential of Dental Hygienists in Oral and Maxillofacial Surgery, *Dent. Hyg., 57,* 30, September, 1983.
Schultz, R.C. and de Camara, D.: Athletic Facial Injuries, *J. Am. Med. Assoc., 252,* 3395, December 28, 1984.
Snyder, B.S.: Oral Surgery, in Steele, P.F., ed.: *Dental Specialties for the Dental Hygienist,* 2nd ed. Philadelphia, Lea & Febiger, 1978, pp. 173–198.
Souba, W.W. and Wilmore, D.W.: Diet and Nutrition in the Care of the Patient with Surgery, Trauma, and Sepsis, in Shils, M.E. and Young, V.R., eds.: *Modern Nutrition in Health and Disease,* 7th ed. Philadelphia, Lea & Febiger, 1988, pp. 1306–1336.
Wood, G.A. and Wadon, A.J.: Nutritional Support for the Oral Surgery Patient, *Br. J. Oral Maxillofac. Surg., 22,* 201, June, 1984.

Fractures

Bailey, B.J. and Clark, W.D.: Management of Mandibular Fractures, *Ear Nose Throat J., 62,* 371, July, 1983.
Bender, I.B. and Donati, R.: Scintigraphic Detection of a Spontaneous Mandibular Fracture with Spontaneous Healing: Report of a Case, *Compend. Contin. Educ. Dent., 6,* 351, May, 1985.
Carroll, M.J., Hill, C.M., and Mason, D.A.: Facial Fractures in Children, *Br. Dent. J., 163,* 23, July 11, 1987.
Finnegan, B.M.: Periodontal Complications Associated with Teeth Involved in the Line of Mandibular Fracture, *Quintessence Int., 14,* 919, September, 1983.
Frame, K.: Conservative Management of a Patient with a Fractured Atrophic Mandible, *Br. Dent. J., 162,* 27, January 10, 1987.
Lindquist, C., Sorsa, S., Hyrkas, T., and Santavirta, S.: Maxillofacial Fractures Sustained in Bicycle Accidents, *Int. J. Oral Maxillofac. Surg., 15,* 12, February, 1986.

49 *The Patient With Oral Cancer*

Care of the cancer patient before, during, and after therapy has as its main purposes attaining and maintaining oral health at the highest possible level and contributing to the patient's general and mental health. The patient may be under the care of a team of medical and dental specialists including the dentist, oral surgeon, dental hygienist, physician, radiation oncologist, and registered nurse. Special rehabilitation personnel, such as a plastic surgeon, speech therapist, psychiatrist, and maxillofacial prosthodontist, are frequently involved after the treatment phase.

DESCRIPTION

A *neoplasm* is an abnormal, uncontrolled new growth generally classified as *benign* or *malignant.* Characteristics of benign and malignant neoplasms are compared in table 49–1.

Of the oral soft-tissue neoplasms, more than 90 percent are malignant squamous cell carcinomas. They spread by local extension and by the lymphatic system.

I. Incidence

Early recognition of suspicious lesions was described on pages 109 and 111. Because the patient suffers no pain or other symptoms from early cancer, detection is dependent on oral examination by a dentist and a dental hygienist during routine examinations.

When discovered early, surgical removal or other treatment can increase the cure rate at the local site, before invasion to adjacent tissues and lymph nodes of the neck. By the early detection of lesions, serious post-treatment sequelae can be prevented or minimized.

A. Number of Oral Cancers

Approximately 4 percent of all cancers in males and 2 percent in females are oral. The tongue and the floor of the mouth are the most common locations for oral tumors. Approximately 17,700 new cancers of the oral cavity proper, 4200 of the lip, and another 8700 of the oropharynx occur annually in the United States.[1] Males between the ages of 40 and 65 have the highest numbers of lip and tongue cancers.

B. Deaths

Cancer is the second ranking cause of death in the United States. Only diseases of the heart rank higher in adults, and accidents in children under 15 years of age. Oral cancers cause approximately 2.2 percent of all cancer-related deaths.

II. Etiology and Predisposing Factors

A neoplasm begins when a cell or group of cells undergoes uncontrolled growth. Although the specific cause of cancer is not known, extensive research is being conducted. Several factors predispose to cancer formation. Implicated have been weakened immunity, a history of syphilis and other infections, herpes simplex and other viruses, diet (particularly in colon cancer), and the factors described here.[2]

A. Long-term Exposure to the Sun's Rays

1. Squamous cell carcinoma of the lower lip has been related to overexposure. A high percentage of patients with lip cancer have occupations that require outdoor activity and work.
2. Pigmentation appears to intervene, so that carcinoma of the lower lip is relatively rare in black people.

B. Heavy Tobacco Use

1. The use of tobacco in any form increases the chances of developing oral cancer. Long-term exposure to the chemical carcinogens of tobacco as well as trauma to the tissues from the heat are significant factors.
2. Holding smokeless tobacco products or snuff on an area of the oral mucosa will lead to tissue changes and premalignant lesions.
3. The risk of developing a second primary oral cancer is greatly increased by continued use of tobacco.[3]

C. Chronic Alcoholism

Chronic alcoholism increases the tendency to develop cancer. Chronic alcoholics have more lesions of the tongue and floor of the mouth than of other locations in the oral cavity.

PREPARATION FOR TREATMENT

Time may be a factor for the patient with advanced malignancy. The aim in preparation of a patient for treatment for cancer is to restore the mouth to optimal health before the surgery, radiation, or chemotherapy. The extent and severity of the after effects of cancer therapy are related to the condition of the teeth and soft tissues before therapy.

Table 49–1. Characteristics of Benign and Malignant Neoplasms

Characteristic	Benign	Malignant
Cell Characteristics	Cells resemble normal cells of the tissue from which the tumor originated	Cells often bear little resemblance to the normal cells of the tissue from which they arose; there is both anaplasia and pleomorphism
Mode of Growth	Tumor grows by expansion and does not infiltrate the surrounding tissues; encapsulated	Grows at the periphery and sends out processes that infiltrate and destroy the surrounding tissues
Rate of Growth	Rate of growth is usually slow	Rate of growth is usually relatively rapid and is dependent on level of differentiation; the more anaplastic the tumor the more rapid the rate of growth
Metastasis	Does not spread by metastasis	Gains access to the blood and lymph channels and metastasizes to other areas of the body
Recurrence	Does not recur when removed	Tends to recur when removed
General Effects	Is usually a localized phenomenon that does not cause generalized effects unless by location it interferes with vital functions	Often causes generalized effects such as anemia, weakness, and weight loss
Destruction of Tissue	Does not usually cause tissue damage unless location interferes with blood flow	Often causes extensive tissue damage as the tumor outgrows its blood supply or encroaches on blood flow to the area; may also produce substances that cause cell damage
Ability to Cause Death	Does not usually cause death unless its location interferes with vital functions	Will usually cause death unless growth can be controlled

From Porth, C.: Pathophysiology: Concepts of Altered Health States, 2nd ed. Philadelphia, J.B. Lippincott Co., 1986.

Basic preparation follows the same general outline as described on pages 589–591 for a patient having oral surgery. Objectives and treatment include steps to reduce the oral microbial count and provide a better environment for surgical procedures, as well as to improve the conditions for healing.

I. Oral Findings

Many patients with oral cancer may not have sought dental treatment for many years. They may have neglected personal care that could have maintained oral cleanliness. Therefore, it is not unusual to find some or all of the following:
A. Broken-down teeth, some with exposed pulps.
B. Severe periodontal involvement.
C. Ill-fitting dentures.
D. Extremely poor oral hygiene.

II. Dental Treatment Plan

When the patient is to have therapy by radiation, particular attention must be paid to eliminating sources of infection in the oral cavity. When consid-

eration is given to proper preparation for treatment and supervision of preventive measures during and after treatment, the incidence of harmful effects can be reduced.

Because of the effect of radiation on the bone and other tissues, dental procedures such as tooth removal, periodontal surgery, and endodontic treatment that could open a channel for infection to reach the bone are contraindicated after therapy. Therefore, the objectives in dental and dental hygiene care prior to radiation are to reduce the incidence of complications of radiation, particularly osteoradionecrosis and postirradiation caries.

The patient's total treatment plan should include at least the following:

A. Prevention
A complete preventive program for bacterial plaque control and fluoride therapy started at the first appointment.

B. Removal of Nonrestorable Teeth
Extensively involved teeth may need extraction because of severity of bone loss, mobility,

and other signs of advanced periodontal disease, large carious lesions with pulpal exposures not conducive to endodontic therapy, or periapical radiographic findings.

In the past, treatment frequently called for complete extraction of all teeth that would be in the pathway of radiation whether or not they were broken down or diseased. Now, only teeth that are definitely beyond salvaging are removed.

Some patients have such badly broken-down teeth that all of them have to be removed. When extractions are needed, trimming of the bone and careful surgical removal of all spicules is necessary. As long a healing period as possible should be allowed before starting radiation, because when bone is irradiated, healing and remodeling stop.

C. Surgical Procedures

Removal of residual root tips and other subsurface pathologic areas that are found in radiographs of edentulous areas.

D. Endodontic Therapy

Endodontic therapy for essential abutment teeth. Treatment planning for prosthetic replacements must be done in advance so that abutment teeth can receive proper treatment before radiation.

E. Periodontal Therapy

1. Complete scaling and planing.
2. Surgical procedures when time permits follow-up for healing.
3. Occlusal adjustment.

F. Restoration of Carious Lesions

SURGICAL TREATMENT

The three forms of treatment for oral cancer are surgery, radiation, and chemotherapy.

Surgical treatment involves the primary lesion and the regional lymph nodes. Small lesions may be removed by simple excision. Some are totally removed when a biopsy is used for diagnosis.

Radical neck dissection is a procedure that includes wide removal of tissues around a tumor. This is necessary when the oropharynx and neck are involved, in order to prevent the spread of the cancer to the lymph nodes.

RADIATION THERAPY

Therapeutic radiation may be the only treatment or it may be used in conjunction with surgery.[4,5]

I. Objectives

A. As a Total Treatment

Exposures are usually given as daily doses, made in fractions of the total dose.

B. In Conjunction with Surgery

1. *Preoperatively.* To reduce the size of the neoplasm as an aid to surgery by limiting the surgical area.
2. *Postoperatively.* To control residual disease.

II. Types

A. External

1. *Orthovoltage.* Low-yield radiation was formerly used for superficial lesions. It has high skin and bone absorption factors and is not used currently.
2. *Mega- or Supervoltage.* High-yield radiation includes cobalt-60 and the linear accelerator. It has a sparing effect on skin and bone and less scatter radiation to surrounding tissues than orthovoltage. Divided doses are given over 6 to 8 weeks on an outpatient appointment plan.

B. Internal Implant

The source of radiation is placed within the body. Less radiation is delivered to surrounding tissues than when an external source is utilized. Radium needles and radioactive radon and gold seeds are used.

III. Effects of Radiation Therapy

Irradiation is the exposure of tissues to x-rays or other forms of radiation. The purpose is to destroy cancerous cells. Damage to surrounding normal tissue cannot be avoided, but the severity of damage can be minimized.

Ionizing radiation induces tissue changes, some of which are apparent during the treatment period and may continue for a few weeks or months after cessation of irradiation. Other changes may not be evident until after treatment and may have long-term significance.

Early changes result from damage to the epithelium and include dermatitis, mucositis, alopecia, and at first, an increased salivary flow. Later changes include atrophy of the salivary glands with diminished salivary flow and diminished bone vascularity.

A. Mucosa

1. *Mucositis.* Inflammation of the mucosa may appear as early as 1 week after radiation therapy is started.
   a. Cellular changes. Initially an inflammatory response occurs with edema. The tissues may become ulcerated and necrotic with sloughing. Later, fibrosis develops.
   b. Clinical signs. Sensitivity to temperature extremes and pressure, an unpleasant odor from the necrotic tissue and plaque collection are commonly found. The patient with dentures may not be able to tolerate wearing them.
   c. Recovery. The severe signs will heal and disappear within a few weeks after radia-

tion is stopped, but the epithelium never completely recovers and tends to be thin and more fragile than normal.

2. *Effects on Patient.* Toothbrushing and other personal care may be neglected because of the sensitivity of the tissues. A flavored dentifrice may not be tolerated. A soft diet may be required.

B. Salivary Glands

Radiation to the salivary glands may be unavoidable, depending on the location of the cancerous lesion. The radiation primarily affects the serous gland cells with a lessening of secretion.

1. *Xerostomia.* A reduced quantity of saliva may be noticed as early as the third or fourth day after the beginning of radiation.

2. *Changes in Saliva.* Saliva is thickened and sticky, which makes swallowing difficult.

3. *Changes in Mucosa.* Dry mucosa may be prone to cracks and bleeding.

4. *Effects on Patient*
   a. Difficulty in speaking and swallowing.
   b. Difficulty in wearing prostheses.
   c. Increased dental caries.

C. Bone

Radiation damages bone cells and blood vessels within the bone. Changes in the endothelial cells lead to sclerosis of the vessels. The result is change in the growth potential of the bone and lowered resistance to infection.

1. *Predisposing Factors.* The lowered resistance to infection predisposes the bone to infection that may reach the bone through an ulcer in the mucosa, deep periodontal pocket, periapical lesion, open socket from tooth extraction, or other potential channel for microorganisms.

   The infection may develop many years after radiation because the bone changes are not reversible. Osteoradionecrosis occurs more frequently in the mandible because of the limitation of the blood supply.

2. *Symptoms.* Osteoradionecrosis is characterized by pain, trismus, exposed bone, sequestration, and pathologic fracture. The infection can be suppurative, and halitosis is usually present.

   Treatment is difficult and may involve extended antibiotic therapy and surgery for the removal of the sequestra, or even part of the mandible.

3. *Prevention.* Correct pre- and postradiation procedures have had a definite effect on lowering the incidence of osteoradionecrosis. Maintenance of oral cleanliness and health are contributing preventive factors.

D. Teeth

1. *"Radiation Caries"*
   a. Description. Teeth with exposed root surfaces are especially susceptible. The le-

sions develop in the cervical thirds and gradually encircle the necks of the teeth (figure 14–6, page 217). The carious lesions appear black or dark brown.
   b. Predisposing factors. Xerostomia, neglect of plaque control measures, soft cariogenic diet, sore mouth, and changes in oral flora are responsible, not radiation directly.
   c. Prevention. Intensified preventive measures for fluoride application and plaque control are needed. The use of a saliva substitute containing fluoride is also indicated (page 188).

2. *Tooth Development.* Radiation in children can affect the odontogenic cells. A tooth bud may be completely destroyed if irradiated before mineralization has started.

3. *Sensitivity of Teeth.* The teeth with marked dental caries are particularly sensitive, but all teeth may react to temperature extremes.

E. Taste

Taste can be altered by degeneration of taste buds or by changes in the quantity of saliva.

F. Loss of Appetite

Because of sore mouth, loss of taste sensation, diminished saliva, and related symptoms, interest in eating fades, and a loss of appetite occurs, followed by weight loss. Denture wearers who cannot wear their dentures have an added eating problem.

G. Trismus

Trismus is spasm of the muscles of mastication. It can result from fibrosis in the muscle fibers that were irradiated. It may occur 3 to 6 months after therapy has stopped, and it makes opening of the mouth very difficult. Exercises and stretching appliances have been used for treatment.

CHEMOTHERAPY[6]

I. Objectives

Chemotherapeutic drugs are used to control widely scattered neoplasms and to supplement treatment by surgery and/or radiation. The objective is to destroy or deactivate the cancer cells with as little destruction of normal cells as possible. Side effects from the drugs are significant and frequently involve the oral tissues.

II. Types of Chemotherapeutic Agents[6]

Chemotherapeutic drugs fall into four major groups; others are used occasionally or are in an experimental category. The drugs may be used singly, but more commonly are used in combinations. The types of drugs are alkylating agents, antimetabolites, antibiotics, and plant alkaloids. Others include hormones, steroids, and enzymes.

III. Side Effects of Chemotherapy

Rapidly proliferating normal cells are susceptible to the suppressive action of chemotherapeutic agents. These include hair, bone marrow, and oral and intestinal mucosal epithelial cells. The drugs are *immunosuppressive* by inhibiting antibody responses and inducing leukopenia. They are *myelosuppressive* by depressing bone marrow activity, which results in leukopenia and thrombocytopenia.

IV. Oral Complications

Whether chemotherapeutic drugs are administered for malignancies of the head and neck or elsewhere in the body, oral effects are common. Nearly 40 percent of adult and 90 percent of child patients with malignancies not of the head and neck were shown to have oral problems.[7] In that study, ulceration was the most common complication.

Loss of appetite, nausea, vomiting, and diarrhea are frequent side effects of chemotherapy. When oral lesions are present and the mouth is sore, eating can be difficult. Oral lesions may become so severe that the patient's health and nutritional state are affected. Chemotherapy may have to be stopped, which changes the degree of success that can be expected from the treatment and, therefore, the patient's chances of survival.[8]

Principal oral effects may be grouped as cytotoxic, hemorrhagic, and infectious, in addition to the nutritional problems mentioned.[6,7,9] Different effects are produced by the various drugs used.

1. *Cytotoxicity.* Toxic effects to the oral mucosal cells result in ulcerations and loss of surface characteristics. The incidence is greater in younger patients. Loss of nutritional support may complicate the problem. Fewer oral lesions develop when bacterial plaque is under control and the tissues show signs of health.[10]

2. *Hemorrhage.* Bone marrow suppression leads to thrombocytopenia; clinically, petechiae may be present and spontaneous gingival bleeding may occur. The frequency and severity of bleeding are directly related to whether the patient already has mucositis and/or periodontitis, and also has received radiation therapy. The state of health of the gingiva is highly significant.

3. *Infections.* As a result of immunosuppression and myelosuppression, chronic infections may increase in severity and become acute. Changes occur in the oral microflora, with a shift to predominantly gram-negative microorganisms and fungi. Candidiasis is the most frequent fungal infection. Viral infections are relatively infrequent except for herpes simplex. Necrotizing ulcerative gingivitis may occur in the neglected mouth.[9]

PERSONAL FACTORS[11,12]

Patient attitudes and feelings may be similar to those of any patient with a major chronic disease or disability. As with other diseases with limited hope for cure, strong feelings of hopelessness and despair predominate.

The very word *cancer* brings fear and anxiety to the patient. The concerns of a patient may differ at different stages of treatment.

I. Patient Problems

A. Early Fears and Anxieties
1. Outcome.
2. Imminent surgery, radiation, or other treatment.
3. Disfigurement, changes in appearance, and pain.
4. Extended hospitalization.
5. Financial stress.

B. During and Following Therapy
1. Preoccupation with details of examinations, treatments, symptoms, or medications.
2. Depression and grief, which may lead to withdrawal and isolation.
3. Major concerns include obvious facial deformity, speech difficulty, swallowing difficulty, drooling, and odors from debris collection and tissue changes.

II. Suggestions for Approach to Patient

A. Provide explanations before and after therapy to prevent misconceptions and apprehensions, and attempt to allay fears.

B. Provide paper and pencil for patient with a speech difficulty to write questions and requests.

C. Show acceptance. Acknowledge the appropriateness of the patient's concerns.

D. Express empathy, but avoid oversolicitousness.

E. Help to direct thoughts and efforts toward restoration of functional activity.

F. Instill trust and security by demonstrating genuine interest.

G. Assist the patient who was an alcoholic, used tobacco products excessively, or had other habits that have to be eliminated. The patient may need the help of psychiatry, Alcoholics Anonymous, or other type of support organization.

DENTAL HYGIENE CARE

In the not too distant past, the patient with oral cancer was doomed to complete tooth removal or at least removal of all teeth in the line of radiation. When the teeth were left in the mouth, severe radiation caries inevitably developed. A high percentage of patients had osteoradionecrosis. Now, many teeth are saved, restored, and preserved by an intensive daily preventive program of bacterial plaque control and self-applied fluoride by gel trays or brush-on.

The dental hygienist's contribution to the preparation of the patient for cancer therapy and the continued supervision of oral health and preventive techniques during treatment and regularly thereafter has special significance. Bacterial plaque control, irrigation, rinsing, fluoride application, dietary factors for general health and dental caries prevention, along with specific instrumentation for the health of the periodontal tissues, are major areas of attention for the dental hygienist.

I. Patient Instruction

A. Bacterial Plaque Control

A complete instruction series (pages 370–374) should be started before cancer treatment, with careful supervision. The patient must understand the reasons for intensive oral health care. Scaling and planing can be accomplished within the same series of appointments. Time is usually an important factor when a malignant tumor is involved.

1. *Toothbrushing.* Sulcular brushing with a soft nylon brush is recommended for the following reasons:
   a. "Radiation caries" occurs primarily at the cervical third, about the necks of the teeth. Emphasis must be placed on keeping the cervical areas plaque-free.
   b. Control of gingival health with prevention of gingivitis is necessary. Fewer side effects develop from chemotherapy when optimum oral health is maintained.[10]
   c. Sensitivity of teeth is associated most frequently with the cervical third. Brushing with a desensitizing dentifrice with fluoride can help alleviate sensitivity and prevent dental caries (pages 499–500).
2. *Tongue Brushing.* Bacteria and debris collect on a dry tongue.
3. *Dental Floss.* Proximal surface plaque must be removed. Other interdental devices may be helpful.

B. Nutrition and Diet

Every possible attempt to improve the general health must be made. If the patient is malnourished and debilitated, a high protein diet is needed. Reduction of cariogenic foods is essential to the dental caries prevention program.

A hospitalized patient will be under the supervision of a physician who gives diet prescription orders to the hospital dietitian. The private or clinic physician may make specific recommendations to the patient. Within the framework of the physician's orders, the dental hygienist may also help the patient and the person who will prepare the patient's food at home. Instructions in the preparation of foods in a blender may be needed (page 598).

Because the mouth may be sore and tender, a topical anesthetic in the form of a troche may be needed before eating. During the treatment phase and immediately following radiation therapy, swallowing may be difficult, and because of xerostomia, liquids are needed with meals to moisten the food for swallowing. Because the patient suffers from a loss of appetite and difficulty in eating, weight loss is common. Diet selection can be very important so that proper nutrients are included within the limited diet.

C. Other Instruction

1. *Reduction of Sources of Irritation to the Mucosa.* The patient must not use alcohol or tobacco.
2. *Care of Dental Prostheses.* Frequently, prostheses are not worn during the period of cancer therapy. The use of a saliva substitute can provide relief and make it possible to wear dentures with comfort.

   Meticulous denture hygiene must be maintained when the dentures are worn. Instruction and frequent supervision of cleansing procedures can be very important to most patients.

II. Instrumentation

A. Mouth Preparation for Radiation and Surgery

Although complete periodontal treatment before treatment of oral cancer is ideal, time frequently contraindicates prolonged procedures. Minimum preparation, therefore, includes complete nonsurgical therapy with calculus removal and root planing. Excessive manipulation of tissues and instrumentation within the few days preceding oral surgery should be avoided.

Whenever possible, the following should be completed:

1. Scaling and planing. These may be accomplished in conjunction with bacterial plaque control instruction in a series of quadrant treatments.
2. Removal of all rough and overhanging margins and finishing all restorations.

B. Continuing Treatment

Repeated scaling and planing are needed at frequent maintenance appointments to supplement plaque control efforts by the patient.

III. Fluoride

A. Dentifrice

Use of a fluoride dentifrice is basic to fluoride therapy. The tissues may not tolerate a highly flavored dentifrice during the period when the mucosa is inflamed. A bland dentifrice with fluoride may be recommended.[13]

B. Gel Tray Applications

The patient must receive daily fluoride applications while receiving radiation therapy. The incidence of postirradiation caries can be reduced by use of a custom tray with a fluoride gel or by brushing with the gel after regular brushing.[14]

1. *Application by Patient.* The patient can be trained to make the application. During radiation therapy, the patient may be preoccupied or too uncomfortable to have interest in carrying out the procedure because it may appear to have no immediate benefit.

    When it seems apparent that the patient may neglect the fluoride, the topical daily application must be made, if possible, by a family member after instruction.

2. *Procedure.* Prepare custom trays before the radiation therapy starts, one for each dental arch. Fluoride gel is placed in the tray and fitted over the teeth for 5 minutes. The patient does not rinse after removal.

3. *Effect on Sensitivity of the Teeth.* Topical fluoride on a daily basis benefits the patient by lessening tooth sensitivity.

IV. Saliva Substitute

A patient undergoing radiation therapy for cancer of the head and neck may have a drop in saliva flow up to 60 percent during the first week and 95 percent by the sixth week.[15] Severe discomfort with drying, cracking, and bleeding of the mucosa, difficulty during mastication and swallowing, which can affect nutritional factors, food particles clinging to the teeth and gingiva with increased bacterial plaque, inability to wear prostheses, and increased susceptibility to dental caries are major effects from xerostomia.

The increase in dental caries following irradiation is caused by a lack of saliva and not by the direct radiation to the tooth. Information about xerostomia is in Chapter 12 on pages 187–188.

Instructions to the patient are simple, and no limitations are placed on the frequency of use. The only contraindication is if a patient is on a low sodium diet. The patient is instructed to place a drop or two in the mouth and spread the gel around with the tongue.

V. Maintenance

A. Preventive Self-care

The importance of prevention and control throughout the patient's life cannot be overemphasized. All the steps for care of the gingiva and teeth should be continued daily.

B. Frequency of Appointments

Examination of the oral mucosa and supervision of gingival and dental health are carried out daily during therapy, weekly following the completion of therapy, and then monthly as indicated by the condition of the oral tissues.

The dental hygiene appointment will include at least the following:

1. Extraoral and intraoral soft tissue examination.

2. Gingival examination with pocket measurements and evaluation of bleeding, tooth mobility, and other signs of periodontal infection.

3. Evaluation of bacterial plaque and plaque removal procedures. Review of techniques to motivate and encourage the patient.

4. Instrumentation. Scaling and planing as needed must be completed. Patients receiving immunosuppressive drugs need antibiotic premedication prior to instrumentation (page 91).

5. Review of fluoride procedures with a check to be certain the patient has refilled the fluoride prescription.

TECHNICAL HINTS

I. Preparation of History

Preparation of a medical and dental history for all patients should include questions relative to radiation therapy received. Radiation during childhood should be recorded as well as that during adulthood.

II. Patient Referral

When a patient is referred to a specialist or specialty clinic, a check must be made to ascertain that the patient arrives for the appointment. Frightened patients may become confused or may postpone the visit if they do not realize the urgency of the condition.

III. Source of Material

American Cancer Society
90 Park Avenue
New York, New York 10016.
    Local cancer society addresses can be obtained from the New York office.

FACTORS TO TEACH THE PATIENT

I. The importance of oral soft tissue screening and complete oral examination at regular frequent intervals.

II. Plaque control methods, gel-tray application, use of saliva substitute, and all other details of personal care.

III. Why use of alcohol and tobacco must be stopped.

IV. Instruction for family members in oral health care for the sick and helpless patient.

References

1. Cancer Statistics, 1989, *CA, 39,* 3, 12, January/February, 1989.
2. Silverman, S. and Shillitoe, E.J.: Etiology and Predisposing Factors, in Silverman, S., ed.: *Oral Cancer,* 2nd ed. New York, The American Cancer Society, 1985, pp. 7–36.
3. Silverman, S., Gorsky, M., and Greenspan, D.: Tobacco Usage in Patients with Head and Neck Carcinomas: A Follow-up Study on Habit Changes and Second Primary Oral/Oropharyngeal Cancers, *J. Am. Dent. Assoc., 106,* 33, January, 1983.
4. Galente, M., Phillips, T.L., Silverberg, I.J., Carter, S.K., and

Cadman, E.C: Treatment, in Silverman, S.: *Oral Cancer,* 2nd ed. New York, The American Cancer Society, 1985, pp. 55–63.

5. O'Sullivan, B.P., Oatis, G.W., and Grisius, R.J.: Osteoradione-crosis: Its Prevention, *Clin. Prevent. Dent., 4,* 8, July-August, 1982.

6. Peterson, D.E. and Sonis, S.T., eds.: *Oral Complications of Cancer Chemotherapy.* The Hague, Martinus Nijhoff Publishers, 1983, pp. 1–12.

7. Sonis, S.T., Sonis, A.L., and Lieberman, A.: Oral Complications in Patients Receiving Treatment for Malignancies Other than of the Head and Neck, *J. Am. Dent. Assoc., 97,* 468, September, 1978.

8. Dreizen, S.: Stomatotoxic Manifestations of Cancer Chemotherapy, *J. Prosthet. Dent., 40,* 650, December, 1978.

9. Peterson and Sonis: op. cit., pp. 125–127.

10. Lindquist, S.F., Hickey, A.J., and Drane, J.B.: Effect of Oral Hygiene on Stomatitis in Patients Receiving Cancer Chemotherapy, *J. Prosthet. Dent., 40,* 312, September, 1978.

11. Allen, J.: The Psychosocial Effects of Cancer and Its Treatment in the Elderly, *Spec. Care Dentist., 4,* 13, January-February, 1984.

12. Turns, D. and Sands, R.G.: Psychological Problems of Patients with Head and Neck Cancer, *J. Prosthet. Dent., 39,* 68, January, 1978.

13. Greenspan, D. and Silverman, S.: Study of a Bland Dentifrice for Persons with Radiation-induced Mucositis and Vesiculoerosive Disease, *J. Am. Dent. Assoc., 99,* 203, August, 1979.

14. Dreizen, S., Brown, L.R., Daly, T.E., and Drane, J.B.: Prevention of Xerostomia-related Dental Caries in Irradiated Cancer Patients, *J. Dent. Res., 56,* 99, February, 1977.

15. Shannon, I.L., Starcke, E.N., and Wescott, W.B.: Effect of Radiotherapy on Whole Saliva Flow, *J. Dent. Res., 56,* 693, June, 1977.

Suggested Readings

Buckingham, R.W.: Dental Care Policies for Treating the Terminal Cancer Patient, *Dent. Hyg., 55,* 23, April, 1981.

Greene, S.L.: Treating the Head and Neck Cancer Patient, *Dent. Hyg., 54,* 23, January, 1980.

Harris, L.L., Vogtsberger, K.N., and Mattox, D.E.: Group Psychotherapy for Head and Neck Cancer Patients, *Laryngoscope, 95,* 585, May, 1985.

Lampe, H.B., Lampe, K.M., and Skillings, J.: Head and Neck Cancer in the Elderly, *J. Otolaryngol., 15,* 235, August, 1986.

Larsen, G.L.: Rehabilitation for the Patient with Head and Neck Cancer, *Am. J. Nurs., 82,* 119, January, 1982.

Niehaus, C.S., Meiller, T.F., Peterson, D.E., and Overholser, C.D.: The Dental Hygienist's Role in a Pediatric Oncology Center, *Dent. Hyg., 61,* 414, September, 1987.

Schweiger, J.W.: Patients with Head and Neck Cancer—Pre- and Posttherapy Dental Care, *Spec. Care Dentist., 7,* 18, January-February, 1987.

Strauss, R.P.: The Patient with Cancer: Social and Clinical Perspectives for the Dentist, *Spec. Care Dentist., 8,* 129, May-June, 1988.

Wheeler, R.L., Logemann, J.A., and Rosen, M.S.: Maxillary Reshaping Prostheses: Effectiveness in Improving Speech and Swallowing of Postsurgical Oral Cancer Patients, *J. Prosthet. Dent., 43,* 313, March, 1980.

Wright, W.E., Haller, J.M., Harlow, S.A., and Pizzo, P.A.: An Oral Disease Prevention Program for Patients Receiving Radiation and Chemotherapy, *J. Am. Dent. Assoc., 110,* 43, January, 1985.

Early Detection

Amsel, Z., Strawitz, J.G., and Engstrom, P.F.: The Dentist As a Referral Source of First Episode Head and Neck Cancer Patients, *J. Am. Dent. Assoc., 106,* 195, February, 1983.

Bhaskar, S.N.: *Synopsis of Oral Pathology,* 7th ed. St. Louis, The C.V. Mosby Co., 1986, pp. 309–364, 520–634.

Chiodo, G.T., Eigner, T., and Rosenstein, D.I.: Oral Cancer Detection. The Importance of Routine Screening for Prolongation of Survival, *Postgrad. Med., 80,* 231, August, 1986.

Hall, G.L., Melrose, R.J., and Abrams, A.M.: Education in Early Detection of Oral Squamous Cell Carcinoma: A Community Outreach Program, *J. Am. Dent. Assoc., 100,* 362, March, 1980.

LePine, E., Kent, K., and Samit, A.: Site-dependent Manifestations of Head and Neck Cancers, *Gen. Dent., 32,* 446, September-October, 1984.

Moyer, G.N., Taybos, G.M., and Pelleu, G.B.: Toluidine Blue Rinse: Potential for Benign Lesions in Early Detection of Oral Neoplasms, *J. Oral Med., 41,* 111, April-June, 1986.

Shafer, W.G., Hine, M.K., and Levy, B.M.: *A Textbook of Oral Pathology,* 4th ed. Philadelphia, W.B. Saunders Co., 1983, pp. 86–229.

Thomas, J.E. and Bell, W.A.: Clinical Aids for the Detection of Oral Cancer in the Elderly, *Gen. Dent., 33,* 492, November-December, 1985.

Tobacco

Baric, J.M., Alman, J.E., Feldman, R.S., and Chauncey, H.H.: Influence of Cigarette, Pipe, and Cigar Smoking, Removable Partial Dentures, and Age on Oral Leukoplakia, *Oral Surg. Oral Med. Oral Pathol., 54,* 424, October, 1982.

Frithiof, L., Anneroth, G., Lasson, U., and Sederholm, C.: The Snuff-induced Lesion. A Clinical and Morphological Study of a Swedish Material, *Acta Odontol. Scand., 41,* 53, Number 1, 1983.

Koop, C.E.: Smoking and Cancer, *Hosp. Pract., 19,* 107, June, 1984.

Massey, J.D., Moore, G.F., and Yonkers, A.J.: Smokeless Tobacco: A Risk Factor in Oral Cancer, *Ear Nose Throat J., 63,* 453, September, 1984.

McGuirt, W.F.: Snuff Dipper's Carcinoma, *Arch. Otolaryngol., 109,* 757, November, 1983.

Radiation Therapy

Al-Tikriti, U., Martin, M.V., and Bramley, P.A.: A Pilot Study of the Clinical Effects of Irradiation on the Oral Tissues, *Br. J. Oral and Maxillofac. Surg., 22,* 77, April, 1984.

Bernhoft, C.-H. and Skaug, N.: Oral Findings in Irradiated Edentulous Patients, *Int. J. Oral Surg., 14,* 416, October, 1985.

Beumer, J. and Seto, B.: Dental Extractions in the Irradiated Patient, *Spec. Care Dentist., 1,* 166, July-August, 1981.

Carl, W.: Managing the Oral Manifestations of Cancer Therapy, Part I: Head-and-Neck Radiation Therapy, *Compend. Contin. Educ. Dent., 9,* 306, April, 1988.

Coffin, F.: The Incidence and Management of Osteoradionecrosis of the Jaws Following Head and Neck Radiotherapy, *Br. J. Radiol., 56,* 851, November, 1983.

Cooper, J.S. and Fried, P.R.: Toxicity of Oral Radiotherapy in Patients with Acquired Immunodeficiency Syndrome, *Arch. Otolaryngol. Head Neck Surg., 113,* 327, March, 1987.

Dodd, D.T., George, D.I., Farman, A.G., Sharma, S., and Wilson, D.: Backscatter Radiation from Restorative Materials During Cobalt 60 Therapy, *J. Oral Med., 40,* 72, April-June, 1985.

Engelmeier, R.L. and King, G.E.: Complications of Head and Neck Radiation Therapy and Their Management, *J. Prosthet. Dent., 49,* 514, April, 1983.

Engelmeier, R.L.: A Dental Protocol for Patients Receiving Radiation Therapy for Cancer of the Head and Neck, *Spec. Care Dentist., 7,* 54, March-April, 1987.

Fleming, T.J. and Rambach, S.C.: A Tongue-shielding Radiation Stent, *J. Prosthet. Dent., 49,* 389, March, 1983.

Gunn, W.G.: Radiation Therapy for the Aging Patient, *CA, 30,* 337, November-December, 1980.

Herring, H.W. and Greene, P.E.: Use of a Complete Denture as a Radiation Carrier, *J. Prosthet. Dent., 49,* 803, June, 1983.

Hutton, J., Koulourides, T., and Borden, L.: Evaluation of Cariostatic Disciplines for Postradiation Caries, *Caries Res., 16,* 390, Number 5, 1982.

Katz, S.: The Use of Fluoride and Chlorhexidine for the Prevention of Radiation Caries, *J. Am. Dent. Assoc., 104,* 164, February, 1982.

Keene, H.J. and Fleming, T.J.: Prevalence of Caries-associated Microflora After Radiotherapy in Patients with Cancer of the Head and Neck, *Oral Surg. Oral Med. Oral Pathol., 64,* 421, October, 1987.

Marx, R.E.: Osteoradionecrosis: A New Concept of Its Pathophysiology, *J. Oral Maxillofac. Surg., 41,* 283, May, 1983.

Murray, C.G., Daly, T.E., and Zimmerman, S.O.: The Relationship Between Dental Disease and Radiation Necrosis of the Mandible, *Oral Surg. Oral Med. Oral Pathol., 49,* 99, February, 1980.

Poole, T.S. and Flaxman, N.A.: Use of Protective Prostheses During Radiation Therapy, *J. Am. Dent. Assoc., 112,* 485, April, 1985.

Reynolds, W.R., Hickey, A.J., and Feldman, M.I.: Dental Management of the Cancer Patient Receiving Radiation Therapy, *Clin. Prevent. Dent., 2,* 5, September-October, 1980.

Ritchie, J.R., Brown, J.R., Guerra, L.R., and Mason, G.: Dental Care for the Irradiated Cancer Patient, *Quintessence Int., 16,* 837, December, 1985.

Strauss, M.: Long-term Complications of Radiotherapy Confronting the Head and Neck Surgeon, *Laryngoscope, 93,* 310, March, 1983.

Sullivan, M.D. and Fleming, T.J.: Oral Care for the Radiotherapy-treated Head and Neck Cancer Patient, *Dent. Hyg., 60,* 112, March, 1986.

Tatcher, M., Kuten, A., Helman, J., and Laufer, D.: Perturbation of Cobalt 60 Radiation Doses by Metal Objects Implanted During Oral and Maxillofacial Surgery, *J. Oral Maxillofac. Surg., 42,* 108, February, 1984.

Toljanic, J.A. and Saunders, V.W.: Radiation Therapy and Management of the Irradiated Patient, *J. Prosthet. Dent., 52,* 852, December, 1984.

Vergo, T.J. and Kadish, S.P.: Dentures as Artificial Saliva Reservoirs in the Irradiated Edentulous Cancer Patient with Xerostomia: A Pilot Study, *Oral Surg. Oral Med. Oral Pathol., 51,* 229, March, 1981.

Chemotherapy

Barrett, A.P.: Clinical Characteristics and Mechanisms Involved in Chemotherapy-induced Oral Ulceration, *Oral Surg. Oral Med. Oral Pathol., 63,* 424, April, 1987.

Carl, W.: Oral and Dental Care for Cancer Patients Receiving Radiation and Chemotherapy, *Quintessence Int., 12,* 861, September, 1981.

Debiase, C.B. and Komives, B.K.: An Oral Care Protocol for Leukemic Patients with Chemotherapy-induced Oral Complications, *Spec. Care Dentist., 3,* 207, September-October, 1983.

DePaola, L.G., Peterson, D.E., Overholser, C.D., Suzuki, J.B., Minah, G.E., Williams, L.T., Stansbury, D.M., and Niehaus, C.S.: Dental Care for Patients Receiving Chemotherapy, *J. Am. Dent. Assoc., 112,* 198, February, 1986.

Dreizen, S., McCredie, K.B., and Keating, M.J.: Chemotherapy-induced Oral Mucositis in Adult Leukemia, *Postgrad. Med., 69,* 103, February, 1981.

Fattore, L.D., Baer, R., and Olsen, R.: The Role of the General Dentist in the Treatment and Management of Oral Complications of Chemotherapy, *Gen. Dent., 35,* 374, September-October, 1987.

McClure, D., Barker, G., Barker, B., and Feil, P.: Oral Management of the Cancer Patient, Part I: Oral Complications of Chemotherapy, *Compend. Contin. Educ. Dent., 8,* 41, January, 1987.

Purdell-Lewis, D.J., Stalman, M.S., Leeuw, J.A., Humphrey, G.B., and Kalsbeek, H.: Long Term Results of Chemotherapy on the Developing Dentition: Caries Risk and Developmental Aspects, *Community Dent. Oral Epidemiol., 16,* 68, April, 1988.

Infections

DePaola, L.G. and Minah, G.E.: Isolation of Pathogenic Microorganisms from Dentures and Denture-soaking Containers of Myelosuppressed Cancer Patients, *J. Prosthet. Dent., 49,* 21, January, 1983.

DePaola, L.G., Minah, G.E., and Elias, S.A.: Growth of Potential Pathogens in Denture-soaking Solution of Myelosuppressed Cancer Patients, *J. Prosthet. Dent., 51,* 554, April, 1984.

Dreizen, S., Bodey, G.P., and Valdivieso, M.: Chemotherapy-associated Oral Infections in Adults with Solid Tumors, *Oral Surg. Oral Med. Oral Pathol., 55,* 113, February, 1983.

Greenberg, M.S., Cohen, S.G., Boosz, B., and Friedman, H.: Oral Herpes Simplex Infections in Patients with Leukemia, *J. Am. Dent. Assoc., 114,* 483, April, 1987.

McElroy, T.H.: Infection in the Patient Receiving Chemotherapy for Cancer: Oral Considerations, *J. Am. Dent. Assoc., 109,* 454, September, 1984.

Periodontal Disease

DePaola, L.G., Peterson, D.E., Minah, G.E., Overholser, C.D., Stansbury, D.M., Williams, L.T., Niehaus, C.S., and Suzuki, J.B.: Acute Periodontal Infection Associated with Dental Prostheses During Cancer Chemotherapy, *Gerodontics, 2,* 212, December, 1986.

Fattore, L.D., Strauss, R., and Bruno, J.: The Management of Periodontal Disease in Patients Who Have Received Radiation Therapy for Head and Neck Cancer, *Spec. Care Dentist., 7,* 120, May-June, 1987.

Suzuki, J.B., DePaola, L.G., and Nauman, R.K.: Periodontal Therapy in a Patient Undergoing Cancer Chemotherapy, *J. Am. Dent. Assoc., 104,* 473, April, 1982.

Wright, W.E.: Periodontium Destruction Associated with Oncology Therapy. Five Case Reports, *J. Periodontol., 58,* 559, August, 1987.

Nutrition

Baredes, S. and Blitzer, A.: Nutritional Considerations in the Management of Head and Neck Cancer Patients, *Otolaryngol. Clin. North Am., 17,* 725, November, 1984.

Jackson, M.J., Vergo, T.J., Palmer, C.A., and Lund, W.: Nutritional Considerations of the Head and Neck Cancer Patient: Some Correlations in a Retrospective Study, *J. Prosthet. Dent., 57,* 475, April, 1987.

Jones, J.A. and Lang, W.P.: Nutrition During Treatment of Head and Neck Cancer, *Spec. Care Dentist., 6,* 165, July-August, 1986.

Samaranayake, L.P.: Nutritional Factors and Oral Candidosis, *J. Oral Path., 15,* 61, February, 1986.

50 Care of Patients with Disabilities

Many types of disabilities or handicaps require special attention and adaptations during dental and dental hygiene appointments. The general term disability refers to any reduction of a person's activity that has resulted from an acute or chronic health condition and affects motor, sensory, or mental functions.

A disability may be permanent or temporary. A temporary disability may be physical, such as a fracture of a leg, or physiologic with physical limitations, such as during pregnancy. Chronic systemic diseases may result in crippling disabilities. The causes of disabilities may be factors of heredity, systemic disease, trauma, or combinations of these.

The Developmental Disabilities Assistance and Bill of Rights Act of 1987 defined the term *developmental disability* as a severe, chronic disability of a person that

A. is attributable to a mental or physical impairment or combination of mental or physical impairments;
B. is manifested before the person attains the age of 22;
C. is likely to continue indefinitely;
D. results in substantial functional limitations in three or more of the following areas of major life activity:
    (i) self-care,
    (ii) receptive and expressive language,
    (iii) learning,
    (iv) mobility,
    (v) self-direction,
    (vi) capacity for independent living, and
    (vii) economic self-sufficiency; and
E. reflects the person's need for a combination and sequence of special, interdisciplinary, or generic care, treatment, or other services that are of lifelong or extended duration and are individually planned and coordinated.[1]

Current trends toward deinstitutionalization have brought alternative living, educational, and work arrangements to many individuals with physical and mental disabilities. Specially staffed community housing for group living has been made available. Children taken out of institutional life and trained for community living in transitional homes are being integrated into regular school and health programs.

The term *normalization* is used to mean the attempt to provide a normal pattern of daily living. *Mainstreaming* is the integration of people with handicaps into their communities. Through a program of rehabilitation, persons with disabilities may receive vocational, educational, placement, medical, and dental services as needed.

DENTAL AND DENTAL HYGIENE CARE

Oral health for the individual with a handicap takes on more than usual significance and presents a challenge to dental personnel. For the patient, the handicap provides enough of a burden without additional oral problems, which can reduce an already lowered potential for normal living. Preventive measures, particularly fluoridation and other means for protecting the teeth with fluoride, must be encouraged and promoted through community effort and personal instruction to minimize oral problems.

Imagination, ingenuity, and flexibility are necessary for those involved in treating people with handicaps. Individualization and modification of usual procedures will be necessary in addition to the material described in this chapter. Patience, calmness, and kindness are keys to approaching the special patient.

I. Objectives

The dental team can make a significant contribution to the well-being, independent mobility, and sense of personal value of a patient with a handicap. Whether employed in private practice, working in an institutional or community clinical and educational setting, or contributing on a volunteer basis, the dental team must have as its objectives to

A. Motivate the patient and those who provide daily care for the patient. Personal oral care practices conducive to maintaining healthy oral tissue with freedom from infection must be developed.
B. Contribute to the patient's general health, of which oral health is an integral part. Prevention of tooth loss increases the ability to masticate food, which, in turn, is essential to prevent malnutrition and to increase resistance to infection.
C. Prevent the need for extensive dental and periodontal treatment that the patient may not be able to undergo because of lowered physical stamina or the inability to cooperate. Dentures or other

removable appliances can be hazardous for certain patients or impossible for others.

D. Aid in the improvement of appearance, thereby contributing to social acceptance. An untidy person with unclean teeth and halitosis (from local causes) is much less acceptable socially than is one with a clean mouth.

E. Make appointments pleasant and comfortable experiences.

II. Types of Conditions

A variety of disabling conditions are found among persons with handicaps. An individual may have more than one type of crippling or limiting problem. The following list is not intended to include all possibilities, but it is representative.[2] Many of the diseases and syndromes that have these symptoms are described in the various chapters throughout Section VI of this book.

A. Mental retardation.

B. Seizure disorders; convulsive states.

C. Sensory impairments
1. Visual.
2. Speech.
3. Hearing.

D. Learning disabilities
1. Perceptual handicaps.
2. Dyslexia.

E. Surgical disfigurement
1. Amputation of limbs.
2. Maxillofacial defects after oral cancer surgery.

F. Congenital defects: cleft lip and/or palate.

G. Paralysis
1. Spastic and athetoid paralysis (cerebral palsy).
2. Brain or spinal cord damage (paraplegia, hemiplegia, quadriplegia).

H. Respiratory problems.

I. Neuromotor/locomotor
1. Muscle dystrophy, weakness.
2. Multiple sclerosis.
3. Myasthenia gravis.
4. Parkinsonism.
5. Joint symptoms (including temporomandibular).

J. Chronic disease limitations
1. Cardiovascular.
2. Blood diseases.
3. Diabetes.
4. Arthritis.
5. Malignancies.

III. Pretreatment Planning

A large majority of patients with disabilities can be treated in the private dental office setting. Only a relatively few need hospitalization because of marked difficulties in management or because of a systemic condition that would require special medical supervision.

A. Preliminary Information

Information about the younger and/or dependent, mentally retarded, or elderly senile patient is obtained from a parent, relative, advocate, or other person responsible. The essential information can be obtained in advance by telephone or interview.

Medical and other record forms can be mailed to the home for completion. Advance information permits the dental team to be prepared for the patient so that valuable appointment time is not wasted and complete attention can be devoted to the patient's needs.

B. Records and Forms

1. *Medical History.* In addition to the usual topics covered by questions (page 83), information relative to the disabling condition is needed. At least the following should be included:
   a. Specific disabling condition. When diagnosed, history of treatments, hospitalizations, current medications and other therapy, names and addresses of specialists involved.
   b. Record of institutionalization.
   c. History of communicable diseases; most recent blood tests; immunizations.
   d. Seizures. History, frequency, treatment.
   e. Muscular coordination. Mobility, dexterity.
   f. Communication. Speech, vision, hearing.
   g. Mental capacities. Schooling, special classes.
   h. Degree of independence. Self-care, ability to dress and feed self, perform own oral care with brush, floss, other aids.
   i. Dietary restrictions.

2. *Dental History*
   a. Previous dental experiences. Patient's attitude, ability to cooperate.
   b. Difficulties in obtaining appointments in other locations.
   c. Most recent care. Scaling, restorations, extractions, other.
   d. Oral infections and oral habits.
   e. Fluoride history. Fluoridation, dietary supplements, self- or professionally applied topical methods, including years, ages, and frequency.
   f. Current home care methods. Aids and special devices, frequency, degree of self-care.
   g. Patient/parent. Concepts of perceived needs, attitudes and apparent emphasis on dental care.

3. *Consent Forms.* Consent forms for minor, dependent, and/or incompetent patient must be signed by parent or legal guardian.

C. Consultations with Physicians and Other Specialists

Medical aspects of the patient's care are integrated into treatment planning for oral care. The physician can supply information the dentist can apply in the selection of antibiotic, sedative, or other necessary pharmaceutical agents. Additional pertinent information may be obtained from other medical specialists and the social worker.

D. Discussion with Parent or Other Direct Care Person

1. Determine familial interrelationships. Many parents devote their lives to the care of their child who is handicapped. Dental personnel must make every effort to learn from the parents or other direct-care providers the capabilities of the patient and the methods most effective for gaining cooperation. The names, ages, and interrelationships of other family members can prove helpful.

   Families may overindulge the special child. Sweets may be used as rewards or bribes to pacify. Poor behavior may be condoned.

2. Describe to the parent the cooperation and assistance needed. Special help may be needed during the appointment and for supervision of oral care on a daily basis in the total preventive care program.

3. Solicit parental help in preparing the patient for the appointments. Ask that procedures and facilities be described in advance in a pleasant and positive manner to reassure the patient.

4. Invite the patient to the office or clinic before the appointment to see the facility and become familiar with the surroundings and staff.

5. List special aids the patient must bring to the appointment, such as a transfer board for transfer into the dental chair, hearing aid, dental prostheses, and bacterial plaque control devices currently in use.

E. Appointment Scheduling

1. *Determine Special Requirements.* Determine whether special requirements of the patient's daily schedule influence time selection.[3] The cooperation of the patient may be decreased if basic routines are disturbed. Some examples follow:
   a. Appointment for the diabetic patient must not interfere with medication, meal, or between-meal eating schedules.
   b. Elderly person who rises early may feel better during a morning appointment.
   c. Arthritic patient may have greater mobility late in the morning or in the afternoon.
   d. Child's nap schedule should be respected.
   e. Early morning appointment may be difficult for a patient who requires a long time for morning preparation, such as a patient with a spinal cord injury or colostomy.

2. *Effect of Transportation Requirements*
   a. A family member who accompanies the patient should not be expected to lose a day's work if the dental appointment can be accommodated otherwise. Families may have limited financial resources because of expenses related to treatment of the person with the disability.
   b. Wheelchair patient may need to reserve a public wheelchair transport vehicle and, thus, may be limited by the schedule.

3. *Time of Appointment*
   a. Arrangement at a time when the patient will not have to wait a long time after arrival. If daily appointments tend to run increasingly off schedule by late morning or afternoon, the patient with a disability should be scheduled for the appointment at the start of the day or for the first appointment in the afternoon.
   b. Schedule a difficult patient when the clinician is at optimum energy or patience.
   c. Allow sufficient time so that the patient does not feel rushed; many persons with disabilities cannot hurry.

4. *Follow-up*
   The frequency of maintenance appointments must be individualized. The time depends on the patient's oral problems and general disabilities. Frequent appointments are encouraged for the following reasons:
   a. To decrease length of single appointment by keeping the oral tissues at an optimum level of health.
   b. To assist the patient whose handicap limits the ability to perform personal oral hygiene techniques.
   c. To provide motivation through monitoring of plaque and review of procedures for the patient and the parent or other direct care person involved.

BARRIER-FREE ENVIRONMENT

A variety of factors can explain the general lack of dental and dental hygiene care of the elderly patient or of individuals of any age who are disabled. One of the more significant reasons is the existence of physical barriers confronting patients who may attempt to keep appointments. Fear of not being able to cope with architectural barriers, fear of falling, or fear of attracting attention in an embarrassing way all can be hindrances to seeking oral care.

In general, a facility that is barrier-free for a patient in a wheelchair will be accessible to all other individuals. The patient in a wheelchair requires more space for turning and positioning than does a patient with crutches or a walker, or than a patient accompanied by another person walking at the side to guide or provide support.

In addition to space requirements, special features are needed for other specific disabilities. For example, braille floor indicators can be installed beside the numbers on elevators. For people with limited vision, doorways, steps, and stairways can be outlined with bright colors that contrast with the background.

Guidelines and specifications for a barrier-free environment are available. The descriptions below represent general features based on governmental regulations for accessibility standards, along with suggested applications for a dental clinic or office.[4,5,6]

I. External Features

A. Parking

A reserved area, clearly marked, should be close to the building entrance and 13 feet wide (8-foot car space with 5-foot access aisle)[5] to permit a person with a handicap to open car doors for exiting and reboarding.

B. Walkways

A 3-foot-wide walkway is needed for wheelchair accommodation. The surface must be solid and nonslip without irregularities. Curb ramps (cuts) from the street and from the parking area are necessary.

C. Entrance

At least one entrance to the building should be on ground level or be accessible by a gently sloping ramp (rise of 1 inch for every 12 inches). An easily grasped handrail (height 30 to 34 inches) is needed on at least one side, and preferably both sides, to accommodate left- and right-handed cane and one-crutch users.

D. Door

The light-weight door with a lever type of handle must open at least 32 inches for a wheelchair and a person using a tall crutch (figure 50–1).

II. Internal Features

Official regulations specify dimensions for accessibility of all aspects, including passageways, floors, drinking fountains, and restrooms. A few will be described.

A. Passageways

The passageways should be at least 3 feet wide with handrails along the sides. They should be free from obstructions, such as hanging signs with which a tall blind person could collide.

B. Floors

Level floors with nonslip surfaces are important. Thick or small unattached movable rugs or carpets present obstacles for wheelchairs or walkers and hazards for a patient with crutches, cane, or leg brace.

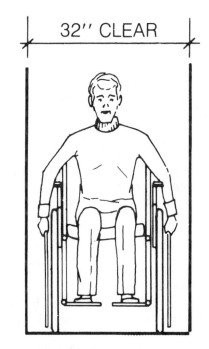

Figure 50–1. Wheelchair Accessibility. Wheelchairs designed for adults vary in width from 2 feet 3 inches to 2 feet 8 inches. A clear door width of 32 inches to accommodate these wheelchairs has been accepted as the official regulation. (From United States General Services Administration, Department of the Defense, Department of Housing and Urban Development, and Postal Service: Uniform Federal Accessibility Standards, *Federal Register*, 49, 31528, August 7, 1984.)

C. Reception Area

At least part of the furniture should permit easy access during seating and rising. Preferred are chairs with 18-inch-high, flat, firm seats and arms for support when pushing oneself up by the arms. Chairs must not slide or tip as the person rises.

III. The Treatment Room

In a group of several treatment rooms in which a limited number of patients in wheelchairs are served, only one room needs to be made accessible. Dental personnel should be versatile in exchanging rooms to serve special patients.

A. Dimensions

Space is needed for both the dental chair and related dental equipment, as well as for the wheelchair. The doorway must be at least 32 inches wide. The wheelchair is placed beside and parallel to the dental chair for patient transfer. In a small facility, the dental chair can be rotated to give room for turning the wheelchair.[6]

When planning or redesigning for wheelchair accessibility, the dental chair selected should be able to be lowered to 19 inches from the floor, and be accessible from both sides for wheelchair transfer. An x-ray machine in the same treatment room can simplify the problems of moving the patient into a separate radiography room.

B. Wheelchair Used During Treatment

The wheelchair of a patient who is unable to transfer easily, if at all, is positioned for direct utilization.

1. *Portable Headrest.*[7] A portable headrest may be attached to the wheelchair handles.
2. *Position of Dental Chair.* The dental chair can be swiveled to permit the wheelchair to be backed up to place the patient's head in a usual operating position. The dental light can then be directed into the patient's oral cavity and adjusted for access to the equipment.
3. *Wheelchair Lift.* An automatic wheelchair lift that tilts the chair back to a usual working position can be obtained for a clinical facility where wheelchair patients are treated frequently.[7]

IV. Patient Instruction

When a teaching area is planned for patient instruction, attention must be given to assure accessibility for a patient in a wheelchair. The same facility can be used by a seated nondisabled patient.

A. Dimensions

The usual 32-inch doorway and turnabout space for a wheelchair would be indicated. The tabletop and washbasin built at a height of 32 to 34 inches permit clearance underneath for knees and wheelchair arms (figure 50–2). The same regulations are used for a lavatory sink.

B. Wash Basin

Lever- or blade-type handles on faucets are usable by patients who cannot grip round handles or who have no hands. Hot pipes under the sink must be covered or insulated, because patients who have no sensation in their legs could be burned. The hot water temperature should be regulated, if possible.

C. Mirror

Mirrors and dispensers are positioned low. A tilt mirror could provide better viewing of the teeth during instruction. A tilt mirror with a hinge has more adaptability for tall and short patients and for patients with bifocal eyeglasses.

An unattached hand mirror, preferably on a pedestal that tilts, is a necessary supplement to the wall mirror. A magnifying mirror can provide an excellent aid for viewing the disclosed plaque and the devices for plaque removal.

PATIENT RECEPTION: THE INITIAL APPOINTMENT

The orientation of a patient with a disability paves the way for long-term dental and dental hygiene supervision and care. When a patient is passive, follows instructions, and possibly has received sedative medication, the situation is different from that of a patient who is apprehensive and fearful, perhaps be-

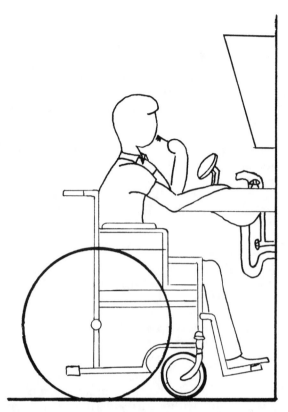

Figure 50–2. Plaque Control Facility. The tabletop and washbasin in a patient instruction area or lavatory should be built at a height of 32 to 34 inches to provide clearance underneath for knees of the patient and arms of the wheelchair. Hot pipes under a sink must be covered or insulated because patients with no sensation could be burned.

cause of past medical and dental experiences. Other patients have difficulties of communication or have limitations of body movement and control. The problems of management and care become greatly intensified for such patients.

I. Orientation

The first appointment includes and, when necessary, is devoted entirely to a basic orientation to the facilities, the dental chair, and the personnel. The examination of the oral cavity is started, and depending on the degree of patient cooperation, various steps in the examination may be completed. Preventive personal care procedures to alleviate gingival inflammation are initiated, and participation of the direct-care person is solicited.

Several orientation visits may be necessary because hurrying or forcing a patient may cause more severe problems. In a long-term care facility where patients live on the premises, daily short visits to the clinic may be possible to condition or desensitize a patient.

II. Communication

Each patient is different, and members of the dental team must watch, listen, and learn procedures that will develop the patient's trust. Parents and others who work with and care for the patient can explain how best to communicate. The parent will help to interpret the changing moods of the patient.

Even for the patient who cannot or will not speak and may appear withdrawn, the ability to understand what is being said should not be underestimated.

Nonverbal communication using facial expression, pointing, body language, and demonstration helps certain patients to respond. Other patients write messages on a pad of paper or use sign language, a language board, or other devices the dental personnel can learn. Suggested procedures for the hearing-impaired patient are described on page 680.

III. Preventive Care Introduction

Whether or not the examination and treatment plan are completed at the initial visit, the personal oral daily care program should be introduced. After finding out what the current daily care has been, instruction for the parent or other direct-care provider is presented along with that for the patient.

The first step in treatment is the elimination of gingival infection. This goal can be accomplished primarily by daily plaque removal. When dental caries is present, or in keeping with routine practice policy, a food diary form is explained in preparation for daily recording at home. The completed form can be brought in or mailed in so that it can be ready for review at the next appointment.

The complete instruction and prevention program is described on pages 620–628.

WHEELCHAIR TRANSFERS[8,9]

Three basic transfer techniques will be described here. The size, weight, and mobility of the patient, along with any special physical conditions, influence the choice. The patient may prefer to transfer from the left or the right side of the dental chair depending on which side of the body is stronger.

When the patient is in a total support wheelchair, transfer to the dental chair may not be advisable. Dental and dental hygiene care may be hampered, however, unless a portable headrest and possibly a wheelchair lift, as described on page 614, are available.

I. Preparation for Wheelchair Transfer

A. Clear the Area

Before starting a transfer, clear the area by moving the operating stool, bracket tray, portable unit, and dental light. After the transfer, release the wheelchair brake to move it aside. In a small treatment room, the wheelchair may be folded and set aside.

B. Special Needs of Patient[6]

1. *Chair Padding.* Special padding is usually used in a wheelchair as a protection from pressure sores. Depending on the length of the appointment, the patient will decide whether the padding should be moved to the dental chair. Pressure sores are described on page 657.

2. *Bags and Catheters.* Patients who do not have control of urine discharge, such as those with paraplegia or quadriplegia, will have a bag with tubing for collection. The bag may be attached to the leg of the patient or to the wheelchair. After transfer, the tubing must be checked to be sure it is not bent or twisted.

3. *Spasms.* Ask the patient about susceptibility to spasms, and what procedures to follow for prevention.

4. *Advice Concerning Transfer.* Ask the patient, family member, or attendant how best the clinician can help during the transfer. The patient must be allowed to do as much as possible.

II. Mobile Patient Transfer

When a patient can support his or her own weight, the "stand and pivot" technique can be used.

A. Position the Wheelchair

Face the wheelchair in the same direction as the dental chair at approximately an angle of 30 degrees; set brakes; remove footrests. The patient will adjust a power-driven chair and set the brakes before turning it off.

B. Prepare Dental Chair

1. Adjust dental chair to same height as or lower than the wheelchair.
2. Clear path for transfer by moving the dental chair arm and removing the arm of the wheelchair.

C. Approach to Patient

1. Face the patient and place feet outside the patient's feet for pivoting. Clinician's knees should be close to or against the patient's knees to prevent buckling.
2. Place hands under the patient's arms and grasp the waist belt in back. Patient places arms around clinician's neck or places hands on wheelchair arms to push up. Clinician lifts patient to standing position.

D. Pivot to Dental Chair

1. Pivot together slowly until the patient is backed up to the side of the dental chair with the backs of the legs touching. The patient is gently lowered to sitting position. Reposition the arm of dental chair.
2. Grasp patient's legs together between the ankles and knees, and lift them onto the dental chair.

E. Repeat in Reverse

After the appointment, the patient is returned to the wheelchair in the reverse order of procedure.

III. Immobile Patient Transfer

When the patient is unable to support his or her own weight, two aides are required. The parent, advocate, or other attendant may serve as the second person.

A. Position the Wheelchair
1. Position wheelchair in the same direction as and parallel with the dental chair; set brakes, remove footrests.
2. Adjust the dental chair to the same height as or lower than the seat of the wheelchair.
3. Move arm of dental chair out of transfer area and remove arm of wheelchair.

B. First Aide
Aide I is positioned behind the wheelchair. Place feet, one on either side of the rear wheel nearest the dental chair; place hands under the patient's arms below the elbows, pressing forearms against the patient's lower thorax area.

C. Second Aide
Aide II may do either of the following, depending on the size and weight of the patient:
1. Face patient and grasp hands under the patient's knees.
2. Face dental chair and place one arm under the thighs and the other under the calves of the lower legs.

D. Transfer
On a prearranged signal, with a steady motion, the patient is lifted and gently transferred to the dental chair.

E. Repeat in Reverse
After the appointment, the patient is returned to the wheelchair in the reverse order of procedure.

IV. Sliding Board Transfer

A patient may bring a sliding board or one may be kept in the office or clinic. Two persons will be needed when the patient is heavy or less mobile.[6]

A. Position the Wheelchair
1. Position the wheelchair in the same direction as and parallel with the dental chair; set the brakes; remove the footrests if they will be in the way of the sliding board.
2. Adjust the seat of the dental chair to slightly lower than the wheelchair seat.
3. Move the arm of the dental chair out of transfer area and remove the arm of the wheelchair.

B. Adjust the Sliding Board
Patient or clinician places the sliding board well under the hip of the patient. The board is extended across the dental chair.

C. Transfer
1. Patient slides by shifting weight, balancing on hands, and walking the buttocks across the board. The clinician who faces the patient can

assist or even do the transfer by holding the patient under the axillae.
2. Board is removed and replaced after the appointment.

D. Repeat in Reverse
Dental chair is positioned slightly higher than the wheelchair seat for the return transfer.

V. Walking Frame, Crutches, Cane

The clinician asks the patient for instructions in how to assist.

A. Walking Frame to the Dental Chair
1. Adjust dental chair upright with arm out of the way and seat to level of back of patient's knees.
2. Patient backs up to dental chair until back of legs touch, then lowers into the chair. Clinician stabilizes the walking frame.
3. Clinician takes patient by the ankles to lift legs and turn patient onto the dental chair.
4. Remove walker to a place out of the way of dental personnel.

B. Walking Frame from the Dental Chair
1. Raise dental chair to upright and ask patient to wait while the walker is positioned. Allow ample time for patient to adjust to upright position to prevent effects of postural hypotension.
2. Move arm of dental chair; position chair to approximate height of patient's knees.
3. Grasp ankles, gently turn patient, and swing legs down.
4. Reposition walker.
5. Patient uses one hand to push up and other to grasp walker. When walker is used for balance, one hand must be in the middle to prevent tipping.
6. If patient wants assistance when rising, clinician can hook an arm under the patient's arm on left side if patient is right-handed. The patient's right hand is used to grasp the walker.

C. Crutches
1. Dental chair is positioned upright at a level with patient's knees. Some patients need the chair higher so seating does not require knees to be bent.
2. Clinician assists, as directed by patient, while patient lowers into the chair; the legs are lifted onto the dental chair.
3. After the appointment, with patient seated on the side of the dental chair, pass the crutches together to one hand. The patient usually will use the other hand to push up. If assistance in rising is requested, the clinician can hook an arm under the patient's arm as directed.

D. Cane
1. Dental chair is positioned at the level of the patient's knees or higher if the patient may have difficulty in bending the knees.

2. Patient may need assistance in lifting the legs onto the dental chair.

3. After the appointment, when the patient is seated on the side of the dental chair, the clinician passes the cane to the patient and assists patient to rise only as directed.

PATIENT POSITION AND STABILIZATION

The objectives in patient positioning and stabilization are to let the patient feel comfortable and secure while the professional person performs in a position that provides adequate illumination, visibility, and accessibility. A hyperactive patient or a patient with involuntary muscle movements can wear a special stabilizing device to enable the clinician to work and to prevent damage to the oral tissues by accidental movement of instruments.

I. Chair Position

A. Tip Chair Back Slowly

Immediately after a patient with cerebral palsy or other condition that involves a lack of muscle control is in the dental chair, start to tip the chair back to provide balance so that the patient cannot fall. While tipping back the chair, place one hand on the patient's shoulder to offer assurance and support. Never place the chair back quickly. Advance in steps to allow the patient to adjust.

B. Chair Up

A patient with a respiratory complication must have the chair back up. A patient with a cardiac disease or a patient wearing a pacemaker should be asked "How many pillows do you use at night?" The chair can be adjusted accordingly.

II. Body Adjustments

During the appointment, patients with a spinal cord injury must do a "push up" and patients with quadriplegia must shift their weight every 20 minutes for 10 to 15 seconds. By doing so, the patient can maintain good circulation and healthy tissue of the buttocks where there is no sensation. The procedure is a preventive measure for decubitus ulcers and should be a consideration during long dental procedures.

III. Body Stabilization

A restraint can be used to limit body movement and provide support for paralyzed limbs. When a restraint of any type is to be used, it should be explained to the patient. The patient must understand that the devices are used to help the dentist and to make the patient more comfortable, and are by no means a form of punishment.

A. Body Enclosure Restraints

Although a small patient may be held by a parent, such positioning can be tiring and insecure. Better cooperation is usually obtained by the use of positive restraints, such as commercial wraps, which are available, or improvised wraps.

1. *Pediwrap.* The *Pediwrap* is made of nylon mesh and encloses the patient from neck to ankles. It is available in 3 sizes to fit infants and children through 10 years of age.[10] It is frequently used with support straps about the patient's legs and arms.

2. *Papoose Board.* A *Papoose board* is a board with padded wraps to enclose a patient (figure 50–3). It is available in three sizes from a small child size to an adult size.[11]

3. *Bedsheet or Blanket.* The parent can bring from home a blanket or sheet that is familiar to the patient. The sheet or blanket is folded firmly around the patient twice and held securely by a Velcro strap around the body. Support straps about the legs and body provide the patient with additional control.

B. Support Straps

Adhesive tape (2 or 3 inches wide), canvas, or Velcro straps may be used with or without a body enclosure restraint. A soft restraint may be made from a soft material, such as flannel, with a padded section to place over the wrists, ankles, or where needed. Ties 4 to 6 inches wide may be

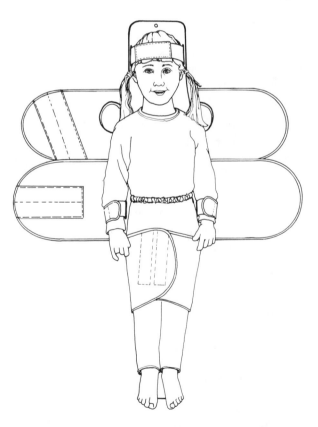

Figure 50–3. Papoose Board. Stabilization is accomplished by three body wraps and a head restrainer. The arms are secured at the wrists, as shown, before the large center wrap is closed. (From King, E.M., Wieck, L., and Dyer, M.: *Illustrated Manual of Nursing Techniques.* Philadelphia, J.B. Lippincott Co., 1977, page 311.)

passed around the dental chair or may be tied to the arms of the chair.

C. Hand Restraint or Support Mitt

A thumbless mitt made from unbleached cotton can have long ties attached at the wrist line. The ties are first tied at the wrist and then looped around the arm of the dental chair and secured.[12]

D. Head Stabilization

1. *Arm of Clinician.* From a working position at 12:00 (top of patient's head), the nondominant arm is placed around the patient's head to hold it in position.
2. *Mouth Prop* (page 631).

CLINIC PROCEDURES FOR EVALUATION OF PATIENT

As many as possible of the procedures for evaluation are accomplished at the first appointment. The goals should be the same for all patients, namely, to prepare the evaluation material to be reviewed and analyzed by the dentist for treatment planning.

The patient may not be able to complete all the steps in the evaluation, and extra time must be spent on orientation. Each clinic procedure is prefaced by an explanation and demonstration. Several trials may be needed.

I. Patient Histories

Certain patients require prophylactic antibiotics prior to instrumentation (pages 85 and 91). Suggestions for preparing the medical history are on page 611.

II. Vital Signs: Blood Pressure Determination

For the patient who will be examined in a body enclosure restraint, blood pressure determination must be accomplished early in the appointment, before application of the restraint.

III. Extraoral and Intraoral Examination

When a mouth prop is needed to perform intraoral procedures, the intraoral pathologic examination can be made in conjunction with the gingival and dental examinations. The mouth prop is placed first on one side and then on the other.

IV. Photographs

Depending on the treatment, photographs may be requested by the dentist. A patient requiring orthodontic therapy, maxillofacial surgery, or other special treatment may need to be photographed.

V. Radiographic Survey

A. *Periapical Survey*

Because the most diagnostic information can be gained from periapical and bitewing surveys, the attempt should be made to obtain as many of the essential exposures as possible.

1. Use a mouth prop, film holder, and much patience. When help is needed, the parent or other attendant can assist.
2. Patient and attendant wear lead aprons; person holding film in mouth can wear a lead glove. Dental personnel never hold film for a patient.

B. *Extraoral, Occlusal, Panoramic*

The overall views provided by occlusal or extraoral surveys can aid in locating anomalies, retained root tips, impactions, and other abnormalities, but such surveys are not substitutes for the detail provided by periapical radiographs. For example, a periapical film is needed to identify root fracture and apical disorders that may be present in the patient with cerebral palsy who bruxes heavily and may traumatize anterior teeth.

VI. Study Casts[13]

Study casts are needed for orthodontic, prosthetic, and phases of restorative therapy or for documentation and recording purposes. With adequate patient preparation and orientation, cooperation can be obtained. Suggestions for technique are listed here.

A. Use a comfortable tray and bead with a soft wax (page 154). A flexible tray may prove easier to insert.
B. Practice the insertion and removal several times to prepare the patient. Practicing tray insertion may be started at one appointment and the actual impression made at another.
C. Apply a topical anesthetic to the intraoral tissues when the patient has a gag reflex.
D. Use fast-setting alginate and warm water.

VII. Gingival Examination

Despite difficulties, a thorough evaluation must be made. Procedures for examination were described on pages 191–210. Clinical aspects, including the degree of inflammation, pockets, mucogingival involvement, frenal attachments, and tooth mobility, are detected and recorded. Information from the radiographs is used to confirm the presence and degree of periodontal destruction.

Evaluation of the amount, extent, and location of calculus is needed so that an appropriate estimate of scaling requirements may be made for the dental hygiene treatment plan. Overall oral cleanliness and the presence of plaque and materia alba provide a prevue to plaque control instruction needs.

VIII. Dental Examination

A. Number, size, color, and occlusion of the teeth.
B. Dental caries.
C. Supernumerary teeth, malformations, and other irregularities that frequently are associated with certain developmental disabilities.

ORAL MANIFESTATIONS

Oral diseases of disabled individuals are not different in kind from those of nondisabled persons. The two principal diseases found are dental caries and periodontal infections. Other oral findings described later include congenital malformations, oral injuries, and malocclusions. In the chapters devoted to describing specific individuals with disabilities, oral characteristics of each are included.

For a majority of patients with disabilities, dental and dental hygiene treatment is not different once the patient is in the dental chair, sedated if needed, and stabilized physically. For a few other patients, an oral manifestation can be caused by, or be a result of, the patient's disabling condition or the treatment for it. Examples are included here.

I. Congenital Malformations

A. Cleft Lip or Palate (page 582)

B. Other Craniofacial Anomalies

C. Tooth Defects

An increased incidence of malformations has been observed with developmental disabilities, for example,

1. Variations in number and structure of teeth.
2. Dentinogenesis imperfecta, amelogenesis imperfecta, enamel hyperplasia, and other abnormalities of tooth structure.

II. Oral Injuries

A. Attrition

Attrition caused by bruxism is particularly common among individuals with cerebral palsy and mental retardation.

B. Trauma to Teeth and Soft Tissues

Trauma to teeth and soft tissues may result from accidents (instability, falling), self-abuse, or seizures. The individual with epilepsy is particularly susceptible to accidents. Chipped and fractured teeth, as well as residual scars in the tongue and lips, may be seen frequently.

Because of personal limitations and living a protected life, many patients with disabilities are not exposed to contact sports, traffic accidents, and other accident-prone situations. The incidence of facial trauma may be expected to be less.

III. Facial Weakness or Paralysis

When a patient has muscle weakness or paralysis of one side of the face, bilateral mastication is not possible. Plaque usually collects more heavily, and food debris is retained on the involved side. Certain patients may have bilateral weakness.

IV. Malocclusion

Malocclusion is frequently found among persons with developmental disabilities. Factors contributing to problems of occlusion include skeletal and muscular deformities, such oral habits as tongue thrust, macroglossia, mouth breathing, and/or congenitally missing teeth.

V. Dental Caries

Survey summaries vary, so generalizations cannot be made concerning the prevalence of dental caries in disabled persons. Studies have shown a high incidence of *untreated* dental caries, as well as many missing teeth, which may be a reflection of the type of dental care the patient has or has not received. The dentist may have been unable to cope with the problems presented by the individual with a handicap and, therefore, more extractions than restorations were performed.[14]

The more fortunate patients with fewer carious lesions and extractions may have lived in a community with fluoridated water or had the benefit of supplements, such as tablets, rinses, or professional topical fluoride applications. They may also have had knowledgeable parents who were able to control the exposures to carbohydrates in the diet.

VI. Gingival and Periodontal Diseases[15]

Gingival and periodontal diseases have been shown to have an increased incidence especially in individuals with mental retardation and those with physical conditions that prevent daily self-care. Patients with Down's syndrome have a greater incidence of severe periodontal disease with bone loss at an earlier age than that of other individuals with mental retardation (pages 650–651).

Many patients with disabilities have poor oral hygiene and heavy calculus deposits. Factors related to plaque control are described on page 621, and calculus is discussed on page 631.

VII. Therapy-related Oral Findings

A. Phenytoin-induced Gingival Overgrowth

Patients whose treatment for seizures requires phenytoin (Dilantin) are susceptible to a slight to severe gingival enlargement. The severity of the enlargement usually depends on the maintenance of healthy gingival tissue associated with adequate daily plaque control. A description of phenytoin-induced gingival overgrowth is included in Chapter 52, pages 642–644.

B. Chemotherapy

Oral ulcerations, mucositis, and susceptibility to infection are frequent manifestations following cancer chemotherapy (page 605). Patients with leukemia have a high incidence of oral manifestations, including lymphadenopathy, gingival changes with bleeding, and petechiae, that are more severe following chemotherapy.

C. Radiation Therapy

When radiation therapy of the head and neck area involves the cells of the salivary glands, xerostomia can result and contribute to an increased incidence of dental caries. The symptoms and treatment aspects of radiation therapy are described on pages 603–604.

DENTAL HYGIENE TREATMENT PLAN

Parts of the total treatment plan that are to be accomplished by the dental hygienist can be identified under preventive, educational, and therapeutic services. Choice of procedures depends on the findings of the clinical examination and includes some or all of the items listed here.

I. Preventive Therapy

A. Bacterial Plaque Control

B. Fluoride Program
1. Supervision of self-applied daily fluoride.
2. Periodic professionally applied topical fluoride.

C. Pit and Fissure Sealants

D. Use of Artificial Saliva for Xerostomia

II. Educational

A. Orientation
Patient orientation to each dental hygiene and dental procedure.

B. Counseling
Parental counseling starting as early as possible after an infant is known to have a disability.

C. Instruction in Disease Control
1. Plaque control for natural teeth and appliances.
2. Daily fluoride, systemic and/or topical.
3. Dietary and nutritional effects.

III. Therapeutic

A. Patient's plaque control for therapeutic purposes until tissue health is attained.
B. Complete scaling and root planing.
C. Removal of overhanging fillings.
D. Reevaluation for additional periodontal therapy.
E. Restorative phase; finishing restorations.

DISEASE PREVENTION AND CONTROL

I. Preventive Program Components[16,17]
A. Bacterial plaque control.
B. Fluorides.
C. Pit and fissure sealants.
D. Diet counseling.
E. Regular professional examinations and treatment at intervals as recommended by the dentist and dental hygienist.

II. Functioning Levels

For a patient who does not have a mental or physical disability, neglect of personal oral hygiene usually can be explained by either a lack of knowledge and understanding about the need for plaque removal and how it is accomplished or a lack of motivation to carry out the necessary daily routines. For certain patients with disabilities, the problem of disease control becomes greatly magnified because of a lack of the necessary mental and/or physical coordination to carry out even the simplest of oral hygiene measures.

Depending on the severity of the disability, many patients need either complete or partial assistance. Assistance must be provided by parents and other family members when living at home, or by an aide or other person responsible for the patient's care in a residence or institutional setting. The dental hygienist has a twofold responsibility to teach and supervise the patient and those who care for the patient. Suggestions for in-service education are on pages 628–630.

A *high, moderate,* or *low* functioning level refers to the daily living skills (bathing, toothbrushing, dressing, for example) an individual can do alone, what range or degree of assistance is needed, or whether the person depends on others for complete care. The functioning levels have also been called *self-care, partial care,* or *total care.*[8] In another concept, the terms *supervised, supervised/assistance,* and *maintenance (by others)* have been used.[19]

A. High Functioning Level
The high functioning, self-care group includes those capable of flossing and brushing their own teeth. Many patients, particularly children and those of all ages who are mentally retarded, need varying degrees of encouragement, motivation, and supervision.

B. Moderate Functioning Level
The moderate functioning, partial-care group includes those capable of carrying out at least part of their oral hygiene needs, but who require considerable training, assistance, and direct supervision. The assistance may be verbal, gestural, or hand-over-hand.

C. Low Functioning Level
The low functioning, total-care group includes those unable to attend to their own care and are therefore dependent. Patients in this group may be bedridden and nonambulatory, although others may be confined to wheelchairs. With training, some may be able to attempt a part of their own care.

III. Preparation for Instruction

A. Basic Planning Questions
1. What is the patient's functioning level?
2. Will the patient do all or part of the plaque removal personally or require partial or total care?
3. Is the patient involved in any community dental health programs (home, school, or day activity) and can the dentist and/or dental hygienist in such a program be contacted to coordinate the instruction given?
4. Will the parent or attendant do part or all of the oral care?

5. What disabilities have the greatest influence on the extent of self-care possible and anticipated success of the overall preventive program? Mental? Physical? Sensory? Learning? Oral?

6. Which techniques and procedures will best fit the situation of the particular patient and the parent or attendant?

7. How can the patient be helped to be as independent as possible?

B. Introduction

For the answers to these questions, an initial plan is made, with the realization that the system is on a trial-and-error basis. As the skills of the patient and parent improve and less plaque is observed and recorded on succeeding appointments, adaptations can be made. In the meantime, communication improves and the patient's trust develops as the sincere concern of the dental team is realized.

For all patients, with or without a disability, the aim is complete daily plaque control. Such an ideal result may seem far from reality with a moderate- or low-functioning person, but with continuing reinforcement and inspiration, progress can be made. Patient and parental attitudes, willingness to participate, and acceptance of the recommended procedures must be taken into consideration.

BACTERIAL PLAQUE REMOVAL

I. Components

General procedures for instruction and methods for toothbrushing, interdental plaque removal, and care of fixed and removable prostheses were described in Chapters 22 through 25. Individualization for each patient's needs and abilities is necessary. Each step must be explained slowly and carefully.

A. Provide Basic Information

Plaque formation and disease development are described on a level at which the patient and parent can learn and be motivated.

B. Disclose and Show Plaque

An on-going record of the extent of plaque in graphic form by which the patient and parent can watch progress may help to motivate many patients.

C. Toothbrushing

1. Provide a soft toothbrush and ask the patient to remove the disclosed plaque from the teeth. For the completely dependent patient, the parent will demonstrate. Alternative positions for the parent are described on page 626, and in figure 50–9.

2. Plaque removal is more important than the specific technique used, as long as damage is not done to the gingiva or teeth. A scrub-brush

or circular Fones method is usually appropriate and within the capability of most patients (pages 309, 310).

3. Explain each step and demonstrate slowly.

4. Adaptations for brush handles and other devices to promote or make possible a patient's independent performance are described on pages 622–625.

5. Patients who are carriers of hepatitis or who have any known communicable disease should keep their toothbrushes and related materials apart from and use a sink separate from the other people in the same residence. The use of a powered brush is contraindicated because of aerosol formation. Nonimmune direct-care personnel should protect themselves with gloves and mask when helping with or performing plaque control for a patient with a communicable disease.

D. Dentifrice

A dentifrice containing fluoride is recommended for patients who can use a dentifrice. An ingestible dentifrice may prove useful. The factors to consider when deciding whether a standard noningestible dentifrice should be used include the following:[16]

1. When a patient cannot rinse or expectorate, a dentifrice should not be used. The person who is institutionalized and severely handicapped may be treated with a suction brush as described on page 638.

2. When a parent or other direct care person is performing the brushing the paste may limit visibility for thorough plaque removal. When a paste is used, only a small amount should be placed on the brush (pea size, figure 29–8, page 410).

3. Dentifrice may increase gag reflex for certain patients.

4. For the patient whose problem is brush manipulation, and for whom special adaptations of the brush are recommended, management of the dentifrice may be awkward and messy.

5. Dentifrice is not essential to plaque removal, and other means for daily fluoride application may prove easier for certain patients. A brush-on gel may be recommended.

E. Dental Floss

With time and repeated instruction, many patients with disabilities can learn to use dental floss, and some can learn to use other interdental aids. The use of a floss holder can make flossing possible for certain patients, such as those with limited digital dexterity or the use of only one hand.

The holder may also be useful for the parent or other person who cares for the patient. Methods for increasing the size of a toothbrush handle may be adapted for the handle of a floss holder.

II. Evaluation

Many patients, parents, and direct care personnel can learn with demonstration and practice how to examine the teeth and gingiva. The signs of healthy gingiva, especially color and absence of bleeding on brushing, can be noted.

For selected patients, the thoroughness of brushing can be improved if a disclosing agent is used at the start. The visible objective then is to remove all the color. Another system is to apply a disclosing agent after brushing to determine completion of plaque removal. Then, any additional plaque noted is brushed and removed.

When a patient brushes first, followed by the parent or direct care person, the disclosing agent might be applied by the parent so the task of removal can be completed. Because the patient is encouraged to do as much as possible and is praised for whatever successes are accomplished, the plaque disclosed for the parent to remove may be a factor of discouragement to the patient who really had done the very best to the extent of individual capability. A better plan could be for the patient to do all the brushing and flossing once a day, and for the parent to do all the brushing and flossing at a different time.

SELF-CARE AIDS

Although a parent or attendant may be willing to brush the patient's teeth, as much as possible should be carried out by the patient. Psychologic benefits to the patient result in feelings of self-esteem and accomplishment when able to manage the important and worthwhile task of brushing.

For patients of all ages whose main deterrent to personal self-care is related to grasp, manipulation, or control of a toothbrush, adaptations of the brush have been devised.[20,21,22] Modifications to accommodate specific needs include enlarged handles, hand attachments, and elongated handles.

I. General Prerequisites for a Self-care Aid

A. Cleanable.
B. Durable. Can withstand exposure to water and saliva.
C. Resistant to absorption of oral fluids.

II. Toothbrushing

A. For Patient with Fingers Permanently Fixed in a Fist

Insert the brush handle into the grasp.

B. For Patient Who Cannot Grasp and Hold

1. *Objective.* To fasten the brush handle to the open hand.
2. *Methods*
   a. Velcro strap around hand has a slit on the palm side into which the brush handle can be inserted. A vinyl pocket with an adjustable Velcro strap is commercially avail-

able. The toothbrush handle fits into the pocket (figure 50–4A). The device is used to hold other utensils for the patient, such as eating utensils.[23]
   b. Handle of fingernail brush attached to toothbrush by adhesive water-resistant tape (figure 50–4B).
   c. Wide rubber strap or a length of small-diameter rubber tubing attached through the hole in the toothbrush handle and tied adjacent to the brush head so the patient's hand can be slipped under the rubber and be held firmly (figure 50–4C).

C. For Patient with Limited Hand Closure (unable to manipulate usual toothbrush handle or floss holder)

1. *Objective.* Enlarge the diameter of the handle.
2. *Methods*
   a. Bicycle handle grip: Insert toothbrush handle (figure 50–5A).
   b. Soft rubber ball or a styrofoam ball. Push brush handle in (figure 50–5B). Styrofoam

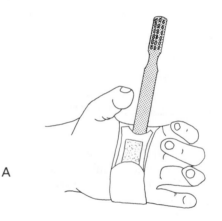

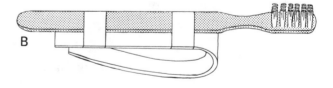

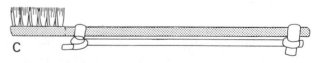

Figure 50–4. Aids for Patient Who Cannot Grasp and Hold. A. Adjustable Velcro strap around hand has a pocket designed to hold the toothbrush handle. **B.** Handle of a fingernail brush attached to toothbrush by adhesive tape. **C.** Rubber tubing attached firmly to toothbrush handle enables patient to hold brush across the palm of the hand. A floss holder also may be held by these methods.

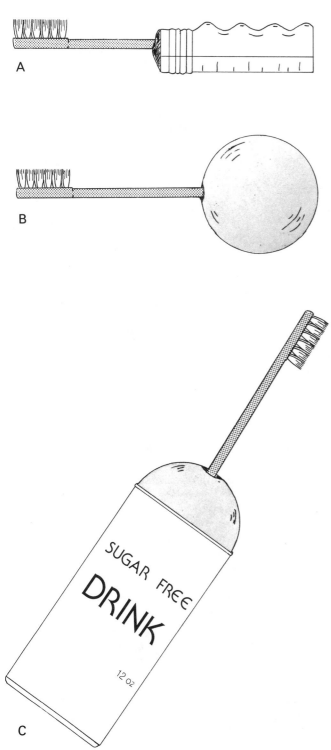

Figure 50–5. Aids for Patient With Limited Grasp. A. Toothbrush inserted into a bicycle handle grip. **B.** Toothbrush inserted into a soft rubber ball. **C.** Toothbrush in soft rubber ball inserted into a juice or soda pop can provide a wide-diametered handle for patients with limited hand closure.

balls are available in various sizes from craft shops.

  c. Juice or soda pop can. Place the rubber ball with toothbrush inside the can (figure 50–5C).

  d. Foam rubber hair roller. Insert brush handle.

  e. Quick-cure acrylic. Obtain an impression of the hand grasp by having the patient grasp a cylinder of base plate wax. Then, fill the wax cylinder with quick-cure acrylic. Insert the toothbrush handle before the acrylic sets. The angle may be adjusted to set the brush head for the patient's convenient use. Polish the acrylic.

D. For Patient Unable to Lift Hand or Arm (with limited shoulder or elbow movement)

  1. *Objective.* Lengthen the handle of the brush.

  2. *Prerequisite.* The material must be strong or rigid enough to maintain the brush contact with sufficient lateral pressure to remove plaque from the tooth surfaces.

  3. *Methods*

    a. Cylinder of wood with brush handle cemented inside.[20]

    b. Two brushes. Cut the head from an old used brush and fasten the handle to the end of the new brush handle (glue, tape, heat).

    c. Tongue depressors taped to the brush handle, then one or two other tongue depressors taped to overlap and provide an extension.

    d. Commercially available stiff metal extender with bolt attachment and wing nut to attach through a hole in the toothbrush. Brush may be used full length or cut off.[23]

    e. Bicycle spoke, coat hanger, or other means for elongation fixed with a handle of acrylic resin. The metal tip may be heated and pushed into the toothbrush handle.[24,25] Use double or triple thickness to avoid flexibility.

E. For Patient Who Can Hold and Position the Toothbrush But Cannot Manipulate To Make Strokes for Plaque Removal

  Guide patient to learn to move the head up and down or from side to side while brush is held against the teeth.[25]

F. Use of a Powered Toothbrush

  A powered brush can serve as a motivational adjunct for selected patients (page 310). For an uncoordinated patient, a powered brush could be harmful. The various models present different characteristics.

  1. *Advantages and Disadvantages*[26]

    a. The extra weight of the handle may prove advantageous for some patients, but disadvantageous for others with limited arm strength.

b. The on/off mechanism may require more strength and finger coordination to operate than certain patients can manage.

c. The brush handle is thick and therefore helpful for a patient with grasping problems.

d. The vibration created during use cannot be tolerated by certain patients.

2. *Suggestions for Use*

a. For use without hands, attach the brush handle by means of a clamp in a stationary upright position lower than the patient's mouth when bending down. Patient can insert the brush and apply to the teeth, moving the head for application to all surfaces. The use of a dentifrice probably would be contraindicated because splashing might be uncontrollable.

b. A Velcro cuff around the hand and the brush can aid in brush control.

3. *Institutional Use.* Although not possible for most institutionalized patients to use for themselves, powered brushes have been found effective by direct-care staffs in certain situations. One handle for 10 or 12 clients has been used. Handles must be replaced promptly when out of order, which may present problems in some institutions.

Cross-contamination is a problem even when individual tips are labeled, washed, and kept apart. Handles must be sanitized and covered for each brushing. Special instruction for the direct care people is necessary, and repeated motivation for any toothbrushing program is important. Using a powered brush is not encouraged by many dental hygienists associated with long-term care institutions.

III. Use of Floss Holder

A. Types

Several types of plastic floss holders are available (figure 50–6).

B. Use

Careful instruction should be provided and supervision given periodically to prevent tissue damage. As threaded into a holder, the floss is in a straight line (figure 50–7A).

To avoid cutting the papilla when applied interproximally:

1. Use a rest or fulcrum to prevent snapping through the contact.

2. Pull the floss mesially (to clean the distal of a tooth) or push distally (to clean mesial surface) to allow floss to be positioned on the side of the papilla (figure 50–7).

IV. Cleaning Removable Dental Appliances[20,27]

The details for cleaning removable appliances were described on pages 346–349. The same mate-

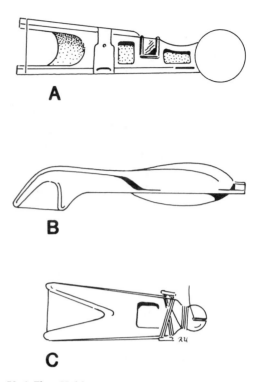

Figure 50–6. Floss Holders. A variety of floss holders are available, including **A.** a holder with a replaceable floss container, **B.** a holder with a replaceable floss cartridge and a thin edge for cleaning the tongue, and **C.** a holder with a threading mechanism for a 24-inch length of floss applied at each use. A fourth type, shown in figure 50–7, is operated in a manner similar to that shown in **C.**

rials and procedures are recommended for the patient with a handicap or for another person who will care for the appliance.

Management of both the appliance and the brush requires attention and skill, and instruction in methods that prevent accidents is necessary. In all procedures, the sink must be partially filled with water and/or a face cloth or small towel should be placed in the sink to serve as a cushion should the denture be dropped.

A. Grasp Problem

For the patient with difficulty grasping or holding the brush, a denture brush handle may be adapted by any of the methods described for the regular toothbrush (figure 50–5). A fingernail brush may be used instead of a standard denture brush, provided all denture surfaces can be reached for plaque removal.

B. One Hand

For the patient handicapped by hemiplegia or for the patient with use of two hands but who needs to grasp the denture with two hands to prevent accidents, the following are recommended:

1. Denture brush with suction cups to attach low inside the sink bowl (figure 50–8B).

2. Fingernail brush with suction cups.

3. Denture brush in mounting that has suction

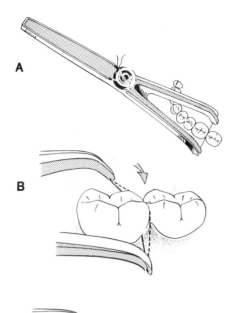

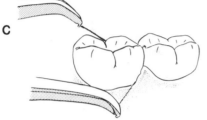

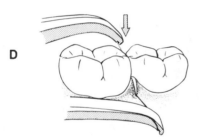

Figure 50–7. Use of a Floss Holder. A. The floss is held over the proximal contact for insertion. A hand rest should be applied on the chin to prevent excess pressure. **B.** As the floss is lowered gently and drawn through the contact area, the holder should be pulled mesially when the floss is applied to the distal surface and pushed distally when the floss is applied to the mesial surface. **C.** Floss is lowered slightly below the gingival margin. **D.** Floss cut in the papilla when used incorrectly.

cups. These are available commercially (figure 50–8A).[23]

INSTRUCTION FOR DIRECT CARE PERSON

Individuals who need partial or total care present with varying degrees of ability to cooperate, depending on the nature of the handicap. The size of the patient and whether the patient is ambulatory, bedridden, or in a wheelchair are among the factors that influence the technique for management.

The instruction for the parents or the other direct

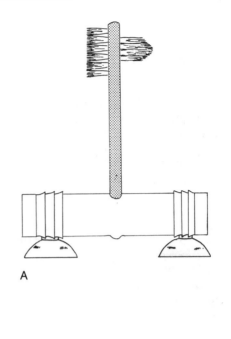

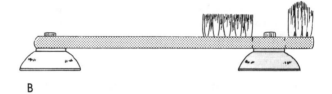

Figure 50–8. Denture Brushes with Suction Cups. A. Denture brush in a commercially available mounting. **B.** Suction cups attached directly to a denture brush. Either brush may be positioned in a sink to aid the person who has one hand or who needs to grasp the denture with two hands to prevent accidental dropping and breakage.

care persons should be given where the specific techniques can actually be demonstrated as they will be done at home. When the patient lies down with the head in the parent's lap, for example, a suitable couch should be used, or chairs can be placed together. Time and repeated practice sessions are needed for successful plaque removal for a difficult patient.

I. Self-care and Attitude

Whenever possible, instruction for the parents, other family members, or direct care persons begins with their own personal oral care. The most success comes when those who care for the patient have knowledge and understanding of the purposes and techniques and can demonstrate their own bacterial plaque removal.

An appreciation for the need for preventive care and for why the health of the teeth and gingiva are of great importance to the well-being and overall health of the patient can help those responsible to develop the patience and take the necessary time from their own busy schedules.

II. General Suggestions

A. Place

The plaque removal procedures must be performed where both the patient and the parent can be comfortable and relaxed. A small bathroom may be the least desirable place because positioning the patient may be awkward except when a standing position can be used.

Good light, easy visibility of the teeth, and control of the head of the person with the disability are prerequisites.

B. Teaching Techniques for Plaque Removal

1. *Use of Finger and Hand Rests.* The person performing the plaque removal must learn how to balance the toothbrush, dental floss, floss aid, or any other implement with a finger or hand rest on the side of the patient's face or chin. Such contact contributes to total patient control and to effective use of the plaque removal device.
2. *Use of a Mouth Prop.* For certain patients, plaque removal is impossible without a mouth prop, and demonstration for insertion on both sides is needed. For home use, a washable, rubber prop is practical.

III. Positions

General positions that involve one or two people are suggested here.[16] When the patient is young, hyperactive, unable to cooperate, and the assistance of a second person is not available, the use of a blanket or sheet wrap may be necessary (page 617).

In the following description, the term "parent" is used to mean the family member or other direct care person who may be performing the plaque removal.

A. Parent Standing

With the parent standing from behind, the arm is brought around the patient's head and the chin is cupped while using the thumb and index finger to retract the lips and cheeks. The other hand applies the toothbrush, floss aid, or other device. This technique requires that the patient be able to bend the head back far enough for the parent to see the maxillary teeth. The procedure may be applicable for the following:

1. Short patient standing in front of and backed up to the parent.
2. Tall patient seated in a chair with the head tipped back to lean against the parent, or seated in a large chair or sofa with the head stabilized against the top of chair back.
3. Patient in a wheelchair leaning back against the parent. Wheelchair brakes are set.

B. Parent Seated

1. Patient seated on pillow on floor in front of parent, with back close to the chair and head turned back into parent's lap (figure 50–9A). The parent may place his/her legs over the shoulders of the patient to restrain arms and body movements (figure 50–9B).
2. Parent is seated at the end of a sofa or couch, and patient is lying down with the head in parent's lap (figure 50–9C).
3. For a bedridden patient, the parent may sit at the patient's head and place the head in the lap. When body and arm movements must be controlled, the parent can sit beside the patient, lean across the patient's chest, and hold the patient's arm against the body with the elbow. The hand of the restraining arm can hold the mouth prop, retract, or whatever is necessary. If the patient is particularly difficult, a sheet or blanket wrap would be indicated.

C. Two People

In any of the positions previously mentioned, the parent may need the assistance of a second person to hold the hands and arms or otherwise restrain the patient.

A small child may be placed across the laps of two persons seated facing each other. One stabilizes the head and brushes and flosses while the other person holds hands, arms, and legs, as needed (figure 50–9D).

FLUORIDES

Selection of a multiple fluoride program for an individual patient depends on the age, the caries status, and the concentration of fluoride in the water supply. In addition, for a patient with a handicap, the abilities to cooperate, to accept the vehicle and mode of application, and to master the technique required for a self-administered preparation dictate the final recommendation. Detailed reference tables have been prepared by a special fluorides task force of the National Foundation of Dentistry for the Handicapped.[28]

I. Fluoridation

A. Community Water Fluoridation

As more communities begin to fluoridate the water supplies, more of the total population, including persons with handicaps, will benefit.

B. Institutional Water Fluoridation

Research has shown the benefits derived from fluoridation of a school water supply when the community in which the school was located could not or did not have fluoridation. These programs were summarized in Chapter 29, page 399.

Institutions where individuals with disabilities reside may have a water supply that could be fluoridated. Installation is a relatively inexpensive procedure when the health benefits and the decreased need for professional care are realized.

II. Dietary Supplements

When the community water supply is deficient in fluoride content, the fluoride level is below opti-

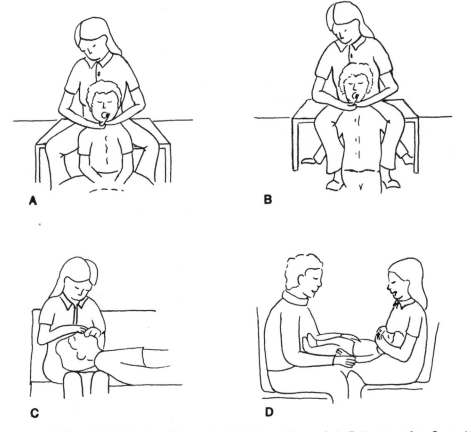

Figure 50–9. Positions for Child or Disabled Patient During Bacterial Plaque Removal. A. Patient seated on floor with head turned back into the lap of parent or direct-care person. **B.** Patient's arms restrained by legs of parent or direct-care person. **C.** Patient reclining on couch with head in lap of parent or direct-care person. **D.** Two people participating with small child between. One holds patient for stabilization while other holds the head for toothbrushing and flossing.

mum, or the water intake by a child is low, a supplement is recommended, as described on pages 400–401. Depending on the masticatory function of the child, whether chewing or rinsing is possible, the fluoride can be prescribed in the form of a chewable tablet, lozenge, drops, or mouthwash to swallow after swishing.

III. Professionally Applied Topical Fluoride

When there is no water fluoridation, or when the benefits of water fluoridation must be supplemented, at least two topical applications per year are indicated, and more frequently if the dental caries rate is high. The method for application and system for isolation of the teeth depend on the patient's ability to cooperate.

IV. Self-applied Procedures

Whether the individual with a disability is a child or an adult, a home fluoride program is indicated.

After disease control techniques for flossing and toothbrushing have been completed before the patient retires, a mouthrinse, for the patient who can rinse, a gel applied by tray or toothbrush, or a chewable tablet, for the patient who can chew and who needs a fluoride supplement, may be advised. For a

young, dependent, low-functioning person, brushing with a gel or swabbing with a fluoride rinse might be most applicable.

Parental supervision and cooperation are essential. Motivation of the parent or direct care person needs regular reinforcement by the dental team.

PIT AND FISSURE SEALANTS

Pit and fissure sealants have been used for children with developmental disabilities with satisfactory results.[29,30] The principles for application are the same as those described for all patients (pages 419–423). The use of a rubber dam is especially important for patients with excess saliva, hyperactivity of the tongue, or other management difficulties.

When a severely disabled patient will be administered general anesthesia for restorative procedures, pit and fissure sealants should be placed in all noncarious occlusal surfaces while the patient is under control. For all young patients, the sealant can be placed as soon after eruption as the tooth will hold a rubber dam.[16]

DIET INSTRUCTION

Efforts to help adults who are disabled and the parents, family members, advocates, and others responsible to understand the general dietary requirements for oral health and how to put the principles into daily practice are a distinct part of the total preventive program. Information from Chapter 28 is applicable to patients with special needs as well as to all patients.

A careful analysis of current habits, extent of knowledge, family customs, and economic factors as they relate to a patient's condition is necessary before specific recommendations can be made. In an institutional setting, efforts can be directed to contact and work with the administrative personnel, teachers, dietitians, and aides. Coordination of plaque control, snack selection, and snack availability, together with the fluoride program, opens the way to caries control.

I. Factors That Influence Diet Habits

For certain patients, diet selection and utilization center around problems of mastication, whereas for others, the transport of food to the mouth is a major undertaking. The problems of the elderly patient were described on page 568.

The following partial list of problems is suggested to help during dietary analysis and counseling. Many of the problems are directly related to increases in plaque accumulation and resultant dental caries and periodontal infections.

A. Masticatory or Feeding Problems
Problems in eating can lead to the use of a soft diet, often composed mainly of carbohydrates.

B. Overindulgence in Sucrose-containing Foods
Sweets are sometimes used as rewards or bribes by unsuspecting family members or teachers involved in behavior modification procedures in training programs.

Nonambulatory or otherwise confined patients may have less access to between-meal foods, and therefore, may eat more regularly, as served. On the other hand, the confined person may have snacks and sweets readily available, which can lead to dental destruction.

C. Inability to Accomplish Personal Plaque Control Measures
Problems of daily bacterial plaque removal can be related to a physical disability or lack of assistance from a parent or aide, combined with a diet high in cariogenic foods, which leads to dental caries development.

D. Lack of Professional Care and Instruction
Many patients do not receive adequate professional care because of unavailability, inability to obtain care because of physical barriers, inadequate financial support, lack of knowledge of the importance of oral health, or preoccupation with other major health problems.

E. Medications
1. Medications with a side effect of xerostomia contribute to dental caries.
2. Medications that diminish appetite as a side effect influence diet habits.
3. Medications contained within a sucrose base designed to mask the flavor of the agent or to pacify the patient contribute to dental caries incidence.

F. Obesity
Obesity is a problem with certain patients who suffer from inactivity, overeating, boredom, or lack of knowledge of proper food selection.

G. Food Preparation
Difficulty of food preparation can be a major limitation to diet selection for adults with neuromuscular disorders. Wheelchair confinement, lack of muscular coordination, hemiplegia or paraplegia, and dependence on others for grocery shopping are examples of problems encountered.

II. Diet Analysis and Counseling

A. Food Diary
A high-functioning patient, except the very young, may be able to keep a food diary, and participation should be encouraged. The parent, advocate, or other responsible person can assist, or in the case of a low- or moderate-functioning person, may complete the entire diary. With the aid of the diary and the information from the medical and dental histories, items for counseling can be selected.

B. Recommendations
General procedures for analysis and counseling were described on pages 383–389. Adaptations involve long-range planning for gradual modification of each patient's diet.

The person who selects and prepares the food must be involved in the planning. Sugarless snacks and sugarless rewards during behavior modification training are especially important to control.

Parents need instruction as early as possible after a newborn is known to be developmentally disabled, so that fluoride, diet, early personal hygiene, and the prevention of nursing bottle caries can be coordinated into the daily program. As described on page 550, the infant's early care should include an oral examination by the dentist and dental hygienist before 12 months of age.

GROUP IN-SERVICE EDUCATION

Dental hygienists are called upon to carry out in-service education in a variety of situations. In-service programs may be provided for teachers, registered nurses, other health professionals, parents, and volunteers in school and community preventive programs. For example, all persons mentioned could be involved in the preparation for a program of classroom weekly rinsing with a fluoride mouthrinse. When a program is citywide and many dental hygienists are involved, in-service preparation for the dental hygienists themselves is necessary.

A special need exists for in-service instruction in oral health measures for the direct care personnel in extended care institutions. Many patients in such facilities are unable to care for their own needs and may require total care, partial assistance, supervision, or regular reminders. The dental hygienist is able to work with the direct care personnel to teach them appropriate techniques and to motivate them to incorporate oral care into the daily routine for each resident or patient.

The general suggestions outlined in the following sections pertain to preparation and content for in-service workshops for the oral care of long-term patients. To supplement this brief introduction, a section of the *Suggested Readings* at the end of this chapter contains references that describe programs where in-service education has been included.

I. Preparation for an In-Service Program

A. Planning

An in-service program needs careful planning. For many groups, time for in-service is taken from an already busy work schedule. Nonmotivated participants require special considerations. The most important factor contributing to the success of a program is the genuine concern and enthusiasm of the program leader in motivating the participants.

The material must be clear and to the point, interestingly presented with appropriate visual aids, and stimulating for learning. Objectives should be defined in writing and serve as a guide to preparation and evaluation.

Problems of the staff must be recognized. Some members may have negative oral health attitudes, minimal educational background, and poor personal oral health.

Initially, basic preparation includes learning about the functioning levels of the clients and assessing the procedures used for their oral care. A survey of the plaque control materials and devices available and in current use, methods for labeling or storing individual brushes, and the frequency of use is important.

B. Use of Clinic Records

Clinic records for each patient should be examined for information relative to the dental status and to those who wear dentures. Medical histories must be reviewed so that special general or oral health problems can be considered and necessary precautions taken.

When a dental hygienist is employed regularly within an institution, a much more complete assessment can be made. The dental hygienist invited to the institution for the specific purpose of presenting the workshop might only have a telephone conversation with the supervisor to determine facts about the residents and their oral health.

C. Gingival/Plaque Index

The use of a gingival or plaque index (pages 262, 273) can provide a baseline of information from which progress can be evaluated. The direct care personnel could carry out the daily plaque control program and see the changes that take place by comparing survey results at a later date. Such continuing participation could provide a real motivation to the group.

II. Program Content

A. The Participants' Own Plaque Control

Based on the premise that persons who are motivated to care for their own mouths have a clearer understanding of the effects and importance of oral care and give a higher priority to the time spent daily, an in-service education group needs to participate in a personal plaque control program. A plaque-free score (page 264) or other evaluation device can be used. A group may be willing to work in pairs and learn to evaluate and score each other, thereby learning the techniques to be applied to their clients.

B. Facts About Etiology and Prevention

Basic information about plaque, its formation, and how gingivitis and dental caries develop are important to most groups. The progress of disease from reversible gingivitis to severe periodontitis can be explained, as can the process of dental caries, which begins with a small cavity and progresses to a diseased pulp. Prevention through plaque control, fluoride, dietary controls, sealants, and early treatment for restorations must be carefully presented. Handout materials and colorful visual aids promote learning.

C. Oral Examination

1. *Oral Mucosa.* Techniques demonstrated and practiced by the participants on each other should include the use of a tongue depressor to retract and a disposable mirror and a light source to see the oral mucosa.
2. *Tongue.* How to hold the tongue, using a sponge to lift and inspect all parts, can be shown.
3. *Gingiva.* Color, size, and bleeding that occurs spontaneously or while brushing can be explained and demonstrated. When projection is possible, slides can be included for all aspects of the instructional material. When a camera is available for intraoral photography, "before" and "after" pictures of the patients can be shown. Changes effected by the plaque control supervised by the direct care aides are more meaningful than are pictures of strangers.

4. *Bacterial Plaque.* Inspection for plaque can be demonstrated when the disclosing agent is used prior to plaque scoring and removal.

5. *Denture Supporting Mucosa.* Patients with dentures need the supporting tissues examined periodically by the dentist, but direct care persons will be able to notice changes that should be called to the dentist's attention as a result of their daily cleaning and massaging of the mucosa under the denture.

6. *Dentures.* Sample dentures may be used to help the participants learn to examine each denture for cracks or sharp edges. Examination for deposits can be made by the patient and the direct care person and compared with the denture after it has been cleaned.

D. Techniques of Mouth Care and Disease Control

Staff members can be trained to work in pairs.[31] Working in pairs is more efficient, particularly in the care of difficult patients.

A plan for each client can be worked out with the aides so that individual problems relative to dental caries prevention, gingival disease control, or complete or partial denture care can be solved. Teaching some or all of the following may be included, depending on the needs of the clients.

1. *Plaque Control.* Instruction includes positioning of the patient (page 626), application of disclosing agent, examination for plaque on the teeth, toothbrush selection and technique, use of a mouth prop, and flossing with or without a floss aid. The use of a portable or bedside suction unit for removing debris from a patient's mouth can be practiced by a paired team.[31]

2. *Fluoride Application.* The objectives and techniques for brushing with a gel, swabbing with a mouthrinse, assisting the patient with a chewable tablet, or applying a gel tray can be included.

3. *Denture Care.* Procedures for care of dentures and of the mucosa under the denture are shown.

4. *Saliva Substitute.* Use of saliva substitute for dry mouth is demonstrated.

E. Denture Marking Procedure

Not all members of the staff need to learn the technique for marking dentures for personal identification. Because dentures should be marked soon after arrival, personnel involved with admissions of new clients are most in need of the instruction.

In a large hospital or rehabilitation center, new dentures made in the dental clinic are marked during processing. The techniques for denture marking are outlined in Chapter 46, pages 578–579.

III. Records

A record form to be completed for each client is essential to follow-up and evaluation. During the instruction periods, the staff can learn how to complete the record and where to file the copies.

The form can be designed with spaces to record information obtained during the oral examination, the functioning level and degree of cooperation, the procedures needed for dental caries control, periodontal health, and/or denture care. In addition, the instruction provided, the implements and materials used, the planned future instruction, the prognosis, and any other personal notes can be included.

IV. Follow-up

After direct care personnel have had an opportunity to try their newly learned procedures, an opportunity to have questions answered should be provided. Direct observation by the dental hygienist of techniques performed with and for the clients, advice concerning oral problems of particular patients, and corrections when necessary can motivate and encourage both client and aide.

Disclosing and recording the plaque for comparison of scores before and after the program can show the progress being made.

V. Continuing Education

A. Individual instruction should be provided for each new employee during the orientation period for that employee.

B. Periodic updating for all employees can be accomplished at regular intervals. Questions and problems can be discussed, and plans can be introduced for changing a certain procedure based on new research evidence.

C. A specific plan for scheduled oral health programs may be a requirement for licensure of a health care facility.[32]

INSTRUMENTATION

Customary techniques must be adapted. With basic knowledge of methods for maintaining patient stability, adequate visibility of working area, secure instrument grasps and finger rests, and well-controlled strokes, instrumentation for calculus removal and root planing can be effectively accomplished.

Patients who are hyperactive, lack muscular control, or have a mental deficiency provide many challenges. With some patients, the tasks of keeping the head and mouth positioned, the profuse saliva controlled, and the oversized or hyperactive tongue held back may seem insurmountable. Patience, a gentle but firm touch, and continuing experience are essential.

I. Preparation For Instrumentation
A. Premedication

1. Antibiotic coverage as indicated for susceptible patients (pages 85 and 91).

2. Sedative for control of selected patients.

B. Plaque Control Instruction Precedes Scaling

1. Disclose and present or review information on plaque.
2. Continue practice on plaque removal methods that were selected for the particular patient. The patient, parent, and attendant demonstrate.

II. Stabilization

For certain patients, opening the mouth is difficult and maintaining the mouth in an open position is impossible. A mouth prop can be used to assist the patient. Verbal encouragement of the patient must continue throughout the appointment.

A. Ratchet Type (Molt's Mouth Gag)

The preferred, most stable mouth prop is a sterilized prop that can be nearly closed for insertion between the teeth. It can be opened gradually to hold the jaws to the necessary position. The tips are covered with rubber tubing and are positioned over the maxillary and mandibular teeth on one side while the clinician treats the opposite side.

B. Rubber Bite Block

A long piece of dental floss should be tied through the holes in a commercially available rubber mouth prop so that, in case of a sudden respiratory change, the prop can be quickly pulled out and breathing normalized.

C. Tongue Depressors

A practical, disposable mouth prop can be made from three to six tongue depressors taped together. A folded sponge should be placed under the tape to provide a cushion.

D. Precautions for the Use of a Mouth Prop

1. Mobile teeth could be knocked out and aspirated.
   a. Loose primary teeth in young patient.
   b. Mobile teeth in advanced periodontal disease.
2. Fatigue of the patient's facial and masticatory muscles and temporomandibular joint.
3. Patient must know that all stabilization devices are for comfort and to make the work easier and that they are in no way meant to hurt or punish.

III. Treatment by Quadrants

For many patients, particularly those with generalized heavy supra- and subgingival calculus, treatment by quadrants under local anesthesia is the procedure of choice. Removal of calculus and overhanging fillings can be completed more efficiently.

A. Scaling Requirements

The occurrence of generalized heavy calculus deposits in disabled patients is not unusual. The reason may be inadequate personal and professional care or factors related to the disabling condition.

Studies of certain groups have suggested that the heavy calculus deposits may be related to metabolic factors. For example, in a group of children aged 10 to 15 years with cystic fibrosis, 90 percent had calculus, and in a group of the same age with asthma, 100 percent had calculus. Only 43 percent of the able-bodied children measured in the study had calculus deposits. The occurrence of calculus in the children with cystic fibrosis and asthma was believed to be related to their elevated salivary calcium and phosphorus.[33]

The objective of the clinical techniques is the complete removal of calculus and planing of root surfaces. The compromising or rationalization of complete treatment neglects the patient's needs and permits advanced periodontal disease to develop.

B. Need for Assistance

A dental assistant is needed while treating many types of patients with disabilities. Many patients have excess saliva, whereas others have uncontrollable tongue and general body movements, all of which can hinder instrumentation.

1. *Stabilization and Visibility.* With assistance for stabilization, visibility, and maintenance of a clear field, the procedure is less traumatic for the patient and less time-consuming for all.
2. *Precaution During Evacuation.* Patients such as those with chronic lung disorders, asthma, or cystic fibrosis and patients with cerebral palsy are considered "aspiration risks." For example, a sudden spasm in the facial, neck, or throat areas could cause a patient with cerebral palsy to aspirate foreign matter from the mouth into the airway.

C. Instruments

1. Unbreakable mirrors are recommended for use with a patient subject to spasm or sudden closure.
2. Use single-end sharp instruments to prevent accidents when a patient moves involuntarily.
3. Use of an ultrasonic scaler is contraindicated for an aspiration risk patient. It also should not be used for patients who over-react to sensory stimuli, such as a patient with autism (pages 651–653).

D. Technique Suggestions

1. *Introduce Each Procedure and Sound to Prevent Startling a Patient.* Follow the basic instruction rule to "show, tell, then do." When a patient is blind or deaf, the rule has double significance.
2. *Finger Rests.* Firm, dependable finger rests are needed. Supplemental or reinforced rests can contribute to instrument stability. With certain

patients, external finger and hand rests may be safer for the clinician.[34]

TECHNICAL HINTS

Sources of Materials

American Dental Hygienists' Association
444 North Michigan Avenue
Chicago, Illinois 60611
   The Power of a Healthy Smile. Dental Care Resource Kit for Serving the Disabled

American Dental Association
Order Department
211 East Chicago Avenue
Chicago, Illinois 60611
   Oral Health Care in the Nursing Facility (J 010)

National Easter Seal Society for Crippled Children and Adults
2023 West Ogden Avenue
Chicago, Illinois 60612
   Casamassimo, P.: *Toothbrushing and Flossing. A Manual of Home Dental Care for Persons Who Are Handicapped*
   Nowak, A.J.: *Helping Handicapped Persons Clean Their Teeth*

National Foundation of Dentistry for the Handicapped and Academy of Dentistry for the Handicapped
1250 14th Street
Denver, Colorado 80202
Request list of available materials.

References

1. United States Developmental Disabilities Assistance and Bill of Rights Act of 1987, P.L. 100–146.
2. American Association of Dental Schools, Section on Comprehensive Care and General Dentistry: Curriculum Guidelines for Dentistry for the Person With a Handicap, *J. Dent. Educ., 49,* 118, February, 1985.
3. Ettinger, R.L., Beck, J.D., and Glenn, R.E.: Eliminating Office Architectural Barriers to Dental Care of the Elderly and Handicapped, *J. Am. Dent. Assoc., 98,* 398, March, 1979.
4. United States General Services Administration, Department of Defense, Department of Housing and Urban Development, and Postal Service: Uniform Federal Accessibility Standards, *Federal Register, 49,* 31528–31613, August 7, 1984.
5. Bill, D.J. and Weddell, J.A.: Dental Office Access for Patients With Disabling Conditions, *Spec. Care Dentist., 6,* 246, November-December, 1986.
6. Hale, J., Snow, M., and Stiefel, D.J.: Providing Office Accessibility to the Disabled Patient, *J. Dent. Handicap., 3, 10,* Summer, 1977.
7. Metal Dynamics Corporation, 9324 State Road, Philadelphia, Pennsylvania 19114.
8. Posnick, W.R. and Martin, H.H.: Wheel Chair Transfer Techniques for the Dental Office, *J. Am. Dent. Assoc., 94,* 719, April, 1977.
9. Stiefel, D.J., Schubert, M.M., Hale, J.M., and Friedel, C.A.: *Wheelchair Transfers in the Dental Office.* Disability Dental Instruction, 4919 Northeast 86th Street, Seattle, Washington 98115, 42 pp.
10. Clark Associates, 370 Park Avenue, Worcester, Massachusetts 01610.
11. Olympic Medical Corporation, 4400 7th Avenue South, Seattle, Washington 98108.
12. Northup, H.L., State of Rhode Island, Department of Mental Health, Retardation and Hospitals, Dr. Joseph H. Ladd Center, North Kingstowne, Rhode Island, personal communication.
13. Koster, S.: Orthodontic Treatment of Handicapped Persons, in Wei, S.H.Y. and Casko, J., eds.: *Orthodontic Care for Handicapped Persons,* Proceedings of a Workshop, University of Iowa, Iowa City, Iowa, 1977, p. 31.
14. Nowak, A.J.: Dental Care for the Handicapped Patient–Past, Present, Future, in Nowak, A.J.: *Dentistry for the Handicapped Patient.* St. Louis, The C.V. Mosby Co., 1976, p. 11.
15. Steinberg, A.D.: Periodontal Evaluation and Treatment Considerations with the Handicapped Patient, in Nowak, A.J.: *Dentistry for the Handicapped Patient.* St. Louis, The C.V. Mosby Co., 1976, pp. 302–328.
16. Nowak, A.J.: *Dentistry for the Handicapped Patient.* St. Louis, The C.V. Mosby Co., 1976, pp. 167–192.
17. Sonnenberg, E.M. and Shey, Z.: A Review of Preventive Dentistry for the Handicapped Individual, *Clin. Prevent. Dent., 1,* 16, July-August, 1979.
18. Troutman, K.C.: Prevention of Dental Disease for the Handicapped, in DePaola, D.P. and Cheney, H.G., eds.: *Preventive Dentistry.* Preventive Dental Handbook Series, vol. 2. Littleton, Massachusetts, PSG Publishing, 1979, pp. 205–224.
19. Meador, H.G.: Toothbrushing: A Sensible Approach for the Mentally Retarded, *Dent. Hyg., 53,* 462, October, 1979.
20. Duncan, J.L.: Incorporating Oral Hygiene Procedures in Geriatric Nursing Homes, *Dent. Hyg., 53,* 519, November, 1979.
21. Price, V.E.: Toothbrush Modifications for the Handicapped, *Dent. Hyg., 54,* 467, October, 1980.
22. Sroda, R. and Plezia, R.A.: Oral Hygiene Devices for Special Patients, *Spec. Care Dentist., 4,* 264, November-December, 1984.
23. Fred Sammons Inc., Box 32, Brookfield, Illinois 60513.
24. Albertson, D.: Prevention and the Handicapped Child, *Dent. Clin. North Am., 18,* 595, July, 1974.
25. Ettinger, R.L. and Pinkham, J.R.: Oral Hygiene and the Handicapped Child, *J. Int. Assoc. Dent. Child., 9,* 3, July, 1978.
26. Mulligan, R.A.: Design Characteristics of Electric Toothbrushes Important to Physically Compromised Patients, *J. Dent. Res., 59,* 450, Abstract 731, Special Issue A, March, 1980.
27. Ettinger, R.L. and Pinkham, J.R.: Dental Care for the Homebound—Assessment and Hygiene, *Aust. Dent. J., 22,* 77, April, 1977.
28. National Foundation of Dentistry for the Handicapped, National Fluorides Task Force: A Guide to the Use of Fluorides for the Prevention of Dental Caries With Alternative Recommendations for Patients With Handicaps, *J. Am. Dent. Assoc., 113,* 506, September, 1986.
29. Ripa, L.W. and Cole, W.W.: Occlusal Sealing and Caries Prevention: Results 12 Months After a Single Application of Adhesive Resin, *J. Dent. Res., 49,* 171, January, 1970.
30. Richardson, B.A., Smith, D.C., and Hargreaves, J.A.: A 5-year Clinical Evaluation of the Effectiveness of a Fissure Sealant in Mentally Retarded Canadian Children, *Community Dent. Oral Epidemiol., 9,* 170, August, 1981.
31. Gertenrich, R.L. and Hart, R.W.: Utilization of the Oral Hygiene Team in a Mental Health Institution, *ASDC J. Dent. Child., 39,* 174, May-June, 1972.
32. Title 22, California Administrative Code, Section 72301 (e) and CFR 405.1129 (a).
33. Wotman, S., Mercadante, J., Mandel, I.D., Goldman, R.S., and Denning, C.: The Occurrence of Calculus in Normal Children, Children With Cystic Fibrosis, and Children with Asthma, *J. Periodontol., 44,* 278, May, 1973.
34. Pattison, G. and Pattison, A.M.: *Periodontal Instrumentation. A Clinical Manual.* Reston, Virginia, Reston Publishing, 1979, pp. 187–189.

Suggested Readings

American Association of Dental Schools, Section on Dental Hygiene Education: Curricular Guidelines for Dental Hygiene Care for the Handicapped, *J. Dent. Educ., 48,* 266, May, 1984.

Bober-Moken, I. and Clark, M.S.: The Handicapped in Dentistry, *Clin. Prevent. Dent., 3,* 15, November-December, 1981.

Braff, M.H.: Dental Treatment for Developmentally Disabled Patients, *Spec. Care Dentist., 5,* 109, May-June, 1985.

Brody, H.A.: A Dental Care System for Patients With Developmental Disabilities, *Spec. Care Dentist., 5,* 124, May-June, 1985.

Chohayeb, A.A.: Prevalent Medical and Dental Conditions Among the Handicapped, *Spec. Care Dentist., 5,* 114, May-June, 1985.

Cluff, L.E.: Chronic Disability of Infants and Children: A Foundation's Experience, *J. Chronic Dis., 38,* 113, Number 1, 1985.

Dudley, A.: Working With Special Patients, *RDH, 7,* 43, November/December, 1987.

Dwyer, B.A.: Professional Tips for the Non-handicapped: Measuring Expectations, *Dent. Assist., 53,* 21, January-February, 1984.

Entwistle, B.: Private Practice Preventive Dentistry for the Special Patient, *Spec. Care Dentist., 4,* 246, November-December, 1984.

Fenton, S.J., Fenton, L.I., Kimmelman, B.B., Shellhart, W.C., Sheff, M.C., Scott, J.P., Staggers, J.A., and Portugal, B.V.: ADH Ad Hoc Committee Report: The Use of Restraints in the Delivery of Dental Care for the Handicapped—Legal, Ethical, and Medical Considerations, *Spec. Care Dentist., 7,* 253, November-December, 1987.

Kostiw, U.: Dental Hygiene Care for the Handicapped Patient, *Dent. Hyg., 55,* 14, January, 1981.

Lancial, L.A.: The Dental Hygienist as Dental Care Advocate for Persons With Disabilities, *Spec. Care Dentist., 4,* 267, November-December, 1984.

Lange, B.M., Entwistle, B.M., and Lipson, L.F.: *Dental Management of the Handicapped: Approaches for Dental Auxiliaries.* Philadelphia, Lea & Febiger, 1983, 169 pp.

Levine, N.: Community Responses to the Disabled and the Dental Profession's Responsibility, *Can. Dent. Assoc. J., 51,* 35, January, 1985.

Lindemann, R.A. and Henson, J.L.: Acceptance of Dental Prophylaxis By the Institutionalized Patient, *Spec. Care Dentist., 4,* 77, March-April, 1984.

Lizaire, A.L., Borkent, A., and Toor, V.: Dental Health Status of Nondependent Children With Handicapping Conditions in Edmonton, Alberta, *Spec. Care Dentist., 6,* 74, March-April, 1986.

Mann, J., Wolnerman, J.S., Lavie, G., Carlin, Y., Meir, S., and Garfunkel, A.A.: The Effect of Dental Education and Dental Treatment on the Dental Status of a Handicapped Population: A Longitudinal Study, *Spec. Care Dentist., 6,* 180, July-August, 1986.

Nelson, L.P., Sweeney, E.A., and Nelson, B.N.: Dental Treatment Times in a Population of Patients With Handicapping Conditions, *Spec. Care Dentist., 7,* 67, March-April, 1987.

Nowak, A.J.: Dental Disease in Handicapped Persons, *Spec. Care Dentist., 4,* 66, March-April, 1984.

Nunn, J.H. and Murray, J.J.: The Dental Health of Handicapped Children in Newcastle and Northumberland, *Br. Dent. J., 162,* 9, January 10, 1987.

Pool, D.M.: Dental Care for the Handicapped Adolescent, *Int. Dent. J., 32,* 194, June, 1982.

Seals, R.R. and Cain, J.R.: Prosthetic Treatment for Chemical Burns of the Oral Cavity, *J. Prosthet. Dent., 53,* 688, May, 1985.

Sinykin, S.G.: The Dental Assistant and the "Special Patient," *Dent. Assist., 53,* 24, January-February, 1984.

Stiefel, D.J., Rolla, R.R., and Truelove, E.L.: Effectiveness of Various Preventive Methodologies for Use With Disabled Persons, *Clin. Prevent. Dent., 6,* 17, September-October, 1984.

Storhaug, K.: Caries Experience in Disabled Pre-school Children, *Acta Odontol. Scand., 43,* 241, Number 4, 1985.

Strauss, R.P., Hairfield, W.M., and George, M.C.: Disabled Adults in Sheltered Employment: An Assessment of Dental Needs and Costs, *Am. J. Public Health, 75,* 661, June, 1985.

Taicher, S. and Sela, M.: Complete Dentures for Handicapped Children Using Custom-made Teeth, *Spec. Care Dentist., 6,* 112, May-June, 1986.

Wasinger, J.L.: A Personal Approach to Dental Care for Patients With Handicapping Conditions, *Spec. Care Dentist., 6,* 156, July-August, 1986.

White, C.S.: Nasogastric Intubation—Oral and Perioral Care, *Spec. Care Dentist., 4,* 19, January-February, 1984.

Willard, D.H. and Nowak, A.J.: Communicating With the Family of the Child With A Developmental Disability, *J. Am. Dent. Assoc., 102,* 647, May, 1981.

Treatment

Adair, S.M. and Durr, D.P.: Modification of Papoose Board Restraint to Facilitate Airway Management of the Sedated Pediatric Dental Patient, *Pediatr. Dent., 9,* 163, June, 1987.

Barker, D.T.: A Motorized Surgery Unit for Treatment of the Handicapped Patient, *Br. Dent. J., 162,* 436, June 6, 1987.

Baycar, R., Aker, F., Serowski, A., and Bailey, G.: Mobile Oral Treatment and Examination Chair, *Spec. Care Dentist., 3,* 224, September-October, 1983.

Bazan, M.T. and Ellard, J.D.: A Combination Mouth Prop-Suction Device, *Spec. Care Dentist., 3,* 164, July-August, 1983.

Casamassimo, P.S.: Radiographic Considerations for Special Patients—Modifications, Adjuncts, and Alternatives, *Pediatr. Dent., 3,* 448, Special Issue 2, 1981.

Dicks, J.L.: Modifications of Treatment for the Severely Handicapped Adult Patient Under General Anesthesia, *Spec. Care Dentist., 1,* 262, November-December, 1981.

Dudley, A.: Treating the Patient With Special Health Needs, *RDH, 4,* 40, March-April, 1984.

Felder, R.S., Gillette, V.M., and Leseberg, K.: Wheelchair Transfer Techniques for the Dental Office, *Spec. Care Dentist., 8,* 256, November-December, 1988.

Kaminsky, S.B., Kaurich, M.J., and Chenderlin, J.: Managing Cooperative Nonambulatory Patients: Transfers to the Dental Chair, *Gerodontics, 4,* 1, February, 1988.

Lejeune, R.C.: Modification of an Ultrasonic Scaler for Portable Use, *Spec. Care Dentist., 6,* 274, November-December, 1986.

McGhay, R.M.: A Simple Headrest for Patients Confined to Wheelchairs, *J. Prosthet. Dent., 44,* 347, September, 1980.

Montanarella, M., McKnight-Hanes, C., and Davila, J.M.: New Device for Dental Radiography for Use With General Anesthesia, *Spec. Care Dentist., 6,* 160, July-August, 1986.

Napierski, G.E.: Positioning Wheelchair Patients for Dental Treatment, *J. Prosthet. Dent., 47,* 217, February, 1982.

Sappington, D.B. and Woehrlen, A.E.: Anesthetic Considerations in the Dental Care of the Patient With Physical and Emotional Handicaps, *Spec. Care Dentist., 3,* 244, November-December, 1983.

Smith, H.P. and King, D.L.: A Postural Support Device for Handicapped Children, *J. Dent. Handicap., 4,* 14, Fall/Winter, 1978.

Bacterial Plaque Control

Arblaster, D.G., Rothwell, P.S., and White, G.E.: A Toothbrush for Patients With Impaired Manual Dexterity, *Br. Dent. J., 159,* 219, October 5, 1985.

Clemens, C. and Taylor, S.: Toothbrushing to Music, *Dent. Hyg., 54,* 125, March, 1980.

Cutter, C.R.: Diet Influences in Dental Care for the Developmentally Disabled Patient, *Spec. Care Dentist., 2,* 106, May-June, 1982.

Entwistle, B.M. and Rudrud, E.H.: Behavioral Approaches to Toothbrushing Programs for Handicapped Adults, *Spec. Care Dentist., 2,* 155, July-August, 1982.

Feigal, R.J. and Jensen, M.E.: The Cariogenic Potential of Liquid Medications: A Concern for the Handicapped Patient, *Spec. Care Dentist., 2,* 20, January-February, 1982.

Francis, J.R., Hunter, B., and Addy, M.: A Comparison of Three Delivery Methods of Chlorhexidine in Handicapped Children. 1. Effects on Plaque, Gingivitis, and Toothstaining, *J. Periodontol., 58,* 451, July, 1987.

Francis, J.R., Addy, M., and Hunter, B.: A Comparison of Three Delivery Methods of Chlorhexidine in Handicapped Children. II. Parent and House-Parent Preferences, *J. Periodontol., 58,* 456, July, 1987.

Goho, C.: A Digital Brushing Technique for Patients With Perceptuomotor Difficulties, *Clin. Prevent. Dent., 5,* 6, March-April, 1983.

Gomes, D.C., Shakun, M.L., and Ripa, L.W.: Effect of Rinsing With a 1.5% Hydrogen Peroxide Solution (Peroxyl) on Gingivitis and Plaque in Handicapped and Nonhandicapped Subjects, *Clin. Prevent. Dent., 6,* 21, May-June, 1984.

Mann, J., Wolnerman, J.S., Lavie, G., Carlin, Y., and Garfunkel, A.A.: Periodontal Treatment Needs and Oral Hygiene for Institutionalized Individuals With Handicapping Conditions, *Spec. Care Dentist., 4,* 173, July-August, 1984.

Mulligan, R. and Wilson, S.: Design Characteristics of Floss-holding Devices for Persons With Upper Extremity Disabilities, *Spec. Care Dentist., 4,* 168, July-August, 1984.

Rommerdale, E.H., Comer, R.W., and Caughman, W.F.: University of Mississippi Dental Care Unit: Toothbrushing for the Handicapped, *Spec. Care Dentist., 3,* 108, May-June, 1983.

von Gonten, A.S. and Albright, L.R.: Prosthesis Cleaning Aid for Manually Handicapped Patients, *J. Prosthet. Dent., 51,* 283, February, 1984.

Programs With Inservice Education

Block, P.L.: An Oral Care Program for Hospitalized Patients: A Project for the Dental Health Committee, *Milit. Med., 145,* 42, January, 1980.

Deal, T.S. and Roppel, A.L.: Evaluation of a Supplemental Dental Booklet for Long-term Facilities, *Spec. Care Dentist., 6,* 162, July-August, 1986.

Duncan, J.L.: Incorporating Oral Hygiene Procedures in Geriatric Nursing Homes, *Dent. Hyg., 53,* 519, November, 1979.

Kass, L.: Dental Health Program for the Institutionally Mentally Retarded, *Dent. Hyg., 53,* 76, February, 1979.

Kowitz, M.D., Ness, J.C., Campbell, J.G., Clapham, E., Moretti, G.M., Gallagher, T.M., and Spate, D.J.: Prosthetic Maintenance Research Program for the Geriatric Patient, *J. Calif. Dent. Assoc., 7,* 37, November, 1979.

Meador, H.G.: Toothbrushing: A Sensible Approach for the Mentally Retarded, *Dent. Hyg., 53,* 462, October, 1979.

Miller, G.I.: Oral Health Care for the Retarded Institutional Patient: One Hospital's Experience, *J. Hosp. Dent. Pract., 13,* 147, Fourth Quarter, 1979.

Schmidt, S.M., Leach, M., Nicolaci, A.B., Sutton, R.B., and O'Donnell, J.P.: The Dental Health Educator and Programs for Institutions With Persons Who Are Mentally Retarded, *Spec. Care Dentist., 1,* 174, July-August, 1981.

Thornton, M.A.: Preventive Dentistry in the Veterans Administration, *Dent. Hyg., 53,* 121, March, 1979.

Wasserman, B.S., Kovler, L., Mandelkorn, W., and Laster, G.E.: Development of an Inpatient Oral Health Education Program in an Acute Care Facility, *Spec. Care Dentist., 3,* 263, November-December, 1983.

HOMEBOUND PATIENTS

Within recent years, efforts have been made through research and organized programming to attend to the oral health needs of the chronically ill and disabled. Patients of all age groups who are confined to hospitals, institutions, nursing homes, skilled nursing facilities, or private homes need special adaptations for dental and dental hygiene care. Portable equipment is available, and special training for dental personnel is encouraged.

Dental care for the chronically ill must be completed in a variety of surroundings. For the hospitalized person, dental clinics frequently are available to provide care for in-patients. Those who are not hospitalized may be confined to their homes or may be able to be transported to the dental office or clinic in a wheelchair, depending on the severity and extent of disability.

Dentists and dental hygienists in private practice have occasion to attend to patients confined to their homes. Dental hygiene techniques lend themselves to care for the bedridden because nearly the entire treatment can be completed with manual instruments. Instruction in personal oral preventive procedures has particular significance for the comfort, as well as the health, of the patient. Suggestions relative to planning and conducting a home visit are included in this chapter.

I. Objectives

A. Aid in preventing dental caries and periodontal infections that require extensive treatment.
B. Assist in preventing further complication of the patient's state of health by lessening oral care problems.
C. Contribute to the patient's comfort, mental ease, and general well-being.
D. Encourage adequate personal care procedures, whether performed by the patient or an attendant.
E. Contribute to general rehabilitation or habilitation of the patient.

II. Preparation for the Home Visit

A. Understanding the Patient
1. Consider the characteristics associated with the particular chronic illness or disease.
2. Consider special problems related to age. (For example, for the gerodontic patient, see Chapter 45.)
3. Review patient's medical history (by telephone, if preliminary visit is not practical) to determine unusual precautions that must be taken. Arrange with physician and dentist when premedication is indicated (page 91).

B. Instruments and Equipment
1. *Protective Barriers.* Mask, eyeglasses, gloves.
2. *Instruction Materials.* Toothbrush, interdental aids (several types, until needs of patient are known).
3. *Sterile Equipment.* Sterile instruments and other items are transported in the sealed packages in which they were sterilized.
4. *Disposable Items.* Gauze sponges, cotton rolls and pellets, wood points, fluoride application trays, and other essential disposable items are prepared in packages that will be convenient to open and use at the bedside.
5. *Pharmaceuticals.* Such substances as the disclosing agent, postoperative antiseptic, polishing agent, and topical fluoride preparation are carried in small, tightly closed bottles.
6. *Coverall.* A large plastic drape is of particular importance, because in certain types of illness the patient's coordination during rinsing may be limited.
7. *Emesis Basin for Patient Rinsing.* Although a small basin undoubtedly would be available at the home, the kidney-shaped basin facilitates the rinsing process.
8. *Lighting.* Adaptation of available possibilities.
   a. Headlight or Reflector. Dentist may have as part of the office equipment; with practice, the dental hygienist can learn to use with ease.
   b. Photography Spot Light. Might be available either from the dentist or from the patient's home; need a type with a narrow, concentrated beam.
   c. Gooseneck Lamp. Might be available in patient's home; need bulb of adequate wattage.
9. *Miscellaneous Items Usually Available at the*

Home. Arrangements must be planned (by telephone) in advance of appointment.

 a. Large Towels. For covering pillows.

 b. Pillows. Types of pillows available that may be firm enough to assist in maintaining patient's head in reasonably stationary position.

 c. Hospital Bed. Can be adjusted most effectively for patient's position.

 d. Container for Prosthesis.

C. Appointment Time

Arrange during the patient's usual waking hours at as convenient a time as possible in relation to nursing care and mealtime schedule.

III. Approach to Patient

Because a majority of patients who come to the dental office are active people with good general health, the adjustment to the relatively helpless, chronically ill person is sometimes difficult. One may tend to be oversolicitous, an attitude that may not contribute to the development of a cooperative patient.

Usually, a direct approach with gentle firmness is most successful. Establishment of rapport with the patient depends in part on whether the patient has requested and anticipated the appointment or whether those caring for the patient have insisted on and arranged for the visit.

A. Personal Factors

Frequently, the well-adjusted chronically ill person may be more appreciative of the care provided than is the patient who comes to the dental office. The ill patient also may be well aware of the difficulties under which the dental hygienist is working. The cooperation obtained frequently depends on the patient's attitude toward the illness or disability.

A prolonged illness that may have been accompanied by suffering is not conducive to a healthy outlook on life. Monotonous confinement contributes to the development of characteristics such as those listed below.

1. Unable to maintain a cheerful attitude.
2. Bored or dissatisfied with sameness of daily routine.
3. Easily depressed.
4. Discouraged about recovery; leads to mental state that may retard recovery.
5. Sensitive and easily offended.
6. Demanding; enjoys being waited on if used to having prompt attention to each request.
7. Indifferent to personal appearance and general rules of personal hygiene.
8. Preoccupied with details of medical examinations, tests, treatment, medications, and symptoms.

B. Suggestions for General Procedure

1. Request that visitors be asked to remain out of the room during the appointment to prevent distraction of patient.
2. Introduce each step slowly to be sure patient knows what is being done.
3. Do not make the patient feel rushed. Listen attentively; socializing is one of the best ways to establish rapport.
4. Regardless of inconvenience of arrangements, plan two or more appointments when extensive scaling is required.

 a. Need to avoid tiring the patient.

 b. Need for observing tissue response.

 c. Need to give encouragement in plaque control procedures.

IV. Dental Hygiene Care and Instruction

A. The Working Situation

Because many patients can sit up in a chair or wheelchair for at least 1 or 2 hours each day, only rarely must procedures be performed while the patient is in bed. For the patient in a chair, a kitchen or large bathroom may be most satisfactory for working. In either situation, ingenuity is needed to arrange patient position, head stabilization, and proper lighting to maintain patient comfort and yet provide access for the clinician.

1. *Patient in Bed*

 a. Hospital Bed. Adjust to lift patient's head to desirable height.

 b. Ordinary Bed. Use firm pillows to support patient.

2. *Patient in Wheelchair*

 a. Portable headrest may be attached to back of plain chair or wheelchair.

 b. Although the chair can be backed against a wall and a pillow inserted for the head, the patient preferably should be moved to a davenport or chair where a more stable headrest could be provided.

3. *Small Patient.* Positions for plaque control described on page 627 and shown in figure 50–9 may be applicable for dental hygienist during treatment.

4. *Suggestions for Lighting*

 a. Overhead Lighting. Turn off to reduce shadows in the mouth.

 b. Headlight. Usually the most convenient and efficient form of lighting because of concentrated beam.

 c. Head Reflector. Reflect light from bed lamp attached to bed behind patient's head.

 d. Gooseneck or Photographer's Light. Care must be taken not to direct the light into patient's eyes.

5. *Instrument Arrangement.* Arrange on towel on table beside bed or chair.

B. Evaluation: Treatment Plan
1. Vital signs.
2. Extraoral/intraoral examination.
3. Periodontal evaluation.
4. Dental examination.

C. Personal Oral Care

Provide specific instruction for attendant of helpless or uncoordinated patient. Demonstrate in patient's mouth. A powered toothbrush may prove valuable for certain patients (pages 310–311).

D. Instrumentation

Scaling is complicated by instability of head. A mouth prop may be needed when patient has difficulty opening mouth.

E. Fluoride Application

Selection of method for fluoride application varies with the patient and the home situation. The use of self-care techniques depends on the patient's handicap and the cooperation of the attendant. The greatest benefit is obtained from a daily mouthrinse, chewable tablet, or gel applied in a mouthguard tray or brushed on (pages 407–410).

F. Dietary Suggestions
1. Consultation with physician concerning prescribed diet is necessary. When significant relationships of diet to oral health are suspected, they should be reported to the dentist. The patient's problem can then be discussed with the physician and dietary adjustments made.
2. Cariogenic foods should be avoided as snacks. The patient and those who provide the patient's food need specific suggestions for food substitutes that are noncariogenic.
3. Factors influencing suggestions for diet
   a. Patient's appetite may be poor, particularly if the patient is discouraged about the state of health.
   b. The patient who is finicky in food selection may have affected the general nutritional state or may have used cariogenic foods in excess.
   c. Monotony of meals may have lessened the desire to eat.

G. Appointment Plan for Maintenance

THE HOSPITALIZED HELPLESS OR UNCONSCIOUS PATIENT

Personal oral care procedures for the hospitalized patient are accomplished by the attendant member of the nursing staff when self-care by the patient is impossible. Planning and conducting an oral health in-service program for the nursing staff and other direct-care persons are described on pages 628–630.

Understanding the possible procedures for oral care of hospitalized patients is important to all dental hygienists, whether or not they are employed in a hospital, if they are to appreciate ramifications of dental hygiene care for the many types of patients with special needs.

Skill is required to carry out routine methods of toothbrushing, rinsing, and cleaning of removable dentures for the conscious patient who is able to cooperate. Methods must be adapted when the patient's head cannot be elevated. When the patient's illness or injury involves the oral cavity, the advice and recommendations of the attending oral surgeon are followed.

Maintenance of oral cleanliness for the acutely ill or unconscious patient requires special procedures because of the complete helplessness of the patient. Objectives and methods described below have application for patients with other special needs, for example, the patient with a fractured jaw (page 592) or severe mental retardation (pages 648–649).

I. Objectives of Care

A. Prevent debris in the mouth from being aspirated and clogging air passages.
B. Minimize the possibility of oral infection.
C. Clean the mouth and provide comfort for the patient.

II. Care of Removable Dentures

A. Remove dentures from the patient's mouth. Usual hospital policy requires removal of dentures when a patient is unconscious.
B. Procedure for removal is described on page 513.
C. Clean the dentures (page 514) and store in water in a covered container by the patient's bedside. Fresh water or denture cleanser must be provided daily to prevent bacterial growth.[1]

III. General Mouth Cleaning

A. Edentulous and Dentulous
1. Clean the mouth at least three times each day to prevent dryness and sordes. Sordes is a crust-like material that collects on the lips, teeth, and gingiva of a patient with a fever or dehydration in a chronic debilitating disease.
2. Toothbrushing and flossing are essential for mechanical plaque removal. Other devices, such as swabs or gauze sponges, are much less effective and more time consuming.[2]

B. Brushing and Flossing
1. *Patient Who Can Rinse.* When unable to manipulate brush or floss but able to rinse and expectorate, a patient can be propped upright and an emesis basin used.
2. *Patient Who Cannot Participate.* Suction is a necessity. When suction is used, an assistant is needed, except for the suction toothbrush described in section IV.
3. *Brush.* A powered brush may be more efficient and thorough than a manual brush when an attendant must brush a helpless patient's teeth. A mouth prop can be placed in one side while the other side is retracted.

IV. Toothbrush with Suction Attachment

The toothbrush with attached suction provides an efficient and safe method for patient care.

A. Description of the Brush[3,4]

1. Soft-textured nylon brush with hole drilled between the bristles in the middle of the head of the brush.
2. Small plastic tubing inserted into hole; end adjusted slightly below level of brushing plane.
3. Other end of tubing passed across back of brush handle and attached to handle by small rubber bands (figure 51–1).
4. Tubing is connected by an adapter to aspirator or suction outlet.
5. Suction brushes are also manufactured commercially (see *Technical Hints* at the end of chapter).

B. Procedure for Use of Brush

The detailed procedure would be outlined for hospital personnel and included in the nursing procedures manual. An abbreviated outline of the basic steps is included here.

1. Prepare patient.
   a. The patient may be aware of what is going on, although may not respond in a usual manner.
   b. Tell patient that the teeth are going to be brushed, and thereafter maintain a one-way conversation despite patient's inability to respond verbally.
   c. Turn patient on a side and place a pillow at the back for support.
   d. Place a face towel under patient's chin and over bedding.
2. Attach toothbrush to suction outlet and lay brush on towel near patient's mouth.
3. Place a rubber bite block on one side of the patient's mouth between the teeth. String tied to bite block is fastened to the patient's gown with a safety pin.
4. Dip brush in fluoride mouthrinse; turn on suction.
5. Gently retract lip and carefully apply the appropriate toothbrushing procedures; apply suction over each tooth surface with particular care at each interproximal area. Moisten brush frequently.
6. Move bite block to opposite side of mouth and continue brushing procedure.
7. Place brush in cup of clear water to allow water to be sucked through to clear the tubing during the procedure, if there is clogging, and after brushing to clean the tube.
8. Remove bite block; wipe patient's lips with paper wipe and apply petrolatum.
9. Wash brush and bite block; prepare materials for next use.

V. Relief for Xerostomia

A. Lubricate Lips

Use petroleum jelly or other appropriate cream. Application may be needed several times each day.

B. Use Saliva Substitute

Swab the oral mucosa using a saliva substitute. Lemon and glycerin swabs formerly were used by hospital personnel, but the acidic effect of the lemon led to demineralization of enamel, and the drying effect of the glycerin was contradictory to the intended outcome.[5,6] Swabs prepared with saliva substitute are available to relieve xerostomia and can be used as frequently as needed throughout the day and night.[7]

TECHNICAL HINTS

I. Sources for Suction Toothbrushes

Ora Genics
5699 S.E. International Way, Unit D
Milwaukie, Oregon 97222
Vac-U-Brush

II. Insurance

Check practice liability insurance for alternate practice settings, such as a private home or nursing care facility.

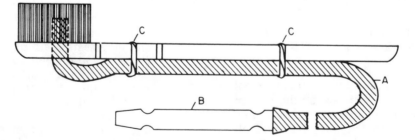

Figure 51–1. Suction Toothbrush. A. Plastic tubing. **B.** Adapter for attachment of the tubing to an aspirator or suction outlet. **C.** Small rubber bands attach the tubing to the brush handle. The plastic tube is inserted through a hole in the head of the brush and extended to a level slightly below the brushing plane.

References

1. DePaola, L.G. and Minah, G.E.: Isolation of Pathogenic Microorganisms from Dentures and Denture-soaking Containers of Myelosuppressed Cancer Patients, *J. Prosthet. Dent., 49,* 20, January, 1983.
2. Seto, B.G., Wolinsky, L.E., Tsutsui, P., and Avera, C.: Comparison of the Plaque-removing Efficacy of Four Nonbrushing Oral Hygiene Devices, *Clin. Prevent. Dent., 9,* 9, March-April, 1987.
3. Capps, J.S.: New Device for Oral Hygiene, *Am. J. Nursing, 58,* 1532, November, 1958.
4. Tronquet, A.A.: Oral Hygiene for Hospital Patients, *J. Am. Dent. Assoc., 63,* 215, August, 1961.
5. Daeffler, R.J.: Oral Care, *Hospice J., 2,* 81, Spring, 1986.
6. Poland, J.M.: Xerostomia in the Oncologic Patient. Combating Complications of Treatment, *Am. J. Hospice Care, 4,* 31, May/June, 1987.
7. *Moi-stir Oral Swabsticks,* Kingswood Laboratories, Inc., P.O. Box 744, Carmel, Indiana 46032.

Suggested Readings

American Dental Association: *Oral Health Care in the Nursing Facility.* Chicago, American Dental Association, (J 010 ADA Catalog).

American Dental Hygienists' Association: *Care for the Homebound Patient.* Chicago, American Dental Hygienists' Association, 1983, 18 pp.

Anderson, J.L.: Dental Treatment for Homebound and Institutionalized Patients, in Nowak, A.J.: *Dentistry for the Handicapped Patient.* St. Louis, The C.V. Mosby Co., 1976, pp. 211–224.

Baycar, R., Aker, F., and Serowski, A.: Portable Dental Chair, *Spec. Care Dentist., 3,* 57, March-April, 1983.

Ettinger, R.L., Rafal, S., and Potter, D.E.: Dental Care Programs for Chronically Ill Homebound Patients, for Residents of Nursing Homes and for Patients in Geriatric Hospitals, in Holm-Pedersen, P. and Löe, H., eds.: *Geriatric Dentistry.* Munksgaard, St. Louis, The C.V. Mosby Co., 1986, pp. 393–412.

Levine, W.A., Hoek, C.B., and Fenster, R.K.: An Occlusal Prosthesis to Assure Airway Patency in the Comatose Patient, *J. Prosthet. Dent., 44,* 451, October, 1980.

Napierski, G.E. and Danner, M.A.: Oral Hygiene for the Dentulous Total Care Patient, *Spec. Care Dentist., 2,* 257, November-December, 1982.

Niessen, L.: Dental Hygiene Caseload in a Chronic Care Facility, *Dent. Hyg., 58,* 164, April, 1984.

Olsen, R.A., Weiss, L.P., and Carlson, M.R.: Fiberoptics in Dentistry for the Homebound, *Spec. Care Dentist., 5,* 34, January-February, 1985.

Peters, T.E.D., Blair, A.E., and Freeman, R.G.: Prevention of Self-inflicted Trauma in Comatose Patients, *Oral Surg. Oral Med. Oral Pathol., 57,* 367, April, 1984.

Shaver, R.O.: Care for the Homebound Aged, *Spec. Care Dentist., 3,* 271, November-December, 1983.

Siskind-Houle, B.: The Dental Hygienist's Role in Care of the Elderly, *Dent. Hyg., 53,* 507, November, 1979.

Stiefel, D.J., Lubin, J.H., and Truelove, E.L.: A Survey of Perceived Oral Health Needs of Homebound Patients, *J. Public Health Dent., 39,* 7, Winter, 1979.

Nursing Care Facility

Benson, B.H., Niessen, L.C., and Toga, C.J.: Dental Treatment and Demand for Services in a Veterans Administration Nursing Home Care Unit, *J. Public Health Dent., 44,* 147, Fall, 1984.

Casamassimo, P.S., Coffee, L.M., and Leviton, F.J.: A Comparison of Two Mobile Treatment Programs for the Homebound and Nursing Home Patient, *Spec. Care Dentist., 8,* 77, March-April, 1988.

Ceridan, B.W.: Dentistry in a Nursing Home, *J. Am. Dent. Assoc., 114,* 302, March, 1987.

Duncan, J.L.: Incorporating Oral Hygiene Procedures in Geriatric Nursing Homes, *Dent. Hyg., 53,* 519, November, 1979.

Empey, G., Kiyak, H.A., and Milgrom, P.: Oral Health in Nursing Homes, *Spec. Care Dentist., 3,* 65, March-April, 1983.

Kamen, S.: The Resolution of Oral Health Care for the Institutionalized Geriatric Patient, *Spec. Care Dentist., 3,* 249, November-December, 1983.

Kimmel, H., Friedman, B., and Bachiman, R.: Outreach—Oral Health Care for Nursing Home Residents, *N.Y. State Dent. J., 46,* 265, May, 1980.

O'Laughlin, J.M.: A Comprehensive Oral Care Plan for Nursing Homes, *Spec. Care Dentist., 5,* 14, January-February, 1985.

Shareff, H.L. and Strauss, R.P.: Behavioral Influences on the Feasibility of Outpatient Dental Care for Nursing Home Residents, *Spec. Care Dentist., 5,* 270, November-December, 1985.

Simpson, R., Cunningham, M., Glenn, R., and Jakobsen, J.: Transportation Problems and Dental Care of Nursing Home Residents, *J. Am. Dent. Assoc., 106,* 178, February, 1983.

Yamagata, P.A.B., Sue, C., and Stiefel, D.J.: Use of Dental Service in a Nursing Home, *Spec. Care Dentist., 5,* 64, March-April, 1985.

Hospital Patient

Benson, C.M., Maibusch, R., and Zimmer, S.E.: Oral Health of Hospitalized Patients. Part I: An Overview of Oral Hygiene Nursing Care, *Dent. Hyg., 54,* 384, August, 1980.

DeLaney, D.F., VanOstenberg, P.R., and Salley, J.J.: A Dental Hygienist in the Hospital, *Dent. Hyg., 57,* 31, November, 1983.

Emery, C.A.: Evaluation of Oral Hygiene in a Hospitalized Population, *Gen. Dent., 28,* 54, January-February, 1980.

Gamble, J.W.: The Hospitalized Dental Patient, in Clark, J.W., ed. *Clinical Dentistry, Volume 1,* Chapter 32, Philadelphia, J.B. Lippincott, 1984, pp. 1–29.

Harris, N.O. and Christen, A.G.: Primary Preventive Dentistry in a Hospital Setting, in Harris, N.O. and Christen, A.G.: *Primary Preventive Dentistry,* 2nd ed. Norwalk, Connecticut, Appleton & Lange, 1987, pp. 503–532.

Miller, M.: Dental Health Education in the Hospital—A Role for the Dental Hygienist, *Can. Dent. Hyg., 13,* 38, Summer, 1979.

Pickard, R.G. and Grigel, M.A.: Provision of Preventive Dentistry in the Hospital Environment, *J. Am. Dent. Assoc., 100,* 881, June, 1980.

Roubenoff, R., Roubenoff, R.A., Preto, J., and Balke, C.W.: Malnutrition Among Hospitalized Patients, *Arch. Intern. Med., 147,* 1462, August, 1987.

Salley, J.J., VanOstenberg, P.R., and Gump, M.L.: Dentistry and Its Future in the Hospital Environment, *J. Am. Dent. Assoc., 101,* 236, August, 1980.

Smith, B.W.: Dentistry in the Hospital Setting, *Spec. Care Dentist., 4,* 56, March-April, 1984.

Zimmer, S. and Maibusch, R.: Oral Health of Hospitalized Patients: Part II. A Clinical Study, *Dent. Hyg., 54,* 423, September, 1980.

52 *The Patient with Epilepsy*

Epilepsy is not a disease entity, but is rather a term used to describe a symptom or group of symptoms of disordered function of the central nervous system. A person with epilepsy may be susceptible to recurrent involuntary loss of consciousness or awareness with or without convulsive movements or spasms. Some patients may have convulsions without loss of consciousness.

The patient's medical history should reveal a susceptibility to seizures, and the physician must be contacted when additional information other than that provided by the patient is required. The well-controlled patient who is under anticonvulsant medication usually presents no specific problems. An uncontrolled patient may require special treatment. A knowledge of symptoms is important in all cases, and dental personnel should know and be able to apply emergency measures in or out of the dental office.

Except for effects left by accidents occurring during a seizure, oral manifestations are limited to certain patients being treated with phenytoin (sodium diphenylhydantoin, Dilantin), which may induce a gingival overgrowth.

Care of the oral cavity becomes important for its relationship both to general health and to oral accidents that may occur during a severe attack. All patients are advised by their physicians to live a moderate lifestyle and pay strict attention to general health rules.

Occupation may be limited because the person with epilepsy cannot be permitted to participate in activities that provide hazards in the event of a seizure. Such limitation is particularly depressing to adults who have acquired epilepsy since reaching the working age and thus may be required to change their vocation.

DESCRIPTION[1,2,3]

A seizure is a convulsive disorder that results from a transient, uncontrolled alteration in brain function. The effect is an abrupt onset of symptoms that may be of a motor, sensory, or psychic nature, depending on which brain cells are involved.

I. Types of Seizures

The two basic types of seizures are *generalized* and *partial.* The international classification of seizures is outlined in table 52–1.

Table 52–1. International Classification of Seizures

Partial Seizures (seizures beginning locally)

A. Simple Partial Seizures (without loss of consciousness)

  1. With motor signs
  2. With somatosensory or special sensory symptoms
  3. With autonomic symptoms
  4. With psychic symptoms

B. Complex Partial Seizures

  1. Simple partial onset followed by impairment of consciousness
  2. With impairment of consciousness at onset

C. Partial Seizures Evolving to Generalized Tonic-clonic Convulsions (secondarily generalized)

Generalized Seizures (bilaterally symmetrical, without local onset)

A. Nonconvulsive Seizures

  1. Absence seizures
  2. Atypical absence seizures
  3. Myoclonic seizures
  4. Atonic seizures

B. Convulsive Seizures

  1. Tonic-clonic seizures
  2. Tonic seizures
  3. Clonic seizures

Unclassified Epileptic Seizures

(From International League Against Epilepsy, Commission on Classification and Terminology: Proposal for Revised Clinical and Electroencephalographic Classification of Epileptic Seizures, *Epilepsia,* 22, 489, August, 1981.)

A seizure that is focal in origin and involves only a part of the brain is called a partial seizure. A generalized seizure, on the other hand, is not specific in area of origin and affects the entire brain at the same time. Terminology used in table 52–1 and in the study of seizures is defined in table 52–2.

II. Etiology[2,3]

Epilepsy is a symptom of a disorder of the central nervous system, the explanation for which is not clear. During infancy, seizures can be related to congenital maldevelopment or a birth injury, whereas in

Table 52–2.   Glossary of Terms for the Study of Seizures

Absence: a generalized seizure of sudden onset characterized by a brief period of unconsciousness. Formerly called petit mal.

Atonic: relaxed; without normal tone or tension.

Aura: warning sensation felt by some people immediately preceding a seizure; may be flashes of light, dizziness, peculiar taste, or sensation of prickling or tingling.

Automatism: involuntary motor activity, such as lip smacking or repeated swallowing.

Autonomic symptoms: pallor, flushing, sweating, pupillary dilation, cardiac arrhythmia, incontinence.

Clonic: alternate contraction and relaxation of muscle.

Consciousness: degree of awareness and/or responsiveness of a person to externally applied stimuli.

Convulsion: a violent spasm.

Grand mal: name formerly used for a generalized or major seizure.

Myoclonic: a spasm or twitching of a muscle or group of muscles; may be generalized or confined to a certain body area; isolated or repetitive.

Paresthesia: an abnormal spontaneous sensation, such as burning, prickling, or tingling.

Petit mal: name formerly used for generalized absence or minor epilepsy.

Psychic symptoms: dreamy states, time distortion, fear, rage, depression, illusions, hallucinations.

Seizure: an episode of abnormal motor, sensory, autonomic, or psychic activity (or combination of these) as a consequence of sudden excessive discharge from cerebral neurons. A part or all of the brain may be involved.

Spasm: an involuntary muscular contraction; may be tonic or clonic.

Status epilepticus: rapid, repetitive recurrence of seizures without regaining consciousness between attacks; life threatening; emergency care urgent.

Tonic: state of continuous, unremitting action of a muscular contraction.

Tonic-clonic: in a seizure, a sudden sharp tonic contraction of muscles; followed by clonic convulsive movements.

---

older children and adolescents, trauma, infections, or idiopathic causes also are possible. In middle age and older, vascular disease, and the other symptomatic factors listed here are predominant.

A. Idiopathic Epilepsy
1. Genetic predisposition to seizures or to other neurologic abnormalities for which seizure may be a symptom.
2. Congenital conditions, such as maternal infection (rubella).
3. Tends to manifest early in life; onset of majority of cases between ages 2 and 14 years.

B. Acquired Epilepsy
1. Known cerebral lesion brings about dysfunction leading to seizures.
   a. Brain tumor.
   b. Trauma (head injury).
   c. Infection (meningitis, encephalitis).
   d. Degenerative brain disease.
2. Alcoholism and drug addiction; seizures are common during drug withdrawal.

III. Clinical Manifestations

A. Possible Precipitating Factors
1. Psychologic stress; apprehension.
2. Fatigue; sleep deprivation.
3. Sensory stimuli: flashing lights, noises, peculiar odors.
4. Alcohol use; withdrawal from alcohol or other substances.

B. Aura
Not all patients have a warning, or aura, before a seizure. A patient with a warning may seek a safe place to sit or lie down in privacy. In the dental environment, the patient can inform the personnel, so that procedures can be terminated and brief preparations made.

The aura may be a special sensory stimulus, a sensation of numbness, tingling, or a twitching or stiffness of certain muscles.

C. Partial Seizures
1. *Simple.* Seizures may include a brief staring spell, a shake of a finger or hand and/or a jerk of muscles about the mouth. Although dizziness and jumbled speech may occur, loss of consciousness does not result.
2. *Complex*
   a. Trance-like state with confusion lasts usually for a few minutes, sometimes for hours.
   b. Consciousness is impaired to varying degrees.
   c. Patient may manifest purposeless movements or actions followed by confusion, incoherent speech, ill humor, bad temper; does not remember what happened during the attack.

D. Generalized Absence
1. Loss of consciousness for 5 to 30 seconds.
2. Patient usually does not fall; posture becomes fixed; may drop whatever is being held.

3. May become pale.
4. May have rhythmic twitching of eyelids, eyebrows, or head.
5. Attack ends as abruptly as it begins. Patient resumes activities; may or may not be aware of attack.

E. Generalized Tonic-Clonic

1. Loss of consciousness is sudden and complete; the patient falls. A patient may slide out of the dental chair.
2. The entire voluntary musculature experiences continuous contraction, which is the *tonic* (tension with rigidity) phase. The *clonic* movements follow, with intermittent muscular contraction and relaxation.
3. Muscles of the chest and pharynx may contract at the same time, thus forcing air out. The result is a peculiar sound known as the "epileptic cry."
4. Color is pale at first, then the superficial veins become gorged. The chest becomes fixed and aeration of blood ceases, leading to cyanosis of the face.
5. Pupils dilate.
6. Intermittent muscular contractions follow, rapidly at first, then less frequently. If the tongue is between the teeth, it may be bitten.
7. The incident lasts from 1 to 3 minutes; the bladder, and rarely the rectum, may be emptied.
8. Respiration begins to return. Saliva, which previously could not be swallowed, may become mixed with air and appear as foam.
9. Postconvulsive coma is characterized by fixed or sluggish pupils, noisy respiration, profuse perspiration, cyanosed lips, and complete relaxation of body muscles.
10. Patient emerges in a cloudy state.
11. Postconvulsive phase includes headache, muscle aches, and drowsiness. Patient usually falls into a deep sleep.

IV. Treatment[2,3]

Anticonvulsant drugs are used to prevent seizures.[4,5]

Patients whose epilepsy is caused by a brain tumor undergo surgery for tumor removal. Anticonvulsant medication is usually necessary following the surgery.

In addition to medication, patients frequently need psychologic or psychiatric support therapy to aid in coping with problems during rehabilitation. Psychologic stress may increase the frequency of seizures.

ORAL FINDINGS

Epilepsy in itself produces no oral changes. Specific effects relate to anticonvulsant therapy using phenytoin and to the results of oral accidents during seizures.

I. Gingival Manifestation

Phenytoin-induced gingival overgrowth occurs in 25 to 50 percent of persons using phenytoin for treatment.[6] No other anticonvulsant drug produces such an unusual side effect. Other drugs that produce a similar gingival enlargement are described on page 186.

Phenytoin has been used in the treatment of many conditions other than epilepsy. These include behavior problems, stuttering, headaches, neuromuscular disturbances, and cardiac conditions. The presence of gingival enlargement and a history of phenytoin use should not lead to the assumption that the patient has epilepsy.

II. Effects of Accidents During Seizures

A. Scars of Lips and Tongue

During generalized tonic-clonic seizures, the oral tissues, particularly tongue, cheek, or lip, may be bitten. Scars may be observed during the extraoral/intraoral examination, and the cause may be differentiated from other types of healed wounds.

B. Fractured Teeth

During the tonic and clonic movements, the teeth may be clamped and bruxing may be forceful enough to fracture teeth.

PHENYTOIN-INDUCED GINGIVAL ENLARGEMENT (OVERGROWTH)

Gingival enlargement is one of several side effects from treatment with phenytoin. The condition is also called Dilantin hyperplasia, Dilantin-induced hyperplasia, diphenylhydantoin-induced hyperplasia, diphenylhydantoin gingival hyperplasia, Dilantin-induced gingival fibrosis, and phenytoin-induced hyperplasia.

I. Side Effects of Phenytoin

In addition to gingival overgrowth, other long-term side effects may influence dental hygiene appointments. During history preparation and the extraoral/intraoral examination, the effects described below can aid in understanding the patient and planning treatment.

A. General Effects That May Occur[7]

Drowsiness, gastric distress, skin rash, ataxia (loss of muscular coordination that may be apparent by an unsteady gait), and restlessness are not uncommon. Increased body and facial hair growth may occur in women.

B. Nutritional Influences

Vitamins K, D, and folic acid are affected by anticonvulsant drugs. A megaloblastic anemia can result from a low folic acid blood level, which is described on page 704. Epithelial changes, such as glossitis, angular cheilitis, and ulcerations of the lips, tongue, and buccal mucosa, may be observed.[8]

C. Fetal Hydantoin Syndrome[7,9]

Children of women receiving anticonvulsant therapy during pregnancy are more susceptible to malformations. They may have craniofacial abnormalities, growth retardation, mental deficiency, congenital heart defects, and cleft lip and/or palate.

II. Occurrence[6]

A. Age

Incidence is greater in younger patients than in older patients just beginning therapy.

B. Initial Enlargement

The gingiva may start to enlarge within a few weeks or even after a few years following the initial administration of the drug.

C. Dosage and Length of Treatment

The size of the dose and the length of treatment are not necessarily factors in the incidence or nature of the gingival enlargement.

D. Sites

The anterior gingiva are usually more affected than the posterior, and the maxillary more than the mandibular. Facial and proximal areas are usually larger than lingual and palatal.

E. Edentulous Areas

Although rare, an overgrowth of tissue may occur in an edentulous area. A source of trauma or irritation from a denture or the presence of retained roots and unerupted teeth usually has been associated with the overgrowth.[10]

III. Tissue Characteristics

A. Early Clinical Features

The overgrowth appears as a painless enlargement of interdental papillae with signs of inflammation. Eventually, the tissue becomes fibrotic, pink, and stippled, with a mulberry- or cauliflower-like appearance (figure 52–1B).

B. Advanced Lesion

With time, the tissue increases in size, extends to include the marginal gingiva, and covers a large portion of the anatomic crown. Often, cleft-like grooves are between the lobules (figure 52–1A).

C. Severe Lesion

Large, bulbous gingiva may cover the enamel, tend to wedge the teeth apart, and interfere with mastication. Note the severe growth about the mandibular left canine in figure 52–1A.

D. Microscopic Appearance

During therapy, phenytoin is present in the saliva, blood, gingival sulcus fluid, and bacterial

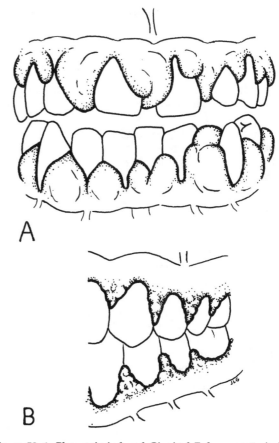

Figure 52–1. Phenytoin-induced Gingival Enlargement. A. Papillary enlargement with cleft-like grooves. Note the effect of the pressure of the fibrotic tissue on the position of teeth. Maxillary incisors and the mandibular left canine have been wedged away from normal positions. **B.** Mulberry-like shape of interdental papillae.

plaque. The number of fibroblasts and the amount of collagen in the tissue are increased. The stratified squamous epithelium is thick, with long rete pegs. Inflammatory cells are in greatest abundance near the base of the pocket.

IV. Complicating Factors

A. Plaque and Gingivitis

Adequate plaque control, particularly if started before the administration of phenytoin, may decrease the extent of gingival overgrowth.[6,11,12] Application of antiplaque agents (stannous fluoride,[13] chlorhexidine[14]) has been effective in decreasing bacterial plaque formation and gingival overgrowth.

B. Other Contributing Factors

Mouthbreathing, overhanging and other defective restorations, large carious lesions, calculus, and other plaque-retaining factors encourage gingival overgrowth. Treatment must include removal of overhangs and calculus and restoration of carious lesions.

V. Treatment of Phenytoin-induced Gingival Overgrowth

A. Conservative Treatment

Scaling with a concentrated program of bacterial plaque control and oral physical therapy may help early lesions to regress. Once the tissue has become fibrotic, however, shrinkage cannot be expected.

A program of prevention and control should be started prior to, or simultaneously with, the initial administration of phenytoin.

B. Change in Drug Prescription

Phenytoin alone or with phenobarbital has been a drug of choice for use with patients subject to generalized seizures since the drug was introduced in 1938. Other drugs in current use do not induce gingival enlargement. When the patient has a severe problem and is faced with embarrassment and social problems because of the appearance of the gingiva, the physician could be approached concerning the possibility of changing the prescription to a different drug. If possible, such a change should be made just prior to gingivectomy or other surgical removal procedure that may be planned.

C. Surgical Removal

Assuming a sufficient band of attached gingiva exists, one surgical procedure that has been used for tissue removal has been gingivectomy. Prior to surgery, a regulated program of plaque control should be introduced and continued as soon as surgical dressings have been removed.[15]

DENTAL HYGIENE CARE

For the patient with epilepsy, general health has special significance, and oral health contributes to general health. For the patient with phenytoin-induced gingival enlargement, emphasis in appointments is on a rigid oral hygiene program if the gingival enlargement is to be kept to a minimum.

I. Patient History

Except in an unusual situation, most patients with epilepsy will have had a thorough medical examination prior to the dental appointment. In preparing the patient history, however, all patients should be asked whether they ever had a seizure or currently have recurrent or occasional seizures. When the answer is positive, additional questioning is indicated.

A. History of Seizures

Questioning includes type, frequency, severity, and duration of episodes. The precipitating factors, need for any special premedication, and all information that may have application during the dental and dental hygiene appointments must be carefully documented.

B. Medications

The type, dosage, effectiveness in seizure control, and known side effects of medication are recorded. Patients using valproic acid may be subject to blood coagulation defects and should be questioned concerning bleeding and ease of bruising.[16] Prior to deep scaling or surgical procedures, when bleeding can be expected, blood testing for platelet count and bleeding time provides important information for the prevention of an emergency situation.

II. Patient Approach

A. Provide a calm, reassuring atmosphere.
B. Treat with patience and empathy; avoid over-solicitousness.
C. Encourage self-expression, particularly if the patient tends to be quiet and withdrawn and has narrowed interests.
D. Recognize possible impairment of memory when reviewing personal oral care procedures.
E. Help patient to develop interest in caring for the mouth; commend all little successes.
F. Drugs used in treatment tend to make patient drowsy.
   1. Be understanding when patient is late or misses an appointment.
   2. Plan telephone reminder at opportune time if patient is chronically late.
   3. Do not mistake drowsiness (effect of drugs) for inattentiveness.

III. Treatment Plan: Instrumentation

The treatment needs of a patient with phenytoin-induced gingival enlargement were described earlier. The dental hygiene treatment, planned within the total treatment plan, is determined by whether the patient is just starting phenytoin therapy or, if already receiving phenytoin, by the severity of the gingival enlargement.

A. Prior To and At the Start of Phenytoin Therapy

A rigorous plaque control program and complete scaling are introduced in preparation for phenytoin therapy. The patient (and parents) must understand that, with controlled oral hygiene and emphasis on all phases of prevention, gingival enlargement can be prevented to a large degree.[11,12,13]

B. Initial Appointment Series for Patient Treated With Phenytoin

Weekly appointments for complete plaque control instruction and scaling are planned with the following objectives:
1. *Slight or Mild Gingival Overgrowth.* Conservative treatment, including frequent thorough scalings, can be expected to lead to tissue reduction, provided the patient cooperates in daily plaque control. Frequent maintenance appointments can contribute to function and

comfort with minimum periodontal involvement.

2. *Moderate Gingival Overgrowth.* After the initial series of weekly plaque instruction and scalings, reevaluation of the tissue can determine whether further procedures are needed. An optimum level of oral health may be attained by changing the medication to another anticonvulsant drug, using surgical pocket removal, and continuing frequent maintenance appointments.

3. *Severe Fibrotic Overgrowth.* Initial scaling and plaque control are carried out to prepare the mouth for surgical pocket removal. Plans for changing the drug or altering the dose should be discussed with the patient's physician.

C. Maintenance Appointment Intervals

Frequent appointments on a 1-, 2- or 3-month plan are indicated, depending on the severity of the gingival enlargement and the ability and motivation of the patient to maintain the oral health. Most patients need continuing assistance and supervision, and their response is influenced by the instruction and devotion of the dental personnel.

IV. Treatment Plan: Prevention

Daily plaque removal and fluoride therapy, the use of pit and fissure sealants, and dietary control all have a vital part in the care of the patient with a convulsive disorder. Initiation of preventive measures as soon as possible after the disorder has been diagnosed can contribute to the total health and well-being of the patient.

EMERGENCY CARE[2]

When a seizure occurs, no attempt should be made to stop the convulsion or to restrain the patient. An outline for procedure appears in table 60–1 on page 752. Some additional suggestions regarding patient care during a generalized seizure that are applicable in a dental office are included here.

I. Objectives

A. To prevent body injury.
B. To prevent accidents related to the oral structures, such as:
  1. Tongue bite.
  2. Broken or dislocated teeth.
  3. Dislocated or fractured jaw.
  4. Broken fixed or removable dentures.
C. To assure adequate ventilation.

II. Preparation for Appointment

When the patient's medical history indicates epilepsy, precautions may prevent complications should a seizure occur.
A. Emergency materials should be readied in a convenient place.

B. Have patient remove dentures for duration of appointment.
C. Provide a calm and reassuring atmosphere.
D. Have other dental personnel available in case of an emergency.

III. First Signs of Seizure

A. Lower the dental chair and tilt back; ease the patient to the floor if space permits.
B. Establish airway.
C. Do not restrain the patient in any way.
D. Clear aside movable dental equipment and sharp, potentially injurious instruments.
E. Turn patient's head gently on side to prevent aspiration of saliva and to prevent the tongue from dropping back. Do not apply force to turn the head while the neck is stiff during the convulsive stage.
F. Check for breathing obstruction.
G. Loosen tight belt, collar, necktie.
H. *Do not* force anything between the teeth. If an instrument becomes clamped between the teeth during a sudden attack, do not attempt to remove it.
I. Monitor vital signs; initiate basic life support if indicated; summon medical assistance.
J. Observe patient's actions and prepare a report for the patient's dental record, as well as for the physician (page 737 and figure 60–1).

IV. Postconvulsive Phase

A. Allow patient to rest.
B. Talk to the patient in a low, reassuring tone. Ask onlookers to leave the patient in privacy.
C. When repeated convulsions occur, promptly obtain medical help.
D. Check oral cavity for trauma to teeth or tissues. Palliative care can be administered. When a tooth is broken, the piece must be located so that aspiration can be prevented.

TECHNICAL HINTS

I. Never use a glass syringe or other breakable instrument when a seizure could occur.
II. When a patient vomits during a seizure, use high-power evacuator with wide tip to remove material from the mouth as a first aid measure against aspiration of vomitus into the airway.
III. Source of Informational Materials

Epilepsy Foundation of America
1828 L Street N.W.
Washington, D.C. 20036

References

1. International League Against Epilepsy, Commission on Classification and Terminology: Proposal for Revised Clinical and Electroencephalographic Classification of Epileptic Seizures, *Epilepsia, 22,* 489, August, 1981.
2. Malamed, S.F.: *Handbook of Medical Emergencies in the Den-*

tal Office, 3rd ed. St. Louis, The C.V. Mosby Co., 1987, pp. 238–252.

3. Brunner, L.S., Suddarth, D.S., Bare, B.G., Boyer, M.J., and Smeltzer, S.C.O.: *Textbook of Medical-Surgical Nursing,* 6th ed., Philadelphia, J.B. Lippincott, 1988, pp. 1489–1495.

4. Requa, B.S. and Holroyd, S.V.: *Applied Pharmacology for the Dental Hygienist.* St. Louis, The C.V. Mosby Co., 1982, pp. 231–238.

5. Snyder, N.C.: *Dental Hygiene Clinical Applications in Pharmacology.* Philadelphia, Lea & Febiger, 1987, pp. 179–188.

6. Hassell, T.M.: *Epilepsy and the Oral Manifestations of Phenytoin Therapy.* Monographs in Oral Science, Volume 9. London, S. Karger, 1981, pp. 116–127.

7. Felpel, L.P.: Anticonvulsants, in Neidle, E.A., Kroeger, D.C., and Yagiela, J.A.: *Pharmacology and Therapeutics for Dentistry,* 2nd ed. St. Louis, The C.V. Mosby Co., 1985, pp. 225–236.

8. Mallek, H.M. and Nakamoto, T.: Dilantin and Folic Acid Status. Clinical Implications for the Periodontist, *J. Periodontol., 52,* 255, May, 1981.

9. Friis, M.L.: Epilepsy Among Parents of Children With Facial Clefts, *Epilepsia, 20,* 69, February, 1979.

10. Dreyer, W.P. and Thomas, C.J.: Diphenylhydantoinate-induced Hyperplasia of the Masticatory Mucosa in an Edentulous Epileptic Patient, *Oral Surg. Oral Med. Oral Pathol., 45,* 701, May, 1978.

11. Pihlstrom, B.L., Carlson, J.F., Smith, Q.T., Bastien, S.A., and Keenan, K.M.: Prevention of Phenytoin Associated Gingival Enlargement—a 15-month Longitudinal Study, *J. Periodontol., 51,* 311, June, 1980.

12. Allan, S.: The Role of the Dental Hygienist in the Prevention, Control and Treatment of Dilantin Hyperplasia, *Can. Dent. Hyg. (Probe), 20,* 139, December, 1986.

13. Steinberg, S.C. and Steinberg, A.D.: Phenytoin-induced Gingival Overgrowth Control in Severely Retarded Children, *J. Periodontol., 53,* 429, July, 1982.

14. O'Neil, T.C.A. and Figures, K.H.: The Effects of Chlorhexidine and Mechanical Methods of Plaque Control on the Recurrence of Gingival Hyperplasia in Young Patients Taking Phenytoin, *Br. Dent. J., 152,* 130, February 16, 1982.

15. King, D.A., Hawes, R.R., and Bibby, B.G.: The Effect of Oral Physiotherapy on Dilantin Gingival Hyperplasia, *J. Oral Pathol., 5,* 1, Number 1, 1976.

16. Hassell, T.M., White, G.C., Jewson, L.G., and Peele, L.C.: Valproic Acid: A New Antiepileptic Drug With Potential Side Effects of Dental Concern, *J. Am. Dent. Assoc., 99,* 983, December, 1979.

Suggested Readings

Addy, V., McElnay, J.C., Eyre, D.G., Campbell, N., and D'Arcy, P.F.: Risk Factors in Phenytoin-induced Gingival Hyperplasia, *J. Periodontol., 54,* 373, June, 1983.

Brunsvold, M., Tomasovic, J., and Ruemping, D.: The Measured Effect of Phenytoin Withdrawal on Gingival Hyperplasia in Children, *ASDC J. Dent. Child., 52,* 417, November-December, 1985.

Church, L.F. and Brandt, S.K.: Phenytoin-induced Gingival Overgrowth Resulting in Delayed Eruption of the Primary Dentition. A Case Report, *J. Periodontol., 55,* 19, January, 1984.

Dahllöf, G. and Modeer, T.: The Effect of a Plaque Control Program on the Development of Phenytoin-induced Gingival Overgrowth. A 2-year Longitudinal Study, *J. Clin. Periodontol., 13,* 845, October, 1986.

Drew, H.J., Vogel, R.I., Molofsky, W., Baker, H., and Frank, O.: Effect of Folate on Phenytoin Hyperplasia, *J. Clin. Periodontol., 14,* 350, July, 1987.

EeG-Olofsson, O., Lundström, A., and Hamp, S.-E.: Oral State of Children With Epilepsy on Treatment with Sodium Valproate, *Scand. J. Dent. Res., 91,* 219, June, 1983.

Hassell, T., O'Donnell, J., Pearlman, J., Tesini, D., Murphy, T., and Best, H.: Phenytoin Induced Gingival Overgrowth in Institutionalized Epileptics, *J. Clin. Periodontol., 11,* 242, April, 1984.

Holmes, G.L., Blair, S., Eisenberg, E., Scheebaum, R., Margraf, J., and Zimmerman, A.W.: Tooth-brushing-induced Epilepsy, *Epilepsia, 23,* 657, December, 1982.

Lundström, A., Eeg-Olofsson, O., and Hamp, S.-E.: Effects of Antiepileptic Drug Treatment With Carbamazepine or Phenytoin on the Oral State of Children and Adolescents, *J. Clin. Periodontol., 9,* 482, November, 1982.

Marshall, W.R., Lattanzi, D.A., Weaver, G.S., and Schmitt, L.J.: Laser Excision of Type III Phenytoin-induced Gingival Hyperplasia, *Spec. Care Dentist., 7,* 207, September-October, 1987.

Modeer, T. and Dahllöf, G.: Development of Phenytoin-induced Gingival Overgrowth in Non-institutionalized Epileptic Children Subjected to Different Plaque Control Programs, *Acta Odontol. Scand., 45,* 81, Number 2, 1987.

Peoples, G.A.: Anesthetic and Surgical Considerations in Children With Dilantin Gingival Hyperplasia, *J. Oral Med., 35,* 97, October-December, 1980.

Pick, R.M., Pecaro, B.C., and Silberman, C.J.: The Laser Gingivectomy. The Use of the CO$_2$ Laser for the Removal of Phenytoin Hyperplasia, *J. Periodontol., 56,* 492, August, 1985.

Reich, D.R., Bernbaum, J., and Moskowitz, W.B.: Passive Delayed Eruption of the Primary Dentition Secondary to Dilantin Administration, *Oral Surg. Oral Med. Oral Pathol., 52,* 599, December, 1981.

Reynolds, N.C. and Kirkham, D.B.: Therapeutic Alternatives in Phenytoin-induced Gingival Hyperplasia. A Case Report and Discussion, *J. Periodontol., 51,* 516, September, 1980.

Roberge, R.J. and Maceira-Rodriguez, L.: Seizure-related Oral Lacerations: Incidence and Distribution, *J. Am. Dent. Assoc., 111,* 279, August, 1985.

Robinson, P.B., Harris, M., and Harvey, W.: Abnormal Skeletal and Dental Growth in Epileptic Children, *Br. Dent. J., 154,* 9, January 8, 1983.

Royer, J.E., Hendrickson, D.A., and Scharpf, H.O.: Phenytoin-induced Hyperplasia of the Pre-eruptive Stage, *Oral Surg. Oral Med. Oral Pathol., 56,* 365, October, 1983.

Rucker, L.M.: Prosthetic Treatment for the Patient With Uncontrolled Grand Mal Epileptic Seizures, *Spec. Care Dentist., 5,* 206, September-October, 1985.

Seymour, R.A., Smith, D.G., and Turnbull, D.N.: The Effects of Phenytoin and Sodium Valproate on the Periodontal Health of Adult Epileptic Patients, *J. Clin. Periodontol., 12,* 413, July, 1985.

Steinberg, A.D.: Office Management of Phenytoin-induced Gingival Overgrowth, *Compend. Contin. Educ. Dent., 6,* 138, February, 1985.

Stinnett, E., Rodu, B., and Grizzle, W.E.: New Developments in Understanding Phenytoin-induced Gingival Hyperplasia, *J. Am. Dent. Assoc., 114,* 814, June, 1987.

53 *The Patient with Mental Retardation*

With trends toward deinstitutionalization and emphasis on special training and education in local agencies and schools, more people with mild and moderate mental retardation have appeared as dental and dental hygiene patients in private dental offices and clinics, as well as in school and community dental facilities. Dental hygienists in all settings have opportunities to contribute to the health and well-being of this special group.

I. Definitions

A. Mental Retardation

Mental retardation refers to significantly subaverage general intellectual functioning that exists concurrently with deficits in adaptive functioning and manifests during the developmental period before the age of 18.[1]

General intellectual functioning is defined by an intelligence quotient (IQ or IQ equivalent) obtained by use of one or more individually administered tests. Significant subaverage intellectual functioning is specified as an IQ of 70 or below and generally is considered within the range of 65 to 75 to meet individual differences.

Adaptive functioning refers to the person's effectiveness in social skills, communication, and daily living skills, as well as to how standards of personal independence and social responsibility characteristic of the age and cultural group are met. Adaptive functioning is influenced by such factors as motivation, education, and social and vocational opportunities and has more chance for improvement by remedial efforts than does IQ, which tends to be more fixed.[1]

B. Mental Deficiency

The term *mental deficiency* may be used interchangeably with mental retardation, although mental deficiency is more frequently used to imply persons of all ages, whether manifested in the developmental period or later.

C. Mental Illness

Mental retardation must not be confused with mental illness. The term mentally ill refers to a person with an emotional disorder. Examples of severe mental illnesses are schizophrenia and psychoses, and examples of less severe mental illnesses are personality disorders and psychoneuroses. The symptoms and methods for treatment of mental illnesses are very different from those of mental retardation.

A person with mental retardation can become disturbed or mentally ill. Special treatment then would be needed, and the attitude and support of professional persons can be especially important.

II. Levels of Mental Retardation

The levels of intellectual functioning are designated *mild, moderate, severe,* and *profound.* Standardized intelligence tests are used to determine individual levels. The Intelligence Quotient (IQ) expresses the test results. A category of *Unspecified Mental Retardation* is used when standard tests cannot be performed because of lack of cooperation, severe impairment, or infancy.

Adaptive functioning is described briefly for each of the categories as they are listed below. An understanding of expected capabilities can help to provide necessary background information for teaching basic oral care procedures.

A. Mild Retardation
1. *IQ.* 50–55 to approximately 70.
2. *Adaptive Functioning*
   a. Child. In special classes for the educable, the child advances to a level of third to sixth grade. Practical skills can be learned.
   b. Adult. At adult level, the individual cares for personal hygiene and other necessities, with reminders. Communication is good, although the attention span and memory are less than average. Activities that do not require involved planning or rapid implementation can be carried out satisfactorily. Most educable individuals can engage in semiskilled or simple skilled work with guidance, and so maintain themselves.

B. Moderate Retardation
1. *IQ.* 35–40 to 50–55.
2. *Adaptive Functioning.*
   a. Child. A marked developmental lag occurs in the early years, but the child can be trained in personal care and hygiene with help. These children attend classes and learn simple habits and skills, but they do not learn to read and write. They speak in short sentences, and understand best when

single-thought, short sentences are used. They participate well in group activities.

   b. Adult. As adults, these individuals attend to personal care, with reminders, and have a relatively short attention span and memory. Although they may have problems of coordination, they perform simple tasks and are conscientious about taking responsibility for errands and helpful duties. Although not completely capable of self-maintenance, many do unskilled work with direct supervision.

C. Severe Retardation
   1. *IQ.* 20–25 to 35–40.
   2. *Adaptive Functioning*
     a. Child. Children at this level can benefit from systematic habit training and may make attempts at personal care and dressing with assistance. They usually walk, use some speech, and respond to directions.
     b. Adult. Adults conform to a daily routine and may help with household and other small tasks, in spite of a limited attention span. Some personal care with supervision is possible.

D. Profound Retardation
   1. *IQ.* Below 20 or 25.
   2. *Adaptive Functioning*
     a. Child. Delays occur in all phases of development, and close supervision and care are necessary.
     b. Adult. Many remain inert and placid throughout the early years and never learn to sit up. A few may learn a few words, but as a group their ability to interact is lacking. Nursing care is needed, and many cannot feed themselves.

ETIOLOGY OF MENTAL RETARDATION[1]

Mental retardation represents a more or less important symptom in well over 200 different conditions. Many of these are rare. A variety of means of classification is found in the literature. It has been convenient to divide the causes into factors operating before birth, at birth, and after birth.

A majority of cases of mental retardation results from prenatal influences; a small number is effected as injuries at birth. Diagnosis may be complicated and difficult, and many cases can only be classified as of unknown origin.

I. Major Causative Factors[1]

A. Hereditary factors.
B. Early alterations of embryonic development.
C. Pregnancy and perinatal problems.
D. Physical disorders acquired in childhood.
E. Environmental influences.
F. Unknown.

II. Examples During Prenatal Period
A. Infections
   Brain damage can result from maternal infection during pregnancy. Serious infections during the first trimester are most likely to cause physical malformations.

   1. *Congenital Rubella Syndrome.* German measles virus infection during the first trimester may result in abnormalities, and mental retardation may occur. The rubella syndrome also may include cataracts, cardiac anomalies, deafness, and microcephaly.

     Immunization with rubella vaccine has reduced the incidence of the disease in the general population. Because more prospective mothers now are immune than were in the past, retardation related to the virus infection has been reduced.

   2. *Congenital Syphilis.* Transfer of syphilis from the mother leads to numerous symptoms, and when the central nervous system is involved, hydrocephalus, convulsions, and mental retardation can result. Hutchinson's triad, which is associated with the late stage of congenital syphilis, includes deafness, interstitial keratitis, and dental defects. Hutchinsonian incisors, which are notched and tapered, mulberry molars, and microdontia are typical (figure 14–2, page 213).

   3. *Neonatal Congenital Toxoplasmosis.* Infection of the fetus transplacentally may lead to miscarriage, stillbirth, or a living baby with severe clinical disease. The effects may include hydrocephalus or microcephalus, blindness, and mental retardation.

B. Metabolic Disorders
   1. *Phenylketonuria (PKU).* Phenylketonuria results from an error of metabolism in which the enzyme necessary for digestion of the amino acid phenylalanine is missing. Severe mental retardation is a consequence. Early recognition of the missing enzyme with early dietary control lessens the severity of retardation. Many states require blood and urine screening tests soon after an infant is born. A diet free from animal and vegetable protein is necessary.

   2. *Congenital Hypothyroidism.* Cretinism is usually the result of partial or complete absence of the thyroid gland at birth. Mental retardation accompanies a variety of physical symptoms related to defective development.

C. Chromosomal Abnormality
   Down's syndrome is described in a separate section on pages 650–651.

III. Examples of Pregnancy and Birth

A. Mechanical Injury at Birth
Damage leading to mental retardation may have a variety of causes, including difficulties of labor and delivery.

B. Hypoxia
Asphyxiation from prolonged oxygen deficiency may result from labor complications.

C. Fetal Alcohol Syndrome (FAS) (page 728)

IV. Examples During Postnatal Period

A. Infections
Cerebral infection may be caused by a wide variety of organisms. Examples of diseases that may have this effect are encephalitis and meningitis.

B. Postnatal Trauma
Accidents may result in a fractured skull or prolonged unconsciousness.

C. Nutritional Disorder
Dietary imbalances and inadequacies, debilitating diseases, or parasitic diseases can lead to slow development and retardation.

GENERAL CHARACTERISTICS

I. Physical Features

Because most individuals with mental retardation are in the borderline and mild categories, no unusual physical characteristics should be expected at initial patient evaluation, other than those present in the usual population of normal intelligence.

Within the low moderate, severe, and profound groups certain physical variations appear more frequently. Facial or other characteristics may be pathognomonic for a particular condition or syndrome; that is, there may be an identifying characteristic that is specific for that condition and rarely occurs in other syndromes.

Skull anomalies include microcephaly (smaller), hydrocephalus (larger, contains fluid), spherical, conical, or otherwise asymmetrical shapes. Other features, such as asymmetries of the face, malformations of the outer ear, anomalies of the eyes, or unusual shape of the nose, may be present. Growth and physiologic development are generally delayed.

II. Oral Findings

A higher incidence of oral developmental malformations has been observed, some specifically associated with particular syndromes or conditions. Oral findings that have been observed to occur more frequently in individuals with mental retardation than in those with normal intelligence include the following:

A. Lips
Thickness of the lips is common.

B. Tooth Anomalies
Teeth may be imperfectly formed; eruption patterns may be delayed or irregular.

C. Periodontal Conditions[2,3]
Gingivitis and periodontitis are common in individuals with mental retardation. Patients with Down's syndrome have more severe disease than do those from other groups with mental retardation.

D. Habits
Incidence of clenching, bruxing, mouth-breathing, and tongue thrusting is increased.

E. Dental Caries[2,3]
The factors that are effective in the prevention of dental caries in the special group are the same as those in a population of normal intelligence. These factors include exposure to fluoridation and other forms of fluoride, form and frequency of cariogenic foods in the diet, and the control of bacterial plaque.

Studies have shown that, when all degrees of retardation are grouped together, dental caries incidence is generally higher for noninstitutionalized than for institutionalized patients, particularly among the profoundly retarded group.[2] Institutionalized individuals have a controlled diet with less food available between meals. They also may have less accessibility to snacks containing refined carbohydrates, except those brought by visitors.

The private water supply for many institutions has been fluoridated. This may be equally true of the community water supply where the noninstitutionalized individuals reside.

When the figures for dental caries incidence are separated according to degree of retardation, the severely and profoundly retarded patients have been shown to have significantly more dental caries.[2]

DENTAL AND DENTAL HYGIENE CARE AND INSTRUCTION

Procedures for management and care of the patient with a disability were described in Chapter 50 with suggestions for various types of adaptations. The patient with mental retardation may have physical and sensory disabilities or systemic disease problems; therefore, information from various chapters can be applied during treatment. Patients with any type of mental retardation need basic periodontal therapy consisting of intensive daily plaque control, scaling, and frequent maintenance supervision.

In the following pages, the special characteristics and problems of patients with Down's syndrome and the syndrome of autism (Kanner's syndrome) are described.

DOWN'S SYNDROME

A special and unique group of individuals with mental retardation has a chromosomal abnormality manifested in Down's syndrome or trisomy 21 syndrome. The incidence of Down's syndrome in the United States is approximately 1 in 1000 live births and stillbirths.[4]

Formerly, the incidence of births of babies with Down's syndrome increased with advancing maternal age. In recent years, however, the average age of mothers of infants with Down's syndrome has decreased.[5] Also, statistical evidence shows that the father can be the source of the chromosomal abnormality.[6]

Patients with Down's syndrome have a combination of characteristic abnormalities that is relatively constant. They tend to resemble one another.

I. Physical Characteristics[7]

A. Stature
Small, with a short neck; awkward, waddling gait; general growth retardation.

B. Head
Microcephaly; flat on facial and occipital sides; short, underdeveloped nose with depressed bridge; scanty hair.

C. Eyes
Oblique slant laterally with narrow opening between eyelids; fold of skin continues from upper eyelid over the inner angle of the eye (epicanthic fold) (figure 53–1). Nearsightedness, eyes crossing inward, and cataracts are common.

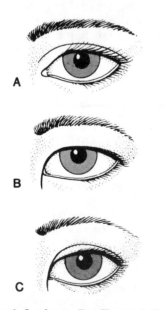

Figure 53–1. Down's Syndrome: Eye Characteristics. A. Absence of an epicanthic fold. **B.** Epicanthic fold in Oriental populations. **C.** Epicanthic fold of person with Down's syndrome. (Redrawn from Smith, G.F. and Berg, J.M.: *Down's Anomaly*, 2nd ed. Edinburgh, Churchill Livingstone, 1976.)

D. Hands
Broad, with short stubby fingers. The little fingers are curved inward. A single transverse palmar crease may also be present (figure 53–2).

II. Oral Findings

A. Lips
Habitually, the young person with Down's syndrome holds the mouth open with the tongue protruded. The lips are often thickened, cracked, and dry, a result of excessive bathing in saliva while the mouth is open.

Mouthbreathing is common. Because respiratory infections frequently exist, and the tonsils and adenoids are often enlarged, breathing through the nose may not be easy.

B. Tongue and Palate
The tongue is generally deeply fissured and appears large. The jaws are narrow and the palate is short and narrow, which tends to force the tongue into protrusion, thereby making it appear larger.

The incidence of cleft lip, cleft palate, or cleft uvula is greater than in the general population.[8]

C. Teeth
Eruption is delayed and irregular in sequence. There may be microdontia and congenitally missing teeth. Such anomalies as fused teeth and peg lateral incisors occur frequently.

D. Occlusion
Angle's Class III and posterior crossbite are common and relate to the flat face and underdevelopment of the mid-facial region. Frequently, the teeth are spaced because certain anomalous teeth are narrow and require less space, and teeth are missing.

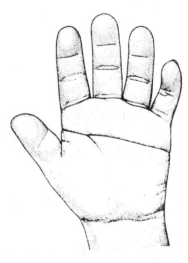

Figure 53–2. Down's Syndrome: Hand. Short stubby fingers with little finger curved inward are characteristic. An identifying feature is the single transverse palmar crease. (From Smith, G.F. and Berg, J.M.: *Down's Anomaly*, 2nd ed. Edinburgh, Churchill Livingstone, 1976.)

E. Periodontal Disease[9]

Increased susceptibility to plaque and bacterial products is apparent. Periodontal conditions are more severe than can be accounted for by local factors alone. Even at early ages, individuals with Down's syndrome show bone loss and other effects of periodontal infection. Disorders of leukocyte function have been shown, and the altered immune system may explain the increased severity of periodontal infection.

Necrotizing ulcerative gingivitis (NUG), superimposed over gingivitis or periodontitis, has been found in more patients with Down's syndrome than with other types of mental retardation.

III. Disease Incidence and Susceptibility

The mortality rate among patients with Down's syndrome is high during their early years because of high susceptibility to respiratory infections, congenital heart lesions, and leukemia. Premature senile dementia is characteristic among older individuals.

A. Susceptibility to Infection

Defects in the body's defense mechanisms lead to early infections of a serious nature.

B. Hepatitis

Patients with Down's syndrome have an unusual response to hepatitis B surface antigen (HBsAg). Residents of institutions for mentally retarded individuals have a high incidence of hepatitis B, especially among children with Down's syndrome.[10,11] The carrier rate is much higher than in the community at large.

Prevention of Hepatitis B is described on pages 19–20. Vaccine immunization is indicated at a very early age for children with Down's Syndrome.

IV. Level of Mental Retardation

Generally, the IQ of patients with Down's syndrome is under 50. Those who have been institutionalized for a long period of time may show lower IQ scores.

Socially, many of the children are more advanced, and may appear to have more intelligence than actually exists. The characteristics of friendliness and personal interaction are described below. Many people with Down's syndrome are fond of music and have a good sense of rhythm. They enjoy singing, playing an instrument, and listening to music. Background music in the dental office or clinic may be helpful in gaining rapport with these special patients.

V. Personal Characteristics[12]

The newborn baby with Down's syndrome is considered a "good" baby by the parents. Later, many of the small children are cheerful, happy, and responsive to learning. Individual differences can be noted, and personality disturbances may occur.

Typical characteristics listed here may suggest management approaches for dental and dental hygiene appointments.
A. Like attention; require affection for feeling of security.
B. Cheerful disposition; rarely irritable; easily amused.
C. Sociable, observant; take initiative.
D. Tendency to imitate; mischievous.
E. Periods of stubbornness; obstinate and determined to have their own way. Parental discipline is necessary. In the dental hygiene appointment, the initial approach can be important to continued control and cooperation.

AUTISTIC DISORDER

Autism is a behavioral developmental disability manifested by limited ability to understand and communicate. Autistic disorder appears during the first 36 months of life, but it is not the result of the baby's environment as was once thought.

Other names commonly used for the condition are Kanner's syndrome, early infantile autism, primary autism, infantile or childhood autism, and childhood psychosis. Because autism is a life-long disability and autistic people live a normal life span, names that refer to infancy or childhood are less accurate.

Children all over the world have been found with autism, and no factor of race, ethnic background, parental intelligence, social class, or parental personality has been shown to be related. In many cases, there is an associated diagnosis of mental retardation. Autism is found in males four times more frequently than in females.

I. Characteristics

Autism is a severely incapacitating condition. It is present at birth, but may not be identified specifically for months or years.

A. Behavioral Features[13]
1. *Impairment in Reciprocal Social Interaction*
   a. Failure to develop interpersonal relationships.
   b. Failure to develop cooperative play, imaginative play, and friendships.
2. *Impairment in Verbal and Nonverbal Communication and Imaginative Activity*
   a. Language may be completely absent or may be immature with use of stereotyped and repetitive speech (echolalia).
   b. Avoids eye-to-eye contact, facial expressions or other nonverbal activity.
3. *Markedly Restricted Repertoire of Activities and Interests*
   a. Stereotyped body movements include rocking, spinning, sniffing, hand clapping, or swaying movements of the body.
   b. Resistance or marked distress over minor changes in the environment or routine.

c. Diet limited to a few foods.
4. *Self-injurious Behavior*
    a. Head banging.
    b. Biting of fingers, hand, or wrist.

B. Other Disorders

Autism may occur alone or with other conditions that also have an influence on the central nervous system, such as metabolic disturbances, Down's syndrome, or epilepsy. Children with autism may develop seizures between ages 11 and 19.

C. Prognosis

Individuals with autism may live a normal life span, and a few become relatively self-sufficient with regular employment. Symptoms may change with age, and periodic reexamination for reassessment is important.

II. Treatment[14]

Because the cause is not known, treatment has not been specific. A variety of approaches has been tried singly or in combination, depending on the individual's needs. In addition to psychotherapy, behavioral modification, and drugs, special education classes for play therapy and speech therapy may be used.

A. Psychotherapy

Parents of an autistic child are under such stress that emotional disorders of the parents may emerge. Along with supportive counseling, the need for psychotherapy may become evident. Psychotherapy and special schooling are often helpful for an autistic child in the near-normal IQ range.

B. Behavior Modification

To provide continuity in behavior modification treatment by a specialist, parents may be trained in the basic procedures and serve as paraprofessionals.[15] The parent has the responsibility for care of an outpatient child for many more hours than does the therapist, and learning needs constant reinforcement.

C. Pharmacotherapy[16]

Various psychotropic drugs, hormones, megavitamins, and other pharmaceutical agents have been tried. Drug therapy depends on the individual needs, and the main objective is to make the child more receptive to education and other therapies.

Patients may have other drugs in their complete treatment regime that need consideration during dental and dental hygiene appointments. The patient with seizures may receive phenytoin. Phenytoin-induced gingival overgrowth is described on page 642.

III. Personal Factors and Dental Hygiene Care[17,18]

For many patients with autism, appointments for health care, medical or dental, are frightening, difficult experiences. Because of language disability, lack of communication, anxiety, and limited social contact, dental care may have been neglected.

Although not all autistic patients are difficult to treat, a few are impossible to treat without sedation, general anesthesia, or physical restraints.[19,20] Hospitalization with general anesthesia is usually considered a last resort because it does nothing to aid in making a cooperative patient for the future.

A. Oral Health Problems

Except when autism is combined with a developmental disability of a different nature, no specific oral manifestation exists. The general health and factors that must be considered for preappointment planning, such as antibiotic premedication, are also not manifestations specifically related to autism. Several factors can contribute to a condition of poor oral health.
1. *Previous Dental Care.* The parent may not have taken the child to obtain care because of fear of the child being hurt, or fear of embarrassment that would result from the behavior of the difficult child. Frustration at home over continuous management of the disabled child could lead a parent to place dental care at a low priority level.

    For the child who had been taken to a dental office or clinic, previous dentists and dental hygienists may not have succeeded in accomplishing treatment of a satisfactory quality.
2. *Dental Caries.* Problems of feeding may have led the parent to lines of least resistance in the serving of foods the child would accept, without regard for nutritive content or dental caries prevention.

    The child's need for sameness may have been applied to dietary selection. A minimal, limited diet may or may not have included excess carbohydrates.

    A second factor is the possibility that the rewards used in behavior modification therapy may be carbohydrates. Frequent repetition of cariogenic rewards over long periods could have had a major effect on dental caries development.
3. *Oral Hygiene.* Even a parent or direct care staff person who is well informed about current plaque control procedures may have had such difficulty in coping with an uncooperative autistic child that daily oral care procedures have never been carried out adequately.

B. Dental Staff Preparation

Advanced review and discussion of the patient's medical, dental, and personal histories, and information from the physician, psychiatrist, teacher, or other persons associated with the patient may be necessary as the dental team members begin to learn how to work with the patient.

Several short orientation appointments may be planned initially.

The same members of the dental team should be involved at each appointment so that the patient will not be disturbed by changes and time will not be lost in reorientation.

C. Structured Environment

1. Provide the child with predictable and consistent experiences.
2. Create a quiet environment free from sensory stimuli. Avoid use of loud, inconsistent background music, noisy dental apparatus, and irrelevant conversations.
3. Begin with orientation to the setting and to each part of the equipment. The first appointment may not include any instruments, as the patient may not be ready. Patience and firmness are necessary elements. Instruction takes the form of "show–tell–do" repeated many times.
4. Use the parent to help to condition the patient. Give the parent a plastic mouth mirror and a few dental films to take home for practice in the mouth each day.
5. Apply behavior modification procedures if the child is trained by that method. Use the parent or therapist-teacher to assist in presenting in a simple step-by-step manner the preventive measures. Reinforcers or rewards are given immediately following each success. By using noncariogenic or, better still, nonedible rewards, the parent or teacher can be educated.

TECHNICAL HINTS

I. Informed Consent

Written approval of the treatment plan is obtained from the parent or legal guardian.[21]

II. Sources of Materials and Information

American Association on Mental Deficiency
1719 Kalorama Road, N.W.
Washington, D.C. 20019

National Society for Autistic Children
Suite 1017
1234 Massachusetts Avenue, N.W.
Washington, D.C. 20005

References

1. American Psychiatric Association: *Diagnostic and Statistical Manual of Mental Disorders* (Third edition—Revised) (DSM-III-R), Washington, D.C., American Psychiatric Association, 1987, pp. 28–33.
2. Tesini, D.A.: An Annotated Review of the Literature of Dental Caries and Periodontal Disease in Mentally Retarded Individuals, *Spec. Care Dentist., 1,* 75, March-April, 1981.
3. Pieper, K., Dirks, B., and Kessler, P.: Caries, Oral Hygiene and Periodontal Disease in Handicapped Adults, *Community Dent. Oral Epidemiol., 14,* 28, February, 1986.
4. Adams, M.M., Erickson, J.D., Layde, P.M., and Oakley, G.P.: Down's Syndrome. Recent Trends in the United States, *JAMA, 246,* 758, August 14, 1981.
5. Holmes, L.B.: Decreasing Age of Mothers of Infants with the Down Syndrome, *N. Engl. J. Med., 298,* 1419, June 22, 1978.
6. Cohen, F.L.: Paternal Contributions to Birth Defects, *Nurs. Clin. North Am., 21,* 49, March, 1986.
7. Smith, G.F. and Berg, J.M.: *Down's Anomaly,* 2nd ed. Edinburgh, Churchill Livingstone, 1976, pp. 14–41.
8. Schendel, S.A. and Gorlin, R.J.: Frequency of Cleft Uvula and Submucous Cleft Palate in Patients with Down's Syndrome, *J. Dent. Res., 53,* 840, July-August, 1974.
9. Reuland-Bosma, W. and van Dijk, J.: Periodontal Disease in Down's Syndrome: A Review, *J. Clin. Periodontol., 13,* 64, January, 1986.
10. Blumberg, B.S., Gerstley, B.J.S., Sutnick, A.I., Millman, I., and London, W.T.: Australian Antigen, Hepatitis Virus and Down's Syndrome, *Ann. N.Y. Acad. Sci., 171,* 486, September 24, 1970.
11. Dicks, J.L. and Dennis, E.S.: Down's Syndrome and Hepatitis: An Evaluation of Carrier Status, *J. Am. Dent. Assoc., 114,* 637, May, 1987.
12. Smith and Berg: op. cit., pp. 72–75.
13. American Psychiatric Association: op. cit., pp. 33–39.
14. Robinson, M.D. and Milius, A.C.: Childhood Autism, in Nowak, A.J.: *Dentistry for the Handicapped Patient.* St. Louis, The C.V. Mosby Co., 1976, pp. 102–120.
15. Freeman, B.J. and Ritvo, E.R.: Parents as Paraprofessionals, in Ritvo, E.R., ed.: *Autism. Diagnosis, Current Research and Management.* New York, Spectrum, 1976, pp. 277–285.
16. Fish, B.: Pharmacotherapy for Autistic and Schizophrenic Children, in Ritvo, E.R., ed.: *Autism. Diagnosis, Current Research and Management.* New York, Spectrum, 1976, pp. 107–119.
17. Burkhart, N.: Understanding and Managing the Autistic Child in the Dental Office, *Dent. Hyg., 58,* 60, February, 1984.
18. Kamen, S. and Skier, J.: Dental Management of the Autistic Child, *Spec. Care Dentist., 5,* 20, January-February, 1985.
19. Braff, M.H., and Nealon, L.: Sedation of the Autistic Patient for Dental Procedures, *ASDC J. Dent. Child., 46,* 404, September-October, 1979.
20. Lowe, O. and Jedrychowski, J.R.: A Sedation Technique for Autistic Patients Who Require Dental Treatment, *Spec. Care Dentist., 7,* 267, November-December, 1987.
21. Snow, M.K. and Stiefel, D.J.: *Dental Treatment of the Mentally Retarded.* Disability Dental Instruction, 4919 Northeast 86th Street, Seattle, Washington 98115, 15 pp.

Suggested Readings

Brayer, L., Goultschin, J., and Mor, C.: The Effect of Chlorhexidine Mouthrinses on Dental Plaque and Gingivitis in Mentally Retarded Individuals, *Clin. Prevent. Dent., 7,* 26, January-February, 1985.

Davila, J.M. and Menendez, J.: Relaxing Effects of Music in Dentistry for Mentally Handicapped Patients, *Spec. Care Dentist., 6,* 18, January-February, 1986.

Davila, J.M. and Jensen, O.E.: Behavioral and Pharmacological Dental Management of a Patient with Autism, *Spec. Care Dentist., 8,* 58, March-April, 1988.

Dawson, L.R. and Hoffman, J.A.: Treatment of a Traumatic Ulcer on a Handicapped Individual: A Case Report, *Spec. Care Dentist., 2,* 207, September-October, 1982.

Dura, J.R., Torsell, A.E., Heinzerling, R.A., and Mulick, J.A.: Special Oral Concerns in People with Severe and Profound Mental Retardation, *Spec. Care Dentist., 8,* 265, November-December, 1988.

Engelmeier, R.L.: Technique for Constructing Custom Thumbchewing Guards, *J. Prosthet. Dent., 54,* 154, July, 1985.

Forsberg, H., Quick-Nilsson, I., Gustavson, K.-H., and Jagell, S.: Dental Health and Dental Care in Severely Mentally Retarded Children, *Swed. Dent. J., 9,* 15, Number 1, 1985.

Garrard, S.D.: Health Services for Mentally Retarded People in Community Residences: Problems and Questions, *Am. J. Public Health, 72,* 1226, November, 1982.

Girgis, S.S.: Dental Health of Persons with Severe Mentally Handicapping Conditions, *Spec. Care Dentist., 5,* 246, November-December, 1985.

Gotowka, T.D., Johnson, E.S., and Gotowka, C.J.: Costs of Providing Dental Services to Adult Mentally Retarded: A Preliminary Report, *Am. J. Public Health, 72,* 1246, November, 1982.

Hamilton, J.: Andy Wants to Be Grown Up: Managing Parental Anxiety, *The Exceptional Parent,* June, 1980. (Reprinted in *J. Am. Dent. Assoc., 101,* 882, November, 1980.)

Indresano, A.T. and Rooney, T.P.: Outpatient Management of Mentally Handicapped Patients Undergoing Dental Procedures, *J. Am. Dent. Assoc., 102,* 328, March, 1981.

Kamen, S.: Dental Management of Patients with Mental Retardation and Related Developmental Disorders, *Can. Dent. Assoc. J., 47,* 663, October, 1981.

Klein, F.K. and Dicks, J.L.: Evaluation of Accumulation of Calculus in Tube-fed, Mentally Handicapped Patients, *J. Am. Dent. Assoc., 108,* 352, March, 1984.

Lange, B.: Effects of Modeling on the Oral Health Care of Persons with Mentally Handicapping Conditions, *Spec. Care Dentist., 5,* 255, November-December, 1985.

Lindemann, R. and Henson, J.L.: Self-injurious Behavior: Management for Dental Treatment, *Spec. Care Dentist., 3,* 72, March-April, 1983.

Lowe, O. and Lindemann, R.: Assessment of the Autistic Patient's Dental Needs and Ability to Undergo Dental Examination, *ASDC J. Dent. Child., 52,* 29, January-February, 1985.

Lu, D.P.: Clinical Investigation of Relative Indifference to Pain Among Adolescent Mental Retardates, *ASDC J. Dent. Child., 48,* 285, July-August, 1981.

Miles, U.: Educationally Sub-normal (mild) Children—the Neglected Ones in Dental Health Education, *Dent. Health (London), 23,* 3, Number 4, 1984.

Miller, M.: Oral Hygiene Management of the Moderate to Severely Mentally Retarded Child, *Dent. Hyg., 53,* 265, June, 1979.

Nicolaci, A.B. and Tesini, D.A.: Improvement in the Oral Hygiene of Institutionalized Mentally Retarded Individuals Through Training of Direct Care Staff: A Longitudinal Study, *Spec. Care Dentist., 2,* 217, September-October, 1982.

O'Donnell, J.P. and Cohen, M.M.: Dental Care for the Institutionalized Retarded Individual, *J. Pedod., 9,* 3, Fall, 1984.

Ohmori, I., Awaya, S., and Ishikawa, F.: Dental Care for Severely Handicapped Children, *Int. Dent. J., 31,* 177, September, 1981.

Seto, B.G. and Lynch, S.: Safety of Hospital Dental Treatment for the High-risk Patient, *Spec. Care Dentist., 4,* 253, November-December, 1984.

Shaw, L., Harris, B.M., Maclaurin, E.T., and Foster, T.D.: Oral Hygiene in Handicapped Children: A Comparison of Effectiveness in the Unaided Use of Manual and Electric Toothbrushes, *Dent. Health (London), 22,* 4, Number 1, 1983.

Tesini, D.A.: Age, Degree of Mental Retardation, Institutionalization, and Socioeconomic Status as Determinants in the Oral Hygiene Status of Mentally Retarded Individuals, *Community Dent. Oral Epidemiol., 8,* 355, October, 1980.

Udin, R.D. and Kuster, C.G.: The Influence of Motivation on a Plaque Control Program for Handicapped Children, *J. Am. Dent. Assoc., 109,* 591, October, 1984.

Vigild, M.: Periodontal Conditions in Mentally Retarded Children, *Community Dent. Oral Epidemiol., 13,* 180, June, 1985.

Vigild, M.: Prevalence of Malocclusion in Mentally Retarded Young Adults, *Community Dent. Oral Epidemiol., 13,* 183, June, 1985.

Wadsworth, C.L., Farrington, F.H., Schroeder, J.R., and Neel, N.L.: The Successes and Failures of Two Approaches to Dental Care in Institutions for Patients Who Are Mentally Handicapped, *Spec. Care Dentist., 6,* 175, July-August, 1986.

Walker, J.D., Crall, J.J., and McDonnell, J.E.: Phenylketonuria and Dentistry: Review of the Literature, *ASDC J. Dent. Child., 49,* 280, July-August, 1982.

Woehrlen, A.E. and Sikora, G.J.: Treatment Planning Considerations for the Patient with Developmentally Disabling Conditions, *Spec. Care Dentist., 7,* 175, July-August, 1987.

Down's Syndrome

Barnett, M.L., Press, K.P., Friedman, D., and Sonnenberg, E.M.: The Prevalence of Periodontitis and Dental Caries in a Down's Syndrome Population, *J. Periodontol., 57,* 288, May, 1986.

Gisel, E.G., Lange, L.J., and Niman, C.W.: Tongue Movements in 4- and 5-year-old Down's Syndrome Children During Eating: A Comparison with Normal Children, *Am. J. Occup. Ther., 38,* 660, October, 1984.

Hunt, N.: *The World of Nigel Hunt; the Diary of a Mongoloid Youth.* New York, Garrett, 1967, 126 pp.

Kroger, J. and Day, V.: Down's Syndrome: Hygienist's Perspective, *Dent. Hyg., 55,* 35, March, 1981.

Latner, L.E.: The Caries Experience in Three Genotypes of Down's Syndrome, *J. Pedod., 7,* 83, Winter, 1983.

MacFarlane, T.W. and Follett, E.A.C.: Serum Hepatitis: A Significant Risk in the Dental Care of the Mentally Retarded, *Br. Dent. J., 160,* 386, June 7, 1986.

Margar-Bacal, F., Witzel, M.A., and Munro, I.R.: Speech Intelligibility After Partial Glossectomy in Children with Down's Syndrome, *Plastic Reconstr. Surg., 79,* 44, January, 1987.

Olbrisch, R.R.: Plastic Surgical Management of Children with Down's Syndrome: Indications and Results, *Br. J. Plastic Surg., 35,* 195, April, 1982.

Reuland-Bosma, W., van Dijk, L.J., and van der Weele, L.: Experimental Gingivitis Around Deciduous Teeth in Children with Down's Syndrome, *J. Clin. Periodontol., 13,* 294, April, 1986.

Rozner, L.: Facial Plastic Surgery for Down's Syndrome, *Lancet, 1,* 1320, June 11, 1983.

Saxén, L. and Aula, S.: Periodontal Bone Loss in Patients with Down's Syndrome: A Follow-up Study, *J. Periodontol., 53,* 158, March, 1982.

Shaw, L. and Saxby, M.S.: Periodontal Destruction in Down's Syndrome and in Juvenile Periodontitis. How Close a Similarity? *J. Periodontol., 57,* 709, November, 1986.

Taicher, S., Sela, M., Lewin-Epstein, J., Wexler, M.R., and Peled, I.J.: Use of Polydimethylsiloxane Subdermal Implants for Correcting Facial Deformities in Down's Syndrome, *J. Prosthet. Dent., 52,* 264, August, 1984.

Williams, C.A., Weber, F.T., McKim, M., Steadman, C.I., and Kane, M.A.: Hepatitis B Virus Transmission in a Public School: Effects of Mentally Retarded HBsAG Carrier Students, *Am. J. Public Health, 77,* 476, April, 1987.

54 *The Patient with a Physical Handicap*

Many diseases of the locomotor system and nervous system have as a symptom or leave as a chronic aftereffect loss of function in the form of a physical handicap.

This chapter contains brief descriptions of selected diseases or conditions to illustrate the types of care necessary and the adaptations that must be made by the patient as well as by the professional person during treatment appointments.

General suggestions that may be adapted to a variety of patients with disabilities were described in Chapter 50. From those descriptions, methods and materials can be selected as they apply in the situations created by the different disorders included in this chapter and encountered in practice. References and suggested readings are included at the end of the chapter for additional information.

SPINAL CORD DYSFUNCTIONS

Among persons disabled by spinal cord dysfunction, paralysis is a common symptom. Paralysis means the loss of power of voluntary movement of a muscle as the result of interruption of one of the motor pathways from the cerebrum to the muscle fiber.

I. Types of Paralysis

A. Paresis

Paresis means partial paralysis. The term may be used to designate weakness rather than complete paralysis.

B. Quadriplegia (Tetraplegia)

Quadriplegia means complete or partial paralysis (paresis) of the trunk and all four extremities.

C. Paraplegia

Paraplegia is complete or partial paralysis of the lower trunk and both lower extremities.

D. Hemiplegia

Hemiplegia means complete or partial paralysis of one side of the body.

E. Triplegia

Triplegia is hemiplegia with the additional paralysis of one limb on the opposite side.

II. Causes of Disruption of Spinal Cord Function

Examples are provided in parentheses.
A. Trauma (spinal cord injury).

B. Neoplasms (within the cord or extradural).
C. Viral or bacterial infections (poliomyelitis).
D. Progressive degenerative disorders (multiple sclerosis).
E. Vascular accidents (hemorrhage, thrombus, embolus, hematoma).
F. Compression from an arthritic spur (spondylytic osteoarthritis).
G. Congenital anomalies or deformities (myelomeningocele, meningocele, spina bifida).

SPINAL CORD INJURY

Spinal cord injury is the impairment of spinal cord function resulting from the application of an external traumatic force. The effect is partial or complete paralysis to a degree related to the spinal cord level and the extent of the injury.

I. Occurrence

At least one half of the trauma cases result from motor vehicle accidents; other causes are falls, diving accidents, and violence, such as from gunshot or stabbing wounds. A large majority of the patients are teenage or young adult men.

II. The Initial Injury

Total or partial loss of sensory, motor, and autonomic function occurs below the level of injury. The injury may be diagonal and leave one side with better function than the other at that particular level.

A. Types of Injury

Damage to the spinal cord may result from one or more of the following:
1. Fracture, dislocation, or both, of one or more vertebrae.
2. Compression, stretching, bending, or severing of the spinal cord.

B. Emergency Patient Care[1,2]

At the scene of an accident, severe damage can be done by inexpert care. The patient should be placed in a supine position, but when back injury is suspected, the arms and legs should be straightened with caution. Any twisting motion may produce irreversible injury to the spinal cord by bony fragments cutting into or severing the cord. When transfer is made, the patient must be moved by at least four persons and placed on a board for transport.

C. Spinal Shock

Immediately after the injury, spinal shock causes a complete loss of reflex activity. The result is a flaccid paralysis below the level of injury. The state of spinal shock may last from several hours to 3 months.

III. Characteristics of Spinal Cord Injury

The pattern of signs and symptoms depends on the nature and level of injury to the spinal cord. There are 7 cervical (C), 12 thoracic (T), and 5 lumbar (L) vertebrae, with paired spinal nerves extending from each.

The areas of the body that are controlled at the different levels are illustrated in figure 54–1. The patient's condition is referred to by the letter C, T, or L, followed by the specific vertebra number where the injury occurred. The most severely handicapped patients have a lesion level above C6, which refers to the sixth cervical vertebral level.

A. Sensorimotor Effects

1. *Complete Lesion.* A complete transection or compression of the spinal cord leaves no sensation or motor function below the level of the lesion.
2. *Incomplete Lesion.* Partial transection or injury of the spinal cord leaves some evidence of sensation or motor function below the level of the lesion. The sensation and motor function may return within a few hours after injury, and maximum return may occur in 6 months to 1 year.

B. Other Possible Effects

1. Impairment of voluntary bladder and bowel control.

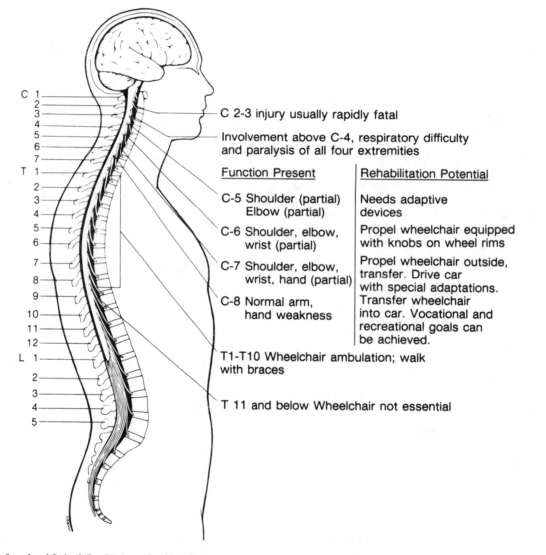

C 1
2
3 — C 2-3 injury usually rapidly fatal
4
5 — Involvement above C-4, respiratory difficulty
6   and paralysis of all four extremities
7

Function Present	Rehabilitation Potential
C-5 Shoulder (partial) Elbow (partial)	Needs adaptive devices
C-6 Shoulder, elbow, wrist (partial)	Propel wheelchair equipped with knobs on wheel rims
C-7 Shoulder, elbow, wrist, hand (partial)	Propel wheelchair outside, transfer. Drive car with special adaptations.
C-8 Normal arm, hand weakness	Transfer wheelchair into car. Vocational and recreational goals can be achieved.

T 1-T10 Wheelchair ambulation; walk with braces

T 11 and below Wheelchair not essential

Figure 54–1. Levels of Spinal Cord Injury. On the left, the vertebrae are designated as C (cervical), T (thoracic), and L (lumbar). The results of spinal cord injury depend on the levels of injury, as shown on the right by function present at the specific level. The most severely handicapped patients have a lesion level above C6. (From Brunner, L.S., Suddarth, D.S., Bare, B.G., Boyer, M.J., and Smeltzer, S.C.O.: *Textbook of Medical-Surgical Nursing,* 6th ed., Philadelphia, J.B. Lippincott Co., 1988.)

2. Impairment of sexual function.

3. Impairment of vasomotor and body temperature regulatory mechanisms.

IV. Secondary Complications That May Occur[3]

Most of the complications described here do not occur in patients with lesions below the T6 level.

A. Respiratory Function

Respiratory difficulties may occur. During dental hygiene therapy, attention to patient position and continuous suction to keep passageways clear are vital. Some quadriplegic patients are unable to elicit a functional cough and need assistance. By placing manual pressure over the abdomen, below the diaphragm, after the patient has inhaled, the patient may be assisted while an attempt to cough is made.[3]

B. Tendency for Pressure Sores[4]

A pressure sore (decubitus ulcer) is caused by pressure exerted on the skin and subcutaneous tissues by bony prominences and the object on which they rest, such as a mattress. The result is tissue anoxia or ischemia. The cutaneous tissue becomes broken or destroyed, thereby leading to destruction in the subcutaneous tissue. An ulcer forms, which may be very slow to heal and may become infected by secondary bacterial invasion. Anemia and poor nutrition may also contribute.

Prevention of pressure can be accomplished by the use of padding and by regular turning of the patient. The dental chair can be positioned to prevent pressure. The patient may be asked to bring special padding to be used during the appointment, and also may be asked to provide instruction for the dental personnel so correct procedures can be followed.

C. Spasticity

As spinal shock subsides, muscle-reflex spasticity develops from a slight to a severe degree. Stimuli, such as pressure sores, infections, and sensory irritation, may bring on a spasm. Before dental hygiene treatment, the patient should be asked about susceptibility to spasms and to describe the procedure to follow should one occur.

D. Body Temperature

High-level quadriplegic patients are unable to regulate body temperature. A blanket may be needed in colder weather and air cooling during summer. When air conditioning is not available, the patient's temperature should be monitored. In the event of a rise in temperature, treatment should be postponed.

E. Vulnerability to Infection

Infections related to elimination, decubitus ulcer, and respiratory problems are the most common.

F. Autonomic Dysreflexia

1. *Definition.* Autonomic dysreflexia, or hyperreflexia, is an *emergency* condition in which the blood pressure increases sharply. It may occur in patients with lesions at T4 or above, but not below that level. A variety of stimuli may precipitate dysreflexia, especially an irritation to the bowel or bladder.

2. *Symptoms*

    a. Increased blood pressure with slowed pulse rate. The blood pressure may rise to 300/160 mm. Hg.

    b. Pounding headache.

    c. Flushing, chills, perspiration, stuffy nose.

    d. Restlessness; increased spasticity.

3. *Emergency Care*[3]

    a. Position chair upright gradually. Do NOT recline the chair, because increased blood pressure in the brain could result.

    b. Monitor the blood pressure.

    c. Call for medical aid.

    d. Check bladder distention and unclamp catheter.

V. Personal Factors

The typical patient is a young man, possibly a former athlete. Depression and discouragement along with the pain and pressures of treatment and rehabilitation make psychiatric therapy necessary for many patients.

Physical and occupational therapists provide self-care training and preparation for discharge from the rehabilitation hospital. As much responsibility as possible is given the patient for personal care. Daily oral care, which at first may have been carried out by the nursing care staff, gradually should become a part of the daily hygiene routine accomplished by the patient, depending on the cord level of injury.

VI. Dental Hygiene Care

Emergency dental care may be needed during the patient's hospital period of recovery and treatment.

By the time the patient is able to be transported to a dental office or clinic, physical and psychologic preparation for daily living will be at a stage where the patient has developed a stable routine.

Most of the information necessary for patient management and instruction is presented in Chapter 50. A few special considerations will be described here.

A. Dental Chair Position

1. Wheelchair transfers (page 615).

2. Chair angle[3]

    a. For the patient with a gravity-drained urinary appliance, the chair may be adjusted to accommodate the drainage, or the patient should be uprighted at intervals to allow drainage to take place. The bag may require emptying during the appointment.

    b. The chair angle should not be changed abruptly because of the patient's susceptibility to postural hypotension.

    c. Change the patient's body position in the

chair by lifting and turning at intervals to prevent pressure sores and pain in muscles and joints. The use of padding was mentioned earlier in this section.

B. Four-handed Dental Hygiene

An assistant is a necessity. Precautions for the patient with spinal cord injury relate to the problems of respiration, pressure sores, spasms, autonomic dysreflexia, temperature control, and other factors that were described earlier. Assistance is definitely needed in many ways, including the following:

1. Assist in wheelchair transfer and in turning the patient at intervals.
2. Monitor vital signs.
3. Watch the patient for signs of body needs, emergencies.
4. Assist with rubber dam. A rubber dam should always be used for appropriate procedures, such as application of topical fluorides, sealants, and polishing of restorations, because of danger of a respiratory complication should materials be inhaled.
5. Suction
   a. Prevent aspiration of foreign materials, such as calculus.
   b. Use ultrasonic instruments with great caution, if at all. When use of such instruments is unavoidable, care must be taken to prevent aspiration of water, to avoid spraying the throat and stimulating a gag or cough, and to make sure the instrument tip does not overheat.
6. Assist with all procedures to make the total treatment time as brief and efficiently used as possible without sacrificing patient comfort.

C. Disease Control

A complete preventive program with bacterial plaque control, fluorides, and diet counseling is essential. Frequent appointments usually are necessary to motivate, follow up with additional instruction, and assist the patient in carrying out the recommended procedures. Instruction for the direct care person for the severely injured patient must be provided.

Care of removable appliances includes cleaning of mouth-held implements.

VII. Mouth-Held Implements

The patient without hands or without the use of hands may utilize the mouth for performing many tasks and the teeth for holding objects. The maintenance of optimum oral health has special significance for these individuals because many of these functions could not be accomplished in an edentulous mouth.

Mouth-held appliances have been fabricated that are effective in carrying out a variety of basic procedures and that contribute to increased independ-ence for a person without the use of hands. A device makes possible such activities as pressing light switches, writing, typewriting, dialing a telephone, pushing an elevator button, or turning the pages of a book.

An *orthosis* is a device added to a person's body to restore function, assist weak muscles, correct a deformity, immobilize a part, or substitute for absent motor power. Criteria for an adequate oral orthosis include the following:[5]

1. Does not harm the oral tissues.
   a. Stabilization of occlusion with contact for all fully erupted teeth and the biting forces distributed to as many teeth as possible.
   b. Is not traumatic to the periodontal supporting structures.
   c. Does not prevent eruption of teeth.
2. Is comfortable, and does not cause fatigue.
   a. Patient can talk, swallow, and moisten the lips.
   b. Orthosis can be inserted and removed by the patient.
   c. Orthosis is adaptable for the various needs of the quadriplegic patient.
3. Can be cleaned and cared for easily.
   a. Taste is pleasant; no odors.
   b. Surface texture is smooth.
4. Is relatively easy to construct; inexpensive.

The formerly used plain mouthsticks required gripping the stick with the teeth. The teeth could be damaged from chipping and undue and uneven pressures that led to periodontal trauma. When the appliance was adapted to anterior teeth only, tipping and extrusion of the incisors resulted.

A minimum requirement for the preparation of an orthosis is that it cannot damage soft or hard oral tissues. One prerequisite is the use of a sanitary material that can be easily cleaned.[5] Before making impressions for constructing a mouthpiece, periodontal and restorative therapy should be completed and the occlusion adjusted. Plaque control procedures must be effective, and the patient must be instructed carefully in the importance and methods of oral hygiene and appliance care.

MYELOMENINGOCELE[6]

Spina bifida is a congenital defect or opening in the spinal cord. A portion of the spinal membranes may protrude through the opening with or without spinal cord tissue. When the spinal cord protrudes through the spina bifida, the condition is called *myelomeningocele.*

Embryologically, a neural tube forms during the first month of pregnancy. From the neural tube, the brain, brain stem, and spinal cord arise, and eventually, the vertebrae form and enclose the spinal cord. When a place in the spinal column fails to close, the result is an open defect in the spinal canal, which is called a spina bifida. The cause of the failure of the tube to develop and close normally by 1 month is not known.

I. Types of Deformities

A. Myelomeningocele

A myelomeningocele is a protrusion or out-pouching of the spinal cord and its covering (meninges) through an opening in the bony spinal column. Because part of the spinal cord and nerve roots protrude, flaccid paralysis of the legs and part of the trunk results, depending on the level of the protrusion (herniation).

B. Meningocele

A meningocele is a protrusion of the meninges through a defect in the skull or spinal column. Because no neural elements are contained in the protrusion, paralysis is uncommon.

C. Spina Bifida

Spina bifida is a congenital cleft in the bony encasement of the spinal cord. When no out-pouching of the meninges or spinal cord exists, the condition is called *spina bifida occulta.* Usually, spina bifida occulta has no symptoms.

II. Physical Characteristics

Depending on the level of the myelomeningocele, some or all of the signs and physical characteristics listed here may be found.

A. Bony Deformities

Muscle imbalance from paralysis can cause dislocation of the hip, club foot, and spinal curvatures, such as humpback (kyphosis), curvature (scoliosis), or swayback (lordosis).

B. Loss of Sensation

Lack of skin sensitivity to pain, temperature, and other sensations can lead to problems of inadvertent burn or trauma unrecognized by the patient or attendant, or to pressure sores, described on page 657. Frequent position changes are necessary.

C. Bladder and Bowel Paralysis

The nerve supplies to bladder and bowel are usually affected. Lack of bowel and bladder control requires continual attention. Kidney infection with loss of kidney function is one cause of shorter life expectancy.

D. Hydrocephalus

Hydrocephalus is a condition characterized by an excessive accumulation of fluid in the brain. The fluid dilates the cerebral ventricles, causes compression of brain tissues, and separates the cranial bones as the head enlarges (figure 54–2). Development is slowed, and mental retardation is present. Many of these patients have seizures.

A high percentage of children with myelomeningocele have hydrocephalus.

III. Medical Treatment

Surgical, orthopedic, medical, urologic, and physical and occupational therapy may constitute a min-

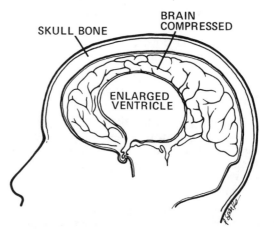

Figure 54–2. Hydrocephalus. The ventricle is enlarged because of the accumulation of fluid. Brain tissues are compressed. (From Bleck, E.E. and Nagel, D.A.: *Physically Handicapped Children. A Medical Atlas for Teachers.* New York, Grune & Stratton, 1975.)

imum of specialties involved in the care of a patient with myelomeningocele.

A. Neurosurgery

1. *Closure of the Myelomeningocele.* Surgical closure helps to prevent infections that may otherwise enter into the spinal cord. Paralysis is not lessened by the surgery.
2. *Treatment of the Hydrocephalus.* Permanent drainage systems may be accomplished in the form of a ventriculoatrial shunt between the cerebral ventricle and the atrium of the heart (figure 54–3). Sometimes, drainage by way of the abdomen in the form of a ventriculoperitoneal shunt is used.

B. Orthopedic Surgery

Bracing to support the trunk and lower limbs is used in accord with the extent of the individ-

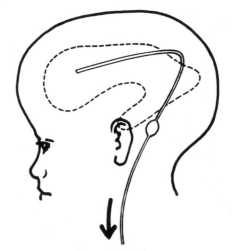

Figure 54–3. Shunt for Hydrocephalus Treatment. Fluid is drained by way of a ventriculoatrial or ventriculoperitoneal shunt. (From Bleck, E.E. and Nagel, D.A.: *Physically Handicapped Children. A Medical Atlas for Teachers.* New York, Grune & Stratton, 1975.)

ual's paralysis. Ambulation varies from dependency on a wheelchair, walker, or use of crutches or cane to near normal with only foot problems. Orthopedic surgical procedures can assist by reducing or correcting deformities.

IV. Dental Hygiene Care

Management for the physical handicaps of the patient with myelomeningocele can be adapted from the information in Chapter 50. Wheelchair transfers and assistance for patients with crutches were described on pages 615–617. Special adaptations for plaque control techniques are needed when the cervical or thoracic body level is involved, and the assistance of a direct care person may be required.

Patients with seizures treated with phenytoin may need gingival treatment for phenytoin-induced gingival overgrowth. The condition is described on page 642.

Patients with shunts need prophylactic antibiotic premedication prior to all dental and dental hygiene instrumentation.[7]

CEREBROVASCULAR ACCIDENT (Stroke)

Cerebrovascular accident (CVA) or stroke is a sudden loss of brain function resulting from interference with the blood supply to a part of the brain. The patient is frequently disabled by changes in motor, communication, and perception functions. Hemiplegia or hemiparesis is common.

I. Etiologic Factors[8]

The stroke may be severe and followed by death within minutes. The less severe attack leaves the patient with symptoms and signs that will be described below. Strokes are usually brought on by one of the following:

A. Thrombosis

A clot within a blood vessel of the brain or neck closes or occludes the vessel and shuts off the oxygen supply to the portion of the brain supplied by that vessel, thus resulting in cerebral infarction.

B. Cerebral Embolism

A blood vessel is blocked by a clot or other material carried through the circulation from another part of the body.

C. Ischemia

The blood flow decreases to an area of the brain, usually as the result of an atheromatous constriction of the arteries supplying the area.

Transient ischemic attack (TIA) is the most common manifestation (see III., A.).

D. Cerebral Hemorrhage

A cerebral blood vessel may rupture and bleed into the brain tissues.

E. Predisposing Factors

Patients with certain conditions may be considered "risk" patients, or persons more susceptible to having strokes. Early diagnosis and treatment for control of the following predisposing factors are necessary in the prevention of stroke and its devastating effects. Risk factors related to atherosclerosis are described on page 689, and to hypertension on page 687.
1. Atherosclerosis.
2. Hypertension, the greatest risk factor that leads to stroke.
3. Drug abuse (especially in adolescents and young adults).
4. Cardiovascular disease (rheumatic heart disease, congestive heart failure, history of TIAs).
5. Diabetes.
6. Use of oral contraceptives (enhanced by hypertension, cigarette smoking, age over 35, and high estrogen levels).

II. Occurrence

A. Cerebral thrombosis is the most common cause of stroke.
B. Stroke is the third leading cause of death in the United States.

III. Signs and Symptoms

The effects of a stroke depend on the location of the damage to the brain, as well as to the degree or extent of involvement.

A. Transient Ischemic Attack (TIA)

"Little strokes" may last a few minutes to an hour, and may leave no damage. A history of transient attacks is a possible risk factor or warning.

B. Acute Symptoms of a Stroke

Acute symptoms and emergency procedures are included in table 60–1, page 749.

C. Residual or Chronic Effects

Approximately two thirds of those who survive have some degree of permanent disability. Temporary or permanent loss of thought, memory, speech, sensation, or motion results. The side of the brain affected influences the symptoms.

The side of the face and body affected is opposite to that of the brain injury (figure 54–4). Persons with right hemiplegia have more difficulty with verbal communication and are more apt to be cautious, anxious, and disorganized. Patients with left hemiplegia have difficulty with action requiring physical coordination, and may respond impulsively with overconfidence.[9]

Common signs and symptoms are described briefly here for application during clinical patient care.
1. *Paralysis.* Hemiplegia (one side of the body) or portions, such as an arm, leg, or the face.
2. *Articulation.* Difficulty of speech, which may

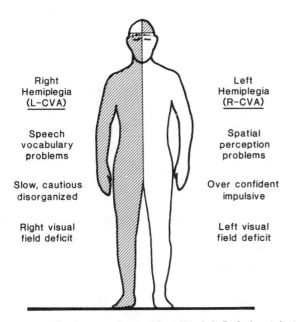

Figure 54–4. Cerebrovascular Accident (Stroke). Right hemiplegia is the result of left-side brain damage; left hemiplegia results from right-side brain damage.

be caused by involvement of the tongue, mouth, or throat as well as by brain damage related to the speech centers.

3. *Salivation.* Difficulty in control of saliva complicated by difficulty in swallowing.
4. *Sensory.* Loss in infected parts with superficial anesthesia, or the opposite may occur with increased sensitivity to pain and touch.
5. *Visual Impairment.* Blurred vision, or diminished visual acuity.
6. *Mental Function.* May be unaffected, but slowness, poor memory, and loss of initiative are common. Brain deterioration may occur over a period of time.
7. *Personal Factors.* Personality changes relate to emotional trauma, fear, discouragement, and dependency. Anxiety neuroses and periods of depression, which are common, may require assistance from a psychiatrist, psychologist, or social worker.

IV. Medical Treatment

A. Surgical

Treatment may include surgical correction of aneurysms, clots, or malformations. Newer developments include surgery in the intracranial arteries using an operating microscope to remove very small clots or to perform minute grafting to bypass blocked vessels and provide collateral circulation.

B. Physical and Occupational Therapy

Rehabilitation techniques are vital to the patient's functioning.

C. Drugs

Careful recording of the medical history includes the listing of medications. The patient may be taking a variety of drugs for some or all of the following purposes:

1. Anticoagulant (to thin the blood).
2. Antihypertensive (to lower the blood pressure).
3. Thrombolytic (to dissolve clots).
4. Vasodilator (to relax the blood vessels of the brain).
5. Steroid (to control brain swelling).
6. Anticonvulsant (to help to control seizures).

V. Dental Hygiene Care

Elective dental treatment is not usually advisable until 6 months or more after a stroke, but when possible, preventive measures and plaque control techniques should be introduced or reinstated early. Regular appointments for preventive care should be initiated as soon as a release can be obtained from the physician.

Patients may be homebound or brought to the clinic or office by wheelchair or walker. Factors described in Chapter 50 apply for the patient who has had a stroke. Every attempt should be made to provide complete care, because temporary care may increase the severity of needs at a later time. The dental hygienist must perform complete scaling and root planing to control the periodontal status.

A. Appointment Procedures

Because of weakness, treatment may best be accomplished in shorter appointments and small increments of instrumentation. The suggestions for appointments (page 612) have already been described. The application of four-handed dental hygiene during instrumentation is necessary for all the same reasons described on page 658 for the patient with a spinal cord injury.

B. Disease Control

Techniques for plaque control may need special adaptations. When the right-handed person is paralyzed on the right side (or the left-handed on the left), development of dexterity for the manipulation of plaque removal implements with the nondominant hand will take time and patience. The patient must be as self-sufficient as possible, but should be encouraged to have the paralyzed side deplaqued daily (brush, floss, and supplementary aids) by a family member or other direct care person for whom instruction has been provided.

The paralyzed side of the face tends to sag or droop, and because of inactivity of the tongue on the same side, self-cleansing is ineffective. Lack of sensation hinders the patient from realizing that collection of food debris and tooth deposits may be extensive.

Rinsing is difficult or impossible. Thus, the

preferred method for daily fluoride application may be the use of a gel tray by the direct care person or the brushing of the teeth with a fluoride gel. When xerostomia is present, substitute saliva can be recommended (page 188).

Modified handles for toothbrushes and floss holders are shown on pages 622–623. The patient who wears dentures requires a suction cup brush to clean the denture with one hand (figure 50–8, page 625).

MUSCULAR DYSTROPHIES[10]

The muscular dystrophies are genetic disorders characterized by progressive severe weakness and loss of use of symmetrical groups of muscles. The term *dystrophy* means degeneration and is associated with atrophy and dysfunction.

At least eight syndromes of muscular dystrophy have been separated by clinical and genetic means. The cause of each type is not known, but the underlying pathologic processes do not differ. Generally, the diseases are limited to skeletal muscles with cardiac muscle only rarely involved.

All muscular dystrophies are rare. The two types described are the more common.

I. Duchenne Muscular Dystrophy (Pseudohypertrophic)

A. Occurrence
The Duchenne type is limited to males and transmitted by female carriers.

B. Age of Onset
The condition becomes apparent during early childhood, between 2 and 5 years; usually before 10 years.

C. Characteristics
1. *Musculature.* Enlargement (pseudohypertrophy) of certain muscles, particularly the calves, is present in early years.
2. *Weakness of Hips.* Child falls frequently, has increasing difficulty in standing erect.
3. *Lordosis.* Abdominal protuberance.
4. *Gait*
   a. Waddling. Either walks on toes or flatfoot as a result of muscle contracture.
   b. Balance. Precarious; patient arches back in attempt to find center of gravity; gait is slow because balance must be attained with each step.
5. *Progressive Muscular Wasting.* Eventual involvement of thighs, shoulders, trunk; inactivity is detrimental and increases the individual's helplessness and dependency.
6. *Intellectual Impairment.* Average IQ in the range of 80 to 90; some patients have normal intelligence and others have a moderate to severe level of retardation.

D. Prognosis
Disablement severe by puberty; child is confined to a wheelchair. Patients rarely live to reach their third decade.

II. Facioscapulohumeral Muscular Dystrophy

A. Occurrence
Males and females are equally affected.

B. Age of Onset
Between 10 and 18 years, with an average at 13 years, after puberty. Mild symptoms may appear at later ages.

C. Characteristics
1. Facial muscles involved, particularly the obicularis oris.
2. Scapulae prominent; shoulder muscles weak; difficulty in raising the arms.
3. Difficulty in closing eyes completely.

D. Prognosis
Progression is slower than that of the Duchenne type. Most patients live a normal life span and become incapacitated late in life.

III. Medical Treatment

A specific treatment is not known. Symptoms may be relieved. The patient is encouraged to lead as full a life as possible and to keep active.

IV. Dental Hygiene Care

Adaptations depend on the patient's disability. Patients may have slight muscular involvement, may be ambulatory but have balancing difficulties, may be in a wheelchair, or may be bedridden. Factors described for general consideration of patients with disabilities have application (Chapter 50). Suggestions listed below are useful for certain patients.

A. Patient Reception and Seating
1. *Assistance for the Walking Patient*
   a. Certain patients do better without assistance, because they have developed their own method of balancing and the slightest touch may upset them.
   b. Many patients gain balance by holding both hands on the partially flexed forearm of person walking beside them.
2. *Seating Preparation.* Raise chair and chair arm. Allow patient to sit directly. Lift patient's legs onto dental chair if such assistance is needed.
3. *Seated Patient.* Tilt chair back gently; balance is precarious while sitting as well as standing; patient may fall forward.
4. *Assistance for Patient While Rising from Chair*
   a. Stand directly in front of patient. Lock arms around lower back and pull forward near hips.
   b. Allow patient to sway upper trunk back while rising to standing position.

c. Provide support until balance is obtained for walking.

B. Patient Instruction

1. *Problems of Oral Cleanliness*
   a. Facial muscle weakness may interfere with self-cleansing mechanisms and prevent adequate rinsing by the patient with facioscapulohumeral dystrophy.
   b. Effect of gaping lips on oral tissues is similar to that of mouthbreathing.
   c. Weakness of arm and shoulder causes difficulty in applying toothbrush. A powered brush or an adapted handle for a regular brush (pages 622–623) may have advantages.

2. *Disease Control*
   a. Instruct parent or other person who cares for patient.
   b. When patient is receiving therapy, solicit assistance and advice from the occupational therapist.

MYASTHENIA GRAVIS

Myasthenia gravis is an autoimmune neuromuscular disease characterized by weakness and fatigability of symmetrical voluntary muscles. It is caused by an autoimmune process that results in a defect in nerve impulse transmission at the neuromuscular junctions. In myasthenia gravis, the numbers of acetylcholine receptors in each neuromuscular junction are reduced markedly when compared to the normal number of receptors.[11]

The patient with myasthenia gravis has a special significance for dental professionals because the facial and oral parts served by certain cranial nerves are involved early. Muscles of the eyes, facial expression, mastication, and swallowing are affected. In advanced severe forms of the disease, muscle involvement may be extensive and result in total paralysis.

I. Occurrence

The onset of myasthenia gravis may occur at any age. The early peak at about age 20 affects females twice as frequently as males. In late adult life, more males than females are affected.

II. Signs and Symptoms

A. Early Signs

Weakness of eye movements with double vision (diplopia) and drooping eyelids (ptosis) may be the initial indicators. In certain patients, the disease may not progress farther.

B. Oral and Facial Problems

Involvement of muscles of the face, mastication, and tongue lead to swallowing difficulties (dysphagia) and a lack of facial expression. Disturbed speech and expression, with a weak voice that sounds tired and muffled, are typical. A patient may support the chin with one hand to help during talking.

C. Progressive Involvement

When the muscles that are used during breathing become involved, serious respiratory complications can result. Because of the lack of facial expression, distress may be difficult for the patient to convey.

Generalized fatigue is usually not so evident in the morning or immediately after rest. Weakness may increase as the day goes by, a factor pertinent to the time selected for dental and dental hygiene appointments.

D. Precipitating Factors

Individual reactions vary, but the more common predisposing, aggravating factors affecting the severity of muscular involvement include emotional excitement, surgical procedures, loss of sleep, alcoholic intake, and, especially, infections. Prevention of oral infections and of the need for dental or periodontal surgery contribute to patient stability. Myasthenic crisis is best avoided by elimination and prevention of infection and all precipitating factors.

E. Types of Crises

1. *Myasthenic Crisis*[12]
   a. Cause. A myasthenic crisis may result from increased severity of the disease, or it may be precipitated by one of the aggravating factors previously mentioned. The relative deficiency of acetylcholine, which leads to the crisis symptoms, can usually be corrected by the physician's administration of anticholinesterase.
   b. Symptoms and signs. The inability to swallow, speak, or maintain a patent airway is sudden. Marked weakness of respiratory and pharyngeal muscles leads to depression of respiration and obstruction. The patient may also have double vision and drooping eyelids.
   c. Emergency care
      i. Suction.
      ii. Provide a patent airway.
      iii. Obtain medical assistance; transport to hospital emergency facility.

2. *Cholinergic Crisis*
   a. Cause. The cholinergic crisis results from overmedication with anticholinesterase.
   b. Symptoms and signs. Increased muscle weakness occurs within 30 to 60 minutes of taking the medication. Excessive pulmonary secretion, cramps, and diarrhea also are characteristic.
   c. Treatment. No further medication should be taken at that time. Medical assistance is needed promptly. When respiratory symptoms develop, ventilation is urgent (page 747).

III. Medical Treatment[12]

Medical treatment may have two purposes: (1) to influence the course of the disease, and (2) to induce disease remission. Anticholinesterase agents are used for most patients at intervals during the day. A sustained-release preparation may be used at bedtime, particularly for the patient who awakens with severe weakness.

Current therapy for attempting to induce remission includes surgical removal of the thymus gland, particularly if a tumor of the gland develops, and drug therapy. Steroids and immunosuppressive medications have been shown to benefit selected patients.[11]

IV. Dental Hygiene Care

A. Appointment Factors

1. *Time and Length.* Short appointments planned early in the day and in conjunction with the patient's medication schedule. Weakness worsens with activity.

2. *Maintenance.* Frequent appointments to aid the patient in obtaining and maintaining freedom from oral infection.

3. *Preparation for the Appointment.* Office emergency equipment for a possible respiratory emergency must be checked and in order. Stress reduction procedures should be followed.

   At the outset, the patient should be asked about medication and whether it has been taken on schedule prior to the appointment.

B. Four-handed Dental Hygiene

For any patient who is a potential respiratory risk, an assistant is needed to aid in observing the patient and to monitor vital signs. Because the patient with myasthenia gravis may have difficulty in providing a warning of distress, the need for supervision is indicated.

1. *Suction.* An assistant is needed to maintain the airway, to assure no problem of aspiration, and to provide a clean field for efficient instrumentation to minimize appointment time. A side effect of the anticholinesterase medication is increased salivation.

2. *Rubber Dam.* Apply for appropriate procedures to prevent aspiration of harmful substances.

C. Patient Instruction for Disease Control

1. *Diet Evaluation.* A dietary survey and instruction are recommended. The patient with myasthenia gravis may have difficulty in masticating and swallowing, and adequate food selection for oral health and dental caries prevention may be difficult.

2. *Plaque Control.* Weakness and fatiguability may have discouraged the patient's routine daily plaque control efforts. A powered brush or other aids (pages 622–624) might be recommended. Instruction for a family member or other direct care person may be needed to provide the severely disabled patient with assistance.

MULTIPLE SCLEROSIS

Multiple sclerosis is a chronic demyelinating disease of the central nervous system characterized by progressive disability. It is also called *disseminated sclerosis.* Sclerosis means hardening, especially by overgrowth of interstitial tissue.

Pathologically, the myelin sheath is destroyed within the white matter of the central nervous system. The sheath degenerates in patches called *MS plaques* and is replaced by sclerotic tissue. There is interference with the transmission of nerve impulses and frequent involvement of the spinal cord and optic nerves.

I. Occurrence

A. Onset

Usually, the onset is between 20 and 40 years of age, rarely before 15 or after 55 years.

B. Geographic

The disease is more prevalent in temperate climates.

II. Characteristics

A. Initial Symptoms: Vary

1. May be visual impairment, difficulty in coordination, tremor, fatigue, weakness, or numbness of a part of the body.

2. May have a sudden onset of severe illness with paralysis or marked weakness.

B. Course of Disease

1. *Relapses and Remissions.* An attack may last several days or weeks and be followed by a symptom-free period. Physical impairment varies, but the condition worsens with each attack.

2. *Precipitating Factors*
   a. Infection. Various types of infection, systemic or local, can stimulate a relapse. Oral infections are no exception.
   b. Stress and emotional trauma.
   c. Injury.
   d. Heavy exercise and fatigue.
   e. Pregnancy. For certain patients, pregnancy may appear to increase the risk and bring on an attack. Because the effect is more likely to be noticed during the first several months after delivery, fatigue and stress may be the direct precipitating effects.

      Effects of multiple sclerosis on the pregnancy should also be recognized. Possible side effects of medications on the developing fetus should be considered because certain medications used may have to be discontinued if they are teratogenic.

3. *Longevity.* People with multiple sclerosis may

live many years. Death is usually the result of an infection, such as of the urinary tract or bronchopneumonia. Fewer than half of those afflicted may eventually become nonambulatory.

C. Physical Symptoms

A wide distribution of areas is affected. Symptoms fluctuate, and several years may elapse between attacks. With extended rest, symptoms usually subside.

1. Involuntary motion of eyes (nystagmus); may later become partially or completely blind.
2. Speech disorders; possible loss of speech in advanced stages.
3. Changes in muscular coordination and gait; loss of balance; spasms.
4. Paralysis of one or more extremities; occasionally, facial paralysis.
5. Autonomic derangements, such as urinary frequency and urgency; later urinary incontinence.
6. Susceptibility to infection, particularly upper respiratory.

D. Personal Factors

1. Optimism and cheerfulness out of proportion to the degree of disability and seriousness of the illness; euphoria or the opposite, leading to depression.
2. Subject to sharp deviations of mood; emotional outbursts with spells of laughing and crying.
3. Poor memory; poor judgment.
4. Passive dependency; lack of responsibility.

III. Medical Treatment

A. No specific treatment because the cause of the disease is unknown.
B. General hygienic care; adequate nutrition, rest, avoidance of strain, prevention of infections, and prevention of injury.
C. Physical and occupational therapy; exercise, but not strenuous exertion, is very important.
D. Psychotherapy for personality problems and morale building is frequently necessary.
E. Drugs are primarily prescribed for alleviation of symptoms. Immunosuppressant drugs have been tried because of the possibility of an immunologic etiologic factor.
F. Patient should continue in a usual occupation as long as possible; activity should be encouraged.

IV. Dental Hygiene Care

Many factors described in Chapter 50 have direct application for the patient with a disability associated with multiple sclerosis. For the patient with paraplegia or quadriplegia, items from the section on patients with spinal cord injuries can be used (pages 657–658).

Because relapses may be precipitated by infections, dental hygiene care for the prevention of periodontal infection assumes particular significance.

A. Appointment Considerations

1. Provide a warm, quiet, comfortable atmosphere. The patient needs to remain relaxed mentally and physically; people nearby cannot be tense, restless, or noisy.
2. Frequent short appointments contribute to the prevention of fatigue, emotional stress, and advanced dental or periodontal conditions.

B. Patient Instruction

1. *Problems of Personal Oral Care*
   a. Involvements of the tongue and facial muscles interfere with the self-cleansing mechanisms.
   b. Paralysis may make grasping and manipulating a toothbrush difficult or impossible. Adaptive aids are described on pages 622–623.
2. *Factors Affecting Teaching*
   a. Slow response of patient; give instruction slowly and simply.
   b. Visual disturbances (pages 674–676).

CEREBRAL PALSY

Palsy means impairment of the ability to control movement, and cerebral palsy means a condition in which injury to parts of the brain has occurred prenatally, natally, or postnatally and has resulted in paralysis or disruption of motor parts. Such a condition can occur at any age as a result of brain injury from a variety of causes.

Cerebral palsy can be caused by anoxia during pregnancy or delivery, maternal infection during pregnancy (for example, rubella), blood type incompatibility, severe nutritional lack during pregnancy, or maternal diabetes endocrine imbalance. Later in infancy, infectious diseases such as meningitis or encephalitis, lead poisoning, direct trauma from accidents, or battering (nonaccidental injury) may be implicated.

Symptoms usually can be observed during the first year after birth, but may not appear for several years. General symptoms that may occur are tense, contracted muscles, uncontrolled movements of limbs, eyes, or head, poor coordination, muscle spasms, problems with hearing and/or seeing, and a lack of manual dexterity.

I. Types of Characteristics[13,14]

Classified by motor activity, six types have been named. In each type, different parts of the brain are damaged, and the symptoms vary respectively. More than 50 percent of those with cerebral palsy are in the spasticity group, 15 to 20 percent are athetoid, and the remainder are divided among the other four types or have mixed types.

A. Spasticity

1. Muscles have increased tone, tension, and activity.
2. Condition characterized by spasms, which are sudden, involuntary contractions of single muscles or groups of muscles.
3. Patient has complete or partial loss of ability to control muscular movement; therefore, movements are awkward and stiff.
4. Lack of control causes patient to fall easily; patient tends to avoid activity and thus may gain weight, particularly during teen years; caloric requirement is therefore low.
5. Brain damage to motor area of cerebral cortex (figure 54–5).

B. Athetosis

1. Condition characterized by constant, involuntary unorganized muscular movement.
2. Patient lacks ability to direct muscles in the motions desired; probably the most difficult dental patient.
3. Grimacing, drooling, and speech defects are common.
4. Factors influencing movements
   a. Effort by patient to control muscle activity results in exaggerated muscle movement.
   b. May be initiated and aggravated by stimuli outside body, such as sudden noises, bright lights, or quick movements by people or things in the area.
   c. Intensity influenced by emotional factors. Patient is least in control in an emotionally charged environment, such as the dental office.
5. Patient constantly in motion; burns up energy; usually very thin; caloric requirement of diet is therefore high.
6. Brain damage to basal ganglia (figure 54–5).

C. Ataxia

1. Loss of equilibrium; balance and orientation difficult; walk uncertain; has difficulty in sitting straight.
2. Lack of coordination; needs time to execute changes.
3. Patient inactive because of balance disturbance; tends to put on weight; caloric requirement in diet is therefore low.
4. Brain damage to cerebellum (figure 54–5).

D. Rigidity

1. Muscles may be rigid and stiff, with resistance to movement and hypertonicity.
2. Tendency to lack of activity.

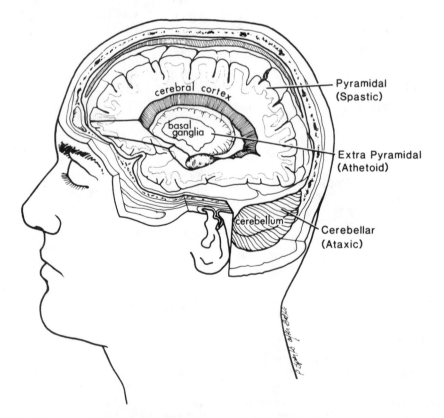

Figure 54–5. Cerebral Palsy. Shown are the major parts of the brain involved in each of the three major types of cerebral palsy—spastic, athetoid, and ataxic. (From Bleck, E.E. and Nagel, D.A.: *Physically Handicapped Children. A Medical Atlas for Teachers.* New York, Grune & Stratton, 1975.)

E. Tremor

Involuntary muscle quivering may affect part or all of the body.

F. Flaccidity

1. Hypotonia or atonia of muscles that are flabby and weak.
2. Unable to stand or raise head.
3. Drooling; difficulty in swallowing and chewing; speech problems.

G. Mixed

Various combinations of the six types occur.

II. Conditions Accompanying Motor Activity

In addition to impaired movement, weakness, and lack of coordination, the handicapping conditions listed below may also occur.

A. Mental Retardation

Approximately 50 percent of individuals with cerebral palsy also have mental retardation.

B. Learning Disabilities

Of the 50 percent who are not mentally retarded, many have problems of learning because of sensory defects, especially hearing and seeing, as well as perceptive-cognitive deficiencies. Speech difficulties and inability to move about freely can also contribute to learning problems.

C. Seizures

Between 25 and 30 percent have seizures and undergo related drug therapy.

D. Sensory Disorders

Seeing and hearing problems are common.

III. Medical Treatment

Surgical, orthopedic, and medical care, as well as speech, physical, and occupational therapy, may constitute a minimum of specialties involved in the care of a patient with cerebral palsy. Bracing to support the lower limbs and the use of canes, crutches, walkers, or wheelchairs help to increase function. Surgery may be needed for orthopedic deformities or for correcting eye or ear difficulties.

Patients may use tranquilizers to reduce tension or aid in limiting problems associated with nerve damage. Other medication may include drugs for seizure control. There is no cure for cerebral palsy.

IV. Oral Characteristics

A. Disturbances of Musculature

Facial grimacing, abnormal muscle function, facial asymmetry, and problems of mastication and swallowing are common. Opening of the mouth may present problems during dental and dental hygiene therapy, as well as during plaque control at home.

B. Malocclusion

The incidence of malocclusion is high. Oral habits of mouth breathing, tongue thrusting, and faulty swallowing contribute to orthodontic needs.

C. Attrition

Severe, constant, involuntary grinding of teeth wears down tooth structure and restorations. Bruxism is most extensive in the athetoid group.

D. Fractured Teeth

Patients fall frequently; accidents to anterior teeth result.

E. Dental Caries

The rate of dental caries may be slightly higher, but the factors that operate for the patient with cerebral palsy are the same as those for the physically normal population. Difficulties in maintaining plaque control and problems of mastication, which lead to the use of a soft diet, may predispose to an environment for bacterial plaque formation.

F. Periodontal Disease

Periodontal or gingival infections are found in a high percentage of patients with cerebral palsy.

1. *Phenytoin-induced Gingival Overgrowth.* When phenytoin is used for the prevention of seizures, the patient is susceptible to gingival enlargement. The condition and its prevention are described on pages 642–644.
2. *Predisposing Factors to Periodontal Involvement.* Mechanical difficulties related to plaque control, mouth breathing, and increased food retention because of ineffective self-cleansing all lead to increased periodontal involvement and plaque collection. Many patients with cerebral palsy have heavy calculus deposits.

V. Dental Hygiene Care

Procedures described in Chapter 50 apply in the management of the patient with cerebral palsy. Many special adaptations are needed, and experience contributes to developing the necessary patience and confidence.

Dental hygiene care is complicated by the difficulties the patient has in cooperating and by the oral manifestations previously listed. Understanding the physical characteristics is particularly necessary to the success of the appointments. Athetoid movements should not be interpreted as lack of cooperation, and a patient's inability to communicate does not mean lack of comprehension.

Dentists occasionally must use general anesthesia in a hospital situation for the unmanageable patient.

Dangers for both the patient and dental personnel may result from the uncontrolled movement of the patient. The sudden forceful closure of the mouth on the finger of the clinician or on a mouth mirror, or movement of the patient that diverts a sharp instrument into the patient's tissues, are examples.

Assistance throughout appointments is important.

Suggestions for management should be solicited from family or direct care attendants. Sedation through premedication may be possible, and various restraining procedures may be used (page 631).

Selected patients with cerebral palsy may use a mouth-held instrument as described on page 658. Oral care and preventive measures are vital to this group of patients.

BELL'S PALSY

Bell's palsy is a paralysis of the facial muscles innervated by the facial or seventh cranial nerve. Although the cause is not known, various possible agents have been implicated, including bacterial and viral infections, particularly herpes simplex, trauma from tooth removal, or surgery of the parotid gland area, such as the removal of a tumor.

I. Occurrence

Although relatively rare, the incidence increases with each decade of life. Women are more frequently affected than men in younger age groups, but after age 50, the disorder is more common in men.

II. Characteristics[15]

A. Signs and Symptoms

Abrupt weakness or paralysis of facial muscles, usually without preceding pain, occurs on one side of the face.
1. *Mouth.* The corner of the mouth droops, and salivation with drooling is uncontrollable.
2. *Eye.* Eyelids cannot be closed. Watering and drooping of the lower lid invite infection.

B. Functional Problems

Speech and mastication are difficult.

C. Prognosis

A majority of patients experience a return to normal within a month; many have a spontaneous recovery. Others may have lasting residual effects or permanent paralysis.

III. Medical Treatment[16]

Without knowledge of the specific cause, treatment has not been definitive. Temporary palliative measures, such as protecting the eye during sleep and massaging the involved muscles, provide some relief.

A. Drugs

Steroids have been used to improve the prognosis.

B. Surgical[17]

The objectives for surgical procedures have been to improve the appearance, provide facial symmetry with voluntary motion, and provide control of the eye and the mouth. Surgery has included repair of the facial nerve, nerve transplantation and grafting, crossover nerve grafts from the uninvolved side of the face, muscle transfers, and free muscle grafts. Prosthetic rehabilitation has been combined with surgical treatment.

C. Prostheses[18]

Surgery may be contraindicated or unsuccessful, and prosthetic treatment may aid in providing tissue support and may assist in speech. Facial symmetry has been improved with the use of removable prostheses.

IV. Dental Hygiene Care

Instruction and frequent appointments to supplement the patient's efforts usually are needed. A removable prosthesis needs daily care because debris and plaque collect readily. The involved side needs meticulous bacterial plaque removal because self-cleansing ability has been lost.

When only the seventh nerve is affected, sensory responses are still intact. When anesthesia is used on the opposite side, special precautions should be provided for postoperative care until the anesthesia has worn off.

Protective goggles should be worn by the patient. Care is necessary to ensure that calculus, polishing paste, or other foreign material does not enter the eye because the eyelid lacks its natural ability to close for protection.

PARKINSON'S DISEASE

Parkinson's disease is a progressive disorder of the central nervous system characterized by loss of postural stability, slowness of spontaneous movement, resting tremor, and muscular rigidity. It is also known as *paralysis agitans, Parkinson's syndrome,* and *Parkinsonism.*

Although the cause is not known, the basis for the specific group of symptoms is degeneration of certain neurons in the substantia nigra of the basal ganglia, where posture, support, and voluntary motion are controlled. In addition, a severe deficiency of dopamine, one of the substances that participates in nerve transmission, occurs.

I. Occurrence

Parkinson's disease affects middle-aged and older persons primarily, with a higher incidence in men than in women.

II. Characteristics

The signs and symptoms center around tremor, rigidity, and loss or impairment of motor function (akinesia). These three factors also occur in other conditions, which must be differentiated by a physician when a diagnosis is made.

A. General Manifestations
1. Body posture bent, with bent head and general stiffness.

2. Motion and responses slowed; difficulty in keeping balance.
3. Gait quick and shuffling.
4. Speech monotonous and slow.
5. Tremor of one or both hands; the fingers may be involved in a pill-rolling motion in which the thumb and index finger are rubbed together in a circular movement. The tremor can be reduced or stopped when the person engages in purposeful action.
6. Intellect is seldom affected except in the very advanced stages.
7. Eventually, after 10 to 20 years, the person may become incapacitated and may require complete care.

B. Face and Oral Cavity
1. Expression is fixed and mask-like with diminished eye blinking.
2. Tremor in lips, tongue, neck, and difficulty in swallowing.
3. Excess salivation and drooling.

III. Treatment

Maintenance of good general health, with plenty of rest and nutritious meals, is encouraged. Professional physical therapy and occupational therapy have particular significance for a patient's well-being.

Although no known cure exists for Parkinson's disease, symptomatic control can be accomplished, at least in part, by replenishing the dopamine shortage with levodopa. Side effects are common, and may indicate an overdose.[19] Orthostatic hypotension and dizziness may be expected and should be considered when adjusting the dental chair.

IV. Dental Hygiene Care

Various adaptations of procedures can be anticipated from knowledge of the physical characteristics previously noted. Personal interest, attention, and encouragement contribute to help the patient to bear the stresses of the disability.

General suggestions for the gerodontic patient in Chapter 45 may prove useful, as well as suggestions related to physical disabilities in Chapter 50. Special adaptations for plaque control may be needed.

ARTHRITIS

Diseases of the joints, including arthritis, are among the most common causes of chronic illness in the United States. In addition to arthritis as a disease entity, arthritic manifestations are produced as part of various other chronic diseases. The disability may be temporary or permanent, partial or complete. A person may suffer from more than one type at a time.

Arthritis means inflammation in a joint. It may occur in an acute or chronic form and may be local-ized or generalized. When many joints are involved, the term *polyarthritis* may be applied.

Factors that have been implicated in the cause of rheumatic and arthritic diseases include infectious agents, traumatic disorders, endocrine abnormalities, tumors, allergy and drug reactions, and inherited or congenital conditions. When the cause is known, specific medical, physical, and surgical therapies may be available to alleviate pain and disability.

I. Rheumatoid Arthritis[20]

Rheumatoid arthritis is a chronic, immunologic systemic disease in which inflammation of the joints occurs in exacerbations and remissions. The cause is unknown, and the means by which the inflammation in the joints is initiated remains a question.

A. Occurrence
The onset usually occurs between ages 20 and 40, although it may occur at any age. More females than males are affected. It is rare in tropical countries.

B. Signs and Symptoms
1. Joint pain and swelling. Rheumatoid arthritis is a polyarthritis with migratory pain, swelling, tenderness, and warmth in symmetrical joints. Fingers, hands, and knees are usually affected first.
2. Morning stiffness and stiffness after periods of inactivity.
3. Weakness, fatigue, loss of appetite and weight, anemia, low grade fever.
4. Subcutaneous nodules in elbows, wrists, or fingers in approximately 20 percent of the patients; nodules may appear in other body organs.
5. Possible temporomandibular joint involvement. There may be pain with jaw movements and difficulty in chewing. Ankylosis may develop but is not a common finding.
6. Progressive deformity with limited motion in the more severely involved joints and muscle atrophy adjacent to the joints.

C. Medical Treatment
Without a specifically known cause, therapy is limited to an individualized program involving pain relief, physical and occupational therapy, and overall health maintenance with adequate nutrition. The most widely prescribed drug is aspirin, which is used for its anti-inflammatory effect. Selected patients have been treated by joint replacement surgery.

II. Juvenile Rheumatoid Arthritis

Rheumatoid arthritis occurring in children under 16 years of age differs from the disease in adults. The onset is usually more acute, with prolonged fever and enlargement of the spleen and lymph nodes. The inflammation of many joints, particularly knees, wrists, and spine, may appear after a few weeks. Figure 54–6 shows the shape of affected fingers. The temporomandibular joint may be involved, with pain and limited oral opening.

Many patients have complete remissions, some have increasing disability, and others may have mild arthritic symptoms that continue for years. Children are encouraged to lead as normal a life as possible. The long-term treatment program includes activity to maintain function and drugs to relieve pain.

III. Degenerative Joint Diseases

Degenerative joint disease (DJD), or osteoarthritis as it is frequently called, affects the weight-bearing joints particularly. Because inflammation is not the basic joint problem, degenerative joint disease is a more accurate term.

No specific cause is known, but predisposing factors may include repeated trauma, obesity, age-related changes in the joint tissues, mechanical stresses to the weight-bearing joints, and genetic predisposition.[21]

A. Occurrence

The onset occurs between 50 and 70 years of age, with the average onset 20 years later than that of rheumatoid arthritis. As many as 85 percent of people over age 70 have evidence of degenerative joint disease.

B. Symptoms

At first insidious, with slight stiffness of a single joint, the eventual condition leads to much pain, deformity, and limitation of movement.
1. Hips, knees, fingers, and vertebrae affected most frequently.
2. Swelling rare; ankylosis does not occur.
3. Stiffness in the morning on rising and after periods of inactivity; diminishes with exercise.

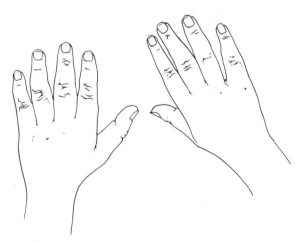

Figure 54–6. Child with Rheumatoid Arthritis. The fingers are tapered from fat central areas. The joint nearest the tip of the finger is the least involved. (From Bleck, E.E. and Nagel, D.A.: *Physically Handicapped Children. A Medical Atlas for Teachers.* New York, Grune & Stratton, 1975.)

4. Pain aggravated by temperature changes and bearing body weight.
5. Temporomandibular joint usually without pain or other clinical symptoms, although crepitation, clicking, or snapping may occur when the joints are exercised.

C. Medical Treatment

Moderate exercise, aspirin or other pain-relieving drug therapy, weight reduction for obese patients, physical therapy, and selected orthopedic surgical procedures comprise the general treatments available. Total hip or knee joint replacement has proved satisfactory for many patients, and has been used more widely for DJD than for rheumatoid arthritis.

IV. Personal Factors

With long-term illnesses, patients are frequently discouraged or apprehensive. Certain patients may be worried, pessimistic, or resigned. Some may be impatient and tend to harm themselves by overexercise. A few are irritable, a characteristic related to the pain that has been suffered.

V. Dental Hygiene Care

A high standard of general health contributes to the well-being of the patient with arthritis. Maintenance of oral health contributes to general health.

Adjustments for physical disabilities of the patient with arthritis may be found in Chapter 50. Assistance with ambulation, chair positioning, and other special adaptations are needed.

A. Patient History

Questions to determine whether the patient has a joint prosthesis should be included in the patient history. Because of the susceptibility to infection at the interface of the bone and the prosthesis, prophylactic antibiotic premedication to prevent bacteremia is essential.[22,23] A patient who is anticipating surgery for a joint replacement should be counseled to complete all needed periodontal and restorative therapy before the surgery to prevent the need for repeated antibiotic premedication.

B. Instrumentation

For the patient with arthritis of the temporomandibular joint, instrumentation may need adaptations to accommodate a minimal opening of the mouth. Fatigue in the joint may be reduced by rest periods, by minimizing the pressure on the mandible, and by overall efficiency to shorten the necessary appointment time. More frequent appointments can contribute to keeping the oral health at a maximum and thus preventing long, difficult scaling sessions.

C. Plaque Control

Because of hand and arm involvement, a patient may have difficulty grasping a toothbrush or lifting the arm for sufficient periods to clean the mouth completely. Adapted brushing procedures may be applied (pages 622–624).

D. Diet and Nutrition

1. No special nutritional factors are known to be associated with the course or treatment of arthritis. Physicians generally recommend a normal, well-balanced diet with a controlled caloric intake for weight control. Encouragement of restriction of sweets and selection of noncariogenic between-meal snacks can help to improve oral health.
2. Obtaining a food diary for several days to a week can be important for dietary analysis and counseling, especially for the gerodontic arthritic patient.

SCLERODERMA
(Progressive Systemic Sclerosis)

Scleroderma is an autoimmune disease of connective tissue characterized by an overproduction of collagen. The most striking physical symptom is the immobility and rigidity of the skin, but inflammation and sclerosis occur throughout the body. Thus, the disease has the full title of *progressive systemic sclerosis.*

The cause is not known, but research has been concerned with studying collagen synthesis irregularities, associated immunologic disorders, and microvascular abnormalities. Hereditary factors are not involved.

I. Occurrence

Scleroderma usually has its onset between ages 30 and 50, but may affect persons of any age, even infants. It may develop over months or years and is two to five times more common in females.

II. Characteristics

Scleroderma may be localized and involve only the skin, or it may be generalized and involve all body organs. The most notable changes are in the skin, gastrointestinal tract, kidneys, heart, muscles, and lungs. Eventual death results from renal failure, cardiac failure, pulmonary insufficiency, or intestinal malabsorption. Symptoms vary, and all individuals do not have all the symptoms and signs listed below.

A. General Manifestations

1. *Joints.* Pain, swelling, and stiffness of the fingers and knee joints.
2. *Polyarthritis.* Symmetrical polyarthritis, similar to rheumatoid arthritis.
3. *Skin.* Hard and fixed; ivory-white, yellow, or gray, sometimes with brown pigmentation in the late stages.
4. *Face.* When affected, the face becomes masklike and expressionless.

B. Oral Characteristics[24]

1. *Lips.* Thin, rigid, with oral stricture and difficulty in opening and closing.
2. *Mucosa.* Thin, pale, tender, rigid, with poor healing capacity.
3. *Gingiva.* Pale and unusually firm.
4. *Teeth.* Mobility is common.
5. *Radiographic Findings.* Marked widening of the periodontal ligament spaces. This finding is sometimes considered pathognomonic for scleroderma.
6. *Mastication.* Difficult; temporomandibular joint movement is limited.
7. *Tongue.* May be immobile; speech difficult.

III. Medical Treatment

Specific therapy is not known. Medications that retard collagen deposition have not yet been effective for scleroderma. Treatment, therefore, has been directed at specific system complications, physical therapy, and attempts to maintain normal activities.

IV. Dental Hygiene Care

The tightening of the skin and lips limits opening of the mouth and complicates all dental and dental hygiene procedures, as well as daily self-care by the patient. Every effort for preservation of the teeth and gingiva in health should be made to prevent the need for extensive treatment. With oral stricture, the preparation and wearing of dentures is difficult or impossible as the disease becomes more severe.[25]

Patients with scleroderma are sensitive to cold and dampness, stress, undue emotional tension, and fatigue. All these factors can be considered for the dental hygiene appointment.

TECHNICAL HINTS

Sources of Materials and Information

National Foundation of Dentistry for the Handicapped
1250 14th Street (Suite 610)
Denver, Colorado 80202

Arthritis Foundation
1314 Spring Street N.W.
Atlanta, Georgia 30309

National Multiple Sclerosis Society
205 East 42nd Street
New York, New York 10017

National Spinal Cord Injury Foundation
149 California Street
Newton, Massachusetts 02158

American Spinal Injury Association
250 East Superior Street (Room 619)
Chicago, Illinois 60611

Spina Bifida Association of America
343 South Dearborn (Suite 317)
Chicago, Illinois 60604

United Cerebral Palsy Associations
66 East 34th Street
New York, New York 10016

References

1. Brunner, L.S., Suddarth, D.S., Bare, B.G., Boyer, M.J., and Smeltzer, S.C.O.: *Textbook of Medical-Surgical Nursing,* 6th ed. Philadelphia, J.B. Lippincott, 1988, pp. 1504–1513.
2. Buchanan, L.E. and Nawoczenski, D.A.: *Spinal Cord Injury: Concepts and Management Approaches.* Baltimore, Williams and Wilkins, 1987, pp. 23–60.
3. Schubert, M.M., Snow, M., and Stiefel, D.J.: *Dental Treatment of the Spinal Cord Injured Patient.* Disability Dental Instruction, 4919 Northeast 86th Street, Seattle, Washington, 98115, 34 pp.
4. Buchanan and Nawoczenski: op. cit., pp. 101–121.
5. Blaine, H.H. and Nelson, E.P.: A Mouthstick for Quadraplegic Patients, *J. Prosthet. Dent., 29,* 317, March, 1973.
6. Bleck, E.E.: Myelomeningocele, Meningocele, Spina Bifida, in Bleck, E.E. and Nagel, D.A., eds.: *Physically Handicapped Children—A Medical Atlas for Teachers.* New York, Grune & Stratton, 1975, pp. 181–192.
7. Croll, T.P., Greiner, D.G., and Schut, L.: Antibiotic Prophylaxis for the Hydrocephalic Dental Patient with a Shunt, *Pediatr. Dent., 1,* 81, June, 1979.
8. Brunner, Suddarth, Bare, Boyer, and Smeltzer: op. cit., pp. 1439–1448.
9. Schubert, M.M., Snow, M.K., Stiefel, D.J., and DeFreece, A.: *Dental Treatment of the Stroke Patient.* Disability Dental Instruction, 4919 Northeast 86th Street, Seattle, Washington 98115, 29 pp.
10. Robbins, S.L., Cotran, R.S., and Kumar, V.: *Pathologic Basis of Disease,* 3rd ed. Philadelphia, W.B. Saunders Co., 1984, pp. 1308–1310.
11. Robbins, Cotran, and Kumar: op. cit., pp. 1310–1312.
12. Brunner, Suddarth, Bare, Boyer, and Smeltzer: op. cit., pp. 1484–1486.
13. Danforth, H.A., Snow, M., and Stiefel, D.J.: *Dental Management of the Cerebral Palsied Patient.* Disability Dental Instruction, 4919 Northeast 86th Street, Seattle, Washington, 98115, 30 pp.
14. Sorenson, H.W.: Physically Handicapped, in Nowak, A.J.: *Dentistry for the Handicapped Patient.* St. Louis, The C.V. Mosby Co., 1976, pp. 23–38.
15. Shafer, W.G., Hine, M.K., and Levy, B.M.: *A Textbook of Oral Pathology,* 4th ed. Philadelphia, W.B. Saunders Co., 1983, pp. 859.
16. Vap, J.G.: Bell's Palsy, *Ear Nose Throat J., 57,* 284, July, 1978.
17. Ewing, J.A. and Endicott, J.N.: Rehabilitation of the Face After Facial-nerve Paralysis, *Ear Nose Throat J., 57,* 288, July, 1978.
18. Larsen, S.J., Carter, J.F., and Abrahamian, H.A.: Prosthetic Support for Unilateral Facial Paralysis, *J. Prosthet. Dent., 35,* 192, February, 1976.
19. Snyder, N.C.: *Dental Hygiene Clinical Applications in Pharmacology.* Philadelphia, Lea & Febiger, 1987, p. 229.
20. Robbins, Cotran, and Kumar: op. cit., pp. 1351–1355.
21. Hahn, B.H.: Arthritis, Connective Tissue Disorders, and Extraarticular Rheumatism, in Steinberg, F.U., ed.: *Care of the Geriatric Patient,* 6th ed. St. Louis, The C.V. Mosby Co., 1983, pp. 47–56.
22. Rubin, R., Salvati, E.A., and Lewis, R.: Infected Total Hip Replacement After Dental Procedures, *Oral Surg. Oral Med. Oral Pathol., 41,* 18, January, 1976.
23. Mulligan, R.: Late Infections in Patients with Prostheses for Total Replacement of Joints: Implications for the Dental Practitioner, *J. Am. Dent. Assoc., 101,* 44, July, 1980.
24. Wood, R.E. and Lee, P.: Analysis of the Oral Manifestations of Systemic Sclerosis (Scleroderma), *Oral Surg. Oral Med. Oral Pathol., 65,* 172, February, 1988.
25. Uthman, A.A., Winkler, S., and Scott, S.J.: The Scleroderma Patient, *J. Oral Med., 33,* 65, April-June, 1978.

Suggested Readings

Basson, M.D. and Burney, R.E.: Defective Wound Healing in Patients with Paraplegia and Quadriplegia, *Surg. Gynecol. Obstet., 155,* 9, July, 1982.

Been, V.C.: Harborview, *Dent. Hyg., 54,* 480, October, 1980.
Corbet, B.: *Options. Spinal Cord Injury and the Future.* Denver, Hirschfield, 1980, 152 pp.
Crinzi, R.A., Palm, N.V., Mostofi, R., and Indresano, A.T.: Management of a Dental Infection in a Patient with Sturge-Weber Disease, *J. Am. Dent. Assoc., 101,* 798, November, 1980.
Kleiman, C.S. and Tadano, P.: Maximum Independence for the SCI Patient, *RDH, 3,* 15, January/February, 1983.
Koster, S.: Orthodontics for the Handicapped Patient, in Nowak, A.J.: *Dentistry for the Handicapped Patient.* St. Louis, The C.V. Mosby Co., 1976, pp. 331–333.
Quart, A.M.: Dental Treatment for Spinal Cord Injury Patients in a Specialized Reclinable Wheelchair, *Spec. Care Dentist., 2,* 252, November-December, 1982.
Swerdloff, M.: The Problems and Concerns of the Handicapped, *J. Dent. Educ., 44,* 131, March, 1980.

Mouth-held Orthosis

Cloran, A.J., Lotz, J.W., Campbell, H.D., and Wiechers, D.O.: Oral Telescoping Orthosis: An Aid to Functional Rehabilitation of Quadriplegic Patients, *J. Am. Dent. Assoc., 100,* 876, June, 1980.
DiPietro, G.J., Warfield, D.K., and Bradshaw, A.J.: A Jaw-operated Proximity Switch for a Paraplegic Patient, *J. Prosthet. Dent., 56,* 711, December, 1986.
Drago, C.J.: Design Considerations for Construction of a Mouthstick Prosthesis, *Quintessence Dent. Technol., 10,* 451, July-August, 1986.
Kozole, K.P., Gordon, R.E., and Hurst, P.S.: Modular Mouthstick System, *J. Prosthet. Dent., 53,* 831, June, 1985.
Mulligan, R.: A Physiologic Bitestick Appliance for Quadriplegics, *Spec. Care Dentist., 3,* 24, January-February, 1983.
Olsen, R.A., Prentke, E.M., and Olsen, D.B.: A Versatile and Easily Fabricated Mouthstick, *J. Prosthet. Dent., 55,* 247, February, 1986.
Rodeghero, P., Claman, L., Cellier, S., and Lotz, J.W.: The Long-term Effect of Mouthsticks on Periodontal Support, *Spec. Care Dentist., 5,* 251, November-December, 1985.
Smokler, J. and Rappaport, S.C.: Mouthstick Prosthesis for a Patient With Arthrogryposis Multiplex Congenita, *J. Prosthet. Dent., 42,* 316, September, 1979.

Cerebrovascular Accident

Imm, L.C.: Dental Management of the Stroke Patient, *Dent. Hyg., 57,* 43, October, 1983.
Kaplan, E.L., ed.: *Cardiovascular Disease in Dental Practice.* American Heart Association, 1986, pp. 14–16.
Kleiman, C.S., Zafran, J.N., and Zayon, G.M.: Dental Care for the Stroke Patient, *Dent. Hyg., 54,* 237, May, 1980.
Veis, S.L. and Logemann, J.A.: Swallowing Disorders in Persons with Cerebrovascular Accident, *Arch. Phys. Med. Rehabil., 66,* 372, June, 1985.
Wertsch, J.J.: Rehabilitation of the Patient After Cerebrovascular Accident, *Spec. Care Dentist., 4,* 177, July-August, 1984.

Muscular Dystrophy

Cherny, I., Lopez, J.I., and Schuman, N.J.: Dental Treatment for a Patient with Duchenne Muscular Dystrophy and Malignant Hyperthermia, *Gen. Dent., 34,* 299, July-August, 1986.
Darras, B.T., Harper, J.F., and Francke, U.: Prenatal Diagnosis and Detection of Carriers with DNA Probes in Duchenne's Muscular Dystrophy, *N. Engl. J. Med., 316,* 985, April 16, 1987.
Leinbach, T.E.: Prosthetic Treatment of Malocclusion in Patients with Muscular Dystrophy, *J. Prosthet. Dent., 58,* 604, November, 1987.
Morinushi, T. and Mastumoto, S.: Oral Findings and a Proposal for a Dental Health Care Program for Patients with Duchenne Type Muscular Dystrophy, *Spec. Care Dentist., 6,* 117, May-June, 1986.
Petty, T.L. and Crespi, P.: Duchenne Muscular Dystrophy: A Report of Case, *Spec. Care Dentist., 7,* 211, September-October, 1987.

Siegel, I.M.: Muscular Dystrophy. Multidisciplinary Approach to Management, *Postgrad. Med., 69,* 124, February, 1981.

Smith, P.E.M., Calverley, P.M.A., Edwards, R.H.T., Evans, G.A., and Campbell, E.J.M.: Practical Problems in the Respiratory Care of Patients with Muscular Dystrophy, *N. Engl. J. Med., 316,* 1197, May 7, 1987.

Stenvik, A. and Storhaug, K.: Malocclusion Patterns in Fourteen Children with Duchenne's Muscular Dystrophy, *ASDC J. Dent. Child., 53,* 215, May-June, 1986.

Myasthenia Gravis

Gallagher, D.M., Erickson, K.L., and Genkins, G.: Current Concepts in the Surgical Treatment of Patients with Myasthenia Gravis, *J. Oral Surg., 39,* 30, January, 1981.

Schneider, P.E.: Dental Management of a Child with Severe Myasthenia Gravis, *Spec. Care Dentist., 3,* 266, November-December, 1983.

Shaw, D.H., Cohen, D.M., and Hoffman, M.: Dental Treatment of Patients with Myasthenia Gravis, *J. Oral Med., 37,* 118, October-December, 1982.

Multiple Sclerosis

Cnossen, M.W.: Considerations in the Dental Treatment of Patients with Multiple Sclerosis, *J. Oral Med., 37,* 62, April-June, 1982.

Fabiano, J.A.: Orofacial Involvement in Multiple Sclerosis, *Spec. Care Dentist., 3,* 61, March-April, 1983.

Garsrud, O.: Therapeutic Dental Aid for Patient with Multiple Sclerosis, *Br. Dent. J., 150,* 356, June 16, 1981.

Lopez, W.M. and Moore, E.M.: Lateral Gaze Deficit Suggesting Multiple Sclerosis, *Oral Surg. Oral Med. Oral Pathol., 62,* 657, December, 1986.

Marra, T.R.: Multiple Sclerosis with Onset After Age 60, *J. Am. Geriatr. Soc., 32,* 16, January, 1984.

Cerebral Palsy

Bourke, L.F. and Jago, J.D.: Problems of Persons with Cerebral Palsy in Obtaining Dental Care, *Aust. Dent. J., 28,* 221, August, 1983.

Hengen, M.: The Role of the Dental Hygienist in the Dental Care of the Cerebral Palsy Patient, *Dent. Hyg., 54,* 472, October, 1980.

Leary, B.A. and Zucker, S.B.: Teaching Preventive Dentistry to Adolescents with Cerebral Palsy, *Spec. Care Dentist., 1,* 13, January-February, 1981.

Oliver, R.G.: Theoretical Aspects and Clinical Experience with the Palatal Training Appliance for Saliva Control in Persons with Cerebral Palsy, *Spec. Care Dentist., 7,* 271, November-December, 1987.

Ray, S.A., Bundy, A.C., and Nelson, D.L.: Decreasing Drooling Through Techniques to Facilitate Mouth Closure, *Am. J. Occup. Ther., 37,* 749, November, 1983.

Bell's Palsy

Adour, K.K., Hilsinger, R.L., and Callan, E.J.: Facial Paralysis and Bell's Palsy: A Protocol for Differential Diagnosis, *Am. J. Otol., 6,* 68, Supplement, November, 1985.

Facer, G.W.: Facial Nerve Paralysis. Is It Always Bell's Palsy? *Postgrad. Med., 69,* 206, February, 1981.

Gates, G.A.: Facial Paralysis, *Otolaryngol. Clin. North Am., 20,* 113, February, 1987.

Hughes, G.B.: Current Concepts in Bell's Palsy, *Ear Nose Throat J., 62,* 6, October, 1983.

Keels, M.A., Long, L.M., and Vann, W.F.: Facial Nerve Paralysis: Report of Two Cases of Bell's Palsy, *Pediatr. Dent., 9,* 58, March, 1987.

Olsen, K.D.: Facial Nerve Paralysis. I. General Evaluation, Bell's Palsy, *Postgrad. Med., 75,* 219, June, 1984.

Arthritis

Altman, R.D.: Osteoarthritis. Aggravating Factors and Therapeutic Measures, *Postgrad. Med., 80,* 151, August, 1986.

Cassidy, J.T.: Treatment of Children with Juvenile Rheumatoid Arthritis, *N. Engl. J. Med., 314,* 1312, May 15, 1986.

Christensen, J.R.: A Soft Tissue Lesion Related to Salicylate Treatment of Juvenile Rheumatoid Arthritis: Clinical Report, *Pediatr. Dent., 6,* 159, September, 1984.

Cohen, S.B.: Arthritis—But What Sort? *Geriatrics, 37,* 49, December, 1982.

Kale, S.A. and Jones, J.V.: Rehabilitating the Elderly Arthritic, *Geriatrics, 36,* 101, June, 1981.

Krane, S.M. and Simon, L.S.: Rheumatoid Arthritis: Clinical Features and Pathogenetic Mechanisms, *Med. Clin. North Am., 70,* 263, March, 1986.

Larheim, T.A., Storhaug, K., and Treito, L.: Temporomandibular Joint Involvement and Dental Occlusion in a Group of Adults with Rheumatoid Arthritis, *Acta Odontol. Scand., 41,* 301, Number 5, 1983.

Ogden, G.R.: Complete Resorption of the Mandibular Condyles in Rheumatoid Arthritis, *Br. Dent. J., 160,* 95, February 8, 1986.

Pliskin, M.E., Lally, E.T., and Quinn, P.: Severe Oral Ulceration in a Patient Taking Low-dose Methotrexate for Rheumatoid Arthritis, *Compend. Contin. Educ. Dent., 7,* 430, June, 1986.

Stern, N.S., Trop, R.C., and Balk, P.: Total Temporomandibular Joint Replacement in a Patient with Rheumatoid Arthritis: Report of Case, *J. Am. Dent. Assoc., 112,* 491, April, 1986.

Stewart, C.L. and Standish, S.M.: Osteoarthritis of the TMJ in Teenaged Females: Report of Cases, *J. Am. Dent. Assoc., 106,* 638, May, 1983.

Tanaka, T.T.: A Rational Approach to the Differential Diagnosis of Arthritic Disorders, *J. Prosthet. Dent., 56,* 727, December, 1986.

Tanchyk, A.P.: Prevention of Tooth Erosion from Salicylate Therapy in Juvenile Rheumatoid Arthritis, *Gen. Dent., 34,* 479, November-December, 1986.

Wigley, F.M.: Osteoarthritis: Practical Management in Older Patients, *Geriatrics, 39,* 101, March, 1984.

Zide, M.F., Carlton, D.M., and Kent, J.N.: Rheumatoid Disease and Related Arthropathies. I. Systemic Findings, Medical Therapy, and Peripheral Joint Surgery, *Oral Surg. Oral Med. Oral Pathol., 61,* 119, February, 1986.

Scleroderma

Alexandridis, C. and White, S.C.: Periodontal Ligament Changes in Patients with Progressive Systemic Sclerosis, *Oral Surg. Oral Med. Oral Pathol., 58,* 113, July, 1984.

Asboe-Hansen, G.: Scleroderma, *J. Am. Acad. Dermatol., 17,* 102, July, 1987.

Eversole, L.R., Jacobsen, P.L., and Stone, C.E.: Oral and Gingival Changes in Systemic Sclerosis (Scleroderma), *J. Periodontol., 55,* 175, March, 1984.

Marmary, Y., Glaiss, R., and Pisanty, S.: Scleroderma: Oral Manifestations, *Oral Surg. Oral Med. Oral Pathol., 52,* 32, July, 1981.

Naylor, W.P.: Oral Management of the Scleroderma Patient, *J. Am. Dent. Assoc., 105,* 814, November, 1982.

Parma-Benfenati, S., Ferreira, P.A., Fugazzotto, P.A., Calura, G., Berdichevsky, M., and Ruben, M.P.: Progressive Systemic Sclerosis (Scleroderma): Oral Mucosal Changes, *Gen. Dent., 34,* 107, March-April, 1986.

Robbins, J.W., Craig, R.M., and Correll, R.W.: Symmetrical Widening of the Periodontal Ligament Space in a Patient with Multiple Systemic Problems, *J. Am. Dent. Assoc., 113,* 307, August, 1986.

Seow, W.K. and Young, W.: Localized Scleroderma in Childhood: Review of the Literature and Case Report, *Pediatr. Dent., 9,* 240, June, 1987.

Wood, R.E. and Lee, P.: Analysis of the Oral Manifestations of Systemic Sclerosis (Scleroderma), *Oral Surg. Oral Med. Oral Pathol., 65,* 172, February, 1988.

55 *The Patient with a Sensory Handicap*

Successful management and treatment of any patient depend to a large extent on the interpersonal communication between the patient and the clinician. When a patient has a vision or hearing impairment, communication assumes a different dimension. Suggestions for adaptations for patients with hearing or visual problems are described in this chapter.

Special skills used to counsel, motivate, and educate a patient with a sensory handicap must be developed and practiced. Although nonverbal channels provide a primary method of communication with the hearing impaired person, verbal and "touch" channels are essential for the person with visual impairment.

VISUAL IMPAIRMENT

Limitations of sight cover a broad spectrum from the slightly affected to the completely blind with no perception of light. Adaptations during the appointment vary then from a procedure as simple as providing a patient's eyeglasses before demonstrating a toothbrushing procedure to those required for the partially sighted or completely sightless as described in this section.

Loss of sight is a major physical deprivation. In many persons, blindness is secondary to a primary condition that may have been the cause of the blindness and in itself may be disabling.

In the United States, "legal blindness" is defined as follows: the central visual acuity is 20/200 or less in the better eye after correction, or visual acuity of more than 20/200 if there is a peripheral field defect in which the widest diameter of the visual field is less than a radius of 10 degrees. Only approximately 3 percent of legally blind persons are totally blind. The term legal blindness is a legal, not a medical, term, but certification of the degree of severity of blindness is obtained from an ophthalmologist.

I. Causes of Blindness

The leading causes of blindness are diabetic retinopathy, senile cataracts, glaucoma, vascular disease, and infections.[1] At least one half of the blindness in children is of prenatal origin particularly resulting from maternal infections (rubella, syphilis, toxoplasmosis). Other causes are injuries, neoplasms, and retrolental fibroplasia. Retrolental fibro-

plasia was once a major cause of blindness in premature infants, but now is rare because it can be prevented by proper control of the oxygen exposure of an infant.

II. Personal Factors

Each person with visual impairment must be considered in relation to individual aptitudes, interests, abilities, and potentialities, with sight as one factor involved. No pattern of patient attitudes and personality characteristics can be described. The only common characteristic this group of patients has is difficulty in seeing. A few suggestions of factors involved are mentioned here.

A. Patient History

Assistance in completing the personal questionnaire may be needed. Specific details of the patient's limitations must be recorded so that adaptations can be made during the appointment.

B. Child

1. *Learning Ability*
   a. Sensory defects often mask a child's intellectual capacity because responses cannot be the same as in other children.
   b. Blind children may learn to speak later than sighted children and may start school when they are a year or two older.
   c. A blind child takes longer than does the sighted child to cover the same amount of material; therefore, the educational level for the blind child may be different from that for the sighted child of the same chronologic age.
   d. Blind children are deprived of the opportunity to learn by imitation.
2. *Personal Factors.* Environment influences the child's adjustment, and parental attitude affects the blind child as it does the sighted child. When the parent is overindulgent and protective, the child may be self-centered, dependent, and emotionally less stable.

C. Adult

The adult who has always been blind or has been so since childhood has made adjustments and may be employed in a limited but useful occupation. The greater number of those who become blind after adulthood experience an immediate natural reaction of depression and feeling of helplessness.

When loss of vision is incipient, the reactions of shock and upheaval usually are less, but dread, worry, and anxiety may be experienced for years in anticipation. When the patient begins to accept the handicap, efforts for rehabilitation are made easier. Independence and self-confidence should be developed, and the patient must be helped to avoid helplessness.

III. Dental Hygiene Care: Totally Blind

A. Factors in Patient Care
1. A blind person can perceive a new experience readily if told about it in detail.
2. Because of the visual handicap, the patient must rely more on other senses and cultivate them.
3. A blind person must be neat and orderly. If something is put down, it must be located readily again.
4. A blind person does things deliberately and slowly to gain perception and prevent accidents.
5. Effective conversation with a blind person can best be accomplished by speaking as on a telephone.
6. A blind person learns to interpret and rely on tone of voice more than do persons with sight who can watch facial expressions.

B. Patient Reception and Seating
1. Lower dental chair prior to receiving patient; move other dental equipment, such as the bracket tray and operating stool, from pathway.
2. Guide to dental chair. Patient holds arm and is led without being pushed or pulled (figure 55–1).
3. Provide forewarnings of potential hazards in the pathway.
4. Instruct patient of step up to conventional dental chair.
5. The patient who has become familiar with office arrangement from previous appointments should be informed of changes to prevent embarrassment.
6. When leaving the treatment room during the appointment, explain absence; prevent embarrassment of patient speaking to someone who is not there; speak when reentering the room.

C. The Dog Guide
1. Do not distract a dog guide on duty by speaking to or touching it.
2. Ask the patient where the best place would be for the dog to stay during the appointment. The dogs are gentle, carefully trained animals, and may lie quietly in a corner of the treatment room as directed by the patient.

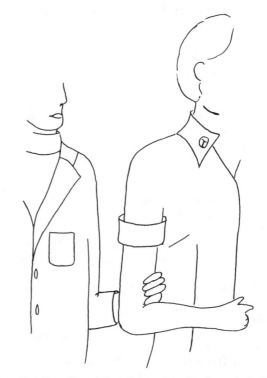

Figure 55–1. Escorting a Blind Person. The blind person holds the arm of the guide just above the elbow and walks beside and slightly behind. The guide verbally gives advance notice of approaching changes. The blind person can sense the body motion of the guide and anticipate changes.

D. Introduce Clinical Procedures
1. Describe each step in detail before proceeding. Explain instruments, materials, and how each will be applied. Mention flavors.
2. Permit patient to handle instruments, such as a mouth mirror. This applies particularly to child patient who is not familiar with dental procedures.
3. Use other instruments of a similar size and shape when describing scalers or explorers because handling sharp instruments would be dangerous for the patient.
4. Prepare patient for power-driven instruments.
   a. Avoid surprise applications of compressed air, water from syringe, or power-driven instruments.
   b. Apply moving rubber cup to child's finger. When power-driven instruments disturb the patient, a porte polisher may be used when polishing is considered necessary.
5. Speak before touching the patient. By maintaining contact of a finger on a tooth or through retraction while changing instruments, repeated orientation can be avoided.
6. Rinsing:
   a. Use evacuator when possible.
   b. Without evacuation, explain the water syringe and place rinsing cup in the patient's

hand each time. Do not expect the patient to pick it up from unit.

c. Help the patient avoid embarrassment if water is spilled.

E. Instructions for Patient
1. Give instructions clearly and concisely.
2. Visual aids, such as models, may be used if described in detail and given to the patient to handle.
3. Demonstrate toothbrushing in patient's mouth.

IV. Dental Hygiene Care: Partially Sighted

Persons with sight often underestimate the degree and fail to realize how useful a little vision can be. Patience in helping a patient to make full use of available vision, without oversolicitousness, is important. Although many of the procedures described for the totally blind person can be applied to the partially sighted person, a few additional hints are suggested below.

Elderly patients with failing sight rarely admit such a handicap. Sight failure in the aged individual or lowered vision in a person of any age may be suspected from the patient's unusual squinting, blinking, or lack of continued attention. Techniques can be adapted without mention of sight to the patient.

A. Patient Position
Adjust for patient comfort. Tilting back a patient with glaucoma may increase pain and pressure in the eyes.

B. Light
Avoid glare of the operating light in the patient's eyes. Sensitivity to light is characteristic of many eye conditions.

C. Patient Instruction
1. Position patient for best vision. For example, a patient with glaucoma has no peripheral vision; thus instruction should be given directly from the front.
2. Do not expect patient to see fine detail such as that in a radiograph or on a small model.
3. Work patiently and give instruction slowly. Patient may have slow visual accommodation.
4. Present the patient's eyeglasses before beginning instruction.

HEARING IMPAIRMENT

When hearing is impaired to the extent that it has no practical value for the purpose of communication, a person is considered deaf. When hearing is defective but functional with or without a hearing aid, the terms "hard of hearing" or "hearing impaired" are used.

I. Causes of Hearing Impairment

Inability to hear may be temporary or permanent. A wide variety of factors contribute to deafness. In young children, heredity; prenatal influences, particularly rubella and blood incompatibilities; perinatal conditions, notably birth trauma and prematurity; and postnatal influences, particularly infectious diseases (meningitis), trauma, and drugs are important causes.

Deafness beginning during school-age years can result from complications of upper respiratory infections. Older people may develop deafness following chronic infection of the middle ear, toxicity from various chemotherapeutic drugs, and trauma. Deterioration of hearing range may occur with aging.

II. Characteristics

A. Major Types
1. *Conductive Hearing Loss*
   a. Part involved. Middle ear, external canal, or drum membrane.
   b. Hearing aid. Plate behind ear; sound is conducted by bone.
   c. Speech. Soft and low; person hears own voice louder than that of others.
2. *Perceptive or Sensorineural Hearing Loss*
   a. Part involved. Inner ear; injury to nerves.
   b. Hearing aid. Button in ear; sound conducted by air. Hearing aids are more helpful to those with conductive hearing loss.
   c. Speech. Loud; person cannot hear own voice.
3. *Combined Conductive and Sensorineural Hearing Loss*
4. *Psychogenic Hearing Loss*
   a. Unrelated to structural changes.
   b. May be a manifestation of an emotional disturbance.

B. Characteristics Suggesting Hearing Impairment
Partial deafness may not have been diagnosed, or certain patients, particularly the elderly person, may not admit hearing limitation. Clues to the identification of a hearing problem are listed as follows.
1. Lack of attention; fails to respond to conversational tone.
2. Intentness; strained facial expression; stares at others.
3. Turns head to one side; hearing may be good on one side only.
4. Gives unexpected answer unrelated to question; does one thing when told to do another.
5. Frequently asks others to repeat what was said.
6. Unusual speech tone.
7. Inaccurate pronunciation, which is characteristic of a child who repeats what is heard. With defective hearing, certain sounds are missing in the hearing range.

C. Personal Factors
People with hearing loss are at a disadvantage because they are not aware of what is being said

(Continued on page 680)

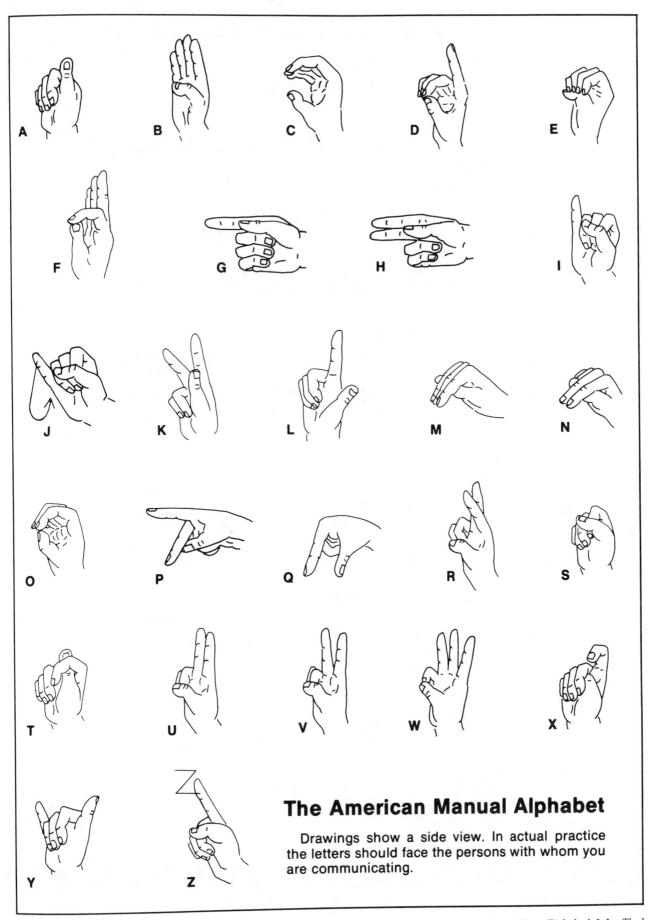

The American Manual Alphabet

Drawings show a side view. In actual practice the letters should face the persons with whom you are communicating.

Figure 55–2. American Manual Alphabet. Fingerspelling is used in combination with signs and lip reading. (From Riekehof, L.L.: *The Joy of Signing*, Second Edition, Gospel Publishing House, Springfield, Missouri. Copyright 1987. Reproduced by permission.)

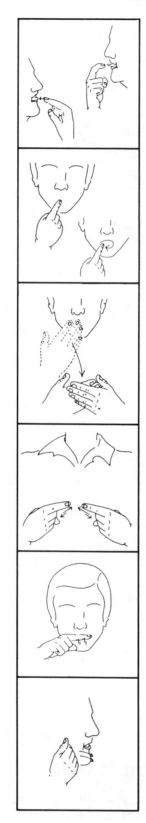

TEETH

Run the tip of the bent index finger across the teeth.
Usage: strong white *teeth*.

TONGUE

Touch the tip of the tongue with the index finger.
Usage: A look at your *tongue* tells the doctor something.

MOUTH

Point to the mouth.
Usage: The dentist looked into my *mouth*.

LIPS

Trace the lips with the index finger.
Usage: Your *lips* are easy to read.

GOOD, WELL

Touch the lips with the fingers of the right hand and then move the right hand forward placing it palm up in the palm of the left hand.
Origin: It has been tasted and smelled and offered as acceptable.
Usage: *good* food; doing *well* at work.

PAIN, ACHE, HURT

The index fingers are jabbed toward each other several times.
Note: This sign is generally made in front of the body but may be placed at the location of the pain, as: headache, toothache, heartache, etc.
Usage: suffered *pain* after the accident; *aching* all over; my knee *hurts;* have an *earache*.

TOOTHBRUSH

Using the index finger as a brush, imitate the motion of brushing the teeth.
Usage: *brushing teeth* twice a day.

DAILY, EVERY DAY

Place the side of the "A" hand on the cheek and rub it toward the chin several times.
Origin: Indicating several tomorrows.
Usage: *daily* bread.
       drive to work *every day.*

Figure 55–3. Examples of Signing. Selected words that may be used during a patient's dental appointment. (From Riekehof, L.L.: *The Joy of Signing*, Second Edition, Gospel Publishing House, Springfield, Missouri. Copyright 1987. Reproduced by permission.)

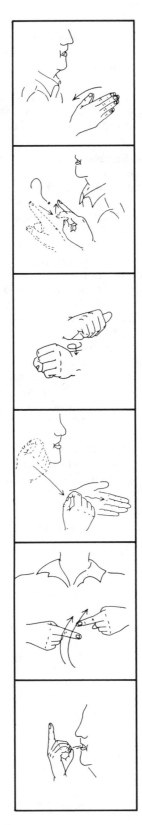

ASK, REQUEST

Place the open hands palm to palm and draw them toward the body.
Origin: Hands held as in prayer.
Usage: *Ask* for help. What is your *request?*

QUESTION

Draw a question mark in the air with the index finger; draw it back and direct it forward as if placing the dot below the question mark.
Usage: That *question* is hard to answer.

ENGAGEMENT, APPOINTMENT, RESERVATION

Make a small circle with the right "A" hand and then place the wrist on the wrist of the left "S" which is facing right.
Origin: Indicating one is bound.
Usage: a dinner *engagement* tonight.
a 4 o'clock *appointment*.
a plane *reservation*.

SECRETARY

Take an imaginary pencil from the ear, write into the left hand and make the "PERSON" ending.
Origin: A person who takes notes.
Usage: Teri is my good *secretary*.

COME

Index fingers rotating once around each other move toward the body. Or, use the open hand in a beckoning motion.
Origin: Using the hands in a natural motion.
Usage: When can you *come* to my home?
Come, I'm waiting for you. (Use second description.)

DENTIST

Place the right "D" at the teeth.
Origin: The initial sign at the teeth.
Usage: Let the *dentist* check your teeth.

Figure 55–3. *Continued.*

around them. Conversation always should be carried on within the sight of the patient. Patients with hearing loss are bothered when they do not know what others are saying. This reaction is especially true of older persons who develop paranoid tendencies and believe that, when they cannot hear, other people are talking about them. Children do not have this problem, but live in their own little world and watch others.

III. Dental Hygiene Care

At the initial appointment, the patient may need to be accompanied by a person who can assist with the preparation of the histories and listen while the treatment plan is presented. Lengthy or involved explanations require an interpreter who is familiar with the communication methods of the patient.

A. Patient With Hearing Aid

1. Be careful not to touch a hearing aid when it is operating.
2. Ask patient to turn off or remove a hearing aid when a power-driven dental instrument, particularly an ultrasonic scaler, will be used. The noise can be amplified many times, much to the discomfort of the patient.
3. Speak slowly. Pause between sentences.

B. Patient With Partial Hearing Ability

1. Speak clearly and distinctly; direct speaking to side of "good" ear, if hearing is impaired on one side only.
2. Eliminate interfering noises from street outside or saliva ejector suction.

C. Lip Reader

1. Be sure patient is looking; do not turn to side; speak directly.
2. Speaker's face must be clearly visible so patient can read lips easily; difficult when dental light is directed to patient's face or the clinician has back to window.
3. Speak in normal tone; do not accentuate words; pause more frequently than usual.
4. Do not raise voice; raising voice aggravates the situation; patient may be inclined to withdraw.
5. When patient cannot understand, use alternate words to express the same thought; many letters and combinations of letters look the same on the lips; others are not visible at all.
6. Keep calm; display of irritation or annoyance over difficulties in conversing discourages or upsets the patient.
7. Write proper names or unusual words the patient fails to understand.
8. When wearing a mask, communication by writing notes will be necessary. If maximum precautions are being observed (page 58), the pencil and paper can be destroyed with the other disposables.

D. Sign Language

All the points previously mentioned for the lip reader apply to patients who use sign language because lips are read along with signs. Learning basic sign language and finger spelling can provide health personnel with an added communication skill.[1] The American manual alphabet is shown in figure 55–2.[2] A few examples of signs are shown in figure 55–3.

E. General Suggestions

1. Written messages. Use a clipboard with a marker-type pen attached and large paper, at least 8½ × 11 inches. Write clearly.
2. Do not startle the patient by tapping to gain attention.
3. Watch for patient's motions and facial expressions to determine reaction or discomfort.
4. Teach by demonstration
   a. Use mirror and show bacterial plaque removal methods directly on teeth.
   b. Younger child may be taught to rinse by watching and imitating.
   c. Provide reassurance and approval by maintaining eye contact and smiling.
5. Person with a hearing impairment should always have a written appointment card to assure complete understanding; appointments made by telephone should be confirmed by mail.
6. Use judgment in prolonging conversation with deaf person. Certain patients are under tension and tire easily, whereas others enjoy the opportunity to communicate.

TECHNICAL HINTS

Sources of Materials and Information

American Foundation for the Blind
15 East 16th Street
New York, New York 10011

National Society to Prevent Blindness and Its Affiliates
79 Madison Avenue
New York, New York 10016

National Academy, Gallaudet College
800 Florida Avenue, N.E.
Washington, D.C. 20002
(Professional Training Program for communication and training in deafness)

References

1. Engar, R.C. and Stiefel, D.J.: *Dental Treatment of the Sensory Impaired Patient.* Disability Dental Instruction, 4919 Northeast 86th Street, Seattle, Washington 98115, 65 pp.
2. Riekehof, L.L.: *The Joy of Signing,* 2nd ed. Springfield, Missouri, Gospel Publishing House, 1987.

Suggested Reading

Bomberg, T.J. and Ernst, N.S.: Improving the Dental Office Environment for the Older Patient, *J. Am. Dent. Assoc., 108,* 789, May, 1984.
Brunner, L.S., Suddarth, D.S., Bare, B.G., Boyer, M.J., and

Smeltzer, S.C.O.: *Textbook of Medical-Surgical Nursing,* 6th ed. Philadelphia, J.B. Lippincott Co., 1988, pp. 1329–1393.

Kanar, H.L.: The Blind and the Deaf, in Nowak, A.J.: *Dentistry for the Handicapped Patient.* St. Louis, The C.V. Mosby Co., 1976, pp. 121–133.

Lange, B.M., Entwistle, B.M., and Lipson, L.F.: *Dental Management of the Handicapped: Approaches for Dental Auxiliaries.* Philadelphia, Lea & Febiger, 1983, pp. 11–38.

Visual Impairment

Grossnickle, K., Lehew, D., Odell, D., and Staub, C.: *Take Time to Communicate.* Cumberland, Maryland, Dental Hygiene Program, Allegany Community College, 1981, 12 pp.

Morsey, S.L.: Communicating With and Treating the Blind Child, *Dent. Hyg., 54,* 288, June, 1980.

Talley, L.: *Let Your Fingers Do the Talking.* Johnson City, Tennessee, Department of Dental Hygiene, Eastern Tennessee State University, 1981, 44 pp.

Hearing Impairment

Clark, C.A., Cangelosi-Williams, P., Lee, M.A., and Morgan, L.: Dental Treatment for Deaf Patients, *Spec. Care Dentist., 6,* 102, May-June, 1986.

Huether, K.J. and Born, D.O.: Dentistry for Hearing Impaired Persons, *Northwest Dent., 61,* 14, January-February, 1982.

Jones, G.A., Dickens, R.L., Armbruster, D.L., and Laughter, J.S.: Dental Xrays Found to Have No Effect on Hearing Aids, *J. Am. Dent. Assoc., 113,* 912, December, 1986.

LoCascio, E., Rubinstein, L., and Aymard, L.L.: Deafness and Dental Health Care, *Clin. Prevent. Dent., 7,* 11, July-August, 1985.

Sweeney, D.-J.: Volunteer Work in Deaf Community Keeps This Dental Hygienist Going, *Can. Dent. Hyg., 21,* 158, December, 1987.

Warner, R.W.: Improving Communication With the Older Patient: Overcoming the Physical Barrier of a Hearing Loss, *Spec. Care Dentist., 6,* 15, January-February, 1986.

56 *The Patient with a Cardiovascular Disease*

Cardiovascular, as the names implies, includes diseases of the heart and blood vessels. Diseases of the heart are the leading causes of death in the United States.

Patients with cardiovascular conditions are encountered frequently in a dental office or clinic and may be from any age group, although the highest incidence is among older people. A heart disease may be present for many years before the symptoms are recognized. The patients seen in the dental office range from those with no obvious symptoms to the nearly disabled. In severe cases, the nonambulatory patient may require care in the home.

I. Classification

Classification of the diseases is made either on an anatomic or etiologic basis. In an anatomic system, diseases of the pericardium, myocardium, endocardium, heart valves, and blood vessels are defined. In an etiologic system, the diseases are named by the cause. The principal causes of heart diseases are infectious agents, atherosclerosis, hypertension, immunologic mechanisms, and congenital anomalies.

II. Major Cardiovascular Diseases

The five major cardiovascular diseases are congenital heart disease, rheumatic heart disease, infective endocarditis, ischemic heart disease, and hypertensive heart disease. Characteristics and symptoms are complex and overlapping. In this chapter, each of the major diseases is described by its principal symptoms and treatments as well as the applications in dental hygiene care.

III. Terminology

The terminology used for describing the cardiovascular diseases is listed and defined in table 56–1. Prefixes, suffixes, and other word derivations to clarify the terminology are listed on pages 757–759.

CONGENITAL HEART DISEASES

Anomalies of the anatomic structure of the heart or major blood vessels result following irregularities of development during the first 9 weeks in utero. The fetal heart is completely developed by the ninth week.

Early diagnosis is important because between one fourth and one half of the infants born with cardio-

vascular anomalies require treatment during the first year. Treatment usually involves surgical correction.

I. Types

Many types of heart defects exist. Those that occur most frequently are the ventricular septal defect, patent ductus arteriosus, atrial septal defect, and transposition of the great vessels.

A diagram of the normal heart is shown in figure 56–1 to provide a comparison with the anatomic changes that may appear in a defective heart. Congenital anomalies either produce abnormal pathways in the blood flow or interfere with the flow itself. The two most common anomalies will be described.

A. Ventricular Septal Defect

In this type of defect, the left and right ventricles are connected through an opening in their dividing wall (septum). The oxygenated blood from the lung, which is normally pumped by the

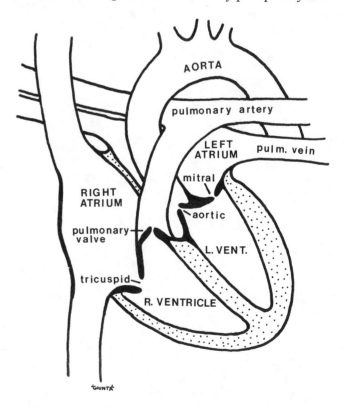

Figure 56–1. The Normal Heart. The major vessels and the location of the tricuspid, pulmonary, aortic, and mitral valves are shown.

Table 56–1.   Glossary of Terms Used in Cardiovascular Diseases

Aneurysm: dilation of an artery.

Angina: severe constricting pain.

Angina pectoris: pain in the chest.

Anoxia: absence of oxygen supply to tissues.

Anticoagulant: medication used to prevent blood coagulation.

Apnea: absence of breathing.

Arrhythmia: irregularity of the heartbeat.

Arterial blood: oxygenated blood carried by an artery away from the heart to nourish the tissues.

Asphyxia: impaired exchange of oxygen and carbon dioxide; suffocation.

Atheroma (atheromatous plaque); lipid (cholesterol) deposit on the intima (lining) of an artery; the lesion of atherosclerosis.

Bradycardia: slowness of heartbeat (less than 60 beats per minute in an adult).

Cyanosis: dark blue color of skin and mucous membranes caused by deficient oxygenation of tissues by the blood.

Dyspnea: shortness of breath.

Dysrhythmia: defective irregular heart rhythm.

Edema: excessive fluid in cells or tissues.

Electrocardiogram: graphic record of the heart's action.

Embolus: detached blood clot; mass of bacteria or other foreign matter blocking a blood vessel.

Hypoxia: reduced oxygen supply to tissues.

Infarct: area of tissue that has undergone necrosis as a result of complete blockage of blood flow; usually from obstruction of the artery supplying the area.

Ischemia: local anemia or oxygen deprivation because of mechanical obstruction of the blood supply.

Lumen: open space inside a tubular structure (blood vessel or intestine).

Murmur: irregularity of heart beat sound caused by a turbulent flow of blood through a valve that has failed to close.

Myocardial: relating to the myocardium, the middle layer of the heart; consists of muscle.

Occlusion: blockage; state of being closed.

Orthopnea: discomfort on breathing in any position except sitting erect or standing.

Prolapse: slide forward, fall down, slip from usual position.

Sclerosis: induration or hardening.

Stenosis: narrowing or stricture.

Aortic stenosis: narrowing of aortic valve opening.

Mitral stenosis: narrowing of mitral valve opening.

Syncope: a sudden transient loss of consciousness; fainting.

Tachycardia: rapid action of the heart.

Tetralogy of Fallot: congenital, cyanotic malformation of the heart which includes pulmonary stenosis, ventricular septal defect, hypertrophy of the right ventricle, and dextroposition of the aorta.

Thrombus: blood clot attached to the intima of a blood vessel; may occlude lumen.

Venous blood: nonoxygenated blood from the tissues; blood pumped from the heart to the lungs for oxygen.

Ventricular fibrillation: dysrhythmia with heart muscle bundles contracting independently without producing effective circulation.

left ventricle to the aorta and then to the entire body, can pass across to the right ventricle as shown in figure 56–2.

When the opening is very small, only a heart murmur and little disability result. If the opening is large, the heart enlarges to compensate for overwork.

B. Patent Ductus Arteriosus

A patent ductus arteriosus means the passageway (shunt) is open between the two great arteries that arise from the heart, namely the aorta and the pulmonary artery. Normally, the opening is closed during the first few weeks after birth. When the opening does not close, blood from the aorta can pass back to the lungs, as shown in figure 56–3. The heart compensates in the attempt to provide the body with oxygenated blood and becomes overburdened.

II. Etiology

Causes are genetic, environmental, or a combination. Many are unknown.

A. Genetic

Heredity is apparent in some types of defects. An example of a chromosomal defect is Down's syndrome, in which congenital heart anomalies occur frequently (page 650).

B. Environmental

Most congenital anomalies originate between the fifth and eighth weeks of fetal life, when the heart is developing.
1. Rubella (German measles).
2. Drugs

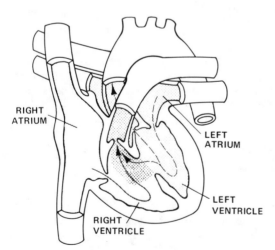

Figure 56–2. Ventricular Septal Defect. The right and left ventricles are connected by an opening that permits oxygenated blood from the left ventricle to shunt across to the right ventricle and then recirculate to the lungs. Compare with figure 56–1 in which the septum separates the ventricles. (From Bleck, E.E. and Nagel, D.A.: *Physically Handicapped Children. A Medical Atlas for Teachers.* New York, Grune & Stratton, 1975.)

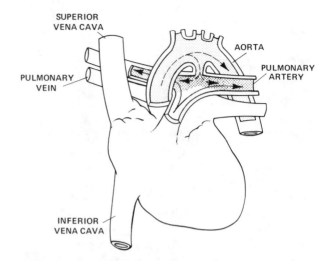

Figure 56–3. Patent Ductus Arteriosus. An open passageway between the aorta and the pulmonary artery permits oxygenated blood from the aorta to pass back into the lungs. Arrows show directions of flow through the patent ductus. Compare with normal anatomy in figure 56–1. (From Bleck, E.E. and Nagel, D.A.: *Physically Handicapped Children. A Medical Atlas for Teachers.* New York, Grune & Stratton, 1975.)

a. Chronic maternal alcohol abuse. The fetal alcohol syndrome is described on page 728.
b. Thalidomide.

III. Prevention

A. Use of rubella vaccine for childhood immunization. Vaccination confers indefinite immunity. Vaccination for women of child-bearing age is highly advised. The vaccine should not be given during pregnancy, and not within 3 months of becoming pregnant, because of potential risks to the fetus.
B. No medications used during pregnancy without prior consultation with the physician.
C. Appropriate use of radiologic equipment. A lead apron should be used when oral radiographs are made.
D. Control of drug and alcohol addictions.
E. Genetic counseling.

IV. Clinical Considerations

A. Signs and Symptoms of Congenital Heart Disease

General conditions that may be present and that influence patient management are
1. Easy fatigue.
2. Exertional dyspnea; fainting.
3. Cyanosis of lips and nailbeds.
4. Poor growth and development.
5. Chest deformity.
6. Heart murmurs.

B. Dental Hygiene Concerns

1. *Prevention of Infective Endocarditis.* Defective heart valves are susceptible to endocarditis from bacteremia produced during oral treatments.

2. *Elimination of Oral Disease.* Maintenance of a high level of oral health.

RHEUMATIC HEART DISEASE[1,2]

Rheumatic heart disease is a complication following rheumatic fever. A rather high percentage of patients with a history of rheumatic fever have permanent heart valve damage. The damaged heart valve, as in congenital heart disease, is susceptible to infective endocarditis.

I. Rheumatic Fever

A. Incidence

Approximately 90 percent of initial attacks occur between ages 5 and 15. The patient is left susceptible to future attacks, which may cause additional damage to previously damaged heart valves. The tendency to recurrence diminishes with age.

B. Etiology

1. The onset of acute rheumatic fever usually appears 2 to 3 weeks after a beta-hemolytic group A streptococcal pharyngeal infection.
2. Rheumatic fever and rheumatic heart disease are believed to be immunologic disorders caused by sensitization to antigens of beta-hemolytic group A streptococci.

C. Prevention

The persistence and severity of the pharyngeal infection are significant factors in whether rheumatic fever follows; therefore, early diagnosis and treatment of streptococcal throat and pharyngeal infections are necessary.

D. Symptoms of Rheumatic Fever

Over a period of several months of low grade fever, the joints, heart muscles, central nervous system, skin, and subcutaneous tissues become involved. All of the symptoms described below disappear with recovery except the cardiac valve damage.

1. *Arthritis.* Migratory polyarthritis is present, which may affect more than one joint at a time. The temporomandibular joint is rarely involved.
2. *Carditis.* In a severe case, death may result from heart failure during the acute stage of rheumatic fever, or valvular damage may be sustained with disability. Severity varies, and many patients do not have heart symptoms at the time of the acute illness, some never, and others may have rheumatic heart disease diagnosed later in life without having had evidence of rheumatic fever.

   The mitral valve is most commonly affected, followed by the aortic valve (figure 56–1). Rheumatic carditis is almost always associated with a significant murmur of insufficiency. The damaged valves are susceptible to infection, leading to infective endocarditis.
3. *Subcutaneous Nodules.* Painless swellings may appear over bony prominences.
4. *Chorea.* Irregular and involuntary actions of muscles, particularly of the extremities and the face, may appear as a late or delayed manifestation.
5. *Erythema Marginatum.* A pink skin rash, which may appear long after the acute stage, tends to be migratory and transient.

II. The Course of Rheumatic Heart Disease

Many factors influence the outlook after rheumatic fever symptoms subside. Usually, no symptoms persist except the effects of the valvular deformity.

A. Symptoms

1. Stenosis or incompetence of valves; most commonly, the aortic and mitral valves.
2. Heart murmur influenced by the amount of scarring of the valves and myocardium.
3. Cardiac arrhythmias.
4. Late symptoms include shortness of breath, elevation of diastolic blood pressure, enlargement of the left ventricle, and increasing signs of cardiac failure.

B. Practice Applications

The significance in dental and dental hygiene practice is the same as for congenital heart disease.

1. Maintenance of a high level of oral health to prevent a need for treatment of advanced disease.
2. Prevention of infective endocarditis by antibiotic premedication.

INFECTIVE ENDOCARDITIS[1,3]

Infective endocarditis is a microbial infection of the heart valves or endocardium that occurs in proximity to congenital or acquired defects. Subacute infective endocarditis, often called subacute bacterial endocarditis (SBE), is of vital concern in the dental and dental hygiene care of high-risk patients with valvular defects.

A bacteremia, or presence of microorganisms in the bloodstream, is necessary for the development of infective endocarditis. A transitory bacteremia usually is created during dental hygiene treatment as well as during surgical procedures involving the upper respiratory tract, genitourinary tract, or lower gastrointestinal tract.

Infective endocarditis is a serious disease, the prognosis of which depends on the degree of cardiac damage, the valves involved, the duration of the infection, and the treatment. Patients are prone to develop heart failure leading to death unless the infection is promptly controlled.

Infective endocarditis is characterized by the formation of vegetations composed of masses of bacteria and blood clots on the heart valves. The vegetations may arise on normal valves, but are most likely to occur on previously damaged valves. When bacteremia occurs, the heart valves may become infected, and infective endocarditis can develop.

I. Etiology

A. Microorganisms

Almost any species of microorganisms may cause infective endocarditis. Streptococci and staphylococci are responsible in a large majority of cases, with alpha-hemolytic streptococci being the most prevalent. Because yeast, fungi, and viruses have been implicated, the choice of the name "infective" endocarditis is more inclusive than "bacterial" endocarditis.

B. Predisposing Factors

1. *Heart Valve Damage.* Approximately 40 to 60 percent of damaged heart valves result from rheumatic heart disease, and another 10 percent are congenital in origin. Other causes include syphilis, atherosclerosis, and degenerative heart disease.
2. *Infection at Portals of Entry.* Infections at sites where microorganisms may enter the circulating blood provide a constant source of potential infectious microorganisms. In the oral cavity, organisms enter the blood by way of periodontal and gingival pockets, where multitudes of many species of microorganisms are harbored. An open area of infection such as an ulcer caused by an ill-fitting denture may also provide a site of entry.

C. Precipitating Factors

1. *Self-induced Bacteremia.* In the oral cavity, self-induced bacteremias may result from eating, bruxing, chewing gum, or any activity that can force bacteria through the wall of a diseased sulcus or pocket.
2. *Trauma to Tissues by Instrumentation.* Bacteremias are created during general or oral surgery, endodontic procedures, periodontal therapy, scaling, and particularly, any therapy that causes bleeding.

II. Disease Process

A. Bacteremia Initiated

1. Trauma from instrumentation can rupture blood vessels in the gingival sulcus or pocket.
2. Pressure from trauma forces oral microorganisms into the blood. Ease of entry of organisms directly relates to the severity of trauma and the severity of the gingivitis or periodontitis.

B. Bacterial Implantation

1. Circulating microorganisms attach to damaged heart valve, prosthetic valve, or other susceptible area.

2. Microorganisms proliferate to form bacterial masses.

C. Subsequent Effects

1. Heart valve becomes inflamed; function is diminished.
2. Clumps of microorganisms (emboli) may break off and spread by way of the general circulation; complications result.

III. Prevention

Three basic areas for attention in dental and dental hygiene care contribute to the prevention of infective endocarditis. These are identification of risk patients, prophylactic antibiotic coverage for appointment procedures, and working with the patient to improve and maintain a high level of oral health to diminish the frequency and severity of bacteremias.

A. Patient History

1. *Special Content.* It cannot be overemphasized that a careful, complete patient history is needed to detect risk patients. Specific questions should be directed to elicit any history of rheumatic fever and its related symptoms, congenital heart defects, cardiac surgery, presence of prosthetic valves, pacemaker, or previous episode of infective endocarditis.
2. *Consultation with Patient's Physician.* Consultation can be assumed necessary for all patients with a history of rheumatic fever, heart defects, and any other condition suggesting the need for prophylactic antibiotic premedication. Instrumentation, including the use of a probe or explorer during evaluation of the patient, must be withheld until the medical status is cleared.

B. Prophylactic Antibiotic Premedication

1. *Recommended Regimens.* The recommendations of the American Heart Association are outlined on page 91. The American Dental Association Council on Dental Therapeutics has approved the recommendations as they pertain to dentistry.[4,5]
2. *Objectives of the Recommended Regimen*
   a. Prevent bacteremia or reduce the severity and magnitude of it.
   b. Administer antibiotic 1 hour before, so the blood level at the time of the actual procedure is adequate to control infection and prevent infective endocarditis.

C. Dental Hygiene Care

Maintenance of a high degree of oral health is very important to each patient susceptible to infective endocarditis.

1. *Instruction.* Instruction in brushing and flossing at initial appointments should be provided while the patient is under antibiotic coverage, particularly if the gingiva shows signs of inflammation and bleeds readily.

2. *Sequence of Treatment.* Plaque removal instruction should precede instrumentation for scaling and root planing, in order to bring the tissues to as healthy a state as possible. The more severe the disease, the higher the incidence of bacteremia during and following instrumentation.
3. *Instrumentation*
   a. Reduce the microbial population about the teeth and oral mucosa prior to instrumentation by having the patient brush, floss, and rinse thoroughly with an antiseptic mouthrinse.
   b. Use particular care in all instrumentation to prevent unnecessary trauma.

HYPERTENSION[6,7]

Hypertension means an abnormal elevation of blood pressure. It is a symptom, not a disease entity. It is a contributing or risk factor in many vascular diseases, or it may be a result or an effect of underlying pathologic changes.

Detection of blood pressure for dental and dental hygiene patients has become an essential step in patient evaluation prior to treatment. Early detection, with referral for additional diagnosis and treatment when indicated, can prove to be life saving for certain people. In addition, knowledge of the health problems of patients is needed so dental and dental hygiene care can be safe and free from dangers of emergencies that may arise.

I. Etiology

A. Primary or Essential Hypertension
1. *Incidence.* Approximately 90 percent of all hypertension is primary or essential.
2. *Cause.* Idiopathic; the etiologic factors are unknown.
3. *Predisposing or Risk Factors.* Combinations of the factors listed are more significant than any one alone.
   a. Heredity.
   b. Overweight.
   c. Race: the incidence is higher among black than among white Americans, the illness is more severe, and the mortality rate is higher at a younger age.
   d. Climate: hypertension is less common in tropical and semitropical countries.
   e. Salt, particularly in excess, in the diet.
   f. Sex: males are more affected before age 45; females slightly more than males in later years.
   g. Age: general increase from birth to age 20; leveling off until 40 years of age, then a slow increase into the older age group.
   h. Cigarette smoking and other risk factors for atherosclerosis are interrelated (page 689).
   i. Oral contraceptives; severe hypertension from contraceptives is uncommon. Increased hypertension over years of using contraceptives has been shown, particularly when other risk factors are also involved.
   j. Environmental conditions that increase stress factors.

B. Secondary Hypertension
About 10 percent of all hypertension is secondary: a specific cause can be identified, in which the pathologic elevation of blood pressure is secondary to a major underlying disease. Examples are disorders of the kidney or of the adrenal or pituitary glands.

II. Blood Pressure Levels

The blood pressure is the pressure exerted by the blood within the arteries. It is determined by the cardiac output, resistance of the capillary bed, and volume and viscosity of the blood. Diseases can alter each of the parts, and thus alter the blood pressure.

Procedures for blood pressure determination are described with other vital signs in Chapter 7, pages 98–101.

Blood pressure fluctuates, so that more than one reading is needed. The blood pressure should be measured two or three times and the average reading entered in the patient's record. When physicians plan treatment for a hypertensive patient, it is customary to study the individual's pattern by making at least three determinations on at least two different days.

A. Low Blood Pressure
Many healthy people have a normal diastolic pressure under 90 mm. Hg or even under 80 mm. Hg, which may be considered "low blood pressure." Such a level is normal for that person and no clinical problems are evident.

A marked sudden drop in blood pressure is usually associated with an emergency such as severe blood loss, shock, myocardial infarction, or other medical problem. Immediate attention, in the category of a medical emergency, is indicated. Referral to specific procedures can be found in table 60–1, pages 748–749.

B. Postural Hypotension
Postural or orthostatic hypotension is a condition in which fainting, nausea, or feelings of faintness or dizziness occur when a person sits up quickly from a supine position. One predisposing factor for postural hypotension is the medication used for hypertension.[8]

III. Clinical Symptoms of Hypertension

Because hypertension frequently goes unrecognized because of the lack of apparent clinical symptoms, determination of the blood pressure takes on added significance. Knowledge of the possible symptoms can aid dental personnel in watching their patients for early signs or for identification from the information the patient presents during the preparation of the patient history.

A. High Blood Pressure

Evidence of the following may be present:
1. Headaches.
2. Dizziness, fainting.
3. Shortness of breath, particularly on effort.
4. Disturbances of concentration or memory impairment.

B. Long-standing Severe Elevation of Blood Pressure

Hypertensive crisis is a life-threatening disorder. The brain, eyes, heart, or kidneys may undergo marked changes in function. In the severe state, if any or all of the following are noted, the patient should be referred immediately:
1. Occipital headaches, more severe in the morning.
2. Mental confusion leading to stupor, coma, convulsions.
3. Blurring of vision; possible loss of sight.
4. Severe dyspnea.
5. Chest pains similar to angina pectoris.

C. Major Sequelae

1. Hypertensive heart disease: enlarged heart with eventual cardiac failure.
2. Cerebral vascular accident (stroke, page 660).
3. Hypertensive renal disease.
4. Ischemic heart disease (page 689).

IV. Treatment

A. Goals

1. *Primary Hypertension*
   a. Achieve and maintain diastolic pressure level at 90 or below with minimal adverse effects.
   b. Lower the risk of serious complications and premature death.
2. *Secondary Hypertension.* Surgical or other correction of the cause is needed.

B. Life Style Changes

1. *Diet.* Salt restriction and weight loss may be all that is needed for the control of mild elevations of blood pressure.
2. *Cigarette Smoking.* All forms of tobacco must be eliminated.
3. *Other Risk Factors.* Factors that contribute to stress and tension must be decreased or minimized. Risk factors were listed on page 687.

C. Antihypertensive Drug Therapy[6,7]

1. *Selection of Therapy.* The decision by the physician to prescribe drug therapy at the various levels depends on the severity of the hypertension as well as all factors related to the patient's health.
2. *Categories of Drugs Used in Therapy*
   a. Diuretics to promote renal excretion of water and sodium ions.

b. Sympatholytic agents to modify the sympathetic nerve activity.
   c. Vasodilators to act directly on the blood vessels.
3. *Duration.* Management of hypertension must be considered a lifelong endeavor. Periodic monitoring is essential every 3 to 6 months. Dental personnel can encourage their patients to continue treatment even when a normal reading is maintained. Because many antihypertensive drugs have undesirable side effects, the patient may become discouraged and discontinue treatment.
4. *Side Effects.* The effects of the different drugs prescribed vary, but some of the problems confronted by patients may actually influence the behavior at dental and dental hygiene appointments. Cancellation of an appointment could be anticipated. Side effects may include some or all of the following:
   a. Fatigue.
   b. Gastrointestinal disturbances including nausea, diarrhea, or cramps.
   c. Xerostomia (potential for dental caries).
   d. Postural hypotension with dizziness and fainting.
   e. Impotence.
   f. Depression.

V. Hypertension in Children

Children 3 years of age and over should have blood pressure determinations made at least annually. A variety of cuff sizes are available, and other procedural suggestions are described on pages 98–101.

When a child between ages 3 and 12 has a diastolic pressure greater than 90 mm. Hg, or if over age 12, greater than 100 mm. Hg, further investigation is indicated.[9] Because hypertension has a familial tendency, determining the pressure levels for children of parents known to have hypertension may reveal important information about the health of the child. In one study, 50 percent of the children with elevated blood pressures had parents with hypertension.[10]

HYPERTENSIVE HEART DISEASE[11]

Hypertensive heart disease results from the increased load on the heart because of elevated blood pressure. When the peripheral arterial resistance to the flow of blood pumped from the heart is increased, the blood pressure rises. The heart attempts to maintain its normal output; to cope with the increased workload resulting from the peripheral resistance, muscle fibers are stretched, and the heart enlarges.

The effect of hypertension on the heart is at first a thickening of the left ventricle. In later stages, the entire heart is enlarged. This may be discerned by radiographic and medical examination.

Cardiac enlargement has no specific symptoms, but the patient may have symptoms of hypertension such as headaches, weakness, and others listed on pages 687–688. When undiagnosed and untreated, the severity increases and left ventricular congestive failure occurs, resulting from the disturbance of cardiac function.

ISCHEMIC HEART DISEASE

Ischemic heart disease is the cardiac disability, acute and chronic, that arises from reduction or arrest of blood supply to the myocardium.

The heart muscles (myocardium) are supplied through the coronary arteries, which are branches of the descending aorta. Because of the relationship to the coronary arteries, the disease is often referred to as *coronary heart disease* or *coronary artery disease.*

Ischemia means oxygen deprivation in a local area from a reduced passage of fluid into the area. Ischemic heart disease is the result of an imbalance of the oxygen supply and demand of the myocardium, which in turn, results from a narrowing or blocking of the lumen of the coronary arteries.

I. Etiology

Other factors may be involved, but the principal cause of the reduction of blood flow to the heart muscle is *atherosclerosis* of the vessel walls, which narrows the lumen, thus obstructing the flow of blood.

A. Definition of Atherosclerosis

Atherosclerosis is a disease of medium and large arteries in which atheromas deposit on and thicken the intimal layer of the involved blood vessel. An atheroma is a fibro-fatty deposit or plaque, containing several lipids, especially cholesterol. With time, the plaques continue to thicken and, eventually, close the vessel (figure 56–4). Some plaques calcify, whereas others may develop an overlying thrombus.

B. Predisposing Factors for Atherosclerosis

Each of the risk factors listed here is significant alone. When these factors occur in combinations, the risk of atherosclerosis is increased, and therefore, of ischemic heart disease. Prevention depends on educational programs along with early identification of persons at risk.[12]

1. Elevated levels of blood lipids; the result of an increased dietary intake of cholesterol, saturated fat, carbohydrate, especially sucrose, alcohol, and calories.
2. Elevated blood pressure.
3. Cigarette smoking.
4. Diabetes.
5. Obesity.
6. Insufficient physical activity.
7. Increased tensions; emotional stress.
8. Family history. Genetic inheritance may not be the factor so much as the perpetuation of familial life-style habits. Diet, smoking habits,

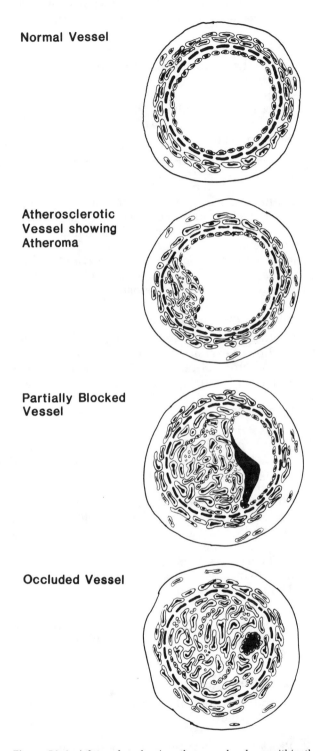

Normal Vessel

Atherosclerotic Vessel showing Atheroma

Partially Blocked Vessel

Occluded Vessel

Figure 56–4. Atherosclerosis. An atheroma develops within the lining of the normal blood vessel. The atheroma is made of a fatty deposit containing cholesterol. At first, the atheroma is small and no symptoms are apparent; but eventually, it enlarges and completely blocks the vessel, thus depriving the area served by the vessel of oxygen. (From *Arteriosclerosis 1981.* Report of the Working Group on Arteriosclerosis of the National Heart, Lung, and Blood Institute, National Institutes of Health, United States Department of Health and Human Services, NIH Publication No. 81–2034, June 1981.)

tensions, and tendencies toward lack of exercise are typical examples.

II. Manifestations of Ischemic Heart Disease

Each of the following manifestations is described in this section:
A. Angina pectoris.
B. Myocardial infarction.
C. Congestive heart failure.
D. Sudden death.

ANGINA PECTORIS

Angina pectoris is a symptom complex or syndrome of discomfort in the chest and adjacent areas, which results from transient and reversible myocardial oxygen deficiency. Although other forms of coronary disease may cause similar pain symptoms, approximately 90 percent of angina attacks are related to coronary artery atherosclerosis.

I. Predisposing Factors

An attack of angina pectoris may be precipitated by exertion or exercise, emotion, or a heavy meal. In the dental office or clinic, a preventive atmosphere of calmness and quiet can do much to alleviate stress.

II. Symptoms

A. Chest Pain

Each person who suffers from angina has a characteristic pattern of pain symptoms. When changes in the usual pains occur, the physician must be notified.

Commonly, the patient has thoracic pain, which is substernal and radiates down the left arm and up to the mandible. It may last for seconds or minutes.

The pain is squeezing or crushing, paroxysmal, or pressing, with a feeling of weight on the chest. The patient stops and tends to stiffen.

B. Other Symptoms

The patient may be pale and also experience faintness, sweating, difficulty in breathing, anxiety, or fear.

III. Treatment

A vasodilator, usually nitroglycerin, is administered sublingually.

IV. Procedure During an Attack in the Dental Office

A. Terminate Treatment

Stop the dental or dental hygiene procedure. Call for assistance and the emergency kit or cart.

B. Position Patient

Seat the patient up to a comfortable position; reassure the patient.

C. Administer Vasodilator

Administer nitroglycerin sublingually. Use of the patient's own supply is preferable. Prior to starting procedures of the appointment, the patient's supply should be placed within reach. The patient can be asked when the nitroglycerin was purchased, because the potency is lost after 6 months out of a sealed storage container.

D. Check Patient Response

Give additional vasodilator. Usually, the first tablet relieves the condition within minutes. When it is suspected that the patient's supply may not be fresh and the first tablet has been ineffective, use of a second tablet from the dental office emergency kit may be advisable.[13]

E. Call for Medical Assistance

When the patient does not respond to the second dose of vasodilator, assume the attack to be a myocardial infarction. Oxygen administration may be indicated.

F. Record Vital Signs

Measure blood pressure, take pulse rate, and count respirations.

G. Observe Recovery

For the patient who recovers without additional medical assistance, allow a rest period before dismissal. Record vital signs again.

V. Subsequent Dental and Dental Hygiene Appointments

Make an entry in the patient's permanent record, noting especially any procedures that may have contributed to the attack.

MYOCARDIAL INFARCTION

Myocardial infarction is the most extreme manifestation of ischemic heart disease. It is also called *heart attack, coronary occlusion,* or *coronary thrombosis.* It results from a sudden reduction or arrest of coronary blood flow.

The most common artery associated with a myocardial infarction is the anterior descending branch of the left coronary artery. That is also the most common site of advanced atherosclerosis.

I. Etiology

The immediate cause often is a thrombosis that blocks an artery already narrowed by atherosclerosis. In turn, the blockage creates an area of infarction, which leads to myocardial necrosis of the area. Necrosis of the area can occur within a few hours.

A few patients die immediately or within a few hours. Sudden death may be caused by ventricular fibrillation.

II. Symptoms

A. Pain

1. *Location.* Pain symptoms may start under the sternum, with feelings of indigestion, or in the

middle to upper sternum. Pain may last for extended periods, even hours. When the pain is severe, it gives a pressing or crushing heavy sensation and is not relieved by rest or nitroglycerin.

2. *Onset.* The pain may have a sudden onset, sometimes during sleep or following exercise. The pain may be radial, similar to angina pectoris, which extends to the left arm and mandible.

B. Other Symptoms

Cold sweat, weakness and faintness, shortness of breath, nausea, and vomiting may occur. Blood pressure is lowered.

III. Management During an Attack

A. Stop dental and dental hygiene treatment, sit the patient up for comfortable breathing, give nitroglycerin, and reassure the patient.

B. Summon medical assistance.
1. When nitroglycerin does not reduce the angina-like pain within 3 minutes, call both a physician and an ambulance with paramedical personnel.
2. Record vital signs.
3. Administer oxygen.
4. Apply cardiopulmonary resuscitation if indicated while waiting for medical assistance.
5. Transport to hospital.

IV. Treatment After Acute Symptoms

A. Medical Supervision

Current medical care for heart attack calls for a shortened rest period with increased activity, in keeping with the strength and progress of the patient. Most patients experience extreme fatigue during their convalescence.

B. Life Style Changes

Limited diet and elimination of smoking and stressful activities are essential. Many patients need considerable education, reassurance, and motivation.

C. Subsequent Appointments

Elective dental and dental hygiene appointments are postponed 3 months to 1 year until the patient's physician has given consent.

CONGESTIVE HEART FAILURE

Heart failure is a syndrome in which an abnormality of cardiac function is responsible for the inability or failure of the heart to pump blood at a rate necessary to meet the needs of the body tissues. Because of the collection of fluids in various body organs, the term *congestive heart failure* is used.

I. Etiology

The many causes for heart failure fall into two categories: underlying and precipitating causes.

A. Underlying Causes

Examples of cardiovascular disease that result in heart failure are
1. Heart valve damage (rheumatic heart disease, congenital heart disease).
2. Myocardial failure as a result of an abnormality of heart muscle or secondary to ischemia.

B. Precipitating Causes

Examples that place an additional load on a chronically burdened myocardium are
1. *Acute Hypertensive Crisis.* Severe symptoms of headache, mental confusion, dizziness, shortness of breath, and chest pain may predispose to heart failure.
2. *Massive Pulmonary Embolism.* A thrombus may form in a lower extremity of an inactive person with low cardiac output and circulatory stasis. The thrombus may break loose and, carried by the blood, lodge in the pulmonary artery to cause a pulmonary embolism. Severe dyspnea, cyanosis, congestive failure, and shock result.
3. *Arrhythmia.* After resuscitation of a person with myocardial infarction, ventricular fibrillation, a type of arrhythmia, is the major risk leading to sudden death.

II. Clinical Manifestations

The clinical manifestations coincide with the parts of the heart involved. Signs and symptoms are different, depending, in general, on whether the left or the right side of the heart or both are affected. The general effects are extreme weakness, fatigue, fear, and anxiety.

A. Left Heart Failure

The left side of the heart receives oxygenated blood from the lungs and pumps the blood into the aorta to the rest of the body. A pathologic condition of the left ventricle or the mitral valve alters output, and causes respiratory difficulty because of the backup of fluid and blood into the lungs.

Clinical symptoms are more prominent at night. The patient rests better in a sitting or semisitting position with more than one pillow.
1. *Subjective Symptoms*
   a. Weakness, fatigue.
   b. Dyspnea, particularly evident on exertion. Shortness of breath on lying supine, relieved when sitting up.
   c. Cough and expectoration.
   d. Nocturia.
2. *Objective Symptoms*
   a. Pallor; sweating, cold skin.
   b. Breathing obviously difficult.
   c. Diastolic blood pressure increased.
   d. Heart rate rapid.
   e. Anxiety, fear.

B. Right Heart Failure

The right heart receives the venous blood from the vena cava and pumps it to the lungs for oxygenation. Right heart failure shows evidence of systemic venous congestion with peripheral edema. When left heart failure precedes right heart failure, the heart is already congested. Resistance to receiving the venous blood is an additional factor.

1. *Subjective Symptoms*
   a. Weakness, fatigue.
   b. Swelling of feet and/or ankles. The edema progresses to the thighs and abdomen (ascites) in advanced stages of heart failure.
   c. Cold hands and feet.
2. *Objective Symptoms*
   a. Cyanosis of mucous membranes and nailbeds.
   b. Prominent jugular veins.
   c. Congestion with edema in various organs: enlarged spleen and liver; gastrointestinal distress with nausea and vomiting; central nervous system involvement with headache and irritability.
   d. Anxiety, fear.

III. Treatment During Chronic Stages

A patient with an appointment in a dental office or clinic may be receiving a variety of medical treatments. These should be revealed by questioning during preparation of histories. Nearly all patients with heart failure complications will have the following in their medical treatment plan:

A. Drug Therapy

Physicians may prescribe many different medications for patients with cardiovascular disease. The general types are listed in table 6–3, page 88.

B. Dietary Control

1. Limited sodium intake to alleviate fluid retention.
2. Weight reduction.

C. Limitation of Activity

Activity should be limited depending on the severity of the health problem and the advice of the physician.

IV. Emergency Care for Heart Failure and Acute Pulmonary Edema

A medical emergency that demands urgent attention may occur anywhere. The patient with heart failure or acute pulmonary edema is usually conscious.

A. Position the patient for comfortable breathing: upright.
B. Administer oxygen.
C. Record and monitor vital signs (blood pressure, respiratory rate, and pulse).
D. Reassure the patient.

E. Obtain medical assistance: physician and ambulance.

SUDDEN DEATH

Clinical death that occurs within 24 hours after onset of symptoms is known as sudden death, whereas death within 30 seconds is instantaneous death. Biologic death occurs when permanent cellular damage has been done, primarily from lack of adequate oxygen supply. Biologic death takes place when oxygen delivery to the brain is inadequate for 4 to 6 minutes.

I. Etiology

Nearly all sudden deaths are from cardiovascular causes, predominantly coronary atherosclerosis. Examples of noncardiac causes are cerebral hemorrhage, drug overdose or toxicity, and pulmonary thromboembolism.

II. Mechanism of Sudden Cardiovascular Death

A. Definition and Description

A majority of sudden deaths is caused by *ventricular fibrillation.* Because of many premature beats in which individual muscle bundles fibrillate or contract independently, the ventricle cannot be refilled. Insufficient blood is pumped into the coronary arteries to supply the myocardium. A severe lack of oxygen to the heart muscles causes ventricular standstill, which is one form of cardiac arrest.

B. Clinical Signs of Death

1. Loss of consciousness.
2. No respiration, no pulse, no blood pressure.
3. Dilated pupils.

III. Emergency Care[14]

A. Immediate Need: Oxygen

Every second counts; only 4 minutes, or 6 at the most, can elapse before enough brain cells die from lack of oxygen to produce biologic death.

B. Basic Life Support

Details of the procedures are described on pages 740–744.
1. Provide artificial ventilation.
2. Provide artificial circulation.
3. Provide transportation to a hospital.

CARDIAC PACEMAKER

The natural pacemaker, or center where the normal heartbeat is initiated, is the sino-atrial (S-A) node located in the right atrium or auricle. From that node, impulses are sent along the muscle walls to stimulate and regulate the contractions of the ventricles, which pump the blood throughout the body.

When the natural pacemaker cells are not able to

maintain a reliable rhythm, or when the impulses are interrupted because of heart block, cardiac arrest, various arrhythmias, or other disease conditions, treatment by a cardiologist may include the placement of an artificial pacemaker.

I. Description

A. Definition

A cardiac pacemaker is an electronic stimulator used to send a specified electrical current to the myocardium to control or maintain a minimum heart rate. It may be single chambered (to ventricle or atrium) or dual chambered, which senses and paces both chambers.

B. Parts and Power

A permanently implanted pacemaker has electrodes inserted transvenously to the endocardium. Less commonly, the leads may go to the pericardium of the external heart wall.

The electrodes are connected to the power source, a plastic- or metal-encased, hermetically sealed pulse generator, containing a lithium anode battery. The pulse generator is implanted under the skin in the thorax or upper abdomen. The area selected depends on the individual condition as determined by the cardiologist (figure 56–5).

C. Types

Research has provided many advancements in pacemaker technology. Current systems involve rate-responsive or physiologic pacing. Sensors may be alert to muscle or physical activity vibrations, body temperature, or respiration rate. The research will have a significant impact on the future of pacing. The two general types are demand and fixed rate.

1. *Demand.* The demand pacemaker stimulates the heart only when the rate varies from a predetermined norm. By sensing a discrepancy in the electrical signals produced by natural means, the pacemaker sends a signal or stimulus, which regulates the heartbeat.

2. *Fixed Rate.* A preset rate of electrical stimuli is provided independent of the natural heart activity when the natural beat is too slow. Each patient is evaluated for the type of pacemaker that is best for the condition of that individual's heart. The fixed rate is currently used infrequently.

II. Interferences and Their Effects

External electromagnetic interferences can stop or alter the function of a pacemaker. Different models of pacemakers and their sensitivities to interference vary. Newer models are made with a special shielding to protect against interference.

Ultrasonic scaling units, electrodesensitizing equipment, pulp testers, electric toothbrushes,[15] electrosurgery machines, certain casting equipment, and the Myomonitor,[16] are among the potential sources of interference with a pacemaker in a dental care setting. Dental devices that apply an electric current directly to the patient are considered those most likely to interfere.

The dental environment has been shown to be a source of moderate electromagnetic interference. All dental equipment should be kept in good repair. Electric devices that contact or can contact the patient should be checked for leakage, because leakage can be a source of interference. Electric appliances must be earth-grounded.

The effect of distance has not been sufficiently researched; hence patients in adjacent dental treatment rooms should be checked before equipment is used.

Although the evidence for interferences in the dental setting is not great, concern must be shown because all pacemakers are not the same.

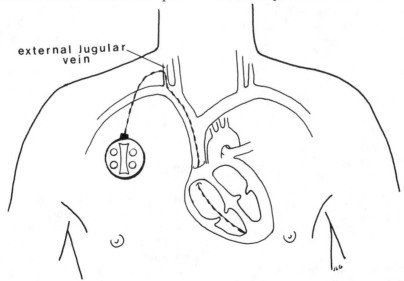

external jugular vein

Figure 56–5. Cardiac Pacemaker. The pulse generator is implanted under the skin in the thorax or upper abdomen. The lead electrodes may go to the ventricle or to the atrium or both to provide the necessary stimulus for regulation of the heartbeat.

III. Pacemaker Malfunction

A. Symptoms

A patient may mention feelings of discomfort. At the same time, the clinician must be aware of possible changes and signs in the event of stopping or altering of a pacemaker.
1. Difficulty in breathing.
2. Dizziness, light headedness, feelings of faintness, or syncope.
3. Changes in pulse rate.
4. Swelling of legs, ankles, arms, wrists.
5. Chest pain.
6. Prolonged hiccoughing.
7. Muscle twitching.

B. Emergency Procedures

In the event a pacemaker should be turned off, immediate action is needed.
1. Turn off all suspected sources of interference.
2. Call for medical assistance; a defibrillator may be needed.
3. Position the patient for cardiopulmonary resuscitation.
4. Open airway, check for breathing, and begin mouth-to-mouth ventilation. The complete procedure is described on pages 740–741.
5. Observe the patient. When the heart is forced to assume its rhythm again as a result of artificial circulation, the pacemaker will be set into action to resume the generation and regulation of the pulse.

IV. Appointment Guidelines for a Pacemaker

General procedures for all patients with cardiovascular involvement as described in this chapter apply to the patient wearing a pacemaker. In addition, certain adaptations are recommended.

A. Informed Consent[17]

The signature of the patient or the patient's parent or guardian on a formal statement is a necessary protection against any legal liability in the event of complications or undesirable effects. The patient should receive careful instruction in the anticipated procedures and materials used. Dental and dental hygiene records should be accurate and all-inclusive with a detailed record for each appointment.

B. Patient Histories

The usual health history should be supplemented with information about the type of pacemaker, how long it has been in use, where it is located, the underlying disease condition, and other information pertinent to the patient's safety during dental and dental hygiene appointments. Consultation with the patient's cardiologist is indicated.

C. Prophylactic Antibiotic Premedication

The underlying cardiovascular disease is the basic determinant for the use of antibiotic prophylaxis. Infective endocarditis has occurred in patients with pacemakers. The pacemaker wires may serve as a predisposing factor.

Antibiotic prophylaxis may be indicated during the first 6 months following placement of the pacemaker. After implantation, the pulse generator and the electrodes are usually covered by endothelium. Although the patient with a pacemaker appears to be at low risk of endocarditis, the dentist and the cardiologist may choose to use antibiotics to cover dental and dental hygiene procedures.[4]

D. Patient Preparation

1. *Chair Position.* Positioning the patient to support breathing and circulation is important. If the patient experiences difficulty in breathing when in the supine position, the chair back should be elevated to reduce stress.

   The patient may experience some discomfort from wire tension or strain at the implant site if the chair is positioned too far back. That depends on the location of the pulse generator.
2. *Lead Apron.* Protection of the pulse generator and the lead wires is indicated. A lead apron can serve to interrupt interferences that may be created by electric devices, including handpieces. A lead apron can be heavy and uncomfortable, however, and therefore, may require some consideration.

E. Radiography

Implantation and monitoring of a pacemaker may have required multiple exposures to radiation. Dental radiation should be limited, when possible, and the patient protected by a full-sized lead apron.

F. Instrumentation

The use of manual procedures is advisable. In the absence of specific information, and until the time when all pacemakers are known to be safely shielded, avoidance of power-driven instruments known to cause interference is recommended.

ANTICOAGULANT THERAPY

Anticoagulants are used in the treatment of many cardiovascular diseases to prevent embolus and thrombus formation. A prescribed drug may be continued indefinitely in the patient's life as a preventive measure.

Drugs most commonly used to prevent or delay blood coagulation are heparin (hospital-administered intravenous) and coumarin derivatives. Although precautions are needed to prevent hemorrhage, discontinuing the drug can be much more hazardous for the patient than performing the dental and dental hygiene therapy with precautions. When extensive surgical procedures are required, the patient may be hospitalized.

I. Clinical Procedures

A. Consultation

Information about the patient's prothrombin time is obtained from the physician during an initial consultation. The prothrombin time is a test of the coagulation phase of blood clotting used to monitor therapy with anticoagulants. A therapeutic range of 1½ to 2 times the normal level is preferred.

B. Treatment Planning

1. *Pretest for Prothrombin Time*
   a. Determine the prothrombin time within 24 hours before an appointment. The patient can have the test made on the day of a dental appointment by preplanning with the physician and the laboratory. Most patients have a routine appointment for monitoring of the blood, and dental appointment dates can be planned to coincide.[18]
   b. Safe level for dental and dental hygiene procedures is considered to be 1½ times the normal, provided precautions are taken during instrumentation and postoperative care.
2. *Quadrant Scaling and Root Planing*
   a. Treat the most healthy quadrant first. The least bleeding will occur.
   b. Teach and emphasize daily bacterial-plaque control procedures in a series of appointments to prepare the gingival tissue for instrumentation. Healthy, healed tissue does not bleed as readily or as profusely.

C. Local Hemostatic Measures

Instrumentation can be performed for most patients without complication, provided precautions are taken to minimize tissue trauma and control bleeding, and not to dismiss the patient until bleeding has stopped.
1. *Pressure.* Pressure with sponges or cotton pellets packed interdentally can aid in control.[19]
2. *Suture.* Sutures may be used to close and adapt the tissue interdentally, following deep scaling and root planing.
3. *Periodontal Dressing.* Placement of a dressing is sometimes advisable to provide pressure and protection from trauma that may initiate postoperative bleeding. Dressing placement is described on pages 490–491.

II. Postoperative Instructions

The practice by oral surgeons of closely observing patients for 6 to 8 hours following a surgical procedure may have application following certain dental and dental hygiene procedures for selected patients. At least, it may be advisable to check with the patient that postoperative instructions are being followed closely.

Postoperatively, the patient is advised to avoid vigorous toothbrushing and rinsing for several hours or until the next day. The use of extraoral icepacks may be helpful. General postoperative instructions may be found on page 592; for the care of an area with a dressing, see table 36–1, page 492.

The use of a soft diet, cool rather than hot foods, and general moderation in activity may be important.

Long-term instruction must emphasize the maintenance of gingival health to prevent future bleeding problems.

CARDIOVASCULAR SURGERY

Cardiac surgery has become widely used. Patients in dental offices and clinics who have had or will have surgery should be identified and need special procedures. Because the patient with a cardiac prosthesis is at risk for infective endocarditis, all possible dental treatment must be completed before the date of cardiac surgery and preventive measures must be emphasized.

I. Presurgical

Before elective cardiac surgery, the patient's mouth should be brought to a state of optimum health, with all sources of infection removed. All restorations and other dental procedures must be completed.

Depending on the type of operation to be performed, antibiotic prophylaxis will be required. So that the resistance of the oral flora is decreased before the cardiac surgery, time should elapse between completion of the dental and periodontal therapy, including dental hygiene procedures, and the cardiac surgery.

Patients requiring cardiac surgery need information and motivation relative to the importance of oral health in eliminating a potential source of infective endocarditis. Vigilance in a preventive program including plaque control and self-applied fluorides is essential.

II. Postsurgical

A. Maintenance Appointments

Frequent appointments are necessary for supervision and maintenance.

B. Prophylactic Antibiotics

1. Antibiotic coverage for all dental and dental hygiene procedures for patients with synthetic prostheses is essential. Because of the high susceptibility to infective endocarditis, the special regimen for high-risk patients includes both penicillin and streptomycin (page 91).
2. Patients with implanted vascular autographs generally do not need antibiotic premedication before dental and dental hygiene appointments.[20] An example of an implanted vascular autograph is the use of a patient's own blood vessel to provide an aortocoronary bypass. The saphenous vein and the internal mammary artery are most commonly used.

TECHNICAL HINTS

I. Record Prescriptions

Record all prescriptions by date, drug, dose, and directions in the patient's permanent record.

II. Determine Status of Prescription

Check that the patient has filled the prescriptions.

III. Prepare for Appointment

Before each appointment for a patient with a cardiovascular disease

A. Determine and record blood pressure.

B. Review patient history and notes relative to previous appointments to prepare adequately for the current appointment.

C. Check with the patient to be sure that prescribed medications have been taken and at the proper time.

    1. Antibiotic premedication must be taken 1 hour before the appointment.

    2. Question the patient concerning drugs that may have been taken on the same day as the appointment, such as a sedative, alcoholic beverage, or other, which may influence the premedication or the effect of an anesthetic to be given.

IV. Source of Materials

Local Heart Association
and
American Heart Association
7320 Greenville Avenue
Dallas, Texas 75231

FACTORS TO TEACH THE PATIENT

I. Hypertension Therapy

Encourage patients who have been diagnosed as hypertensive to continue their prescribed therapy.

II. Stress Reduction Procedures[21]

A. Select an appointment time that is optimum with respect to time of day when the patient is feeling best and may be less fatigued. Most anxious patients prefer a morning appointment.

B. Get adequate sleep and rest, and engage in nonfatiguing activities during the 24 hours before the appointment.

C. Use premedication as prescribed for sleeping the night before. A sedative may be prescribed to be taken 60 minutes before an appointment; at the dental office, if possible. When taken at home 1 hour before, the patient should not drive a car.

D. Allow time to get to the dental office or clinic; bring own reading material, knitting or sewing, or other relaxing activity in the event waiting is unavoidable.

E. Eat breakfast, lunch, or other usual between-meal food and take usual medications on schedule.

F. When other family members, especially children, have dental or dental hygiene appointments, do not add to their stress by relaying personal negative feelings.

References

1. Robbins, S.L., Cotran, R.S., and Kumar, V.: *Pathologic Basis of Disease,* 3rd ed. Philadelphia, W.B. Saunders Co., 1984, pp. 571–596.
2. Brunner, L.S., Suddarth, D.S., Bare, B.G., Boyer, M.J., and Smeltzer, S.C.O.: *Textbook of Medical-Surgical Nursing,* 6th ed. Philadelphia, J.B. Lippincott Co., 1988, pp. 549–555.
3. Sonis, S.T., Fazio, R.C., and Fang, L.: *Principles and Practice of Oral Medicine.* Philadelphia, W.B. Saunders Co., 1984, pp. 125–136.
4. Shulman, S.T., Amren, D.P., Bisno, A.L., Dajani, A.S., Durack, D.T., Gerber, M.A., Kaplan, E.L., Millard, H.D., Sanders, W.E., Schwartz, R.H., and Watanakunakorn, C.: Prevention of Bacterial Endocarditis. A Statement for Health Professionals by the Committee on Rheumatic Fever and Infective Endocarditis of the Council on Cardiovascular Disease in the Young, *Circulation, 70,* 1123A, December, 1984.
5. Dajani, A.S.: Endocarditis Prophylaxis (Letter to Editor), *J. Am. Dent. Assoc., 116,* 154, February, 1988.
6. Little, J.W. and Falace, D.A.: *Dental Management of the Medically Compromised Patient,* 2nd ed. St. Louis, The C.V. Mosby Co., 1984, pp. 103–115.
7. Sonis, Fazio, and Fang: op. cit., pp. 45–57.
8. Malamed, S.F.: *Handbook of Medical Emergencies in the Dental Office,* 3rd ed. St. Louis, The C.V. Mosby Co., 1987, pp. 112–113.
9. National Heart, Lung, and Blood Institute, Task Force on Blood Pressure Control in Children: Recommendations of the Task Force on Blood Pressure Control in Children, *Pediatrics, 59,* 799, Number 5, Supplement, May, 1977.
10. Kowalski, C.I., Randolph, M.F., and Macko, D.J.: A Study of Blood Pressure in Children, *J. Am. Dent. Assoc., 97,* 966, December, 1978.
11. Robbins, Cotran, and Kumar: op. cit., pp. 567–569.
12. Sonis, Fazio, and Fang: op. cit., pp. 35–44.
13. Malamed: op. cit., p. 348.
14. Malamed: op. cit., pp. 366–390.
15. Escher, D.J., Parker, B., and Furman, S.: Pacemaker Triggering (Inhibition) by Electric Toothbrush, *Am. J. Cardiol., 38,* 126, July, 1976.
16. Martinis, A.J., Jankelson, B., Radke, J., and Adib, F.: Effects of the Myo-monitor on Cardiac Pacemakers, *J. Am. Dent. Assoc., 100,* 203, February, 1980.
17. Dreifus, L.S. and Cohen, D.: Implanted Pacemakers: Medicolegal Implications, *Am. J. Cardiol., 36,* 266, August, 1975.
18. Rooney, T.P.: General Dentistry During Continuous Anticoagulation Therapy, *Oral Surg. Oral Med. Oral Pathol., 56,* 252, September, 1983.
19. Carranza, F.A.: *Glickman's Clinical Periodontology,* 6th ed. Philadelphia, W.B. Saunders Co., 1984, pp. 568–569.
20. Lindemann, R.A. and Henson, J.L.: The Dental Management of Patients with Vascular Grafts Placed in the Treatment of Arterial Occlusive Disease, *J. Am. Dent. Assoc., 104,* 625, May, 1982.
21. Malamed: op. cit., pp. 40–41.

Suggested Readings

Abraham-Impijn, L., Borgmeijer-Hoelen, A., and Gortzak, R.A.T.: Changes in Blood Pressure, Heart Rate, and Electrocardiogram During Dental Treatment with Use of Local Anesthesia, *J. Am. Dent. Assoc., 116,* 531, April, 1988.

Bisno, A.L.: The Rise and Fall of Rheumatic Fever, *JAMA, 254,* 538, July 26, 1985.

Caccamo, L.P.: The Cardiovascular Patient: A Review of Pathophysiology and Dental Implications, *Spec. Care Dentist., 1,* 88, March-April, 1981.

Chapman, N.L.: Alteration of Nutrition Habits in Ischemic Heart Disease, *Clin. Prevent. Dent., 2,* 9, January-February, 1980.

Dalen, J.E. and Hickler, R.B.: Oral Contraceptives and Cardiovascular Disease, *Am. Heart J., 101,* 626, May, 1981.

Dionne, R.A.: The Pharmacological Basis of Pain Control in Dental Practice: Local Anesthetics, *Compend. Contin. Educ. Dent., 1,* 229, July-August, 1980.

Ellrodt, A.G., Ault, M.J., Reidinger, M.S., and Murata, G.H.: Efficacy and Safety of Sublingual Nifedipine in Hypertensive Emergencies, *Am. J. Med., 79,* 19, October 11, 1985.

Farkas, J.A. and Goebel, W.M.: Assessing the Risk of Angina for Dental Therapy, *Oral Surg. Oral Med. Oral Pathol., 58,* 253, August, 1984.

Friedlander, A.H.: Risk Assessment of the Older Dental Patient: A Review of the Pathophysiology of the Cardiovascular System, *Spec. Care Dentist., 7,* 41, January-February, 1987.

Friedlander, A.H. and Gorelick, D.A.: Panic Disorder: Its Association with Mitral Valve Prolapse and Appropriate Dental Management, *Oral Surg. Oral Med. Oral Pathol., 63,* 309, March, 1987.

Gaidry, D., Kudlick, E.M., Hutton, J.G., and Russell, D.M.: A Survey to Evaluate the Management of Orthodontic Patients with a History of Rheumatic Fever or Congenital Heart Disease, *Am. J. Orthod., 87,* 338, April, 1985.

Garfunkel, A.A., Massot, S., and Galili, D.: Oral Treatment Needs for Patients Requiring Heart Surgery, *Spec. Care Dentist., 7,* 167, July-August, 1987.

Gillum, R.F., Folsom, A.R., and Blackburn, H.: Decline in Coronary Heart Disease Mortality. Old Questions and New Facts, *Am. J. Med., 76,* 1055, June, 1984.

Hancharik, S.D.: At Risk: Hypertensive Patients, *RDH, 4,* 23, March/April, 1984.

Harms, K.A. and Bronny, A.T.: Cardiac Transplantation: Dental Considerations, *J. Am. Dent. Assoc., 112,* 677, May, 1986.

Hasse, A.L., Heng, M.K., and Garrett, N.R.: Blood Pressure and Electrocardiographic Response to Dental Treatment with Use of Local Anesthesia, *J. Am. Dent. Assoc., 113,* 639, October, 1986.

Henry, H. and McCarron, D.: Diet and Hypertension: An Update on Recent Research, *ASDC J. Dent. Child., 50,* 145, March-April, 1983.

Hondrum, S.O.: Hypertensive Episode in the Dental Office, *Gen. Dent., 33,* 134, March-April, 1985.

Knapp, J.F. and Fiori, T.: Oral Hemorrhage Associated with Periodontal Surgery and Hypertensive Crisis, *J. Am. Dent. Assoc., 108,* 49, January, 1984.

Lynch, M.A.: Diseases of the Cardiovascular System, in Lynch, M.A., Brightman, V.J., and Greenberg, M.S., eds.: *Burket's Oral Medicine,* 8th ed. Philadelphia, J.B. Lippincott, 1984, pp. 663–688.

Milam, S.B. and Giovannitti, J.A.: Digitalis Toxicity, *J. Periodontol., 55,* 414, July, 1984.

Mulligan, R.: Pretreatment for the Cardiovascularly Compromised Geriatric Dental Patient, *Spec. Care Dentist., 5,* 116, May-June, 1985.

Mulligan, R.: Response to Anticoagulant Drug Withdrawal, *J. Am. Dent. Assoc., 115,* 435, September, 1987.

Niebergall, C., Giglio, J.A., and Campbell, R.L.: Evaluation and Management of the Cardiac Patient for Office Oral Surgery, *Anesth. Prog., 30,* 67, May-June, 1983.

Parker, J.O., Vankoughnett, K.A., and Farrell, B.: Nitroglycerin Lingual Spray: Clinical Efficacy and Dose–Response Relation, *Am. J. Cardiol., 57,* 1, January, 1986.

Quinn, T.W.: The President's Corner. Mitral Valve Prolapse, *Anesth. Prog., 29,* 101, July-August, 1982.

Reuben, B.M.: A Current Practical Review of Local Anesthesia, *Dent. Surv., 56,* 38, July, 1980.

Spuller, R.L.: The Central Indwelling Venous Catheter in the Pediatric Patient—Dental Treatment Considerations, *Spec. Care Dentist., 8,* 74, March-April, 1988.

Infective Endocarditis

Cawson, R.A.: Infective Endocarditis as a Complication of Dental Treatment, *Br. Dent. J., 151,* 409, December 15, 1981.

Ehrmann, E.H.: Infective Endocarditis and the Dentist, *Aust. Dent. J., 31,* 351, October, 1986.

Friedman, M.L.: Antibiotic Therapy in a Dental Patient with Recent Mitral Valve Replacement, *Gen. Dent., 34,* 397, September-October, 1986.

Guntheroth, W.G.: How Important are Dental Procedures As a Cause of Infective Endocarditis? *Am. J. Cardiol., 54,* 797, October 1, 1984.

Littner, M.M., Kaffe, I., Tamse, A., and Buchner, A.: New Concept in Chemoprophylaxis of Bacterial Endocarditis Resulting from Dental Treatment, *Oral Surg. Oral Med. Oral Pathol., 61,* 338, April, 1986.

McKinsey, D.S., Ratts, T.E., and Bisno, A.L.: Underlying Cardiac Lesions in Adults with Infective Endocarditis. The Changing Spectrum, *Am. J. Med., 82,* 681, April, 1987.

Sadowsky, D. and Kunzel, C.: Clinician Compliance and the Prevention of Bacterial Endocarditis, *J. Am. Dent. Assoc., 109,* 425, September, 1984.

Stimmel, H.M., Orchen, J.J., Skaff, D.M., Brown, A.T., and Spedding, R.H.: Penicillin-resistant Alpha-hemolytic Streptococci in Children with Heart Disease Who Take Penicillin Daily, *ASDC J. Dent. Child., 48,* 29, January-February, 1981.

Sullivan, B.V. and Blong, M.A.: The Cardiac Patient. Chemoprophylaxis Considerations, *Dent. Hyg., 60,* 462, October, 1986.

Tzukert, A.A., Leviner, E., and Sela, M.: Prevention of Infective Endocarditis: Not by Antibiotics Alone. A 7-year Follow-up of 90 Dental Patients, *Oral Surg. Oral Med. Oral Pathol., 62,* 385, October, 1986.

Vose, J.M., Smith, P.W., Henry, M., and Colan, D.: Recurrent *Streptococcus mutans* Endocarditis, *Am. J. Med., 82,* 630, March 23, 1987.

Pacemaker

American Heart Association: *Living With Your Pacemaker.* American Heart Association, National Center, 7320 Greenville Avenue, Dallas, Texas 75231.

Griffiths, P.V.: The Management of the Pacemaker Wearer During Dental Hygiene Treatment, *Dent. Hyg., 52,* 573, December, 1978.

Purcell, J.A. and Burrows, S.G.: A Pacemaker Primer, *Am. J. Nurs., 85,* 553, May, 1985.

Sager, D.P.: Current Facts on Pacemaker Electromagnetic Interference and Their Application to Clinical Care, *Heart Lung, 16,* 211, March, 1987.

Rosengarten, M.D. and Chiu, R.C.J.: Artificial Cardiac Stimulation: A Current View of Physiologic Pacemakers, *Can. Med. Assoc. J., 128,* 1377, June 15, 1983.

Oral soft tissue changes, lowered resistance to infection, and bleeding tendencies are major factors to be considered for patients with blood diseases. Oral manifestations of blood disorders are generally exaggerated in the presence of bacterial plaque and local predisposing factors.

In this chapter, anemias, leukemias, and hemorrhagic disorders are described. Table 57–1 lists and defines terminology used to describe hematologic conditions. Prefixes, suffixes, and other word derivatives to clarify the terminology are listed on pages 757–759.

ORAL FINDINGS SUGGESTIVE OF BLOOD DISORDERS

Early signs of systemic conditions frequently appear in the oral soft tissues. The patient's medical history may not reveal the existence of a blood disorder, but clinical examination may reveal tissue characteristics suggestive of disease. An important referral for medical examination may lead to diagnosis and treatment of a serious disease. In addition, the findings of laboratory blood examination may provide essential information for safe and effective dental and dental hygiene therapy.

Oral soft-tissue changes that may occur in patients with blood diseases are not necessarily exclusive to systemic blood disorders. The important thing is to recognize change in a previously healthy patient, or what appears to be an exaggerated response in a patient being examined at an initial appointment.

Findings that may suggest a blood disorder including the following:

A. Gingival bleeding, spontaneously or upon gentle probing.
B. History of difficulty in controlling bleeding by usual procedures.
C. History of bruising easily, with large ecchymoses.
D. Numerous petechiae.
E. Marked pallor of the mucous membranes.
F. Atrophy of the papillae of the tongue.
G. Persistent sore or painful tongue (glossodynia).
H. Acute or chronic infections, such as candidiasis, that do not respond to usual treatment.
I. Severe ulcerations associated with a lack of response to treatment.
J. Exaggerated gingival response to local irritants, sometimes with characteristics of necrotizing ulcerative gingivitis (ulceration, necrosis, bleeding, pseudomembrane).

NORMAL BLOOD[1]

I. Composition

The blood is composed of 55 percent plasma fluid and 45 percent formed elements. The formed elements are categorized by type into *erythrocytes* (red blood cells or corpuscles), *leukocytes* (white blood cells), and *thrombocytes* (platelets). The cell forms and nuclei are shown in figure 57–1.

The red blood cells comprise about 44 percent and the white blood cells 1 percent of the 45 percent total formed elements.

The *hematocrit* is the percentage of packed volume of blood cells, the normal value for which approximates 45 percent, as shown in table 57–2. The test for the hematocrit is commonly used in general health evaluations.

II. Origin

In adults, all blood cells originate in the bone marrow. The erythrocytes and granulocytes pass through a series of transformations from the stem cell (cell of origin), the *hemocytoblast,* and leave the bone marrow as mature cells to enter the circulating blood.

The bone marrow also produces the stem cells for the agranulocytes. The lymphocytes and monocytes leave the bone marrow in immature forms and go to the lymphoid tissues for later maturing. In certain blood diseases and cancers, the immature cell forms predominate.

III. Plasma

The constituents of the fluid portion of the blood are similar to the fluid constituents of the connective tissue. The plasma is comprised 90 percent of water and 10 percent of the following:

A. Plasma Proteins

1. Albumin (functions to maintain tissue fluid pressure).
2. Gamma globulins (circulating antibodies essential in the immune system).
3. Beta globulins (transport of hormones, metallic ions, and lipids).
4. Fibrinogen and prothrombin (blood clotting).

Table 57–1. Glossary of Terms Used in Hematology

Anaplasia: loss of structural differentiation with reversion to a more primitive cell type.

Aplasia: defective development or congenital absence of an organ or tissue.

Differential cell count: record of the number of white blood cells, including determination of the percent of each type of white cell present, in a given sample.

Ecchymoses: large purplish patches caused by bleeding under (into) the skin.

Epistaxis: nosebleed.

Erythropoietic: pertaining to the formation of erythrocytes (red blood cells).

Glossitis: inflammation of the tongue.

Glossodynia: painful tongue with sensations of burning.

Hematocrit: fraction of the blood occupied by red blood cells.

Hematologic system: consists of the blood and the sites where blood is produced, including bone marrow and lymph nodes.

Hematopoietic: producing blood.

Hemoglobin: oxygen-carrying protein component of the red blood cell.

Hemolysis: dissolution or destruction of red blood cells with liberation of hemoglobin.

Infiltration: the act of passing into or penetrating a substance, cell, or tissue.

Leukocytosis: increase in the total number of white blood cells.

Leukopenia: decrease in the total number of white blood cells.

Lysis: disintegration or dissolution of cells.

Macrocyte: a large-sized red blood cell (opposite of microcyte, a small-sized cell).

Megaloblast: large nucleated, embryonic cell; precursor of an erythrocyte in an abnormal erythropoietic process, as observed in pernicious anemia.

Myelogenous: produced by or originating in the bone marrow.

Myelocyte: young cell of the granulocyte series; occurs normally in bone marrow; found in circulating blood in certain diseases.

Neutropenia: reduction in the number of neutrophils (polymorphonuclear leukocytes or PMNs).

Petechiae: pinhead-sized hemorrhages in the skin and mucous membranes.

Phagocytosis: process of ingestion and digestion of bacteria and foreign particles by white blood cells.

Purpura: hemorrhage into the skin and mucous membranes; larger areas than petechiae.

Thrombocytopenia: reduced number of platelets.

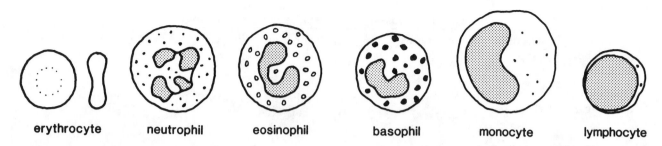

erythrocyte   neutrophil   eosinophil   basophil   monocyte   lymphocyte

Figure 57–1. Red and White Blood Cells. Diagram to show normal cell forms drawn to scale for comparison of cell size. Note the shape of nuclei in each of the white blood cells. The erythrocyte or red blood cell does not have a nucleus; its biconcave disc shape is shown in the lateral view second from the left.

Table 57–2. Tests Used for Blood Evaluation

Test	Normal Range*	Causes of Deviations
Hemoglobin	Males: 14–18 g./100 ml. Females: 12–16 g./100 ml.	Increased in Polycythemia Dehydration Decreased in Anemias Hemorrhage Leukemias
Hematocrit (volume of packed red cells)	Males: 40–54% Females: 37–47%	Increased in Polycythemia Dehydration Decreased in Anemias Hemorrhage Leukemias
Bleeding Time	Duke: 1–3½ minutes Ivy: less than 5 minutes Modified Ivy: 2½–10 minutes (Mielke template)	Prolonged in Disorders of platelet function Thrombocytopenia von Willebrand's disease Leukemias Aspirin and certain other drug use
Clotting Time	Glass tube: 4–8 minutes	Prolonged in Vitamin K deficiency Severe hemophilia Anticoagulant therapy Liver diseases
Prothrombin Time (P.T.)	11–15 seconds	Prolonged in Polycythemia vera Prothrombin deficiency Anticoagulant therapy Vitamin K deficiency Liver diseases Aspirin use
Partial Thromboplastin Time (P.T.T.)	68–82 seconds	Prolonged in Hemophilia A and B von Willebrand's disease Anticoagulant therapy

*The normal range varies with the specificity of the technique used. There is also a range variation, depending on the health facility and the laboratory.

B. Inorganic Salts

Sodium, potassium, calcium, bicarbonate, chloride.

C. Gases

Dissolved oxygen, carbon dioxide, and nitrogen.

D. Substances Being Transported

Hormones, nutrients, waste products, enzymes.

IV. Red Blood Cells (Erythrocytes)

A. Description

Although usually called red blood cells, they are more properly termed corpuscles because they have no nuclei (figure 57–1). They are biconcave discs that contain hemoglobin. The cells are sensitive and flexible and change shape readily as they pass through small capillaries.

Table 57–3 contains reference values for blood cells and the names of conditions in which increases or decreases in the normal values occur.

B. Functions

Hemoglobin carries oxygen to the body cells in the form of oxyhemoglobin. Carbon dioxide is transported from the cells.

The hemoglobin is measured in grams (g.) per 100 milliliters (ml). Normal values are shown in table 57–2 and range from 12 to 18 g. per 100 ml. The values reflect the anemic state when the hemoglobin is lowered. They also reflect pathologic conditions in which the hemoglobin is increased to a level higher than normal.

V. White Blood Cells (Leukocytes)

A. Types

White blood cells are divided into two general groups, the granulocytes and the agranulocytes. Granulocytes have granules in their cytoplasm, whereas the agranulocytes do not. They are further subdivided as shown in figure 57–2.

B. Functions

All white cells are amoeboid or motile, which permits them to pass through the walls at the terminal ends of capillaries and into the connective tissue. Their work is done within the connective tissue, where they have phagocytic, immunologic, and other functions related to the inflammatory process.

The cells respond to an injury or invasion of microorganisms and migrate into the area in large numbers. Neutrophils arrive first and are active in the phagocytosis of foreign material and microorganisms.

The blood functions as a transport medium for the white cells as they pass to areas in the connective tissue where they are needed. Their numbers and proportions in the blood maintain a constant level in health, as shown in table 57–3.

A differential cell count of the white blood cells is used in the detection and monitoring of diseased states. Increases and decreases of each cell type can be associated with certain conditions.

C. Agranulocytes

1. *Lymphocytes.* A mature lymphocyte is a small round cell with a round nucleus that nearly fills the cell, leaving only a narrow rim of cytoplasm (figure 57–1). Less mature forms are larger, with more cytoplasm.

   In the connective tissue, certain lymphocytes may differentiate into plasma cells, which produce and secrete antibody. The *plasma cell* is a relatively large oval cell with an eccentric nucleus. Lymphocytes and plasma cells are common in areas of chronic inflammation.

2. *Monocytes.* A monocyte is a large cell with a bean-shaped or indented nucleus. It is actively phagocytic. In the connective tissue, monocytes differentiate into macrophages, which are important in immunologic processes.

D. Granulocytes

1. *Neutrophils.* Neutrophils are the most numerous of all the white blood cells. They are also named polymorphonuclear leukocytes and referred to as "PMNs" or "polys." The nucleus of a neutrophil has three to five lobes connected by thin chromatin threads.

   In circulation, the cells are round, but in the tissues they are more or less amoeboid as they function in phagocytosis. Neutrophils are part of the first line of defense of the body.

2. *Eosinophils.* An eosinophil usually has a two-lobed nucleus and larger, coarser granules than those of a neutrophil. The granules stain a distinct bright pink, so that microscopically the cells can be readily recognized, even though they are few in number. The numbers increase markedly during allergic conditions.

3. *Basophils.* In contrast to the eosinophil or neutrophil, the nucleus of a basophil is usually in "U" or "S" form. The functions of the basophil are related to increasing vascular permeability

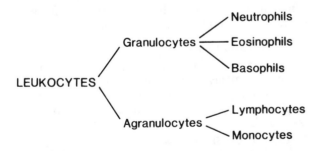

Figure 57–2. Types of Leukocytes. Leukocytes are of two general types, the granulocytes and the agranulocytes. They are subdivided as shown.

Table 57–3.   Blood Cells Reference Values

Cell Type	Normal Value	Causes of Increase	Causes of Decrease
Red Blood Cells	Male 4.5–6.0 Female 4.3–5.5 million per cu. mm.	Polycythemia Dehydration	Anemias Leukemias Hemorrhage
Platelets	150,000–400,000 per cu. mm. Wintrobe method: 140,000–440,000 per cu. mm.	Polycythemia vera Chronic myelocytic leukemia Sickle cell anemia Rheumatic fever Hemolytic anemias Bone fractures	Acute severe infections Cirrhosis of the liver Thrombocytopenic purpura Acute leukemias Aplastic anemias Pernicious anemia
White Blood Cells	5,000–10,000 per cu. mm.	Inflammation Overexertion Polycythemia vera	Aplastic anemia Granulocytopenia Drug poisoning Thrombocytopenia Radiation Severe infections

DIFFERENTIAL
  White Cell Count
 	
Granulocytes
 	
**1. Neutrophils
  (PMNs)**
	60–70%	Acute infections
		Myelogenous leukemia
		Poisoning
		Erythroblastosis
			Aplastic anemia
			Granulocytopenia

2. Eosinophils	1–3%	Allergic diseases Dermatitis Hodgkin's disease Scarlet fever	Aplastic anemia Typhoid fever
3. Basophils	1%	Certain chronic infections	Aplastic anemia
Agranulocytes **1. Lymphocytes**	20–35%	Lymphocytic leukemia Chronic infections Viral diseases	Aplastic anemia Myelogenous leukemia Radiation
2. Monocytes	2–6%	Monocytic leukemias Tuberculosis Infective endocarditis Hodgkin's disease	Aplastic anemia

during inflammation, thus permitting phagocytic cells to pass into the area.

VI. Platelets

A platelet is a small round or oval formed element without a nucleus. It is approximately one fourth the size of a red blood cell. Platelets are active in the blood clotting mechanism and essential in the maintenance of the integrity of blood capillaries by closing them at a time of injury. After healing, the platelets participate in clot dissolution.

ANEMIAS

Anemia means a reduction of the hemoglobin concentration, the hematocrit, or the number of red blood cells to a level below that which is normal for the individual. As a result of anemia, oxygen-carrying capacity to the cells is diminished. Oxygen is essential in all body tissues for normal maintenance.

I. Classification by Cause

Anemias are usually classified into three groups by general causes. The categories and an example of each are listed here. Later in the chapter, selected specific anemias with their oral implications will be described.

A. Caused by Blood Loss

1. *Acute.* Blood loss from trauma or disease.
2. *Chronic.* An internal lesion with constant slow bleeding, usually of gastrointestinal or gyne-

cologic origin can lead to a chronic loss of blood. An *iron deficiency anemia* can result.

B. Caused by Increased Hemolysis

Hemolysis means the destruction of red blood cells. These types of anemias are called "hemolytic anemias" because of the cell destruction.

1. *Hereditary Hemolytic Disorders*

    Example: *Sickle cell anemia,* which belongs to the group of hereditary disorders called the hemoglobinopathies.

2. *Acquired Hemolytic Disorders*

    Examples: drugs, infections, and certain physical and chemical agents that may cause red cell destruction. In the category of antibody-mediated anemia, *erythroblastosis fetalis* occurs when a mother is Rh negative and develops antibodies against a fetus that is Rh positive. It is sometimes called hemolytic disease of the newborn.

C. Caused by Diminished Production of Red Blood Cells

A nutritional deficiency or bone marrow failure may be the reason for diminished production.

1. *Nutritional Deficiency*

    a. Inadequate dietary choices or inadequate intake.

    b. Defective absorption from the gastrointestinal tract.

        Example: *pernicious anemia,* which results from a B_{12} vitamin absorption deficiency.

    c. Increased demand for nutrients.

        Example: *iron deficiency anemia,* which may occur during pregnancy or during a growth spurt.

2. *Bone Marrow Failure*

    Example: *aplastic anemia,* which may result from bone marrow failure because of drug use, irradiation, or chemicals. In aplastic anemia, a combination occurs of anemia, neutropenia, and thrombocytopenia, which means a quantitative decrease in all cells formed in the bone marrow.

II. Clinical Characteristics of Anemias

When a patient's medical history shows the presence of anemia, certain general characteristics may be anticipated for which clinical adaptations may be needed.

The general signs and symptoms are

A. Pale and thin skin.

B. Weakness, malaise, easy fatigability.

C. Dyspnea on slight exertion, faintness.

D. Headache, vertigo, tinnitus.

E. Dimness of vision, spots before the eyes.

F. Brittle nails with loss of convexity.

IRON DEFICIENCY ANEMIA

Iron deficiency anemia is a hypochromic microcytic anemia, which means that the hemoglobin is deficient (hypochromic) and the red blood corpuscles are smaller than normal and deficient in hemoglobin (microcytic). In general, it is found more in younger than in older people, and more in females than in males.

I. Causes

A. Malnutrition or malabsorption.

B. Chronic infection.

C. Increased body demand for iron over and above the daily intake. Example: during pregnancy.

D. Chronic blood loss. When iron deficiency anemia occurs in men or in postmenopausal women, it usually indicates internal bleeding, and tests are needed to find the source.

1. Causes of internal bleeding

    a. Gastrointestinal diseases such as ulcer, cancer.

    b. Drugs, notably aspirin.

    c. Hemorrhoids.

2. Excessive menstrual flow.

3. Frequent blood donations.

II. Signs and Symptoms

A. General

Clinical manifestations of iron deficiency anemia include general weakness, headache, pallor, and fatigue on slight exertion.

B. Oral[2]

1. Pallor of the mucosa and gingiva.

2. Tongue changes

    a. Atrophic glossitis with loss of filiform papillae. In moderate and severe anemia, when the hemoglobin is at 10 or below, the tongue is smooth and shiny. The patient may have burning, painful sensations (glossodynia).

    b. Secondary irritations to the thinned, atrophic mucosa may result from smoking, mechanical trauma, or hot, spicy foods.

III. Therapy

Iron deficiency anemia is treated with oral ferrous iron tablets. Liquid preparations, which are sometimes used for children, may stain the teeth. Administering the medicine by way of a straw is advised.

MEGALOBLASTIC ANEMIAS

Megaloblastic anemias are characterized by abnormally large (megalo-) red blood cells, many of which are oval shaped. The two principal types of megaloblastic anemias are *pernicious anemia* and *folate deficiency anemia.*

Pernicious anemia is caused by a deficiency of vitamin B_{12} and folate deficiency anemia is from a deficiency of folate, or folic acid. These two vitamins are essential in red blood cell production in the bone marrow. When one or the other is deficient, the basic precursor cell ("-blast") is altered, which leads to a derangement in the formation of red blood cells, and abnormal, megaloblastic cells result.[3] A megaloblastic anemia can result from a deficiency of either vitamin B_{12} or folate, or both together.

I. Pernicious Anemia

The implication of "fatality" when the word "pernicious" is used can be misleading, because synthetic vitamin B_{12} is now available for treatment and disease control. The traditional name is still in use, however.

A. Etiologic Factors

Vitamin B_{12} deficiency can be caused by decreased intake (inadequate diet or impaired absorption) or increased requirement (pregnancy, hyperparathyroidism, disseminated cancer). Pernicious anemia is caused by *impaired absorption* of B_{12} because of failure of production of *intrinsic factor* (IF) by the gastric mucosa.

Pernicious anemia is primarily a disease of people over 40 years of age. Frequently, the reason for lack of production of *intrinsic factor* is either chronic atrophic gastritis or surgical removal or partial removal of the stomach.

In the childhood form of the disease, other causes are in effect; no gastric abnormality exists. Although more research is needed, the cause may be either a hereditary inability to produce intrinsic factor, or the intrinsic factor produced may be ineffective.

B. Clinical Findings

1. *General.* Weakness, tingling or numbness of fingers and toes, and weight loss are usually found. Central nervous system involvement may be manifested by difficulty in walking, some lack of coordination, loss of position sense, and mental confusion.

2. *Oral*
   a. Tongue (atrophic glossitis, burning tongue). The tongue may be painful and inflamed, flabby, red, smooth, and shiny, with loss of filiform papillae. Secondarily, sensitivity to hot or spicy foods and other irritants and painful swallowing may be expected.
   b. Gingiva and mucosa. Soft tissues may be pale and atrophic and appear similar to those in a general vitamin B deficiency.

C. Treatment

Vitamin B_{12} is administered by injection twice weekly until the condition is controlled, and then monthly, indefinitely.

The main sources of vitamin B_{12} are meat and dairy products, that is, all foods containing animal protein. Liver is a rich source and was originally used in therapy before the development of synthetic B_{12}.

II. Folate Deficiency Anemia

Folate deficiency anemia has the same characteristics as pernicious anemia, except clinically, no neurologic changes are evident.

A. Etiologic Factors[3]

Folate deficiency can be caused by decreased intake (inadequate diet, impaired absorption), increased requirement (pregnancy, disseminated cancer), or blocked activation (certain drugs impair the utilization of folate).

B. Dietary Factors

Folates are abundant in green vegetables (spinach, lettuce, cabbage, asparagus), yeast, and liver. Only minimal subsistence diets or special diets influenced by factors such as poverty, food faddism, or alcoholism, when the use of alcohol takes precedence over food, are likely to be deficient in folates. Folate deficiency anemia is not uncommon, but it may be more frequently related to malabsorption than to inadequate intake.

SICKLE CELL ANEMIA[4]

Sickle cell anemia is a hereditary form of hemolytic anemia, resulting from a defective hemoglobin molecule. The name is derived from the crescent or "sickle" shape the red corpuscles assume when they become deoxygenated.

The disease occurs primarily in the black population and in white populations of Mediterranean origin. Tests are available for screening and diagnosis of those with sickle cell trait. Genetic counseling can play an important role in prevention. Detection of the presence of sickle cell anemia is possible before birth, so that proper observation and supervision of the infant and young child can be provided.

I. Disease Process

Signs and symptoms do not appear until after approximately the sixth month, when hemoglobin has matured. Growth and development may be impaired during the early years. Young children are markedly susceptible to communicable diseases and especially to pneumococcal infections.

The disease abnormality is in the type and solubility of hemoglobin. The defective hemoglobin loses oxygen and the red blood cells become distorted into sickled shapes (figure 57–3). Increases in blood fluid viscosity result, and blood stasis occurs, which can lead to thrombosis formation and infarction. The sickled cells may collect in the vital organs and lead to serious involvement and organ enlargement, particularly of the liver and spleen. Chronic changes may occur in any organ system of the body.

II. Clinical Course

A. Severe Hemolytic Anemia

In adults, chronic hemolytic sickle cell disease can be severe. The hematocrit may range between

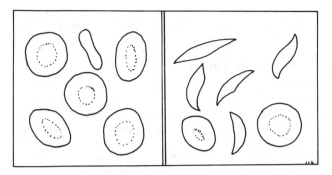

Figure 57–3. Sickle Cell Anemia. Left, diagrammatic drawing of normal red blood cells. **Right,** sickle shapes of red blood cells of a patient with sickle cell anemia.

18 and 30 percent. The life span of red blood cells normally is from 90 to 120 days, whereas in hemolytic anemia such as sickle cell anemia, the red blood cell survival rate is about 10 to 15 days.

B. Sickle Cell Crisis

Periodic recurrences of clinical exacerbations of the disease with periods of remission characterize childhood and adolescence. The acute form of the disease is called the sickle cell crisis.

1. *Precipitating Factors.* Crises may appear at any time with or without stimuli. However, viral or bacterial infections, other systemic diseases, exertion, trauma, temperature changes (dehydration in summer, reflex vasospasm in cold weather) may be specific precipitating factors.

2. *Clinical Signs and Symptoms.* A crisis is characterized by severe pain. Infarctions occur in various tissues and organs. When the central nervous system becomes involved, symptoms of seizure, stroke, or coma may develop.

The effects of a crisis may be reversible to some degree, severe physical conditions can result, or a crisis can be fatal. The high mortality rate in young children may be the result of the effects of crisis or of severe infections.

C. Systemic Changes That May Occur

Chronic changes may occur in any organ system at any age. The kidney is a major organ affected; changes in the cardiopulmonary system can result in enlargement of the heart, heart murmurs, and coronary insufficiency. Ocular disturbances are not uncommon in adults, even leading to blindness. Certain patients may be susceptible to cerebrovascular accidents with hemiplegia.

Changes that occur in all bones, including the mandible result from thrombosis and infarction, and infection.

D. Treatment

1. *Preventive Procedures*
   a. Use folate supplements daily to cope with increased need by the bone marrow.
   b. Avoid and/or promptly treat infections; ad-

minister pneumococcal polyvalent vaccine to children.
   c. Obtain genetic counseling for those with sickle cell trait.

2. *Treatment for Disease State*
   Supportive and palliative treatments include those for specific symptoms during crises, such as pain relief and the use of antibiotics for infectious diseases. Oxygen therapy and blood transfusions have limited selective use.

III. Oral Implications

A. Radiographic Findings[5,6]

Although radiographic findings of bone changes cannot be considered exclusive to sickle cell anemia, the high incidence of characteristics listed here provides a relationship that may, in time, contribute to diagnosis. The bone changes can be observed in patients with sickle cell trait as well as in those with sickle cell anemia.

1. Decreased radiodensity; increased osteoporosis.
2. Coarse trabecular pattern with large marrow spaces.
3. Significant bone loss in children, indicating the presence of periodontitis.

B. Oral Soft Tissues

The tissues may show the pallor typical of anemias, and because of the specific destruction of tissues in the liver of the patient with sickle cell anemia, the gingiva may have a jaundiced color.

Periodontal evaluation for all ages is likely to reveal pockets, infection, bleeding, and the need for a strict preventive and treatment program.

C. General Suggestions for Appointment Management[7,8]

The objective during therapy is to provide care without precipitating a sickle cell crisis. In general, during a sickle cell crisis, treatment should be limited to emergency relief.

1. Prepare or review the comprehensive medical history.
2. Use prophylactic antibiotics. For a patient so highly susceptible to infection, antibiotics should be considered routine, because any form of tissue manipulation can create a bacteremia.
3. Obtain a hematocrit and a hemoglobin determination immediately prior to each treatment appointment. The patient's physician can provide the interpretation and advise whether the patient is able to have a dental or dental hygiene appointment that day.
4. Teach and supervise a comprehensive preventive program to minimize oral infection and control etiologic factors.

POLYCYTHEMIAS

Polycythemia means an increase in the number and concentration of red blood cells above the normal level. Hemoglobin and hematocrit values are raised. The three general categories are described in the following.

I. Relative Polycythemia

When a loss of plasma occurs without a corresponding loss of red blood cells, the concentration of cells increases and a relative polycythemia results. The causes of fluid loss may be conditions such as dehydration, diarrhea, repeated vomiting, sweating, or loss of fluid from burns.

Other contributing factors may be smoking, hypertension, obesity, and stress, particularly in middle-aged males.

II. Polycythemia Vera (Primary Polycythemia)[9]

In contrast to "relative" polycythemia, which results from fluid loss, in primary, "absolute" or "true" polycythemia, an actual increase occurs in the number of circulating red blood cells. In addition to an increased red blood cell count and hemoglobin value, the white cell and platelet counts are also elevated. The viscosity of the blood is increased, which affects the oxygen transport to the tissues.

A. Cause

Polycythemia vera is a neoplastic condition resulting from a bone disorder in which the primitive red cells or stem cells proliferate. It occurs more frequently after age 40 and more in males.

B. Clinical Signs and Symptoms

Clinical manifestations relate to increased blood volume and viscosity and the tendencies to thrombosis and hemorrhage.

1. *General.* Hemorrhagic spots such as petechiae or ecchymoses appear on the skin. The patient suffers from headaches, dizziness, nasal and gastric bleeding, and abdominal pain. Elevated blood pressure and enlarged spleen are found along with high blood test values. A few cases transform into leukemia.
2. *Oral*
   a. The tongue, mucous membranes, and gingiva are deep purplish-red.
   b. The gingiva are enlarged, with bleeding on slight provocation.

C. Treatment

1. Chemotherapy or radiation.
2. Phlebotomy, to reduce the total volume, and particularly, the red cell volume, of the blood.

D. Dental Hygiene Treatment Considerations

Increased health of the gingival tissues can result from frequent maintenance appointments for the supervision of personal daily plaque removal procedures. When supplemented by professional treatment, especially calculus removal, bleeding tendencies can be lessened.

III. Secondary Polycythemia[9]

Secondary polycythemia is also called erythrocytosis, which simply means an increase in numbers of red blood cells. The increased red cell production can result from hypoxia, such as occurs in residents of high altitudes.

Another cause for increased numbers of red blood cells is an increase in the body's production of erythropoietin, a hormone essential to stimulate the development of the red blood cells in bone marrow. A variety of diseases and tumors can cause excess erythropoietin production. Treatment of the underlying condition is necessary to correct the secondary polycythemia.

WHITE BLOOD CELLS

Disorders of the white blood cells may occur because of a decrease (leukopenia) or an increase (leukocytosis) in cell numbers. The types of white blood cells were described in table 57–3 and illustrated in figure 57–1.

I. Leukopenia

A decrease in the total number of white blood cells results when cell production cannot keep pace with the turnover rate or when an accelerated rate of removal of cells occurs, as in certain disease states.

A. Conditions in which Leukopenia Occurs

1. *Specific Infections.* Typhoid fever, influenza, malaria, measles (rubeola), and German measles (rubella) are examples.
2. *Disease or Intoxification of the Bone Marrow.* Chronic drug poisoning, radiation, and autoimmune or drug-induced immune reactions may be implicated.

B. Agranulocytosis[10]

Agranulocytosis, or malignant neutropenia as it is sometimes called, is a rare, serious disease involving the destruction of bone marrow. Drugs or an autoimmune process are the usual causes.

1. *Clinical Course.* With a sharp drop in white blood cells, bacterial invasion may be rapid, and acute illness may develop. Malaise, chills, and fever are followed by extreme weakness. With complete depression of the bone marrow, blood cells cannot be produced, and death can occur within a few days.

   Initial therapy involves terminating the use of a toxic drug that may have caused the condition and using antibiotics and other symptom-relieving measures. Bone marrow transplants may be the only possible, definitive treatment, assuming that a compatible donor is available.
2. *Oral Lesions.* Ulceration in the mouth and

pharynx is common in agranulocytosis. Symptoms also include gingival bleeding, increased salivation, and a fetid odor. During the severe illness, only palliative relief is possible, using a soft diet and attempts at cleaning the mouth with a soft toothbrush, possibly a suction brush (page 638).

II. Leukocytosis

An increase in the numbers of circulating white blood cells may be caused by inflammatory and infectious states, trauma, exercise, and other conditions listed in table 57–3. The most extreme abnormal cause of leukocytosis is leukemia.

LEUKEMIAS

Leukemias are malignant neoplasias of immature white blood cells. They are characterized by abnormally large numbers of specific types of leukocytes and their precursors, located within the circulating blood and bone marrow and infiltrated into other body tissues and organs.

I. Classification[11]

Leukemias are first named by whether they are acute or chronic and then subdivided by the maturity and type of white cell predominating, whether lymphocytic, myelocytic, or myelogenous.

A basic classification of leukemias includes the following types:

1. Acute lymphocytic (lymphoblastic) leukemia (ALL).
2. Chronic lymphocytic leukemia (CLL).
3. Acute myelocytic (myeloblastic) leukemia (AML).
4. Chronic myelocytic leukemia (CML).

II. Etiology

Specific causes are not known, and extensive research continues. Viral causes have been demonstrated in laboratory research with animals.

Predisposing factors, or leukemogenic agents, which have been shown to influence the development of certain types of leukemias, are ionizing radiation, environmental chemical agents, and genetic factors.

III. Disease Process and Effects

Leukemias are characterized by (1) generalized replacement of bone marrow with proliferating leukemic cells, (2) large numbers of immature white cells in the circulating blood, and (3) widespread infiltrates of white cells throughout the body. The changes that result may be divided into primary and secondary. Tertiary effects also are associated with the treatment given.

A. Primary Changes

The primary changes are those directly related to the increase in numbers of white blood cells.

1. *Bone Marrow.* All of the active red marrow is affected; the marrow is replaced by the neoplastic cells.
2. *Lymph Nodes.* Nodes throughout the body are usually enlarged in all forms of leukemia, because of the accumulation of increased numbers of leukemic cells.
3. *Spleen and Liver.* Both liver and spleen are enlarged, the spleen to the greater degree.
4. *Other Leukemic Infiltrates.* Many organs and tissues become involved, for example the kidneys, adrenals, thyroid and myocardium. Infiltrates in the gingiva are described under Oral Manifestations.

B. Secondary Changes

Secondary changes are the result of complications that arise from the destructive effects of the leukemic infiltrates.

1. *Anemia.* Red cells cannot develop because of the infiltrated bone marrow. Severe anemia can result.
2. *Thrombocytopenia.* Abnormal bleeding tendency is a significant characteristic of all forms of leukemia. The platelet count is very low.
3. *Susceptibility to Bacterial Infection.* Circulating white cells do not have their usual defense capacities.
4. *Osteoporosis.* Expansion of the marrow spaces and changes in the bone by the leukemic infiltrate lead to osteoporosis and radiographic radiolucency. Osseous changes in the maxilla and mandible are not uncommon.

IV. Clinical Signs and Symptoms

A. Onset

Marked differences exist between the clinical findings of acute and chronic forms of leukemia. The acute diseases appear suddenly and severely, whereas the chronic types are insidious.

B. Physical Symptoms: Acute

1. Fatigue, pallor, weakness (from anemia).
2. Purpura and ecchymoses of the skin, bleeding from the nose and gingiva (from thrombocytopenia).
3. Lymphadenopathy, splenomegaly, hepatomegaly.
4. Fever, indicating an infection (from lowered resistance).
5. Headache, nausea, vomiting, and sometimes seizures and coma (from leukemic infiltration of the meninges).

C. Physical Symptoms: Chronic

1. Low-grade fever, night sweats.
2. Weight loss, weakness, easy fatigability.
3. Anemia with exertional dyspnea.
4. Lymphadenopathy, splenomegaly, hepatomegaly.

V. Treatment for Leukemia[12,13]

A. Induction of Remission

The objective at the outset is to return the blood and bone marrow at least to minimally normal blood test levels.

1. Chemotherapy
2. Irradiation.

B. Preventive Central Nervous System Therapy

Cranial radiation supplemented by chemotherapy is administered for central nervous system infiltration.

C. Stabilization Therapy

Treatment for anemia, bleeding, infections, and other complications is needed.

D. Continuation Therapy

During remission, therapy must be continued to prevent bone marrow relapse. Therapy may be stopped after 2 to 4 years of remission.

Children in remission go to school and participate in normal activities. Physically, the only difference is the loss of hair, a side effect of chemotherapy, which is often reversible if chemotherapy is completed. Remission periods are used for routine dental and dental hygiene therapy.

E. Bone Marrow Transplant[14]

When indicated, transplants may be performed during remission, while the patient is stronger and the numbers of cancer cells may be fewer. Chemotherapy and total body radiation precede the marrow transplant to eradicate leukemic cells and suppress immunoreactivity.

Marrow from an identical twin or matched sibling to prevent graft-versus-host complications is administered intravenously. Autologous bone marrow has been used, which has been obtained from the patient during a remission period.

VI. Oral Manifestations

A high percentage of patients with leukemia have oral complications. Patients with acute leukemias have more oral problems than do those with chronic disease.

The oral lesions may be described as those that result from the effects of the infiltration, of treatment, and of the depression of bone marrow and lymphoid tissue.[15,16]

A. Leukemic Infiltrate of the Gingiva

Patients with monocytic leukemia tend to have more pronounced gingival lesions than do patients with other forms of leukemia.

The gingiva is grossly enlarged and bluish red, has blunted papillae and a soft, spongy consistency. The enlargement may be great enough to cover a large portion of the anatomic crowns of the teeth.

B. Effects of Treatment: Direct Drug Toxicity

Oral complications that result from the use of chemotherapeutic agents include painful ulcerations, spontaneous gingival bleeding, tongue desquamation, xerostomia, and secondary infections. Chemotherapy and its effects are described on pages 604–605.

C. Depression of Bone Marrow and Lymphoid Tissue

1. *Hemorrhagic Manifestations*
   a. Petechiae and ecchymoses may be observed on the lips, soft palate, floor of the mouth, and buccal and labial mucosa.
   b. Gingival bleeding appears spontaneously or on gentle provocation.
2. *Increased Susceptibility to Infection.* Bacterial, fungal, viral. Many types of organisms may be found in the local areas of infection, which are often associated with severe ulceration. Candidiasis is a common finding, with white plaques covering varying degrees of the mucosal surfaces.[15]

VII. Dental Hygiene Care

Selection of procedures centers around the patient's problems of susceptibility to infection and bleeding. During acute exacerbations, the patient is usually very ill, and certain suggestions described here may apply to hospital care. Consultation with the patient's physician, hematologist, or oncologist is mandatory to explain the oral treatment needed and to obtain information about the hematologic status.

A. Preparation for Appointments

1. *Prophylactic Antibiotic Premedication* (page 91). The patient with leukemia is susceptible to infection, and drugs used in therapy are immunosuppressive.
2. *Blood Evaluation.* Complete blood evaluation tests, including a minimum of those listed in table 57–2, are essential shortly before dental and dental hygiene treatment.
3. *Aseptic Techniques.* Patients with leukemia who have had multiple blood transfusions may be carriers of hepatitis and other communicable diseases (pages 18, 22). Because the patient is also very susceptible to infection, a two-way emphasis on high-level aseptic technique exists.

B. Oral Examination

A careful, thorough examination is needed. Dental and periodontal conditions without symptoms may become acute problems during chemotherapy.

C. Acute Problems During Exacerbation Periods

1. *Gingival Inflammation.* Palliative treatment for grossly enlarged, bleeding, ulcerated gingiva includes frequent warm saline rinses, a nutritious liquid diet with dietary supplements, and plaque removal procedures using a soft toothbrush. A suction toothbrush may be of value in the hospital setting (page 638).

2. *Scaling.* When the platelet and white blood cell counts permit, scaling can be started.

3. *Post-treatment Instructions.* The objective is to control bleeding. The diet should consist of cold, clear liquids for the first 24 hours, and then cool, soft foods. Because suction can disturb clotting, the use of straws should be avoided. Smoking or other use of tobacco is prohibited, and medications that suppress platelet function, such as aspirin, should be avoided. A close follow-up is indicated: the patient should be seen as frequently as possible. A healing time two or three times longer than normal may be expected.

4. *Candidiasis and Other Oral Infections.* Rinsing with nystatin is usually indicated for Candida infection. Treatment for oral lesions associated with chemotherapy is limited and nonspecific. A mouthrinse containing a topical anesthetic may be necessary to relieve the pain and discomfort from oral mucosal ulcerations while eating.

D. Oral Care During Remission

Complete preventive care with a supervised plaque removal program, daily self-applied fluoride, sealants, dietary control, and any other measure deemed necessary to obtain and maintain optimum oral health for the individual should be instituted during the remission period. Complete scaling, planing, and all periodontal therapy must be completed along with dental treatments. Although it may be doubtful that all severe tissue reactions during periods of chemotherapy can be alleviated, much suffering can be prevented if the oral cavity is in a state of health at the outset.

HEMORRHAGIC DISORDERS

Hemorrhagic disorders have in common tendencies to spontaneous bleeding and moderate to excessive bleeding following trauma or a surgical procedure. Spontaneous bleeding occurs as small hemorrhages into the skin or mucous membranes and other tissues, and appears as petechiae or purpura. Moderate to excessive bleeding or prolonged bleeding may follow dental hygiene therapy, including scaling and root planing. A history or suspicion of a bleeding problem should be fully evaluated before treatment is started.

I. Detection

A. Patient's Medical and Dental Histories

A carefully prepared medical history can provide specific information about bleeding disorders and the treatment received by the patient. When no specific disease is mentioned, clues to possible hemorrhagic tendencies must be sought out through interview.

A basic health questionnaire (pages 80–81) should include items related to bleeding, bruising, blood transfusions (and for what reasons they were needed), blood disorders, familial blood disorders, and previous abnormal bleeding that may have followed past dental or dental hygiene appointments. Follow-up conversational questioning after "yes-no" answers on a written questionnaire can delve into sufficient detail to determine the need for blood tests before treatment is started.

Additional information is also obtained by consultation with the patient's physician. When blood tests have been made in the past but are not recent, new reports can be requested.

B. Laboratory Blood Tests

Selected basic tests are listed in table 57–2 with their normal values. Additional tests are frequently needed for a thorough evaluation of specific conditions.

Certain tests may be needed on the same day as treatment, because blood values may fluctuate. For example, the patient using anticoagulants is required to have a prothrombin time determination within 24 hours of appointment time (page 695). A patient with leukemia also needs immediate preevaluation, as described on page 708.

The types and numbers of tests vary. For example, the information required prior to subgingival instrumentation and periodontal surgery depends on the severity of the patient's condition. The opinions of dentists and physicians may differ, depending on their previous experiences. For a patient with leukemia, the tests recommended may include a prothrombin time, partial thromboplastin time, thrombin time, fibrinogen level, and platelet count, in addition to routine blood counts and a differential white count.[15]

II. Types of Hemorrhagic Disorders

A. Abnormalities of the Blood Capillaries

In this type of disorder, vascular fragility is increased, which leads to petechial and purpuric hemorrhages in the skin or mucous membranes, including the gingiva. A variety of conditions may cause bleeding as a result of an abnormality of the blood vessel walls, including the following:

1. Severe infections (septicemias, severe measles, typhoid fever).
2. Drug reactions (sulfonamides, phenacetin).
3. Scurvy or vitamin C deficiency (impaired collagen of vessel wall).

B. Platelet Deficiency or Dysfunction

1. *Thrombocytopenia.* A lowered number of platelets may be caused by decreased production in the bone marrow. The cause of bone marrow depression may be invasive disease such as leukemia or deficiencies such as folate or vitamin B_{12} deficiency anemias.

2. *Platelet Dysfunction.* A defect in platelet function interferes with the blood clotting mechanism and leads to a prolonged bleeding time. Defects occur as a result of certain hereditary states, uremia, certain drugs, and von Willebrand's disease. An example of drugs that affect blood clotting is the salicylates (aspirin).[17,18]

C. Blood Clotting Defects

A possible irregularity or disorder is associated with each of the many clotting factors.
1. *Acquired Disorders*
   a. Vitamin K deficiency. Vitamin K is essential for prothrombin synthesis and factors VII, IX, X.
   b. Liver disease. Nearly all of the clotting factors are produced in the liver. When the liver is not functioning properly, the clotting factors may be altered.
2. *Hereditary Disorders.* At least 30 hereditary coagulation disorders exist, each resulting from a deficiency or abnormality of a plasma protein. Clinically, their signs and symptoms are similar. The following three are described in detail in the next section:
   a. Hemophilia A (factor VIII abnormality).
   b. Hemophilia B (factor IX abnormality).
   c. von Willebrand's disease (von Willebrand factor, which chemically forms a large part of the factor VIII complex. One component affects platelet function).

HEMOPHILIAS[19]

The hemophilias are a group of congenital disorders of the blood clotting mechanism. The three most common types are classic hemophilia A, hemophilia B or Christmas disease, and von Willebrand's disease.

Hemophilias A and B are inherited by males through an X-linked recessive trait carried by females, and von Willebrand's disease is transmitted by an autosomal codominant trait. Rarely is a female affected by hemophilias A or B, but von Willebrand's disease occurs in males and females.

I. General Characteristics

A. Level of Clotting Factor

The severity of the disease can be related directly to the level of the clotting factor in the circulating blood. Normal concentrations of the clotting factors are between 50 and 100 percent.

Patients with severe hemophilia have a clotting factor VIII or IX less than 1 percent. They have spontaneous bleeding into muscles, joints, and soft tissues, and severe, prolonged bleeding after minor trauma.

When the hemophilia is less severe, the clotting factor is in the 2 to 5 percent range. Spontaneous bleeding may be only occasional; gross bleeding occurs after light but definite trauma.

The accepted minimal surgical level of clotting factor is 30 percent. The same percentage applies for any procedure that causes bleeding, notably subgingival scaling and planing. Consultation with the patient's hematologist is mandatory.

B. Effects and Long-term Complications

1. *Effects of Minor Trauma.* Bleeding and bruising from minor trauma vary, depending on the severity of the disease.
2. *Hemarthroses.* Bleeding into the soft tissue of joints (knees, ankles, elbows) begins in the very young with severe hemophilia. Much swelling, pain, and incapacitation are created.
3. *Joint Deformity and Crippling.* Permanent joint damage can result, and the patient may need splints, braces, or orthopedic surgery.
4. *Intramuscular Hemorrhage.* Hemorrhage into the muscles is accompanied by pain and limitation of motion.
5. *Oral Bleeding.* Bleeding from the gingiva is common and more extensive when periodontal infection is more severe. Because of fear of bleeding, patients may neglect toothbrushing and flossing, which can lead to increased plaque accumulation and inflammation. Small children may injure the oral area when they tumble, and severe bleeding can result.

II. Treatment[19]

Recent developments in therapy have changed the quality of life and possibly the life span for many people with hemophilia. The use of outpatient clinics and home therapy have nearly eliminated the long and expensive hospitalizations of years past.

A. Factor Replacement Therapy

Clotting factor preparations include *cryoprecipitate* (containing factor VIII and fibrinogen) and *concentrates* of a variety of products available for reconstitution.

B. Home Infusion Program

Hemophilia care-center teams work with health personnel in the patient's home community to plan and carry out an individual program of instruction for the parents of a young patient and self-care by the patient by age 10, or as soon as the child is capable. The prescribed concentrates of clotting factor can be stored in the home refrigerator and reconstituted as needed for infusion.

The parents and child are taught to recognize the symptoms of the beginning of a bleeding episode or bleeding from injury, and how to administer the treatment. For patients who have bleeding episodes often, such as more than once each week, a prophylactic schedule may be appropriate. Many patients do not require more than one infusion each month, so that routine prophylaxis is not needed.

A sense of security for a patient is provided through contacts with a social worker and local health personnel. Telephone consultations are available on a 24-hour basis with the hemophilia care center, which may be located at a distance. Precautions are taken to arrange for infusion if necessary during school or working hours.

C. Complications of Frequent Replacement Therapy

a. Hepatitis and cirrhosis.

b. Acquired immunodeficiency syndrome (AIDS). Factor replacement concentrates are made from pooled donated plasma. A patient with hemophilia who receives replacement therapy can be exposed to thousands of donors a year. In the early years of the AIDS epidemic, before positive testing for AIDS antibody was required for all donated blood, many patients with hemophilia were exposed. Hemophilia is included with the high-risk AIDS list (page 22).

D. Immunizations

As part of preventive therapy, each patient should receive hepatitis vaccine at the time of diagnosis of hemophilia. When vaccines are available for non-A, non-B hepatitis and AIDS, the hemophilia patients should be among the early recipients.

III. Dental Hygiene Care

Although prevention and control of bleeding are the central issues when planning appointments for a patient with hemophilia, other factors also require adaptations and attention. A few of these patients are multihandicapped as a result of internal hemorrhages, which have led to mental and physical problems. Suggestions for appointments from Chapter 50 may prove useful for the patient who has had hemarthroses and orthopedic treatment.

A few patients have suffered brain damage as a result of cerebral hemorrhage and may be limited intellectually. Others have emotional stresses related to the disease and its treatment. New channels for adjustment have opened since patients have been able to develop the responsibility for self care. This is in contrast to previous requirements of long hospitalizations, childhood separations from family and school, and dependency on others.

A. Preparation for Appointments

1. *Preliminary Evaluation.* The patient's medical and dental histories must include the pertinent hemophilic history with information about the type, severity, treatment, medications used for pain and other symptoms, and family history. Additional information from the hematologist contributes to planning safe and effective appointments. Thorough and complete oral care can contribute in every respect to the health and well-being of the patient.

2. *Premedication*
   a. Factor replacement therapy. In preparation for local anesthetic administration, subgingival instrumentation, surgical procedures, or any procedure likely to cause bleeding, replacement therapy is given just prior to the appointment in accord with medical consultation.
   b. Prophylactic antibiotic premedication is usually indicated because of the susceptibility to infection. Patients with joint prostheses require antibiotic premedication.[20]

B. Preventive Program

The prevention and control of gingival and dental diseases constitute important aspects of care for patients with hemophilia. Not only are dental and periodontal treatments complicated by necessary special precautions, but spontaneous oral bleeding problems can be at least partially controlled by the elimination of oral diseases.

1. *Parental Instruction.* All possible preventive measures should be started while the child is very young, including fluorides, sealants, plaque control, diet for caries control, and early professional supervision.

2. *Bacterial Plaque Removal.* Complete instruction is given as for any patient. A soft brush is indicated.
   a. Flossing. Teach flossing carefully and correctly to prevent cutting the gingiva and inducing proximal bleeding.
   b. Aids for handicaps. Patients with limited range of motion may benefit from the special adaptations described on pages 622–625.

C. Local Anesthesia

1. *Prevention of Hematomas.* Hematomas may be produced following administration of local anesthesia into loose connective tissue that is highly vascularized. The incidence of hematoma is greatly lessened by the current use of factor replacement therapy.

2. *Procedure for Local Anesthesia.* Use a continuous aspirating technique as the needle is advanced. Medical supervision is needed, because additional replacement therapy may be indicated.

   Instructions for postoperative care must include a request for parental supervision to be sure a young patient does not bite or chew the soft tissues during the time when the anesthesia is wearing off.

D. Instrumentation

All instrumentation is performed carefully but thoroughly to minimize tissue trauma and prevent bleeding. Treatment planning for a series of appointments as described on pages 294–295 is appropriate.

1. *Tissue Conditioning.* When oral care has been neglected and the gingiva are soft, spongy, and bacterial plaque is abundant, a tissue conditioning program is advised. Patient instruction in plaque control procedures is given, practiced, and repeated as necessary over a series of appointments. All possible motivational devices can be employed (pages 298, 371).

   Scaling can be accomplished in small segments. As the tissue begins to shrink, heal, and become more firm, subgingival scaling and root planing can be completed.

2. *Probing and Periodontal Treatment Planning.* Depending on the bleeding tendencies of the gingival tissues, probing and charting for complete periodontal treatment planning may need to be postponed for a few appointments while tissue conditioning is carried out.

   Many patients can be brought to a state of periodontal health through conservative measures of subgingival scaling, and root planing. Complete treatment should be accomplished, including periodontal surgery. As with all oral surgery for a patient with hemophilia, coordination with the medical team and hospitalization when indicated can provide the patient with safe and effective treatment.

E. Miscellaneous Treatment Suggestions

Techniques and procedures should be analyzed to make sure that all excess trauma to the patient is prevented. The same procedures should be applied to all patients, but they are more significant with a patient who has a bleeding problem.

1. *Rubber Dam.* A thin rubber dam may be more gentle to the oral tissues than a heavy one. The use of a Young's frame may eliminate pressure, especially at the corners of the mouth. Rubber dam clamps can be checked for sharp corners and placed carefully without damage to the gingival tissues.

2. *Film Placement.* Films can cut and press on the mucous membranes. Care in placement must be exercised.

3. *Impressions.* Beading the rims of the trays protects the mucosa from pressure and damage from a hard, possibly rough, surface (page 154).

4. *Evacuation.* High-vacuum suction tips may be sharp. Caution in the use of suction is necessary to prevent pulling the sublingual or other mucosal tissues into the suction tip and causing hematomas.

   Selection of a saliva ejector is important. The use of a soft, rubber-padded tip may prevent injury to the sublingual mucosa.

5. *Periodontal Dressing.* After subgingival scaling and planing, a periodontal dressing can provide pressure and adapt the tissue against the teeth as an aid for the prevention of post-appointment bleeding.

6. *Treatment for Hematoma.* Ice pack application may limit the spread of a hematoma as a temporary measure. Prompt replacement therapy may be needed.

7. *Aspirin.* Never suggest the use of aspirin for pain relief of a patient with a bleeding disorder. The bleeding tendency is greatly increased by drug-induced platelet dysfunction.

8. *Frequency of Maintenance Care.* Frequent appointments can aid in keeping the oral tissues in an optimum state of health and help prevent the need for complex dental treatments.

TECHNICAL HINT

Sources of Materials

National Hemophilia Foundation
110 Green Street (Room 406)
New York, New York 10012

Leukemia Society of America
733 Third Avenue
New York, New York 10017

National Leukemia Association
Roosevelt Field, Lower Concourse
Garden City, New York 11530

National Association for Sickle Cell Disease
4221 Wilshire Boulevard (Suite 360)
Los Angeles, California 90010

References

1. Borysenko, M. and Beringer, T.: *Functional Histology,* 2nd ed. Boston, Little, Brown, 1984, pp. 67–81.
2. McCarthy, P.L. and Shklar, G.: *Diseases of the Oral Mucosa,* 2nd ed. Philadelphia, Lea & Febiger, 1980, p. 405.
3. Robbins, S.L., Cotran, R.S., and Kumar, V.: *Pathologic Basis of Disease,* 3rd ed. Philadelphia, W.B. Saunders Co., 1984, pp. 630–635.
4. Robbins, Cotran, and Kumar: op. cit., pp. 618–622.
5. Sanger, R.G. and Bystrom, E.B.: Radiographic Bone Changes in Sickle Cell Anemia, *J. Oral Med., 32,* 32, April-June, 1977.
6. Sanger, R.G. and McTigue, D.J.: Sickle Cell Anemia—Its Pathology and Management, *J. Dent. Handicap., 3,* 9, Winter-Spring, 1978.
7. Smith, D.B. and Gelbman, J.C.: Dental Management of the Sickle Cell Anemia Patient, *Clin. Prevent. Dent., 8,* 21, March-April, 1986.
8. Smith, H.B., McDonald, D.K., and Miller, R.I.: Dental Management of Patients with Sickle Cell Disorders, *J. Am. Dent. Assoc., 114,* 85, January, 1987.
9. Robbins, Cotran, and Kumar: op. cit., pp. 641–643.
10. Shafer, W.G., Hine, M.K., and Levy, B.M.: *A Textbook of Oral Pathology,* 4th ed. Philadelphia, W.B. Saunders Co., 1983, pp. 732–734.
11. Robbins, Cotran, and Kumar: op. cit., pp. 674–685.
12. Smithson, W.A., Gilchrist, G.S., and Burgert, E.O.: Childhood Acute Lymphocytic Leukemia, *CA, 30,* 158, May/June, 1980.
13. Simone, J.V.: The Treatment of Acute Lymphoblastic Leukaemia, *Br. J. Haematol., 45,* 1, May, 1980.
14. Fefer, A.: Bone Marrow Transplants in Leukemic Patients in Remission, *CA, 30,* 45, January/February, 1980.

15. Segelman, A.E. and Doku, H.C.: Treatment of the Oral Complications of Leukemia, *J. Oral Surg., 35,* 469, June, 1977.

16. Barrett, A.P.: Gingival Lesions in Leukemia. A Classification, *J. Periodontol., 55,* 585, October, 1984.

17. Snyder, N.C.: *Dental Hygiene Clinical Applications in Pharmacology.* Philadelphia, Lea & Febiger, 1987, pp. 84–85.

18. American Dental Association, Council on Dental Therapeutics: *Accepted Dental Therapeutics,* 40th ed. Chicago, American Dental Association, 1984, pp. 233–234.

19. Mosher, D.F.: Disorders of Blood Coagulation, in Wyngaarden, J.B. and Smith, L.H., eds.: *Cecil Textbook of Medicine,* 18th ed. Philadelphia, W.B. Saunders Co., 1988, pp. 1060–1072.

20. Mulligan, R.: Late Infections in Patients with Prostheses for Total Replacement of Joints: Implications for the Dental Practitioner, *J. Am. Dent. Assoc., 101,* 44, July, 1980.

Suggested Readings

Adler, S.S.: Anemia in the Aged: Causes and Considerations, *Geriatrics, 35,* 49, April, 1980.

Drummond, J.F., White, D.K., and Damm, D.D.: Megaloblastic Anemia with Oral Lesions: A Consequence of Gastric Bypass Surgery, *Oral Surg. Oral Med. Oral Pathol., 59,* 149, February, 1985.

Fernandez, A.J. and Flaxman, N.A.: Common Laboratory Tests, Values, and Interpretations, *Spec. Care Dentist., 5, 264,* November-December, 1985.

Greenberg, M.S. and Lynch, M.A.: Hematologic Disease, in Lynch, M.A., Brightman, V.J., and Greenberg, M.S., eds.: *Burket's Oral Medicine,* 8th ed. Philadelphia, J.B. Lippincott, 1984, pp. 727–764.

Pindborg, J.J.: *Atlas of Diseases of the Oral Mucosa,* 4th ed. Copenhagen, Munksgaard, 1985, pp. 94–98.

Sickle Cell Anemia

Charache, S., Lubin, B., and Reid, C.D., eds.: *Management and Therapy of Sickle Cell Disease.* Bethesda, Maryland, United States Department of Health and Human Services, National Institutes of Health, NIH Publication No. 85–2117, September, 1985, 34 pp.

Cox, G.M. and Soni, N.N.: Pathological Effects of Sickle Cell Anemia on the Pulp, ASDC *J. Dent. Child., 51,* 128, March-April, 1984.

Crawford, J.M.: Periodontal Disease in Sickle Cell Disease Subjects, *J. Periodontol., 59,* 164, March, 1988.

Daramola, J.O.: Massive Osteomyelitis of the Mandible Complicating Sickle Cell Disease: Report of Case, *J. Oral Surg., 39,* 144, February, 1981.

Grodecki, E.Z. and Friedman, J.M.: Mandibular Osteomyelitis Secondary to Infarcts Associated with Sickle Cell Anemia, *Spec. Care Dentist., 5,* 217, September-October, 1985.

Rada, R.E., Bronny, A.T., and Hasiakos, P.S.: Sickle Cell Crisis Precipitated by Periodontal Infection: Report of Two Cases, *J. Am. Dent. Assoc., 114,* 799, June, 1987.

Sears, R.S., Nazif, M.M., and Zullo, T.: The Effects of Sickle-cell Disease on Dental and Skeletal Maturation, *ASDC J. Dent. Child., 48,* 275, July-August, 1981.

Zvolanek, J.W., Everingham, J., and Towns, C.: Histology of the Gingiva in Sickle Cell Anemia, *J. Oral Med., 42,* 138, July-September, 1987.

White Blood Cell Disorders

Barrett, A.P.: Oral Changes As Initial Diagnostic Indicators in Acute Leukemia, *J. Oral Med., 41,* 234, October-December, 1986.

Barrett, A.P.: A Long-term Prospective Clinical Study of Orofacial Herpes Simplex Virus Infection in Acute Leukemia, *Oral Surg. Oral Med. Oral Pathol., 61,* 149, February, 1986.

Berkowitz, R.J., Jones, P., Barsetti, J., Cheung, N.K., and Coccia, P.F.: Stomatologic Complications of Bone Marrow Transplantation in a Pediatric Population, *Pediatr. Dent., 9,* 105, June, 1987.

Charon, J.A., Mergenhagen, S.E., and Gallin, J.I.: Gingivitis and Oral Ulceration in Patients with Neutrophil Dysfunction, *J. Oral Pathol., 14,* 150, February, 1985.

Connolly, S.F., Lockhart, P.B., and Sonis, S.T.: Severe Oral Hemorrhage and Sepsis Following Bone Marrow Transplant Failure, *Oral Surg. Oral Med. Oral Pathol., 56,* 483, November, 1983.

Dreizen, S., McCredie, K.B., and Keating, M.J.: Chemotherapy-associated Oral Hemorrhages in Adults with Acute Leukemias, *Oral Surg. Oral Med. Oral Pathol., 57,* 494, May, 1984.

Dreizen, S., McCredie, K.B., Keating, M.J., and Luna, M.A.: Malignant Gingival and Skin "Infiltrates" in Adult Leukemia, *Oral Surg. Oral Med. Oral Pathol., 55,* 572, June, 1983.

Felix, D.E. and Lukens, J.: Oral Symptoms as a Chief Sign of Acute Monoblastic Leukemia: Report of Case, *J. Am. Dent. Assoc., 113,* 899, December, 1986.

Goldman, L.J., Seitz, S.J., and Peterson, D.E.: Dental Considerations for the Patient with Acute Leukemia, *Gen. Dent., 31,* 398, September-October, 1983.

Gordon, M.R., O'Neal, R.B., and Woodyard, S.G.: A Variation from Classic Oral Manifestations Associated with Acute Myeloblastic Leukemia. A Case Report, *J. Periodontol., 56,* 285, May, 1985.

Greenberg, M.S., Cohen, S.G., Boosz, B., and Friedman, H.: Oral Herpes Simplex Infections in Patients with Leukemia, *J. Am. Dent. Assoc., 114,* 483, April, 1987.

Heimdahl, A., Johnson, G., Danielsson, K.H., Lönnquist, B., Sundelin, P., and Ringden, O.: Oral Condition of Patients with Leukemia and Severe Aplastic Anemia. Follow-up 1 Year After Bone Marrow Transplantation, *Oral Surg. Oral Med. Oral Pathol., 60,* 498, November, 1985.

Long, L.M., Jacoway, J.R., and Bawden, J.W.: Cyclic Neutropenia: Case Report of Two Siblings, *Pediatr. Dent., 5,* 142, June, 1983.

McGaw, W.T. and Belch, A.: Oral Complications of Acute Leukemia: Prophylactic Impact of a Chlorhexidine Mouth Rinse Regimen, *Oral Surg. Oral Med. Oral Pathol., 60,* 275, September, 1985.

Nelson, L. and Pliskin, M.E.: Dental Considerations in Children with Leukemia, *Compend. Contin. Educ. Dent., 5,* 538, July/August, 1984.

Pritchard, J.F., Ferguson, D.M., Windmiller, J., and Hurt, W.C.: Prepubertal Periodontitis Affecting the Deciduous and Permanent Dentition in a Patient with Cyclic Neutropenia. A Case Report and Discussion, *J. Periodontol., 55,* 114, February, 1984.

Rakocz, M., Serota, F.T., Nelson, L.P., Reich, D.R., Werther, P.L., and August, C.S.: Dental Management of the Child Undergoing Bone Marrow Transplantation, *J. Am. Dent. Assoc., 104,* 485, April, 1982.

Scully, C. and Gilmour, G.: Neutropenia and Dental Patients, *Br. Dent. J., 160,* 43, January 25, 1986.

Scully, C. and MacFarlane, T.W.: Orofacial Manifestations of Childhood Malignancy: Clinical and Microbiological Findings During Remission, *ASDC J. Dent. Child., 50,* 121, March-April, 1983.

Seto, B.G., Kim, M., Wolinsky, L., Mito, R.S., and Champlin, R.: Oral Mucositis in Patients Undergoing Bone Marrow Transplantation, *Oral Surg. Oral Med. Oral Pathol., 60,* 493, November, 1985.

Smith, G.: Initial Oral Signs of Acute Leukemia, *Dent. Hyg., 55,* 16, April, 1981.

Sonis, A.L. and Sonis, S.T.: The Presence of Lymphoblasts in the Gingival Crevice of Children with Acute Lymphoblastic Leukemia, *J. Periodontol., 52,* 276, May, 1981.

Stafford, R., Sonis, S., Lockhart, P., and Sonis, A.: Oral Pathoses as Diagnostic Indicators in Leukemia, *Oral Surg. Oral Med. Oral Pathol., 50,* 134, August, 1980.

Vandesteen, G.E., Altman, L.C., and Page, R.C.: Peripheral Blood Leukocyte Abnormalities and Periodontal Disease, *J. Periodontol., 52,* 174, April, 1981.

Williams, L.T., Peterson, D.E., and Overholser, C.D.: Leukemia and Dental Treatment, *Dent. Hyg., 55,* 29, April, 1981.

Zeni, T.M. and Zach, G.A.: Neutropenic State and Its Periodontal Manifestations, *Gen. Dent., 34,* 223, May-June, 1986.

Bleeding Disorders

Ah Pin, P.J.: The Use of Intraligamental Injections in Haemophiliacs, *Br. Dent. J., 162,* 151, February 21, 1987.

Dugdale, M. and Smith, R.M.: The Patient with Bleeding Problems, *Dent. Clin. North Am., 27,* 271, April, 1983.

Evian, C.I., Corn, H., Guernsey, L.H., and Rosenberg, E.S.: Complications of Severe Bleeding in a Patient with Undiagnosed Factor XI Deficiency, *Oral Surg. Oral Med. Oral Pathol., 52,* 12, July, 1981.

Hasson, D.M., Poole, A.E., delaFuente, B., and Hoyer, L.W.: The Dental Management of Patients with Spontaneous Acquired Factor VIII Inhibitors, *J. Am. Dent. Assoc., 113,* 633, October, 1986.

Hobson, P.: Dental Care of Children with Haemophilia and Related Conditions, *Br. Dent. J., 151,* 249, October 20, 1981.

Larson, C.E., Chang, J.-L., Bleyaert, A.L., and Bedger, R.: Anesthesia Considerations for the Oral Surgery Patient with Hemophilia, *J. Oral Surg., 38,* 516, July, 1980.

Lynch, M.A.: Bleeding and Clotting Disorders, in Lynch, M.A., Brightman, V.J., and Greenberg, M.S., eds.: *Burket's Oral Medicine,* 8th ed. Philadelphia, J.B. Lippincott Co., 1984, pp. 765–783.

Monsour, P.A., Kruger, B.J., and Harden, P.A.: Prevalence and Detection of Patients with Bleeding Disorders, *Aust. Dent. J., 31,* 104, April, 1986.

Prince, S.: An Alternative to Blood Product Therapy for Dental Extractions in the Mild to Moderate Haemophiliac Patient, *Br. Dent. J., 162,* 256, April 11, 1987.

Redding, S.W.: Evaluation of Bleeding Disorders, *Compend. Contin. Educ. Dent., 5,* 25, January, 1984.

Rindum, J.L., Schiødt, M., Pindborg, J.J., and Scheibel, E.: Oral Hairy Leukoplakia in Three Hemophiliacs with Human Immunodeficiency Virus Infection, *Oral Surg. Oral Med. Oral Pathol., 63,* 437, April, 1987.

Saunders, S.D.: A Management Perspective in the Treatment of Hemophilia, *Dent. Hyg., 56,* 32, October, 1982.

Staffileno, H. and Ciancio, S.: Bleeding Disorders in the Dental Patient: Causative Factors and Management, *Compend. Contin. Educ. Dent., 8,* 501, July/August, 1987.

Sydney, S.B. and Ross, R.: Periodontal Surgery in a Patient with von Willebrand's Disease, *J. Am. Dent. Assoc., 102,* 660, May, 1981.

Toy, L., Williams, T.E., and Young, E.A.: Nutritional Status of Patients with Hemophilia, *J. Am. Dietet. Assoc., 78,* 47, January, 1981.

Vinckier, F. and Vermylen, J.: Dental Extractions in Hemophilia: Reflections on 10 Years' Experience, *Oral Surg. Oral Med. Oral Pathol., 59,* 6, January, 1985.

White, C.A., Rees, T.D., and Hurt, W.C.: Factor XII (Hageman Factor) Deficiency in a Periodontal Surgery Patient, *J. Oral Med., 41,* 105, April-June, 1986.

Zakrzewska, J.: Gingival Bleeding as a Manifestation of von Willebrand's Disease. A Review of the Literature and Management, *Br. Dent. J., 155,* 157, September 10, 1983.

58 *The Patient with Diabetes Mellitus*

A preventive dental hygiene program is vital for the patient with diabetes mellitus. The patient with diabetes, particularly one whose condition is unstable or uncontrolled, has a lowered resistance to infection and a delayed healing process. Gingival reactions to bacterial plaque are frequently exaggerated. Periodontal diseases tend to develop with increased severity at an earlier age than in the nondiabetic patient.

The presence of infection, including infection in the oral cavity, may intensify the diabetic symptoms and contribute to difficulty in insulin regulation. The dental team, therefore, has a significant responsibility to provide the patient with oral care and instruction for self-care aimed at maintaining health and preventing gingival and periodontal infections.

Modifications of dental and dental hygiene procedures for the diabetic patient may be indicated, depending on the severity and control of the diabetes. No treatment involving tissue manipulation, including subgingival probing and scaling, should be attempted until the diabetic state has been confirmed with the patient's physician.

THE DIABETIC SYNDROME: CLASSIFICATION[1,2]

Diabetes mellitus is defined as a genetically heterogeneous group of disorders that are characterized by glucose intolerance. Terminology related to the disorders is listed in table 58–1 with definitions.

I. Diabetes Mellitus (DM)

A. Insulin-dependent diabetes mellitus (IDDM).
B. Noninsulin-dependent diabetes mellitus (NIDDM)
   1. Nonobese NIDDM.
   2. Obese NIDDM.
C. Associated with other conditions and syndromes (e.g., pancreatic disease, hormonally, drug- or chemically-induced).

II. Impaired Glucose Intolerance (IGI)

A. Nonobese.
B. Obese.
C. Associated with other conditions and syndromes (e.g., pancreatic disease, hormonally, drug- or chemically-induced).

III. Gestational Diabetes (GDM)

IV. Previous Abnormality of Glucose Tolerance (PrevAGT)

Return to normal glucose tolerance: gestational diabetes, after parturition; obese diabetes, after weight loss.

V. Potential Abnormality of Glucose Tolerance (PotAGT)

Increased risk: family history, obesity, mother of neonate weighing more than 9 pounds, identical twin of diabetic person.

DESCRIPTION

I. Type I. Insulin-Dependent Diabetes Mellitus (IDDM)

A. Characteristics
   1. Insulin deficiency.
   2. Dependence on injected insulin to sustain life and prevent ketosis.
   3. Usually arises in childhood or puberty, but may occur at any age.
   4. Abrupt onset of symptoms.
      a. Weight loss, weakness.
      b. Polyuria, polydipsia, polyphagia.
      c. Hyperglycemia from body's inability to utilize glucose.

B. Former Names
IDDM has been known as juvenile diabetes, juvenile-onset diabetes, ketosis-prone diabetes, and brittle diabetes.

II. Type II. Noninsulin-Dependent Diabetes Mellitus (NIDDM)

Types I and II are compared in table 58–2.

A. Characteristics
   1. Not dependent on insulin for prevention of ketonuria and not prone to ketosis.
   2. Minimal or no symptoms; asymptomatic for years, with slow disease progression.
   3. Onset typical after 35 to 40 years of age, but may occur in younger individuals.
   4. Obese type: represent 80 percent of the diabetic population; condition improves with weight reduction and diet control.

Table 58–1. Glossary of Terms Used in Diabetes Mellitus

Brittle diabetes: term used formerly to describe very unstable juvenile diabetes.

Gestational diabetes: diabetes that occurs during pregnancy.

Glyconeogenesis (gluconeogenesis): formation of glycogen from noncarbohydrates, such as protein or fat, by conversion of the fat to glucose.

Glucose level (of blood): normal level is 80 to 110 mg/dl (milligrams per deciliter).

Hyperglycemia: high level of glucose in the circulating blood; contrast with hypoglycemia when blood sugar level is below normal.

Hyperpnea: respiration deeper and more rapid than normal.

Insulin: a powerful hormone secreted by the beta cells in the islets of Langerhans of the pancreas.

Ketoacidosis: diabetic coma; too little insulin (see text page 717).

Ketosis: enhanced production of ketone bodies; excess production leads to ketoacidosis.

Ketone: end product of fat metabolism.

Ketone body: acetone body.

Ketonuria: increased urinary excretion of ketone bodies.

Oral glucose tolerance test (OGTT): a test used for diagnosis of diabetes. After ingestion of a specific amount of glucose solution, the fasting blood glucose rises promptly in a nondiabetic, then falls to normal within 2 hours. In diabetes, the blood glucose rise is greater and the return to normal is prolonged. (Fasting blood glucose means the glucose determination on a specimen of blood drawn after at least 10 hours of fasting.)

Polydipsia: excessive thirst.

Polyphagia: excessive ingestion of food.

Polyuria: excessive excretion of urine.

Pruritus: itching.

Retinopathy: degenerative disease of the retina. Called diabetic retinopathy when it occurs with diabetes of long standing.

Table 58–2. Comparison of Characteristics of Insulin-dependent and Noninsulin-dependent Diabetes Mellitus

Characteristic	Insulin-dependent Diabetes Mellitus	Noninsulin-dependent Diabetes Mellitus
Age of Onset	Usually under 25 years; may appear later	Adulthood, particularly over 40 years; may appear at younger ages
Body Weight	Normal or thin	High percent obese at the time of diagnosis
Onset of Clinical Symptoms	Rapid/abrupt	Slow/insidious
Severity	Severe	Mild
Diabetic Emergency (Ketoacidosis)	Common	Rare
Stability	Unstable	Stable
Insulin Treatment Required	Almost all	Less than 25 percent
Chronic Manifestations	Uncommon before 20 years; prevalent and severe by age 30	Develop slowly with age

5. Nonobese type: represent 10 percent of the diabetic population.

B. Former Names

NIDDM has been called adult-onset diabetes, maturity-onset diabetes, ketosis-resistant diabetes, maturity-onset type diabetes of the young.

III. Type III. Gestational Diabetes (GDM)

A. Characteristics

1. Begins or is recognized during pregnancy; diabetic women who become pregnant are not included in this category.
2. Above-normal risk of perinatal complications; increased frequency of fetal loss.
3. Glucose intolerance may be transitory; patient motivation to maintain normal glucose and body weight influences health of baby.

B. Postpartum

1. In the majority of patients, glucose tolerance returns to normal, and is reclassified into Class IV: previous abnormality of glucose tolerance.
2. Others go on to develop overt diabetes in 15 to 20 years, particularly postmenopausally.

ACTION OF INSULIN

Normally, insulin is released from the pancreas in proportion to the amount of glucose in the blood. The beta cells of the pancreas stimulate or inhibit insulin secretion directly in accord with the blood glucose level.

I. Functions of Insulin

As a powerful hormone, insulin directly or indirectly affects every organ in the body.
A. Facilitates conversion of glucose to fat in adipose tissue.
B. Speeds the conversion of glucose to glycogen in the liver and muscles.
C. Facilitates the transmission of glucose into cells.
D. Speeds the oxidation of glucose within the cells for energy.

II. Effects of Decreased Insulin

In diabetes, insulin is decreased in amount or function.
A. With decreased insulin, less glucose is transmitted through cell walls into the cells.
B. Glucose increases in the circulating blood until a threshold is reached when glucose spills over into the urine.
C. Without glucose in the cells to use for energy, the cells utilize fats.
   1. End products of fat metabolism (ketones) accumulate in the blood.
   2. Ketones are acid. Usually, when they accumulate, they are neutralized in the blood. When the quantity is large, the neutralizing

effect is depleted rapidly and an acid condition (acidosis) results.
3. In severe, untreated, or inadequately controlled diabetes, acidosis leads to diabetic coma (ketoacidosis).

III. Insulin Complications

With earlier diagnosis, improved treatment procedures, and better informed patients and their families, emergencies have decreased. Recognizing the earliest symptoms in order to arrest the development of a crisis stage is increasingly important.

A. Insulin Reaction

Too much insulin (hyperinsulinism), with lower levels of blood glucose.

B. Diabetic Coma (Ketoacidosis)

Too little insulin (hypoinsulinism). See table 58–3 for a comparison of the characteristics of insulin reaction and diabetic coma, and the respective treatment procedures.

EFFECTS OF DIABETES

I. Infection and Diabetes

A. Patients with diabetes, particularly those whose disease is inadequately controlled, are more susceptible to infections.
B. Failure to treat an infection increases the severity of the diabetic state and intensifies the symptoms; it can precipitate diabetic coma.
C. With infection present, insulin requirements may increase; with elimination of the infection, it may be possible to decrease the prescribed insulin.
D. Frequently encountered infections involve the urinary tract, skin, lungs (pneumonia or tuberculosis), and the oral cavity, particularly the periodontium.
E. Factors involved are impaired circulation, alterations in carbohydrate and protein metabolisms, altered nutritional state, or abnormal immunologic response.

II. Diabetes in Pregnancy

A. Effects on Mother

Insulin adjustment, carefully supervised prenatal care, and improved obstetric practices have lessened much of the potential danger for the mother.

B. Effects on Offspring

1. Infants are larger; premature births more frequent; incidence of congenital malformations is high.
2. High perinatal death rate; lower rate with improved prenatal care.

III. Long-term Complications

Patients with controlled diabetes may develop complications later than those whose disease is less

Table 58–3.   Comparison of Insulin Reaction and Diabetic Coma

	Insulin Reaction (Hypoglycemia)	Diabetic Coma (Ketoacidosis)
History (Predisposing Factors)	Too much insulin Too little food: delayed or omitted Loss of food by vomiting or diarrhea Excessive exercise	Too little insulin: omission of medication or failure to increase dose when requirements increased Too much food Infection Stress Illness of any sort
Cause	Lowered blood glucose with excess insulin in proportion	Decreased glucose utilization when insufficient insulin leads to prolonged increasing acidosis
Occurrence	In insulin-dependent diabetics particularly the unstable, severe type	Insulin-dependent person who is poorly controlled, unstable, who omits or reduces insulin for emotional or other reasons
Onset	Sudden Slower when long-acting insulin is used	Gradual, over many hours, even days
Physical Findings	Skin: moist, increased perspiration Hunger Headache Tremor Pallor Dilated pupils Dizziness, staggering gait Weakness	Skin: flushed and dry Nausea, vomiting Lack of appetite Dry mouth, thirst Soft, sunken eyeballs Increased urination Abdominal pain
Vital Signs		
Temperature	Normal or below	Elevated when infection
Respirations	Normal	Hyperpnea; acetone breath odor
Pulse	Fast; irregular	Weak; rapid
Blood Pressure	Normal or slightly elevated	Lowered; person may be in shock
Behavior	Drowsiness Restlessness, anxiety, irritability Incoordination Stupor, confusion Eventual coma, with or without convulsion	Progressive drowsiness Confusion Lethargy Weakness Eventual coma
Treatment	Give sugar to raise the blood glucose level (orange juice, candy, sugar cubes) Revival: prompt Unconscious or unresponsive: treated by injection of glucagon* or may require intravenous glucose	Immediate professional care, hospitalization Keep patient warm Fluids for the conscious patient Insulin injection
Prevention	Smooth regulation of diabetes with steady diet, insulin, exercise	Early diagnosis of diabetes Well-indoctrinated, regulated patient

*Glucagon is a hormone produced by the alpha cells of the pancreas, which increases blood glucose.

well controlled. The principal involvements are in the nervous system (neuropathy), kidney (nephropathy), retina (retinopathy), and blood vessels (arteriosclerosis and atherosclerosis).

Kidney disease is most severe in insulin-dependent diabetes, whereas atherosclerotic coronary disease is common in older persons with diabetes. Retinopathy occurs frequently, and diabetes is a leading cause of blindness in the United States.

IV. Personal Factors

A. Impact of Personality on Diabetes

1. Problems during treatment may be related to an imbalance between diet and insulin, but often can be influenced by the patient's conscious or subconscious attempt to resist the treatment.
2. Periods of emotional distress bring on alterations in the blood glucose.
3. Changes that lead to acidosis and coma may start during periods of depression, hostility, or anxiety, particularly when such symptoms lead to neglect of diet or insulin.

B. Impact of Diabetes on Personality

1. Reaction to an initial diagnosis may be extremely traumatic, with long-term effects, particularly in a child. An adult patient may suffer fear, frustration, and confusion. Less mature adults show less acceptance, and may reject the diagnosis and try to control their treatment.
2. Adult behavior during the course of treatment can vary from reckless neglect of treatment to the opposite extreme of obsession with details and preoccupation with weighing of foods and extreme attention to personal hygiene.
3. Adolescents may find the restrictions nearly intolerable and their hopes for the future seemingly destroyed. Growing independence and rejection of authority figures (parents and physician) makes diabetes control difficult.
4. Younger children may exhibit feelings of oppression, restriction, or suppressed emotions because of subordination and control by the diabetic regimen.
5. Parents' attitudes influence the diabetic child's adjustment.
   a. Overanxious, overprotective parent may precipitate anxiety states or complete dependence of the child.
   b. Overindulgent parent may indirectly lead the child to exploitation or even complete control.
   c. Indifferent or nonchalant parent may give the child feelings of desertion, neglect, or depression.

TREATMENT FOR DIABETES CONTROL

Objectives in patient care are to correct metabolic disturbances, attain the best possible state of general health, and prevent or postpone complications or chronic effects of diabetes. Treatment methods depend on the severity of the disease and the age, activity, vocation, and psychologic needs as well as the nutritional and weight problems of the patient.

I. General Procedures

A. Methods Used

1. Immediate treatment to manage the acute symptoms.
2. Elimination of sources of infection, including oral diseases.
3. Patient education for self-care.
4. Diet and exercise.
5. Medication: insulin for the insulin-dependent patient. Oral antidiabetic agents may be used for selected patients.
6. Personal hygiene: physical and mental.

B. Self-care

No known cure exists for diabetes. The success of treatment depends on the knowledge, understanding, and attitude of the patient, and on how well the condition is managed on a day-to-day basis throughout life.

1. *Instruction.* Continuing instruction must be provided the patient by the health team, including the physician, registered nurse, dietitian, and other specialists. The dentist and dental hygienist participate to instruct and supervise the patient's oral health practices for the prevention and control of oral diseases.
2. *Components of Self-care*
   a. Objectives: to prevent infections and injuries; prevent glycosuria; and maintain the best possible general health.
   b. Specific instruction; the elements of treatment learned and carried out by the individual include diet management; urine testing; technique of insulin injection and sites for it; care of syringe and of insulin; care of the feet to prevent lesions and infections; and what to do in case of acute complications.
   c. Instruction materials: a number of excellent books and other printed materials have been prepared specifically for the patient with diabetes. Review of some of these materials can provide the dental team members with greater insight into the background and knowledge of the patient in preparation for oral health instruction. Addresses for sources of informational materials are included in Technical Hints at the end of this chapter.

II. Diet and Exercise

Diet planning is basic to all diabetic therapy. Exercise is an essential part of the treatment program and contributes to lowering insulin requirements.

A. Fundamentals of the Diabetic Diet

1. *Carbohydrates.* Elimination of concentrated carbohydrates (sugar, frostings, pastries, candy, syrup, and others).
2. *Total Food Intake.* The daily intake may be identical with normal for the patient's age and stature, with appropriate adjustments for growth in the young patient, degree of activity, and occupation. The obese patient needs a weight-reduction diet.
3. *Diet Selection*
   a. Individual quantitative need. As the treatment schedule is planned by the physician and dietitian, the individual needs are determined within the framework of the patient's customary diet. The adequate diabetic diet is calculated so that ideal body weight can be obtained and maintained.
   b. Food exchange system. This widely used system groups foods into six categories, namely, bread, meat, vegetable, milk, fruit, and fat. Each patient is instructed in specific selections from each list. Only the specific amounts are to be eaten and other additions cannot be made. Food exchange means that a certain serving from one group can be exchanged only with an equivalent from the same group.

      At first, all patients are expected to measure and weigh their food so that the size of proper servings can be learned. Patients with severe diabetes may need to weigh and measure for a longer period or indefinitely.

B. Eating Habits

1. *Distribution of Food.* Daily regimen of eating a prescribed caloric intake is essential to balance insulin and blood glucose.
2. *Meals.* Three spaced, on time, meals and three interval feedings are usually indicated. All food, including that used between meals, is counted into the day's total intake.
3. *Intake of Food.* Patient must eat all the food prescribed at the prescribed times. Rejected foods or foods lost through vomiting must be reported because these may explain changes in glucose balance.

III. Medication

A. Insulin Therapy

1. *Types of Insulin.* Insulin is classified as short-acting, intermediate-acting, or long-acting.
2. *Dosage.* Depends on the individual.
   a. Objective is to attain optimum utilization of glucose throughout each 24 hours.
   b. Factors affecting the need for insulin are food intake, illness, stressful events, variations in exercise, or infections.

B. Oral Antidiabetic Agents

Oral antidiabetic (hypoglycemic) agents are used less than in past years because research has revealed significant detrimental side effects. They may still be used when diet control has proved unsuccessful or insulin cannot be used for a reason such as allergy or immune reaction. One group of antidiabetic agents, the sulfonylureas, acts by stimulating insulin release from the beta cells.

ORAL RELATIONSHIPS

The oral mucosa, tongue, and periodontal tissues of a patient with diabetes mellitus may show unusual susceptibility and a tendency toward more marked reactions to injury, infections, and all local irritants than do tissues of nondiabetics. Such a response is related to generally lowered resistance and delayed healing processes.

I. Periodontal Involvement[3,4,5]

A. Clinical Findings

Marked periodontal disease may be observed at early ages, particularly in patients with insulin-dependent diabetes. Oral findings may include alveolar bone resorption, loss of attachment, pocket formation, and increased tooth mobility, sometimes accompanied by pathologic tooth migration and other signs of trauma from occlusion. Patients with diabetes are more susceptible to periodontal abscess formation.

B. Contributing Factors

1. Diabetes acts as a conditioning, modifying, and accelerating factor, with local irritants having an important role in the development of periodontal symptoms.
2. Inadequate plaque control contributes to more severe tissue response because of decreased resistance.

II. Dental Caries

A. Uncontrolled Diabetes

The dental caries rate is generally consistent with the patient's own age group or may be slightly higher related to diminished saliva and dry mouth or to a high carbohydrate diet in the obese.

B. Controlled

With a well-regulated diet, necessarily low in or free of sugar-containing foods, and with a regular eating pattern that excludes permissive and unaccounted-for between-meal snacks, a reduced dental caries rate is frequently observed.

III. Other Oral Findings

In addition to the signs and symptoms of periodontal disease, certain other oral findings may be noted. These occur primarily when diabetes is uncontrolled or poorly controlled. These signs can be important for identifying a previously undiagnosed case of diabetes.

Diabetes does not cause oral disease. The conditions listed here relate to or secondarily result from the lowered resistance and susceptibility to infection that is characteristic of the tissues of patients with diabetes.

A. Lips
Drying, cracking, angular cheilitis.

B. Xerostomia
Alteration in microflora, increased plaque formation.

C. Mucosa
Edematous, red, possibly ulcerated; burning sensations; poor tolerance for removable prostheses.

D. Dry, Sore Mouth
May lead to diet alterations incompatible with diabetic diet requirements.

DENTAL HYGIENE CARE

Because infection in the oral cavity can alter the course of diabetes and its treatment, the control of oral diseases has a vital role in the maintenance of the patient's health. Frequent and thorough care, with regular supervision of the patient's self-care, is required. This, in turn, requires gaining the patient's utmost cooperation and confidence.

I. Patient History

To supplement the basic medical history obtained from a patient with diabetes, additional questioning will provide essential information, such as the type and schedule of medication, dietary requirements, meal schedule, and frequency of medical appointments. History updating at each maintenance appointment can provide significant new information.

Pertinent questions for an undetected diabetic condition apply to weight loss, excess thirst, hunger, and family history of diabetes.

II. Consultation with Physician

Consultation between the dentist and the physician is necessary before any instrumentation involving tissue manipulation is performed.

A. Information Obtained
1. Degree of control, stability, and severity of the diabetes, susceptibility of the patient to emergency reactions.
2. Other health problems that may influence oral care.
3. Advice relative to a prescription for prophylactic antibiotic therapy.
4. Instructions that have been given the patient about diet, personal care, medication adjustment, or other.

B. Use of Information
The dental hygienist should study and apply information from the patient history and the physician-dentist consultation in order that dental hygiene phases of care and instruction be conducted in accord with the health requirements of the patient.

III. Appointment Planning

Stress, including that created during a dental or dental hygiene appointment, increases glycemia and a tendency toward diabetic acidosis and coma. Appointment planning centers around stress prevention.

A. Antibiotic Premedication
Consultation with the patient's physician or specialist in diabetes is necessary.

In general, the patient with well-controlled diabetes can be treated the same as a patient without diabetes. When the patient is first examined and periodontal infection is evident, however, antibiotic premedication may be advisable.

Uncontrolled, unstable diabetes mellitus requires prophylactic antibiotic premedication because of the reduced ability to resist infection.

B. Time
1. Choice: morning, 1½ to 3 hours after the patient's normal breakfast and medication, during the descending portion of the blood glucose level curve.
2. Long-acting medication: adjust time accordingly.

C. Precautions
1. The patient should not be kept waiting unduly.
2. Do not interfere with the patient's regular meal and between-meal eating schedule.
3. Avoid long periods of stressful procedures: dental and dental hygiene care should be divided into units for short appointments appropriate to the individual's needs.
4. Additional precautions are indicated for the patient with long-term diabetes with complications related to atherosclerosis and other cardiovascular diseases (Chapter 56). The needs of the gerodontic patient may be applied (Chapter 45).
5. Prepare for diabetic emergency when the patient's history reveals diabetic instability or susceptibility to emergencies. Keep sugar cubes or canned orange juice available for the conscious patient as part of the office emergency supplies (page 737 and table 60–1, pages 750–751).

IV. Clinical Procedures

A. Instrumentation
1. *Quadrant or Area Scaling.* When a patient is known to have a healing problem, limiting the number of teeth to be completed at each ap-

pointment is recommended. For each area, scaling should be completed insofar as possible. A plaque check and review of personal oral hygiene procedures prior to each scaling will improve the health of the tissues and condition them for succeeding scalings.

With complete scaling and root planing in deep pockets, particularly in areas of furcation involvement, the possibility for periodontal abscess formation may be kept to a minimum.

2. *Postoperative Healing.* Undue trauma to tissues must be avoided to encourage postoperative healing without complications.

B. Fluoride Application

When the gingival tissue has been inflamed or scaling has been extensive, a topical fluoride application should be postponed until the gingival tissue shows improvement following healing and personal oral care by the patient.

V. Patient Instruction

A. Influence of Diabetes Instruction

Many patients with diabetes are already education-oriented because instruction relative to diabetes and self-care procedures by the physician, nurse, and dietitian is an integral part of therapy. Some emphasis on the care of the mouth may have been made. The interrelation of oral tissue infection and the control of diabetes can be reinforced as personal instruction is given.

B. Bacterial Plaque Control

Self-care measures for plaque control are selected on the basis of individual needs (pages 370–371). Continuing supervision with review of recommended procedures is critical to the patient with diabetes because of increased susceptibility to periodontal tissue involvement.

C. Diet

1. Correlate information about dental caries prevention with the elimination of cariogenic foods. Because a diabetic diet contains no concentrated sweets, cooperation in caries control measures can be expected.
2. Reinforce principles of a nutritious diet in accord with the instruction provided by the physician.

VI. Maintenance Phase

A. Appointment for supervision and examination on a regular 2- to 3-month basis.
B. Probe carefully to detect early gingival bleeding and evidence of pocket formation.
C. Soft-tissue examination with attention to areas of irritation related to fixed and removable prosthesis must be carried out at each appointment.
D. Calculus cannot be permitted to accumulate; therefore, routine scaling and planing are required.

PREVENTION OF DIABETES

When diabetes is detected and treated early, complications may be minimized, postponed, or possibly prevented. Mass screening has been used for many years to locate those persons who may have diabetes. Both blood and urine tests have been used for screening, but blood tests have been shown to be the most reliable.

In the universal effort of the health professions and community groups to find early diabetes, it is becoming increasingly evident that dental offices and clinics may become important screening centers. The history-taking and oral examination procedures for dental patients can be extremely useful for singling out diabetic suspects. Suspects can then be referred for a blood test, or an initial screening test can be performed in the dental office.

In addition to the objectives related to the health and well-being of individuals and the community health aspects of case finding, the dentist and dental hygienist have a responsibility to seek out diabetic patients in order that safe and successful dental and periodontal treatment, including the phases of care assigned the dental hygienist, may be carried out. Before proceeding with traumatic, stress-creating treatment in an infection-prone patient, every effort should be made to discover the true systemic condition of each patient.

I. Diabetic Suspects Among Dental Patients

A. Patients in a Diabetes-Risk Group[2]

From observation and through questions in the patient history, the following may be identified:

1. Individuals with close relatives who have diabetes.
2. Women with abnormal obstetric history; such as multiple spontaneous abortions or stillbirths; or babies over 9 pounds at birth.
3. Obese persons, particularly in the over-40 age group.
4. Those with eye, kidney, or coronary artery disease.
5. Persons with early-onset arteriosclerosis
   a. Premenopausal women with myocardial infarction.
   b. Men having myocardial infarctions before the age of 40.
6. Persons with frequent or chronic infections.

B. Patients with Symptoms Suggestive of Diabetes

Questions in the patient history can be directed to obtain information such as the following:

1. Weight changes: weight loss with increased appetite.
2. Thirst; frequent urination.
3. Slow-healing cuts, bruises, or skin infections such as boils.
4. Pain in extremities: fingers and toes.
5. Fatigue and drowsiness.

6. Most recent blood tests; whether test was made for blood glucose.

C. Repeat of Patient History

With long-standing patients, it is not unusual for the history to have been completed at an initial visit without follow-up reviews being made periodically. Illnesses, hospitalizations, or other involvements, including a diagnosis of diabetes, may have occurred subsequent to the original history record. At each maintenance appointment, a review history is indicated (pages 83, 540).

TECHNICAL HINTS

Sources of Materials and Information

American Diabetes Association
National Service Center
P.O. Box 25757
1660 Duke Street
Alexandria, Virginia 22313

Canadian Diabetic Association
1491 Yonge Street
Toronto, Ontario, M4T 1Z5 Canada

International Diabetes Federation
10, Queen Anne Street
London W1 M OBD, England

Juvenile Diabetes Foundation International
60 Madison Avenue
New York, New York 10010

References

1. National Diabetes Data Group, Harris, M. and Cahill, G., Chairmen: Classification and Diagnosis of Diabetes Mellitus and Other Categories of Glucose Intolerance, *Diabetes, 28,* 1039, December, 1979.
2. Brunner, L.S., Suddarth, D.S., Bare, B.G., Boyer, M.J., and Smeltzer, S.C.O.: *Textbook of Medical-Surgical Nursing,* 6th ed. Philadelphia, J.B. Lippincott Co., 1988, pp. 898–909.
3. Saadoun, A.P.: Diabetes and Periodontal Disease: A Review and Update, *J. West. Soc. Periodont. Periodont. Abstr., 28,* 116, Number 4, 1980.
4. Cianciola, L.J., Park, B.H., Bruck, E., Mosovich, L., and Genco, R.J.: Prevalence of Periodontal Disease in Insulin-dependent Diabetes Mellitus (Juvenile Diabetes), *J. Am. Dent. Assoc., 104,* 653, May, 1982.
5. Manouchehr-Pour, M. and Bissada, N.F.: Periodontal Disease in Juvenile and Adult Diabetic Patients: A Review of the Literature, *J. Am. Dent. Assoc., 107,* 766, November, 1983.

Suggested Readings

Anderson, J.W.: Nutrition Management of Diabetes Mellitus, in Shils, M.E. and Young, V.R., eds.: *Modern Nutrition in Health and Disease,* 7th ed. Philadelphia, Lea & Febiger, 1988, pp. 1201–1229.
Chait, A.: Dietary Management of Diabetes Mellitus, *ASDC J. Dent. Child., 51,* 455, November-December, 1984.
Faulconbridge, A.R., Bradshaw, W.C.L., Jenkins, P.A., and Baum, J.D.: The Dental Status of a Group of Diabetic Children, *Br. Dent. J., 151,* 253, October 20, 1981.
Firkin, D.J. and Ferguson, J.W.: Diabetes Mellitus and the Dental Patient, *N.Z. Dent. J., 81,* 7, January, 1985.
Galea, H., Aganovic, I., and Aganovic, M.: The Dental Caries and Periodontal Disease Experience of Patients with Early Onset Insulin Dependent Diabetes, *Int. Dent. J., 36,* 219, December, 1986.
Goteiner, D.: Glycohemoglobin (GHb): A New Test for the Eval-

uation of the Diabetic Patient and Its Clinical Importance, *J. Am. Dent. Assoc., 102,* 57, January, 1981.
Leeper, S.H., Kalkwarf, K.L., and Strom, E.A.: Oral Status of "Controlled" Adolescent Type I Diabetics, *J. Oral Med., 40,* 127, July-September, 1985.
Levin, M.E., Rigg, L.A., and Marshall, R.E.: Pregnancy and Diabetes. Team Approach, *Arch. Intern. Med., 146,* 758, April, 1986.
Lynch, M.A.: Diabetes, in Lynch, M.A., Brightman, V.J., and Greenberg, M.S., eds.: *Burket's Oral Medicine,* 8th ed. Philadelphia, J.B. Lippincott Co., 1984, pp. 842–851.
Malamed, S.F.: *Handbook of Medical Emergencies in the Dental Office,* 3rd ed. St. Louis, The C.V. Mosby Co., 1987, pp. 198–214.
Munroe, C.O.: The Dental Patient and Diabetes Mellitus, *Dent. Clin. North Am., 27,* 329, April, 1983.
Murrah, V.A.: Diabetes Mellitus and Associated Oral Manifestations: A Review, *J. Oral Path., 14,* 271, April, 1985.
O'Malley, B.C.: Recent Advances in Managing the Complications of Diabetes, *Geriatrics, 35,* 51, June, 1980.
Rhodus, N.L.: Detection and Management of the Diabetic Patient, *Compend. Contin. Educ. Dent., 8,* 73, January, 1987.
Rizza, R.A.: New Modes of Insulin Administration: Do They Have a Role in Clinical Diabetes? *Ann. Intern. Med., 105,* 126, July, 1986.
Rothwell, B.R. and Richard, E.L.: Diabetes Mellitus: Medical and Dental Considerations, *Spec. Care Dentist., 4,* 58, March-April, 1984.
Ryan, D.E. and Bronstein, S.L.: Dentistry and the Diabetic Patient, *Dent. Clin. North Am., 26,* 105, January, 1982.
Salans, L.B.: Diabetes Mellitus. A Disease that is Coming Into Focus, *JAMA, 247,* 590, February 5, 1982.
Sarnat, H., Eliaz, R., Feiman, G., Flexer, Z., Karp, M., and Laron, Z.: Carbohydrate Consumption and Oral Status of Diabetic and Nondiabetic Young Adolescents, *Clin. Prevent. Dent., 7,* 20, July-August, 1985.
Tenovuo, J., Alanen, P., Larjava, H., Vilkari, J., and Lehtonen, O.-P.: Oral Health of Patients with Insulin-dependent Diabetes Mellitus, *Scand. J. Dent. Res., 94,* 338, August, 1986.
Tsutsui, P., Rich, S.K., and Schonfeld, S.E.: Reliability of Intraoral Blood for Diabetes Screening, *J. Oral Med., 40,* 62, April-June, 1985.
Zoeller, G.N. and Kadis, B.: The Diabetic Dental Patient, *Gen. Dent., 29,* 58, January-February, 1981.

Periodontal Disease

Aleo, J.J.: Diabetes and Periodontal Disease. Possible Role of Vitamin C Deficiency: An Hypothesis, *J. Periodontol., 52,* 251, May, 1981.
Barnett, M.L., Baker, R.L., Yancey, J.M., MacMillan, D.R., and Kotoyan, M.: Absence of Periodontitis in a Population of Insulin-dependent Diabetes Mellitus (IDDM) Patients, *J. Periodontol., 55,* 402, July, 1984.
Bartolucci, E.G. and Parkes, R.B.: Accelerated Periodontal Breakdown in Uncontrolled Diabetes, *Oral Surg. Oral Med. Oral Pathol., 52,* 387, October, 1981.
Bissada, N.F., Manouchehr-Pour, M., Haddow, M., and Spagnuolo, P.J.: Neutrophil Functional Activity in Juvenile and Adult Onset Diabetic Patients with Mild and Severe Periodontitis, *J. Periodont. Res., 17,* 500, September, 1982.
Carranza, F.A.: *Glickman's Clinical Periodontology,* 6th ed. Philadelphia, W.B. Saunders Co., 1984, pp. 461–465, 565–566.
Gislen, G., Nilsson, K.O., and Matsson, L.: Gingival Inflammation in Diabetic Children Related to Degree of Metabolic Control, *Acta Odontol. Scand., 38,* 241, Number 4, 1980.
Goteiner, D., Vogel, R., Deasy, M., and Goteiner, C.: Periodontal and Caries Experience in Children with Insulin-dependent Diabetes Mellitus, *J. Am. Dent. Assoc., 113,* 277, August, 1986.
Gusberti, F.A., Syed, S.A., Bacon, G., Grossman, N., and Loesche, W.J.: Puberty Gingivitis in Insulin-dependent Diabetic Children. 1. Cross-sectional Observations, *J. Periodontol., 54,* 714, December, 1983.
Harrison, R. and Bowen, W.H.: Periodontal Health, Dental Caries,

and Metabolic Control in Insulin-dependent Diabetic Children and Adolescents, *Pediatr. Dent., 9,* 283, December, 1987.

Manouchehr-Pour, M., Spagnuolo, P.J., Rodman, H.M., and Bissada, N.F.: Impaired Neutrophil Chemotaxis in Diabetic Patients with Severe Periodontitis, *J. Dent. Res., 60,* 729, March, 1981.

Manouchehr-Pour, M., Spagnuolo, P.J., Rodman, H.M., and Bissada, N.F.: Comparison of Neutrophil Chemotactic Response in Diabetic Patients with Mild and Severe Periodontal Disease, *J. Periodontol., 52,* 410, August, 1981.

Mashimo, P.A., Yamamoto, Y., Slots, J., Park, B.H., and Genco, R.J.: The Periodontal Microflora of Juvenile Diabetics. Culture, Immunofluorescence, and Serum Antibody Studies, *J. Periodontol., 54,* 420, July, 1983.

McMullen, J.A., Van Dyke, T.E., Horoszewicz, H.U., and Genco, R.J.: Neutrophil Chemotaxis in Individuals with Advanced Periodontal Disease and a Genetic Predisposition to Diabetes Mellitus, *J. Periodontol., 52,* 167, April, 1981.

Rylander, H., Ramberg, P., Blohme, G., and Lindhe, J.: Prevalence of Periodontal Disease in Young Diabetics, *J. Clin. Periodontol., 14,* 38, January, 1987.

Tervonen, T. and Knuuttila, M.: Relation of Diabetes Control to Periodontal Pocketing and Alveolar Bone Level, *Oral Surg. Oral Med. Oral Pathol., 61,* 346, April, 1986.

Zambon, J.J., Reynolds, H., Fisher, J.G., Shlossman, M., Dunford, R., and Genco, R.J.: Microbiological and Immunological Studies of Adult Periodontitis in Patients with Noninsulin-dependent Diabetes Mellitus, *J. Periodontol., 59,* 23, January, 1988.

59 *The Patient with Alcoholism*

The use of alcohol is common in a large percentage of the population. Some people are considered light drinkers; some, moderate; and others, heavy or problem drinkers. A small percent are chronically dependent on alcohol and suffer from *alcoholism*. Alcoholism is a chronic, progressive disease that is treatable and can be arrested. Treatment for this illness implies control, not complete cure. The *recovering alcoholic* must be dedicated to life-long abstinence.

People from each category of alcohol use appear as patients needing dental and dental hygiene care. Knowledge of their social and physical health histories and the effect alcohol use may have on oral health is essential to treatment planning.

DESCRIPTION

I. Terminology

Terminology to describe the use and abuse of alcohol is defined in table 59–1. Alcohol used for drinking purposes is ethyl alcohol or ethanol. Other alcohols are methyl, an industrial solvent, and isopropyl, used for rubbing alcohol.

II. Clinical Pattern of Alcohol Use

Alcohol dependency develops after periods of use of alcohol followed by pathologic abuse. In the early period, the person functions appropriately in work, family, and social situations.

As drinking continues in the alcoholic, episodes may occur of alcohol intoxication with amnesia and blackouts. Early evidences of withdrawal symptoms require more alcohol for self-treatment, which creates a vicious cycle leading to dependency.

A. Signs of Alcohol Intoxication[1]

Intoxication results from recent ingestion of excessive amounts of alcohol. It is characterized by behavioral changes that tend to alter the usual behavior of the individual.

1. *Behavioral Changes.* Aggressiveness, impaired judgment, and impaired social or occupational functioning.
2. *Physical Characteristics.* Slurred speech, incoordination, unsteady gait, and flushed face.
3. *Complications*
   a. Irresponsible actions in work and family settings.
   b. Accidents with resultant bruises, fractures, or brain trauma.
   c. Suicide.

B. Signs of Alcohol Abuse[2]

1. *Adult*
   a. Health problems.
   b. Arrest, accident involvement.
   c. Impairment of job performance.
   d. Difficulties in personal relationships.
2. *Adolescent*
   a. Poor school performance.
   b. Trouble with parents.
   c. Involvement with law enforcement personnel.

C. Signs of Alcohol Dependence

1. Inability to stop drinking before intoxication occurs; inability to cut down or limit drinking in spite of repeated attempts; binge drinking.
2. Amnesia for events happening during a period of intoxication.
3. Continuation of drinking in spite of other serious physical disorder that is aggravated by alcohol use.
4. Increased tolerance; increased amount of alcohol ingested.
5. Withdrawal leads to withdrawal symptoms such as morning-after "shakes"; relief obtained by use of more alcohol.

III. Etiology

Both genetic predisposition and environmental influences have been implicated as causes for alcoholism. Children of alcohol-dependent parents have a significantly higher incidence of alcoholism than do children of nonalcoholics.

Various precipitating factors may be involved when considering environmental influences. Included are psychologic stress, social contacts, being raised in a setting where heavy drinking is encouraged or tolerated as acceptable, and current lifestyle.

SYSTEMIC EFFECTS

I. Metabolism of Alcohol

A. Ingestion and Absorption

1. Upon intake, alcohol is promptly absorbed from the stomach and small intestine; less rapidly in the presence of food.

Table 59–1. Glossary of Terms Used in Alcoholism

Abstinence: refrain from use: hold back.

Abuse: general term applied to substance misuse, resulting in one or more problems for the individual.

Acne rosacea: a facial skin condition usually characterized by a flushed appearance; often accompanied by puffiness and a "spider-web" effect of broken capillaries.

Addiction: implies a physical dependence on the effects of a drug or other substance.

Alcohol dependence: an illness characterized by significant impairment directly associated with persistent and excessive use of alcohol; impairment may involve physiologic, psychologic, and/or social dysfunction.

Alcoholism: a progressive, chronic disease with physiologic, psychologic, and behavioral implications.

Amnesia: impairment of long- and/or short-term memory.

Analgesia: loss of sensibility to pain without loss of consciousness.

Antabuse: brand name of generic drug disulfiram; used to deter consumption of alcohol by persons being treated for alcohol dependency by inducing vomiting.

Blackout: temporary amnesia occurring during periods of intensive drinking; person is not unconscious.

Delirium: extreme mental and usually motor excitement marked by a rapid succession of confused and unconnected ideas; often with illusions and hallucinations; may be accompanied by tremors.

Delirium tremens: "DTs"; a serious, dramatic condition associated with the last stages of alcohol withdrawal.

Dementia: condition of deteriorated mentality characterized by a marked decline of intellectual level.

Detoxification: a treatment process used when a substance to which a person is addicted is withdrawn under medical supervision.

Euphoria: feeling of well-being, elation, without fear or worry.

Fetal alcohol syndrome (FAS): an abnormal pattern of growth and development in some children born to chronically alcoholic mothers.

Hallucination: a sensory perception without external stimulation of the relevant sensory organ.

Illicit: illegal; not authorized; not sanctioned by law, rule, or custom.

Polysubstance dependence: addiction to at least three categories of psychoactive substances (not including nicotine or caffeine) but in which no single psychoactive substance has predominated.

Psychoactive drug: a drug possessing the ability to alter anxiety, behavior, cognitive processes, or mental tension.

Psychotropic drug: a drug used in the treatment of mental illness.

Recovering alcoholic: a person afflicted with the disease of alcoholism who is abstaining from the use of alcohol. Recovering alcoholics prefer the term to reformed, cured, "ex," or recovered, because recovering implies an on-going process.

---

2. Alcohol is quickly diffused into all cells and intercellular fluid of the body.
3. Less than 10 percent is excreted directly through the breath, sweat, and urine. The rest is metabolized in the liver.

B. Blood Alcohol Concentration (BAC)[3,4]
1. Within 5 minutes after ingestion, alcohol can be detected in the blood. BAC is measured in milligrams per deciliter (mg/dl).
2. BAC is used in the legal testing of automobile drivers. In most states in the United States, 100 mg/dl or less is the maximum legal driving level. The blood level usually is not measured; it is estimated from the amount present in the expired air and expressed in percent.

C. Effects of BAC at Various Levels

1. The tolerance level varies among individuals. Whereas the inexperienced drinker may lose self control and become nauseated with low levels of alcohol, the experienced drinker tolerates a higher level of alcohol without nausea.
2. Ethanol is a powerful depressant of the central nervous system. In low doses, alcohol can act as a disinhibitor and as a relaxant. Euphoria may be produced. In high doses, alcohol can produce analgesic effects, with reduction of anxiety generally accompanied by reduced alertness and reduced judgment.
3. Blood alcohol concentrations at various levels produce the following characteristic effects:[3,4]

50 mg/dl	sedation, tranquility fine motor coordination reduced unsteadiness on standing
50–100 mg/dl	reduced anxiety enhanced self-esteem reduced critical judgment reduced alertness; slowed reaction time impulsive risk-taking behavior
100—200 mg/dl	intoxication memory deficits possible blackouts increased aggressive behavior
300–400 mg/dl	dilated pupils lowered blood pressure lowered body temperature loss of consciousness
400–500 mg/dl	possibly fatal

D. Liver Metabolism

Over 90 percent of ingested alcohol is converted into acetaldehyde, then into acetone, and finally into carbon dioxide and water, by action of various liver enzymes. High acetaldehyde levels and chronic alcohol consumption impair liver function and lead to liver damage.

II. Health Hazards[5,6]

Prolonged alcohol use causes many serious medical disorders. The alcohol-dependent person is most seriously afflicted, but even less heavy drinkers may have complications. Alcohol-related illnesses may involve any body system. A few are mentioned here.

A. Immunity and Infection[7,8]
1. Alcoholics have diminished immune response: suppression of immune system defense and disturbed function of neutrophils.
2. There is an increased risk for many infections particularly pulmonary diseases (pneumonia, tuberculosis), and viral infections (hepatitis B).
3. Alcoholic liver disease leads to a depressed responsiveness to vaccines, notably hepatitis B vaccine.[9]

B. Digestive System
1. Alcohol ingestion alters the stomach mucosa, stimulates gastric acid secretion, and affects gastric function.
2. Bleeding lesions may develop with desquamation of the stomach lining (acute gastritis).

C. Nutritional Deficiencies
1. The diet of a person who consumes large quantities of alcohol regularly may be limited, because the person loses interest in food and

because the alcohol provides an excess of caloric intake.
2. Marked deficiencies can result from the lack of vitamins, minerals, and other essential nutrients.
3. Secondary malnutrition develops because of the direct effects of alcohol on the gastrointestinal tract. Malabsorption and maldigestion occur following cellular changes in the intestinal wall.

D. Liver Disease
1. Alcohol ingestion causes serious damage to the liver, which influences the health of the entire body.
2. Alcoholic hepatitis and cirrhosis are the most common liver complications. Alcohol abuse is the leading cause of cirrhosis, and cirrhosis is a leading cause of death.

E. Cardiovascular Diseases
1. Cardiomyopathy, heart failure, and enlarged heart occur in greater frequency in long-time alcohol consumers.
2. Significant increases in blood pressure are not unusual.
3. Heavy alcohol consumption increases the death rate from cardiovascular disease.

F. Blood Disorders
1. Reduced formation of new blood cells, megoblastic anemia (page 703), and abnormal iron storage are related to damaged liver function and nutritional deficiencies.
2. Leukopenia is relatively common in alcohol-dependent people.

G. Neoplasms
1. Alcohol use increases the risk of many types of cancers including those of the esophagus, stomach, liver, lung, pancreas, colon, and rectum.[6]
2. Alcohol combined with tobacco use has long been associated with increased neoplasms of the oral cavity, pharynx, and larynx (page 601).
3. A higher risk of breast cancers in women is associated with even moderate drinking.[10]

H. Brain Damage[1,5,11]

Long-term alcohol abuse combined with malnutrition leads to severe damage to both central and peripheral nervous systems. Early changes affect intellectual actions such as judgment and learning ability. With prolonged and heavy alcohol consumption, chronic brain damage results. The two major disturbances are the following:
1. *Dementia Associated with Alcoholism.* Dementia is a severe impairment second only to Alzheimer's disease as a major cause of mental deterioration. It has many symptoms similar to Alzheimer's disease (page 563).
2. *Alcohol Amnestic Disorder (Korsakoff's syn-*

drome). This disorder involves severe and persistent memory impairment with other intellectual functions staying relatively intact. It is a result of nutritional deficiency, specifically thiamine deficiency, in conjunction with chronic alcoholism.

I. Reproductive System[12]

Alcohol affects every branch of the endocrine system, directly and indirectly, through the body's organization of the endocrine hormones. Possible effects are listed here.

1. *Female.* Menstrual disturbances, loss of secondary sex characteristics, infertility, and early menopause. Fetal alcohol syndrome is described in the next section III.
2. *Male.* Atrophy of testicular tubules, suppression of testosterone, loss of mature sperm cells, feminization, and failure of gonadal function.

III. Fetal Alcohol Syndrome[5,13,14]

A. Alcohol Use During Pregnancy

The use of alcohol during the prenatal period can be seriously threatening to the health of the baby. Even children born to mothers who have been occasional drinkers but not alcoholics may have alcohol-related developmental or behavioral problems. The amount of alcohol, if any, that might be considered "safe" to consume during pregnancy has not been established.

Many women who abuse alcohol have poor health habits and inadequate nutritional intake, use tobacco regularly, and abuse other substances. These other factors may also influence the health of the baby.

Alcohol passes freely across the placenta. Increased incidence of spontaneous abortions and stillbirths has been related to alcohol intake. The most severe effects result in the fetal alcohol syndrome (FAS).

B. Signs and Symptoms

A characteristically abnormal pattern of growth and development can be found in children with fetal alcohol syndrome. The signs and symptoms may be grouped under central nervous system dysfunctions, growth deficiency, facial abnormalities, and other disturbances.[5,15]

Individually, the signs or symptoms cannot be considered specific for alcohol because they appear in other conditions; but grouped together, they form this syndrome.

1. *Central Nervous System*
   a. Mental retardation; learning disabilities.
   b. Poor motor coordination.
   c. Irritability; hyperactivity.
2. *Growth Deficiency*
   a. Prenatal and postnatal growth abnormalities in both length and weight.
   b. Microcephaly.

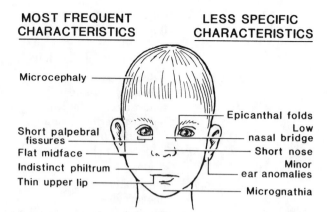

| MOST FREQUENT CHARACTERISTICS | LESS SPECIFIC CHARACTERISTICS |

Microcephaly — Short palpebral fissures — Flat midface — Indistinct philtrum — Thin upper lip — Epicanthal folds — Low nasal bridge — Short nose — Minor ear anomalies — Micrognathia

Figure 59–1. Fetal Alcohol Syndrome. The characteristic abnormal facial features of a child born to a mother who is alcohol-dependent. Growth deficiency is also a recognized feature as are many other signs of developmental and behavioral problems. (Adapted from Little, R.E. and Streissguth, A.P.: Alcohol, Pregnancy and the Fetal Alcohol Syndrome Unit in Alcohol Use and Its Medical Consequences: A Comprehensive Teaching Program for Biomedical Education. Project Cork of Dartmouth Medical School. Milner-Fenwick, Inc., 2125 Greenspring Drive, Timonium, MD 21093.)

   c. Reduced adipose tissue: underweight.
3. *Facial Characteristics* (figure 59–1)
   a. Eyes: short palpebral fissures, epicanthal folds, ptosis.
   b. Nose: short, upturned, with sunken nasal bridge.
   c. Mouth: thin upper lip, smooth philtrum, cleft lip with or without cleft palate.
   d. Midface: depressed, underdeveloped maxilla.
   e. Micrognathia.
   f. Ear: anomalies of shape and position.
4. *Other Disturbances.* Major organ system malformations include cardiac, hepatic, muscular, skeletal, and renal.[15]

WITHDRAWAL SYNDROME[1]

Withdrawal consists of the disturbances that occur after abrupt cessation of alcohol intake in the alcohol-dependent person. Withdrawal signs appear within a few hours after drinking has stopped. Even a relative decline in blood concentration can precipitate the syndrome.

I. Predisposing Factors

Malnutrition, fatigue, depression, and physical illnesses aggravate withdrawal symptoms.

II. Features

A. Tremor of hands, tongue, eyelids.
B. Nervousness and irritation.
C. Malaise, weakness, headache.
D. Dry mouth.
E. Autonomic hyperactivity: sweating, rapid heart beat, elevated blood pressure.

F. Transient hallucinations.

G. Insomnia.

III. Complications

A. Alcohol Withdrawal Delirium (Delirium Tremens, "DTs")

1. May occur within 1 week of cessation of heavy alcohol intake.
2. Features
   a. Marked autonomic hyperactivity: rapid heart beat, sweating.
   b. Vivid hallucinations (visual, auditory, tactile).
   c. Delusions and agitated behavior; tremor.
   d. Confusion and disorientation.

B. Alcohol Hallucinosis

1. Auditory and visual hallucinations develop within 48 hours after abruptly stopping or reducing heavy alcohol intake of long-standing dependency.
2. Features
   a. May last weeks or months.
   b. Impairment is severe, with schizophrenic symptoms, although schizophrenia is not a predisposing factor.
   c. Delirium is not present.

TREATMENT[16]

The overall objective of treatment for the alcoholic is to help the person achieve and maintain total abstinence. An alcohol-dependent person probably can never drink even small amounts of alcohol without eventually resuming dependency.

Treatment includes a combination of medical and psychiatric therapy with self help. Patients are encouraged not to take other psychoactive drugs, including minor tranquilizers and caffeine.

I. Early Intervention

When problem drinkers who are not yet dependent can be identified, counseling may help to reduce and perhaps eliminate the use of alcohol.

II. Detoxification

The term detoxification applies to the management of acute intoxication and the withdrawal syndrome. A variety of treatments may be involved.

A. Treatment for Immediate Emergencies

An alcoholic may have been in an accident or have a medical emergency other than that of the alcohol withdrawal syndrome. Fractures, head injury, internal bleeding, or other problems may require initial attention. In fact, alcohol dependency may be revealed after a patient is admitted for other reasons and withdrawal symptoms appear within a few hours or days.

B. Removal from Source of Alcohol: Abstinence

One of the advantages of hospitalization is that supervision is available. The patient does not have access to usual sources of alcohol.

C. Rest, Sleep, and Proper Diet

One goal of therapy is to restore general physical health by treating nutritional deficiencies and encouraging a normal daily pattern of sleep and meals.

D. Treatment for Medical Complications

Possible medical complications were described with their systemic effects earlier in this chapter. Most alcoholics have additional illnesses.

E. Relief from Acute Withdrawal Signs

Tranquilizers may be prescribed for short-term use. Vitamins, particularly thiamine, are usually administered.

III. Rehabilitation

A. Counseling and Education

The patient must recognize that alcoholism is a serious disease and must be willing to be helped. Family and work associates may be recruited to cooperate with the program. Behavior therapy and psychotherapy have been used.

B. Disulfiram (Antabuse)[3,16]

The drug disulfiram interferes with the metabolism of alcohol by acting on the enzyme that converts acetaldehyde to acetone in the liver. As a result, acetaldehyde accumulates in the tissues. When both alcohol and disulfiram are taken at the same time, nausea and vomiting with hypotension result, and the patient becomes very ill. The drug acts as a deterrent to provide an adjunct to comprehensive therapy in selected patients.

C. Group Therapy

Alcoholics Anonymous (AA) is one source of possible help for motivated individuals. Other people prefer special clinics and centers for treatment.

AA is a fellowship of men and women who help themselves and others to recover from alcoholism. Al-Anon is a separate program for parents, adult children, siblings, and spouses, as well as other persons concerned with the recovering alcoholic. Alateen is a program for the teenage children. Addresses for these special organizations are included in the Technical Hints at the end of this chapter.

D. Psychiatry

Treatment is needed for patients with psychiatric diseases. An increased frequency of schizophrenia, psychoneurosis, sociopathy, and manic-depressive diseases is being recognized among alcohol-dependent people.

E. Aftercare Services

Because recovery takes a long time, an extended period of aftercare is needed. Early relapse is more likely when a recovering alcoholic leaves a treatment system too early. A typical follow-up includes weekly aftercare group meetings for 9 to 12 months.

DENTAL HYGIENE CARE

Only a small percentage of individuals with an alcohol-consumption problem are incapacitated, homeless, shabbily dressed, or socially disoriented. Most alcohol-dependent people continue to maintain home, work, and social relationships, at least initially, and many for a span of years.

In dental and dental hygiene practice, patients who consume alcohol include the occasional social drinker, the light to moderate drinker, the problem drinker, the alcohol abuser, and the alcohol-dependent person. The abstainer or "teetotaler" is particularly important to identify because that patient may be a recovering alcoholic.

Many alcoholics are polysubstance abusers. They may use other psychoactive drugs such as cocaine, heroin, amphetamines, marijuana, or assorted sedatives or hypnotics.

I. Patient History

The quality of the content and the frequent updating of the medical history are essential to patient care because of the many general health-related problems of alcohol ingestion that can influence oral health and treatment procedures.

A. Obtain Patient Confidence

Information about substance use and abuse must be obtained from patients of all age levels. Adolescents of all socioeconomic groups may be involved.[17] The number of elderly alcohol consumers is ever increasing; some of these are alcoholics.[18]

Unfortunately, people are hesitant to reveal personal information about alcohol use because of the social stigma attached to alcoholism. A patient first needs to understand the reasons for obtaining the information as a health-safety measure. More than that, the patient must know that personal information will remain confidential.

B. Present Questions Carefully

Questions must be asked privately and without sign of disapproval or judgment. A patient's family members may provide an alert to the patient's problem.

The basic questionnaire or interview format must have a few leading questions to provide basic facts. Care must be taken not to place the patient on the defensive.

1. *Suggested Content for Routine Questions*
   a. Pattern of alcohol consumption, frequency, amount on an average day.
   b. Systemic conditions, suggestions of alcohol-related diseases.
   c. Hospitalizations suggestive of alcohol-related accidents or detoxification program.
   d. Information about medications; self-prescribed, over-the-counter, and prescribed drugs. A relationship to polydrug abuse, alcoholism, or treatment for alcoholism may be evident.
   e. History of drinking problem.

2. *Screening for Alcohol Abuse or Dependency.* Various questionnaires have been used in the attempt to detect alcoholism. One of these, the **CAGE,** has four selected questions. Although these questions may not provide a positive diagnosis, research has shown that they can alert the interviewer and provide a high index of suspicion. One positive reply can lead to further inquiry. The four questions are as follows:[19]
   a. Have you ever felt you ought to **C**ut down on your drinking?
   b. Have people **A**nnoyed you by criticizing your drinking?
   c. Have you ever felt bad or **G**uilty about your drinking?
   d. Have you ever had a drink first thing in the morning to steady your nerves or to get rid of a hangover (**E**yeopener)?

II. Patient Examination[20]

Except for the increased risk of oral cancer in persons who use alcohol heavily, no specific oral finding can be attributed directly to alcohol as the etiologic agent. The characteristics listed here have been observed frequently. When present, they assist in patient evaluation and treatment planning.

A. Extraoral Examination

1. *Breath and Body Odor of Alcohol and of Tobacco.* Many alcohol users are also heavy tobacco users.
2. *Tremor of Hands, Tongue, Eyelids.* Signs of withdrawal.
3. *Skin.* Redness of forehead, cheeks, nose; acne rosacea; dilated blood vessels produce spider petechiae on the nose.
4. *Face Color.* Light yellowish brown may indicate jaundice from liver disease.
5. *Eyes.* Red, baggy eyes or puffy facial features; bloated appearance.
6. *Evidences of Trauma.* Facial injuries related to falls when intoxicated. Alcohol abusers are especially prone to traumatic accidents.
7. *Lips.* Angular cheilitis related to poor nutrition.

B. Intraoral Examination

1. *Mucosa, Lips, Tongue.* Dry; xerostomia.
2. *Tongue.* Coated; glossitis related to nutritional deficiencies.
3. *Periodontal Infection*
   a. Generalized poor oral hygiene; heavy plaque not unusual.
   b. Calculus deposits may be generalized, depending on patient neglect.
   c. Gingiva: bleeding spontaneous or on probing.

4. *Teeth*
   a. Chipped and fractured from falls and injuries; stained from tobacco use.
   b. Attrition secondary to bruxism.
   c. Erosion secondary to frequent vomiting.
   d. Dental caries: except for neglect of dental care, dental caries incidence may be no different than for the usual population of the age level. An alcoholic who uses primarily wine or sweetened cocktails and frequently snacks on cariogenic foods is likely to have more carious lesions, particularly if gingival recession and root exposures have occurred. Lack of bacterial plaque removal also favors increased incidence of dental caries.

5. *Evidence of Minimal Dental Care.* Although subject to great variation, the overall tendency is for the alcoholic patient to put off dental and dental hygiene care, sometimes in the interest of money needed to purchase alcohol, or for the polysubstance abuser, additional drugs.

   The alcohol-dependent person also tends to use dental care primarily for emergency purposes for pain relief. The evidence may be noted in a patient who has more missing teeth than treated teeth. The indication can be that dental caries was neglected to the point where extraction was requested.

6. *Dentures.* Chipped, missing; may require frequent repairs.

III. Consultation

Information in the patient history may not reveal accurately the extent of a patient's alcohol use, but clinical observations along with the medical history may provide a high degree of suspicion. From that, further inquiry and consultation with the patient's physician may help to confirm precautions needed during clinical procedures.

When a patient does not have a regular physician and has not had a recent medical evaluation, referral to a physician should be made.

IV. Vital Signs

Routine recording of vital signs is indicated. Blood pressure is frequently increased in the alcoholic. Fluctuations can be particularly significant.

V. Clinical Treatment Procedures

The clinical procedures for dental hygiene care are greatly influenced by the many health problems that can result from chronic ingestion of alcohol. Some of the effects were described earlier in this chapter.

A. Scaling and Root Planing

The usual oral tissue response expected following periodontal scaling and root planing may be limited by the changes in the patient's tissues. These can be summarized as follows:

1. Decreased overall reserve that has resulted from degeneration of multiple organ systems.
2. Impaired healing
   a. Prolonged bleeding time: impaired clotting mechanism from chronic liver disease.
   b. Interference with collagen formation and deposition.
   c. Decreased immune system function.
3. Increased susceptibility to infection.

B. Power-driven Instruments

The patient with chronic alcohol abuse or dependency, particularly one who also inhales tobacco smoke, most likely has pulmonary complications. Lung infections are common. Lung abscesses can be caused by bacteria taken into the lungs from the oral cavity or by abnormal breathing during intoxication. Power-driven instruments, particularly ultrasonic scalers and air-brasive stain-removal devices, must be used with caution to prevent inhalation of oral microorganisms by the patient. High-powered suction applied by an assistant is essential.

PATIENT INSTRUCTION

I. Bacterial Plaque Control

Oral health and cleanliness can be especially important for the patient because of the susceptibility to infection and the high incidence of oral cancer. Motivation may be difficult because many patients with alcohol or polysubstance dependency are preoccupied with alcohol or drugs and place less priority on personal hygiene.

A preventive care program for a recovering alcoholic should become part of the total rehabilitation process.

Antibacterial agents, mouthrinses, or any oral hygiene product that contains alcohol must be avoided for all patients suffering from alcoholism. This is absolutely necessary for the recovering alcoholic because recovery depends on a medication-free lifestyle. The most minute amount of alcohol ingested by a patient being treated with disulfiram can cause an emergency.

II. Diet and Nutrition[21]

A. Relation of Diet to Alcoholism

1. Alcoholic beverages contain calories; a day's allotment of calories may be ingested when alcohol is used in excess.
2. The calories of alcohol are "empty" calories without nutritional elements, and the balance of the diet can be very limited.
3. Alcohol unfavorably affects the absorption and digestion of many nutrients by the changes it produces in the mucosa of the gastrointestinal tract.
4. Liver damage has a major detrimental influence on the metabolism of nutrients.

B. Dietary Deficiencies

Malnutrition has been associated for many years with alcoholism. The severe malnutrition that has been described applies primarily to the derelict or "skid row" alcoholic who has limited resources for proper food.

Many middle and upper class alcoholics do not consume an acceptable "balanced" diet, but they cannot be considered with the severely malnourished group.

C. Instruction

After a dietary analysis is reviewed with the patient, help can be provided by reviewing the basic dietary needs and encouraging the use of foods from the four food groups (table 28–1, page 382).

TECHNICAL HINTS

Sources of Information and Materials

Al-Anon Family Group Headquarters
One Park Avenue
New York, New York 10016

Alcoholics Anonymous World Services
P.O. Box 459, Grand Central Station
New York, New York 10163

National Association for Children of Alcoholics
31706 Coast Highway (Suite 201)
South Laguna, California 92677

National Association of Recovered Alcoholics
P.O. Box 95
Staten Island, New York 10305

United States Department of Health and Human Services
Public Health Service
Alcohol, Drug Abuse, and Mental Health Administration
National Institute on Alcohol Abuse and Alcoholism
NIAAA National Clearinghouse for Alcohol Information
P.O. Box 2345
Rockville, Maryland 20852

FACTORS TO TEACH THE PATIENT

I. Alcohol abuse is a great risk to overall health.

II. Incidence of oral cancer is increased by the use of alcohol and tobacco.

III. Mixing alcohol with other drugs (prescription or over-the-counter) can lead to medical emergencies. Always check each drug and its actions before using it in combination with alcohol.

IV. Alcoholism is a disease with serious implications. Advise young people of the dangers involved and discourage them from drinking alcohol.

V. Commercial antibacterial and fluoride mouthrinses may contain up to 30 percent alcohol. Labels must be read carefully. Keep mouthrinse bottles out of reach of children.

VI. Use of alcohol during pregnancy should be avoided because of possible devastating effects on the baby. Be alert to the alcohol content of certain foods and drugs.

VII. Alcohol readily enters breast milk and is transmitted to the infant during nursing.

References

1. American Psychiatric Association: *Diagnostic and Statistical Manual of Mental Disorders* (Third edition—Revised) (DSM-III-R). Washington, D.C., American Psychiatric Association, 1987, pp. 127–134, 173–175.
2. United States Department of Health and Human Services, Secretary of Health and Human Services: *Sixth Special Report to the U.S. Congress on Alcohol and Health.* Rockville, Maryland, National Institute on Alcohol Abuse and Alcoholism, January, 1987, p. 12.
3. Aston, R.: Aliphatic Alcohols, in Neidle, E.A., Kroeger, D.C., and Yagiela, J.A.: *Pharmacology and Therapeutics for Dentistry*, 2nd ed. St. Louis, The C.V. Mosby Co., 1985, pp. 620–627.
4. Berkow, R. and Fletcher, A.J., eds.: *The Merck Manual of Diagnosis and Therapy,* Vol. 1, General Medicine, 15th ed. Rahway, New Jersey, Merck Sharp & Dohme Research Laboratories, 1987, pp. 1141–1144.
5. Eckardt, M.J., Harford, T.C., Kaelber, C.T., Parker, E.S., Rosenthal, L.S., Ryback, R.S., Salmoiraghi, G.C., Vanderveen, E., and Warren, K.R.: Health Hazards Associated with Alcohol Consumption, *JAMA, 246,* 648, August 7, 1981.
6. United States Department of Health and Human Services: op. cit., pp. 60–79.
7. MacGregor, R.R.: Alcohol and Immune Defense, *JAMA, 256,* 1474, September 19, 1986.
8. Adams, H.G. and Jordan, C.: Infections in the Alcoholic, *Med. Clin. North Am., 68,* 179, January, 1984.
9. Lybecker, L.A., Mendenhall, C.L., Marshall, L.E., Weesner, R.E., and Myre, S.A.: Response to Hepatitis B Vaccine (HBVac) in the Alcoholic, *Hepatology, 3,* 807, Abstract 36, May, 1983.
10. Graham, S.: Alcohol and Breast Cancer, *N. Engl. J. Med., 316,* 1211, May 7, 1987.
11. United States Department of Health and Human Services: op. cit., pp. 48–55.
12. United States Department of Health and Human Services: op. cit., pp. 66–70.
13. Streissguth, A.P., Landesman-Dwyer, S., Martin, J.C., and Smith, D.W.: Teratogenic Effects of Alcohol in Humans and Laboratory Animals, *Science, 209,* 353, July 18, 1980.
14. United States Department of Health and Human Services: op. cit., pp. 80–96.
15. Clarren, S.K.: Recognition of Fetal Alcohol Syndrome, *JAMA, 245,* 2436, June 19, 1981.
16. United States Department of Health and Human Services: op. cit., pp. 120–142.
17. MacDonald, D.I.: Drugs, Drinking, and Adolescence, *Am. J. Dis. Child, 138,* 117, February, 1984.
18. Friedlander, A.H. and Solomon, D.H.: Dental Management of the Geriatric Alcoholic Patient, *Gerodontics, 4,* 23, February, 1988.
19. Ewing, J.A.: Detecting Alcoholism. The CAGE Questionnaire, *JAMA, 252,* 1905, October 12, 1984.
20. Friedlander, A.H., Mills, M.J., and Gorelick, D.A.: Alcoholism and Dental Management, *Oral Surg. Oral Med. Oral Pathol., 63,* 42, January, 1987.
21. Shaw, S. and Lieber, C.S.: Nutrition and Diet in Alcoholism, in Shils, M.E. and Young, V.R., eds.: *Modern Nutrition in Health and Disease,* 7th ed. Philadelphia, Lea & Febiger, 1988, pp. 1423–1449.

Suggested Readings

Arrison, E.: Alcoholism: The Dental Assistant's Role in Intervention, *Dent. Assist., 56,* 9, July-August, 1987.
Bush, B., Shaw, S., Cleary, P., Delbanco, T.L., and Aronson, M.D.:

Screening for Alcohol Abuse Using the CAGE Questionnaire, *Am. J. Med., 82,* 231, February, 1987.

Christen, A.G.: Dentistry and the Alcoholic Patient, *Dent. Clin. North Am., 27,* 341, April, 1983.

Cyr, M.G. and Wartman, S.A.: The Effectiveness of Routine Screening Questions in the Detection of Alcoholism, *JAMA, 259,* 51, January 1, 1988.

Elwood, J.M., Pearson, J.C.G., Skippen, D.H., and Jackson, S.M.: Alcohol, Smoking, Social and Occupational Factors in the Aetiology of Cancer of the Oral Cavity, Pharynx and Larynx, *Int. J. Cancer, 34,* 603, November 15, 1984.

Giangrego, E., ed.: Chemical Dependency: the Road to Recovery, *J. Am. Dent. Assoc., 115,* 17, July, 1987.

Klatsky, A.L., Friedman, G.D., and Armstrong, M.A.: The Relationships Between Alcoholic Beverage Use and Other Traits to Blood Pressure: A New Kaiser Permanente Study, *Circulation, 73,* 628, April, 1986.

Molina, M.P.: Treating the Alcoholic Dental Patient, *Dent. Hyg., 55,* 29, March, 1981.

Powell, A.H. and Minick, M.P.: Alcohol Withdrawal Syndrome, *Am. J. Nurs., 88,* 312, March, 1988.

Ratcliff, J.S. and Collins, G.B.: Dental Management of the Recovered Chemically Dependent Patient, *J. Am. Dent. Assoc., 114,* 601, May, 1987.

Roe, D.A.: Nutritional Concerns in the Alcoholic, *J. Am. Dietet. Assoc., 78,* 17, January, 1981.

Schuckit, M.A.: Overview of Alcoholism, *J. Am. Dent. Assoc., 99,* 489, September, 1979.

Sherlock, S.: Nutrition and the Alcoholic, *Lancet, 1,* 436, February 25, 1984.

Szymaitis, D.W.: Dental Considerations for Treatment of the Alcohol-consuming Patient, *J. Am. Dent. Assoc., 95,* 592, September, 1977.

Visocan, B.J.: Nutritional Management of Alcoholism, *J. Am. Dietet. Assoc., 83,* 693, December, 1983.

Williams, G.D., Dufour, M., and Bertolucci, D.: Drinking Levels, Knowledge, and Associated Characteristics, 1985 NHIS Findings, *Public Health Rep., 101,* 593, November-December, 1986.

Fetal Alcohol Syndrome

Barnett, R. and Shusterman, S.: Fetal Alcohol Syndrome: Review of Literature and Report of Cases, *J. Am. Dent. Assoc., 111,* 591, October, 1985.

Barrison, I.G. and Wright, J.T.: Moderate Drinking During Pregnancy and Foetal Outcome, *Alcohol Alcohol., 19,* 167, Number 2, 1984.

Clarren, S.K. and Smith, D.W.: The Fetal Alcohol Syndrome, *N. Engl. J. Med., 298,* 1063, May 11, 1978.

Ouellette, E.M.: The Fetal Alcohol Syndrome, *ASDC J. Dent. Child., 51,* 222, May-June, 1984.

Rosenlicht, J., Murphy, J.B., and Maloney, P.L.: Fetal Alcohol Syndrome, *Oral Surg. Oral Med. Oral Pathol., 47,* 8, January, 1979.

Webb, S., Hochberg, M.S., and Sher, M.R.: Fetal Alcohol Syndrome: Report of Case, *J. Am. Dent. Assoc., 116,* 196, February, 1988.

Wood, N. and Turner, J.W.: Fetal Alcohol Syndrome: A Review, *ASDC J. Dent. Child., 48,* 198, May-June, 1981.

Adolescence and Alcohol

Bradford, D.E.: Alcohol and the Young Child, *Alcohol Alcohol., 19,* 173, Number 2, 1984.

Brook, D.W. and Brook, J.S.: Adolescent Alcohol Use (Editorial), *Alcohol Alcohol., 20,* 259, Number 3, 1985.

Schwartz, R.H.: Management of a Drug-using Adolescent, in Gellis, S.S. and Kagen, B.M., eds: *Current Pediatric Therapy 12.* Philadelphia, W.B. Saunders Co., 1986, pp. 745–748.

Stephenson, J.N., Moberg, D.P., Daniels, B.J., and Robertson, J.F.: Treating the Intoxicated Adolescent. A Need for Comprehensive Services, *JAMA, 252,* 1884, October 12, 1984.

Alcohol in Mouthrinses

Goepferd, S.J.: Mouthwash—A Potential Source of Acute Alcohol Poisoning in Young Children, *Clin. Prevent. Dent., 5,* 14, May-June, 1983.

Leung, A.K.: Acute Alcohol Toxicity Following Mouthwash Ingestion [letter], *Clin. Pediatr., 24,* 470, August, 1985.

Selbst, S.M., DeMaio, J.G., and Boenning, D.: Mouthwash Poisoning, *Clin. Pediatr., 24,* 162, March, 1985.

Tipton, G.A. and Scottino, M.A.: Acute Alcohol Toxicity Following Mouthwash Ingestion in a Child, *Clin. Pediatr., 24,* 164, March, 1985.

Weller-Fahy, E.R., Berger, L.R., and Troutman, W.G.: Mouthwash: A Source of Acute Ethanol Intoxication, *Pediatrics, 66,* 302, August, 1980.

60 *Emergency Care*

It is relatively easy to be skillful in techniques that are repeated frequently. Emergency care is performed only occasionally, and in instances that involve life-saving measures, may be performed once in many years. To be prepared for that rare moment is difficult, but the public expects an individual trained in a health profession to be able to act in an emergency. Periodic review of procedures is necessary if application is to be effective.

Emergencies may occur within or in the vicinity of a dental office or clinic. Readiness involves not only having knowledge of proper procedures, but equipment kept in a convenient place. A quick, handy reference of emergency measures is important, which may be in the form of a posted chart with characteristic symptoms and related treatment.

The information included in this chapter is basic and is presented with no attempt to mention all types of emergencies that may arise, particularly those of complex traumatic injuries. The principal objectives are to list the symptoms and treatment of the more common emergencies that can occur and to provide a list of the equipment that should be readily available. It is assumed that other up-to-date references will be kept in the dental office and that all dental personnel will familiarize themselves with such sources of information.

All dental personnel should be familiar with all procedures required in emergencies. Resuscitation involving techniques such as drug injection or tracheotomy would be carried out by the dentist. Knowledge of procedures and required equipment or materials is necessary to provide the dentist with immediate and efficient assistance.

PREVENTION OF EMERGENCIES

The permanent records of all patients are handled in a confidential manner. Any identification of a health problem should be within the folder. Prior to each appointment, the record should be reviewed so that preparatory steps can be taken.

Prevention of emergencies requires preparedness, alertness, and anticipation. Some of the procedures that contribute to meeting the requirements are described here.

I. The Patient History

The carefully prepared and regularly updated medical and personal history, with adequate follow-up consultation with the patient's physician for integration of dental and medical care, can prevent many emergencies by alerting dental personnel to the individual patient's needs and idiosyncrasies. Factors that should be included in the patient's history have been listed on pages 79–83 and include information concerning:

A. Specific physical conditions that may lead to an emergency.
B. Diseases for which the patient is or has been under the care of a physician and the type of treatment, including medications.
C. Allergies or drug reactions.

II. Rapport and Stress Minimization

Stress and anxiety are the basis for many of the common emergencies that occur in a dental office or clinic. The office atmosphere and the warmth and sincerity of the personnel can help a patient feel accepted and secure.

Reduction of stress includes the following:[1]

A. Appointment Scheduling
1. Time of appointment planned in accord with personal health requirements.
2. Waiting time minimized.
3. Usual meal time and previous meal checked to prevent hunger anxiety or hypoglycemia.
4. Length of appointment limited to the patient's durability.

B. Medication
1. Premedication when indicated and recommended by the physician and dentist.
2. Pain control during treatment.
3. Patient's own prescriptions. Patients who are subject to emergencies should be instructed to bring their own prescribed medicines; for example, the patient with asthma or one who is subject to attacks of angina pectoris.
4. Postoperative instructions for prevention and/or relief of discomfort.

III. Observation and Vital Signs

A. Extraoral Examination
The general appearance of the patient on the day of the appointment may suggest indicators that encourage preparation for emergencies.

B. Vital Signs Monitored and Recorded in the Patient's Record (pages 94–101)

IV. Prevention of Accidents to Face and Eyes[2,3]

Protective eyeglasses are recommended for every patient and for the clinician and assistants at all appointments (page 35). Face and eye accidents that occur during dental and dental hygiene procedures can result in serious disability and loss of working time; an injured patient may justifiably take legal action. The effects of the preventive measures listed here apply to either a patient or a member of the dental staff.

A. Protective full-coverage glasses should be worn by all dental personnel and patients at each appointment.

B. Instruments, medications, and materials being transferred must be carried around the periphery, never over a patient's face.

C. Attention and care must be paid during the use of handpieces, ultrasonic scalers, and other power-driven instruments or implements that create aerosols, splatter, and ejected debris. Handpieces and ultrasonic scalers should be turned on and off only inside the oral cavity. Power-driven instruments should not be in operation while they are being inserted or removed from the patient's mouth. Aerosol production was described on pages 10–11.

D. Appropriate working distance from the operating field to the faces of dental and dental hygiene clinicians should be maintained. A distance of 14 to 16 inches from the patient's mouth to the clinician's eyes is recommended (page 65). The faces and eyes of clinician and assistant should not be positioned within the danger zone close to the patient's mouth.

E. Rubber dam should be used for all appropriate procedures to protect the patient's tissues, prevent aspiration, and provide the clinician with improved access and visibility.

EMERGENCY MATERIALS AND PREPARATION

Organization is a key concept in being prepared for an emergency. Group planning and individual acceptance of responsibility can provide the team with efficiency, composure, and freedom from fear at the time of crisis.

I. Communication: Telephone Numbers for Medical Aid

Telephone numbers should be posted near each extension from which outside calls can be made.

A. Rescue squads with paramedics (fire, police, flying squad, or 911 in many cities in the United States).

B. Ambulance service.

C. Nearest hospital emergency room.

D. Poison information center.

E. Physicians
1. Patient's physician should be listed in the permanent record in a standard, convenient place.
2. Physicians available for emergency calls.

II. Equipment for Use in an Emergency

Every dental office or clinic should have an emergency kit or cart,[4] and everyone in the office must be familiar with its contents. The kit should be in order, its contents replenished and old materials replaced as needed.

The emergency equipment should be portable and kept in a place readily accessible to all treatment rooms. Materials are plainly marked, and kept separate from other office supplies. Materials included are selected to accomplish emergency treatment by current methods.

The items listed below imply proper training in their use. A team should work out additions to the list in keeping with their training and abilities.

A. Basic Equipment
1. Portable positive pressure oxygen delivery system with clear face masks (child and adult sizes).
2. Simple face mask with one-way valve (pocket mask).
3. Bag-valve-mask (Ambu).
4. Plastic oral airways (adult and child sizes) for a team trained in their correct use.
5. Blood pressure cuff and stethoscope.
6. Cricothyrotomy needle.
7. Suction tips with large diameter, such as tonsil and adenoid tips. Tips must have rounded edges so they may be placed into the pharynx without danger of cutting the mucous membrane.
8. Disposable sterile syringes: 2-, 5-, and 10-ml. capacities with disposable needles for intravenous, intramuscular, and subcutaneous injections.
9. Packaged alcohol wipes or swabs.
10. Thermometer.
11. Tourniquets made of rubber or latex tubing. The blood pressure cuff also may be used as a tourniquet.
12. Penlight or flashlight.
13. Scissors.
14. Commercial cold pack (nonrefrigerated quick-forming cold bag.)
15. Brown paper bags.
16. Blanket.
17. Board: 12 × 24 inches to place under patient in a soft dental chair for cardiopulmonary resuscitation.
18. Blank forms: *Record of Emergency* (figure 60–1) with pen.

B. Bandages and Dressings
Dressings are purchased in individual packages and maintained in the sealed sterile state.

RECORD OF EMERGENCY

NAME _____ DATE _____ TIME _____

ADDRESS _____

Onset of Emergency _____
CPR Started _____
Ambulance Called _____
Ambulance Arrived _____
Hospital Called _____
Physician Called _____
Patient Left Office _____
Attended by: Self _____
            Relative _____
            Other _____

Pertinent Medical History _____

Description of Emergency _____

Time							
Blood Pressure							
Pulse							
Respiration							
Pupils							
Skin—color —temperature							
Level of Consciousness							
Medication (specify)							
Other Treatment (specify)							

Comments and Summary

Personnel Attending

Signature of Team Director:

Figure 60–1. Record of Emergency. The form is prepared in duplicate. One copy accompanies the patient to the emergency department, and the second copy is retained in the patient's dental record file.

1. Adhesive bandages.
2. Sterile dressings in sealed envelopes: 2 × 2 inches, and 4 × 4 inches.
3. Rolled bandage: 1-inch (5 yards); 2-inch (5 yards).
4. Adhesive tape.
5. Gauze sponges: 4 × 4 inches.
6. Inflatable splints (assorted sizes).

C. Noninjectable Treatment Items[4]

1. Oxygen: portable E cylinder.
2. Vasodilator: nitroglycerin tablets (0.3 mg.) or amyl nitrite vaporoles (yellow wrapper).
3. Respiratory stimulant: aromatic ammonia in vaporoles (gray wrapper). Because this may be a frequently used item, additional vaporoles kept in each treatment room in a universally selected place can facilitate action for a patient with syncope.
4. Antihypoglycemic: sugar cubes or packages, hard candies.
5. Bronchodilator: metaproterenol (inhaler).
6. Sterile eye irrigating solution.
7. Bicarbonate of soda.
8. Ipecac

D. Drugs[4]

All dental personnel must be familiar with the emergency drugs maintained in the particular office or clinic.

1. *Identification.* The purpose and method of administration for each should be clearly identifed with the container. A compartmentalized clear plastic cabinet or box can be particularly useful for this purpose, because the labels and instructions can be seen from the outside and efficient selection can be made.

    The replacement date must appear clearly on each item with a limited shelf life. When narcotics are included in the list of drugs available for emergencies, storage in a less accessible place than an emergency kit and purchase in small amounts are indicated to prevent them from being stolen easily.

    Drug categories and examples of each that may be kept in a dental office or clinic for use by the dentist are listed here.

2. *Record of Drugs.* A complete record of each available drug is kept. Recorded are the name, dosage, date purchased, address of source if different than the usual local pharmacy, and each itemized record signed by the staff member responsible.

    As each drug is used, a specific entry is made. Expiration dates can be checked at routine intervals. Drug categories and examples of each that may be kept in a dental office or clinic for use by the dentist are listed below.

3. *Essential Injectable Drugs*[4]
    a. For acute allergic reaction: epinephrine 1:1000.
    b. Anticonvulsant: diazepam (Valium 5 mg./ ml.) or a barbiturate such as pentobarbital.
    c. Antihistamine: chlorpheniramine or diphenhydramine HCl (Benadryl).
    d. Narcotic antagonist: naloxone (Narcan 0.4 mg./ml.).

4. *Secondary Injectable Drugs*
    a. Analgesic: morphine sulfate or meperidine (Demerol).
    b. Vasopressor: methoxamine.
    c. Corticosteroid: hydrocortisone sodium succinate (Solu-Cortef).
    d. Antihypoglycemic: 50% dextrose solution (for unconscious patient).

5. *Drugs for Advanced Cardiac Life Support*
    a. Sodium bicarbonate (50-ml. ampule).
    b. Calcium chloride (10% in 10-ml. preloaded syringe or 10-ml. ampule).
    c. Lidocaine (cardiac) (10 mg./ml. in 10-ml. preloaded syringe).
    d. Atropine: atropine sulfate (0.5 mg. in preloaded syringe).

III. Record of Emergency

Figure 60–1 shows an example of a form that can be used to record the essential information during an emergency. Such a form can be printed into pads for the convenience of having a carbon copy to place in the patient's permanent record when the original accompanies the patient to a hospital or other medical facility.

A. Purposes

1. Organize data collected during the emergency.
2. Serve as a time reference during the monitoring of vital signs.
3. Prepare a record from which the medical personnel can interpret the patient's condition at the time of transfer from the dental facility.

B. Uses

1. Evaluation for planning dental and dental hygiene appointments so that future emergencies for the patient can be avoided.
2. Provide a reference in the event legal questions arise. A well-kept record can be vital, and each emergency, however insignificant the incident may seem, should be recorded.[5,6]

IV. Practice and Drill

A. Staff Instruction

Each member of the clinic or office staff must be thoroughly familiar with the location, purpose, effect, and application of each item of equipment and its source.

B. Assignments

Specific responsibilities must be assigned to each staff member to prevent confusion. However, each must know the order of procedures in all types of emergencies and be able to assume

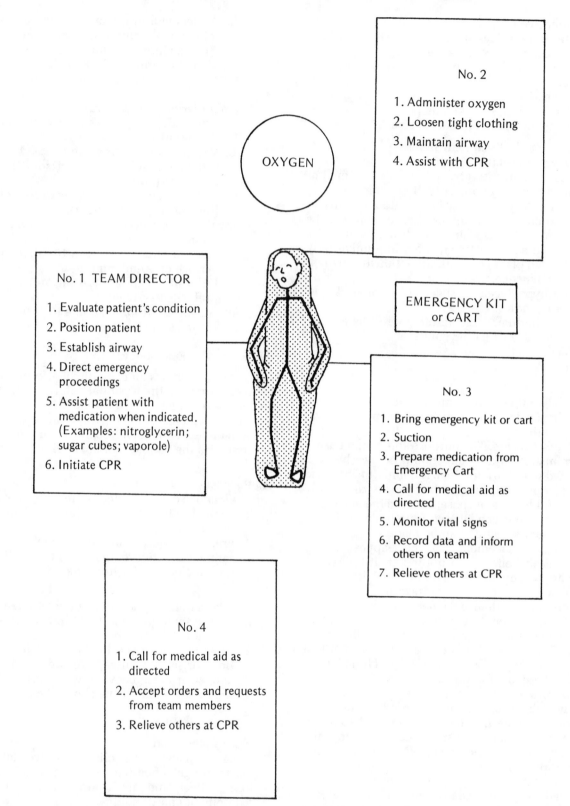

No. 2

1. Administer oxygen
2. Loosen tight clothing
3. Maintain airway
4. Assist with CPR

OXYGEN

No. 1 TEAM DIRECTOR

1. Evaluate patient's condition
2. Position patient
3. Establish airway
4. Direct emergency proceedings
5. Assist patient with medication when indicated. (Examples: nitroglycerin; sugar cubes; vaporole)
6. Initiate CPR

EMERGENCY KIT or CART

No. 3

1. Bring emergency kit or cart
2. Suction
3. Prepare medication from Emergency Cart
4. Call for medical aid as directed
5. Monitor vital signs
6. Record data and inform others on team
7. Relieve others at CPR

No. 4

1. Call for medical aid as directed
2. Accept orders and requests from team members
3. Relieve others at CPR

Figure 60–2. Emergency Team Flow Chart: Four People. Suggested distribution of responsibilities to be memorized and practiced by the dental personnel who form the emergency team. Compare with figure 60–3, flow chart for three people.

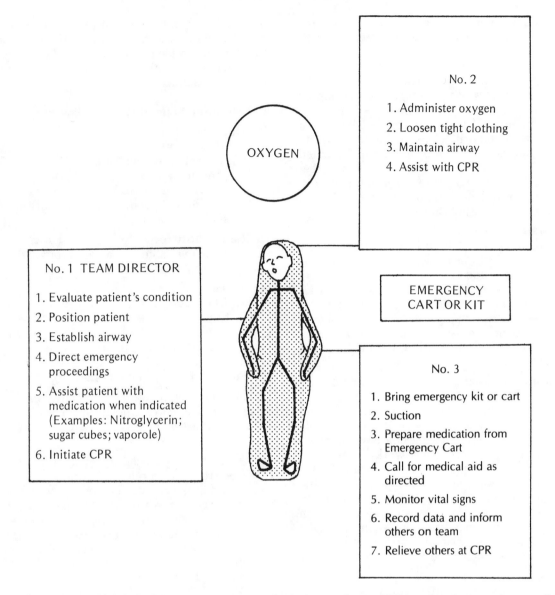

No. 2

1. Administer oxygen
2. Loosen tight clothing
3. Maintain airway
4. Assist with CPR

OXYGEN

No. 1 TEAM DIRECTOR

1. Evaluate patient's condition
2. Position patient
3. Establish airway
4. Direct emergency proceedings
5. Assist patient with medication when indicated (Examples: Nitroglycerin; sugar cubes; vaporole)
6. Initiate CPR

EMERGENCY CART OR KIT

No. 3

1. Bring emergency kit or cart
2. Suction
3. Prepare medication from Emergency Cart
4. Call for medical aid as directed
5. Monitor vital signs
6. Record data and inform others on team
7. Relieve others at CPR

Figure 60–3. Emergency Team Flow Chart: Three People. Suggested distribution of responsibilities when three people are available during an emergency. Compare with figure 60–2, flow chart for four people.

any role when needed. Moments count, and there is no time for fumbling or discussion.

C. Flow Chart

Figure 60–2 shows an example of possible distribution of duties when four people are available to attend the patient, and figure 60–3 shows the distribution when three people are available. Although the chart can be posted for study, it must be memorized by the persons concerned. In a real emergency, no one would have time to consult a flow chart.

1. *Advantages*
   a. Organization efficiently uses personnel.
   b. Sharing responsibility relieves pressure.
   c. Duties can be carried out quietly, without excess discussion.
   d. Necessary work gets done without duplication and without omissions.
2. *Preparation.* The preparation of a flow chart and the assignment of all duties related to emergencies should be a result of planning by the whole team.
3. *Substitutions.* Because a staff member may be absent from the scene at the time of an emergency, each person should know the duties for all positions so that substitutions can be made and duties doubled with a minimum of discussion and no confusion.

D. Drills

1. Regular reviews and rehearsals for each type of emergency should be conducted, preferably on a "surprise" basis, at least once a month.

The dentist can use a specific code call when an intercom or other message system is available.

2. Practice in the use of all procedures, including oxygen administration, resuscitation, and airway maneuvers, as well as specific positioning of a patient for all emergencies, is indicated.

3. Equipment and materials can be checked at the time of the drill to assure their availability and that each is in working order. Outdated supplies can be replaced. One staff member should be in charge of the emergency supplies.

4. Keep a record of drills by making a diary of dates and names of those present.

E. New Staff Member
1. Assignment of duties and practice for the new member should be a part of the first working day's orientation.
2. New members must be expected to renew CPR certificates by taking necessary refresher courses within a specified time. Such a procedure is not necessary in a state where a renewal certificate is required for annual licensure.

F. Procedures Manual
A loose-leaf manual, reviewed and updated three or four times each year, can provide a valuable study and work reference. It is particularly useful during the orientation of a new member.

The notebook can contain work assignments and check lists for equipment and resources. Direct reference information concerning specific emergencies with their symptoms and initial treatment, may be placed in alphabetic order in a specially color-coded section. Members of the team can keep the manual current by bringing references and notes from readings and courses.

BASIC LIFE SUPPORT[7]

Sudden cessation of effective respiration and circulation must be treated immediately. Without breathing and heart action, oxygen cannot be carried to the cells and a deficiency occurs quickly.

Irreversible brain tissue damage may occur within 4 to 6 minutes in the absence of oxygenated blood. After 6 minutes, brain damage nearly always occurs.

Basic patient care in an emergency is defined by the letters A-B-C (figure 60–4). A "D" is sometimes included in the alphabet run to designate definitive care that is required. Examples of definitive care are defibrillation or drug administration by the emergency medical care team or the physicians at a hospital.

It is necessary to keep calm and act promptly, but not hastily. The incorrect procedure may be more harmful than none at all. It is assumed that each member of the dental team will have participated in courses in emergency procedures and resuscitation

techniques while in school and periodically since graduation for refresher, renewal, and updating. This section is intended to provide an outline for reference and review. The steps described are carried out in rapid succession.

I. Determine State of Consciousness

A. Unconscious Patient
1. *Shake the Shoulder and Shout.* If fractures are suspected, the shake must be gentle. The unconscious patient will not respond.
2. *Apply Sensory Stimulation.* The unconscious patient will not respond to sensory application such as pinching.

B. Call Loudly for Help
When available, use an alert (buzzer) system of an office or clinic.

C. Proceed to Treat
1. *Unconscious Patient.* Position for resuscitation.
2. *Conscious Patient.* Determine specific conditions (table 60–1).

II. Position Unconscious Patient

The four basic positions are shown in figure 5–2 (page 65). The correct position for each emergency situation must be learned.

A. Supine
The head is placed on level with the heart; the feet are slightly raised (figure 5–2C). Supine is also defined as completely horizontal, which is the correct position for the patient while cardiopulmonary resuscitation is performed.

The supine position is most frequently used in emergency situations. The exceptions for particular types of emergencies are included in table 60–1.

B. Exceptions for Special Consideration
1. *Pregnancy.* During the third trimester, place patient on her left side to prevent pressure on the vena cava.
2. *Severe Facial Injury.* Turn on side to lessen danger of blood, debris, and displaced parts from falling into the throat and to permit drainage of fluids.

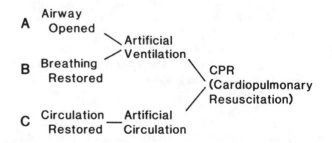

Figure 60–4. Basic Life Support. A. Airway; B. Breathing; C. Circulation. D may be added to indicate Definitive care or treatment.

AIRWAY

I. Open Airway

A. Remove Dental Chair Head Support
A round or wedge-shaped accessory head or shoulder support should be removed to permit the head to lie flat and the chin to be raised without resistance.

B. Tilt Head Back
1. *Head Tilt.* Place palm of hand on patient's forehead to apply backward pressure.
2. *Head Tilt with Chin Lift.* Place palm of hand on forehead to apply backward pressure; place fingertips (not thumb) of other hand under the chin with light pressure on the mandible to bring the chin up (figure 60–5).

II. Check Breathing

A. From beside patient at the shoulder (kneeling if patient is on floor), place ear over the patient's mouth and nose while looking at the chest.
B. LOOK for chest movement.
C. LISTEN for and FEEL air from nose and mouth.
1. Unconscious with no breathing: continue airway procedures.
2. Unconscious and breathing: monitor vital signs, determine other specific conditions (jaw thrust not used).

III. Jaw Thrust

A. Indications
1. First procedure when a neck injury is suspected. It can be done without extending the neck.
2. Second procedure when breathing does not start after airway is opened by the chin lift.

B. Procedure
1. From the top of the patient's head, grasp angles of the mandible, lift and displace it forward; tilt head back.
2. Open lips to allow mouth breathing.
3. Pain from this maneuver may bring response from the patient.

IV. Recheck Breathing (Repeat Step II.)

A. Listen for Possible Obstruction
1. *Partial Obstruction.* Noisy air flow.
2. *Complete Obstruction*
   a. Cannot hear or feel airflow.
   b. No inflation during ventilation.

B. Obstruction Present
Proceed with Airway Obstruction, pages 744–745.

V. Check Pulse

A. Location
1. *Adult.* Carotid pulse in neck (figure 60–6).
2. *Child.* Carotid pulse in neck.

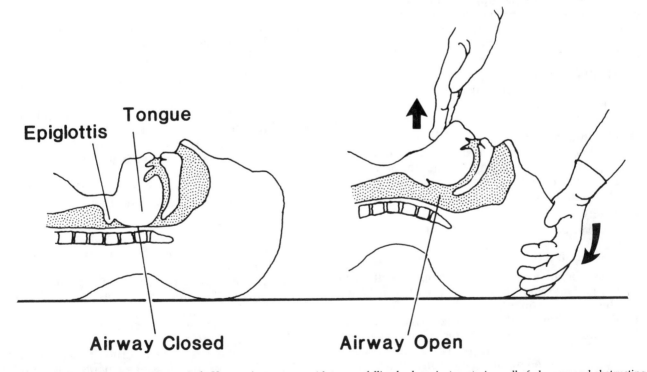

Epiglottis **Tongue**

Airway Closed **Airway Open**

Figure 60–5. Chin Lift to Open Airway. Left, Unconscious person with tongue falling back against posterior wall of pharynx and obstructing the air passage. **Right,** Head is tilted back and chin is lifted by light pressure under the mandible. When neck injury is suspected, a jaw thrust is used. See text for instructions. (After Malamed, S.F.: *Handbook of Medical Emergencies in the Dental Office,* 3rd ed. St. Louis, The C.V. Mosby Co., 1987, page 87.)

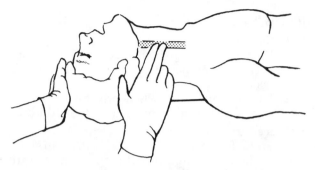

Figure 60–6. Carotid Pulse. To locate the pulse, two or three fingers are placed on the patient's pharynx. The fingers are then slid down into the groove between the trachea and the neck muscles. With gentle pressure, the pulse can be detected.

    3. *Infant:** Brachial pulse of the upper inner arm (figure 7–3, page 97).

B. Determine Need for Cardiopulmonary Resuscitation (CPR)
    1. *Pulse Present.* Patient not breathing: proceed with rescue breathing.
    2. *Pulse Absent.* Proceed with CPR.

RESCUE BREATHING

I. Clear the Mouth

Turn the patient's head to the side to clear the mouth of mucus, vomitus, and other foreign material. Use suction, gauze, and finger. Dentures should be left in place to provide support for mouth-to-mouth ventilation unless the dentures are very loose and could cause throat obstruction if displaced.

II. Position

A. Mouth-to-Mouth
    Pinch the nose closed with thumb and index finger of hand resting on the patient's forehead. Continue to maintain chin lift.

B. Mouth-to-Nose
    When necessary because of oral condition or impossibility of opening the mouth, or when a tight seal cannot be made, the mouth is held closed and the nose is used.

C. Mouth-and-Nose
    Cover both for small child and infant.*

III. Rescue Breathing

A. Take a breath and apply a wide-open mouth over the patient's mouth to make a tight seal. Watch chest for movement.
B. Deliver 2 breaths (1 to 1½ seconds each breath).
C. Remove mouth and take in fresh air between each breath. The rescuer must take care not to become hyperventilated by taking too many deep breaths.
D. When resuscitating an infant or child, the breath

*For purposes of basic life support, an infant is under 1 year of age and a child is a person between 1 and 8 years.

is delivered with only enough volume to make the chest rise and fall.

IV. Repeat the Ventilations

A. For an adult, repeat every 5 seconds (12 per minute).
B. For a child, repeat every 4 seconds (15 per minute).
C. For an infant, repeat every 3 seconds (20 per minute).
D. Rescue breathing is considered effective when the patient's chest rises with each ventilation.

CARDIAC COMPRESSION
(Circulation)

The principle is that rhythmic pressure applied over the lower half of the sternum compresses the heart to produce artificial circulation. The procedure is also called *external cardiac compression.*

Chest compressions are always accompanied by rescue breathing.

I. Position

The patient is in a supine position. When working in a dental chair, lower the chair to its lowest position and place a cardiac arrest board or other firm flat object under the patient's back to provide a solid surface for compression.

II. Adult

A. Locate Point for Compression
    1. Run the middle finger of hand I along the lower edge of the rib cage to the notch in the midline.
    2. With the middle finger in the notch and the index finger beside it, place the heel of hand II next to the index finger on the midline of the sternum.
    3. Place the heel of hand I on top of hand II with the fingers in the same direction. Link and close the fingers.
    4. Turn the fingers up so that only the heel of hand II is on the patient (figure 60–7).

B. Compression
    1. Lean forward over the positioned hands, arms straight, until shoulders are directly over the sternum.
    2. Use a firm, steady, vertical pressure (not a blow). The sternum moves down 1½ to 2 inches (figure 60–7).
    3. Release pressure but maintain contact and position of the hands.
    4. Repeat at a rate of 80 to 100 times per minute.
    5. Make the compressions smooth and uninterrupted; with compression and relaxation of equal duration.
    6. Use the natural weight of the upper body to

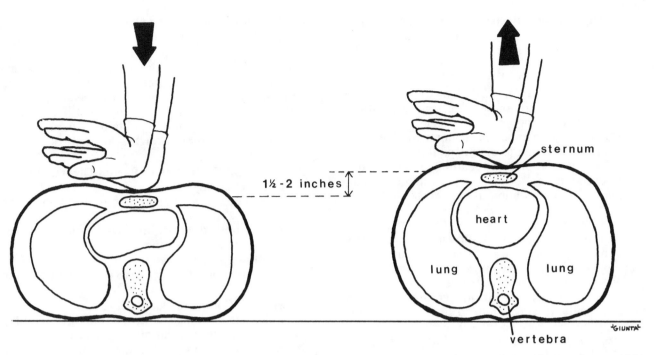

Figure 60–7. External Cardiac Compression. Right, Hands in position on the sternum with fingers turned up. **Left,** Application of firm vertical pressure compresses the heart. The sternum should be compressed 1½ to 2 inches and then released. Hands are held in position for the next compression. For an adult, compressions are repeated at a rate of 80 to 100 per minute.

prevent pushing from the shoulders or depending on arm strength.

7. As the heart is compressed between the sternum and the spine, blood is forced out of the heart into the circulation.
8. Release of pressure allows blood to flow into the heart.
9. An interruption in compression results in a return of blood flow to zero.

III. Child

A. Locate Point for Compression

1. Follow the lower edge of the rib cage to the notch where sternum and ribs meet.
2. Place the middle finger in the notch with the index finger beside it.
3. Place the heel of the other hand next to the index finger.

B. Compression

1. Use one hand only; compress to a depth of 1 to 1½ inches.
2. Release to allow chest to return to normal level.
3. Repeat at a rate of 80 to 100 per minute, using a smooth, even rhythm.
4. Keep fingers up, off the chest.

IV. Infant

A. Locate Point for Compression

1. Place fingers along the sternum with the index finger just below an imaginary line between the nipples.
2. Use the area under the middle and ring fingers.

B. Compression

1. Compress with 2 or 3 fingers to a depth of ½ to 1 inch; release to allow chest to return to normal after each compression.
2. Repeat at a rate of at least 100 per minute, using a smooth rhythm.

V. Coordinated Activity for CPR

A. Lone Rescuer

1. Provide ventilation and compressions.
2. *Adult Patient*
   a. Use ratio 15 to 2: 15 compressions followed by 2 lung inflations.
   b. Compress at the rate of 80 to 100 per minute (count "one and, two and, three and . . .").
   c. Check carotid pulse after 4 cycles of compressions and ventilations; continue if no pulse; check regularly.
3. *Child and Infant*
   a. Use a 5 to 1 ratio, with 5 compressions with a slight pause for 1 ventilation.
   b. Compress at the rate of 80 to 100 per minute for a child; minimum of 100 for an infant.
   c. Reassess after 10 cycles, and every few minutes.

B. Two Rescuers

1. First person begins airway, breathing, and circulation treatment as has been described.
2. Second person calls for medical assistance and ambulance, then promptly takes over either ventilation or circulation.
3. Use coordinated rhythm of 1 to 5: 1 lung inflation after 5 compressions.

4. The rescuer at the patient's head maintains the open airway, monitors the carotid pulse, and provides rescue breathing.

VI. Length of Treatment

A. Signs of recovery: normal skin color returns, patient may gasp or show other sign of breathing, and the body may move or wiggle.
B. Do not stop heart compressions while patient is being transported to the hospital.
C. When circulation and breathing appear to have returned, do not leave patient; watch for need to continue resuscitation in case of relapse.

VII. Sequelae

Cardiopulmonary resuscitation must be continued until medical assistance arrives or the patient begins to recover. When the patient is transported to a hospital, resuscitation must continue.

For emergencies that do not require hospitalization, the patient can be moved to a couch for rest, but must be watched carefully. The cause of the emergency must be determined and additional treatment provided when indicated.

The *Record of Emergency* with monitored vital signs should accompany the patient to the medical care facility for reference by the persons assuming responsibility. The carbon copy for the patient's dental files is marked clearly with recommendations for prevention of future emergencies.

AIRWAY OBSTRUCTION[7]

A procedure of subdiaphragmatic abdominal thrusts, the Heimlich maneuver, is recommended for removal of a foreign body obstructing an airway in adults and children.

I. Prevention

With thought and planning, care can be exercised to prevent aspiration of objects by a patient during a dental or dental hygiene appointment. A few of the procedures that contribute to this are as follows:
A. Place the patient in supine position during examination and treatment. The throat is closed (figure 60–5).
B. Use a rubber dam for all appropriate procedures.
C. Use a length of floss to tie to small objects such as a rubber dam clamp or a bite block. Floss hangs out from angle of lips.
D. Use low-speed handpiece to prevent splashing or spinning masses of agents into the throat.
E. Have assistant use aspirator for various procedures that involve large pieces of calculus, copious blood clots, excess saliva, excess water for ultrasonic scaling, restorative materials, and other potentially inhalable items.
F. Pay attention to mobile permanent or exfoliating primary teeth that could be inadvertently displaced.

II. Recognition of Airway Obstruction

Immediate recognition is essential. Differentiation from other emergencies such as fainting, heart attack, or stroke, in which a sudden respiratory failure may also occur, may be necessary when no object or material was involved that could have been inhaled.

When no doubt exists that an object has been inhaled, medical aid must be obtained. A radiograph may be needed to confirm the location of a radiopaque object.

A. Signs and Symptoms of Partial Obstruction
1. Air exchange
   a. Poor air exchange with gasping and noisy respirations.
   b. Good air exchange with wheezing and forceful coughing.
2. Patient's face is red or cyanotic.
3. Treat poor air exchange as a complete obstruction.

B. Signs of Complete Obstruction
1. No air exchange with attempts at breathing; no sounds from larynx or pharynx.
2. Patient demonstrates the *universal distress signal* (clutches neck with hand).
3. Cyanosis and unconsciousness follow unless emergency care is provided quickly.

III. Outline of Treatment

An airway must be established within 4 to 6 minutes to prevent possible brain damage from oxygen deficiency. With total obstruction, the patient may become unconscious within a few seconds.

Treatment begins with the A-B-C of Basic Life Support, unless inhalation of a specific item was observed. When the inspiration is known, the rescuer may proceed directly to attempt to dislodge the obstruction.

A. Conscious Adult Patient
1. Good air exchange: let patient cough.
2. Poor air exchange or complete obstruction: apply Heimlich maneuver.
3. Patient may become unconscious: proceed for unconscious patient.

B. Unconscious Adult Patient
1. Initiate A-B-C of Basic Life Support (page 740).
2. When breathing attempt is not successful: readjust airway and attempt again.
3. Proceed with airway obstruction management
   a. Heimlich maneuver: 6 to 10 abdominal thrusts.
   b. Examine mouth for object: apply finger sweep.
   c. Repeat steps a and b until object is expelled.

C. Obtain Medical Assistance as Necessary.

IV. Heimlich Maneuver: Abdominal Thrust

Manual thrusts are made to the upper abdomen, or in selected cases, the chest. The abdominal thrust should not be used for a woman during pregnancy.

The thrusts are given to provide pressure against the diaphragm that compresses the lungs. In turn, the pressure in the lungs is increased, which forces air through the trachea and may force out the obstructing object.

A. Patient Standing or Sitting

1. From behind, wrap the arms around the waist of the patient. Make a fist.
2. Hold thumb side of the fist on the patient's upper abdomen above the navel and below the xiphoid. Grab the fist with the other hand.
3. Press the fist into the abdomen with quick upward thrusts.

B. Patient in Supine Position

1. Open the airway.
2. Stand beside and facing the head of the chair when the patient is in the dental chair. On the floor, a more direct thrust can be applied from astride the patient.
3. Hold the heel of one hand over the upper abdomen, with the other hand on top.
4. Apply quick upward thrusts until object is expelled.

V. Chest Thrust

The chest thrust is not used routinely, but is recommended only when it is not possible to use the abdominal thrust, such as during pregnancy and for very obese individuals.

A. Patient Standing or Sitting with Clinician Behind

1. From behind, wrap arms around the chest of the patient at level of armpits.
2. Make a fist. Position the thumb side of the fist on the sternum. The thrust should definitely not be made on the ribs or on the xiphoid because fracture is possible.
3. Grasp the fist with the other hand and apply quick backward thrusts.

B. Patient in Supine Position

1. Open the airway.
2. Position hands on the lower sternum in the same position as for external cardiac compression (page 742 and figure 60–7).
3. Apply quick downward thrusts.

VI. Finger Sweep

After each series of abdominal thrusts, an attempt should be made to remove the offending object by examination of the mouth and throat and by using the fingers, gauze, or suction appropriately. Care must be taken not to force the object deeper.

Finger sweeps are not used for children and infants unless the object is visible.

A. Open the Mouth

Lift the tongue and mandible with the thumb and index finger.

B. Index Finger Sweep

1. Slide the index finger along the buccal mucosa and deep into the throat to the base of the tongue.
2. Anticipate contact with an object, move slowly, with care not to push the object farther into the throat.
3. Hook the end of the finger under and around to remove the object.

C. Repeat

Repeat abdominal thrusts, mouth examination, and finger sweep until object is expelled.

VII. Infant

A. Conscious

1. Good air exchange: encourage coughing.
2. Poor air exchange or complete obstruction: proceed with airway obstruction management.
3. Hold infant face down over the forearm, with the head supported in the hand. Head is lower than the body.
4. Apply four back blows with the heel of the hand, between the infant's shoulder blades.
5. Turn the infant over by placing the free arm over the back and supporting the infant's head with the hand. Place the infant across the thigh with the infant's head lower than its body.
6. Apply four chest thrusts. The point of pressure is the same as for external cardiac compression in the infant (page 743).
7. Repeat back blows and chest thrusts as needed.

B. Unconscious

1. Initiate A-B-C of Basic Life Support (page 740).
2. When breathing attempt is not successful: reposition airway and attempt again.
3. Proceed with airway obstruction management: same as for conscious infant, with four back blows and four chest thrusts.
4. Examine mouth for object: if visible, use a finger sweep to remove it.
5. Repeat steps 3 and 4 until object is expelled.

C. Obtain Medical Assistance as needed.

OXYGEN ADMINISTRATION

Oxygen is an important agent, useful in most emergencies when respiratory difficulty is apparent. Oxygen is not indicated for chronic obstructive lung diseases, especially emphysema. Oxygen is also not indicated in the presence of hyperventilation because the patient is receiving increased amounts of air and is in need of carbon dioxide.

The use of oxygen depends on the breathing status of the individual. When breathing is weak, shallow, or labored, *supplemental oxygen* is used. When the patient is not breathing, *positive pressure oxygen* delivery is needed.

I. Equipment

A. Parts

Oxygen resuscitation equipment consists of an oxygen tank, a reducing valve, a flow meter, tubing, mask, and a positive pressure bag. The E cylinder, which can provide oxygen for 30 minutes, is the minimum size recommended. Smaller tanks provide too little oxygen for a real emergency, and larger tanks are less portable.

B. Directions

Clear, readable directions should be permanently attached to the tank. Practice is a definite part of team drills.

II. Patient Breathing: Use Supplemental Oxygen

A. Apply a full-face clear mask: must fit with a good seal.

B. Supplemental oxygen is started at 4 to 6 liters per minute.

C. Monitor breathing: if breathing stops, proceed with positive pressure oxygen.

III. Patient Not Breathing: Use Positive Pressure

For persons not trained in the use of the bag-valve-mask delivery, a mouth-to-mask procedure should be used.

A. Apply full-face clear mask: must fit with a tight seal.

B. Adjust oxygen flow so that positive pressure bag remains filled.

C. Compress the bag manually at 5-second intervals to provide 12 respirations per minute for an adult. For a child, use 4-second intervals.

D. Watch chest rise and fall. When the chest does not rise and fall, recheck airway for obstruction: proceed with airway obstruction management.

E. Obtain medical assistance.

SPECIFIC EMERGENCIES

Certain systemic disease conditions and physical injuries require specific treatment during an emergency. In table 60–1, the *Emergency Reference Chart*, several conditions are listed with their symptoms and treatment procedures. Some of the same conditions have been described in detail in Section VI of this book.

TECHNICAL HINTS

I. Precautions During Mouth-to-Mouth Ventilation

Infection may be transmitted or acquired.[11] Dental personnel may gain proficiency in the use of face mask with one-way delivery to prevent unnecessary contact with ill, debilitated patients or those known or suspected to be carriers of a disease.[12]

II. Care of Drugs

A. Label each with information about shelf-life and due-date for replacement. Nitroglycerin, for example, must be changed at 6 months.

B. Check weekly to maintain emergency kit in workable order.

C. Test oxygen equipment daily to guard against leaks in tubing and to ensure a supply of oxygen.

D. Dispose of an out-of-date narcotic drug in the presence of a witness to prevent question that the drug may have been stolen.

III. Eye Safety

In addition to eye protection during working hours, professional people should wear protective glasses for activities outside the practice area, such as for sports, hobbies, and other potentially harmful activities.

IV. Medic Alert Identification

Identification for patients with medical problem: a metal emblem worn as a bracelet or a pendant is available to provide specific information pertinent to an emergency that may arise. Information about the emblems is available by writing the Medic Alert Foundation International, Turlock, California, 95380. In addition to noting patients who are wearing the identification and recording the fact along with other information in the patient history, other patients can be given information about the service.

V. Sources of Material and Information:

American Heart Association
7320 Greenville Avenue
Dallas, Texas 75231

American National Red Cross
17th and D Streets N.W.
Washington, D.C. 20006

Table 60–1. Emergency Reference Chart

Emergency	Signs/Symptoms	Procedure

All Cases		1. Determine consciousness (shake and shout)
		2. Place in supine position
		3. Identify major problem
		    A. Airway
		    B. Breathing
		    C. Circulation
		4. Act in accord with findings
		5. Summon assistance

Respiratory Failure	Labored or weak respirations or cessation of breathing Cyanosis or ashen-white with blood loss Pupils dilated Loss of consciousness	Position: supine (not breathing) upright (breathing) Check for and remove foreign material from mouth Establish airway Mouth-to-mouth breathing Monitor vital signs: blood pressure, pulse, respirations Administer oxygen
Airway Obstruction	Good air exchange, coughing, wheezing	Sit patient up Loosen tight collar, belt No treatment: let patient cough
Partial	Poor air exchange, noisy breathing, weak, ineffective cough, difficult respirations, gasping Patient is panicky	Reassure patient Treat for complete obstruction (page 744)

Complete	Gasping with great effort; no noises
	Patient clutches throat
	Unable to speak, breathe, cough
	Cyanosis
	Dilated pupils
		Conscious patient
		    Perform Heimlich maneuver
		    Patient becomes unconscious: proceed for unconscious

		Unconscious patient
		    Initiate A-B-C of Basic Life Support
		    Unsuccessful breathing attempts: proceed with airway obstruction management
		    Perform Heimlich maneuver: 6 to 10 thrusts
		    Examine mouth: apply finger sweep
		    Repeat manual thrusts and finger sweep until object is expelled
		    Try rescue breathing again
		Obtain medical assistance

Table 60–1. Emergency Reference Chart *Continued*

Emergency	Signs/Symptoms	Procedure
Hyperventilation Syndrome	Lightheadedness, giddiness Anxiety, confusion Dizziness Overbreathing (25 to 30 respirations per minute) Feelings of suffocation Deep respirations Palpitations (heart pounds) Tingling or numbness in the extremities	Terminate oral procedure Remove rubber dam and objects from mouth Position upright or best for comfortable breathing Loosen tight collar Reassure patient Ask patient to breathe deeply (7 to 10 per minute) into a paper bag adapted closely over nose and mouth. Carbon dioxide is indicated, NOT oxygen

Hemorrhage	Prolonged bleeding
	  a. Spurting blood: artery
	  b. Oozing blood: vein
		Compression over bleeding area
		  a. Apply gauze pack with pressure
		  b. Bandage pack into place firmly where possible
		Severe bleeding: digital pressure on pressure point of supplying vessel
		Watch for shock symptoms

	Bleeding from tooth socket	Pack with folded gauze; do not dab Have patient bite down firmly Do not rinse
	Bleeding of an extremity	Elevate the part: support with pillows or substitute Apply tourniquet only when limb is amputated, mangled, or crushed
	Nosebleed	Tell patient to breathe through mouth Apply cold application to nose Press nostril on bleeding side for a few minutes Advise patient not to blow the nose for an hour or more
Syncope (fainting)	Pale, gray face, anxiety Dilated pupils Weakness, giddiness, dizziness, faintness, nausea Profuse cold perspiration Rapid pulse at first, followed by slow pulse Shallow breathing Drop in blood pressure Loss of consciousness	Position: Trendelenburg Loosen tight collar, belt Place cold, damp towel on forehead Crush ammonia vaporole under patient's nose Keep warm (blanket) Monitor vital signs: blood pressure, pulse, respirations Keep airway open May require oxygen Keep in supine position 10 minutes after recovery to prevent nausea and dizziness Reassure patient, especially during recovery

Table 60-1. Emergency Reference Chart *Continued*

Emergency	Signs/Symptoms	Procedure
Shock	Skin: pale, moist, clammy Rapid, shallow breathing Low blood pressure Weakness and/or restlessness Nausea, vomiting Thirst, if shock is from bleeding Eventual unconsciousness if untreated	Position: Trendelenburg Keep quiet and warm Monitor vital signs: blood pressure, respirations, pulse Keep airway open Administer oxygen Summon medical assistance

Stroke
(cerebrovascular accident)
	Premonitory
	  Dizziness, vertigo
	  Transient paresthesia or weakness on one side
	  Transient speech defects
	Serious
	  Headache (with cerebral hemorrhage)
	  Breathing labored, deep, slow
	  Chills
	  Paralysis one side of body
	  Nausea, vomiting
	  Convulsions
	  Loss of consciousness
	    (slow or sudden onset)
		Conscious patient
		  Turn patient toward affected side; semiupright
		  Loosen clothing about the throat
		  Reassure patient; keep calm, quiet
		  Monitor vital signs: blood pressure, pulse, respirations
		  Administer oxygen when patient has respiratory difficulty
		  Do not give stimulant, sedative, or narcotic
		  Clear airway; suction vomitus because the throat muscles may be paralyzed
		  Seek medical assistance promptly
		
		Unconscious patient
		  Position: supine
		  Basic life support
		  Cardiopulmonary resuscitation if indicated

Cardiovascular Diseases	Symptoms vary depending on cause	*For all patients*
		  Be calm and reassure patient
		  Keep patient warm and quiet; restrict effort
		  Call for medical assistance

Angina Pectoris (page 690)	Sudden crushing, paroxysmal pain in substernal area Pain may radiate to shoulder, neck, arms Pallor, faintness Shallow breathing Anxiety, fear	Position: upright, as patient requests, for comfortable breathing Place nitroglycerin sublingually Administer oxygen if needed Reassure patient Without prompt relief after a second nitroglycerin, treat as a myocardial infarction
Myocardial Infarction (heart attack) (page 690)	Sudden pain similar to angina pectoris, which also may radiate, but of longer duration Pallor; cold, clammy skin Cyanosis Nausea Breathing difficulty Marked weakness Anxiety, fear Possible loss of consciousness	Position: with head up for comfortable breathing Symptoms are not relieved with nitroglycerin Monitor vital signs: blood pressure, pulse, respirations Administer oxygen if needed Alleviate anxiety; reassure Call for medical assistance for transfer to hospital

(continued next page)

Table 60–1. Emergency Reference Chart *Continued*

Emergency	Signs/Symptoms	Procedure
Cardiovascular Diseases continued **Heart Failure** (page 691)	Difficult or labored breathing Pulmonary congestion with cough May cough up blood Rapid, weak pulse Dilated pupils May have chest pain	Urgent medical assistance needed Place patient in upright position Make patient comfortable: cover with blanket Administer oxygen Reassure patient
Cardiac Arrest	Skin: ashen gray, cold, clammy No pulse No heart sounds No respirations Eyes fixed, with dilated pupils; no constriction with light Unconscious	Position: supine Basic life support Check oral cavity for debris or vomitus; leave dentures in place for a seal Begin cardiopulmonary resuscitation: minutes count (pages 742–744)
Adrenal Crisis (cortisol deficiency)	Anxious, stressed Mental confusion Pain in abdomen, back, legs Muscle weakness Extreme fatigue Nausea, vomiting Lowered blood pressure Elevated pulse	*Conscious patient* Terminate oral procedure Call for help and emergency kit Place patient in supine position with legs slightly raised Request telephone call for medical assistance Administer oxygen Monitor blood pressure and pulse Administration of glucocorticosteroid as determined by dentist
	Loss of consciousness Coma	*Unconscious patient* Place patient in supine position with legs slightly raised Basic life support Try ammonia vaporole when cause is undecided Administer oxygen Summon medical assistance Administration of glucocorticosteroid as determined by dentist Transport to hospital
Insulin Reaction (hyperinsulinism) (hypoglycemia)	Sudden onset Skin: moist, cold, pale Confused, nervous, anxious Bounding pulse Salivation Normal to shallow respirations Convulsions (late)	*Conscious patient* Administer oral sugar (cubes, orange juice, candy) Observe patient for 1 hour before dismissal Determine time since previous meal, and arrange next appointment following food intake
		Unconscious patient Basic life support Position: supine Maintain airway Administer oxygen Monitor vital signs Summon medical assistance Administer intravenous glucose

Table 60–1. Emergency Reference Chart *Continued*

Emergency	Signs/Symptoms	Procedure

Diabetic Coma (ketoacidosis) (hyperglycemia)	Slow onset
	Skin: flushed and dry
	Breath: fruity odor
	Dry mouth, thirst
	Low blood pressure
	Weak, rapid pulse
	Exaggerated respirations
	Coma
		Conscious patient
		  Terminate oral procedure
		  Obtain medical care; hospitalization
		    indicated
		  Keep patient warm
		
		Unconscious patient
		  Basic life support
		  Urgent medical assistance needed

Allergic Reaction
1. Delayed[s]
	Skin
	  Erythema (rash)
	  Urticaria (wheals, itching)
	  Angioedema (localized swelling of
	    mucous membranes, lips, larynx,
	    pharynx)
	
	Respiration
	  Distress, dyspnea
	  Wheezing
	  Extension of angioedema to larynx:
	    may have obstruction from swelling
	    of vocal apparatus
		Skin
		  Administer antihistamine
		
		Respiration
		  Position: upright
		  Administer oxygen
		  Epinephrine
		
		Airway obstruction
		  Position: supine
		  Airway maintenance
		  Epinephrine
		Summon medical assistance

2. Immediate
 	
  Anaphylaxis (anaphylactic shock)
	Skin
	  Urticaria (wheals, itching)
	  Flushing
	Nausea, abdominal cramps, vomiting,
	  diarrhea
	Angioedema
	  Swelling of lips, membranes, eyelids
	  Laryngeal edema with difficult
	    swallowing
	Respiration distress
	  Cough, wheezing
	  Dyspnea
	  Airway obstruction
	  Cyanosis
	Cardiovascular collapse
	  Profound drop in blood pressure
	  Rapid, weak pulse
	  Palpitations
	Dilation of pupils
	
	Loss of consciousness (sudden)
	  Cardiac arrest
		Rapid treatment needed
		Position: supine (except when dyspnea
		  predominates)
		Administer oxygen
		Basic life support
		Monitor vital signs
		Epinephrine
		Cardiopulmonary resuscitation
		
		Summon medical assistance; transfer to
		  hospital

**Local Anesthesia
Reactions**
1. Psychogenic
	Reaction to injection, not the anesthetic
	Syncope
	Hyperventilation syndrome
		See earlier in this table
		  Page 748 (syncope)
		  Page 748 (hyperventilation)

2. Allergic (very rare)	Anaphylactic shock Allergic skin and mucous membrane reactions Allergic bronchial asthma attack	See earlier in this table

(continued next page)

Table 60–1. Emergency Reference Chart *Continued*

Emergency	Signs/Symptoms	Procedure
Local Anesthesia Reactions continued 3. Toxic Overdose	Effects of intravascular injection rather than increased quantity of drug are more common	

	a. Stimulation phase
	   Anxious, restless, apprehensive, confused
	   Rapid pulse and respirations
	   Elevated blood pressure
	   Tremors
	   Convulsions
		Mild reaction
		   Stop injection
		   Position: supine
		   Loosen tight clothing
		   Reassure patient
		   Monitor blood pressure, heart rate, respirations
		   Administer oxygen
		   Summon medical assistance

	b. Depressive phase
	   Follows stimulation phase
	   Drowsiness, lethargy
	   Shock-like symptoms: pallor, sweating
	   Rapid, weak pulse and respirations
	   Drop in blood pressure
	   Respiratory depression or respiratory arrest
	   Unconsciousness
		Severe reaction
		   Basic life support: maintain airway
		   Continue to monitor vital signs
		   Cardiopulmonary resuscitation
		   Administration of anticonvulsant

Epileptic Seizure 1. Generalized tonic-clonic (page 642)	Anxiety or depression Pale, may become cyanotic Muscular contractions Loss of consciousness	Position: supine. Do not attempt to move from dental chair Make safe by placing movable equipment out of reach Do not force anything between the teeth; a soft towel or large sponges may be placed while mouth is open Open airway; monitor vital signs Allow patient to sleep during postconvulsive stage Do not dismiss the patient if unaccompanied
2. Generalized absence (pages 641–642)	Brief loss of consciousness Fixed posture Rhythmic twitching of eyelids, eyebrows, or head May be pale	Take objects from patient's hands to prevent their being dropped

Burns[9]
 	
1. First degree
 	
2. Second degree (partial thickness)
	
	Skin reddened
	Swelling
	Pain
	
	Skin reddened, blisters
	Swelling
	Wet surface
	Pain (more than third degree)
	Heightened sensitivity to touch
		First- and Second-Degree Burns
		   Do not give food or liquids. Anticipate nausea
		   Be alert for signs of shock
		   Do not apply ointment, grease, or bicarbonate of soda
		   Immerse in cool water to relieve pain. Do not apply ice
		   Gently clean with a mild antiseptic
		   Dress lightly with bandage
		   Elevate burned part
		   Obtain medical assistance

(continued next page)

Table 60–1. Emergency Reference Chart *Continued*

Emergency	*Signs/Symptoms*	*Procedure*

Burns continued
3. Third degree
    (full thickness)
	Leathery look
	Insensitive to touch
		Request medical assistance and
		    transport system
		Treat for shock
		Basic life support: maintain airway
		Check for other injuries
		Wrap in clean sheet; transport

4. Chemical burn	Reddened, discolored	Immediate, copious irrigation with
		    water for one-half hour
		Check directions on container from
		    which the chemical came, for antidote
		    or other advice
		Burn caused by an acid may be rinsed
		    with bicarbonate of soda; burn caused
		    by alkali may be rinsed in weak acid
		    such as acetic (vinegar)
		Medical assistance advised or obtained

Internal Poisoning[10]	Signs of corrosive burn around or in
	    oral cavity
	Evidence of empty container or
	    information from patient
	Nausea, vomiting, cramps
		Be calm and supportive
		Basic life support: airway maintenance
		Artificial ventilation (inhaled poison)
		Record vital signs
		Conscious patient
		    Dilute poison in the stomach with 1
		        or 2 glasses of water or milk.
		    Induce vomiting by giving 1
		        tablespoon of syrup of ipecac
		        followed by 1 to 2 glasses of water.
		    Do not induce vomiting if caustic,
		        corrosive, or petroleum products
		        have been ingested
		Avoid nonspecific and questionably
		    effective antidotes, stimulants,
		    sedatives, or other agents, which may
		    do more harm
		Obtain medical assistance

Foreign Body in Eye	Tears
	Blinking
		Wash hands
		Ask patient to look down
		Bring upper lid down over lower lid for
		    a moment; move it upward
		Turn down lower lid and examine: if
		    particle is visible, remove with
		    moistened cotton applicator
		Use eye cup: wash out eye with plain
		    water
		When unsuccessful, seek medical
		    attention: prevent patient from
		    rubbing eye by placing gauze pack
		    over eye and stabilizing with adhesive
		    tape

**Chemical Solution in
Eye**
	Tears
	Stinging
		Irrigate promptly with copious amounts
		    of water. Turn head so water flows
		    away from inner aspect of the eye.
		    Continue for 15 to 20 minutes

Table 60–1.   Emergency Reference Chart *Continued*

Emergency	Signs/Symptoms	Procedure
Dislocated Jaw	Mouth is open: patient is unable to close	Stand in front of seated patient Wrap thumbs in towels and place on occlusal surfaces of mandibular posterior teeth Curve fingers and place under body of the mandible Press down and back with thumbs, and at same time pull up and forward with fingers (figure 60–8) As joint slips into place, quickly move thumbs outward Place bandage around head to support jaw
Facial Fracture	Pain, swelling Ecchymoses Deformity, limitation of movement Crepitation on manipulation Zygoma fracture: depression of cheek Mandibular fracture: abnormal occlusion	Place patient on side Basic life support Support with bandage around face, under chin, and tied on the top of the head (Barton) Seek prompt transport to emergency care facility
Tooth Forcibly Displaced (avulsed tooth)	Swelling, bruises, or other signs of trauma, depending on the type of accident	Instruct patient or parent to rinse tooth gently in cool water and place in water or wrap in wet cloth Bring to the dental office or clinic *immediately* The longer the time lapse between avulsion and replantation, the poorer the prognosis

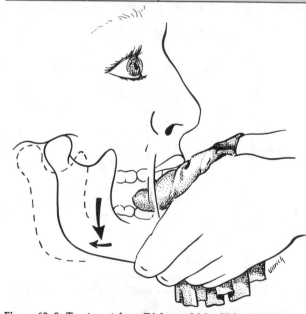

Figure 60–8. Treatment for a Dislocated Mandible. With thumbs wrapped in toweling and placed on the buccal cusps of the mandibular teeth, the fingers are curved under the body of the mandible. The jaw is pressed down and back with the thumbs while pulling up and forward with the fingers to permit the condyle to pass over the articular eminence into its normal position in the glenoid fossa. As the jaw slips into place, the thumbs must be moved quickly aside.

References

1. Malamed, S.F.: *Handbook of Medical Emergencies in the Dental Office*, 3rd ed. St. Louis, The C.V. Mosby Co., 1987, pp. 40–44.
2. Cooley, R.L., Cottingham, A.J., Abrams, H., and Barkmeier, W.W.: Ocular Injuries Sustained in the Dental Office: Methods of Detection, Treatment, and Prevention, *J. Am. Dent. Assoc.*, *97*, 985, December, 1978.
3. Hartley, J.L.: Eye and Facial Injuries Resulting from Dental Procedures, *Dent. Clin. North. Am.*, *22*, 505, July, 1978.
4. Malamed: op. cit., pp. 49–72.
5. American Dental Association, Council on Dental Therapeutics: *Accepted Dental Therapeutics*, 40th ed. Chicago, American Dental Association, 1984, pp. xxv-xxvii.
6. Robbins, K.S.: Medical-legal Considerations, in Malamed, S.F.: *Handbook of Medical Emergencies in the Dental Office*, 3rd ed. St. Louis, The C.V. Mosby Co., 1987, pp. 73–83.
7. American Heart Association: Standards and Guidelines for Cardiopulmonary Resuscitation and Emergency Cardiac Care, *JAMA*, *255*, 2841, June 6, 1986.
8. Malamed: op. cit., pp. 301–322.
9. Heimbach, D.M.: Burns, in Rakel, R.E., ed.: *Conn's Current Therapy*, 1988. Philadelphia, W.B. Saunders Co., 1988, pp. 989–994.
10. Mofenson, H.C., Caraccio, T.R., and Greensher, J.: Acute Poisonings, in Rakel, R.E., ed.: *Conn's Current Therapy*, 1988. Philadelphia, W.B. Saunders Co., 1988, pp. 1005–1040.
11. Hendricks, A.A. and Shapiro, E.P.: Primary Herpes Simplex

Infection Following Mouth-to-mouth Resuscitation, *JAMA*, *243*, 257, January 18, 1980.

12. United States Centers for Disease Control: Recommendations for Prevention of HIV Transmission in Health-care Settings, *MMWR*, *36*, 6s, Supplement, August 21, 1987.

Suggested Readings

American Dental Association, Council on Dental Therapeutics: Office Emergencies and Emergency Kits, *J. Am. Dent. Assoc.*, *101*, 305, August, 1980.

American Dental Association, Council on Dental Therapeutics: *Accepted Dental Therapeutics*, 40th ed. Chicago, American Dental Association, 1984, pp. 89–110.

Braun, R.J.: The Dental Assistant's Role in Medical Emergencies, *Dent. Assist.*, *54*, 19, September/October, 1985.

Cavaillon, J.P.: Neurological and Cardio-pulmonary Problems: Methods of Resuscitation, *Int. Dent. J.*, *36*, 87, June, 1986.

Chapman, P.J.: The Hyperventilation (Overbreathing) Syndrome, *Aust. Dent. J.*, *29*, 321, October, 1984.

Chernega, J.B.: *Emergency Guide for Dental Auxiliaries.* Albany, New York, Delmar Publishers, 1987, pp. 11–48.

Croll, T.P., Brooks, E.B., Schut, L., and Laurent, J.P.: Rapid Neurologic Assessment and Initial Management for the Patient with Traumatic Dental Injuries, *J. Am. Dent. Assoc.*, *100*, 530, April, 1980.

Fast, T.B., Martin, M.D., and Ellis, T.M.: Emergency Preparedness: A Survey of Dental Practitioners, *J. Am. Dent. Assoc.*, *112*, 499, April, 1986.

Fischman, S.L.: Prevention, Management and Documentation of Swallowed Dental Objects, *J. Am. Dent. Assoc.*, *111*, 464, September, 1985.

Goldman, H.S.: Hazards in the Dental Workplace, *Clin. Prevent. Dent.*, *2*, 18, September-October, 1980.

Gray, N.A.: Management of Intraoral Hemorrhage, *Gen. Dent.*, *35*, 116, March-April, 1987.

Hardwick, F.K.: Eye Protection in the Dental Surgery, *J. Dent. Assoc. S. Afr.*, *37*, 29, January, 1982.

Josell, S.D., Owen, D., Kreutzer, L.W., and Goldberg, N.H.: Extraoral Management for Electrical Burns of the Mouth, *ASDC J. Dent. Child.*, *51*, 47, January-February, 1984.

Karras, D.C.: Don't Panic! Here Are Six Ways To Prevent Office Emergencies, *RDH*, *7*, 22, June, 1987.

Ledford, J.R.: A Closer Look at Vision Problems, *RDH*, *8*, 27, January/February, 1988.

Lewis, J.E.S.: A Simple Technique for Reduction of Long-standing Dislocation of the Mandible, *Br. J. Oral Surg.*, *18*, 52, March, 1981.

Lockhart, P.B., Feldbau, E.V., Gabel, R.A., Connolly, S.F., and Silversin, J.B.: Dental Complications During and After Tracheal Intubation, *J. Am. Dent. Assoc.*, *112*, 480, April, 1986.

Milam, S.B., Giovannitti, J.A., and Israelson, H.: Faint in the Supine Position. Selective Review of the Literature and A Case Report, *J. Periodontol.*, *57*, 44, January, 1986.

Morrow, G.T.: Designing a Drug Kit, *Dent. Clin. North Am.*, *26*, 21, January, 1982.

O'Riordan, M.W., Ralstrom, C.S., and Doerr, S.E.: Treatment of Avulsed Permanent Teeth: An Update, *J. Am. Dent. Assoc.*, *105*, 1028, December, 1982.

Schneider, P.E.: Foreign Body Aspiration and Ingestion During Dental Treatment, *Compend. Contin. Educ. Dent.*, *3*, 173, May/June, 1982.

Vincent, J.W.: Reduction of Luxation of the Temporomandibular Joint—An Extraoral Approach, *J. Prosthet. Dent.*, *44*, 445, October, 1980.

Yurino, M.: New Method for Reduction of Acute Anterior Dislocation of the Mandible, *J. Oral Maxillofac. Surg.*, *41*, 751, November, 1983.

Cardiopulmonary Resuscitation

Brand, M.K.: CPR for Oral Health Professionals: A Dental Team Training Course, *Dent. Hyg.*, *54*, 475, October, 1980.

Donegan, J.H.: New Concepts in Cardiopulmonary Resuscitation, *Anesth. Analg.*, *60*, 100, February, 1981.

Glaser, J.B. and Nadler, J.P.: Hepatitis B Virus in a Cardiopulmonary Resuscitation Training Course. Risk of Transmission from a Surface Antigen-positive Participant, *Arch. Intern. Med.*, *145*, 1653, September, 1985.

Hanashiro, P.K. and Wilson, J.R.: Cardiopulmonary Resuscitation, A Current Perspective, *Med. Clin. North Am.*, *70*, 729, July, 1986.

Johnson, L.M.: Giving a CPR Form New Life, *Am. J. Nurs.*, *86*, 60, January, 1986.

Lado, E.A. and Fast, T.B.: Evaluation of a Prototype CPR Assist-tool, *Oral Surg. Oral Med. Oral Pathol.*, *62*, 280, September, 1986.

Mannis, M.J. and Wendel, R.T.: Transmission of Herpes Simplex During CPR Training, *Ann. Ophthalmol.*, *16*, 64, January, 1984.

March, N.F. and Matthews, R.C.: New Techniques in External Cardiac Compressions. Aquatic Cardiopulmonary Resuscitation, *JAMA*, *244*, 1229, September 12, 1980.

Markarian, S.: CPR in a Dental Setting: A Step-by-step Sequence, *Gen. Dent.*, *34*, 134, March-April, 1986.

Martin, M.D. and Fast, T.B.: Skills in Cardiopulmonary Resuscitation: A Survey of Dental Practitioners, *J. Am. Dent. Assoc.*, *112*, 501, April, 1986.

Anesthetics

Bennett, C.R.: *Monheim's Local Anesthesia and Pain Control in Dental Practice*, 7th ed. St. Louis, The C.V. Mosby Co., 1984, pp. 211–266.

Burke, R.H.: Management of a Broken Anesthetic Injection Needle in the Maxilla, *J. Am. Dent. Assoc.*, *112*, 209, February, 1986.

Cawson, R.A., Curson, I., and Whittington, D.R.: The Hazards of Dental Local Anaesthetics, *Br. Dent. J.*, *154*, 253, April 23, 1983.

Crumpton, M.W., Thornton, J.B., and Mackall, L.L.: Anaphylactoid Reaction to Vancomycin During General Anesthesia in a Child Patient, *Pediatr. Dent.*, *5*, 276, December, 1983.

Duncan, G.H. and Moore, P.: Nitrous Oxide and the Dental Patient: A Review of Adverse Reactions, *J. Am. Dent. Assoc.*, *108*, 213, February, 1984.

Giovannitti, J.A.: Evaluation of Local Anesthetic Hypersensitivity Reactions, *Clin. Prevent. Dent.*, *3*, 20, January-February, 1981.

Goodson, J.M. and Moore, P.A.: Life-threatening Reactions After Pedodontic Sedation: An Assessment of Narcotic, Local Anesthetic, and Antiemetic Drug Interaction, *J. Am. Dent. Assoc.*, *107*, 239, August, 1983.

Johnson, W.T. and DeStigter, T.: Hypersensitivity to Procaine, Tetracaine, Mepivacaine, and Methylparaben: Report of a Case, *J. Am. Dent. Assoc.*, *106*, 53, January, 1983.

Levy, S.M. and Baker, K.A.: Considerations in Differential Diagnosis of Adverse Reactions to Local Anesthetic: Report of Case, *J. Am. Dent. Assoc.*, *113*, 271, August, 1986.

Milgrom, P. and Fiset, L.: Local Anaesthetic Adverse Effects and Other Emergency Problems in General Dental Practice, *Int. Dent. J.*, *36*, 71, June, 1986.

Rogo, E.J. and Lupovici, E.M.: Nitrous Oxide. An Occupational Hazard for Dental Professionals, *Dent. Hyg.*, *60*, 508, November, 1986.

Miscellaneous Drugs

De Martino, B.K. and Steinberg, B.J.: The Pharmacologic Aspects of Emergency Drugs in Dental Practice, *Compend. Contin. Educ. Dent.*, *4*, 231, May-June, 1983.

Freas, G.C.: General Approach to the Poisoned Patient, *U.S. Navy Med.*, *77*, 5, May-June, 1986.

Gill, C. and Michaelides, P.L.: Dental Drugs and Anaphylactic Reactions, *Oral Surg. Oral Med. Oral Pathol.*, *50*, 30, July, 1980.

Kloberdanz, B., Bennett, C.R., and McDonald, A.E.: Management of Anaphylactic Shock After a Single Oral Dose of Penicillin: Report of Case, *J. Am. Dent. Assoc.*, *112*, 60, January, 1986.

Maseman, D.: Recognizing Adverse Drug Reactions, *RDH*, *4*, 42, May/June, 1984.

Mittleman, R.E. and Wetli, C.V.: Death Caused by Recreational Cocaine Use. An Update, *JAMA*, *252*, 1889, October 12, 1984.

Roberts, J., Bianco, M.M., and Fine, J.: Fatal Anaphylactic Reaction to Oral Penicillin: Report of Case, *J. Am. Dent. Assoc.*, *110*, 505, April, 1985.

Prefixes, Suffixes, and Combining Forms

a-, an- absence, lack, without, e.g. *a*morphous
ab- from, away, e.g. *ab*normal
ad- (change d to c,f,g,p,s, or t before words beginning with those consonants) to, toward, e.g. *ad*hesion, *ac*-cretion
adeno- gland, e.g. *adeno*fibroma
-algia pain, e.g. neur*algia*
ambi- all (both) sides, round, e.g. *ambi*dexterity
amphi-, ampho- on both sides, double, e.g. *ampho*di-plopia
ana- up, excessive, again, e.g. *ana*bolism
andro- masculine, male, e.g. *andro*gen
angio- vessel, e.g. *angio*ma
anti- against, e.g. *anti*dote
aqu- aqua- water, e.g. *aqu*eous
arthro-, arth- joints, e.g. *arthr*itis
-ase denotes an enzyme, e.g. dextrin*ase*
-asthenia weakness, e.g. my*asthenia* gravis
auto-, aut- self, e.g. *auto*transplant

bi- two, twice, double, e.g. *bi*furcation
bio-, bi- life, living, e.g. *bio*psy
-blast formative cell, e.g. osteo*blast*
-brachy- short, e.g., *brachy*dactylic
brady- slow, e.g. *brady*cardia
bucc- cheek, e.g. *bucc*inator

calc- stone, calcium, lime, e.g. *calc*ification
cardio-, cardi- heart, e.g. *cardio*vascular
cata- down, against, e.g. *cata*bolism
-cele swelling, protrusion, hernia, e.g. meningo*cele*
cephalo-, cephal- head, e.g. *cephalo*metry
cerebro-, cerebr- brain, e.g. *cerebr*al palsy
cheilo-, cheil- lip, e.g. *cheil*itis
chloro-, chlor- pale green, e.g. *chloro*phyll
chromo-, chromat- color, pigmentation, e.g. *chromo*-genic
-cidal killing, e.g. bacteri*cidal*
-clast break up, divide into parts, e.g. osteo*clast*
-clus shut, e.g. oc*clus*ion
co-, com-, con-, cor- with, together, e.g. *con*genital
coll- glue, e.g. *coll*oid
contra- opposite, e.g. *contra*lateral
cryo, cry- cold, freezing, e.g. *cryo*therapy
cuti- skin, e.g. *cuti*cle
cyan- blue, e.g. *cyan*otic
-cyto-, -cyt- cell, e.g. leuko*cyte*

-dactyl, dactylo- fingers, e.g. *dactyl*edema
de- down, away from, separation, e.g. *de*calcification
denti-, dent- tooth, e.g. *dent*ition
-derm-, derma- skin, e.g. hypo*derm*ic
dextr-, dextro- right, toward right, e.g. *dextro*cardia
di- twice, two, e.g. *di*plopia
dia- (drop *a* before words beginning with a vowel) through, apart, e.g., *dia*phragm
dis- separation, opposite, taking part, e.g. *dis*infect
disto-, dist- posterior, distant from center, e.g. *disto*buc-cal
-drome course, e.g. syn*drome*
dur- hard, e.g. in*dur*ation
dys- bad, ill, difficult, e.g. *dys*trophy

ecto-, ect- without, outer side, e.g. *ecto*derm
-ectomy surgical removal, e.g. gingiv*ectomy*
-emia (-aemia) blood condition, e.g. bacter*emia*
en- in, on, into, e.g. *en*demic
encephal-, encephalo- brain, e.g. *encephalo*meningitis
endo- inside, e.g. *endo*dontics
entero-, enter- intestine, e.g. *entero*toxin
epi- upon, after, in addition, e.g. *epi*dermis
erythro-, eryth- red, e.g. *eryth*ema
esthesio-, esthesia (-aesthesia) sensation, perception, e.g. an*esthesia*
ex- beyond, from, out of, e.g. *ex*udate
extra- outside of, beyond the scope of, e.g. *extra*cellular

faci- face, e.g. *faci*al
-facient causes or brings about, e.g. rube*facient*
-ferent carry, bear, e.g. af*ferent*
fibro-, fibr- fibers, fibrous tissue, e.g. *fibro*blast
fract- break, e.g. *fract*ional

galacto-, galact- milk, e.g. *galac*tose
gastro-, gastr- stomach, e.g. *gastr*itis
-gen- produced, e.g. glyco*gen*
genio- chin, lower jaw, e.g. *genio*plasty
germ- bud, early growth, e.g., *germ*inal
gero- old age, e.g. *gero*dontics
glosso-, gloss- tongue, e.g. *gloss*itis
gluco-, gluc- glucose, e.g. *gluco*neogenesis
glyco-, glyc- sweet, e.g. *glyc*erin
gnatho-, gnath- jaw, e.g. *gnatho*dynamometer
-gnosis knowledge, e.g. prog*nosis*
-gram, -graph write, draw, e.g. radio*graphic*
gran- grain, particle, e.g. *gran*uloma

gyn-, gyne-, gynec- woman, e.g., *gyne*cology

hemi- half, e.g., *hemi*section
hemo-, (haemo-) blood, e.g., *hemo*rrhage
hepato-, hepat- liver, e.g. *hepat*itis
hetero-, heter- other, different, e.g. *hetero*geneous
histo-, hist- tissue, e.g., *histo*logy
homo-, homeo- like, similar, e.g. *homeo*stasis
hydro-, hydr- water, e.g. *hydro*cephalic
hygro-, hygr- moisture, e.g. *hygro*phobia
hyper- abnormal, excessive, e.g. *hyper*trophy
hypno-, hypn- sleep, e.g. *hypno*tic
hypo- hyp- deficiency, lack, below, e.g. *hypo*tonic
hystero-, hyster- uterus or hysteria, e.g. *hyster*ectomy

-ia state or condition, e.g. glycosur*ia*
-ic of, pertaining to, e.g. gastr*ic*
idio- one's own, separate, distinct, e.g. *idio*pathic
in- not, without, e.g. *in*activate
infra- beneath, below, e.g. *infra*orbital
inter- between, among, e.g. *inter*cellular
intra- within, into, e.g. *intra*oral
ischo-, isch- suppression, stoppage, e.g. *isch*emia
iso- equality, similarity, e.g. *iso*tonic
-ist one who practices, holds certain principles, e.g. hygien*ist*
-itis inflammation, e.g. dermat*itis*

-ject- throw, e.g. in*ject*ion
juxta- next to, near, e.g. *juxta*position

karyo-, kary- nucleus of a cell, e.g. *karyo*lysis
kerato-, kerat- horny, keratinized tissue, e.g. *kerat*inization
kin- move, e.g. *kin*etic

labio- lip, e.g. *labio*version
lacto-, lact- milk, e.g. *lact*ation
laryngo-, laryn- larynx, e.g. *laryn*gitis
later- side, e.g. *later*oversion
leuko-, leuk- white, e.g., *leuko*plakia
linguo, lingu- tongue, e.g. *lingu*al
lipo-, lip- fat, fatty, e.g. *lip*oma
-logy doctrine, science, e.g. periodonto*logy*
lympho-, lymph- lymph, e.g. *lymph*angioma
-lysin, -lysis, -lytic dissolving, destructive, e.g. hemo*lysis*

macro-, macr- enlargement, elongated part, e.g. *macro*dontia
mal- bad, ill, e.g. *mal*nutrition
mast-, mastro- breast, e.g. *mast*ectomy
-megalo-, -megal- large, great, e.g. *megalo*blast
melano- dark-colored, relating to melanin, e.g. *melano*genesis
meningo-, mening- meninges, e.g. *mening*itis
meno- month, e.g. *meno*pause
mes-, medi, mesio- middle, intermediate, e.g. *meso*derm
meta-, met- over, beyond, transformation, e.g. *meta*bolism
metro-, metra- uterus, e.g. *metro*fibroma

-metry measure, e.g. cephalo*metry*
micro-, micr- small, e.g. *micro*organism
mono- one, single, e.g. *mono*saccharide
morpho-, morph- form, shape, e.g. *morpho*logy
muco-, muc- relating to mucous membrane, e.g. *muco*gingival
myel-, myelo- bone marrow, spinal cord, e.g. *myelo*blast
myo-, my- muscle, e.g. *myo*cardium

naso- nose, e.g. *naso*palatine
necr- death, e.g. *necr*otic
neo-, ne- new, recent, e.g. *neo*plasm
nephro-, nephr- kidneys, e.g. *nephr*itis
neuro-, neuri-, neur- pertaining to nerves, e.g. *neur*asthenia
nucleo-, nucle- pertaining to nucleus, e.g. *nucleo*protein

ob- (change b to c before words beginning with c) against, toward, e.g. *oc*clusion
odonto-, odont- tooth, e.g. *odont*algia
-oid like, resembling, e.g. ameb*oid*
-oma swelling, tumor, e.g., lip*oma*
-opia, -opy sight, eye defect, e.g. my*opia*
oro- mouth, oral, e.g. *oro*nasal
ortho-, orth- straight, normal, e.g. *ortho*dontics
-osis condition, state, e.g. cyan*osis*
osteo-, oste- bone, e.g. *osteo*porosis
oto-, ot- ear, e.g. *oto*plasty
-ous full of, having, e.g. aque*ous*
ovi-, ovo-, ovu- egg, e.g. *ovu*lation

pan- all, every, general, e.g. *pan*acea
para- beyond, beside, near, e.g. *para*site
patho-, path- disease, e.g. *patho*gnomonic
pedia-, pedo- (paedo-) child, e.g., *pedo*dontics
-penia deficiency, e.g. leukopenia
per- throughout, completely, e.g. *per*cussion
peri- around, near, e.g. *peri*apical
phago- to eat, e.g. *phago*cytic
-phile, -phil loving, e.g. hemo*phil*ia
phlebo-, phleb- vein, e.g. *phleb*itis
-phobe, -phobia fear, dread, e.g. photo*phobia*
pilo- hair, e.g. *pilo*erection
-plas- mold, shape, e.g. gingivo*plas*ty
plasmo-, plasm form, e.g. cyto*plasm*
-plegia, -plexy paralysis, stroke, e.g. hemi*plegia*
pleo- more, e.g. *pleo*morphism
-pnea, (-pnoea) breathing, e.g. dys*pnea*
pneumo- air, lung, e.g. *pneumo*thorax
-poiesis, -poietic production, e.g. erythro*poietic*
poly- many, much, e.g. *poly*saccharide
pont- bridge, e.g. *pont*ic
poro-, -por- opening, pore, duct, e.g. *por*ous
post- behind, after, e.g. *post*natal
pre- before, in front of, e.g. *pre*maxilla
pro- before, in front of, e.g. *pro*gnathic
proprio- one's own, e.g. *proprio*ceptive
proto- first, e.g. *proto*plasm
pseudo- false, deceptive, e.g. *pseudo*membrane

psycho-, psych- mind, mental processes, e.g. *psycho*somatic

pulmo- lung, e.g. *pulmo*nary

pur-, pyo- pus, e.g. *pur*ulent, *pyo*rrhea

pyro- fever, heat, e.g. *pyro*genic

re- back, again, e.g. *re*gurgitate

-renal kidney, e.g. ad*renal*

retro- back, backward, behind, e.g. *retro*molar

-rhage breaking, bursting forth, profuse flow, e.g. hem*orrhage*

-rhea, (-rhoea) flow, discharge, e.g. pyor*rhea*

rhino-, rhin- nose, e.g. *rhin*itis

rube- red, e.g. *rub*ella

sarco- flesh, muscle, e.g. *sarco*ma

-sclero- hard, e.g. *sclero*derma

-scopy examination, inspection, e.g. micro*scopy*

semi- half, partly, e.g. *semi*permeable

sero- serum, serous, e.g. *sero*purulent

sial-, sialo- saliva, e.g. *sialo*graphy

somat-, somato-, -some body, e.g. chromo*some*

-squam- scale, e.g. de*squam*ative

stomat- mouth, e.g. *stomat*itis

sub- beneath, under, deficient, e.g., *sub*acute

super- above, upon, excessive, e.g. *super*numerary tooth

syn- with, together, e.g. *syn*drome

tachy- swift, e.g. *tachy*cardia

tact- touch, e.g. *tact*ile

tera-, terato- monster, malformed fetus, e.g. *terato*genic

thermo- heat, e.g. *thermo*phile

thrombo-, thromb- clot, coagulation, e.g. *thromb*in

trans- beyond, through, across, e.g. *trans*plantation

tropho-, trophic nutrition, nourishment, e.g. hyper*trophic*

-tropic turning toward, changing, e.g. hydro*tropic*

-ule diminutive, small, e.g. tub*ule*

-uria urine, e.g. gluco*suria*

vaso- blood vessels, e.g. *vaso*dilation

vita- life, e.g. *vita*min

xero- dry, e.g. *xero*stomia

Glossary

This brief glossary includes primarily the words that have been used but not defined in the text. Individual glossaries have been prepared for chapters 52, 56, 57, 58, and 59. Many other words are defined in the text and may be located through the Index.

The meaning of words from the basic medical and dental sciences frequently can be determined from the list of word prefixes, suffixes, and combining forms on the previous pages. A medical dictionary is an important adjunct to guide professional reading.

A

Abscess (ab′ses). a localized, circumscribed collection of pus.

Absorption (ab-sorp′shun). taking up of fluids or other substances by the skin or mucous surfaces; passage of substances to the blood, lymph, and cells from the alimentary canal after digestion.

Abutment (ah-but′ment). a tooth or implant used for the support or retention of a fixed or removable prosthesis.

Accessory (ak ses′ō rē). subordinate, attached, or added for convenience.

Acid (as′id). a chemical substance that undergoes dissociation with the formation of hydrogen ions in aqueous solution; pH less than 7.0.

Acidogenic (as ĭ dō jen′ik). acid-forming or producing.

Acne vulgaris (ak′nē vul-ga′ris). a chronic inflammatory disease of the sebaceous glands that appears on the face, back, and chest in the form of eruptions.

Acquired characteristics: those obtained after birth, as a result of environment.

Acuity (ă-ku′ĭ tē). sharpness or clearness, especially of the special senses.

Acute (ă kūt′). having rapid onset, short, severe course, and pronounced symptoms; opposite of chronic.

Adenopathy (ad ĕ-nop′ah-thē). swelling or enlargement of lymph nodes.

Adsorption (ad-sorp′shun). the attachment of one substance to the surface of another substance.

Agar (ah′gar). gelatin extracted from seaweed, used as a nutrient solidifying agent in bacteriologic culture media; constituent of a reversible hydrocolloid impression material.

Agglutination (ă-glu′tĭ-nā′shun). state of being united; adhesion of parts; clumping, as of bacteria or other cells.

Alkali (al′kah-li). a strong water-soluble base; see **Base.**

Allergen (al′er-jen). an antigenic substance that produces hypersensitivity; may be inhaled, ingested, or injected or may produce a reaction upon contact with the skin.

Allergy (al′er jē). a hypersensitive state gained from exposure to a specific substance or allergen, re-exposure to which causes a heightened capacity to react.

Alloplast (al′lo-plast). a graft of an inert metal or plastic material.

Alloy (al′loi). a substance composed of a mixture of two or more metals.

Alopecia (al′ō-pē′shĭ-ah). loss of hair.

Amalgam (ah-mal′gam). an alloy of two or more metals, one of which is mercury.

    Dental amalgam: an alloy of silver, tin, copper, zinc, and mercury, used for dental restorations.

Amelia (ah-mēl′ē ah). congenital absence of a limb or limbs.

Ameloblast (ah-mel′-ō-blast). epithelial cell of the enamel organ; functions in the formation of enamel.

Amniocentesis (am′nĭ-ō-sen-tē′sis). aspiration of fluid from the amniotic sac (around an embryo); used for prenatal testing to reveal chromosomal abnormalities and metabolic disorders.

Amorphous (ă-mor′fus). lacking specific form or shape; unorganized.

Amylase (am′ĭ laze). an enzyme that converts starch into sugar.

Analgesia (an-al-je′zĭ ah). absence of sensibility to pain; loss of sensibility to pain without loss of consciousness; first stage of general anesthesia.

Anaphylaxis (an-ah-fĭ lak′sis). an acute, severe, allergic reaction characterized by sudden collapse, shock, or respiratory and circulatory failure following the injection of an allergen; increased susceptibility to an allergen resulting from previous exposure to it.

Anaplasia (an-ah-plā′sĭ-ah). loss of structural differentiation as seen in many malignant neoplasms; reversion of a cell to a more primitive embryonic type.

Anesthesia (an′es-thē′zĭ ah). loss of feeling or sensation.

    General anesthesia: reversible depression of the cells of higher centers of the central nervous system that makes the patient unconscious and insensible to pain.

    Local anesthesia: loss of sensibility to pain in a specific area, not accompanied by loss of consciousness.

    Topical anesthesia: a form of local anesthesia, whereby

free nerve endings in accessible structures are rendered incapable of stimulation by application of an anesthetic drug directly to the surface of the area.

Aneurysm (an'ū-rizm). dilation of an artery.

Anhydrous (an-hī'drus). containing no water.

Ankylosis (ang kĭ-lō'sis). union or consolidation of two similar or dissimilar hard tissues previously adjacent but not attached, as a tooth and its surrounding bone.

Anlage (ahn'lah-gheh). earliest primary stage in the development of an organ.

Anodontia (an-o-don'shĭ-ah). congenital absence of teeth; failure of teeth to form; may be partial or complete.

Anodyne (an'ō-dīne). any agent that neutralizes or relieves pain.

Anomaly (ă nom'ă-lē). deviation from the normal.

Anorexia (an'o-rek'sĭ-ah). diminished appetite; aversion to food.

Anoxia (an-ok'sĭ-ah). oxygen deficiency; a condition in which the cells of the body do not have or cannot utilize sufficient oxygen to perform normal functions

Antibiotic (an'tĭ-bi-ot'ik). a chemical substance derived from fungi or microorganisms; in dilute solutions, can destroy or inhibit the growth of bacteria and other microorganisms; used in the treatment of infectious diseases of man, animals, and plants.

Antidote (an tĭ-dōte). a medicine or other remedy for counteracting the effects of a poison.

Apatite (ap'ah-tīte). inorganic compound with a complex formula containing calcium and phosphate; makes up the inorganic portion of bones and teeth.

   Fluorapatite (flu'or-ap'ah-tite). containing fluoride radical.

   Hydroxyapatite (hī drok'se-ap'ah-tīte). containing hydroxyl radical.

Aphasia (ă fa'zĭ-ah). loss of the power of expression by speech, writing, or signs or of comprehension of spoken or written language, as a result of injury or disease of the brain centers.

Aphtha (af'thah). a little ulcer.

Aphthous ulcer (af'thus ul'ser). aphthous stomatitis; canker sore, vesicle that ruptures after 1 or 2 days and forms a depressed, spherical, painful ulcer with elevated rim.

Aqueous (a'kwē-us). water; prepared with water.

Armamentarium (ar'mah-men-ta'rē-um). the equipment, such as books, materials, and instruments essential to professional practice.

   Dental hygiene armamentarium: all the instruments and equipment used during a dental hygiene procedure.

   Dental hygiene instrumentarium: set of instruments used for a particular clinical procedure by the dental hygienist.

Articulation (ar-tik'ū-la'shun). the place where two or more bones of the skeleton join or unite; bony joint that may or may not be movable.

Artifact (ar'tĭ fact). caused by the technique used, not a natural occurrence; in radiography, a structure, blemish, or an unintended radiographic image that may result from the faulty manufacture, manipulation, exposure, or processing of an x-ray film.

Ascites (ă-sī'tēz). accumulation of fluid in the abdominal cavity.

Asepsis (ă-sep'sis). condition in which septic, infective, putrefactive material is absent; exclusion of microorganisms.

Asphyxia (as-fik'sĭ-ah). suffocation or a temporary state of lifelessness as a result of cessation of breathing.

Aspirator (as pĭ-ra'tor). an apparatus employing suction.

Astringent (as-trin'jent). a substance that causes contraction or shrinkage and arrests discharges.

Ataxia (ă-tak'sĭ-ah). loss of the power of muscular coordination.

Atom (at'om). the small particle of an element that is composed of protons, neutrons, and electrons.

Atrophy (at'rō-fē). a degenerative process characterized by diminution in size and wasting away of cells or of an organ, generally associated with an interference in nutrition.

Attenuation (ah-ten ū-a'shun). reducing, thinning, or weakening; reduction of the virulence of a virus or pathogenic microorganism, as by successive culture or repeated inoculation; in radiography, the process by which a beam of radiation is reduced in energy when passing through some material.

Attrition (ă trish'un). gradual wearing away of tooth structure, resulting from mastication.

Audiologist (aw de-ol'ō-jist). a specialist in evaluation and rehabilitation of those whose communication disorders center, in whole or in part, in the hearing function.

Autogenous (aw-toj'en-us). originating within the body; for example, autogenous vaccine prepared from bacteria obtained from the infected person.

Autograft (aw'tō-graft). a graft in which the tissue is obtained from the same individual.

Autonomic (aw tō-nom'ik). a division of the nervous system that supplies the sensory innervation for the smooth muscles, heart, and glands. It is divided into the parasympathetic (craniosacral) and the sympathetic (thoracolumbar) systems.

Auxiliary (awk-sil'ē-ar-ē). giving support; helping; aiding; assisting.

B

Bacteremia (bak'ter-ē mĭ-ah). presence of bacteria in the blood. It may be transient, intermittent, or continuous.

Bacterial spore: a resistant form of bacteria encapsulated by a thick cell wall that enables the cell to survive in environments unfavorable to immediate growth and division; not a reproductive mechanism.

Bactericide (bak'ter i sīd). capable of destroying bacteria.

Bacteriostatic (bak ter i-o-stat'ik). capable of inhibiting the growth and multiplication of bacteria.

Barodontalgia (aerodontalgia) (bar ō don tal'jĭ ah). the sudden acute pain response in a tooth under reduced atmospheric pressure, notably during high-altitude flying.

Base (bās). a chemical substance that in solution yields hydroxyl ions and reacts with an acid to form a salt and water. A base turns red litmus paper blue and has a pH higher than 7.0.

Bevel (bev′el). the inclination a line or surface makes with another when they are not at right angles.

Bifid (bī′fid). cleft into two parts or branches.

Biocompatible (bi′ō-kom-pat′ĭ b′l). harmonious with life; no toxic or injurious effects on biologic function.

Bruxism (bruk′sizm). a neurogenically related habit of grinding, clenching, or clamping the teeth. Damage to the teeth and attachment apparatus can result.

Buffer (bŭf′er). any substance in a fluid that tends to lessen the change in hydrogen ion concentration (reaction) that otherwise would be produced by adding acids or alkalis.

C

Cachexia (kă kek′sĭ-ah). lack of nutrition; wasting; may occur in the course of chronic disease.

Calcification (kal sĭ-fĭ-ka′shun). the process by which organic tissue becomes hardened by a deposit of calcium and other inorganic salts within its substance.

Cancer (kan′ser). malignant and invasive neoplasm; see **Neoplasm: Precancerous lesion.**

Canker sore: see **Aphthous ulcer.**

Carbohydrate (kar bō-hi′drāte). organic compound of carbon, hydrogen, and oxygen: includes starches, sugars, cellulose; formed by plants and used for growth and source of energy.

Carcinoma (kar-sĭ-no′mah). a malignant neoplasm of epithelial origin.

Caries: see **Dental caries.**

Cariogenic (kār ē-ō jen′ik). caries producing; conducive to caries.

Carious (kă′rē-us). affected with caries or decay; in dentistry, a carious lesion is a cavity in a tooth that is the result of dental caries.

Cartilage (kar′tĭ lij). firm, elastic, flexible connective tissue that is attached to articular bone surfaces and that forms certain parts of the skeleton.

Cassette (kă-set′). light-tight container in which x-ray films are placed for exposure to x-radiation; usually backed with lead to eliminate the effect of back-scatter radiation.

Cataract (kat′ah-rakt). a clouding or opacity of the lens of the eye that leads to blurring of vision and eventual loss of sight.

Caustic (kaws′tik). an agent that burns or corrodes; destroys living tissue; having a burning taste.

Cauterize (kaw′ter īze). to burn, corrode, or destroy living tissue by means of a caustic substance, heated metal, or an electric current.

Cementicle (cē men′ti-k′l). small globular mass of cementum (diameter 0.2 to 0.3 mm.); may lie free within the periodontal ligament or be attached to the cementum of the root surface.

Cephalometer (sef ah-lom′ĕ ter). an orienting device for positioning the head for radiographic examination and measurement.

Cephalometry (sef ah-lom′ĕ trē). measurement of the bony structure of the head using reproducible lateral and anteroposterior radiographs.

Cheilosis (kē lo′sis). a condition marked by fissuring and dry scaling of the surface of the lips and angles of the mouth; characteristic of riboflavin deficiency.

Chemotaxis (kē mō tak′sis). attraction of living protoplasm to chemical stimuli; for example, movement of neutrophils to an area of inflammation; a host defense mechanism.

Chorea (kō-rē′ah). a nervous disorder characterized by irregular and involuntary action of the muscles of the extremities and the face.

Chronic (kron′ik). characterized by a long, slow course; opposite of acute.

Clean (klēn). freedom from or removal of all matter in which microorganisms may find favorable conditions for continued life and growth.

Cleidocranial dysostosis (klī′dō krā′nĭ-al dĭs-os-tō′sis). developmental defect characterized by absence of development of clavicles and abnormal shape of skull.

Coagulation (kō-ag-ū-lā′shun). changing of a soluble into an insoluble protein; process of changing into a clot.

Coaptation (kō-ap-tā′shun). proper adaptation or union of parts to each other, such as the ends of a fractured bone or the edges of a wound without overlap.

Col (kawl). concavity of the interdental gingiva; ridge-shaped depression between two peaks formed by the facial and lingual or palatal papillae.

Comatose (kō′mah-tos). in a state of coma; profound unconsciousness.

Commissure (kom′ĭ-shur). angle or corner of eye or lips.

Communicable (ko-mu′nĭ-kah b′l). capable of being transmitted from one person to another.

Congenital (kon-jen′ĭ-tal). existing at or before birth.

Contagious (kon-tā′jus). communicable; transmissible by contact with an infected or sick person.

Contracture (kon-trak′chūr). shortening or distortion; permanent, as from shrinkage of muscles, or temporary, from sudden stimulus.

Corrosion (ko-rō′zhun). the slow destruction of the texture or substance of a tissue, as by the action of a corrosive or destructive substance.

Crepitation (krep ĭ-ta′shun). a crackling sound; noise made by rubbing together the ends of a broken bone.

Cryosurgery (krī ō-ser′jerē). surgery performed with the use of extremely low temperature.

Cryotherapy (krī ō-ther′ah pē). therapeutic application of cold.

Cryptogenic (krip tō-jen′ik). of obscure, doubtful, or undeterminable origin.

Current (kur′rent). the number of electrons per second passing a given point on a conductor. Electrons are negatively charged and move toward the positive.

Cuticle, primary (kū′tĭ k′l). a delicate membrane covering the crown of a newly erupted tooth: produced by the ameloblasts after they produce the enamel rods. Also called Nasmyth's membrane.

Cyst (sĭst). a sac, normal or pathologic, containing fluid or other material.

  Dentigerous cyst: formed by a dental follicle, containing one or more well-formed teeth.

Radicular cyst: an epithelial-lined sac, formed at the apex of a pulpless tooth, containing cystic fluid.

Cystic fibrosis (sis'tik fĭ-brō'sis). a generalized hereditary disorder of young children primarily; characterized by signs of chronic pulmonary disease (as a result of excess mucus production in the respiratory tract) and pancreatic deficiency.

D

Debridement (dā brēd'-mon). removal of debris, foreign material, or devitalized tissue.

Defibrillator (dē fib'rĭ lā tor). an agent or measure, for example an electric shock, that arrests fibrillation of the ventricular muscle and restores the normal beat.

Fibrillation: exceedingly rapid contractions that replace normal contractions.

Deglutition (deg'loo tish'un). the act of swallowing.

Dehiscence (dē-his'ens). isolated area in which a root is denuded of bone when the denuded area extends to the margin of the bone. Compare with **Fenestration.**

Dehydration (dē hī dra'shun). removal of water; the condition that results from undue loss of water.

Dental caries (den'tal kar'ēz). a disease of the calcified structures of the teeth, characterized by decalcification of the mineral components and dissolution of the organic matrix.

Dental prosthetic laboratory procedures: the steps in the fabrication of a dental prosthesis that do not require the presence of a patient for their accomplishment.

Dental public health: see under **Public health.**

Denticle (den'tĭ k'l). a pulp stone; relatively large body of calcified substance in the pulp chamber of a tooth.

Dentition (den tish'un). the kind, size, and arrangement of the teeth.

Mixed dentition: combination of both primary and permanent teeth present in the oral cavity; state occurs when the first permanent molars erupt and extends until the last primary tooth is exfoliated.

Permanent dentition: the natural teeth that must function throughout adult life.

Primary (deciduous [dē-sĭd'ū-ŭs]) dentition: the first teeth; normally will be shed and replaced by permanent teeth.

Succedaneous (sŭk sē-dā'nē-ŭs) **dentition:** permanent teeth that erupt in positions of exfoliated primary teeth.

Denudation (den'ū dā shun). laying bare; surgical or pathologic removal of epithelial covering.

Desensitization (dē-sen'sĭ tĭ zā'shun). process of removing reactivity or sensitivity.

Desquamation (des kwah-mā'shun). shedding or casting off, as of the superficial epithelium of mucous membrane or skin; a normal physiologic process.

Detritus (dē trī'tus). debris that adheres to tooth, gingival, and mucosal surfaces.

Diagnosis (dī-ag-nō'sis). a scientific evaluation of existing conditions; the process of determining by examination the nature and circumstances of a diseased condition; the decision reached as to the nature of a disease.

Differential diagnosis: the art of distinguishing one disease from another.

Diastema (dī ă'stĕ mah). a space or cleft; in dentistry, a space between teeth.

Diet (dī'et). the customary allowance of food and drink taken by a person from day to day.

Bland diet: meal plan in which all food that can cause chemical, mechanical, or thermal irritation is avoided.

Digital (dij'ĭ-tal). of, pertaining to, or performed with a finger.

Diplopia (dĭ-plo'pĭ-ah). double vision: single object perceived as two.

Dislocation: see **Luxation.**

Distilled water: water that has been subjected to a process of vaporization and subsequent condensation for purification.

DNA (Deoxyribonucleic Acid) (dē ok'sĭ-rĭ-bō nu-kle'ik as'id). occurs in nuclei (chromosomes) of all animal and vegetable cells; repository of hereditary characteristics.

Donor site (dō'nor sīt). area from which tissue is obtained during surgical procedures such as for a graft.

Dorsum (dor'sum). the back surface or a part similar to the back in position; opposite of ventral surface.

Duct (dukt). a passage with well-defined walls; especially a tube for the passage of excretions or secretions.

Dysarthria (dis-ar'thrĭ-ah). disturbance of articulation as a result of emotional stress or paralysis, incoordination, or spasticity of the muscles used for speaking.

Dyslexia (dis lek'sĭ-ah). impairment of the ability to read.

Dysmorphism (dis-mor'fizm). abnormality of shape.

Dysplasia (dis-plā'zĭ-ah). abnormal development or growth; an alteration in adult cells characterized by variations in their size, shape, and organization.

Dyspnea (disp-ne'ah). difficult or labored breathing.

Dystrophy (dis'trō-fē). degeneration associated with atrophy and dysfunction.

E

Ecology (ē-kol'ō ji). the science that deals with the study of the environment and the life history of organisms.

Ectopic (ek-top'ik). out of place. An **ectopic pregnancy** is one that occurs elsewhere than in the cavity of the uterus.

Edema (ĕ-dē'mah). collection of abnormally large amounts of fluid in the intercellular spaces, causing swelling.

Pitting edema: pressure on edematous area causes pits, which remain for prolonged period after pressure is released.

Edentulous (e-den'tu-lus). without teeth.

Emaciation (ē-mā sē-ā'shun). condition of excessive leanness or wasted body tissues.

Embryo (em'brē-ō). the fetus in its earlier stages of development, before the end of the second month.

Emesis basin (em'ē-sis). a basin, usually kidney shaped, used for receiving material expectorated or vomited.

Emollient (e-mōl'yent). softening or soothing; an agent used to soften the skin or other body surface.

Emphysema (em-fĭ sē′mah). presence of air in spaces of the connective tissue; in pulmonary emphysema, an increase in size of air spaces at terminal bronchioles.

Endemic (en dem′ik). present in a community or among a group of people; the continuing prevalence of a disease as distinguished from an epidemic.

Endodontics (en′dō-don′tiks). that branch of dentistry concerned with the etiology, diagnosis, and treatment of diseases of the dental pulp and their sequelae.

Endometrium (en dō-mē′trĭ-um). the mucous membrane lining the uterus.

Enzyme (en′zīm). an organic compound, frequently protein in nature, that can accelerate or produce by catalytic action some change in a specific substance.

Ephebodontics (e-fē bō don′tiks). dentistry for the individual undergoing the transition from childhood to adulthood; that is, the period of life known as adolescence.

Epidemic (ep′ĭ-dem′ik). the occurrence in a community or region of a group of illnesses of similar nature, clearly in excess of normal expectancy and derived from a common source.

Epithelialization (ep ĭ thē lē al ĭ zā′shun). growth of epithelium over a denuded surface.

Eruption (ē rup′shun). the act of breaking out, appearing, or becoming visible; a visible pathologic lesion of the skin, marked by redness, swelling, or both.

Tooth eruption: the combination of movements of a tooth both before and after the emergence of its crown into the oral cavity, which serves to bring the tooth and maintain it in occlusion with the tooth or teeth of the opposing arch.

Erythema (er ĭ thē′mah). abnormal redness of the skin as a result of local congestion; may result from inflammation or excess exposure to radiation.

Erythrocyte (ē rith′rō sīte). red blood cell; specialized cell for the transportation of oxygen.

Erythroplakia (ē-rith rō pla′kē ah). lesions of the oral mucosa that appear as bright red patches or plaques that cannot be characterized clinically or pathologically as any other disease.

Erythropoiesis (ē-rith rō-poy ē′sis). formation of red blood cells.

Escharotic (es kă rot′ik). corrosive; capable of producing sloughing.

Ethics (eth′iks). the science of right conduct; a system of rules or principles governing the conduct of a professional group, planned by them for the common good of man; the principles of morality.

Etiology (ē ti ol′o-jē). the science or study of the cause of disease; that which is known about the causes of a disease.

Exfoliate (eks fō′lē āte). to fall off in scales or layers; in dentistry, to shed primary teeth.

Exodontics (eks-ō-don′tiks). that branch of dentistry concerned with the removal of teeth; see **Oral and maxillofacial surgery.**

Exostosis (eks-os-tō′sis). a bony outgrowth from the surface of bone.

Extirpation (eks-tir-pā′shun). complete removal or eradication of a part; in dentistry, the removal of the dental pulp from the pulp chamber and root canal.

Exudate (eks′ū dāt). the material composed of serum, fibrin, and white blood cells in variable amounts, formed as a reaction to injury of tissue and blood vessels.

F

Febrile (fe′bril). pertaining to fever; feverish.

Fenestration (fen es-trā′shun). isolated area in which a root is denuded of bone when the marginal bone is intact. Compare with **Dehiscence.**

Fermentable (fer men′ta b′l). term applied to a substance that is capable of undergoing chemical change as a result of the influence of an enzyme; usually applied to substances that break down to an acid or an alcohol; applied to carbohydrate breakdown to form acid in bacterial plaque.

Fetus (fē′tus). the unborn offspring in the uterus, after the second month.

Fibrosis (fī bro′sis). formation of fibrous tissue usually as a reparative or reactive process.

Fistula (fis′tū-lah). commonly used term for a narrow passage or duct leading from one cavity to another, as from a periapical abscess to the oral cavity; see **Sinus tract.**

Flora (flō′rah). the entire plant life of a geographic area; used to indicate the microorganisms that live together in a specific location.

Oral flora: the microorganisms that inhabit the oral cavity of an individual, that are usually saprophytic, and that live together in a symbiotic relationship.

Focal infection: infection caused by bacteria or toxins carried in the blood from a distant lesion or focus.

Follicle (dental) (fol′ĭ k′l). the sac that encloses the developing tooth before its eruption.

Forensic dentistry (fo rĕn′sik). the aspect of dental science that relates and applies dental facts to legal problems; encompasses dental identification, malpractice litigation, legislation, peer review, and dental licensure.

Frenectomy (fre-nek′tō-me). complete removal of a frenum.

Frenotomy (fre-not′ō-me). partial removal of a frenum.

Frenum, pl. frena (fre′num) (fre′na). a narrow fold of mucous membrane passing from a more fixed to a movable part, as from the gingiva to the lip, cheek, or undersurface of the tongue, serving in a measure to check undue movement of the part.

Friable (frī′a b′l). easily broken or crumbled.

G

Germicide (jer′mĭ sīd). anything that destroys bacteria; applied especially to chemical agents that kill disease germs but not necessarily bacterial spores; applied to both living tissue and inanimate objects.

Gerodontics (jer ō-don′tiks). that branch of dentistry which treats all problems peculiar to the oral cavity in old age and the aging population. Also called geriatric dentistry.

Gestation (jes-tā′shun). pregnancy.

Gingivectomy (jin′jĭ vek′tō-mē). the surgical removal of diseased gingiva to eliminate periodontal pockets.

Gingivoplasty (jin′jĭ-vō-plas′tē). the surgical contouring of the gingival tissue to produce the physiologic architectural form necessary for the maintenance of tissue health and integrity.

Glaucoma (glaw kō′mah). a disease of the eye marked by intense intraocular pressure, which can result in hardness of the eye, atrophy of the retina, cupping of the optic disk, and blindness.

Gnathodynamometer (nath′ō-dĭ nah-mom′ĕ ter). an instrument for measuring the force exerted in closing the jaws.

Graft (grăft). tissues transferred from one site to replace damaged structures in another site.

    Free graft: tissue for grafting is completely removed from its donor site.

    Pedicle graft: the graft remains attached to its donor site. See also **Autograft; Heterograft; Homograft.**

H

Habilitation (hă-bil ĭ-tā′shun). application of measures that will assist a person in obtaining a state of health, efficiency, and independent action.

Halitosis (hal-ĭ tō′sis). offensive or bad breath, may be related to systemic disease or uncleanliness of the oral cavity.

Health (helth). state of complete physical, mental, and social well-being, not merely the absence of disease.

Hemangioma (hē-man′jĭ-ō mah). a benign tumor composed of newly formed capillaries filled with blood.

Hemorrhage (hem′ŏ rij). bleeding; an escape of blood from the blood vessels.

Hemostat (hē′mo-stăt). an instrument or other agent used to arrest the escape or flow of blood.

Heredity (hĕ-red′ĭ-tē). the inheritance of resemblance, physical qualities, or diseases from a familial predecessor; the passage of characteristics from one generation to its progeny by genetic linkage.

Heterograft (het′er-ō-graft). a heterologous graft in which the tissue is obtained from another species.

Homeostasis (hō mē-ō-stā′sis). the state of equilibrium in the living body with respect to various functions and to the chemical compositions of the fluids and tissues.

Homograft (hō′mō-graft). a homologous graft in which the tissue is obtained from a different individual of the same species.

Hydrophilic (hī drō-fil′ik). having a strong affinity for water; as opposed to hydrophobic, repelling water.

Hygiene (hī′jēn). the science that deals with the preservation of health.

Hygroscopic (hī grō-sco′pik). capable of readily absorbing and retaining moisture.

Hyperkeratosis (hī′per-kĕr ŭ tō′sis). abnormal increase in the thickness of the keratin layer (stratum corneum) of the epithelium. **Benign hyperkeratosis** is one of the most common white lesions of the oral mucous membrane.

Hyperkinesis (hī per-kĭ nē′sis). excessive motility; excessive muscular activity.

Hyperplasia (hī per-plā′zi-ah). increase in size of a tissue or organ caused by an increase in the number of cells in normal arrangement.

Hyperthermia (hī per ther′mĭa). therapeutically induced hyperpyrexia (high fever).

    Malignant hyperthermia: rapid onset of extremely high fever with muscle rigidity.

Hypertonic (hī per-ton′ik). having excessive tone, tonicity, or activity.

    Hypertonic solution: one that has a higher molecular concentration than another with which it is compared; of greater concentration than isotonic.

Hypertrophy (hī-per′trō-fē). increase in size of a tissue or organ caused by increase in the size of its cells.

Hyperventilation (hī per ven′til ā′shun). increased alveolar ventilation with carbon dioxide pressure below normal.

Hypnotic (hĭp-not′ik). inducing sleep.

Hypocalcification (hī′pō-kal sĭ-fi-kā′shun). deficiency in the mineral content of a calcified tissue, for example in the enamel, results from disturbance in the maturation phase during development; may be caused by systemic, local, or hereditary factors.

Hypodontia (hī pō-don′shĭ-ah). condition of congenitally missing teeth; partial anodontia.

Hypoplasia (hī pō-plā′zĭ-ah). defective or incomplete development; enamel hypoplasia results when the enamel matrix formation is disturbed.

Hypotonic (hĭ-pō-ton′ik). having diminished tone, tonicity, or activity.

    Hypotonic solution: one that has a lesser molecular concentration than another to which it is compared; of less concentration than isotonic.

Hypoxia (hī-pok′sē-ah). insufficient oxygen in the air, blood, or tissue.

I

Iatrogenic (ī-at′rō-jen ik). caused by inadvertent or erroneous diagnosis and/or treatment by a professional.

Idiopathic (id′ē-ō-path′ik). self-originated; of unknown cause.

Idiosyncrasy (ĭd ē-ō-sin′krah-sē). any tendency, characteristic, or the like, peculiar to an individual.

Immunity (ĭ mu′nĭ-tē). an inherited, congenital, or naturally or artificially acquired ability to resist the occurrence and effects of a specific disease.

    Acquired immunity: that possessed as a result of having and recovering from a disease or from building up resistance against vaccines, toxins, or toxoids.

    Natural immunity: that inherited by the child from the mother or from the race.

    Passive immunity: that possessed as a result of injection of antibodies or antitoxins of serum from an immune individual or from an animal.

Implant (im′plant). a material or body part that is grafted or inserted within body tissues.

Implantation (im plan-tā′shun). the placement within

body tissues of a foreign substance, for example metal or plastic, for restoration by mechanical means. In dentistry, a foreign material placed into or onto the jawbone to support a crown, partial or complete denture.

Incipient (in-sip′ē-ent). beginning to exist; coming into existence.

Incubation (in kū-bā′shun). the keeping of a microbial or tissue culture in an incubator to facilitate development.
> **Incubation period:** used to denote the time between exposure to a communicable disease and the appearance of clinical symptoms.

Inert (in-ert′). without intrinsic active properties; no inherent power of action, motion, or resistance.

Infection (in-fek′shun). invasion of the body by pathogenic microorganisms and the body's response to the microorganisms and their toxic products; transfer of disease from one part to another or one person to another.

Infectious (in-fek′shus). capable of being transmitted; producing an infection.

Inflammation (in flah-mā′shun). reaction of living tissue to injury; a defense reaction of the body characterized by heat, redness, swelling, pain, and loss of function.

Inhibitor (in-hib′ĭ-tor). a substance that arrests or restrains physiologic, chemical, or enzymatic action or the growth of microorganisms.

Inoculation (i-nok ū-la′shun). introduction of microorganisms or some substance into living tissues or culture media: introduction of a disease agent into a healthy individual to induce immunity.

Inorganic (in or-gan′ik). not characterized by organization of living bodies or vital processes; also, pertaining to compounds not containing carbon, except cyanides and carbonates.

Insidious (in-sid′ē-us). coming on gradually or almost imperceptibly; as in a disease, the onset of which is gradual, with a more serious effect than is apparent.

Intermaxillary (in ter-mak′sĭ-lar ĕ). between the maxilla and the mandible.

In vitro (in vē′tro). outside the living body: in a test tube or other artificial environment.

In vivo (in vē′vo). in the living body of a plant or animal.

Ion (ī′on). an electrically charged atom or group of atoms.
> **Anion** (an′ī-on). negatively charged ion, which passes to the positive pole in electrolysis.
> **Cation** (kat′ī-on). positively charged ion, which passes to the negative pole in electrolysis.

I.Q.: Intelligence Quotient; the relationship between intelligence and chronologic age.

Irrigation (ir-ĭ-gā′shun). the flushing or washing out of anything with water or other liquid for the purpose of making it moist, diluting another substance present, or cleaning the area.

Ischemia (ĭs-kē′mĭ-ah). local decrease in the blood supply to tissues because of obstruction of inflow of arterial blood.

Isotonic (ī sō-ton′ik). having a uniform tonicity or tension.
> **Isotonic solution:** one which has the same molecular concentration as another with which it is compared.

Isotope (ī′sō tōp). any of two or more forms of a chemical element, which have different mass numbers because their nuclei contain different numbers of neutrons. Radioactive isotopes are widely used as tracers in research.

J

Jaundice (jawn′dis). condition in which there are bile pigments in the blood and deposition of bile pigments in the skin and mucous membranes, with resulting yellowish appearance.

Jurisprudence (joor ĭs-proo′dens). the science of law, its interpretation and application.

K

Kaolin (kā′ō-lin). a fine white clay; used in pharmacy in ointments and for coating pills.

Keratin (ker′ah-tin). a protein material formed as a transformation product of the cellular proteins of the flat cells on the surface of the epithelium; form of protective adaptation to function.

Keratinization (ker ah-tin ĭ-zā′shun). process of formation of a horny protective layer on the surface of stratified squamous epithelium of certain body surfaces, including the epidermis and masticatory oral mucosa.

L

Laceration (las er-ā′shun). a wound produced by tearing or irregular cutting.

Latent (lā′tent). concealed, not apparent, potential.

Lesion (lē′zhun). an alteration of structure or of functional capacity as a result of injury or disease.

Lethargy (leth′ar-jē). condition of drowsiness or sleepiness.

Leukocyte (lu′ko-sīt). white blood cell; a formed element of the blood consisting of a colorless mass of protoplasm, having ameboid movements and involved in the destruction of disease-producing microorganisms.

Leukoplakia (lu-kō-plā′kē-ah). a white patch or plaque that cannot be characterized clinically or pathologically as any other disease and is not associated with any physical or chemical causative agent except the use of tobacco.

Local (lō′k′l). restricted to one spot or area; not generalized.

Luxation (luk -sā′shun). a dislocation. For example, dislocation of the temporomandibular joint occurs when the head of the condyle moves anteriorly over the articular eminence and cannot be returned voluntarily.

Lymphadenopathy (lim-fad ĕ nop′ah thē). disease process affecting a lymph node or lymph nodes.

M

Macroglossia (mak rō-glos′ē-ah). enlargement of the tongue.

Maintenance phase: series of appointments after initial therapy for periodic reexamination and additional therapy as needed to keep the teeth and periodontal tissues in health without recurrence of disease.

Malaise (mal āz'). any vague feeling of illness, uneasiness, or discomfort.

Malnutrition (mal nū-trish'un). a condition of the body resulting from an inadequate supply or impaired utilization of one or more food constituents.

Mandrel (man'drel). a spindle, axle, or shaft designed to fit a dental handpiece for the purpose of supporting a revolving instrument.

Manifestation (man'ĭ fĕ-stā'shun). that which is made evident, especially to the sight and understanding.

    Oral manifestation: a symptom or sign of a disease in the oral cavity.

Manikin (man'ĭ-kin). model of the human body or a part; used for teaching purposes.

Massage (mah-sahzh'). manipulation of tissues for remedial or hygienic purposes with the hand or other instrument; the systematic application of frictional rubbing and stroking to the gingival tissues for increasing the circulation of blood through the tissues and for increasing the keratinization of the surface epithelium.

Mastication (mas tĭ-ka'shun). a series of highly coordinated functions that involve the teeth, tongue, muscles of mastication, lips, cheeks, and saliva, in the preparation of food for swallowing and digestion.

Matrix (mā'triks). the form or substance within which something originates, takes form, or develops; intercellular substance of a tissue.

    Amalgam matrix: a thin metal form, usually stainless steel, adapted to a prepared cavity to supply the missing wall so the amalgam will be confined when condensed into the cavity preparation.

Maxillofacial (mak-sil ō fā'shal). pertaining to the jaws and the face.

    Maxillofacial prosthetics: the art and science of anatomic, functional, and cosmetic reconstruction, utilizing nonliving substitutes, of those regions in the maxilla, mandible, and face that are missing or defective.

Medication (med ĭ-kā'shun). use of medicine or medicaments for treatment of a disease.

Metabolism (mĕ-tab'ō lizm). the sum total of the chemical changes occurring in the body; chemical process of transforming foods into complex tissue elements and of transforming complex body substances into simple ones, along with the production of heat and energy.

    Anabolism (ah-năb'ō-lizm). the building up of tissue; maintenance and repair of the body.

    Catabolism (kah-tăb'ō-lizm). the breaking down of tissue into simpler constituents for energy production and excretion.

Microcephaly (mī'krō sef'ah lē). abnormal smallness of the head; frequently associated with mental retardation.

Micron (mī'kron). unit of linear measurement; one-thousandth of a millimeter.

Milliliter (mil ĭ-lē'ter). one-thousandth part of a liter, usually abbreviated **ml.** It is approximately equal to 1 cubic centimeter.

Miscible (mis'ĭ-b'l). capable of being mixed.

Monitoring (mon'i tŏr ing). the overall surveillance of a patient by methods employing the senses of touch, sight, hearing, or smell or by means of devices that operate chemically, physically, or electronically to measure the adequacy of the various physiologic functions.

Morbidity (mor-bid'ĭ tē). the morbidity rate is the ratio to the total population of individuals who are ill or disabled.

Mortality (mor-tal'ĭ tē). the mortality rate is the death rate; the ratio of the number of deaths to the total population.

Morphology (mor-fol'ō-je). the science that deals with form and structure without regard to function.

Mucin (mu'sin). secretion of the mucous or goblet cell; a polysaccharide protein which, combined with water, forms a lubricating solution called mucous; contained in saliva.

N

Nasmyth's membrane: see **Cuticle, primary.**

Necrosis (nĕ-kro'sis). cell or tissue death within the living body.

Neoplasm (nē'ō-plazm). a new growth comprised of an abnormal collection of cells, the growth of which exceeds and is uncoordinated with that of the normal tissues; see **Cancer; Precancerous lesion.**

Nidus (nī'dus). the point of origin or focus of a process.

Nosocomial (nōs ō-kō'mĭ-al). denotes a disorder associated with being treated in a hospital, which is unrelated to the primary reason for being in the hospital.

Nostrum (nos'trum). a quack, patent, or secret remedy.

Nutrition (nu-trish'un). sum of processes by which an animal or plant absorbs or takes in and utilizes food substances; ingestion, digestion, absorption (of products of digestion) of food materials through mucous membranes of the alimentary tract, transportation by blood and lymph to body cells where they are used or stored.

Nystagmus (nĭs tag'mus). involuntary rapid movement of the eyeballs.

O

Obstetrician (ob'stĕ-trish'un). a physician who specializes in the management of pregnancy, labor, and the period of confinement after delivery.

Obtundent (ob-tun'dent). having the power to dull sensibility or soothe pain; a soothing or partially anesthetic medicine.

Odontalgia (ō-don-tal'je-ah). toothache; pain in a tooth.

Odontoblast (ō-don'tō-blast). connective tissue cell that functions in the formation of dentin.

Odontolysis (ō don tol'ĭ-sis). dissolution or resorption of tooth structure.

Olfactory (ol-fak'tō-re). pertaining to the sense of smell.

Oncology (ong-kol'ō-jē). study or science of neoplastic growth.

Ophthalmologist (of thal mol'ō-jist). physician with specialized training and experience in the diagnosis and treatment of eye diseases; one versed in **ophthalmology,** the sum of knowledge concerning the eye and its diseases. (Obsolete term: oculist.)

Optician (op-tish′an). technician who grinds and fits lenses; a maker of optical instruments or glasses.

Optometrist (op-tom′ĕ-trist). one who practices **optometry,** the measurement of visual acuity and the fitting of glasses to correct visual defects; a term adopted by opticians.

Oral and maxillofacial surgery: that part of dental practice which deals with the diagnosis and surgical and adjunctive treatment of the diseases, injuries, and defects of the oral and maxillofacial region.

Orthodontics (or thō-don′tiks). the specialty area of the health science of dentistry concerned with the diagnosis, supervision, guidance, and treatment of the growing and mature dentofacial structures, including those conditions that require movement of the teeth and the treatment of malrelationships and malformations of the craniofacial complex.

Orthopedics (orthopaedics) (or-thō-pē′diks). the medical specialty concerned with the preservation, restoration, and development of form and function of the extremities, spine, and associated structures by medical, surgical, and physical methods.

Orthopnea (or′thop-nē′ah). difficulty in breathing in a horizontal position.

Orthosis (or tho′sĭs). a device added to a person's body to substitute for absent motor power, restore function, assist weak muscles, position or immobilize a part, or correct deformities.

Osmosis (oz mo′sĭs). the passage of a solvent through a semi-permeable membrane into a solution of higher molecular concentration, thus equalizing the concentrations on either side of the membrane.

Osteoblast (os′tē-ō-blast). cell whose activity initiates the formation of new bone.

Osteoclast (os′tē-ō-klast). large multinucleated cell that brings about the resorption of bone; found only during the process of active bone or root resorption.

Osteoectomy, ostectomy (os-tē-ō-ek′tō-mĭ) (os-tek′tō-mĭ). removal of tooth-supporting bone for correction of pockets and nonphysiologic bony contours.

Osteomyelitis (os-tē-ō-mĭ-ĕ-lĭ′tis). acute or chronic inflammation of the bone marrow or of the bone and marrow.

Osteoplasty (os′tē-ō-plas′tē). reshaping of bone; **alveoloplasty,** plastic contouring of the alveolar process to achieve physiologic contours in the bone and gingival tissues.

Osteoporosis (os tē-ō-pō-rō′sis). abnormal decrease in density of bone by the enlargement of its canals or the formation of abnormal spaces.

Otolaryngologist (ō tō-lar-in-gol′ō jist). medical specialist who treats the ears, throat, pharynx, larynx, nasopharynx, and tracheobronchial tree.

Otology (ō-tol′ō-jē). the branch of medical science that embraces the study, diagnosis, and treatment of diseases of the ear and related structures.

P

Palliative (pal′ē-ā tĭv). affording relief but not cure.

Pallor (pal′or). paleness.

Palpation (pal pa′shun). examination by means of the hands; perceiving by the sense of touch.

Palpitation (pal-pĭ-ta′shun). rapid beating of the heart with or without irregularity in rhythm.

Parasympathetic (par ah-sim pah-thet′ik). craniosacral division of the autonomic nervous system.

Parenteral (pah-ren′ter-al). route of administration other than by the alimentary canal, that is, by intravenous, intramuscular, or subcutaneous means.

Pathogenesis (path ō-jen′ĕ sis). the course of development of disease, including the sequence of processes or events from inception to the characteristic lesion or disease.

Pathogenic (path-ō-jen′ik) causing disease: disease-producing.

Pathognomonic (path og-nō-mōn′ik). a sign or symptom significantly unique to a disease to distinguish the disease from other diseases.

Pathosis (path-ō′sis). a disease entity.

Pediatric dentistry (pē dē-at′rik). the practice and teaching of, and research in, comprehensive preventive and therapeutic oral health care of children from birth through adolescence; includes care for special patients beyond the age of adolescence who demonstrate mental, physical, and/or emotional problems.

Pedodontics: see **Pediatric Dentistry.**

Periapical (per ē ap′ĭ-kal). around the apex of a tooth.
 Periapical tissues: the tissues surrounding the apex of a tooth, including the periodontal ligament and the alveolar bone.

Pericoronitis (per ĭ kor-ō-ni′tis). inflammation of the soft tissues surrounding the crown of an erupting tooth; frequently seen in association with erupting mandibular third molars and usually accompanied by infection.

Periodontics (per ē ō-don′tiks). the branch of dentistry that deals with the diagnosis and treatment of diseases and conditions of the supporting and surrounding tissues of the teeth or their implanted substitutes.

Periodontology (per ē ō-don tol′ō jē). the scientific study of the periodontium in health and disease.

Periodontopathic (per ē ō-don tō path′ik). refers to an agent able to induce and/or initiate periodontal pathosis.

Periradicular (per ĭ rah-dik′ū-lar). around or surrounding the root of a tooth.

Petechia (pe-tē′kĭ-ah). minute hemorrhagic spot, of pinhead to pinpoint size, in the skin.

Petri plate (pā trē). a small, shallow dish of thin glass with a loosely fitting, overlapping cover, used for plate cultures in microbiology.

pH: symbol commonly used to express hydrogen ion concentration, the measure of alkalinity and acidity. Normal (neutral) pH is 7.0. Above 7.0 the solution is alkaline; below, acidic.

Phosphorescence (fos-fo-res′ens). emission of radiation by a substance as a result of previous absorption of radiation of shorter wave length; contrasts with fluorescence in that the emission may continue for a time after cessation of the ionizing radiation.

Physiologic saline solution: a 0.9% sodium chloride solution, which exerts an osmotic pressure equal to that exerted by the blood, and thus is compatible with blood.

Pipette (pī pet'). a slender, graduated tube for measuring and transferring liquids from one vessel to another.

Placebo (plah-sē'bō). an indifferent substance in the form of a medicine, given for the suggestive effect; an inert compound, identical in appearance with material being tested in experimental research, of which the participants or researchers may or may not know the identity.

Pleomorphism (plē'ō-mor'fizm). occurrence in more than one form.

Precancerous lesion: a morphologically altered tissue in which cancer is more likely to occur than in its apparently normal counterpart. A **precancerous condition** is a generalized state associated with a significantly increased risk of cancer.

Precipitate (prē-sip'ĭ tāte). to cause a substance in solution to separate out in solid particles (verb); that which is separated out is called the precipitate (noun).

Predisposition (prē-dis-pō-zish'un). a concealed but present susceptibility to disease, which may be activated under certain conditions.

Premaxilla (prē'mak-sil'ah). the intermaxillary bone situated in front of the maxilla proper; carries the incisor teeth.

Premedication (prē med-ĭ-kā'shun). preliminary treatment, usually with a drug, to prevent untoward results that may be effected by the treatment to be performed.

Prescribe (prĕ skrīb'). to designate or recommend a remedy for administration; to direct in writing the dosage, preparation, and dispensing of a remedy or drug.

Primate space (prī'māt). diastema or gap in tooth row occasionally observed in primary dentition. Characteristic of almost all species of primate except man. Maxillary primate spaces accommodate mandibular canines and mandibular primate spaces accommodate maxillary canines when teeth are in occlusion. Reduced length of canines accompanied man's evolution, so canines no longer protruded beyond occlusal level and diastema was no longer functional.

Prodrome (prō'drōm). early or premonitory symptom of a disease.

Prognosis (prog-no'sis). a forecasting of the probable course and termination of a disease and the response to treatment; the prospect of recovery from a disease as indicated by the nature and symptoms of the case.

Proliferation (prō-lif ĕ-rā'shun). reproduction or multiplication of similar forms.

Prone (prōn). flat, prostrate; **prone position,** lying flat.

Prosthesis (pros-thē'sis). artificial replacement for a missing part.

Prosthodontics (pros thō-don'tiks). the branch of dentistry pertaining to the restoration and maintenance of oral function, comfort, appearance, and health of the patient by the restoration of natural teeth and/or the replacement of missing teeth and contiguous oral and maxillofacial tissues with artificial substitutes.

Protein (prō'tēn). any one of a group of complex organic nitrogenous compounds widely distributed in plants and animals that form the principal constituents of cell protoplasm. They are essentially combinations of alpha amino acids and their derivatives.

Proteolytic (prō tē-ō-lit'ik). effecting the digestion of proteins.

Protoplasm (prō'tō-plazm). the only known form of matter in which life is apparent; it composes the essential material of all plant and animal cells.

Psychiatry (sī kī'ah-trē). that branch of medicine which deals with the diagnosis and treatment of mental diseases.

Psychosomatic (sī kō-sō-mat'ik). pertaining to the mind-body relationship; having body symptoms of a psychic, emotional, or mental origin.

Ptosis (tō'sis). falling or sinking down; drooping of the upper eyelid.

Ptyalin (tī'ah-lin). an enzyme occurring in the saliva that converts starch into maltose and dextrose.

Public health: the science and art of preventing disease, prolonging life, and promoting physical health and efficiency through organized community efforts.

Dental public health: art of preventing and controlling dental diseases and promoting oral health through organized community efforts.

Pulp stone: see **Denticle.**

Pulpectomy (pul-pek'tŏ me). removal of the pulp chamber and root canals of a tooth.

Pulpotomy (pul-pŏt'o-me). the removal of a portion of the pulp of a tooth, usually meaning the coronal portion.

Purulent (pū'roo-lent). containing, consisting of, or forming pus.

Pus (puhs). a fluid product of inflammation, which consists of a liquid containing leukocytes and the debris of dead cells and tissue elements liquified by the proteolytic and histolytic enzymes that are elaborated by polymorphonuclear leukocytes.

Pyorrhea (pī ō-rē'ah). a purulent discharge; discharge of pus. Formerly a name for advanced, severe periodontal disease.

Q

Quadrant (kwod'rant). any one of the four parts or quarters of the dentition, with the dividing line of the maxillary or mandibular teeth at the midline between the central incisors.

R

Raphe (rā'fē). a ridge, furrow, or seam-like union between two parts or halves of an organ or structure.

Rarefaction (rār ē fak'shun). being or becoming less dense.

Recurrent (rē kur'ent). returning after intermissions.

Refractory (rē-frak'tō-rī). obstinate; not yielding readily to treatment.

Rehabilitation (rē-hă-bil ĭ-tā'shun). restoration to former state of health, efficiency, and independent action; regeneration.

Remission (rē-mish'un). a decrease or arrest of the symptoms of a disease; also the period during which such decrease occurs.

Replantation (rē plăn-tā′shun). replacement into its own alveolar socket of a traumatically or otherwise removed tooth.

Replication (rĕp lĭ kā′shun). repeating a process or duplicating; viral replication: process by which viruses multiply.

Resection (rē-sek′shun). operation in which a part of a tissue or an organ is removed.

Root resection: removal of a root from a multirooted tooth.

Hemisection: removal of half of a tooth.

Resorption (rē-sorp′shun). removal of bone or tooth structure by pressure; gradual destruction of dentin and cementum of the root, as the primary teeth prior to shedding; in orthodontic tooth movement, bone formation on one side compensates for resorption of bone on the other side.

Resuscitation (rē-sus ĭ-ta′shun). restoration of life or consciousness; restoration of heartbeat and respiration.

Rh factor: agglutinogens of red blood cells responsible for isoimmune reactions such as occur in erythroblastosis fetalis and incompatible blood transfusions; erythroblastosis fetalis results when a mother is Rh negative and develops antibodies against the fetus which is Rh positive.

Rheostat (rē′ō-stat). an appliance for regulating the resistance and thus controlling the amount of current entering an electric circuit; the dental unit control is located in a device operated by the foot.

Rheumatic (roo-mat′ik). pertaining to or affected with **rheumatism,** which is a general term pertaining to conditions characterized by inflammation or pain in muscles or joints.

RNA (ribonucleic acid) (rī bō-noo-klā′ik as′id). occurs in nuclei and cytoplasm of all cells; stores and transfers genetic information.

Rubefacient (roo bĕ-fā′shent). reddening of the skin; an agent that reddens the skin by producing active or passive hyperemia.

Ruga (roo′gah). ridge, wrinkle, fold.

Palatal rugae (roo′gī). the irregular ridges in the mucous membrane covering the anterior part of the hard palate.

S

Sarcoma (sar-kō′mah). malignant neoplasm of connective tissue elements.

Sclerosis (skle-ro′sis). abnormal hardening or thickening of tissue, especially as a result of inflammation or disease of the interstitial substance.

Scoliosis (skō lē ō′sis). curvature of the spine.

Senescence (se-nes′ens). process or condition of growing old; physiologic aging not necessarily related to chronologic age.

Senile (se′nīl). of or pertaining to old age; characteristic of old age.

Senility (sĕ-nĭl′ĭ-tē). old age; feebleness of body and mind occurring with old age.

Septum (sep′tum). a dividing wall, partition, or membrane.

Sequestrum (sē-kwes′trum). a piece of necrosed bone that has become separated from the surrounding bone; usually the necrosed bone is being expelled from the body.

Serrated (ser′āt-ed). having a sawlike edge.

Serum (se′rŭm). the clear, liquid part of blood separated from its more solid elements after clotting; the blood plasma from which fibrinogen has been removed in the process of clotting.

Shelf-life: the length of time a substance or preparation can be kept without changing its chemical structure or other properties.

Sinus tract (si′nus trakt). a pathologic sinus or passage leading from an abscess cavity or hollow organ to the surface, or from one cavity to another; formerly known as a fistula.

Slough (sluf). a mass of dead tissue in, or cast out of, living tissue.

Sordes (sor′dēz). filth, dirt, especially crusts that accumulate on the lips, mucosa, and teeth in fever.

Splint: any apparatus, appliance, or device used to prevent motion or displacement of fractured or movable parts.

Dental splint: appliance designed to immobilize and stabilize mobile teeth.

Spore: see **Bacterial spore.**

Stabile (sta′bīl). not moving, stationary, resistant; opposite of labile.

Heat stabile (thermostabile): resistant to moderate degrees of heat.

Stenosis (stĕ-nō′sis). a narrowing of a channel or an aperture, especially a narrowing of one of the cardiac valves.

Stomatitis (stō mă-tī′tis). inflammation of the oral mucosa, because of local or systemic factors.

Subclinical (sŭb-klĭn′ĭ k′l). without clinical manifestations; said of early stages of a disease.

Subluxation (sŭb-lŭk-sā′shun). partial or incomplete dislocation; see **Luxation.**

Submerged tooth (sŭb-merjd′). one which is below the line of occlusion and may be ankylosed; intrusion; infraocclusion.

Supernumerary tooth (sū per-nu′mer-ăr ē). extra tooth; one which is in excess of the normal number.

Suppuration (sŭp ū-rā′shun). formation of pus.

Sympathetic nervous system: that part of the autonomic (involuntary) nervous system which arises in the thoracic and the first three lumbar segments of the spinal cord.

Syndrome (sin′drom). a group of symptoms and signs which, when considered together, characterize a disease or lesion.

Synergistic (sin er-jis′tik). acting jointly; enhancing the effect of another drug, force, or agent.

Systemic (sis-tem′ik). pertaining to or affecting the whole body.

T

Tactile (tak′til). pertaining to the touch; perceptible to the touch.

Tarnish (tar'nish). surface discoloration on a metal, usually the result of oxidation.

Technician, dental laboratory: a technician who performs any type of dental laboratory procedure not requiring the presence of a patient; see also **Dental prosthetic laboratory procedures.**

Teratogenic (ter ah-to-jen'ik). causing abnormal development.

Teratoma (tĕr ă tō'mah). a neoplasm composed of multiple tissues, including tissues not normally found in the organ in which it arises.

Therapeutic (ther ah-pū'tik). pertaining to the treating or curing of disease; curative.

Therapy (ther'ah-pē). the treatment of disease.

Threshold (thresh'old). that amount of stimulus which just produces a perceptible sensation.

   Pain threshold: that amount of stimulus which just produces a sensation of pain.

Tic: an involuntary purposeless movement of muscle, which usually occurs under emotional stress; a twitching, especially of facial muscles.

Tincture (tingk'chur). an alcoholic solution of a drug or other chemical substance.

Tone (tōn). the normal degree of vigor and tension; a healthy state of a part.

Tonguetie (tung'tī). abnormal shortness of the frenum of the tongue, resulting in limitation of the motion of that organ.

Topical (tŏp'ĭ-k'l). on the surface; pertaining to a particular spot; local.

Topography (tō-pog'rah-fē). the detailed description and analysis of the features of an anatomic region or of a special part.

Toxic (tok'sik). poisonous.

Toxicity (toks-ĭs'ĭ-tē). the state or quality of being poisonous; degree of virulence of a toxic microbe or of a poison; the capacity of a drug to damage body tissue or seriously impair body functions.

Toxin (tok'sin). any poisonous substance of microbial, vegetable, or animal origin that causes symptoms after a period of incubation; can induce the elaboration of specific antitoxins in suitable animals.

Tracheotomy (trā kē-ot'ō-me). surgical operation to provide an artificial opening into the trachea.

Transdermal medication: drug delivered by patch on skin; a mode for slow release over extended time.

Transmissible (trans mis'sĭ b'l). capable of being carried across from one person to another.

Transplant (trans'plant). tissue removed from one part of the body and placed at a different site.

Transplantation (trans-plan-ta'shun). implanting a tissue or organ that has been taken from another part of the same body or from another person.

   Autotransplant: transfer of a tissue or organ to another place in the same person.

Trauma (traw'mah). an injury; damage; impairment; external violence, producing body injury or degeneration.

Trauma from occlusion (traumatic occlusion): the injury to periodontal tissues caused by occlusal forces.

Treatment (trēt'ment). the management and care of a patient for the purpose of curing a disease or disorder.

Tremor (trĕm'or). involuntary trembling or quivering.

Trendelenburg position: supine, inclined at an angle of 45 degrees so that the head is slightly lower than the heart.

Trismus (triz'mus). motor disturbance of the trigeminal nerve, especially spasm of the masticatory muscles, which causes difficulty in opening the mouth.

U

Urticaria (ur tĭ-kā'rē-ah). hives; nettle rash; an eruption of itching wheals usually of systemic origin. It may be caused by a state of hypersensitivity to foods or drugs, foci of infection, physical agents (heat, cold, light, friction), or psychic stimuli.

V

Vehicle (vē'ĭ k'l). a substance possessing little or no medicinal action, used as a medium to confer a suitable consistency or form to a drug.

Ventral (ven'tral). anterior, front surface; opposite of dorsal surface.

Virulent (vir'ū-lent). capable of causing infection or disease.

Viscosity (vis-kos'ĭ-tē). stickiness; ability of a fluid to resist change in shape or arrangement during flow.

Volatile (vol'ah-tīl). tending to evaporate readily.

Vulcanite (vul'kan-īt). a hard rubber prepared by vulcanizing India rubber with sulfur; formerly used for making removable dentures.

W

Wheal (hweel, wēl). an acute circumscribed transitory area of edema of the skin; an urticarial lesion; see **Urticaria.**

Whitlow (hwit'lo). a purulent infection or abscess involving the end of a finger; also called a felon.

X

Xerostomia (zē rŏ-stō mē-ah). dryness of the mouth caused by functional or organic disturbances of the salivary glands.

Appendix

Table A–1. Tooth Development and Eruption: Primary Teeth

		Hard Tissue Formation Begins (weeks in utero)	Enamel Completed (months after birth)	Eruption (months)	Root Completed (year)
Maxillary	Central Incisor	14	1½	10 (8–12)	1½
	Lateral Incisor	16	2½	11 (9–13)	2
	Canine	17	9	19 (16–22)	3¼
	First Molar	15½	6	16 (13–19 boys) (14–18 girls)	2½
	Second Molar	19	11	29 (25–33)	3
Mandibular	Central Incisor	14	2½	8 (6–10)	1½
	Lateral Incisor	16	3	13 (10–16)	1½
	Canine	17	9	20 (17–23)	3¼
	First Molar	15½	5½	16 (14–18)	2¼
	Second Molar	18	10	27 (23–31 boys) (24–30 girls)	3

From Lunt, R.C. and Law, D.B.: A Review of the Chronology of Eruption of Deciduous Teeth, *J. Am. Dent. Assoc., 89*, 872, October, 1974.

Table A–2. Tooth Development and Eruption: Permanent Teeth

		Hard Tissue Formation Begins	Enamel Completed (years)	Eruption (years)	Root Completed (years)
Maxillary	Central Incisor	3–4 mos.	4–5	7–8	10
	Lateral Incisor	10 mos.	4–5	8–9	11
	Canine	4–5 mos.	6–7	11–12	13–15
	First Premolar	1½–1¾ yrs.	5–6	10–11	12–13
	Second Premolar	2–2¼ yrs.	6–7	10–12	12–14
	First Molar	at birth	2½–3	6–7	9–10
	Second Molar	2½–3 yrs.	7–8	12–13	14–16
	Third Molar	7–9 yrs.	12–16	17–21	18–25
Mandibular	Central Incisor	3–4 mos.	4–5	6–7	9
	Lateral Incisor	3–4 mos.	4–5	7–8	10
	Canine	4–5 mos.	6–7	9–10	12–14
	First Premolar	1¾–2 yrs.	5–6	10–12	12–13
	Second Premolar	2¼–2½ yrs.	6–7	11–12	13–14
	First Molar	at birth	2½–3	6–7	9–10
	Second Molar	2½–3 yrs.	7–8	11–13	14—15
	Third Molar	8–10 yrs.	12–16	17–21	18–25

From Ash, M.M.: *Wheeler's Dental Anatomy, Physiology, and Occlusion*, 6th ed. Philadelphia, W.B. Saunders Co., 1984, page 24.

Table A–3.   Average Measurements of the Primary Teeth (in millimeters)

		Overall Length	Length of Crown	Length of Root	Width of Crown (mesial-distal at widest point)
Maxillary	Central Incisor	16.0	6.0	10.0	6.5
	Lateral Incisor	15.8	5.6	11.4	5.1
	Canine	19.0	6.5	13.5	7.0
	First Molar	15.2	5.1	10.0	7.3
	Second Molar	17.5	5.7	11.7	8.2
Mandibular	Central Incisor	14.0	5.0	9.0	4.2
	Lateral Incisor	15.0	5.2	10.0	4.1
	Canine	17.5	6.0	11.5	5.0
	First Molar	15.8	6.0	9.8	7.7
	Second Molar	18.8	5.5	11.3	9.9

From Black, G.V.: *Descriptive Anatomy of the Human Teeth*, 4th ed. Philadelphia, The S.S. White Dental Manufacturing Company, 1897, according to Ash, M.M.: *Wheeler's Dental Anatomy, Physiology, and Occlusion*, 6th ed. Philadelphia, W.B. Saunders, Co., 1984, p. 51.

Table A–4.   Average Measurements of the Permanent Teeth (in millimeters)

		Overall Length	Length of Crown	Length of Root	Width of Crown (mesial-distal at widest point)
Maxillary	Central Incisor	23.5	10.5	13.0	8.5
	Lateral Incisor	22.0	9.9	13.0	6.5
	Canine	27.0	10.0	17.0	7.5
	First Premolar	22.5	8.5	14.0	7.0
	Second Premolar	22.5	8.5	14.0	7.0
	First Molar	B* 19.5 L 20.5	7.5	B 12 L 13	10.0
	Second Molar	B 17.0 L 19.0	7.0	B 11 L 12	9.0
	Third Molar	17.5	6.5	11.0	8.5
Mandibular	Central Incisor	21.5	9.0	12.5	5.0
	Lateral Incisor	23.5	9.5	14.0	5.5
	Canine	27.0	11.0	16.0	7.0
	First Premolar	22.5	8.5	14.0	7.0
	Second Premolar	22.5	8.0	14.5	7.0
	First Molar	21.5	7.5	14.0	11.0
	Second Molar	20.0	7.0	13.0	10.5
	Third Molar	18.0	7.0	11.0	10.0

From Ash, M.M.: *Wheeler's Dental Anatomy, Physiology, and Occlusion*, 6th ed. Philadelphia, W.B. Saunders Co., 1984, p. 13.
*B = Buccal measurement; L = Lingual measurement

Index

Page numbers in *italics* refer to illustrations; page numbers followed by "t" refer to tables

Abdominal thrust
  procedure for, 744-745
Abrasion, *216,* 216
  defined, 216, 313, 506
  factors to teach patient about, 223
  toothbrushing and, 313-314
Abrasive agent(s)
  characteristics of particles of, 506-507
  commercial, 508
  defined, 506
  examples of, 507
  factors affecting action of, 506-507
  preparation of, 507-508
Abscess
  defined, 485, 761
  gingival
    defined, 485
  periapical
    periodontal abscess vs., 486-487
  periodontal, 485-487
Absence. *See also* Seizure(s)
  clinical manifestations of, 641-642
  defined, 641t
Absorption
  defined, 761
Abstinence
  defined, 726t
Abstinence syndrome. *See* Withdrawal
  syndrome
Abuse
  alcohol. *See also* Alcoholism
    screening for, 730
    signs of, 725
  child. *See* Child abuse
  drug. *See* Substance abuse
Abutment
  defined, 341, 344, 761
Accessory
  defined, 761
Accident(s)
  to face and eyes
    prevention of, 735
Acid(s)
  defined, 761
  denture cleaning with, 346-347
Acid etching
  cleansing effect of conditioner for, 421
  findings in exposed surfaces after, 525
  in bonding, 522
  in sealant application, *419,* 419, 421-422
Acidogenic
  defined, 761
Acidulated phosphate-fluoride (APF)
  topical application of, 402t, 402
Acne rosacea
  defined, 726t
Acne vulgaris
  defined, 761
Acquired characteristics
  defined, 761

Acquired immunodeficiency syndrome
    (AIDS), 14t, 21-24
  clinical management in, 24
  disease process of, *21,* 22
  head and neck findings in, 23
  hemophilia and, 711
  in children, 23-24
  individuals at risk for, 22
  progression of, *21,* 22-23, *23*
  signs and symptoms of, 23
  testing for, 22
    in infants, 24
    in women of childbearing age, 24
  transmission of, 21-22
Actinomyces viscosus
  in root surface caries, 217
Acuity
  defined, 761
Acute
  defined, 411, 761
Acute necrotizing ulcerative gingivitis. *See*
    Necrotizing ulcerative gingivitis
Acyclovir
  for herpes simplex infections, 26
ADA. *See* American Dental Association
Adaptation, 433, *434*
Adaptive functioning
  in mental retardation, 647-648
  defined, 647
Addiction. *See also* Alcoholism; Substance
    abuse
  defined, 726t
Addis, William, 301
Adenopathy
  defined, 761
Adolescence
  characteristics of, 553-554
  defined, 553
  dental hygiene care in, 554-556
  oral conditions in, 554
  personal factors in, 554
Adrenal crisis
  emergency treatment of, 750t
Adsorption
  defined, 761
Aerobe
  defined, 236
  facultative
    defined, 236
  obligate
    defined, 236
Aerodontalgia
  defined, 762
Aerosol(s)
  contents of, 11
  defined, 10
  disease transmission by, 10-11
  production of
    during polishing, 503
Agar
  defined, 761

Agglutination
  defined, 761
Aging, 561. *See also* Gerodontic patient
  diseases common with, 562-563
  general physiologic changes in, 561-562
Agranulocyte(s), 701
Agranulocytosis, 706-707
AIDS. *See* Acquired immunodeficiency
    syndrome
AIDS dementia, 23
AIDS-related complex (ARC), 23
  head and neck findings in, 23
Air
  instruments for application of, 192
  microorganisms of, 9-10
  purposes and uses of, 192
Airborne infection, 9-11
Airbrasive
  defined, 512
  polishing with, *512,* 512-513
Airway
  obstruction of
    emergency treatment of, 744-745, 747t
    prevention of, 744
    recognition of, 744
  procedure for opening
    in unconscious patient, *741,* 741-742
ALARA concept, 125
Alcohol. *See also* Alcoholism
  abuse of
    screening for, 730
    signs of, 725
  blood concentration of, 726-727
  dependence on
    defined, 726t
    screening for, 730
    signs of, 725
  effects on fetus, 726t, 728, *728*
  intoxication with
    signs of, 725
  metabolism of, 725-727
Alcohol amnestic disorder, 727-728
Alcohol hallucinosis, 729
Alcoholic
  recovering
    defined, 726t
Alcoholic liver disease, 727
Alcoholics Anonymous (AA), 729
Alcoholism, 725-733
  brain damage in, 727-728
  clinical patterns of alcohol use in, 725
  defined, 726t
  dental hygiene care in, 730-731
  diet in, 731-732
  etiology of, 725
  examination in, 730-731
  factors to teach patient about, 732
  health hazards of, 727-728
  oral cancer and, 601
  patient instruction in, 731-732